CW00618156

Bentley's

Textbook of Pharmaceutics

Bentley's

Textbook of Pharmaceutics

edited by E A RAWLINS MSc PhD FPS

formerly Head of the Department of Pharmacy, Brighton Polytechnic
with the assistance of 15 contributors

Eighth Edition

Baillière Tindall . London

A BAILLIÈRE TINDALL book published by
Cassell & Collier Macmillan Publishers Ltd
35 Red Lion Square, London WC1R 4SG
and at Sydney, Auckland, Toronto, Johannesburg
an affiliate of
Macmillan Publishing Co. Inc.
New York

First published 1926
Seventh edition 1971
Eighth edition 1977

ISBN 0 7020 0391 3

Printed by Cox & Wyman Ltd,
London, Fakenham and Reading

Preface

When A. C. Bentley wrote his *Textbook of Pharmacy*, the first edition of which was published in 1926, he intended it to be an adequate and complete substitute for college lectures and he found the warrant for its existence largely in the requirements of those students who were incapable of taking adequate lecture notes and of those pertinacious individuals who needs must pre-empt the efforts of their tutors by learning it all beforehand. In common with most textbooks of the day it was intended to fulfil the requirements of a given syllabus and it reflected the teaching method of the time. Much of this involved learning pharmaceutical data by rote and although Bentley was among the first to include a consideration of the basic principles underlying pharmacopoeial operations, he still devoted a portion of his book to transcripts of the official monographs. To these, however, he added notes giving reasons for the methods used; his textbook was often the only repository of such information and many an examination candidate had reason to be grateful for it.

At that time, pharmacy was rather more of an art than a science, and progress was leisurely, but by the time he published his fourth edition in 1937, the production of synthetic drugs had begun which was to burst into an explosion of effort in succeeding years which was to revolutionize the practice of pharmacy. Bentley died in 1943 and the next revision of his text was carried out by Dr Harold Davis, who incorporated in it the fruit of his extensive experience of hospital pharmacy; he expanded a great deal the section on microbiology and added a new section on pharmaceutical manufacturing. Significantly, he abandoned the objective of covering a given syllabus, aiming simply to assist pharmaceutical students and to provide a work of reference for practising pharmacists. In the next two editions he added new topics such as radio-pharmacy and reduced considerably the amount of material transcribed from the pharmacopoeia, while at the same time commencing the move towards a more generalized approach which has now become the underlying concept of pharmaceutical teaching.

This process has been continued in the present volume and new material has been added to bring it into line with modern requirements. The practice of pharmacy has changed very greatly in the past two decades. Extemporaneous dispensing has been greatly reduced in favour of medicaments presented in unit dosage forms; even so the unique contribution of the pharmacist is central to the provision of clinically efficient modern dosage forms, and is now well recognized. No textbook can be expected to present within a modest extent all that is required for the education and information of the modern pharmacist, even in one field of study. It is hoped, however, that this new edition will help supplement the student's formal teaching, consolidate his knowledge, and at the same time stimulate further reading. We hope too that this edition, like its predecessors, will become recognized as an essential textbook for the student and a valuable work of reference for the practising pharmacist.

In working to this end, I have been fortunate in having the assistance of a group of distinguished contributors. In the last edition Dr Davis pointed out that 'with the rapid growth of new medicaments and the almost continuous flow of new pharmaceutical products, standard works of reference must continually lag behind practice'. The production of a new edition after a long period has served to confirm this view and I am very grateful to my colleagues who, though burdened with heavy duties, have endeavoured to make this book as up-to-date and comprehensive as possible.

June 1975   E. A. Rawlins

The Publishers regret to have to announce to the readers of this book the death of Dr E. A. Rawlins which took place just as the final portions of the book were being passed for press. They would like to pay tribute to the courage of Dr Rawlins and to express their gratitude to him for all the time and effort that he had devoted over a long period to the editing of this book.

Contents

Part III   Pharmaceutical Practice

Part IV   Radioactivity

Part V   Microbiology and Animal Products

Part VI   Formulation and Packing

Index   711

Contributors

M. G. Aiken BPharm, MPS (Chapters 30 & 31)
Senior Lecturer in Pharmaceutics, Brighton Polytechnic

J. E. Carless PhD, FPS (Chapters 1, 2, 3, 5, 6, 7, 8, 9, 12, 13, 14, 15 & 16)
Professor of Pharmaceutics, Chelsea College, University of London

J. O. Dawson BSc, FPS (Chapter 36, with C. C. Yates)
Technical Director Ethicon Sutures Ltd., Edinburgh

R. P. Enever BPharm, PhD, ARIC, MPS (Chapter 10)
Senior Lecturer in Pharmaceutics, School of Pharmacy, University of London

J. W. Hadgraft FPS, FRIC (Chapters 20, 21, 22, 23, 24, 25, 26 & 27)
Regional Pharmaceutical Officer, East Anglia Regional Health Authority

J. P. Hall MSc, FPS, MInst Pkg (Chapter 38)
Reader in Pharmaceutics, Chelsea College, University of London

N. D. Harris PhD, FPS, DIC (Chapters 28 & 29)
Reader in Pharmaceutics, Chelsea College, University of London

J. d'A. Maycock *CBE*, MD (Chapter 35)
The Lister Institute of Preventive Medicine, Elstree, Herts

F. T. Perkins MSc, PhD, MIBiol, FRSA (Chapter 33)
Chief of Biological Research, World Health Organization, Geneva, Switzerland

J. M. Pickett PhD, MPS (Chapters 4, 11, 18)
Senior Lecturer in Pharmaceutics, Brighton Polytechnic

M. N. Pilpel BSc, PhD, DSC (Chapter 17)
Reader in Pharmaceutical Technology Chelsea College, University of London

E. A. Rawlins MSc, PhD, FPS (Chapters 31 & 32)
Formerly *Head of the Department of Pharmacy, Brighton Polytechnic*

M. J. Soulal BSc, PhD, FRIC (Chapter 34)
New Products Development, Beecham Pharmaceuticals, Research Division, Betchworth, Surrey

F. A. J. Talman BSc, FPS (Chapters 19, 37 & 39)
Principal Lecturer in Pharmaceutics, Brighton Polytechnic

C. C. Yates ARIC (Chapter 36, with J. O. Dawson)
Consultant, 34 Roebuck Lane, Buckhurst Hill, Essex

Part I

PHYSICOCHEMICAL PRINCIPLES

1

Solutions

A solution is a homogeneous molecular dispersion of two or more substances, the relative proportions of which may vary between certain limits. These limits are expressed most concisely by the Phase Rule derived by J. W. Gibbs in 1876.

COMPOSITION OF SOLUTIONS

The component which forms the major constituent of a solution is called the *solvent* and the gas, liquid or solid dissolved in it is known as the *solute*. The terms are convenient but do not imply any difference in the role of the two constituents and cease to have any value for pairs of liquids that are miscible in all proportions, e.g. alcohol and water.

The composition of a solution may be expressed in various ways, of which the following are the more common:

(1) The amount of solute in grams (g) or milligrams (mg) in a unit volume of solution.

(2) The amount of solute in gram molecules (moles) in 1 litre of solution. This expresses the concentration as a *molarity*. All solutions of the same molarity contain the same number of molecules in a definite volume of solvent.

(3) The amount of solute is given as a percentage by weight (per cent w/w).

(4) For liquid mixtures, the solute is given as percentage by volume (per cent v/v).

(5) The ratio of moles of solute to the total moles present (solvent and solute). This is known as the *mole fraction* and is most suited to theoretical treatment of solutions. If a solution contains $n_A, n_B, \ldots n_I$, mols of A, B etc., the concentration of each constituent expressed by its molar fraction N is:

$$N_A = n_A/(n_A + n_B \cdots n_I)$$
$$N_B = n_B/(n_A + n_B \cdots n_I)$$
$$N_A + N_B \cdots N_I = 1.$$

MECHANISM OF SOLVENT ACTION

A true solution is formed when two or more previously separated phases are brought together and form one phase. In the gaseous state there is complete miscibility since gases consist of widely separated molecules moving at great speed, occasionally colliding, so that molecules of one gas move freely among molecules of a second gas. Liquids differ from gases in that the molecules of the liquid are always in close proximity due to the forces of attraction between the molecules, and this results in liquids being considerably denser than gases and occupying a definite volume. Thermal energy causes the molecules in a liquid to be constantly on the move so that neighbours are constantly changing. Since a change in neighbour occurs, it is also possible for changes of kind of neighbour to occur when different substances, say A and B, in the liquid state, are brought together, i.e. the liquids mutually dissolve. However, since the forces of attraction between A molecules for themselves may be greater than A molecules for B molecules, the liquids may not be completely miscible. Exact prediction regarding solubility requires a knowledge of the size and shape of molecules and of the short range forces acting between neighbours. Experimentally it is found that some pairs of liquids are miscible in all proportions, some over a limited range of composition and others have no tendency for mixing at all. As a rough guide, we can expect substances that are chemically similar to show mutual solubility and hence the adage 'like dissolves like'. Hartley (1956) has expressed this very clearly—'liquids are mutually soluble to an extent depending on the difference between the force of attraction between unlike molecules and the mean of those between the like pairs. In general the attraction between unlike molecules is less than the mean of the attraction of like molecules and so the attractive forces are best separated by dissociation of the molecules, like with like, in separate phases'.

Unlike liquids, crystalline solids have their molecules in an orderly arrangement of units, i.e. atoms, molecules or ions. These units are in fixed positions so that their neighbours remain individually the same. The insolubility of unionized solids can be explained by the stable crystalline arrangement and low intra-molecular forces between solvent and solute. The melting point of the solute reflects the strength of the intramolecular forces in the solute and so the higher the melting point the less the tendency for it to dissolve in a liquid, provided of course that one is comparing solutes of similar chemical structure, e.g. hydroquinone, melting point 170°, is less soluble than phenol, melting point 41°.

The solubility of electrolytes is largely governed by the electrostatic forces of attraction and repulsion, the most important single property of a solvent being its dielectric constant. Water with a high dielectric constant is said to be a polar solvent and is a good solvent for other polar substances, e.g. electrolytes. When an electrolyte dissolves in water, the cations are attracted to the negative ends of the water dipoles

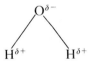

and become associated with a shell of strongly attracted water molecules. A similar though smaller effect occurs with the anions and the $O^{\delta-}$. Hydrocarbons with low dielectric constants are poor solvents for electrolytes due to their non-polar nature.

The immiscibility of water and non-polar substances is due to the strong attraction of water molecules for each other and the absence of attraction of a water molecule for a non-polar molecule; the non-polar substance is thus 'squeezed' out of the water leading to phase separation. The use of the term 'hydrophobic' is often applied to non-polar substances and tends to suggest that the immiscibility between solute and solvent is due to repulsion between the different species of molecules. The term is misleading in so far as it suggests a mechanism that is incorrect.

The polarity of organic substances containing groups such as $-OH$, $-COOH$, $-NH_2$, is due to the unequal sharing of the electron of the covalent bond. Attractions exist between the molecules containing these polar groups and the water molecules and consequently they are readily distributed between the water molecules.

Ethanol is miscible in all proportions with water, but the higher alcohols, e.g. propyl, butyl, etc., become increasingly less soluble due to the increasing size of the non-polar part of the molecules which tends to be expelled from solution. Long chain alcohols such as cetyl alcohol, $C_{15}H_{31}OH$ are sparingly soluble in water and orientate themselves at an air–water interface with the OH group in the water and the hydrocarbon chain directed towards the air. This behaviour at an air–water interface is discussed more fully in Chapter 4.

MIXED SOLVENTS

The solvent properties of mixed solvents that show no association effects, e.g. benzene–cyclohexane; ethylene chloride–ethylene dibromide, is a mean of the properties of the two liquids, when a solute is present in fairly low concentration. There is a complication if large amounts of solute are added especially if it is very soluble in only one phase since the effect may be to bring about separation of the two liquid phases.

As a general guide, the log solubility of fairly low solubility solutes is a linear function of the mol fraction composition of the mixed solvent (Hartley 1956). This relationship helps us to predict the solubility when a very bad solvent is added to a very good solvent as is frequently done in order to precipitate a product from solution. If, for example, a crystalline organic substance is soluble in 10 parts of alcohol but only soluble in 100 000 parts of water, it will only be soluble in 1000 parts of 0.5 M (molar) solution of alcohol in water. This concentration of alcohol expressed as a percentage is approximately 75 per cent so that the addition of as little as 25 per cent water results in almost complete precipitation.

The behaviour of mixed solvents where one solvent tends to associate in the presence of the second differs from this previous case. The association or clustering of molecules tends to give local regions of relatively high solvent concentration which exert considerably higher solvent effect than do the homogeneously distributed non-associated mixed solvents. The clustering tendency of methanol, ethanol and propanol increases in this order and this correlates with the solvent power of 50 per cent solutions of these alcohols in water. A solution containing a high concentration of sodium benzoate in water acts as a good solvent for a number of organic substances particularly phenols, due to the association of benzoate ions providing a liquid hydrocarbon region which is able to exert its solvent effect. Aqueous solutions of surface active agents can dissolve many water insoluble substances due to similar aggregation behaviour, the aggregates in these instances being known as micelles (see Chapter 4).

A detailed discussion of the thermodynamics of solutions is outside the scope of this chapter and the reader should refer to the standard textbooks of physical chemistry to appreciate the concepts of 'ideal behaviour' of solutions. An ideal solution has been defined as one which obeys Raoult's law over the whole range of concentration and at all temperatures. Deviations from ideal behaviour may be due to association or solvation effects. Association refers to a specific interaction between the molecules of the solute, e.g. dimerization of benzoic acid in certain solvents. Solvation refers to the interaction between solute and solvent molecules such as hydrogen bonding. The majority of pharmaceutical solutions, particularly solutions of weak electrolytes are not dilute enough to come within the classification of ideal solutions and thus the colligative properties, e.g. freezing point, osmotic pressure and vapour pressure of these solutions cannot be accurately calculated theoretically. There is however comprehensive freezing point data on drug solutions which can be used to compute the composition of isotonic solutions with a degree of accuracy which is adequate for most pharmaceutical solutions.

FACTORS WHICH INFLUENCE THE RATE AND EXTENT OF SOLUBILITY

TEMPERATURE

The solubility of a solid in a liquid is dependent on the temperature, nature of the solute and the nature of the solvent. If a solute absorbs heat during the process of solution, i.e. has a negative *heat of solution*, its solubility is increased with increase in temperature. Most solutes show this behaviour (Fig. 1.2). If the solute has a positive heat of solution as in the case of calcium hydroxide and calcium sulphate (above 50°), the solubility will be decreased by increasing the temperature.

For an *ideal* solution the variation in solubility of a solid with temperature can be expressed as :

$$\frac{d \ln S}{dT} = \frac{-\Delta H}{RT^2}$$

where S is the solubility (mole fraction), R is the gas constant, T is the absolute temperature and ΔH is the heat of solution. Assuming that ΔH is constant between temperatures T_1 and T_2, integration of the equation between these two limits gives:

$$\log \frac{S_1}{S_2} = \frac{-\Delta H}{2.303R} \left[\frac{1}{T_2} - \frac{1}{T_1} \right]$$

where S_1 and S_2 are the solubilities at temperatures T_1 and T_2 respectively. In an ideal solution the heat of solution ΔH is equal to the heat of fusion of the solid. The equation can also be written in the form:

$$\log S = \frac{-\Delta H}{2.303R} \frac{1}{T} + \text{constant}$$

where the plot of $\log S$ versus $1/T$ is a straight line with a slope of $-\Delta H/2.303R$, enabling the heat of fusion to be calculated. This treatment is not applicable to *non-ideal* solutions or to solutions whose temperatures are considerably above or considerably below the melting point. Polymorphic forms of a solute will have different solubility characteristics and the temperature at which one form reverts to another may be estimated from the point of intersection of the $\log S$ versus $1/T$ plots for the different forms. Shefter and Higuchi (1963) determined the transition temperature of the hydrated form of succinyl sulphathiazole and the pentanol solvate of hydrocortisone acetate using this method.

PARTICLE SIZE

The rate of solution under conditions of constant agitation and temperature is proportional to the surface area of the solid in contact with the solvent. Thus the rate of solution can be increased by using finely divided solids which have a high surface area per unit weight. During dissolution, the rate of solution will decrease due to the decrease in surface area of the particles. If allowances are made for this, the calculation of change of surface area with time becomes very complicated (Higuchi & Hiestand 1963). An alternative approach used by Edmundson and Lees (1965) was to regard solution as an etching process in which a given surface recedes in depth at a rate proportional to time. These two approaches are equivalent, as solution rate measured as volume/unit area/unit time is in fact equivalent to length/time. By dimensional analysis:

$$L^3 L^{-2} T^{-1} = L T^{-1}.$$

Edmundson and Lees (1965) used the Coulter Counter to follow the dissolution of hydrocortisone acetate particles and found that in agreement with the data above, the diameters of the particles decreased linearly with time.

If the particles are reduced to colloidal dimensions (<1 μm) the solubility itself may be affected to a limited degree. This effect is only of practical significance in the case of sparingly soluble solids and can be explained on the basis of increased free energy of the solid. Consider a cube of 1 cm edge; the surface area is 6 cm^2 and the surface energy 6γ ergs if γ is the surface energy (ergs/cm) of the solid. Subdivision of this cube into cubes of 0.1 cm side would produce 10^5 cubes and resultant surface energy of $6 \times 10^5 \gamma$ (ergs). This extra energy over and above that possessed by the original solid is responsible for producing an increase in solubility. The relationship between solubility Sr of a particle of radius r and the bulk solubility $S\infty$ is given by:

$$\ln \frac{Sr}{S\infty} = \frac{2\gamma}{\rho r} \frac{M}{RT}$$

where ρ and γ are respectively the density and surface energy of the solid and M its molecular weight. The substitution of typical values in the equation indicates that a solubility increase of about 8 per cent demands a reduction in particle size from coarse crystals to about 0.1 μm (Higuchi 1958). Barium sulphate particles 0.1 μm diameter have been reported as being twice as soluble as coarse particles (Alexander & Johnson 1949). The experimental verification of the previous equation is difficult as slight contamination of the solid surface by adsorbed impurities could cause a significant reduction in the surface energy and thus solubility changes could be less than predicted. The difference in solubility between small and large crystals is responsible for the coarsening of crystals in suspension (Ostwald ripening).

SOLUBILITY AND DEGREE OF SATURATION

Noyes and Whitney in 1897 studied the rate of solution of cylinders of benzoic acid and lead chloride in water. The surface area of solid and degree of agitation was kept constant. They obtained the following relationship between change of concentration with time and concentration of dissolved solute:

$$\frac{dC}{dt} = K(C_s - C)$$

where C_s = concentration of the saturated solution, C = concentration in the bulk solution and K = a rate constant. Later workers considered the process of dissolution took place, firstly by the formation of a saturated solution at the solid interface and then diffusion from this through the stationary layer of solvent surrounding the solid particle. The saturated film was assumed to form instantaneously and the limiting rate would be the diffusion across the stationary film. Agitation rates would influence the thickness of the film, high rates reducing its thickness. The previous equation could thus be written:

$$\frac{dC}{dt} = \frac{DA}{V\delta}(C_s - C)$$

where D = diffusion coefficient; A = area of interface; δ = thickness of stationary film; V = volume of the solvent. The term 'stationary film' is somewhat misleading as this is the streamline layer in contact with the solid when the solvent is moving in streamline flow. The solute can only pass through this film by the relatively slow process of diffusion. The diffusion coefficient increases with temperature and is inversely proportional to viscosity.

It follows from the Noyes–Whitney equation that in the initial stages of solution the rate of solution is directly proportional to solubility:

$$\frac{dC}{dt} = KC_s$$

Hamlin, Northram and Wagner (1965) found this equation to be applicable to a wide range of drugs although deviations are to be expected if the compounds undergo a reaction with the solvent or if the diffusion coefficient is affected by the nature and concentration of other ions present.

The rate of solution of sparingly soluble drugs in tablet or capsule dosage form controls the rate of absorption of the drug from the gastro-intestinal tract, if the solution rate is the rate-limiting step.

The importance of dissolution rate studies has been discussed by Wagner (1961) and Wurster and Taylor (1965).

SOLUTIONS OF SOLIDS IN LIQUIDS

When a solid is placed in contact with a liquid, particles leave the surface of the solid and pass into the liquid. The particles formed initially consists of blocks of a few molecules which formed the lattice blocks of the crystal; these ultimately break down into molecules or ions. The dissolved material diffuses through the liquid in all directions and some of it returns to the surface of the solid and passes out of solution. The solid continues to dissolve until an equilibrium is established between particles leaving the solid and those returning to it. At this point the solution is said to be *saturated*, and the concentration of the solute in the solution is termed its *solubility* at the temperature of the mixture.

THE DETERMINATION OF SOLUBILITY

The determination of solubility involves the preparation and analysis of a saturated solution. The determination is usually carried out by one of the following methods:

Analytical Method
Excess of the finely divided solid is agitated continuously with the solvent at the required temperature until equilibrium is attained. Most of the available solubility data have been derived from experiments based on this principle. The apparatus shown in Fig. 1.1 is convenient for the determination and is capable of yielding very accurate results (Campbell 1930). Filter tube A, which is about 3 mm bore and is packed with glass wool, is constricted at the upper end; tube B is capillary tubing. The lower bottle is charged with solute and solvent and agitated in a thermostat until solution is complete; up to 24 hours or more may be required for this. The apparatus is then inverted in the thermostat to allow the solution to filter through A into the empty bottle, the expelled air being returned by tube B. Tube B discharges a small quantity of pure solvent into the solution–solid mixture, but with a fine bore capillary this quantity is negligible. The S bend in B prevents the transference of solid into the empty bottle. The apparatus is removed from the thermostat and the filtered saturated solution is analysed. This method avoid inaccuracies due to differences in tempera-

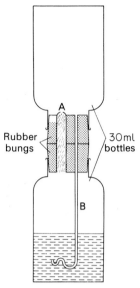

FIG. 1.1. Apparatus for solubility determinations.

ture between the saturated solution and the apparatus used for removal of the test portion.

In the determination of the solubility of finely powdered materials of low solubility, it is essential that the filter is capable of retaining the fine particles otherwise erroneously high results will be obtained when the filtrate is analysed. This difficulty may be overcome by the use of membrane filters which can be obtained in pore sizes down to about 0.2 μm. Filtration is rapid and there is negligible absorption of solute. Commercially available membrane filters include the Oxoid cellulose acetate filters (0.5 μm) and the Millipore filters (0.2 μm upwards). They are not affected by alcohol, ether or hydrocarbons but are soluble in certain esters and ketones. The membranes are fragile and need to be supported on a porous disc during filtration under reduced pressure. For the rapid filtration of small volumes, a syringe type holder is very convenient when the solution is forced through the membrane by the plunger in the syringe. No special thermostatic control of the syringe is necessary for solubility measurements at temperatures near to ambient.

The analysis of the saturated solution is performed by any suitable quantitative chemical analysis or by the determination of such physical characteristics as specific gravity or refractive index. For rough determinations, a measured quantity of the solution may be evaporated to dryness and the residue weighed. The concentration of very sparingly soluble salts, such as barium sulphate, may be calculated from the electrical conductivity of the solution; sparingly soluble lead salts may be determined in a manner similar to that used in the official lead limit tests. If radioisotopes of suitable half life are available, the technique of *isotope dilution analysis* may be applied. This can be illustrated by reference to the determination of barium sulphate solubility. Radioactive barium chloride is added to $BaCl_2$ in solution, in the form of $^{140}BaCl_2$, and on the addition of sulphuric acid, $^{140}BaSO_4$ and $BaSO_4$ are precipitated simultaneously. The specific activity (i.e. counts/min/mg) of the barium sulphate is determined. A saturated solution is then prepared and after evaporation to dryness, the radioactivity of the residue is measured. If both counts are done under standard conditions, the weight of residue in mg will be equal to the counts/min of the residue divided by the specific activity of the barium sulphate. In the case where solubility increases with temperature, the time taken for preparing a saturated solution can be reduced by heating the solvent with an excess of the solute. The solution is cooled to the desired temperature, in contact with the solid, to prevent the formation of a supersaturated solution.

Synthetic Method
A known quantity of solute is mixed with a known quantity of solvent in a stoppered vessel and the mixture is slowly heated in a water bath, with constant agitation, until the last crystal disappears. The temperature is noted. The heating bath is allowed to cool and the temperature at which the first crystal reappears is noted. If a supersaturated solution is not produced, the two temperatures should differ very little. From the proportion of solute and solvent, the solubility at the mean of these two temperatures can be calculated. In a modification of this method, a series of mixtures of solute and solvent of graduated proportions are shaken at a constant temperature until equilibrium is attained. The solubility then lies between the concentration of two mixtures; in one of these all the solute has disappeared and in the other a trace of solute remains. These methods are valuable in cases where accurate methods are not available for the analysis of the saturated solution or where the solvent is not very volatile. For example, the solubility of antioxidants in oils could be most conveniently determined by trial in this way.

SOLUBILITY CURVES

Solubility may be stated in any of the units available for representing concentrations. Usually it is expressed in g or ml of solute per 100 ml or 100 g of solvent or 100 ml or 100 g of saturated solution. In the *British Pharmacopoeia*, the solubility is expressed by stating the number of parts of solvent in which one part of solute will remain in solution at 20°. The solubility of sparingly soluble substances is occasionally given in mg/100 ml or mg per cent. Hence the statement that the solubility of sulphadiazine is 12 mg per cent at 37° means that 12 ml of sulphadiazine will form a saturated solution in 100 ml of water at 37°. For most pharmaceutical purposes the method for the statement of solubility used in the pharmacopoeia is the most convenient.

A solubility curve is a graph relating solubility to temperature (Fig. 1.2). Usually the curve is continuous, but in some cases abrupt changes in the direction of the curve are observed. Generally solubility increases appreciably with rise in temperature so that curves similar to that given for

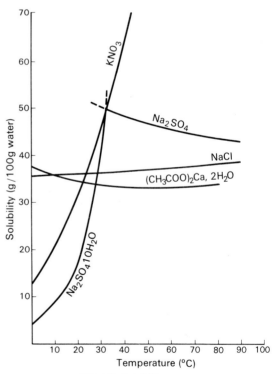

FIG. 1.2. Solubility curves.

potassium nitrate in Fig. 1.2 are most common. Sodium chloride has the unusual property of exhibiting only a slight increase in solubility with temperature; whereas some substances, notably calcium salts of organic acids, are less soluble in hot water than in cold water. The solubility of calcium sulphate is exceptional in that it gradually increases to a maximum at a certain temperature and then it decreases with further increase in temperature.

An abrupt change in direction of a solubility curve is due to a change in the character of the solid phase in contact with the solution, and the curve is better regarded as being made up of two intersecting curves which represent the solubilities of two distinct substances. In the case of sodium sulphate, the break in the curve is due to a change in the degree of hydration of the solid in contact with the saturated solution; up to 32°, the curve represents the solubility of the decahydrate, $Na_2SO_4, 10H_2O$; above 32°, it represents the solubility of anhydrous sodium sulphate, Na_2SO_4, and at 32°, it represents the equilibrium conditions between a saturated solution, the decahydrate and the anhydrous salt. The solubility curve of ammonium nitrate exhibits a break owing to a change of the solid into a second polymorphic form.

Normally when a saturated solution is cooled it deposits crystals. In some cases, when no undissolved solid is present, a solution may be cooled to a temperature which is below saturation temperature, and fail to deposit crystals. Such a solution is said to be *supersaturated*. In the absence of dust particles or undissolved solid, the transformation of a supersaturated solution to a saturated solution may be suspended indefinitely. This *metastable* state is readily broken down by the addition of a small crystal of the solute; dust particles, which can form nuclei for crystallization, or mechanical disturbances frequently cause deposition of the excess of solute hitherto held in solution.

Salts which crystallize with water of crystallization are most frequently capable of producing supersaturated solutions, e.g. sodium thiosulphate, potassium acetate and sodium sulphate. Calcium Gluconate Injection is a notable example of a supersaturated solution; calcium gluconate forms a saturated solution in about 30 parts of water, whereas in the injection it may remain in solution indefinitely in about 10 parts of water.

From a consideration of the properties of saturated solutions, it is apparent that the following rapid methods are available for their preparation:
(1) An excess of solid is dissolved in the solvent at a higher temperature than that at which the solution is required to be saturated and the solution is allowed to cool in contact with undissolved solute.

(2) The quantity of solid necessary to saturate the solution at the required temperature is ascertained from a work of reference. This quantity is dissolved in the solvent, with the aid of heat, and as the solution cools solvent is added to produce the required volume.

Since saturated solutions usually deposit crystals on cooling below saturation temperature, it is often advantageous to take quantities of solvent or solute so that the solution is saturated at a temperature slightly below that at which the solution is to be stored. Then under normal storage conditions no solid is deposited.

THE DISTRIBUTION OF A SOLUTE BETWEEN IMMISCIBLE LIQUIDS

A dissolved solid is distributed between two immiscible liquids in a manner very similar to the distribution of a gas between a liquid and a gas phase, and similar rules apply in both cases. The rules applying to the distribution of a solute between two immiscible solvents are as follows:

(1) *The Distribution Law.* If a solute is in the same molecular condition in both solvents, the ratio in which the solute distributes itself between the two solvents, called the *distribution coefficient*, or *partition coefficient* is constant at constant temperature (cf. Henry's Law, p. 14).

(2) In the presence of several solutes, the distribution of each solute takes place independently of the others (cf. Dalton's Law of partial pressures, p. 14).

If the solute is associated or dissociated or undergoes chemical combination in the two solvents, it is possible to determine the extent to which these changes take place by applying the distribution law to the molecular species which are identical in the two solvents.

When a substance is distributed between two immiscible solvents, A and B:

$$\frac{\text{Concentration in A}}{\text{Concentration in B}} = \text{the distribution coefficient,}$$

or briefly, $\dfrac{C_A}{C_B} = K$

Since saturated solutions of the same solute in two immiscible solvents are in equilibrium, the distribution (or partition) coefficient is equal to the ratio of the solubility of the solute in solvent A to its solubility in solvent B. In most cases, however, K is not strictly constant for all ranges of concentration in the two solvents. The value of K derived from solubilities is therefore only approximate.

EXTRACTION WITH IMMISCIBLE SOLVENTS

Consider a substance, S, soluble 10 g in 100 ml of water and 80 g in 100 ml of chloroform:

$$\frac{C_{chloroform}}{C_{water}} = K = \frac{80}{10} = 8$$

The distribution coefficient (K) is therefore 8.

(1) *Extraction with one quantity of Immiscible Solvent*

Assume that 5 g of substance S is shaken with 100 ml of water and 100 ml of chloroform and let x g be the weight dissolved in the chloroform. Then $(5 - x)$ g will be present in the water layer:

$$\therefore C_{chloroform} = \frac{x}{100} \quad and \quad C_{water} = \frac{(5-x)}{100}$$

But $\quad \dfrac{C_{chloroform}}{C_{water}} = K \quad \therefore \dfrac{x/100}{(5-x)/100} = 8$

$$\therefore \frac{x}{(5-x)} = 8, \text{ or } x = 4.44 \text{ g and } (5-x) = 0.56 \text{ g.}$$

Hence the chloroform will extract 4.44 g of S and 0.56 g will remain in the water layer.

(2) *Extraction with two successive quantities of Immiscible Solvent*

(a) If the volume of chloroform had been 50 ml, then, if y g is the weight of S dissolved in the chloroform:

$$C_{chloroform} = \frac{y}{50} \quad and \quad C_{water} = \frac{(5-y)}{100}$$

Then $\dfrac{C_{chloroform}}{\cdot C_{water}} = \dfrac{y/50}{(5-y)/100} = 8$

$$\therefore \frac{2y}{(5-y)} = 8, \text{ or } y = 4 \text{ g and } (5-y) = 1 \text{ g.}$$

Hence the chloroform layer contains 4 g of S and the water layer 1 g. The amount of S dissolved in the layer of 50 ml of chloroform is nearly as much as that dissolved in the layer of 100 ml of chloroform.

(b) If the chloroform layer is run off, 1 g of S remains in 100 ml of water. On shaking with a further 50 ml of chloroform, if z g is the weight of S dissolved in the chloroform:

$$C_{chloroform} = \frac{z}{50} \quad and \quad C_{water} = \frac{(1-z)}{100},$$

then $\dfrac{C_{chloroform}}{C_{water}} = \dfrac{z/50}{(1-z)/100} = 8$

$$\therefore \frac{2z}{(1-z)} = 8, \text{ or } z = 0.8 \text{ g and } (1-z) = 0.2 \text{ g.}$$

Hence the chloroform layer contains 0.8 g of S and the water layer 0.2 g. By taking two successive quantities, each of 50 ml of chloroform 4.8 g of S is extracted by the chloroform, whereas with a single quantity of 100 ml only 4.44 g is extracted. In the same way, it can be shown that a still more complete extraction would be effected if the chloroform was used in three successive quantities of 50, 25 and 25 ml.

The extraction of a solute from solution by shaking with an immiscible solvent is frequently used in the preparation and assay of materials containing alkaloids. If an aqueous solution of an alkaloidal salt is made alkaline and shaken with chloroform, the alkaloidal base distributes itself in favour of the chloroform phase. Successive extractions will deplete the aqueous phase of alkaloid. If the separated chloroform layers are combined and extracted with an acidic solution, the alkaloid (as a salt) passes into the aqueous phase and is relatively free from extraneous material such as plant pigments and tannins, which do not possess the same solubility characteristics. An extension of this liquid–liquid extraction method is counter-current extraction which is used for the fractionation of mixtures of solutes.

COUNTER-CURRENT EXTRACTION

This technique was developed by L. C. Craig and has been used for the separation of antibiotics, alkaloids, glycosides, etc. The theory and practice of this method has been authoritatively reviewed by Craig and Craig (1956). The apparatus consists essentially of a series of tubes in which the material to be fractionated is successively distributed between two immiscible liquids. Consider an extraction using chloroform and water as solvents. Equal volumes of chloroform are first added to each tube; the solute is dissolved in water and added to tube 1. The tube is shaken to achieve equilibrium and after settling, the upper phase (aqueous) is transferred to tube 2. An equivalent volume of water is then added to tube 1. Tubes 1 and 2 are shaken and when the phases have settled out, the aqueous phase of each tube is transferred to the next tube, i.e. 2 into 3, 1 into 2, and water into 1. In this way a stepwise transfer of aqueous phase occurs after separation of the two phases. A solute whose partition coefficient favours the aqueous phase will be transferred more quickly along the train of extraction tubes than a solute which is more soluble in chloroform. Thus, the partition coefficient of each solute determines its final position in the tubes at the end of a distribution run. The number of distributions and transfers may be fifty or more when it is required to separate solutes of similar solubilities. The amount of solute in each tube is determined and if this is plotted against the tube number, the resultant graph will indicate whether or not a separation has been obtained. It is possible from a knowledge of the partition coefficients, to predict the amount of solute that should be present in each tube. Agreement between theoretical and experimental results is often used as a criterion of purity of the solute being examined. Counter-current machines are available in which provision is made for the automatic shaking and transfer of the phases. The tubes are arranged in pairs and mounted so that equilibration is achieved by gentle rocking. The transfer from one equilibration tube to the next is obtained by the appropriate tilting of the tube (Fig. 1.3). Paper chromatography is a technique based on similar counter-current principles; filter paper acts as an inert support for the aqueous phase and the second liquid phase is an immiscible organic solvent which flows through the

paper by capillary action. The solute which is added to the paper, is subjected to continuous counter-current extraction and its rate of movement along the paper is a function of the partition coefficient.

SOLUTIONS OF LIQUIDS IN LIQUIDS

Water and alcohol mix in all proportions, whereas water and mercury do not mix at all. Between these extremes of complete miscibility and complete immiscibility all degrees of partial *miscibility* or *solubility* may exist. When water is added to ether, or ether is added to water, solution in both cases is limited. A point is reached when the ether will dissolve no more water and the water no more ether. Further addition of water in the first case or of ether in the second results in the formation of two liquid layers, one, the upper layer, consisting of ether containing about 3 per cent of water, the other, the lower layer, consisting of water containing about 10 per cent of ether.

THE DETERMINATION OF SOLUBILITY

An analytical or synthetic method may be used as previously described for the determination of solubility of solids in liquids. In many instances the synthetic method is the most convenient one; oversaturation of the solvent is evident when the solution is turbid and a saturated solution is taken to be that solution lying between the unsaturated and the oversaturated solutions. If the solubility curve is required, the method described below may be employed.

Weighed amounts of the two liquids are placed in hard glass tubes which are sealed by fusion. The tubes are placed in a thermostat and the presence of two phases is shown by a turbidity on shaking. The end point is determined by inspection. The solubility curve of phenol–water can be determined by this method; the tubes of phenol plus water are placed in a water bath which is slowly heated and the temperature at which the turbidity in a tube shows signs of disappearing is noted. The results are then plotted as percentage amounts of one component against the temperature at which homogeneity exists.

An analytical method that involves no manipulative techniques such as filtration or dilution, which may introduce errors, is based on the accurate measurement of refractive index of solutions containing increasing concentrations of solute. The solubility of benzaldehyde in water has been determined by this method (Carless & Swarbrick 1964).

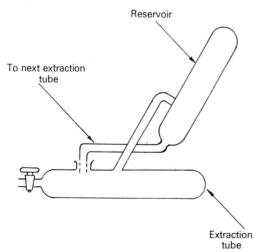

Fig. 1.3. Counter-current extraction tube.

SOLUBILITY CURVES

Temperature has a pronounced effect upon the mutual solubility of liquids and the following solubility curves may be observed:

Type 1: Mutual Solubility Increases with Temperature

When phenol is mixed with water it dissolves up to the limit of its solubility at the prevailing temperature. On adding more phenol a second layer is produced. There is then a solution of phenol in water and a solution of water in phenol. The mutual solubilities increase with increase in temperature until at a certain temperature the two layers merge into one. The temperature at which this occurs is called the *critical solution temperature* or *consolute temperature*. The phase diagram is shown in Fig. 1.4.

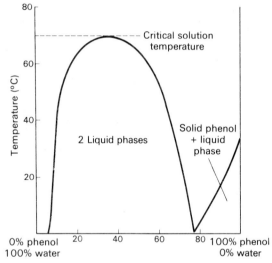

FIG. 1.4. Solubility of phenol in water and water in phenol.

The critical solution temperature of phenol–water is 66° and the critical concentration at this temperature is 34 per cent phenol. At all temperatures above the critical solution temperature, phenol and water are miscible in all proportions.

Type 2: Mutual Solubility Decreases with Temperature

Triethylamine and water are completely miscible below 18.5°; above this temperature they are partially miscible. Paraldehyde and water shows a similar lower critical solution temperature.

Type 3: Closed Solubility Curve

Besides those pairs of liquids which show an upper and those that show a lower critical solution tem-perature, other pairs are known which show both an upper and a lower critical solution temperature; the equilibrium curve takes the form of a closed curve. Thus in the case of nicotine and water; below 61° they are completely miscible, between 61° and 210° they are partially miscible, and they are completely miscible above 210°. Mixtures of *n*-butyl cellosolve (ethylene glycol monobutylether) and water show a similar behaviour. Theoretically all liquid pairs may be considered to have both upper and lower critical solution temperatures but either a solid phase appears or at the other end, one liquid is converted to vapour before complete miscibility occurs.

The critical solution temperature (CST) of a pair of liquids is extremely sensitive to the presence of a third substance, and it may provide an excellent criterion of purity for the liquids. If the third substance is soluble in only one of the liquids the mutual solubilities are decreased, e.g. potassium carbonate will cause alcohol to separate from a water–alcohol mixture. The temperature at which the liquids become completely miscible is raised, in systems having an upper CST and lowered in systems having a lower CST. In the phenol–water system the addition of 1 per cent of potassium chloride to the mixture of critical composition, raises the CST by 12° (Findlay, 1933). A substance soluble in both liquids increases the mutual solubility; an upper CST will be lowered and a lower CST will be raised.

THREE COMPONENT SYSTEMS

For three component systems at constant temperature and pressure, the composition can be expressed in terms of the coordinates of an equilateral triangle. In Fig. 1.5, each corner of the triangle represents a

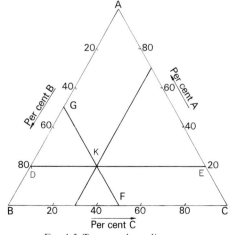

FIG. 1.5. Ternary phase diagram.

pure component, i.e. 100 per cent A, 100 per cent B and 100 per cent C. Each side represents a binary mixture and the interior represents all ternary compositions. A line parallel to one side of the triangle represents a constant percentage of one component, e.g. DE represents 20 per cent of A with varying amounts of B and C. Similarly line FG represents all mixtures containing 50 per cent of B. These lines intersect at K which must be 20 per cent A, 50 per cent B and therefore 30 per cent C. This must be the case since in the construction of an equilateral triangle the sum of the distances from the point K drawn parallel to the three sides is always the same and equal to the length of any one side of the triangle.

In the formulation of pharmaceutical solutions containing two immiscible liquids plus a mutually soluble liquid (cosolvent or blending agent) the triangular diagram provides a convenient means of expressing the data. Consider a mixture of chloroform, acetic acid and water. Acetic acid is miscible with both chloroform and water and its addition to the mixture will cause more water to dissolve in the chloroform and more chloroform to dissolve in the water. In Fig. 1.6 over the concentration range Ba

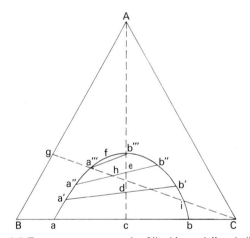

FIG. 1.6. Ternary system: one pair of liquids partially miscible.

and bC the mixture of chloroform and water forms true solutions. Between a and b the system will consist of two liquid layers of varying volumes but of compositions a and b. Point c represents two layers in the ratio:

$$\frac{\text{Weight of layer of composition a}}{\text{Weight of layer of composition b}} = \frac{cb}{ca}$$

If acetic acid is added to this two layer system the overall composition will follow the line cA.

At point d the two conjugate solutions present have the composition a'b'. The line a'b' is known as a tie line and will be parallel to the base only if the acetic acid distributes itself equally between the chloroform and the water. At point e the conjugate solutions will have compositions a"b", respectively. The tie lines usually rotate as they shorten and finally disappear at point f, the *plait point* of the system. To determine the tie line the two layers of a system must be analysed and their composition points joined.

The effect of adding water to the miscible mixture of chloroform and acetic acid of composition g can be followed by inspection of line gC which represents the changing compositions of the ternary mixture. When the ternary composition reaches a''' a second layer appears of composition b''' on the tie line a'''b'''. As the amount of water is increased further to h, the layers alter in composition to a" and b" and finally at i the system reverts to a single phase system. Systems which behave similarly include volatile oils in the presence of propylene glycol and water. Loran and Guth (1951) have studied the castor oil–ethanol–water system in order to determine suitable proportions for use in lotions and hair preparations. The blending agent that promotes miscibility may be a simple solvent such as alcohol or glycols or it may be a surface active agent that exerts its solvent effect due to micelle formation.

The ternary system cresol–soap–water (Lysol) has been studied by Burt (1965) who found that the nature of the cresol isomer affected the position of the regions of immiscibility in the triangular

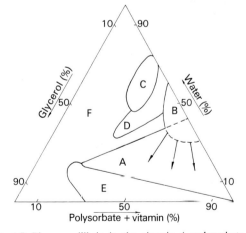

FIG. 1.7. Phase equilibria in the vitamin A–polysorbate 80–glycerol–water system (after Boon et al. 1961). A, Transparent single phase; B, semi-solid; C, faintly opalescent; D, markedly opalescent; E, two transparent phases; F, emulsions. Arrows denote decreasing viscosity in region A.

diagram. The ternary diagram approach was also used by Boon, Coles and Tait (1961) in studying the formulation of solubilized vitamin A preparations. Four components were used but by keeping the concentration of the vitamin constant the results were expressed as shown in Fig. 1.7. From the diagram it was possible to select the range of compositions that produced the required single phase system. These workers found considerable batch to batch variation in the solubilizing properties of the surfactant and this emphasizes the need for careful quality control of materials used in solubility studies.

SOLUTIONS OF GASES IN LIQUIDS

The solubility of gases in liquids is dependent upon the pressure exerted on the gas–liquid system as well as the temperature of the system. These relations are summarized in *Henry's Law*, which states that the solubility by weight of a gas in a liquid at constant temperature is proportional to the pressure of the gas. For example, if 0.028 g of a gas is dissolved by 1000 ml of water at 1 atmosphere pressure, 3×0.028 g will dissolve at 3 atmospheres pressure, provided the temperature is unchanged. As regard their solubilities, gases may be divided into three groups. Gases of the first group, which comprises sparingly soluble gases such as oxygen and nitrogen, obey Henry's Law; gases of the second group, which comprises slightly soluble gases such as carbon dioxide and chlorine, combine partially with water and show considerable deviations from Henry's Law; the third group comprises very soluble gases, such as hydrogen chloride and ammonia, which do not obey Henry's Law. The solubility of gases decreases with increase in temperature and with certain exceptions, such as the hydrogen halides, they are practically completely expelled from solution by prolonged boiling.

The solubility of gases is often expressed by the Bunsen *absorption coefficient* (α) which represents the volume of gas, reduced NTP, dissolved by one volume of liquid at a fixed temperature and 760 mm pressure. The absorption coefficient for nitrous oxide in blood is 0.415 at 37.5°. This means that at 760 mm pressure 1 ml of blood at 37.5° dissolves a volume of nitrous oxide which measures 0.415 ml at 0° and 760 mm pressure.

In a mixture of gases, Henry's Law applies to each gas considered separately and the pressure is then the partial pressure of the gas in question, not the total pressure of the mixture. The partial pressure is the pressure the gas would exert if it occupied the same volume as the mixture of gases. The total pressure is equal to the sum of the partial pressures (Dalton's Law).

METHODS OF DISSOLVING GASES

When a liquid is merely exposed to a gas, the surface layer of the liquid becomes saturated, and then the gas permeates the rest of the liquid by diffusion. More rapid solution is effected by spraying the liquid into the gaseous atmosphere or bubbling the gas through the liquid, because the rate of solution increases rapidly with the increase of surface per given volume of liquid.

Commercially, solutions of gases are made either by spraying the solvent into the gas, or by bubbling the gas under pressure into the solvent, which is kept constantly agitated, or by means of 'coke towers' or 'scrubbers'; these consist of towers loosely packed with coke over which the solvent trickles and dissolves the gas as it is forced up the tower.

METHODS OF REMOVING DISSOLVED GASES

The fact that the solubility of a gas is proportional to its partial pressure can be utilized for the removal of dissolved gases from solution. For instance oxygen can be removed from aqueous solution by bubbling an indifferent gas, e.g. nitrogen, through the solution. The partial pressure of the oxygen is lowered by the nitrogen and it is, therefore, less soluble. Removal of the oxygen will also be hastened by its diffusion into the bubbles of nitrogen which are carried away. A similar explanation can be given of the expulsion of a dissolved gas by boiling the solution. In this case the bubbles of vapour take the place of the indifferent gas. Water can thus be freed of dissolved oxygen and carbon dioxide by boiling.

SOLVENTS USED IN PHARMACY

It is important to distinguish between solvents which are acceptable for inclusion in the final product and those which are suitable only for use in the intermediate states of manufacture or in analytical operations. Obviously the former, being administered with the drug itself, must be non-toxic and non-irritant and must not interfere in any way with the normal absorption. In the case of injectable preparations this is often a severe limitation since the number of available solvents is small. For chemical or pharmaceutical processing, the limiting factors become cost, toxicity (to operators) and inflammability hazards. In some operations it may be difficult to remove the final traces of solvent from a drug, even with vacuum drying; if so, it is important to control the residual volatile matter by a suitable limit test. A trace of methyl alcohol in an injectable drug, for example, might have serious effects on the patient. In analytical operations there are no restrictions on solvents. Thus a water-insoluble drug which is normally given by injectable suspension may be dissolved in benzene to check that it contains no extraneous matter.

The following classication is given only as a guide to the solvents in common use:

Solvents used in manufacture of pharmaceuticals
Methyl, ethyl and isopropyl alcohols; industrial methylated spirit; glycols; ethyl ether and higher ethers; chloroform; acetone; benzene; petroleum ether; acetic acid; etc.

Solvents for oral and external preparations
Water; ethyl alcohol; glycerin; propylene glycol; arachis oil; olive oil; ethyl oleate; liquid paraffin.

Solvents for external preparations
Industrial methylated spirit; isopropyl alcohol; benzyl alcohol; polyethylene glycols; hexylene glycol; ethyl, isopropyl and butyl esters of palmitic, myristic and sebacic acids.

Solvents for injectable preparations
Water for injection; ethyl oleate; arachis oil; olive oil; propylene glycol; benzyl alcohol.

Water has a more extensive range of solubility than any other liquid, and has the advantage of cheapness. It is, therefore, the most commonly employed solvent. One outstanding disadvantage of the use of water as a medium of extraction is connected with its wide range of solubility; it dissolves not only those substances that are required, such as glycosides, but often those which are not, such as gums, albuminous, pectinous and colouring matters, sugars, tannins, vegetable acids, mineral salts and, in the case of hot water, starch. These substances may be favourable to the growth of moulds and bacteria, or in other ways bring about the decomposition of the preparation. The presence of sugars or other carbohydrates in a solution may result in alcoholic fermentation with evolution of carbon dioxide; while the presence of protein matter may lead to nitrogenous fermentation with liberation of ammonia. The addition of 0.25 per cent v/v of chloroform to water, i.e. Chloroform Water, prevents the growth of micro-organisms and is used in preference to water in pharmaceutical mixtures liable to support bacterial growth. Pharmacopoeial preparations are directed to be made with Purified Water which is prepared by distillation or by ion-exchange methods. The B.P.C. and the B.N.F. allow the use of potable water, i.e. water freshly drawn direct from the public water supply ('mains' water) and suitable for drinking. It should be replaced by freshly boiled and cooled Purified Water when the potable water in a district is unsuitable for a particular preparation.

Ethyl Alcohol is widely used in pharmacy as a solvent. It will dissolve resins, glycosides, free alkaloids and their salts but will not dissolve gums, albumins, starch and many inorganic salts. Most fixed oils, with the exception of castor oil, are sparingly soluble in alcohol. Alcohol is a valuable solvent for extracting vegetable drugs on account of its *selective action* and preservative properties. At strengths of 20 to 25 per cent and above, ethyl alcohol inhibits the growth of bacteria, moulds, yeasts and other fungi.

A heavy excise duty is levied on pure ethyl alcohol. Its cost for most pharmaceutical preparations would be prohibitive if a rebate of duty was not allowed. Rebate can be claimed for alcohol used in preparations intended solely for medical purposes. The increased use of industrial methylated spirit, which is duty free, has relieved this situation. Industrial methylated spirit contains commercial methyl alcohol (wood naphtha) and therefore cannot be allowed in internal preparations. Its use is permitted in a number of preparations made according to B.P. and B.P.C. formulae and in special formulae approved by Customs and Excise.

Isopropyl Alcohol (specific gravity 0.788 to 0.793; boiling point 80° to 83°) is more toxic than ethyl alcohol and cannot be used for preparations taken internally. It is often used in lotions and cosmetic perfumes.

Glycerin (specific gravity 1.26; boiling point 290°) is a good solvent for many substances which are not very soluble in water, e.g. borax and phenol. It also acts as a preservative but to a lesser degree than alcohol. Glycerin suffers from the same disadvantage as water in that it dissolves gummy and albuminous matter. It also extracts large quantities of tannins and their oxidation products when these are present in a drug, a property which is sometimes used in preventing the precipitation of tannin-oxidation products from preparations made with other solvents.

Its low volatility and hygroscopic character are of value in maintaining preparations such as kaolin poultice in a moist condition.

Glycols are alcohols containing two hydroxyl groups and are intermediate in their properties between alcohol and glycerin. With the exception of propylene glycol, they are toxic and not employed in preparations intended for internal administration. Large quantities are used in cosmetic preparations. They are hygroscopic, soluble in water and excellent solvents for resins, gums and essential oils.

Ethylene Glycol $CH_2OH.CH_2OH$ (specific gravity 1.113; boiling point 197°) has been used as a solvent of terpeneless oils.

Diethylene Glycol $HOCH_2CH_2.O.CH_2CH_2OH$ (specific gravity 1.117; boiling point 244°) is used as a solvent for nitrocellulose, resins and oils.

Diethylene Glycol Monoethyl Ether (Carbitol) $C_2H_5O.CH_2CH_2.O.CH_2OH$ (specific gravity 1.00; boiling point 200°) is used as solvent of fats and waxes.

Ethylene Glycol Monethyl Ether (Cellosolve) $C_2H_5O.CH_2CH_2OH$ (specific gravity 0.93; boiling point 134°) is used as solvent for insecticidal sprays containing derris and pyrethrum. It is an effective solvent for nitrocellulose.

Propylene Glycol $CH_3CH(OH).CH_2OH$ (specific gravity 1.036; boiling point 187°) resembles glycerin in physical properties but is less viscous. It is miscible in all proportions with water, alcohol, chloroform and with 10 volumes of ether, but immiscible with light petroleum and fixed oils. As a preservative and solvent it can be used in place of glycerin since its toxicity is fairly low. Vitamin D, progesterone, sodium phenobarbitone and chloramphenicol are stable in solution in propylene glycol. Penicillin rapidly decomposes in this solvent.

Polyethylene Glycols known as the *Macrogols*, are mixtures of condensation polymers of ethylene oxide and water, and represented by the formula $HOCH_2(CH_2CH_2O)_nCH_2OH$. They range from liquids where *n* varies from 4 to 15, to waxy solids where *n* may lie between 60 and 80. In naming these glycols, the average molecular weight is indicated by a number immediately following the name. Thus Macrogol 400 is a liquid of approximate molecular weight 400; Macrogol 4000, molecular weight 4000, is a waxy solid. Macrogols of intermediate consistency can be prepared by mixing together appropriate proportions of high and low molecular weight material. They are miscible with water, alcohol, acetone and other glycols. Water-insoluble medicaments can often be dissolved in a macrogol which may form the basis of a 'washable' ointment base.

Ether (specific gravity 0.72; boiling point 34.5°) is an excellent solvent for certain oils, fats and alkaloids. It is not generally suitable for the production of liquid preparations which are to be taken internally owing to its pronounced therapeutic action, or which are to be kept for any length of time, owing to its inflammability and its volatility; it is used, however, in collodions where the volatility makes it particularly valuable and in cases such as male fern extract in which no ether remains in the final preparation.

Chloroform (specific gravity 1.49; boiling point 61°) is a good solvent for many alkaloids and fats, and is frequently used, either alone or with ether, in alkaloidal determinations; it is not inflammable and only sparingly soluble in water. Chloroform has a sweet taste, and is an excellent preservative, hence the frequent use of its aqueous solution in pharmaceutics. An unusual solvent effect is its ability to dissolve certain alkaloidal hydrochlorides; this has been applied in the selective extraction of strychnine hydrochloride from a mixture of strychnine hydrochloride and quinine hydrochloride.

Acetic Acid (specific gravity 1.05; boiling point 118°; melting point 16.6°) is capable of dissolving many of the active principles of crude drugs, and preparations made with it keep well. Its use is limited, however, owing to its acid properties, which make it incompatible chemically with many substances; in some conditions acids are contraindicated therapeutically.

Acetone (specific gravity 0.79; boiling point 56°) will dissolve many resins and fats, and is employed as a solvent for cantharidin in preparations for external use, where its volatility is of value and its odour not of importance. It is unsuitable for preparations for internal use. It is particularly valuable for defatting animal tissues.

Light Petroleum (petrol ether) (specific gravity 0.65; boiling point 40° to 60°) is a fraction of petroleum consisting mainly of hexane; it is very volatile and highly inflammable and is a good solvent for oils, fats and resins. Since it will not dissolve alkaloids or their salts it is a useful solvent for defatting alkaloidal drugs such as ergot. Unlike acetone it is immiscible with water which makes it unsuitable for defatting wet tissue.

Ethyl Oleate (specific gravity 0.88; boiling point 204° at 6 mm) is a good solvent for steroid hormones and other oil-soluble medicaments. It has a relatively low viscosity which makes it a useful vehicle for oily intramuscular injections; vegetable oils, which have similar solvent properties, are more viscous.

Isopropyl Myristate (specific gravity 0.85; boiling point 137–175° at 5 mm) is less greasy than mineral or vegetable oils which it can replace in creams and oily applications. Its miscibility with a wide range of hydrocarbons, vegetable oils, fats and waxes, makes it a useful blending agent for mixtures of these substances. Unlike vegetable oils it shows no tendency to become rancid on storage since it is a saturated fatty acid ester.

Light Liquid Paraffin has been used for preparing oily nasal drops containing oil-soluble substances such as camphor, menthol, etc.

MIXED SOLVENTS

The solubility of a solid in a mixture of solvents is usually intermediate between the values of the constituent solvents, although the actual solubility is not directly proportional to the quantities of solvents present. Alcohol 25 per cent differs only slightly from water as a solvent and it is not until the alcohol content is increased to 60 to 70 per cent that the characteristic solvent action of alcohol is apparent. Some mixed solvents do not follow this pattern; a solute only sparingly soluble in either solvent alone, may be readily soluble in a mixture of the two solvents. This has been termed *cosolvency*,

and may be explained by each solvent dissolving a different part of the molecule. An example is nitrocellulose which is readily soluble in an alcohol–ether mixture but only sparingly soluble in the separate solvents.

Strong solutions of certain solutes such as sodium benzoate and sodium salicylate are capable of dissolving water-insoluble materials, e.g. 30 per cent sodium benzoate readily dissolves chlorocresol (Reeds 1956). This phenomenon is termed *hydrotrophy* and has been discussed by McKee (1946). Large concentrations of a solute are required to cause this effect and it should be distinguished from the solubilizing effect produced by dilute solutions of soap.

When a solution of a substance in one solvent is added to another solvent in which the substance is sparingly soluble, most of the solute will be precipitated. This precipitation due to a change of solvent, occurs in the dispensing of mixtures containing resinous tinctures, e.g. Compound Benzoin Tincture added to water causes precipitation of the water-insoluble resin. Inorganic salts, e.g. ferrous sulphate, in aqueous solution are precipitated on the addition of a large proportion of alcohol.

Recovery of Solvents is essential for reasons of economy in manufacturing processes. When mixed solvents of similar boiling-points are used, the recovery of the individual solvents may be difficult or impossible. If the mixed solvent can be used again in the process then this is unimportant. Large losses may be encountered in the recovery of extremely volatile solvents such as ethyl ether; the use of a higher boiling-point solvent with similar solvent properties may be advantageous, e.g. isopropyl ether. The recovery of solvents whose vapours, mixed with air, form highly inflammable mixtures, should be treated with caution. Ethers are liable to develop peroxides on storage which can explode during heating. It is advisable to decompose these peroxides by chemical treatment. e.g. by shaking with ferrous sulphate solution, before proceeding with the distillation.

REFERENCES

ALEXANDER, A. E. & JOHNSON, P. (1949) *Colloid Science*, 36. London: Oxford University Press.

BOON, P. F. G., COLES, C. L. J. & TAIT, M. (1961) *J. Pharm. Pharmacol.* **13**, 200T.

BURT, B. W. (1965) *J. Soc. Cosm. Chem.* **16**, 465.

CAMPBELL, A. N. (1930) *J. Chem. Soc.* 179.

CARLESS, J. E. & SWARBRICK, J. (1964) *J. Pharm. Pharmacol.* **16**, 633.

CRAIG, L. C. & CRAIG, D. (1956) Laboratory extraction and countercurrent distribution. *Technique of Organic Chemistry* (Ed. by Weissberger), Vol. 3, Part I. New York: Interscience.

EDMUNDSON, I. C. & LEES, K. A. (1965) *J. Pharm. Pharmacol.* **17**, 193.

FINDLAY, A. (1933) *Introduction to Physical Chemistry*, p. 518. London: Longmans, Green.

HAMLIN, W. E., NORTHRAM, J. I. & WAGNER, J. G. (1965) *J. pharm. Sci.* **54**, 1651.

HARTLEY, G. S. (1956) *Progress in the Chemistry of Fats and Other Lipids* (Ed. by R. T. Holman, W. O. Lundberg and T. Malkin), Chapter 2. London: Pergamon Press.

HIGUCHI, T. (1958) *J. Am. pharm. Ass. (Sci. Ed)*, **47**, 657.

HIGUCHI, W. I. & HIESTAND, E. N. (1963) *J. pharm. Sci.* **52**, 67.

LORAN, M. R. & GUTH, E. P. (1951) *J. Am. pharm. Ass. (Sci. Ed)*, **40**, 465.

MCKEE, R. H. (1946) *Ind. engng Chem.* **38**, 382.

REEDS, D. (1956) *Pharm. J.* **177**, 233.

SHEFTER, E. & HIGUCHI, T. (1963) *J. pharm. Sci.* **52**, 781.

WAGNER, J. G. (1961) *J. pharm. Sci.* **50**, 359.

WURSTER, D. E. & TAYLOR, P. W. (1965) *J. pharm. Sci.* **54**, 169.

2

pH EMF and Redox Potentials

Hydrogen ion concentrations are determined over a very wide range and, to avoid the inconvenience of using very small numbers, Sörenson introduced the concept of pH in 1909. He defined pH as the negative logarithm of the hydrogen ion concentration, viz:

$$pH = -\log [H+]$$

A similar notation can be applied to hydroxyl ion concentrations:

$$pOH = -\log [OH^-]$$

where $[H^+]$ and $[OH^-]$ represent the concentrations of hydrogen and hydroxyl ions, respectively.

On thermodynamic grounds these relationships are often modified to:

$$pH = -\log a_{H+}$$

and

$$pOH = -\log a_{OH-}$$

where a_{H+} and a_{OH-} are the 'activity' or effective concentrations of hydrogen and hydroxyl ions, respectively. However, for dilute solutions, one can usually assume:

$$a_{H+} = [H^+]$$

$$a_{OH-} = [OH^-]$$

The pH scale nominally covers the range 0 to 14 but it is possible, under special circumstances, to have pH values outside these limits. A neutral solution has a pH of 7; acid solutions have pH values less than 7 and alkaline solutions greater than 7.

IONIZATION CONSTANTS

Strong acids and bases are, for all practical purposes, completely ionized in aqueous solution so that it is not possible to write any equilibrium expressions. For weak electrolytes, however, equilibrium expressions can be written and, by applying the Law of Mass Action, values of K_a or K_b can be calculated. Ionization constants, often loosely referred to as dissociation constants, are usually expressed in terms of pK_a or pK_b where $pK_a = -\log K_a$ and $pK_b = -\log K_b$. Low values of pK_a or high values of pK_b are characteristic of relatively strong acids or weak bases, whereas high values of pK_a or low values of pK_b indicate relatively weak acids or strong bases. The Lowry Brönsted theory (details of which are outside the scope of this volume) enables the ionization constants of acids, bases and their salts to be verified on the pK_a scale by using the expression:

$$pK_a + pK_b = pK_w = 14 \text{ (at } 25°)$$

Ionization constants vary with temperature, and for purposes of comparison it is essential to record pK_a values at the same temperature.

Ionization constants may be determined by several methods, e.g. conductimetrically, potentiometrically or spectrophotometrically.

The conductimetric method for determining ionization constants requires knowledge of the degree of ionization which can be calculated from the formula:

$$\alpha = \frac{\Lambda_c}{\Lambda_\infty}$$

where Λ_∞ is the equivalent conductance at infinite dilution and is a measure of the complete dissociation of the solute into its ions and Λ_c is the equivalent conductance of the solution being examined and is a measure of the number of solute particles present as ions at concentration c. The ratio Λ_c/Λ_∞ is known as the *conductance ratio*. To obtain K_a it is now necessary to substitute in the equation:

$$K_a = \frac{\alpha^2 c}{(1-\alpha)}$$

where c is the concentration.

The potentiometric determination of ionization constants involves the titration of the acid or base and application of the Henderson equation:

$$pH = pK_a + \log \frac{[salt]}{[acid]}$$

or

$$pK_a = pH - \log \frac{[salt]}{[acid]}$$

There are certain limitations in the use of this equation which need not concern us here but it is of interest to note that at 50 per cent neutralization, i.e. when $[salt] = [acid]$ then $pK_a = pH$. This means that the ionization constant can be read directly from a titration curve simply by recording the pH at 50 per cent neutralization.

The spectrophotometric determination of pK_a also involves the use of the Henderson equation and the application of it to the graph obtained when absorbance versus pH is plotted at a suitable wavelength.

BUFFER SOLUTIONS

Buffer solutions are usually solutions of weak acids (or bases) and their corresponding salts, e.g. acetic acid and sodium acetate. Such solutions resist changes of pH upon the addition of small quantities of acid or alkali and this phenomenon is known as buffer action. In solutions where the buffer action is absent or very low, the pH can change considerably due to the absorption of carbon dioxide from the air or extraction of alkali from the material of the glass container. In the example quoted above, the addition of a small quantity of strong acid (e.g. HCl) results in only a small decrease in pH because the hydrogen ions react with the sodium acetate to liberate the very much weaker acetic acid according to the reaction:

$$CH_3COONa + HCl \rightleftharpoons CH_3COOH + NaCl$$

This equation can be expressed more generally as:

$$Ac^- + H_3O^+ \rightleftharpoons HAc + H_2O$$

If a strong base (e.g. NaOH) is added to the buffer solution, the acetic acid neutralizes the hydroxyl ions:

$$HAc + OH^- \rightleftharpoons Ac^- + H_2O$$

Buffer solutions are not usually prepared from weak bases and their salts since not only are many bases volatile but the solutions often have high temperature coefficients.

The pH of a buffer solution can be determined by applying the Henderson equation. If the salt and acid concentrations are known together with the pK_a of the acid concerned then the pH may be calculated.

Example: What is the pH of the buffer solution prepared by mixing 5 ml $N/100$ acetic acid (pK_a 4.76) with 15 ml $N/10$ sodium acetate?

Total volume = 20 ml

$$\therefore [salt] = \frac{15}{20} \times \frac{1}{10} \text{ g-equiv/l,}$$

$$[acid] = \frac{5}{20} \times \frac{1}{100} \text{ g-equiv/l,}$$

$$pH = pK_a + \log \frac{[salt]}{[acid]}$$

$$= 4.76 + \log \frac{15 \times 1 \times 20 \times 100}{20 \times 10 \times 5 \times 1}$$

$$= 4.76 + \log 30$$

$$= 4.76 + 1.48$$

$$\therefore pH = 6.24$$

DETERMINATION OF pH VALUES

The two most important methods of measuring pH are by the use of coloured indicators or of special electrodes.

COLORIMETRIC METHOD FOR DETERMINING pH

Indicators are either weak acids or bases which exist in two *tautomeric* forms; these two forms differ in colour and the distribution of their valency electrons, e.g. phenolphthalein:

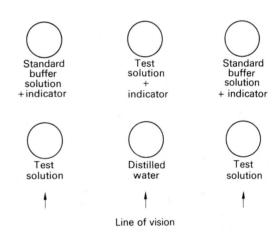

Unionized acid form
(colourless)

Ionized red forms
(red)

The colour of any indicator added to a test solution depends on the ratio of the ionized: unionized forms present and this, in turn, depends on the pH of the solution. Maximum sensitivity to pH change occurs when the concentrations of unionized and ionized forms are equal, i.e. when the pH equals the pK_a of the indicator. The usable range of a single indicator varies by about ± 1.5 pH units on either side of the pK_a value of the indicator; e.g. phenolphthalein has a $pK_a = 9.4$ and a useful pH range of pH 8.2 to 10.0. Mixtures of indicators can be made which can cover most of the range of the pH scale; these 'Universal' indicators are available as liquids or as test papers and are useful in determining pH to approximately ± 1 unit.

To determine the pH correct to about ± 0.2 units, a small sample of the test solution should be mixed with an equal volume of an indicator solution whose working range covers the pH of the test solution. Samples from buffer solutions made up in 0.2 pH intervals are treated in a similar manner and the pH of the test solution determined by direct colour comparisons. Sets of these buffer solutions already admixed with the indicator and in sealed capillary tubes, known as Capillators, are available commercially so it is possible to measure pH values of test solutions within a minute or two. It is important that these standard colours are protected from light to prevent fading.

For larger volumes of test liquid, comparators are used. Essentially these are test tubes used in a manner similar to capillators but are particularly useful when turbid or coloured solutions are being examined. Tubes of distilled water or test solutions only can be placed in front of the tubes being compared (see Fig. 2.1) so that the same total depth of liquid is viewed in each case and compensation

is made for turbidity or colour not due to the indicator.

Standard buffer solution + indicator

Test solution + indicator

Standard buffer solution + indicator

Test solution

Distilled water

Test solution

Line of vision

FIG.2.1. *Comparator* (diagrammatic).

ELECTROMETRIC METHODS FOR DETERMINING pH

Numerous indicator electrodes are available for the determination of pH and, without doubt, the glass electrode is the most widely used. The glass electrode consists of a thin glass bulb of special glass blown at the end of a glass tube and the bulb is filled with dilute acid, e.g. decinormal hydrochloric acid. A silver–silver chloride electrode (a silver wire electrolytically coated with silver chloride) makes the necessary electrical connection with the acid whose pH remains constant (pH_k). Several types of glass are used to make the pH-sensitive glass bulb and those made of lithia glass are suitable over most of the range pH 0 to 14. When the glass bulb is immersed in a solution of unknown pH (pH_x) a potential E_H is set up across the glass according to the equation:

$$E_H = K - 0.0592\,(\mathrm{pH}_x - \mathrm{pH}_k) \qquad (\text{at } 25°)$$

or, by combining constants:

$$E_H = K - 0.0592\,\mathrm{pH}_x \qquad (\text{at } 25°)$$

K is known as the *asymmetry potential* and varies from time to time although it is usually reasonably constant over the period of a working day unless the electrode is subjected to extremes of pH.

To measure the pH of a solution, the bulb of the glass electrode and a suitable reference electrode is immersed in a sample of the solution and the two electrodes connected to a pH meter. The reference electrode is essential for the second electrical contact with the solution and must, of course, have a constant potential irrespective of the pH of the solution (see Fig. 2.2).

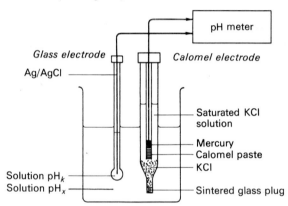

FIG. 2.2 Electrode system for pH measurement.

A simple potentiometer cannot be used to measure the potential difference between the two electrodes because the glass electrode has an exceptionally high resistance ($> 100\ \text{M}\Omega$). This means that any current flowing in the circuit would be insufficient to affect any ordinary galvanometer without some form of electronic amplification.

All pH meters are operated in essentially the same way. The electrical zero of the pH meter is adjusted, if necessary, and, with the electrodes immersed in a buffer solution of standard pH, the asymmetry potential control altered until the meter reads the known pH value of the buffer solution. These standardized electrodes, after rinsing with distilled water, are then immersed in the test solution and the pH value of the solution read from the meter either directly in the case of deflection meters, or after adjusting to a null balance in the case of potentiometric type meters.

Several standard pH solutions are available for the calibration of pH meters, the most popular being 0.05 M potassium hydrogen phthalate solution. Table 2.1 shows the pH of this and some other solutions over a wide temperature range.

TABLE 2.1

pH OF STANDARD SOLUTIONS AT VARIOUS TEMPERATURES

$t(°C)$	I	II	III	IV	V	VI
0	4.011	1.67	—	6.98	9.46	9.51
5	4.005	1.67	—	6.95	9.39	9.43
10	4.001	1.67	—	6.92	9.33	9.36
15	4.000	1.67	—	6.90	9.27	9.30
20	4.001	1.68	—	6.88	9.22	9.25
25	4.005	1.68	3.56	6.86	9.18	9.20
30	4.010	1.69	3.55	6.85	9.14	9.15
35	4.020	1.69	3.55	6.84	9.10	9.11
40	4.031	1.70	3.54	6.84	9.07	9.07
45	4.045	1.70	3.55	6.83	9.04	9.04
50	4.061	1.71	3.55	6.83	9.01	9.01
55	4.080	1.72	3.56	6.84	8.99	8.98
60	4.101	1.73	3.57	6.84	8.96	8.96

I Potassium hydrogen phthalate, $KO_2C.C_8H_4.CO_2H$, (0.05 M). The figures in this column indicate values which are the specifications of the British standard 1947: 1950. The third decimal place is not significant, but is included for interpolation purposes. The salt may be dried at temperatures below 135°.

II Potassium tetroxalate, $KH_3(C_2O_4)_2.\,2H_2O$, (0.05 M). The salt may be purified by crystallization from an aqueous solution below 50°. It must not be dried above 55°.

III Potassium hydrogen tartrate, $KO_2C.(CHOH)_2:CO_2H$: saturated solution at 25°, decanted from excess salt.

IV Potassium dihydrogen phosphate KH_2PO_4, (0.025 M), and disodium hydrogen phosphate. Na_2HPO_4, (0.025 M). The latter should be dried at 110 to 130° for 2 hours.

V Borax, $Na_2B_4O_7.IOH_2O$ (0.01 M).

VI Borax, $Na_2B_4O_7.IOH_2O$ (0.05 M).

The following points should be noted:
(1) Good distilled water (pH 6 to 7) should be used for acid buffer solutions. Freshly boiled and cooled distilled water (i.e. CO_2-free) must be used for alkaline buffer solutions.
(2) The pH values change slightly on dilution with water. The above solutions when diluted with an equal volume of water increase in pH value: I, +0.052; II, +0.186; III, +0.049; IV, +0.049; V, +0.01.
(3) Standard buffer solutions may be stored for up to 2 months in well-closed hard glass or polythene bottles. It is advisable to discard solutions if mould or sediment is visible.

SIGNIFICANCE OF pH IN PHARMACY

The pH of many pharmaceutical preparations must be controlled to ensure optimum stability or physiological activity of the medicament. During the course of manufacture, the pH of the product can be influenced in various ways and a knowledge of the more important factors is useful in the formulation of such products.

Glass is a very useful material for storage but it imparts alkalinity to products stored in glass containers. Special glasses are available and the containers used for pharmaceutical purposes have to comply with tests which limit the alkalinity to acceptable proportions. Solutions which come into contact with filter materials of cotton and paper, for example, tend to make the solutions more alkaline. Distilled water, on the other hand, is usually acid (pH 4.5 to 6) due largely to dissolved carbon dioxide. Even when the dissolved gases are boiled off, the pH can become alkaline, rather than neutral, due to the alkalinity of the glass container.

Precipitation can sometimes occur if the pH of a solution is changed significantly and use can be made of this fact in the preparation of pharmaceutical products. When solutions of the salts of insoluble acids are acidified, the corresponding insoluble acids are precipitated, e.g. sodium benzoate or salicylate will deposit benzoic or salicyclic acids, respectively.

The purification of proteins is simplified by the knowledge that amphoteric compounds are least soluble at the isoelectric point, e.g. insulin precipitates from aqueous solutions at pH 5 to 6. These examples illustrate how solubility is influenced by the degree of ionization which is controlled by pH, as shown by the following relationship:

$$\text{Percentage of ionized molecule}$$

$$= \frac{100}{1 + \text{antilog}(\text{pH} - \text{p}K_a)}$$

where pH refers to the pH of the solution and $\text{p}K_a$ to the weak acid or base under consideration.

The above formula is of particular interest when considering the biological activities of medicaments, since the unionized molecule and ionic species usually have difference activities. Unionized molecules penetrate cell membranes (which are lipid in character) more readily than ions and this accounts for the increased antimicrobial action of benzoic acid ($\text{p}K_a$ 4.2) and salicylic acid ($\text{p}K_a$ 2.97) in acidic solutions. On the other hand the antibacterial activity of the acridines depends on the amount of drug present as the cation, so for maximum effectiveness the $\text{p}K_a$ of these molecules should be numerically as near the pH of the body fluids (about pH 7.4) as possible to ensure that a large amount of the drug is in the ionized form.

Enzymes have maximal activity and stability at definite pH values and outside certain limits they are rendered inactive and may even be destroyed. Thus pepsin has maximal activity at pH 1.5, and is, therefore, effective in the gastric fluid but is rendered inactive in the duodenum where the pH is about 8.

Many compounds are unstable in aqueous solution because hydrolysis takes place. Often, however, the solutions can be stabilized by adjustment of the pH. Basic esters such as amethocaine, amylocaine and procaine require acid conditions to achieve stability. Vitamins are often stable only over a narrow pH range and many B.P. injections are adjusted to a definite pH to ensure stability of the product.

REDOX POTENTIALS

When an ion is oxidized it donates electrons to another ion which is simultaneously reduced by accepting the donated electrons. Thus ferrous iron loses an electron on oxidation to ferric iron:

e.g. $$Fe^{2+} - e \rightleftharpoons Fe^{3+},$$

the converse is also true:

e.g. $$Fe^{3+} + e \rightleftharpoons Fe^{2+},$$

this can be expressed in more general terms, thus:

$$\text{Red} \rightleftharpoons \text{Ox} + ne,$$

where Red refers to the reduced state (reductant) and Ox refers to the oxidized state (oxidant) of the ion; ne is the number of electrons involved in the reaction.

Oxidation–reduction (redox) systems which are under equilibrium conditions can be studied in a similar manner to pH systems but by using an inert (e.g. platinum) indicator electrode together with a reference electrode (e.g. calomel electrode). A potential is set up under these conditions which depends on the relative concentrations of oxidant and reductant. This potential (E_h) is given by the Nernst equation:

$$E_h = E^0 + \frac{0.0592}{n} \log \frac{[\text{Ox}]}{[\text{Red}]} \text{ at } 25°$$

where n is the number of electrons transferred per ion and E^0 is the *standard oxidation–reduction potential*. It will be observed that when the concentrations of oxidant and reductant are equal, then $E_h = E^0$. The potential E_h can be determined by use of a potentiometer to measure the potential difference (E_{cell}) between the indicator electrode (whose potential is E_h) and the reference electrode (E_{ref}) according to the following relationship:

$$E_{cell} = E_{ref} - E_h$$

The E^0 of a redox system is a characteristic constant and gives a measure of its oxidizing or reducing *tendency*. The higher the E^0 value the greater is the oxidizing ability of the system: the lower the E^0 value, the greater is the reducing power of the system, i.e. a system of higher E^0 value will oxidize a second system of lower E^0. Where Redox reactions occur which involve the hydrogen ion, then its concentration must be considered. Thus in the reaction:

$$H_2Q + 2H_2O = Q + 2H_3O^+ + 2e$$

Hydroquinone	Quinone
(reductant)	(oxidant)

the potential at 25° is:

$$E_h = E^0 - \frac{RT}{2F} \ln \frac{[Q][H_3O^+]}{[H_2Q]}$$

or, expressed more generally:

$$E_h = E^0 - \frac{RT}{2F} \ln \frac{[Ox]}{[Red]} - \frac{RT}{F} \ln [H_3O^+]$$

This equation shows that E_h is reduced if the hydrogen ion concentration (activity) is increased or the pH decreased. It is sometimes convenient in systems of a definite pH to combine the last term of the equation with the E^0 to give a standard potential E^0 characteristic of the system at a fixed pH. The standard potentials E^0 for some redox systems of pharmaceutical interest are given in Table 2.2.

TABLE 2.2

STANDARD POTENTIALS OF SPECIFIED pH AT 30°

Redox system	E^0(V)	pH
Adrenalin	0.380	7.0
Ascorbic acid	0.115	5.2
	0.136	4.58
2,6-Dichlorphenolindophenol	0.217	7.0
Methylene blue	0.011	7.0
Riboflavin	−0.208	7.0
	−0.117	5.0

As in the determination of pH, it is possible to use certain dyes to determine the value of E_h approximately as the colour of such dyes varies with their state of oxidation. Methylene blue for example, changes from almost colourless to a deep blue (at pH 7) as E_h varies from 0.040 to −0.062 V. Redox indicators can also be used effectively to determine the equivalence point in redox titrations.

3

Crystalline Solids

The process of crystallization involves a reversal of the changes which occur when a solid melts or dissolves. Except when mixed crystals form, crystalline forms are very pure, and commercially provide a material which is in an attractive physical form. A typical crystal has a regular geometric form with sharp, straight edges and plane surfaces. When fractured, it breaks into pieces with plane faces meeting in sharp edges, whereas a supercooled liquid fractures as easily in one direction as another. The crystalline nature of powders and metals is revealed only by microscopic examination, and in the case of metals the individual crystals are seen to be arranged in a disorderly manner.

The regular external form of a crystal is determined by a regular assembly of atoms or ions arranged in a space lattice having a uniform geometrical form. The arrangement of these units is the most important characteristic of a crystal, for, even if the external form is destroyed by powdering, the internal structure remains. Crystals may vary in size and in the development of different faces owing to the conditions under which they are formed. The constant geometrical form of the units composing the crystal is exhibited in the constancy of the angles between similar faces (Law of constancy of interfacial angles).

The symmetry possessed by crystals is expressed in terms of their symmetry about certain planes and axes of the crystal. An *axis of symmetry* is an axis on which the crystal can be rotated through 360° and occupy the same position more than once. If a crystal possesses a suitable number of axes of symmetry, three of them may be chosen as

crystallographic axes, e.g. alum; in crystals possessing less than three axes of symmetry, e.g. copper sulphate, other axes are chosen as the crystallographic axes. For classification all crystals are referred to seven groups, e.g. cubic (alum), triclinic (copper sulphate), which are defined by the disposition of the crystallographic axes.

The shapes of crystals are often described in general terms which are almost self-explanatory; needle-shaped crystals are often termed acicular, and plate-like crystals, laminar. Such terms give no indication as to the position of the crystals in the system of classification based on crystallographic axes; for example, the prism occurs in several groups.

POLYMORPHISM

Many substances exist in two or more crystalline forms and are said to be *polymorphic*. The differences are due primarily to differences in crystalline structure which give rise to differences in physical properties, e.g. solubility. Red mercuric iodide crystallizes as octahedra when prepared by mixing dilute solutions of mercuric chloride and potassium iodide, washing with cold water and drying below 40°. When heated to above 126°, it changes into the yellow variety which exists as laminar crystals; on cooling the yellow form reverts to the red form. The two official varieties of sulphur are different forms of the same substance. This variety of polymorphism exhibited by elements is termed *allotropy*.

When the change from one polymorphic form is reversible it is said to be *enantiotropic* but when the transition takes place in one direction only, i.e.

25

from a metastable form to a stable form, it is said to be *monotropic*. Polymorphism is known to occur in many steroids, in sulphonamides and barbiturates, the occurrence being frequent in complex molecules, particularly if hydrogen bond formation is possible within the molecule. Detection of different polymorphic forms has been achieved by X-ray diffraction and infra-red adsorption of the crystalline solid. When a crystalline solid is dissolved in solvent, the crystalline structure is lost so that different polymorphs of the same substance will show the same absorption spectra in solution. Sulphathiazole exists in at least two polymorphic forms, one of which (Form I) undergoes a change in crystal structure at about 174° to Form II that melts at 180°. Form I can be prepared by crystallization of sulphathiazole from boiling water or 95 per cent ethanol and seems to be the form commonly met in practice. Cortisone acetate exists in several crystalline forms, only one of which is suitable for preparing stable aqueous suspensions. The unstable forms undergo a polymorphic change in the presence of water which results in crystal growth. The biological activity of chloramphenicol palmitate has been correlated with polymorphic behaviour (Aguiar et al. 1967). Four different polymorphic forms of oil of theobroma have different melting points. Heating it to 38° completely liquefies the fat but destroys the beta stable crystals (m.p. 34.5°), the crystals that are formed being the meta stable gamma, alpha and beta forms melting at 18°, 22° and 28°, respectively, so that the suppositories tend to melt at room temperature. By melting the oil of theobroma at the lowest possible temperature (about 33°) the stable beta form is not lost and a suppository stable at room temperature is produced. Hydrogenated vegetable oils, are also used as suppository bases but as they are unlikely to exist in polymorphic forms they are not affected by slight overheating.

Transitions of unstable to stable forms during heating can often be detected by measuring the volume expansion of a sample confined in a *dilatometer*. Ravin & Higuchi (1957) performed dilatometric analyses of theobroma oil and other waxy materials. Another technique is *differential thermal analysis* which involves the controlled heating of sample and inert reference substance the temperature of each being measured by sensitive thermocouples. If thermal energy is absorbed during crystal rearrangement, the difference in temperature between sample and reference can be detected and displayed on a recording millivoltmeter. Thermal transitions of sulphathiazole and cortisone acetate have been detected with this technique (Carless, Moustafa & Rapson 1966; Guillary 1967).

In the formulation of drugs known to exist as polymorphs, it is essential that the form present in the final preparation should be stable. The form most suitable for preparing stable suspensions will not necessarily be that most stable in the dry state. Infra-red methods for identifying polymorphic forms of steroids and sulphonamides have been described by Mesley & Johnson (1965) and Mesley & Houghton (1967).

Other methods used to identify polymorphic phases of a compound include measurement of refractive index and X-ray diffraction of single crystals or of powders (Haleblian & McCrone 1969).

ISOMORPHOUS CRYSTALS

Many chemical substances of similar chemical constitution form crystals of similar shape, and are said to be *isomorphous* (the same shape). Examples of isomorphous substances are magnesium sulphate, $MgSO_4,7H_2O$ and zinc sulphate, $ZnSO_4,7H_2O$; disodium hydrogen phosphate, $Na_2HPO_4,12H_2O$ and disodium hydrogen arsenate, $Na_2HAsO_4,12H_2O$.

The *alums* form a characteristic group of isomorphous compounds. When equal proportions of the gramme-molecular weights of potassium sulphate, K_2SO_4, and aluminium sulphate, $Al_2(SO_4)_3,18H_2O$ are dissolved in water and the solution is concentrated and allowed to crystallize, a *double salt, potash alum*, is obtained. This consists of homogeneous crystals containing one molecular proportion of potassium sulphate and one molecular proportion of aluminium sulphate combined with 24 molecular proportions of water. If ammonium sulphate is used in place of potassium sulphate, the product is *ammonia alum*.

If a solution which is about to crystallize is seeded with a crystal of a substance, *isomorphous with the substance in solution*, an *isomorphous overgrowth* is obtained; the solute crystallizes round the crystal that has been immersed in the solution. This behaviour is well illustrated by seeding a solution of (colourless) potash alum with a crystal of (purple) chrome alum, when a colourless crystal with a purple centre is obtained.

Another property of isomorphous substances is the formation of *mixed crystals*, which are essentially solid solutions. When solutions of potash alum and chrome alum are mixed and allowed to crystallize, a crop of pale violet crystals consisting of a homogeneous mixture of the two double salts is obtained.

It is not uncommon for substances to have very similar crystalline forms without being similar in chemical constitution or isomorphous. True isomorphous substances exhibit similar crystalline forms and normally form isomorphous overgrowths and mixed crystals.

MECHANISM OF CRYSTALLIZATION

A solution must be saturated before any solid matter can crystallize out. If the temperature of a saturated solution is lowered, or solvent allowed to evaporate from such a solution, then the excess of solid material separates out. On lowering the temperature of a saturated solution very carefully, it is often possible to cool it considerably without the separation of crystals. Such a solution is said to be supersaturated.

The formation of crystals from solution involves two steps; firstly the creation of crystalline nuclei, and secondly the growth of these nuclei into crystals. Nuclei may arise spontaneously, although in actual practice this is thought to be rare, or they may arise by the introduction of minute crystals of the dissolved substance. This operation is known as seeding. The driving force for the nucleation and subsequent growth of the crystals is the supersaturation of the solution. The theory of Miers postulates that a definite relationship exists between the concentration and the temperature at which crystals will spontaneously form in an initially unseeded solution. The form of that relationship is a supersolubility curve roughly parallel to and above the normal solubility curve. Such a curve may be imagined as the solubility for exceedingly fine particles which can be shown to have a solubility appreciably greater than larger crystals. The solubility curves are shown in Fig. 3.1. The theory states that in the region between the two curves (metastable zone) there will be no appreciable spontaneous nucleation, but above the supersolubility curve there is copious spontaneous nucleation. A solution of compositions E will spontaneously crystallize and the solution concentration falls to that given by the normal solubility curve at the prevailing temperature, i.e. point G. A solution represented by point F in the metastable region will remain unchanged unless seeds are added and when nucleation occurs the concentration will again drop to point G.

In crystallization processes the nuclei formation should be under control since the number of nuclei will control the size of the crystal. Large crystals

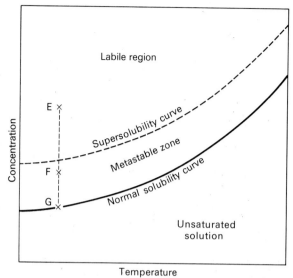

FIG. 3.1. Solubility curves.

may be obtained as a result of slow cooling of solutions just above saturation point, due to the reduction in number of spontaneous nuclei; crystals grow from these few nuclei and will then grow to the desired size before new nuclei appear. Conversely, rapid cooling increases the degree of supersaturation (beyond Miers' supersaturation curve) resulting in a large number of nuclei and a crop of small crystals.

Nuclei may originate in the following ways:

(a) Spontaneously due to cooling an unseeded solution into the labile region.
(b) Deliberate seeding with minute crystals.
(c) Fortuitous seeding by crystals left from previous batch.
(d) Attrition of existing crystals giving rise to fragments that act as seeds. The degree of stirring will affect this factor.

Nucleation may be inhibited by the presence of impurities, especially if of high molecular weight, in the solution.

The most important crystallization technique involves crystallization from a solvent. For this purpose a solvent, in which the crystals are sparingly soluble in the cold and readily soluble in the hot is chosen. The solid is added in portions to a suitable quantity of the hot solvent, until a hot saturated solution is obtained; the hot solution is filtered into a wide-mouthed conical flask and set aside to cool. Usually crystals separate during cooling. Some substances, particularly organic compounds, form supersaturated solutated solutions, and no crystals are deposited on cooling the hot saturated solution. Crystallization, in such cases, may usually be initiated by seeding the supersaturated liquid with a crystal of the solid substance, by stirring or by scratching the sides of the vessel with a glass rod. Crystallization is sometimes effected by strongly cooling a solution saturated at room temperature, or by allowing such a solution to evaporate spontaneously in a desiccator over a substance which will absorb the solvent, e.g. anhydrous calcium chloride for water and alcohol.

The size of crystals usually depends upon the conditions of crystallization.

Very small crystals are obtained by the rapid cooling, with frequent stirring, of solutions almost saturated at their boiling point. Generally the production of very small crystals of a substance is to be avoided, because they tend to cohere into masses which are difficult to wash, and consequently the substance may be less pure than when obtained in crystals of medium size.

Medium-sized crystals are obtained, when crystallizing from water, from solutions saturated at about 60° to 80°. The hot solution is allowed to cool slowly and without mechanical disturbance in a warm room. When a satisfactory strength of solution at a given temperature has been found by experience, it is customary on the large scale to note the specific gravity at that temperature by means of a hydrometer. In future crystallizations the solution is adjusted to the required strength corresponding to the observed temperature and specific gravity.

On the large supersaturated solutions may be induced to crystallize by artificial cooling. Brine from a refrigerating plant is circulated round the pan or tank, which has an outer jacket; or brine may be passed through a coiled tube within the solution. The liner of the pan or tank is made of good conducting material, such as copper or tinned copper, in order that the maximum effect of the brine may be secured. The temperature gradient between parts of the solution near to and remote from the cooling surface ensures that some portion of the solution is at the temperature of the maximum rate of formation of crystal nuclei.

Uniformity in size of crystals of substances, such as sodium sulphate or magnesium sulphate, is obtained by crushing and sifting the large, irregular crystalline masses obtained from the tanks.

Very large crystals are obtained by setting aside a large volume of a solution and allowing it to evaporate spontaneously. The liquid should have been rendered perfectly clear by filtration, and the access of dust must be guarded against. The formation of large crystals may be facilitated by seeding, that is suspending a well-formed crystal of the solute in the solution, the crystal acting as a nucleus.

The mother liquor is the term applied to the liquid remaining after a crop of crystals has been obtained. The mother liquor is not discarded, but is subjected to further concentration and again set aside to crystallize; the second quantity of mother liquor is concentrated and a further crops of crystals is obtained. This process is repeated until practically the whole of the dissolved substance has been recovered. Crops of crystals obtained by concentration of the mother liquor are usually less pure than the first crop and may require recrystallization. The treatment of the mother liquor is very important on the commercial scale, particularly in the crystallization of expensive substances, such as alkaloids, to avoid serious financial loss.

CRYSTAL GROWTHS IN SUSPENSIONS

In suspensions of finely divided solids an increase in crystal size is undesirable since there is a tendency for the crystals to bind together forming a hard cake which is difficult to redisperse. Crystal growth may also lead to other undesirable changes; large particles tend to produce a gritty texture and make them unsuitable for topical, especially ophthalmic, use. The causes of crystal growth in suspensions have been discussed by Higuchi (1958) and are summarized as follows:

(1) Temperature fluctuation; a rise causing increased solubility and a fall causing supersaturation and hence crystallization.
(2) Solid present in a metastable state which has a greater solubility than the stable state, so that the solution is supersaturated with respect to the latter.
(3) Small crystals have a greater solubility than large crystals so that the solution is supersaturated with respect to the latter.
(4) Change of crystal structure due to presence of dispersing solvent.

Crystal growth of drugs can be accelerated by temperature cycling (Carless & Foster 1966).

Possible methods of preventing crystal growth include the use of particles of narrow size range, grinding the solid in the presence of the dispersing fluid (change of crystal structure?), addition of surface active agents which are adsorbed on to the crystal surface and so inhibit the rate of deposition of solute molecules.

A simple suspension of cortisone acetate powder for use as eye-drops is liable to crystal growth; grinding with hydrated aluminium hydroxide and inclusion of methyl cellulose produces a stable aqueous suspension (Flitcroft & Birchall 1957).

Suspensions should, if possible, be confined to insoluble solids, or at least to solids with a flat solubility curve, to minimize the undesirable effects produced by temperature fluctuation.

PRECIPITATION

Substances produced by precipitation are usually microcrystalline. The process involves the mixing of solutions of the reactants and the interaction of these substances to form a sparingly soluble substance. When chemically equivalent quantities of the reactants are used, the order of mixing is not usually of importance. When an excess of one reactant is required for complete precipitation of the product, this reactant is usually gradually added to the other reactant until no further precipitate is produced. This procedure avoids waste of materials and the precipitate will require less washing in order to obtain it in a pure condition. The process of precipitation in the laboratory is best performed in a conical beaker flask, the form of which is most convenient for washing the precipitate by decantation before collecting it on a filter.

The character of a precipitate often depends upon the conditions under which it has been produced. When the reacting substances are mixed at temperatures near to their boiling-point, the precipitate is usually granular and heavy, whereas a precipitate of the same substance produced by mixing cold solutions may be light, take a long time to settle and to wash, and will, perhaps, pass through the filter. Similarly, concentrated solutions produce a precipitate in larger particles than do dilute solutions. A very fine precipitate, once formed, can often be caused to coagulate or form larger particles by boiling or by digesting for some time on a water-bath, e.g. silver bromide and barium sulphate. Some substances can be precipitated only from cold solutions, because of their solubility; acid potassium tartrate and magnesium ammonium phosphate normally crystallize only from cold solutions. Such precipitates can often be induced to form more rapidly by scratching the sides of the vessel with a glass rod, or by vigorous shaking.

The theory of von Weimarn relates the degree of supersaturation with the particle size of the precipitate; the initial velocity of precipitation is proportional to $(Q - S)/S$, where Q is the total concentration of the substance to be precipitated and S is its equilibrium solubility. $Q - S$ will be the amount of material thrown out of solution. For the formation of fine particles $(Q - S)/S$ should be large. This may be achieved by making Q large and/or S small. The use of concentrated solutions will result in a large value for Q, although too high a concentration may produce a gelatinous precipitate. To make the value of S small, the solubility may be reduced by using a solvent in which the product is only slightly soluble. For instance, barium sulphate of colloidal size can be precipitated, by double decomposition, from aqueous alcohol solution in which barium sulphate is less soluble than in water (see Alexander & Johnson 1949).

The preparation of microcrystalline sulphathiazole (Chambers et al. 1942), involves a novel process; a solution of sulphathiazole sodium is neutralized with acid at a low temperature, the mixture being agitated violently by ultrasonic vibrations, or with a high speed stirrer; the precipitated sulphathiazole is centrifuged, washed with water and suspended in normal saline. The precipitate formed under the influence of violent agitation is in a very finely divided condition and yields a stable suspension in normal saline.

FRACTIONAL CRYSTALLIZATION

The process of crystallization affords a method for the purification of crystalline substances. Advantage is taken of the different solubilities of a substance and associated impurities. The impure substance is dissolved by the aid of heat in a solvent, found by experiment to be the most suitable, and the solution is filtered while still hot and set aside to crystallize. If the solvent has been properly selected, the desired substance will crystallize out, while the impurity will remain in solution, since it is unlikely that the solution will be saturated with respect to both the required substance and the impurity. If impurity is still present the process of recrystallization is repeated until the product has attained the desired degree of purity as shown by physical and chemical tests (e.g. melting point, boiling point, density, solubility, crystalline form, optical properties, assay and specific tests for impurities).

Isomorphous substances which form mixed crystals cannot be separated by fractional crystallization, even if their solubilities are widely different.

WATER OF CRYSTALLIZATION

Solid compounds of salts with water of definite composition are called *hydrates* and the combined water is termed *water of crystallization*. For example, when anhydrous copper sulphate ($CuSO_4$), a white powder, is dissolved in water and the solution is set aside to crystallize, the product consists of blue prisms of copper sulphate pentahydrate ($CuSO_4, 5H_2O$).

Water of crystallization forms part of the structure of the crystals and may be attached to the anion or to the cation. In hydrated copper sulphate four of the water molecules, which are readily expelled on heating, are attached to the copper cation and the fifth is attached to the sulphate anion. The fifth molecule of water is held more firmly and is sometimes referred to as *water of constitution*. The nature of the bond linking the water molecules to the salt is as yet not clearly understood, but in certain instances, it has been shown that bonds of the same type as those linking hydrogen to oxygen in water (covalent bonds) are involved.

Some substances are capable of forming crystals with different proportions of water of crystallization; sodium carbonate, for example, can, by various means, be obtained as $Na_2CO_3,10H_2O$, $Na_2CO_3,8H_2O$, $Na_2CO_3,6H_2O$, $Na_2CO_3,5H_2O$ and Na_2CO_3,H_2O. It should not be thought that water of crystallization is essential in order that a salt may be crystalline; no water of crystallization is present in crystals of, for instance, potassium chlorate, potassium dichromate, potassium bromide or sodium chloride. Many organic compounds crystallize with solvent of crystallization; citric acid crystallizes with one molecule of water, $CH_2(COOH).C(OH)(COOH).CH_2COOH,H_2O$; crystalline ergometrine may contain one molecule of acetone of crystallization.

VAPOUR PRESSURE OF HYDRATES

The water present in solids containing water of crystallization exerts a vapour pressure. The magnitude of this vapour pressure is a measure of the tendency of the substance to lose water. If the vapour pressure of the water in the surrounding atmosphere differs from the vapour pressure of the water in the hydrate, the hydrate will tend to gain or lose water until an equilibrium is established with the water vapour in the atmosphere. The loss of water of crystallization by a hydrate to form an anhydrous salt or a hydrate containing fewer molecules of water of crystallization is termed *efflorescence*. The water in sodium sulphate, $Na_2SO_4,10H_2O$, exerts a vapour pressure of 16.3 mm at 20°; the water vapour pressure in the atmosphere is often below this value and then the hydrate effloresces to yield an anhydrous powder. Other examples of efflorescent substances are borax, $Na_2B_4O_7,10H_2O$, and sodium phosphate, $Na_2HPO_4,12H_2O$.

With some substances, the aqueous vapour pressure of a saturated solution is lower than the usual aqueous vapour pressure of the atmosphere. Under these conditions, the solid absorbs atmospheric moisture, forms a hydrate if such can exist, and continues to absorb moisture until a solution is formed; this phenomenon is termed *deliquescence*. A saturated solution of calcium chloride exerts a vapour pressure of 4 to 5 mm at ordinary temperatures; more dilute solutions exert higher vapour pressures up to the vapour pressure of pure water (12 to 17 mm at 15° to 20°). The vapour pressure of the water in the atmosphere may rise as high as about 15 mm. Hydrated calcium chloride or calcium chloride will therefore readily absorb atmospheric moisture and ultimately form a solution of below the concentration of a saturated solution. It will be seen that sodium sulphate may effloresce in an atmosphere in which calcium chloride or its hexahydrate deliquesces. All deliquescent substances are very soluble in water, notable examples being potassium hydroxide, sodium iodide, sodium lactate, trichloracetic acid and zinc chloride.

Many substances which absorb water do not form liquid mixtures or definite compounds with the water. Such substances are said to be *hygroscopic*. In these substances, it is probable that the water is attracted to the solids by the forces responsible for adsorption (Chapter 6). Many chemical and vegetable drugs are hygroscopic, e.g. exsiccated sodium sulphate, and dry extracts. This term is also applied to liquid substances such as sulphuric acid, glycerin and dehydrated alcohol which absorb moisture from the air. There is no doubt, however, that sulphuric acid forms definite compounds with water.

EXSICCATION

The process of removing water of crystallization from hydrated substances is termed *exsiccation*. Exsiccated ferrous sulphate, exsiccated sodium carbonate, exsiccated alum (burnt alum) and anhydrous sodium arsenate are noteworthy examples of substances prepared by exsiccation; magnesium sulphate, sodium phosphate and sodium sulphate are exsiccated as a preliminary step in preparing their respective effervescent granules. The principles underlying the process of exsiccation are the same as those underlying the phenomenon of efflorescence. Substances capable of forming more than one hydrate may be exsiccated in stages. For instance, copper sulphate, $CuSO_4,5H_2O$, on heating may be successively converted into the trihydrate, $CuSO_4,3H_2O$, the monohydrate, $CuSO_4,$

H_2O, and the anhydrous substance, $CuSO_4$. Exsiccated substances are not necessarily anhydrous. Anhydrous ferrous sulphate cannot be prepared by heating the hydrate in air, since basic sulphate is formed before all the water is driven off, but if exsiccation is suitably effected in a vacuum the anhydrous substance, $FeSO_4$, is obtained. Substances containing a large proportion of water of crystallization, e.g. sodium sulphate, Na_2SO_4, $10H_2O$, are usually liquefied on heating by dissolving in the water present.

Exsiccation is effected by weighing the substance into a tared dish and heating, with frequent stirring, until there is no further loss in weight, or until the calculated loss in weight has taken place. A water-bath or steam-oven may be used as a source of heat in some cases, but often a sand-bath or air-oven must be used.

REFERENCES

ALEXANDER, A. E. & JOHNSON, P. (1949) *Colloid Science*, 561. London: Oxford University Press.

AGUIAR, J. A., KRE, J., KINKEL, A. W. & SAMYU, J. C. (1967) *J. pharm. Sci.* **56**, 847.

CARLESS, J. E. & FOSTER, A. A. (1966) *J. pharm. Pharmacol.* **18**, 697.

CARLESS, J. E., MOUSTAFA, M. A. & RAPSON, H. D. C. (1966) *J. Pharm. Pharmacol.* **18**, 190S.

CHAMBERS, L. A., FERGUSON, L. K., HARRIS, T. N. & SCHULMAN, F. (1942) *J. Am. med. Ass.* **119**, 324.

FLITCROFT, J. & BIRCHALL, M. E. (1957) *Pharm. J.* **178**, 79.

GUILLARY, J. K. (1967) *J. pharm. Sci.* **56**, 72.

HALEBLIAN, J. & McCRONE (1969) *J. pharm. Sci.* **58**, 911.

HIGUCHI, T. (1958) *J. Am. pharm. Ass. (Sci. Edn)* **47**, 657.

MESLEY, R. J. & HOUGHTON, E. E. (1967) *J. pharm. Pharmacol.* **19**, 295.

MESLEY, R. J. & JOHNSON, C. A. (1965) *J. pharm. Pharmacol.* **17**, 329.

RAVIN, L. J. & HIGUCHI, T. (1957) *J. Am. pharm. Soc.* **46**, 732.

4

Interfacial Phenomena

INTERMOLECULAR FORCES

All atoms and molecules attract one another due to *van der Waals forces* which arise because of an uneven distribution of electrons around an atom or a group of atoms so that the positive and negative centres do not coincide. The result is the production of a dipole whose behaviour can accurately be described only by recourse to quantum mechanics. The van der Waals forces may be classified into three types:

(a) *Keesom attraction* between polar groups, that is between permanent dipoles. This results from the preponderence of attractive over repulsive orientations since, during rapid thermal motion, dipoles are closer when under attractive orientation.

(b) *Debye attraction* between a permanent dipole and the dipole which it induces in another group.

(c) *London attraction* between individual atoms whereby even non-polar molecules attract each other. Although such atoms or molecules do not possess a dipole moment, they do possess a dipole which is rapidly fluctuating due to the motion of the electrons and whose frequency is about 10^{15} to 10^{16} s^{-1}. Since the time average of the electron distribution is symmetrical, the effect of these transitory dipoles would be self-cancelling were it not for the fact that they induce an in-phase relationship with neighbouring transitory dipoles. It is this effect which enables even the inert gases to liquefy and is responsible for the refractive dispersion of light. Because of the latter phenomenon, the London force is frequently referred to as the *dispersion force*.

All three components therefore have an electromagnetic origin which gives rise to a potential energy field U around the atoms. Because the attraction (negative by convention) *potential* varies inversely as the sixth power of the distance r between the interacting atoms or groups, the attractive force varies inversely as the seventh power since the force F is the gradient

$$-\frac{\partial U}{\partial r}$$

(Fig. 4.1). At close distances of approach, interpenetration of the electron clouds produces a very large repulsive energy (Born repulsion) which varies approximately with r^{-12}. The potential energy function may therefore be written (Lennard-Jones 6–12 potential)

$$U = -Ar^{-6} + Br^{-12}$$

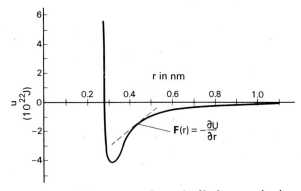

FIG. 4.1 Potential energy curve for a pair of hydrogen molecules.

32

where A and B depend on the nature of the molecules. Because the *force* of attraction varies with r^{-7}, the influence is felt over only a fraction of a nanometre. The van der Waals forces are therefore short-ranged.

The relative contributions of the three components are listed for a few simple molecules in Table 4.1. Generally, the London component pre-

TABLE 4.1

RELATIVE MAGNITUDES OF INTERMOLECULAR INTERACTIONS

Molecule	Dipole Moment $(10^{30}C.m)$	Potential $\times r^6 (10^{41} J.m^6)$		
		Orientation (Keesom)	Induction (Debye)	Dispersion (London)
H_2	0	0	0	11.3
He	0	0	0	1.2
N_2	0	0	0	62
CH_4	0	0	0	117
CO	0.40	0.0034	0.057	67.5
HCl	3.44	18.6	5.4	105
NH_3	4.94	84	10	93
H_2O	6.14	190	10	47

dominates but the Keesom component is excessive with highly polar molecules such as water. In such cases the Keesom force is particularly strong because the hydrogen atom shares only two electrons in the molecule so that it can approach very close to the electronegative atom of a neighbouring molecule thereby forming a *hydrogen bond*. The close approach of the hydrogen proton allows it to pull closer to itself the electron cloud around the electronegative atom of the other molecule. The resulting hydrogen bond strength will depend on the electronegative atoms (generally oxygen, nitrogen or fluorine) on either side of the hydrogen proton and upon the inductive effect of other groups. Its magnitude is usually between 10 and 30 kJ.mol^{-1} and is therefore appreciable although still only a fraction of the strength of covalent bonds which are mostly 200 to 800 kJ.mol^{-1}.

Hydrogen bonding produces molecular association which, in the case of hydrogen fluoride and formic acid, is strong enough to persist even in the vapour state if the temperature is not too high. Water would boil at about 203K were it not for its association into aggregates of higher molecular weight. Since each oxygen atom of water has two lone pairs of electrons, it can form two hydrogen bonds in addition to its two covalent bonds. These four bonds are disposed around the oxygen atom towards the corners of a tetrahedron and enable the production of polymeric clusters of water molecules which continually break and reform under

thermal agitation with a life time of about 10^{-11}s. This structuring of water confers upon it various anomalous properties such as a high surface tension and dielectric constant and the abnormal effect of temperature and pressure upon its density and viscosity.

Besides producing intermolecular association, the hydrogen bond can form intramolecular bridges. Thus o-nitrophenol forms a bond between the nitro-oxygen and phenol-hydrogen atoms and consequently it remains unassociated and boils at 214K. Because the hydrogen bond is internal the compound is only sparingly soluble in cold water but volatile in steam. The groups of p-nitrophenol, on the other hand, are not close enough to form a hydrogen bond. This compound therefore self-associates and boils at the higher temperature of 295K. Since it can form hydrogen bonds with water it is moderately soluble in cold water but it is only slightly volatile in steam. Internal hydrogen bonds play a major role in maintaining the specific configuration of many proteins and their rupture by chemical or thermal means leads to denaturation.

The van der Waals forces are directly involved in the existence of liquid and solid states whereby molecules are held close together and occupy some specific volume depending upon the prevalent temperature and pressure. Because of this a boundary must exist between a condensed phase and a gas or between two condensed phases. Generally speaking, a boundary with a gas is known as a *surface*, other boundaries being referred to as *interfaces*. There is however no strict terminology and any boundary may be referred to either as a surface or as an interface.

LIQUID–GAS AND LIQUID–LIQUID INTERFACES

SURFACE TENSION AND SURFACE ENERGY

A brief consideration of the kinetic energy of molecules will lead one to realize that the surface of a liquid is in a state of violent agitation with molecules leaving and entering from both the bulk liquid and vapour phases. Calculations show that, for water at any rate, the average residence time of a molecule in the surface is of the order of microseconds. Notwithstanding this, strong cohesion between the molecules causes the position of the surface to be definable to within a few molecular thicknesses (Davies & Rideal 1961).

Molecules within the bulk of a liquid are subjected to attractive forces equally in all directions whereas those at the surface have very little attraction from the vapour and so experience a net pull into the liquid. Molecules very near the surface also experience a small net inward attraction and so the surface should be considered more as a region about two or three molecules thick rather than a monomolecular layer. The imbalance of forces results in some molecules being withdrawn into the bulk, thereby slightly increasing the intermolecular distance within the surface giving the latter the character of a stretched elastic membrane, that is the surface is under tension. Such a surface will therefore tend to contract spontaneously and cause droplets or air bubbles to assume a spherical shape.

The *surface tension* γ is defined as the force, in mN, acting within the surface in a direction normal to any line of length 1 m. A force of γ mN.m^{-1} must therefore be applied tangentially to part that surface.

If the surface area of a given volume of liquid is increased isothermally, work must be done to bring molecules into the surface against the inward pull of the bulk liquid. The work required to expand the surface by 1 m^2 is γ mJ and therefore the *excess free surface energy* of a liquid is γ mJ.m^{-2} which is numerically equal to the surface tension. At constant pressure, the free surface energy per m^2 is the excess Gibbs free energy G_s, where the subscript denotes the extra energy of the molecules by virtue of being in the surface. Thus $\gamma = G_s$. Although both the surface tension and the excess free surface energy are numerically equal and have the same dimensional units of MLT^{-2}, they are not identical in a qualitative sense since the tension may be considered as the *result* of the excess energy.

Because surface molecules are not attracted away from the bulk as strongly as they are into it, there is a residual potential attraction energy which constitutes the surface enthalpy H_s mJ.m^{-2}. The molecules in the region of the surface, however, have a greater freedom of movement and so there is an excess entropy in the surface of S_s mJ.m^{-2}.deg^{-1}. Thus if the surface were destroyed, not all of the surface enthalpy would be free to do work and therefore:

$$G_s = \gamma = H_s - TS_s$$

G_s is therefore a measure of the thermodynamic instability of the surface and is that part of the surface enthalpy capable of doing mechanical work. At very high viscosities, however, the relationship between surface free energy and surface tension no longer holds.

Relationship of Surface Tension and Temperature
The surface tension of almost all liquids decreases with a rise in temperature, an almost linear relationship being found. It follows that the surface tension must vanish at some finite temperature this being the critical temperature T_c above which the cohesive forces are no longer capable of maintaining the integrity of a distinct vapour phase. Since surface tension is a function of the distance between the molecules it is dependent upon the liquid density and Eötvös (1886) suggested the relationship:

$$\gamma \left(\frac{M}{\rho}\right)^{2/3} = K_1(T_c - T) = K_1 T_c \left(1 - \frac{T}{T_c}\right)$$

where M is the molecular weight, ρ is the liquid density and K_1 is a constant. van der Waals (1894) proposed a power law of the type:

$$\gamma \left(\frac{M}{\rho_c}\right)^{2/3} = K_2 T_c \left(1 - \frac{T}{T_c}\right)^B$$

where B is a constant for a given liquid. B was given a value of 1.5 but this has been shown to vary for different liquids, a value of 1.2 being appropriate for some.

The linear extrapolation of $\gamma(M/\rho)^{2/3}$ versus T however does not cut the T axis for zero γ at T_c but at a lower temperature $(T_c - d)$ where d is about 6 degrees. The Eötvös equation was therefore modified by Ramsey and Shields (1893) as:

$$\gamma \left(\frac{M}{\rho}\right)^{2/3} = K_3(T_c - T - d)$$

This correction was shown by Katayama (1916) to be unnecessary if the influence of the vapour upon the surface tension of a liquid is taken into account so that:

$$\gamma \left(\frac{M}{\rho_l - \rho_g}\right)^{2/3} = K_4(T_c - T)$$

where ρ_l and ρ_g are the orthobaric densities of the liquid and vapour respectively. The constant K_4 has a value of about 210 nJ.deg^{-1} unless there is strong association between molecules when a lower value is found which varies widely between different liquids. Water, for example, gives a value of about 89 nJ.deg^{-1} at room temperature.

By combining the equations of van der Waals and Katayama and giving B a value of 1.2, Ferguson (1923) deduced that:

$$\frac{\gamma^{1/4}}{\rho_l - \rho_g} = C$$

where C is a constant for a given liquid. Such an equation was also found by Macleod who confirmed the constancy of C experimentally. If both sides of this last equation are multiplied by the molecular weight and ρ_g is neglected as being small compared with ρ_l, the following expression is obtained which is independent of temperature:

$$\frac{M\gamma^{1/4}}{\rho} = MC = [P]$$

where $[P]$ is known as the parachor (Sugden 1924b). The parachor may be regarded as the molar volume when the surface tension is unity and affords a useful means of comparing the molar volumes of different liquids since the comparison is made under conditions where the molecular attractions are approximately equal. An important property of the parachor is its additivity since it has been found to be composed of sets of constants which relate both to the atoms composing the molecule and to the way in which the atoms are bonded together. Its importance in elucidating molecular structure has now, however, been completely superseded by other techniques.

Effect of Surface Curvature
The tension forces in a planar surface are balanced within the plane of the surface. Any curvature to the surface produces a resultant normal force which becomes balanced by a pressure change ΔP within the liquid such that

$$\Delta P = \gamma\left(\frac{1}{r_1} + \frac{1}{r_2}\right)$$

This is the Young-Laplace equation where r_1 and r_2 are the principal radii of curvature.

Curvature of a liquid surface influences the vapour pressure since it alters the distribution of the attractive forces around the molecules in the surface. A difference in chemical potential can readily be shown to exist between liquid drops of different size since there is a decrease in free surface energy upon mass transfer from a smaller to a larger drop via the vapour phase. Assuming ideal behaviour, the vapour pressure P_r of a spherical drop of radius r compared with that (P) over a plane surface is given by the Kelvin equation:

$$\ln\left(\frac{P_r}{P}\right) = \frac{2\gamma M}{RT\rho r}$$

ρ being the liquid density and M the molecular weight of the *vapour*. Values calculated for water are given in Table 4.2.

TABLE 4.2

CALCULATED EFFECT OF DROP SIZE ON VAPOUR PRESSURE OF WATER AT 293K

Radius of drop (nm)	$\dfrac{P_r}{P}$
1000	1.001
100	1.01
10	1.11
1	2.94

It will be noted that the vapour pressure is affected appreciably only at high surface curvature, that is with very small drops. This however is sufficient to render vapour condensation in a dust-free atmosphere very difficult unless the atmosphere is highly supersaturated, any condensate nuclei tending to evaporate rather than to grow.

Derivation of the Kelvin equation assumes that the surface tension remains independent of surface curvature. It is to be expected that high curvature, measurable in terms of molecular dimensions, would diminish the surface attraction of molecules thereby resulting in a decrease in the tension. This decrease however is probably small even with droplets consisting of only a few molecules.

INTERFACIAL TENSION

When a two component system separates into two liquid phases an interfacial region will exist in which the molecules are subjected to unbalanced forces. This leads to an interfacial tension in just the same way as surface tensions are produced. Incomplete miscibility of the two components arises because of a difference in the attraction forces between the two kinds of molecules and it is this difference which results in the imbalance of attraction forces across the interface.

All spontaneous processes result in a decrease in free energy. It has already been noted that the integrity of the condensed state is due to the van der Waals forces and that these arise due to the loss of energy as molecules come together. Further, it was seen that in some liquids such as water, intermolecular attraction greatly exceeds that due to the London interaction owing to the additional strong Keesom interaction in the form of the hydrogen bond. Interference with hydrogen bond formation by non-dipoles would therefore prevent the attainment of the minimum energy state and so the spontaneous process would be a rejection of apolar molecules causing them to occupy some position not interfering with the hydrogen bonds. This means that a separate phase will be formed when water is 'mixed' with a hydrocarbon such as octane or liquid paraffin.

Tetrahedral hydrogen bonding which occurs in ice is retained to a lesser extent in liquid water giving rise to 'flickering-clusters' of structured water (Davies & Litovitz 1965; Erlander 1969; Blandamer 1970). When a solute molecule is dissolved in water it may either (a) substitute for a water molecule in the lattice-like network when there will be competition with solvent molecules for the 'lattice sites' or (b) occupy a cavity in the solvent structure. The latter type of 'interstitial solution' occurs when non-polar solutes are dissolved in highly polar solvents, water molecules forming polyhedral structures around the solute molecules. This means that small hydrocarbon molecules can have a slight solubility in water, the solubility being governed by the size of the solute molecule and that of the cavities in the water structure (Abu-Hamdiyyah 1965). The mean size of the cavities in water is about the size of a C_4 or C_5 hydrocarbon. However, the 'microscopic iceberg' of structured water which forms around non-polar molecules (Frank & Evans 1945) involves a decrease in entropy which overrides the negative enthalpy of dissolution thereby producing an unfavourable positive free energy of dissolution.

If there was no attraction across a water–paraffin oil interface, the interfacial tension γ_{ow} would be given by the sum of the separate surface tensions since these act together, that is $\gamma_{ow} = \gamma_o + \gamma_w$. Water and paraffin molecules do however attract each other by London interaction, the attraction being given by the geometric mean of the London dispersion force components γ^d of the surface tension (Fowkes 1964). Thus for paraffin and water the attraction across the interface is $(\gamma_o \gamma_w^d)^{1/2}$ where $\gamma_o = \gamma_o^d$ and $\gamma_w = \gamma_w^h + \gamma_w^d$, γ_w^h denoting the polar interaction component. The separate tensions are thereby reduced to:

$$\gamma_o - (\gamma_o \gamma_w^d)^{1/2} \quad \text{and} \quad \gamma_w - (\gamma_o \gamma_w^d)^{1/2}$$

for the oil and water sides of the interface respectively and the interfacial tension is given by their sum:

$$\gamma_{ow} = \gamma_{ow}^d = \gamma_o + \gamma_w - 2(\gamma_o \gamma_w^d)^{1/2} \quad (4.1)$$

The superscript in γ_{ow}^d denotes that only the dispersion force interaction across the interface is taken into account.

Consider now an aqueous solution of a solute whose molecules possess both apolar and polar groups, e.g. a fatty acid or alcohol: the solute and solvent will be miscible in all proportions provided

that the apolar group is small as in acetic acid or ethanol (C_2). If the hydrocarbon group is larger it will interfere more with hydrogen bond formation and cause a greater structuring of the water around it. Butyric acid and butanol (C_4) are therefore only partially miscible with water at room temperature and a mixture where neither component is in large excess will separate into two phases. Longer hydrocarbon chains curl-up in order to decrease their contact with water. This effect leads to a decreased entropy of dissolution per CH_2 group with increasing chain length.

Since there is polar interaction between the different molecules, the tension of the interface within a two-phase system will be considerably lower than that predicted by equation 4.1. Some computed values are given in Table 4.3.

TABLE 4.3

EFFECT OF INTERFACIAL INTERACTION ON THE TENSION BETWEEN WATER AND VARIOUS ORGANIC LIQUIDS AT 293K
(Values in mN.m^{-1})

Organic liquid	γ_o (expt)	$2(\gamma_o \gamma_w^d)^{1/2}$ (calc)	γ_{ow}^d (calc)	γ_{ow} (expt)	polar interaction component (calc)
Hexane	18.4	40.1	51.1	51.1	0.0
Octane	21.8	43.6	51.0	50.8	0.2
Decane	23.9	45.7	51.0	51.2	−0.2
Tetradecane	25.6	47.2	51.2	52.2	−1.0
Cyclohexane	25.5	47.2	51.1	50.2	0.9
Benzene	28.9	50.2	51.5	35.0	16.5
Octanol	27.5	49.0	51.3	8.5	42.8
Cyclohexanol	32.7	53.4	52.1	3.9	48.2
Di-n-butylamine	22.0	43.8	51.0	10.3	40.7

$$\gamma_w = 72.8 \qquad \gamma_w^d = 21.8$$

Within experimental error, there is seen to be no polar interaction with saturated hydrocarbons. In the case of benzene, a dipole is induced in the π-bonds giving a further lowering of 16.5 mN.m^{-1} and a resultant interfacial tension of 35.0 mN.m^{-1}. With the last three compounds of Table 4.3, hydrogen bonding involves a much stronger polar interaction with water and consequently leads to low interfacial tensions.

Since an enhanced polar interaction leads to a greater tendency for miscibility of an oil with water, the interfacial tension will parallel the mutual insolubility of the two components. An approximate means of calculating interfacial tensions from surface tensions is afforded by *Antonoff's rule* which states that the interfacial tension is equal to the difference of the surface tensions of the mutually saturated phases:

$$\gamma_{ow} = \gamma_{w(o)} - \gamma_{o(w)}$$

While the rule holds for slightly polar oils such as benzene or chloroform against water, it does not hold for more polar oils such as octanol nor for systems with a negative spreading coefficient (see below).

COHESION, ADHESION AND SPREADING

If two halves of a column of pure liquid were to be pulled apart, two new liquid–air surfaces would be created. The free energy of the system is therefore increased by 2γ mJ for each m^2 cross-section of original column, this increase being known as the *work of cohesion*. For oil and for water the work of cohesion is respectively:

$$W_o = 2\gamma_o \quad \text{mJ.m}^{-2}$$

and

$$W_w = 2\gamma_w \quad \text{mJ.m}^{-2} \qquad (4.2)$$

When an oil and a water surface are brought together, there is a residual energy, γ_{ow} mJ.m^{-2}, at the interface. To separate these two surfaces, *work of adhesion* must be supplied for each m^2 of interface, that is:

$$W_{ow} = \gamma_o + \gamma_w - \gamma_{ow} \quad \text{mJ.m}^{-2} \qquad (4.3)$$

this being known as the *Dupré equation.*

If a drop of pure liquid paraffin is placed on water, it forms a coherent lens (Fig. 4.2). Let A_o and

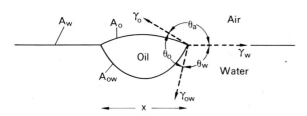

FIG. 4.2. Oil lens–water system parameters.

A_w be the oil–air and water–air surface areas, A_{ow} the oil-water interfacial area and x the horizontal diameter of the lens. Suppose the lens expands over the water surface by an infinitesimal amount dx. The increase in surface energy at the oil–air and oil–water interfaces are respectively $\gamma_o dA_o$ and $\gamma_{ow} dA_{ow}$ and the *increase* at the water–air surface is $\gamma_w dA_w$. *In the latter case dA_w is negative* since water–air surface is being lost at the expense of the expanding oil lens.

The total surface energy gained by the lens expanding dx is therefore:

$$dG^s = \gamma_w dA_w + \gamma_o dA_o + \gamma_{ow} dA_{ow}$$

It follows that if there is a net loss in surface energy upon expansion of the lens:

i.e.
$$\gamma_w \frac{dA_w}{dx} + \gamma_o \frac{dA_o}{dx} + \gamma_{ow} \frac{dA_{ow}}{dx} < 0$$

and the process of expansion will be spontaneous.

As the diameter x of the lens increases however, the oil–air and oil–water interfacial curvatures decreases so that dA_o/dx and dA_{ow}/dx increase as x increases. In the case of liquid paraffin on water, a droplet of the oil would expand into a lens until the energy gained by increasing A_o and A_{ow} just balanced that lost by decreasing A_w:

i.e.
$$\gamma_w \frac{dA_w}{dx} + \gamma_o \frac{dA_o}{dx} + \gamma_{ow} \frac{dA_{ow}}{dx} = 0 \qquad (4.4)$$

Further expansion of the liquid paraffin lens would increase dA_o/dx and dA_{ow}/dx still more and involve a net increase in surface energy. The lens therefore acquires an equilibrium diameter with a minimum energy.

Since a lens involves curvature of the oil–air and oil–water surfaces and since also most of the oil floats below the free water–air surface level:

$$\frac{-dA_w}{dx} > \frac{dA_o}{dx} > \frac{dA_{ow}}{dx}$$

Therefore for a lens to occupy a finite equilibrium diameter in accordance with equation 4.4, $\gamma_w - \gamma_o - \gamma_{ow} < 0$. For liquid paraffin on water we have $72.8 - 31.8 - 55.6 = -14.6$ mJ.m^{-2}, clearly a condition for the formation of a stable lens.

Suppose a drop of a polar oil such as octanol is placed on water. For octanol on water at 293K we have: $\gamma_w - \gamma_o - \gamma_{ow} = 72.8 - 27.5 - 8.5 = +36.8$ mJ.m^{-2}. Such a lens will continue to expand given enough water surface to do so since the condition for minimum surface energy (equation 4.4) cannot be reached. As the lens expands, the oil–air and oil–water surface curvatures approach zero and tend towards the condition $-dA_w/dx = dA_o/dx = dA_{ow}/dx$. Equilibrium in the form of an extremely thin lens would therefore require the condition (from equation 4.4) $dA/dx(\gamma_w - \gamma_o - \gamma_{ow}) = 0$ then:

$$\gamma_w \quad \gamma_o \quad \gamma_{ow} = 0 \qquad (4.5)$$

Clearly this situation is not achieved with octanol on water and so the oil will spread to form a *monolayer*, that is a film one oil molecule thick.

The condition given by equation 4.5 therefore forms the dividing line between those systems where immediate spreading towards a monolayer occurs and those whose immediate tendency is to form a lens. The *initial spreading coefficient* S_{init} is defined as:

$$S_{init} = \gamma_w - \gamma_o - \gamma_{ow} \qquad (4.6)$$

If S_{init} is positive there is an immediate tendency to spread whereas if S_{init} is negative as with liquid paraffin on water, spreading does not occur. Table 4.4 lists a few values for the initial spreading coefficient on water.

TABLE 4.4

INITIAL SPREADING COEFFICIENTS ON WATER AT 293K
(values in $mJ.m^{-2}$)

Organic liquid	γ_o	γ_{ow}	S_{init}
Hexane	18.4	51.1	+3.3
Octane	21.8	50.8	+0.2
Decane	23.9	51.2	−2.3
Tetradecane	25.6	52.2	−5.0
Liquid paraffin	31.8	55.6	−14.6
Benzene	28.9	35.0	+8.9
Chloroform	27.1	32.6	+13.0
Octanol	27.5	8.5	+36.8
Oleic acid	32.5	15.6	+24.7

Combination of equations 4.2, 4.3 and 4.6 gives $S_{init} = W_{ow} - W_o$ showing that an oil will spread on water only if it is sufficiently polar to adhere to the water more strongly than it coheres to itself.

The values quoted in Table 4.4 refer only to the initial condition of the system. However the two liquids tend to become mutually saturated, with the result that γ_w is often found to decrease significantly. Thus although benzene is initially capable of spreading on water, γ_w becomes reduced to 62.4 $mJ.m^{-2}$ and γ_o becomes 28.8 $mJ.m^{-2}$. Thus $S_{final} = 62.4 - 28.8 - 35.0 = -1.4$ $mJ.m^{-2}$ and the benzene-rich phase forms flat lenses with the rest of the water covered by a monolayer of benzene having a surface film pressure π of 10.4 $mN.m^{-1}$ i.e. $\gamma_{w(o)} = \gamma_w - \pi = 72.8 - 10.4 = 62.4$ $mN.m^{-1}$.

So far only the energetics of the system have been considered but reference to Fig. 4.2 will show that there must also be a balance of forces at the triple-point where the three phases, air–oil–water, meet. A condition for equilibrium is:

$$\frac{\gamma_w}{\sin \theta_o} = \frac{\gamma_o}{\sin \theta_w} = \frac{\gamma_{ow}}{\sin \theta_a}$$

If it is assumed that the water–air surface is flat and that the oil–air and oil–water interfaces have spherical curvature since this presents the least surface area for a given diameter of the lens, then there will almost certainly be an imbalance of forces

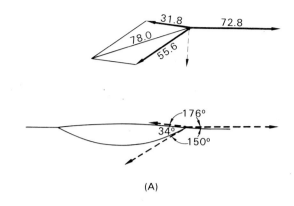

(A)

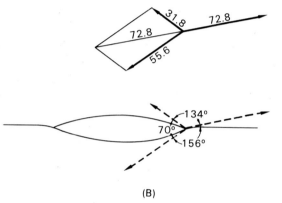

(B)

FIG. 4.3. Liquid paraffin lens floating on water showing necessity for edge distortion. (A), Non-equilibrium; (B), Equilibrium.

as depicted in Fig. 4.3(A). For liquid paraffin on water, $\theta_o = 70°$, $\theta_w = 156°$ and $\theta_a = 134°$ therefore there must be some considerable distortion around the edge of the lens as shown in Fig. 4.3(B).

It has been seen that a good sample of liquid paraffin cannot spread on water. However, if its trace impurities are oxidized by heating it may spread to a multilayer and show interference colours. This multilayer is known as a *duplex film*, so called because the oil–water and oil–air interfaces are still sufficiently apart to act independently. Similar behaviour is observed if sufficient 'spreader' such as a fatty acid or fatty alcohol is dissolved in liquid paraffin. Thus with 0.5 per cent cetyl alcohol (tetradecanol) the condition for initial spreading is achieved: $S_{init} = 72 - 32 - 24 = +16$ $mJ.m^{-2}$ and given a large water surface, the drop will spread to a duplex film. The high spreading power of fatty alcohols leads to monolayer formation of the alcohol in advance of the spreading oil and if the water surface area is small, the monolayer soon covers the water surface and reduces its tension to 48 mN.m^{-1}. This produces a negative spreading coefficient: $S_{final} = 48 - 32 - 24 = -8$ mJ.m^{-2} which results in the oil contracting into one or more lenses surrounded by a monolayer of the alcohol. The sudden lowering of the surface tension around the spreading lens will cause the forces at the edge to become unbalanced. This produces a sudden distortion of the surface around the edge which may be so violent that the distortion is propagated as a wave throughout the lens causing it to shatter into several hundred small lenses which may subsequently coalesce.

MEASUREMENT OF SURFACE AND INTERFACIAL TENSION

Methods for measuring surface and interfacial tension differ in their suitability for particular purposes. Although the surface of a simple liquid attains an equilibrium tension within a few milliseconds of its formation, the surface of some solutions continues to age for a long time due to slow diffusion of molecules to the surface or molecular reorientation at the surface. It follows that those methods which involve enlargement and breakage of the surface cannot always be used to measure equilibrium tensions. The methods summarized below have been discussed in detail by Adamson (1967).

Capillary Rise

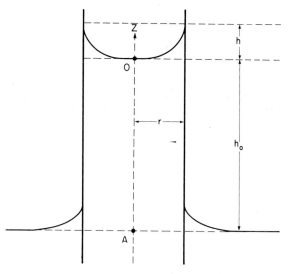

FIG. 4.4. Capillary rise parameters.

The difference in pressure ΔP between the bottom of the meniscus O and point A is given by

$$\Delta P = \Delta\rho g h_o = \frac{2\gamma}{b} + \qquad (4.7)$$

where $\Delta\rho$ is the density difference of the liquid and the air and b is the radius of curvature at O. The term on the right hand side is given by the Young–Laplace equation. At some other point on the meniscus of elevation z above O

$$\Delta P = \Delta\rho g(h_o + z) = \frac{2\gamma}{b} + \Delta\rho g z$$

$$= \gamma\left(\frac{1}{R_1} + \frac{1}{R_2}\right) \qquad (4.8)$$

R_1 and R_2 being the principal radii of curvature.

Because ΔP varies with z, the curvature of the meniscus is not uniform and only for very narrow capillaries, when $h \ll h_o$ can γ be calculated from equation 4.7 since then $b \approx r$. Usually measurement of h_o still leaves b unknown and in order to determine γ from equation 4.7, a relation between b and r is required. Use is made of the so-called capillary constant a^2 defined as $a^2 = bh_o$. For zero contact angles, Sugden (1921) compiled tables of r/b versus r/a and a method of successive approximations may be used to arrive at the value of b.

Although the theory is simple, there are a number of experimental difficulties. Thus it is necessary to ensure that:

 (i) determination of h_o is accurate,
 (ii) glass capillary tubing is absolutely clean,
 (iii) the capillary is vertical,
 (iv) the capillary is of uniform bore,
 (v) only a very small departure from circularity of cross-section exists,
 (vi) the liquid is not very viscous.

A zero contact angle may not be achieved with some solutions due to adsorption of solute on to the glass. With very fine capillaries a further complication due to adsorption is reduction in solute concentration and a consequent change in surface tension.

The necessary condition for zero contact angle may be tested by approaching the equilibrium height h_o with a succession of rising and falling menisci. If h_o is the the same in each case there is perfect wetting. Even so, a rising meniscus may give rise to a non-zero contact angle (see p. 80) and therefore it is best to use data from falling menisci.

In order to eliminate errors due to slight variation

in the bore of the capillary, the tube may be immersed in the liquid to a depth sufficient to locate the meniscus at a position where the area of cross-section is accurately known. Alternatively, the hydrostatic pressure needed to restore the bottom of the meniscus to the level of the external plane surface may be determined. The method may be adapted for the measurement of interfacial tensions.

Maximum Bubble Pressure

A capillary tube dips into the liquid to an accurately known depth and the minimum pressure is determined at which bubbles of an 'inert' gas are just able to grow and detach from the tip. If the bubble formed a surface of spherical curvature, the curvature would be a maximum when a hemispherical bubble had formed and at this point the maximum pressure would be recorded. Equation 4.7 would therefore be applicable. The pressure difference across the bubble surface however, varies with variation in depth of the meniscus and so the bubble surface will not have spherical curvature. As in the case of capillary rise, Sugden (1922) has published correction factors.

The technique has the advantage that zero contact angle is not necessary. It is however necessary to know whether or not the liquid wets the tube, that is, whether the bubble forms upon the internal or external cross-section. Since the method involves an expanding surface, surface ageing cannot be studied, a bubble rate of about 1 s^{-1} being used. A variation in which two tubes of different diameter are used has also been described by Sugden (1922, 1924a).

Sessile Drop

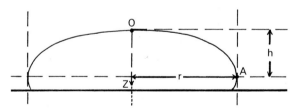

FIG. 4.5. Sessile drop of water in liquid paraffin.

Fig. 4.5 represents a drop of liquid resting on a non-wetting surface (contact angle greater than 90°). The external fluid may be air or another liquid phase. Alternatively, the figure may be visualized in an inverted position where it represents either a drop of a less dense liquid or a bubble of air.

Given that b is the radius of curvature at the vertex O, and that R_1 and r are the radii of curvature at point A in the vertical and equatorial planes respectively, then from equation 4.7:

$$\Delta P = \frac{2\gamma}{b} + \Delta\rho gh = \gamma\left(\frac{1}{R_1} + \frac{1}{r}\right)$$

Although neither b nor R_1 are known, it has been shown that:

$$\frac{\gamma}{\Delta\rho gr^2} = \frac{1}{2}\frac{h^2}{r^2} + \Delta$$

where Δ is a non-dimensional correction factor which varies with h and r. The variation of Δ with drop size was determined by Porter (1933) who found that the curve (Fig. 4.6) was fitted by the empirical equation:

$$\Delta = 0.3047\left(\frac{h}{r}\right)^3\left(1 - 4\left(\frac{h}{r}\right)^2\right)$$

whence

$$\gamma = \Delta\rho gh^2\left[0.5 + 0.3047\frac{h}{r}\left(1 - 4\left(\frac{h}{r}\right)^2\right)\right]$$

The correction term is zero when $r = 2h$.

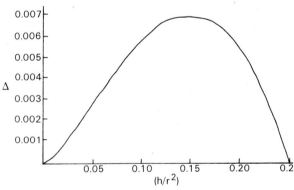

FIG. 4.6. Curve of correction factor versus shape factor for the sessile drop method (Porter 1933).

In order to determine h and r, the drop may be photographed or projected on to a screen. Whilst the correction term only requires determination of the ratio h/r, the absolute value of h is also required. A convenient method is to suspend a rod of known diameter over the vertex of the drop and from the diameter of the image to calculate the enlargement, whence h can be calculated from the size of the drop image (Shotton 1955).

Significant errors can arise from inaccurate measurement of the drop size parameters but these errors can be minimized using large drops. The main sources of error arise from the difficulty in accurately locating the equatorial plane and from deficiencies in the optical system employed.

Another source of error may be inherent in the liquid being examined. If it is a solution which possesses some sort of structure (exhibits plastic flow), the drop may not flatten to the shape corresponding to the true surface tension. Evidence for this was found by Shotton and Kalyan (1960) when determining the interfacial tensions between benzene and gelatin or sodium alginate solutions. An apparently higher tension was found if a drop of solution was formed in benzene instead of a drop of benzene in solution.

Pendant Drop

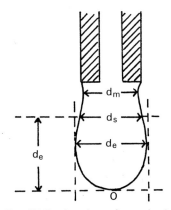

FIG. 4.7. Pendant drop of water in air.

Various ways of calculating surface and interfacial tensions from the shape and size of pendant drops, as shown in Fig. 4.7, have been suggested. Equation 4.8 may be written

$$\frac{1}{r_1/b} + \frac{1}{r_2/b} = \beta\left(\frac{z}{b}\right) + 2$$

where
$$\beta = -\Delta\rho g b^2/\gamma, \qquad (4.9)$$

b being the radius of curvature at O, the vertex of the drop. β is a dimensionless quantity which depends upon the shape of the drop as does the ratio $S = d_s/d_e$ defined in Fig. 4.7. Therefore S is a function of β. For a given value of S, d_e is proportional to b and so equation 4.9 leads to

$$\gamma = \Delta\rho g d_e^2/H$$

where H is a function of S. Measurement of d_e and d_s allows calculation of S from which H may be calculated by the method of Fordham (1948) or read from tables given by the same author and

extended by Stauffer (1965). The latter author has shown that greatest accuracy is achieved with S values close to unity.

Small errors in estimating d_e can lead to considerable errors in d_s. This can be minimized by determining the ratio R of the maximum (d_e) and minimum (d_m) diameters which are less dependent on height than is d_s. H may then be calculated or read from tables (Winkel 1965).

Photographic or projection methods are used to determine the shape and size parameters (Douglas 1950; Campbell Christian & Eaton 1955). The pendant drop is more suitable than the sessile drop method for viscous liquids since there is only a small fraction of the drop area in contact with a solid surface. Compared with the sessile drop, viscous drag has less effect in slowing the attainment of hydrodynamic equilibrium. A check for such an equilibrium can be made by measuring the pendant drop diameters at several heights and comparing the drop shape with that predicted by theory (Roe, Bachetta & Wong 1967).

Drop Volume

If the pendant drop shown in Fig. 4.7 is slowly enlarged, it will grow to a critical length at which it becomes unstable and the waist collapses. Figure 4.8 shows successive stages in the growth of a drop

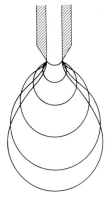

FIG. 4.8. Girth of a drop of water in liquid paraffin. (Diameter of needle tip is 1.06 mm giving $Y_{ow} = 57$ mNm^{-1}).

up to the point of instability, detachment of the drop being illustrated in Fig. 4.9. The extra small drop which is produced arises because of the mechanical instability of the neck. It is evident that not all of the drop becomes detached and as much as 40 per cent may remain attached to the tip.

If it is assumed that the surface tension acts

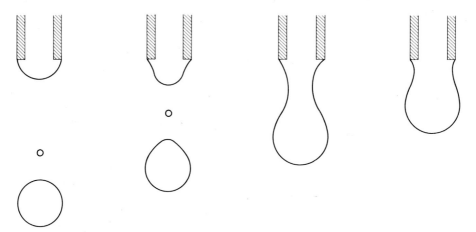

FIG. 4. 9. Successive stages in detachment of a drop.

vertically, then at the moment preceding detachment $mg = v\Delta\rho g = 2\pi r\gamma$ where m and v are the effective mass and the volume of the drop respectively and r is the radius of the tip of the tube. This equation, however, fails to recognize that the volume of the drop is also a function of its shape and that only part of the drop becomes detached.

The shape depends on the ratio between some linear dimension of the tip of the tube such as r and a linear dimension of the drop such as $v^{1/3}$. Thus:

$$v\Delta\rho g = 2\pi r\gamma \; f\left(\frac{r}{v^{1/3}}\right) \qquad (4.10)$$

where $f(r/v^{1/3})$ is the fraction of the 'ideal drop' which actually falls. Harkins and Brown (1919) determined experimentally the correction values plotted in Fig. 4.10. In the case of surface tension measurements, the mean weight of a number of drops may be used to calculate the drop volume v; alternatively, as in the case of interfacial tension measurements, the volume is measured directly by means of a micrometer syringe. Thus $r/v^{1/3}$ can be calculated and the correction factor read from the graph. Substitution in equation 4.10 gives γ. Since the correction factor varies only slightly with change in v near the minimum of the curve (Fig. 4.10), tubes should be selected so that $r/v^{1/3}$ is as close to the minimum as possible.

If the drop is formed too rapidly it becomes too heavy because the waist of the detaching drop gets expanded by the stream of liquid issuing from the tube. The drop must therefore be formed slowly, at least three minutes being required. In practice, when using a micrometer syringe, a rough estimate of the drop volume is obtained rapidly

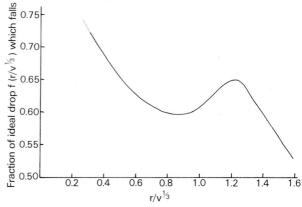

FIG. 4.10. Curve of correction factor versus versus drop shape factor for the drop volume method (Harkins & Brown 1919).

and subsequently about 95 per cent or more of the drop is quickly formed and the process completed slowly over a period of about a minute.

In order to know the effective diameter of the tip when determining interfacial tensions, one must make sure that it is completely wetted by one of the liquids. If the tip is wetted by the external liquid, care must be taken to ensure that the interior of the tube is sufficiently wetted by the liquid forming the drop or the point of detachment of the drop may be inside the tube instead of at the tip. Where the drop liquid wets the tip, care must be taken that it does not climb up the outside of the tube and to prevent this, tubes with sharp edges should be used. Whatever the shape of the tip, smoothness is important. Stainless steel hypodermic needles with the ends ground flat are generally suitable. If necessary, they may be rendered hydrophobic by being coated with a film of ferric stearate or silicone.

du Noüy Ring Tensiometer

This method involves measurement of the force required to detach a platinum wire ring from the liquid surface or from the interface between two liquids. In the latter case the ring must be preferentially wetted by the denser liquid. Careful cleaning of the ring in strong acid or by flaming is essential when it will be preferentially wetted by water. For the determination of γ_{ow} with an oil as the denser phase, the ring may be rendered hydrophobic with silicone. A pull P exerted on the ring results in some of the liquid being raised (Fig. 4.11), the

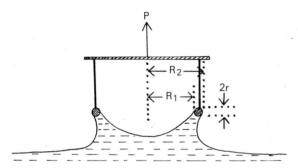

FIG. 4.11. du Noüy ring parameters.

pull being balanced by the weight of liquid. When the upward pull and the weight of liquid exceed the surface tension force, the ring will become detached. If it is assumed that the surface tension acts vertically on the ring with zero contact angle

$$P_{max} = mg = (\text{inner} + \text{outer perimeter})\gamma$$
$$= 2\pi(R_1 + R_2)\gamma \qquad (4.11)$$

where P_{max} is the maximum pull on the ring, m is the mass of liquid raised above the free surface of the liquid and R_1 and R_2 are the radii of curvature of the inner and outer perimeter of the ring.

However, Fig. 4.11 clearly shows that the surface tension does not act vertically on the ring and Harkins and Jordan (1930) showed that equation 4.11 gives values of γ which may be in error by up to 45 per cent. They determined experimentally the correction factor F so that:

$$\gamma = \frac{P_{max}}{2\pi(R_1 + R_2)} \cdot F$$

which reduces to:

$$\gamma = \frac{P_{max}}{4\pi R} \cdot F$$

if r, the radius of the wire, is small so that $R_1 = R_2 = R$.

The volume V of liquid upheld by the ring becomes a maximum at the moment of detachment when it will possess a certain shape which is determined by a function of the three variables R, r and V. Determination of F therefore involves the calculation of the two dimensionless quantities R^3/V and R/r. Zuidema and Waters (1941) found an empirical relationship which enables the tabulated values of F given by Harkins and Jordan (1930) to be extended for conditions frequently met when determining interfacial tensions. Fox and Chrisman (1952) have also extended the correction tables in the other direction, that is for liquids of low tension but high density where the empirical relationship of Zuidema and Waters was found to be invalid.

In order to obtain accurate data the following conditions must be met:

(i) the ring must lie in a flat plane,

(ii) the plane of the ring must be horizontal, a tilt of only 1° causing an error of 0.45 per cent,

(iii) the diameter of the dish must be not less than 8 cm since curvature of the meniscus due to the edge of the dish leads to low determined values of γ. When determining interfacial tensions in circumstances where the ring is unavoidably wetted by the upper liquid the force required to push the ring down through the interface may be measured.

Wilhelmy Plate

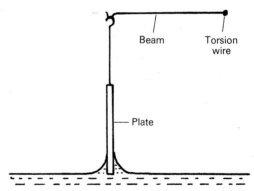

FIG. 4.12. Plate in null position seen edge on.

A thin rectangular plate of glass or mica is suspended vertically from a torsion balance. A dish of liquid is raised under the plate until the liquid surface just contacts the bottom edge of the latter when the surface forces will drag it downwards. The force exerted around the perimeter of the plate may then be measured by the rotation of the torsion wire required to restore the plate to its null position, that is, so that the bottom edge of the plate is coincident with the plane of the free liquid surface (Fig. 4.12).

Provided that the liquid makes zero angle of contact with the plate

$$P_{max} = mg \approx \text{perimeter} \times \gamma = 2(L + T)\gamma$$

$$(4.12)$$

where L and T are respectively the length and thickness of the plate in the horizontal plane and mg is the weight of meniscus liquid. To ensure that L is the measured length of the bottom edge of the plate, the edge must lie in a horizontal plane. This is readily checked when the liquid is raised close to the plate since the edge and its reflection in the liquid surface will then appear to be parallel.

An alternative method, which is particularly useful for following changes in surface tension, is to immerse the plate partially in the liquid and to record the depth of immersion by means of an optical lever. A change in rotation of the torsion wire may then be corrected for the change in buoyancy of the plate to give an accurate measure of the change in the surface force.

A zero contact angle is essential. This may be promoted by careful roughening of the surface of the plate so that the very fine grooves are orientated in all directions (Jordan & Lane 1964). For oils, a roughened mica plate coated with lamp-black is suitable. It is always best to use a receding contact angle (see p. 80) and so, for following decreases in interfacial tension, the lower (denser) phase should be made to wet the plate preferentially.

It is also necessary to use very thin plates since the effective perimeter will tend to differ slightly from $2(L + T)$ due to the meniscus being continuous around the corners of the plate. For plates not much thicker than 100 μm, however, equation 4.12 is sufficiently accurate that it may be used without correction.

SURFACTANTS

If a single molecule or ion contains localized regions one of which is lyophilic and the other is lyophobic, the lyophilic part will favour dissolution (affinity for solvent) and the lyophobic part will favour immiscibility (antipathy for solvent). Both of these characters existing in the same molecule or ion led Hartley to coin the term *amphipathy*. The amphipathic character becomes particularly pronounced if the lyophilic and lyophobic groups are well separated. When considering water as the solvent the groups are termed *hydrophilic* and *hydrophobic*. The latter term does *not* indicate repulsion between the group and water since there is attraction due to dispersion forces, but rather it implies that interference with hydrogen bonding of the water produces a tendency for the hydrophobic group to be expelled to form a separate phase. Since hydrophobic groups tend to be dissolved by non-polar solvents they are also termed *lipophilic*. Thus an amphipathic compound contains both hydrophilic and lipophilic groups and therefore may also be called *amphiphilic*. As a result of the amphipathic character, such compounds will tend to concentrate at the surface of a solution or at the interface between two immiscible liquids or between a liquid and a solid. Such compounds are therefore frequently referred to as *surface-active agents* or *surfactants*. Those surface-active agents which are used for removing dirt from solid surfaces are also commonly referred to as *detergents*. Under suitable conditions of solvent, temperature and concentration, amphipathic compounds spontaneously aggregate to form colloidal structures known as micelles. This spontaneous tendency for association has led to the term *association colloid*.

CLASSIFICATION OF SURFACTANTS

This is made according to the nature of the polar group, which may or may not ionize. There are therefore *ionic* and *non-ionic* surfactants. Ionic surfactants are further divided into *anionic*, *cationic* and *ampholytic* (or *amphoteric*) according to the charge carried by the surface-active ion. The charge of an ampholytic ion depends upon the pH, the zwitterion being shown in Table 4.5.

SURFACE ACTIVITY

In dilute aqueous solutions of amphipaths, the hydrophobic group of those solute molecules in the region of the surface will not always be able to re-enter the bulk solution as readily as it entered the surface. Thus if random motion brings the hydrophobic group into the surface, the amphipathic molecule will stick there (Fig. 4.13) until it is supplied with sufficient suitably directed kinetic energy for it to re-enter the bulk solution. The strength and direction of the force or 'kick' needed for desorption will depend on the structure and orientation of the amphipathic molecule and the structure of its immediate environment at that particular instant in time. During the time of residence of the molecules at the surface, other

TABLE 4.5

EXAMPLES OF SURFACE-ACTIVE AGENTS

Compound	Surfactant Ion or Molecule	Type	Solvent
Potassium stearate	$CH_3(CH_2)_{16}COO^-$	Anionic	Water
Sodium dodecyl sulphate	$CH_3(CH_2)_{11}OSO_3^-$	Anionic	Water
Sodium dioctyl sulphosuccinate	$C_8H_{17}OOCCH_2$ $\mid$ $C_8H_{17}OOCCH_2$ $\mid$ SO_3^-	Anionic	Water
Tetradecyltrimethylammonium bromide	$CH_3(CH_2)_{13}N^+(CH_3)_3$	Cationic	Water
Dodecylpyridinium chloride	$C_{12}H_{25}N^+$	Cationic	Water
N-dodecyl 2-aminoacetic acid	$C_{12}H_{25}N^+H_2CH_2COO^-$	Ampholytic	Water
Lecithin (R_1, R_2 are C_{11} to C_{17})	R_1COOCH_2 $\mid$ $\quad\quad$ O $R_2COOC \quad CH_2OPOCH_2N^+(CH_3)_3$ $H \quad\quad O - H_2O$	Ampholytic	Oil
Cetyl alcohol (Hexadecanol)	$CH_3(CH_2)_{15}OH$	Non-ionic	Oil
Cholesterol		Non-ionic	Oil
Polyethylene glycol 1000 monocetyl ether (Cetomacrogol 1000: m is 15 or 17 and n is 20 to 24)	$CH_3(CH_2)_m(OCH_2CH_2)_nOH$	Non-ionic	Water
Sorbitan mono-oleate	$CHOHCH_2OOC(CH_2)_7CH$ $\quad\quad\quad\quad\quad\quad\quad\quad\quad \parallel$ $\quad\quad\quad\quad\quad\quad\quad CH(CH_2)_7CH_3$	Non-ionic	Oil

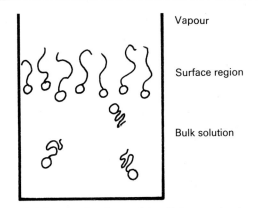

FIG. 4.13. Diagram of surface activity. (Solvent molecules not depicted.)

molecules will also arrive there and so there will be an excess of solute molecules at the surface compared with those in a similar volume of bulk solution containing no surface region.

An increase in size of the hydrophobic group results in increased difficulty of desorption. This means that the average time of residence of solute molecules at the surface becomes longer and the surface excess will be greater as a result. Indeed, long-chain fatty acids and alcohols (C_{10} and above), even in extremely dilute systems, reside almost entirely at the surface forming a surface film one molecule thick (monolayer) which can be considerably compressed by a mechanical barrier (see p. 70) before it will collapse into a surface multilayer.

Adsorption must involve a certain degree of orientation within the surface this being opposed by random rotational motion which favours desorption. Perfect orientation will therefore not be achieved. Although the entropy change of adsorption is negative with very short hydrocarbon chains, thus favouring desorption, it becomes increasingly positive with longer chains (Table 4.6). This shows

TABLE 4.6

THERMODYNAMICS OF ADSORPTION OF FATTY ACIDS IN THE WATER AT 293K
(Ward & Tordai 1946a, b)

Acid	m	ΔG° (kJ.mol^{-1})	$\Delta G^\circ_{m+1} - G^\circ_m$ (kJ per CH$_2$ group)	ΔS° (kJ.deg^{-1}. mol^{-1})	ΔH° (kJ.mol^{-1})
Propionic	3	−6.8		−0.060	−24.7
Butyric	4	−10.3	−3.43	−0.026	−18.0
Pentanoic	5	−13.3	−3.06	+0.005	−7.5
Hexanoic	6	−15.6	−2.26	+0.028	−7.1
Heptanoic	7	−18.9	−3.35	+0.030	−10.0
Octanoic	8	−22.6	−3.68		
Nonanoic	9	−25.5	−2.93		
Decanoic	10	−29.6	−3.94		

that factors other than orientation of the solute molecules in the surface are important. When surfactant molecules are in bulk solution, interference with hydrogen bonding by hydrocarbon chains increases the structuring of the water and the coiling of the chains. Elimination of these effects upon adsorption of long-chain surfactants results in a net increase of entropy.

Traube's rule states that *the concentrations for equal lowering of the surface tension in dilute solutions decrease by about one third for each additional CH$_2$ group in an homologous series.* This concept was extended by Langmuir who showed that if $-\Delta G^\circ$ is the work done in transferring one mol of soap molecules from the bulk to the surface, then

$$\Delta G^\circ_{m+1} - \Delta G^\circ_m$$
$$= -RT \ln 3 = -2.68 \text{ kJ.mol}^{-1} \text{ at } 293\text{K}$$
$$(4.13)$$

where suffix m denotes the number of carbon atoms in the paraffin chain. This arises partly from the increase in molecular orientations available to the chain as each CH$_2$ group is brought above the surface from which one may conclude that the average configuration of the paraffin chains is in the form of the most probable random coil. Traube's rule is only approximate and this is borne out by comparison of equation 4.13 with the fourth

column of Table 4.6. Langmuir found a value of 3.4 in equation 4.13 whilst Ward found 3.72 by an improved method of calculation giving −3.18 kJ.mol^{-1} for the methylene group; a value more in accord with Table 4.6 than that from Traube's rule.

It has been observed that weak attraction of solvent for a substantial part of a solute molecule leads to an accumulation of solute at the surface. On the other hand, if solute–solvent attraction exceeds solvent–solvent attraction, the solute concentration at the surface will be less than in the bulk solution and there will exist a state of negative adsorption leading to an increased surface tension. Such a situation arises with polar organic compounds such as sucrose and with inorganic electrolytes where the effect of the ions follows the lyotropic series (p. 97). The effect of solute concentration upon surface tension is illustrated in Fig. 4.14.

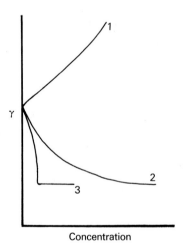

FIG. 4.14. Qualitative effect of various solutes upon the surface tension of water. 1, Inorganic electrolytes and sugars, e.g. NaCl, sucrose; 2, Short-chain acids and alcohols, e.g. tetranoic acid, ethanol; 3, Long-chain ions, e.g. dodecanoate, tetradecyltrimethylammonium.

The Gibbs Equation

Fig. 4.15 represents a solution of a surface-active compound whose surface is located somewhere between AA' and BB', i.e. AA' is above the liquid phase and BB' is below the region of surface irregularity. Region AB therefore contains the whole of the surface whereas region BC consists entirely of bulk solution of ordinary composition.

Let U joules be the total (internal) energy of region BC. The internal energy is a function of the extensive (quantity) factors, viz. entropy S, volume

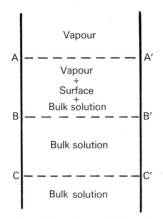

FIG. 4.15. Hypothetical boundaries defining the surface excess.

V and number of mols of solvent (component 1) n_1 and of solute (component 2) n_2. Thus:

$$U = f(S, V, n_1, n_2)$$

Region AB will have a different internal energy from region BC, since the boundaries at A, B and C cannot readily be chosen so as to equate them. The extra energy of region AB is denoted by U^s and may be positive or negative. The excess energy U^s arises because of
  (i) excess entropy per mol S^s,
  (ii) excess volume of liquid V^s,
  (iii) the surface of area A,
  (iv) excess number of mols of solvent and solute, n_1^s and n_2^s respectively, where S^s, V^s and n^s may be positive or negative. Thus:

$$U^s = f(S^s, V^s, A, n_1^s, n_2^s)$$

It follows that:

$$dU^s = T dS^s - P dV^s + \gamma dA + \mu_1 dn^s + \mu_2 dn_2^s \tag{4.14}$$

Since the system is assumed to be at equilibrium the intensive factors are uniform throughout so that there is no need to add the superscript s to temperature T, pressure P or chemical potential μ. The surface tension γ is restricted to the surface so there is likewise no need for the superscript. The reason for the term γdA being positive is that the tension γ acts to contract the surface unlike the pressure P which tends towards expansion.

Since equation 4.14 is derived from a homogeneous function of the first degree, then by Euler's theorem:

$$U^s = T S^s - P V^s + \gamma A + \mu_1 n_1^s + \mu_2 n_2^s$$

whence by differentiation and subtraction of equation 4.14:

$$0 = S^s dT - V^s dP + A d\gamma + n_1^s d\mu_1 + n_2^s d\mu_2$$

so that at constant temperature and pressure:

$$0 = A d\gamma + n_1^s d\mu_1 + n_2^s d\mu_2 \tag{4.15}$$

Considering now each m^2 of surface and defining the *surface excess per m^2*, Γ as:

$$\Gamma = \frac{n^s}{A} \, \text{mol.m}^{-2}$$

then from equation 4.15:

$$-d\gamma = \Gamma_1 d\mu_1 + \Gamma_2 d\mu_2$$

This may be extended for a multicomponent system to:

$$-d\gamma = \sum_i \Gamma_i d\mu_i$$

and so

$$-\frac{d\gamma}{RT} = \sum_1 \Gamma_i \, d \ln a_i \tag{4.16}$$

n^s and hence Γ may be defined in several ways. For example, C of Fig. 4.15 can be located so that regions BC and AB contain the same volume of liquid ($\Gamma^{(V)}$), the same total number of mols ($\Gamma^{(N)}$) or the same total mass ($\Gamma^{(M)}$). For the purpose considered here however, it is best to define BC and AB as containing *the same mass of solvent* this being the convention due to Gibbs and denoted by Guggenhein and Adam as $\Gamma^{(1)}$. Thus $\Gamma_1^{(1)} = 0$.

For a two component system, i.e. one solvent and one solute, equation 4.16 becomes:

$$-\frac{d\gamma}{RT} = \Gamma_2^{(1)} d \ln a_2$$

whence for dilute solutions, where the activity coefficient is almost unity,

$$\Gamma_2^{(1)} \approx -\frac{1}{RT} \frac{d}{d \ln c_2} \tag{4.17}$$

c being the concentration. This is the familiar form of the Gibbs equation and enables the surface excess to be determined from the slope of a plot of surface tension versus the logarithm of the solute concentration (Fig. 4.16).

Fig. 4.16 demonstrates that the slope becomes increasingly negative up to the critical micelle concentration (p. 49) showing that the surface excess increases as the solute concentration increases. It also demonstrates that the Gibbs equation is not valid above the critical micelle concentration.

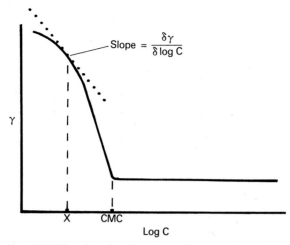

FIG. 4.16. Effect of amphipath concentration on surface tension.

Application of the Gibbs Equation to Real Aqueous Systems

The form of the Gibbs equation given by equation 4.17 is valid only for a two component system and is therefore inapplicable to aqueous solutions since every species must be taken into account. It must be replaced by the general equation 4.16 with the adoption of the Gibbs convention, $\Gamma_{\text{H}_2\text{O}}^{(1)} = 0$.

For a single univalent surface-active strong electrolyte (MA) in water:

$$-\frac{d\gamma}{RT} = \Gamma_{M^+}^{(1)} d\ln a_{M^+} + \Gamma_{A^-}^{(1)} d\ln a_{A^-}$$
$$+ \Gamma_{H^+}^{(1)} d\ln a_{H^+} + \Gamma_{OH^-}^{(1)} d\ln a_{OH^-}$$

The first requirement is therefore to maintain a constant pH such that:

$$d\ln a_{H^+} = -d\ln a_{OH^-} = 0$$

when

$$-\frac{d\gamma}{RT} = \Gamma_{M^+}^{(1)} d\ln a_{M^+} + \Gamma_{A^-}^{(1)} d\ln a_{A^-}$$

(4.18)

According to Pethica the surface concentration of the counter-ion (M^+) is much less than that of the amphipathic ion (A^-) at low concentrations but it may equal it at higher concentrations when a complete monolayer is formed. The effect of this is seen from the two limits (equation 4.19 for very dilute solutions and equation 4.20 for less dilute solutions) to equation 4.18:

if $\Gamma_{M^+}^{(1)} = 0$ $\quad -\dfrac{d\gamma}{RT} = \Gamma_A^{(1)} d\ln c_{MA} f_{\pm}$

(4.19)

if $\Gamma_{M^+}^{(1)} = \Gamma_A^{(1)}$ $\quad -\dfrac{d\gamma}{RT} = 2\Gamma_A^{(1)} d\ln c_{MA} f_{\pm}$

(4.20)

In either case the surface may be considered to be a monolayer of A^- with the diffuse part of the double layer preponderant M^+ and H^+. The Gibbs equation may thus be written (assuming $f_{\pm} = 1$)

$$\Gamma_A^{(1)} \approx -\frac{1}{X\,RT} \cdot \frac{d\gamma}{d\ln c_{MA}}$$

(4.21)

where X varies between 1 and 2 according to the concentration of surfactant. Shinoda and Nakayama (Shinoda, 1954) however, have noted that the surface excess of counter-ions is always less than that of the surface-active ions.

With a surface-active weak electrolyte such as a soap, hydrolysis occurs:

$$A^- + H_2O = HA + OH^-$$

so $\quad \dfrac{a_{HA} \cdot a_{OH^-}}{a_{A^-}} = \text{constant}$

At constant pH:

$$a_{OH^-} = \text{constant}$$

so; $\quad \dfrac{a_{HA}}{a_{A^-}} = \text{constant}$

and; $\quad d\ln a_{HA} = d\ln a_{A^-}$ (4.22)

For a soap, equation 4.18 becomes:

$$-\frac{d\gamma}{RT} = \Gamma_{M^+}^{(1)} d\ln a_{M^+} + \Gamma_{A^-}^{(1)} d\ln a_{A^-}$$
$$+ \Gamma_{HA}^{(1)} d\ln a_{HA}$$

from this and equation 4.22:

$$-\frac{d\gamma}{RT} = \Gamma_{M^+}^{(1)} d\ln a_{M^+}$$
$$+ (\Gamma_{A^-}^{(1)} + \Gamma_{HA}^{(1)})$$
$$\times d\ln(a_{A^-} + a_{HA})$$

(4.23)

Since there is a concentration dependence of the effect of the counter-ions comparison with equation 4.21 gives that:

$$\Gamma_{(A^- + HA)}^{(1)} \approx -\frac{1}{X\,RT} \cdot \frac{d}{d\ln c_{MA}}$$

For aqueous solutions of potassium oleate, for example, equation 4.23 would be:

$$-\frac{d\gamma}{RT} = \Gamma_{K^+}^{(1)} d\ln a_{K^+}$$
$$+ \Gamma_{(\text{oleate} + \text{oleic acid})}^{(1)} d\ln a_{(\text{oleate} + \text{oleic acid})}$$

In order to remove the concentration dependence of the effect of the counter-ions (K^+), a constant excess concentration of another electrolyte such as KCl may be added to each soap solution so that:

$$a_{K^+} \gg a_{(\text{oleate + oleic acid})}$$

and the effect of changing the soap concentration will be that:

$$\text{d} \ln a_{K^+} \ll \text{d} \ln a_{(\text{oleate + oleic acid})}$$

Under these circumstances

$$-\frac{\text{d}\gamma}{RT} \approx \Gamma^{(1)}_{(\text{oleate + oleic acid})} \, \text{d} \ln a_{(\text{oleate + oleic acid})}$$

This is nothing more than the simple form of the Gibbs equation 4.17 for dilute solutions provided that a pure soap is used and the solutions are all of the same pH and contain a constant amount of counter-ion, thus:

$$\Gamma^{(1)}_{\text{soap}} \approx -\frac{1}{RT} \cdot \frac{\text{d}}{\text{d} \ln c_{\text{soap}}}$$

Because of the relatively high concentration of electrolyte, the electrical double layer is thin and so $\Gamma^{(1)}_A$ applies to a very thin surface and may be used to calculate surface packing where the area (m^2) per mole of a monolayer is given by $1/\Gamma^{(1)}_A$. It has been shown that very little additional electrolyte is in fact required and so an equation of the form of equation 4.20 holds only for solutions of extremely pure surface-active electrolytes.

Hydrolysis of soap leads to the formation of free fatty acid which being less soluble than the ion will be more strongly held at the solution surface. If the soap was prepared from impure fatty acid, there will be other anions and free fatty acids present as well, whose area of packing may be different from that of the main constituent. Further, unless very careful purification is accomplished, fatty acids prepared from natural sources will contain traces of fatty alcohols which are very water-insoluble.

Hydrolysis of soaps will be enhanced by a drop in pH. This may occur extensively if solutions are exposed to atmospheric carbon dioxide. If the surfactant is an anion, then these will attract counter-cations some of which will be hydrogen ions. The pH of the surface is therefore lower than that of the bulk and surface hydrolysis is very marked unless the pH is maintained sufficiently high. Conversely, a surface excess of long-chain amines produces a surface with an excess of counter-anions and a consequent higher pH than in the bulk solution.

As the concentration of soap in the very dilute solution is increased, the potential for adsorption will also increase because the soap anions, free acids and alcohols will be more strongly competing for a place in the surface. There is therefore a surface pressure π tending to increase the surface area in order to accommodate more solute. This pressure competes against the cause of the surface tension (which is a negative surface pressure) and results in a lower tension than before; consequently:

$$\gamma = \gamma^0 - \pi \qquad mN.m^{-1} \qquad (4.24)$$

where γ^0 is the surface tension of the solvent alone.

The surface of a soap solution is not filled with soap molecules at low soap concentrations (say at 10^{-4} molar) but becomes progressively filled as the bulk concentration is increased. Not until the surface is fairly well packed with soap molecules does π increase very much. Then further increase in soap concentration causes a marked reduction in γ with little change in the surface excess (see Fig. 4.16 where the slope of the steep portion remains virtually constant).

When a certain degree of packing at the surface is achieved, the energy required to push more soap into the surface approaches that given up on adsorption. A greater lowering of free energy can now take place by the soap molecules in the bulk aggregating with their paraffin chains together and their polar groups orientated towards the water (Fig. 4.20A). These aggregates are known as *spherical micelles* and the lowest concentration at which they form in appreciable numbers is called the *critical micelle concentration* (CMC). The micelles will be formed from all the different amphipathic molecules present and so mixed micelles form in impure systems. Hydrolysis products and other uncharged impurities generally cause formation of micelles to occur at lower concentrations since they are less soluble than soap ions and their lack of a charge lessens the disruptive effect which occurs when like charges are brought together in *ionic micelles*. Above the CMC there is therefore dynamic equilibrium between three pseudophases; the surface, bulk and micelles. The micellar pseudophase is much larger than the surface pseudophase and will tend to accommodate most of the less soluble components. As a result the surface will become depleted of impurities such as fatty alcohol above the CMC. These impurities will not be replaced in the surface by an equivalent amount of soap because the latter is more soluble and so there will be lowering of π and an increase in γ as the soap concentration is increased a little above the CMC.

Further increase in soap concentration will cause increased packing at the surface until the surface tension has decreased again to a constant value.

In theory, the surface is not necessarily one molecule thick, neither does the definition of surface excess require this although studies of the behaviour of dilute surfaces have shown them to be virtually monolayers or at least to act like them. Surface multilayers may occur at concentrations above the CMC. The surface excess will then be underestimated because the Gibbs equation depends on the change in surface tension which resides mainly in the surface molecular layer and amphipathic molecules layered under this will have little influence. Thus $d\gamma/d\,ln\,c$ is not a function of Γ for surface excesses more than one molecule thick so that a γ versus $ln\,c$ plot has zero slope when the monolayer is complete.

Verification of the Gibbs Equation

Some of the first attempts at a direct estimation of the surface excess were made by bubbling air through the solution and collecting the foam. The concentration of solute in the collapsed foam should be greater than that in the solution from which the foam was derived and if the surface area of the bubbles could be accurately estimated then the surface excess could be readily calculated. The results so obtained were unreliable for two reasons; the estimate of the surface area was uncertain and the lifetime of the bubbles was too short for surface equilibrium to be established (Fig. 4.17).

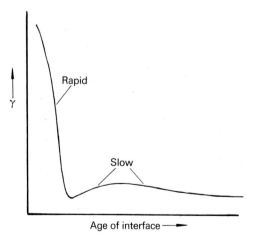

FIG. 4.17. Change of interfacial tension with age.

Successful verification of the Gibbs equation was achieved by McBain and his co-workers who propelled a microtome blade at high speed across the solution surface thereby shaving off a sample to a depth of about 100 μm. Analysis of this layer and of the underlying bulk solution enabled the surface excess to be calculated.

They also compressed solution surfaces by a known amount in a special trough and estimated the surface excess after determining the increase in bulk concentration produced by desorption. Similar observations have been made in reverse by calculating surface excess from the decrease in bulk concentration on producing a stable foam of known surface area. Both of these methods have shown good agreement with the Gibbs equation but indicate that factor X of equation 4.21 cannot always be ignored.

Radioactive tracer techniques have also been used by a number of workers, involving the use of amphipaths tagged with ^3H, ^{14}C and ^{35}S. Low energy radiation is absorbed by water after travelling only a short distance so that a detector placed just above the solution surface will register particles coming only from the surface and a thin layer underlying the surface. In order to correct for the emission received from the thin layer of bulk solution, similar measurements are made using solutions with the same concentration of the isotope contained in non-surface-active compounds. Co-adsorption of counter-ions may similarly be investigated using unstable metal ions. The accumulation of data appears to support equation 4.21.

Surface Ageing

At the instant that a surface is created, the surface will have the same composition as the bulk solution. Attainment of an equilibrium surface excess will therefore exhibit time dependence. Moilliet, Collie and Black (1961) considered two distinct phenomena:

(a) rapid ageing controlled by diffusion, and
(b) slow ageing controlled by steric factors.

One or both of these may be evident with a given surfactant solution depending upon the solute concentration, presence of electrolyte and temperature. A generalized picture is given in Fig. 4.17.

Diffusion towards the surface is rapid but becomes slower as surfactant ions approach the vicinity of the surface due to electrostatic repulsion from ions already adsorbed there. Thus there is rapid diffusion to the subsurface followed by 'activated' adsorption. Diffusion is also adversely affected if much of the surfactant is aggregated into micelles which, being much larger than single ions or molecules, are relatively slow moving. Surface ageing therefore becomes slowed by substances which encourage aggregation into mixed micelles, such as free acids produced by the hydrolysis of soaps. The rate of diffusion of hydrolysable surfactants is thus increased if the pH is adjusted in the direction which suppresses hydrolysis, e.g. to higher pH with soap solutions.

Diffusion to the surface is also more rapid at higher temperatures and greater surfactant concentrations. Electrolytes also facilitate the diffusion of ionic surfactants but they have little effect upon non-ionic surfactants such as methylcellulose. The minimum in the γ-time curve occurs earlier as the concentration is increased, but subsequent ageing effects are little influenced by this factor, leading to the conclusion that only the rapid initial decrease in γ is rate-controlled by diffusion.

The subsequent slower ageing effect appears to be controlled by steric factors such as reorientation and penetration of molecules in the surface. The rise in surface tension is probably associated with a surface phase transition to a condensed state (p. 74) this having been noted with sodium dodecyl sulphate when the area per molecule is reduced to about 0.4 nm². Electrolytes assist the penetration of the surface by both ionic and non-ionic surfactants since expulsion of hydrocarbon chains results in a larger free energy decrease than that resulting from expulsion from a relatively less polar simple aqueous solution (cf. salting out of soaps). Time dependence with surfactants in non-polar solvents may also arise due to slow breakdown of associated molecules such as dimers.

BULK PROPERTIES OF SURFACTANT SOLUTIONS

Most physical properties of *aqueous* solutions of an amphipath change rapidly in magnitude over a limited range of concentration (Figs 4.18 and 4.19). To account for this, McBain and others postulated the existence of aggregates of amphipathic molecules which, if ionized, are closely associated with a large proportion of the counter-ions (otherwise known as *gegenions*). The abrupt nature of the changes in magnitude of the various properties over a limited concentration range suggests that at lower concentrations the molecules are mostly single whereas at higher concentrations they are almost all present as micelles.

Hartley suggested that these are essentially spherical: however, at much higher amphipath concentrations than the CMC, other shapes can exist (p. 59). In aqueous solutions micelles have a

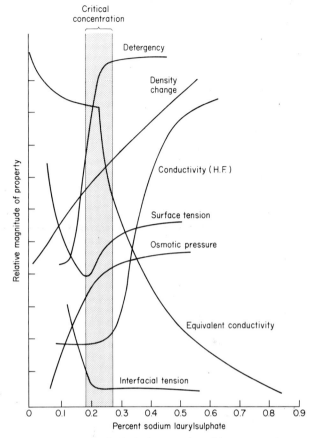

FIG. 4.18. Change of physical properties with concentration (Preston 1948).

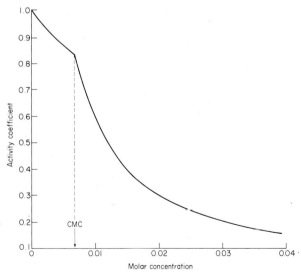

FIG. 4.19. Relationship between activity coefficient and concentration for aqueous solutions of sodium dodecylsulphate (from data of Clayfield & Matthews 1957).

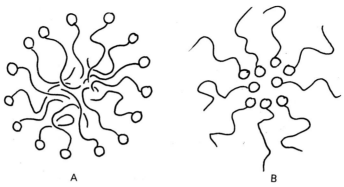

Fig. 4.20. Diagrammatic cross-section of spherical micelles in A, aqueous; and B, non-aqueous solvents.

non-polar liquid-like interior whereas in non-aqueous solvents inverted micelles are formed, held together by polar interaction of the 'head' groups (Fig. 4.20).

Theoretical Treatment of Micelle Formation
When amphipathic molecules associate, they form micelles with a narrow size distribution, the mean number of molecules per micelle being known as the *aggregation number*. The influence of amphipath concentration c, aggregation number n and charge p of the micelle upon the proportion of aggregated molecules may then be predicted by the law of mass action.

For non-ionic molecules, $p = 0$ and

$$nA \rightleftharpoons \underset{cx \quad c(1-x)/n}{A_n}$$

where c is the concentration in terms of single molecules and x is the unaggregated fraction. Although the activity coefficient does not remain at unity with increasing concentration (Fig. 4.21) yet, assuming its constancy for simplicity, then:

$$\frac{[A_n]}{[A]^n} = \frac{c(1-x)}{n(cx)^n} = k$$

and

$$\frac{1-x}{x^n} = k.n.c^{n-1}$$

The CMC may now be defined less ambiguously than in the previous section in the following terms:

$$\text{CMC} = (k.n)^{1/1-n} \qquad (4.25)$$

that is, at the CMC:

$$k.n.c^{n-1} = 1$$

hence:

$$\frac{c^{n-1}}{\text{CMC}} = \frac{1-x}{x^n} \qquad (4.26)$$

Equation 4.26 would also be applicable to ionic molecules provided they were completely dissociated whether present singly or as aggregates. In such a circumstance, however, a large coulomb attraction would exist between the micelles and their counter-ions and consequently dissociation of the micellar molecules is incomplete. Thus if M^+ is a monovalent counter-ion, $p = n - m$ and

$$mM^+ \quad + nA^- \rightleftharpoons M_m A_n^{(n-m)-}$$
$$c - \frac{m}{n}c(1-x) \quad cx \quad c(1-x)/n$$

so that

$$\frac{[M_m A_n]}{[M]^m [A]^n} = \frac{c(1-x)/n}{(cx)^n \left(c - \dfrac{m}{n}c(1-x)\right)^m} = k_{n,m}$$

and

$$\frac{1-x}{x^n \left(1 - \dfrac{m}{n}(1-x)\right)^m} = k_{n,m}.n.c^{(m+n-1)}$$

Generally defining (cf. equation 4.25) the CMC as

$$(k_{n,m}.n)^{1/(1-m-n)} \qquad (4.27)$$

that is,

$$k_{n,m}.n.c^{(m+n-1)} = 1$$

at the CMC, then

$$\frac{c^{m+n-1}}{\text{CMC}} = \frac{1-x}{x^n \left(1 - \dfrac{m}{n}(1-x)\right)^m} \qquad (4.28)$$

from which the concentration relative to the CMC may be computed for all values of x, m and n.

Curves related to equations 4.26 and 4.28 are

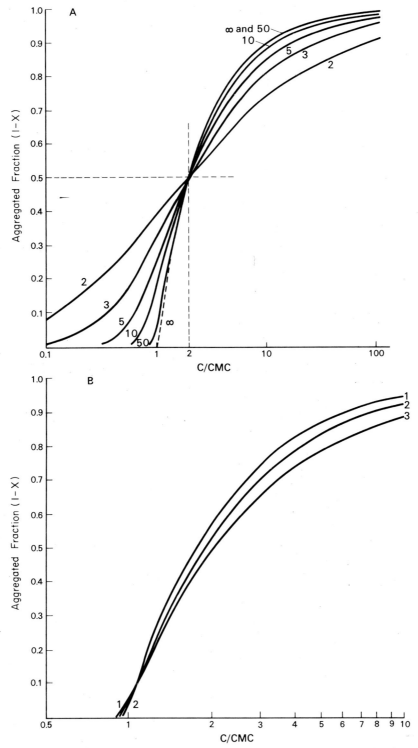

FIG. 4.21. Effect of amphipath concentration upon aggregation into micelles calculated from equations 4.26 and 4.28; A, Non-ionic or completely ionized micelles (for given aggregation numbers); B, Micelles (aggregation number 50) in different states of ionization $(1 = (A_{50}M_{25})^{25-}, 2 = (A_{50}M_{43})^{7-}, 3 = A_{50}$ and $(A_{50})^{50-})$.

plotted in Fig. 4.21 showing that formation of micelles with an aggregation number in excess of about ten produces an abrupt change in aggregated fraction around the CMC. It will also be observed that partial ionization of micelles enhances this abruptness.

Equations 4.25 and 4.27 defining the CMC imply that $d^2x/dc^2 = 0$ at the CMC, that is, aggregation is most abrupt at the CMC. An analogous method of defining the CMC is to take the point corresponding to the maximum curvature in an ideal solution property/concentration plot as in Fig. 4.18, that is $d^3\phi/dc^3 = 0$ where ϕ represents the magnitude of a given property such as conductivity.

An alternative approach is to consider micelle formation as a process of phase separation. This theory supposes that micelles begin to form only at the CMC which is then the saturation concentration for single molecules. Consequently the addition of further surfactant produces an equal amount of micellar pseudophase.

Determination of the Critical Micelle Concentration
Reference to Fig. 4.18 will indicate that a plot of any physical property against amphipath concentration gives a rough indication of the CMC of aqueous solutions. Generally the CMC is taken at the point of intersection of the extrapolated straight lines on either side of the break in the curve. Other properties not indicated in the figure which have been applied, include vapour pressure, refractive index, pH and diffusion coefficient. In order to obtain significant data, good temperature control is often essential particularly with refractive index measurements.

The CMC may also be estimated by the addition of traces of a third component whose absorption spectrum depends upon the state of aggregation of the amphipath. Marked spectral changes are frequently observed with ionic amphipaths when a dye of opposite ionic character is used with it. Thus pinacyanol chloride is commonly used for anionic amphipaths and eosin for cationic compounds. Using pinacyanol chloride, the colour change is from blue above to red below the CMC. The technique is to dissolve a small amount of dye in a solution of the amphipath which is above its CMC and to titrate this with an aqueous solution of the dye. The CMC is taken as the concentration of amphipath at which a colour change is first noticed.

Dyes may also be used with non-ionic compounds but the colour changes are much less pronounced and instead absorption in the ultraviolet region is followed. Another method which is suitable for use with non-ionic compounds is the iodine method. The technique is similar to that using dyes except that a trace of iodine is used and the change in light absorbance with amphipath concentration is followed at a suitable wavelength in the ultraviolet region. A sharp change in the slope of a plot of absorbance versus the logarithm of amphipath concentration indicates the CMC.

Because the interior of micelles in aqueous solution is essentially hydrophobic, water-insoluble compounds are able to dissolve in it. This behaviour is known as *solubilization* (p. 63). Thus the solubility of the added compound increases markedly at concentrations of amphipath above the CMC. In practice an excess of an oil-soluble dye such as Orange OT may be used, the amount taken into solution being determined colorimetrically. Alternatively, solutions of varying amphipath concentration may be titrated with the third component when observation of turbidity may be all that is necessary to detect the limit of solubility. Care must however be exercised in order to ensure that equilibrium has been attained.

For further details the reader is referred to the review by Mulley (1964). There is not always perfect agreement between the various methods, particularly when comparing those which do not involve the addition of a third component with those which do. The third component might well be expected to affect micelle formation, the CMC frequently being lowered.

Factors Affecting Micelle Formation
Thermodynamic factors. Hartley suggested that small aggregates begin to form at the CMC and that these grow rapidly over a small concentration range to a limiting size which is then independent of further increase in concentration. Mass action theory (Fig. 4.21) shows that slight aggregation is to be expected below the CMC. Association between hydrocarbon chains reduces the free energy which results from the disruption of hydrogen bonds in aqueous solution. However, formation of large aggregates in very dilute solutions would be most improbable but dimer formation is known to occur with sodium dodecylsulphate and some soap solutions.

Micelle formation is encouraged by those factors which produce a decrease in the free energy when hydrocarbon–water contact is reduced (p. 35) namely, a decreased water structuring ($+\Delta S$) and a decreased interference with hydrogen bonding ($-\Delta H$). Micellization may be accompanied by an

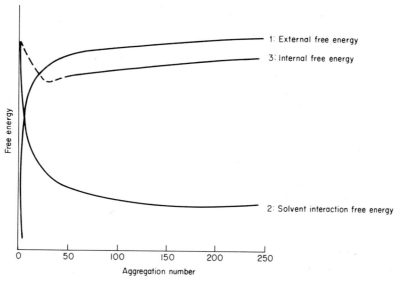

FIG. 4.22. Contribution of various factors to the free energy of an aqueous amphipath solution (not to scale: from Poland & Scheraga 1965).

increase in enthalpy but this is more than compensated by a relatively larger entropy increase. Some workers have shown the enthalpy change to decrease as the alkyl chain is lengthened for a homologous series of amphipaths, possibly reflecting an increase in cohesion between alkyl groups in the micelle. Others, however, have reported an increasing enthalpy of micelle formation with increasing alkyl chain length. These differences reflect a different choice of standard state.

Clearly, entropy plays a dominant role in micellization, the overall mechanism being termed 'hydrophobic bonding' (Abu-Hamdiyyah 1965). Ions however, draw water molecules to themselves and reduce their tendency to form hydrogen bonds with neighbouring water molecules. The effect is to reduce the water structure and therefore there tends to be a lower entropy contribution with ionic micelles. This effect would be influenced by the hydration of the counter-ion and of the polar head group. Various workers have found that counterions higher in the lyotropic series (p. 97) produce higher CMC values and an increase in the size of the polar group of non-ionic amphipaths has a similar effect.

Factors other than those due to hydrophobic bonding contribute to the free energy of micelle formation. Poland and Scheraga have considered the influence of aggregation upon (a) the loss of translational and rotational entropy when a molecule enters a micelle and (b) the entropy of the hydrocarbon chain within the micelle. As will be

seen from Fig. 4.22, factor (a), curve 1, would favour the molecules remaining in a monomeric form, whereas hydrophobic bonding, curve 2, would favour an aggregate of infinite size. However, when the free energy contribution of factor (b), curve 3, is taken into account, the total free energy curve of the system has a minimum at a finite aggregation number but the free energy in an aggregated form is less than that in the unaggregated form only above the CMC (Fig. 4.23). If the solute is ionic, then formation of micelles will involve bringing like charges together against their mutual repulsion. The general result of this is to cause ionic micelles to have smaller aggregation numbers and larger CMC values than non-ionic micelles.

The hydrocarbon group. Increase in the size of the hydrophobic group leads to a greater decrease in

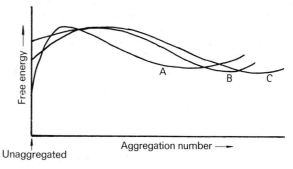

FIG. 4.23. Effect of concentration of amphipath showing a finite aggregation number for a minimum free energy. A, below CMC; B, at CMC; C, above CMC (from Poland & Scheraga 1965).

the free energy upon micellization, thereby promoting micelle formation. This results in a decreased CMC and an increased aggregation number. The free energy change is however less for branched chains then for straight chains and so the former have larger CMC values for a given number of carbon atoms. For a homologous series, the CMC decreases logarithmically with an increase in the number of carbon atoms. The presence of a double bond increases the CMC three or four times.

The polar group. In contrast to the effect of the hydrophobic group, an increase in length of polar chains (e.g. polyoxyethylene) decreases the free energy change upon micellization thereby increasing the CMC and decreasing the aggregation number. Hydration of the polar group of polyoxyethylene alkyl ethers occurs through hydrogen bonding between the ether oxygens and water. Increasing the length of the oxyethylene chain increases the hydration and solubility, thereby opposing the formation of micelles. When a non-ionic molecule is transferred to a micelle, the motion of the oxyethylene chains is restricted to a spiral within the envelope of a truncated cone (Fig. 4.24). This would be expected to reduce the entropy

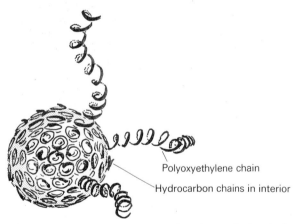

Polyoxyethylene chain

Hydrocarbon chains in interior

Fig. 4.24. Diagrammatic representation of a non-ionic micelle with all but three of the polar groups cut away.

of micelle formation. Since the entropy increase is in fact large, this has been interpreted to mean that micelle formation involves some dehydration of the polar groups. These groups are still however, considerably hydrated in the micelle. Water molecules are probably trapped both within and between the spirals, the proportion of water to number of oxyethylene groups increasing as the chain length increases.

Compared with the large effect that the length of a non-ionic polar group has upon the CMC, the type of an ionic group has little effect. The CMC does however increase slightly with increased hydration of the counter-ions, e.g. $Li^+ > Na^+ > N^+(CH_3)_4$, since hydration causes them to be less closely attached to the micelle and therefore to contribute less to its formation. The influence of the ions upon the water structure (see below) also affects the CMC. Compared with Li^+ and Na^+ which break water structure, tetramethyl ammonium ions enhance water structure thereby producing an appreciably lower CMC.

The position of the polar group in the molecule influences the CMC since moving this group towards the middle of a hydrocarbon chain is equivalent to increasing the branching of the chain which results in an increase in the CMC. The presence of a second polar group also increases the CMC particularly if it is ionized; the magnitude of the effect also depends upon the position of the group.

Electrolytes. The addition of salts increases the aggregation number and decreases the CMC of ionic amphipaths. This effect is due mainly to the reduced repulsion between the head groups as a result of the screening action of the counter-ions but is slightly modified by counter-ion hydration and the effect on the water structure. The effective degree of dissociation of the enlarged micelles is little influenced. Although ionic micelles appear to be predominantly monodisperse in low salt concentrations, there is evidence of a wider size distribution in the presence of higher salt concentrations.

Salts have a relatively small effect upon nonionic amphipaths, its magnitude probably depending upon the hydration of the salt ions, i.e. a salting out effect, where the more hydrated ions depress the CMC the most. The anions are more effective in this than are the cations. Competition for water of hydration by the salt reduces the hydration of the amphipathic molecule thereby increasing the latter's tendency to aggregate.

If the added electrolyte is also capable of forming micelles, the CMC of the mixture lies between those of the pure components. There is however preferential aggregation of the longer chain ions so that there is a larger mol fraction of these in the micelle than in the equilibrium unaggregated fraction.

Hydrogen Ion Concentration. Free fatty acids are less ionized and less soluble than their alkali metal salts, so that a reduction in the pH of a soap solution is accompanied by a reduction in the CMC. As a consequence, the effect of neutral electrolyte upon the CMC is less at a lower pH where the micelles have fewer charges. In contrast to this, the effect of the addition of strong acids to amphipathic strong acids such as dodecylsulphate is comparable to that of neutral electrolytes, the effect of added salts being similar over a wide pH range. Strong acids increase the hydrophilic character of polyoxyethylene groups by oxonium ion formation of the ether oxygens. This effect predominates over the salt effect and results in an increase in the CMC of non-ionic compounds.

Non-electrolytes. The addition of water-soluble compounds such as urea and glycerol generally raises the CMC. The tendency for micelle formation is reduced not only by a decreased structuring of water but also by a decreased dielectric which increases the repulsion between charged head groups, and by an increased solvation of the amphipathic monomer which reduces the enthalpy change of micellization. The overall influence of a particular additive will be governed by a combination of these factors. Such effects are modified if the additive is incorporated into the micelle since this may tend to increase micelle stability at low additive concentrations. Thus a *trace* of ethanol is shown (Fig. 4.25) to decrease the CMC only slightly while longer chain alcohols have a much more pronounced effect (Fig. 4.26). Small amounts of ethanol increase the solubility and lower the Krafft-

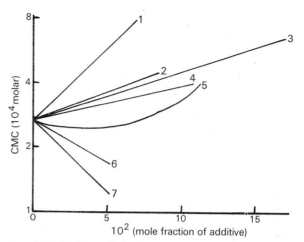

FIG. 4.25. Stability of dodecyltrimethylammonium micelles in aqueous organic solvents at 25°C (from Emerson & Holtzer 1967). 1, dioxane; 2, propan-1:3-diol; 3, ethylene glycol; 4, methanol; 5, ethanol; 6, propan-2-ol; 7, propan-1-ol.

point (see below) but large quantities suppress micelle formation. The hydrocarbon chains of the alcohols penetrate the micelle interior while the polar groups remain on the outside (Fig. 4.34). Long chains in particular enhance the micelle stability since the dispersion force interaction in the micelle interior is increased and the charge density on the micelle surface is probably slightly decreased. The effect of polar compounds which form mixed micelles is both concentration and temperature dependent and as a result the minimum in the

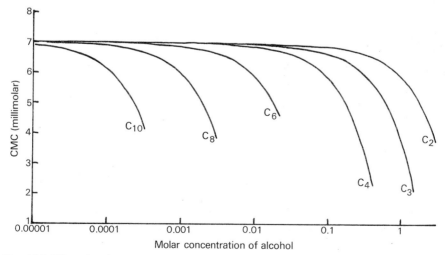

FIG. 4.26. Effect of various normal alcohols on the CMC of potassium tetradecanoate at 18°C (from data of Shinoda 1954).

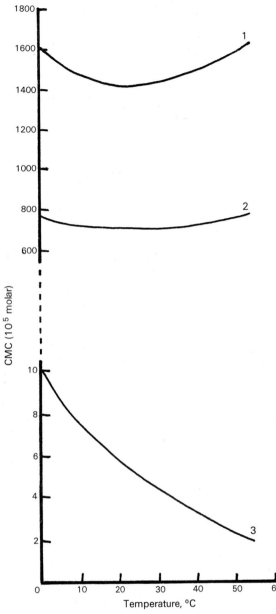

FIG. 4.27. Variation of CMC with temperature for 1, $CH_3(CH_2)_{11}N(CH_3)_3Br$; 2, $CH_3(CH_2)_{11}SO_4Na$; 3, $CH_3(CH_2)_{11}(OCH_2CH_2)_7OH$ (adapted from Schick 1963).

Temperature. An increase in temperature influences the stability of micelles by the following means. First, transfer of hydrocarbon groups from an aqueous to a non-polar environment is normally endothermic and so micelles tend to become more stable by the hydrophobic bond effect. Secondly, the dielectric constant is decreased so that ionic micelles become less stable. Thirdly, thermal agitation increases, resulting in an enhanced disruptive effect. With non-ionic compounds the second factor is non-operative and the first factor outweighs the last. An increase in temperature decreases the hydration of the molecule with a resulting increase in aggregation number and a decrease in the CMC. In the case of ionic compounds, the hydrophobic effect is probably dominant at lower but not at higher temperatures. Such an effect produces a shallow minimum CMC near room temperature. An increase in temperature above that producing the minimum CMC has been shown to decrease the aggregation number and to increase the dissociation of micelles of sodium dodecylsulphate, a sign of the disruptive effect of thermal agitation.

The solubility of an amphipath is influenced by temperature. At low temperatures, solid ionic-type amphipath is in equilibrium with a solution whose concentration is below the CMC. As the temperature is raised the solubility increases until it reaches the CMC at which temperature, called the *Krafft-point*, the solubility begins to increase very rapidly (Fig. 4.28). If micelles are treated as a separate (pseudo-) phase, then the Krafft-point may be considered as the melting-point of the hydrated amphipath above which it becomes dispersed in

CMC–temperature plot with ionic micelles (Fig. 4.27) is eliminated, the CMC decreasing continuously as the temperature falls.

The solubility of sodium dodecylculphate is also increased by traces of short (C_6 to C_8) chain alcohols but large amounts of alcohol, which itself has only a small solubility, cause an alcohol–surfactant gel to separate as a new phase.

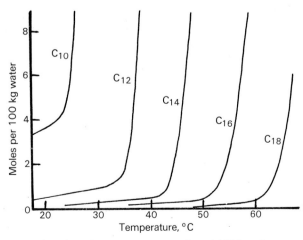

FIG. 4.28 Effect of temperature upon the solubilities of some alkyl sulphonates (after Tartar & Wright 1939).

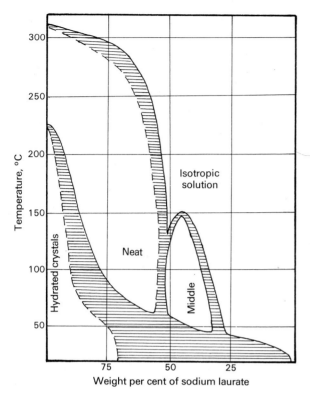

FIG. 4.29. Effect of temperature upon aqueous sodium laurate systems (shaded areas indicate the existence of more than one condensed phase) (after McBain et al. 1938).

solution as micelles. The solubility of ionic compounds is limited at higher temperatures by the separation of liquid crystals (see below and Fig. 4.29). Many non-ionic compounds do not show a Krafft-point, since the saturated solution is in equilibrium with a liquid crystalline phase (Fig. 4.30). High temperatures however suppress hydrogen bonding thereby reducing the hydration of the polar chains and cause the solution to become turbid, the upper consolute temperature being called the *cloud-point*. The turbidity is caused by the separation of an amphipath-rich phase which is not surprising since the micelles grow rapidly below the cloud-point. The dilute aqueous phase has a concentration roughly that of the CMC and contains few, if any, micelles.

STRUCTURE OF MICELLES AND LIQUID CRYSTALS

Above but close to the CMC, micelles are spherical but as the concentration of amphipath is increased the micelles may grow into cylindrical or rod-shaped structures whose diameter is slightly less than twice the fully extended length of the monomers. The tendency to form rod-shaped micelles depends upon the nature of the hydrocarbon chain, with such factors as length, branching and degree of unsaturation. It is also influenced

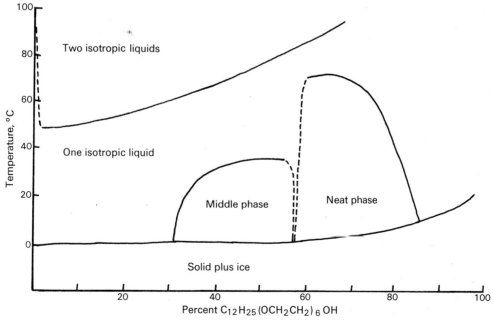

FIG. 4.30. Effect of temperature upon the system dodecyl-hexaoxyethylene glycol monoether plus water (dashed lines are estimated boundaries; after Balmbra et al. 1962).

by the polar group and the counter-ion and pH of ionic compounds while with the non-ionic hexadecylpolyoxyethylene glycol monoether a decrease in polar chain length leads to increased asymmetry of the micelles.

These long micelles often have a random orientation but, as their concentration increases, their freedom of motion becomes restricted producing visco-elastic solutions. Further increase in concentration causes some of them to become closely packed in hexagonal array (Fig. 4.31A) and to separate out as another phase in equilibrium with a more dilute solution containing randomly orientated rods. This new phase which contains the oriented rods is known as the *middle phase*. Progressive increase in concentration results first in a single middle phase and finally in the separation of solid hydrated amphipath. It should be pointed out however, that the micelles of some compounds, such as cetyltrimethylammonium chloride (but not bromide) remain spherical at concentrations below that necessary for the separation of a middle phase. With many compounds a further phase may separate before solid is produced; this is the *neat phase* which has a lamellar structure (Fig. 4.31C). Both the middle and neat phases form what are known as *liquid crystals* and are termed *mesomorphous* (*meso* = between, *morph* = form) because they have a structure intermediate between that of true liquids and crystals.

Other mesomorphic states are known. When a water-soluble amphipath, such as sodium octanoate, is dissolved in decanol containing a trace of water, inverted micelles are produced, that is, the non-ionized polar groups of the fatty acid salt are orientated inwards around a few water molecules and the hydrocarbon chain extends outwards into the alcohol. If the proportion of decanol is now reduced while maintaining a constant proportion of 'soap' and water, an inverted middle phase (Fig. 4.31B) will eventually separate. Continuous decrease of decanol concentration with increase of the 'soap' and water produces, in order, invert middle phase, lamellar phase and finally middle phase.

With some systems a face-centered cubic arrangement of spherical aggregates seems to occur. Such structures are generally observed over only a narrow concentration between the lamellar (neat) and the hexagonal (middle) phases. It is probable that with lipids and potassium soaps, the cubic structure is formed from invert spherical aggregates with the hydrocarbon chains filling the gaps between the water 'cores'. With alkyltrimethyl-

ammonium bromide the aggregates are probably not spherical.

It will be observed that the structure of the middle and neat phases is *anisotropic*, that is, it varies with direction. The middle phase is plastic and too stiff to flow under gravity since the close-packed regular arrangement of the cylindrical aggregates gives it solid character in two dimensions. In the long direction however, there is liquid-like behaviour since the cylinders probably vary in length and are not regularly arranged. The layered structure of the neat phase gives this a greater fluidity. There is no regular arrangement in the two dimensions parallel to the layers but in the direction normal to the layers there is a crystal-like periodic arrangement. The neat phase is therefore solid in one dimension and liquid in two dimensions. It is the ability of the layers to slip over each other that makes the neat phase more mobile than the middle phase. Often, drops of neat phase, which are mobile enough to flow under their own weight, exhibit a stepped surface, each step height being a multiple of the layer thickness.

X-ray diffraction patterns have been used in an attempt to confirm postulated micellar structures. Besides a weak diffraction due to solvent, three bands have been identified in the more concentrated amphipath solutions. The short-spacing (S) band corresponds to the repeat distance of about 0.45 nm for the hydrocarbon chain in the liquid state; the micelle-thickness (M) band has a repeating distance slightly less than twice the length of the hydrocarbon chains and the long-spacing (I) band corresponds to the separation distance of the structures composing the mesomorphous phase (Fig. 4.32).

Liquid crystals are birefringent (have a different refractive index for the two components of the electric vector of light) and may be detected and identified by their effect upon polarized light. Rotation of plane polarized light occurs for light travelling in any direction other than along the optic axis of the uniaxial crystal, so that liquid crystals remain visible when placed between crossed polarizers, whereas light passing through an isotropic phase would be extinguished. Under a polarizing microscope, neat and middle phases may be distinguished by the patterns or 'textures' which are produced (Rosevear 1968).

Mesomorphism as previously described involves the addition of a solvent to the amphipath; this is termed *lyotropic mesomorphism*. *Thermotropic mesomorphism*, on the other hand, involves the production of a liquid crystalline phase merely by

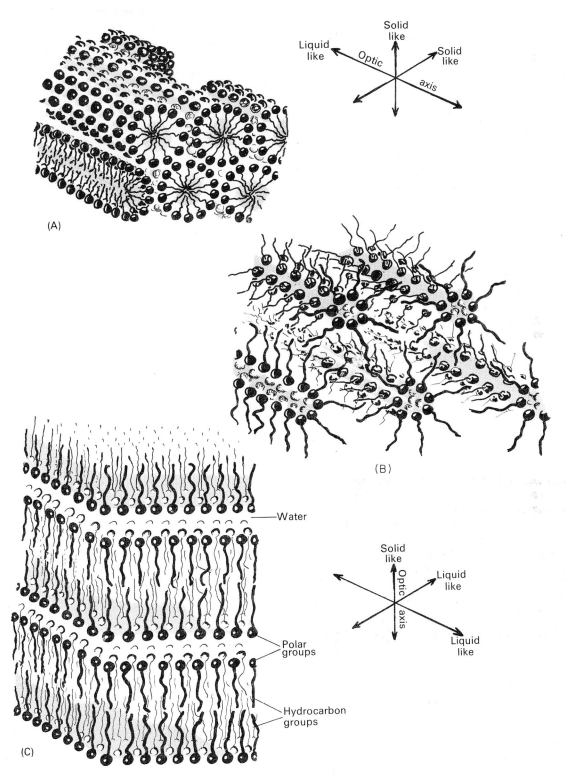

FIG. 4.31. A, Section of middle phase; B, Section of invert middle phase; C, Section of neat phase.

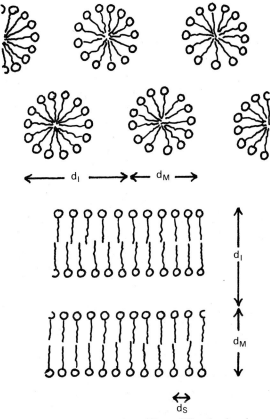

FIG. 4.32. Interpretation of X-ray diffraction bands.

The neat phase is an example of a lyotropic smectic state. The thermotropic smectic state has a similar layered structure except that the molecules may be arranged as single rather than double layers since one end of the molecules may fit neatly to the opposite end of a molecule in an adjacent layer. Smectic crystals are not orientated in a magnetic field but if formed by cooling the isotropic liquid in such a field, orientated crystals are produced. Examples of compounds exhibiting the smectic state are ethyl *p*-azoxybenzoate and octyl *p*-azoxycinnamate.

A nematic structure is occasionally observed with amphipathic solutions which then have a soft, often stringy, consistency. The thermotropic nematic state is produced by heating such compounds as *p*-azoxyanisole whilst N-(4-methoxybenzylidene)-4-butylanilene is nematic at room temperature. Nematic crystals are less ordered than smectic ones since the elongated molecules are arranged parallel to one another without the formation of a layered structure. Normally they are not optically active but, if twisted between a microscope slide and coverslip, they exhibit characteristic microscopic textures somewhat different from those given by smectic or lyotropic middle phases. Molecules in the nematic crystal are readily orientated parallel to a weak magnetic field. The viscosity is therefore dependent on the direction of the field in relation to the direction of flow.

Cholesteric phases are produced by a number of cholesteryl esters but not by cholesterol itself. These have a layered structure quite different from the smectic type. The elongated molecules lie parallel to each other within the plane of a layer, their orientation in adjacent layers being slightly displaced. This displacement arises because the shape of the molecules influences their fit in

warming a crystalline, generally organic, solid. This is a transition phase between the solid crystal and isotropic liquid and gives the compound the appearance of having two melting points. Three types of mesomorphous phase have been distinguished, namely *smectic* (soap-like), *nematic* (thread-like) and *cholesteric* (Chapman 1965).

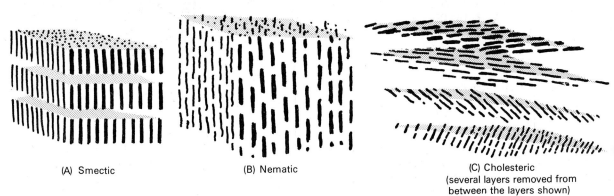

(A) Smectic   (B) Nematic   (C) Cholesteric
                                                      (several layers removed from
                                                      between the layers shown)

FIG. 4.33. Types of thermotropic liquid crystals.

adjacent layers and so these latter trace out a helical path which causes rotation of polarized light. With non-polarized light, circular dichromism is observed giving rise to a multicoloured effect.

Some compounds can exhibit more than one type of mesophase. Ethyl anisal-*p*-aminocinnamate, for example, forms smectic crystals which change to nematic at a higher temperature. A number of cholesteryl fatty acid esters also form smectic crystals but these become cholesteric on further warming.

Stability of Micelles

The equilibrium between micelles and monomers is a dynamic one. When suddenly diluted to below the CMC, some ionic micelles have been shown to have a half-life of a centisecond or even less. Micelle stability is slightly increased by an increase in alkyl chain length and is affected to a small extent by the nature of the counter-ion. Traces of hydrocarbon dissolved in the micelle interior appear to reduce the rate of micelle breakdown but the formation of mixed micelles by the addition of long-chain alcohol may not have an appreciable effect. Micelles formed from mixed anionic and cationic amphipaths however do appear to breakdown less easily. Micelle stability increases with increasing concentration of amphipath above the CMC but decreases with increasing temperature.

SOLUBILIZATION

The interior of a micelle has a different dielectric, from the surrounding solvent. Solutions of amphipaths therefore have the ability of dissolving substances which are insoluble or at best only sparingly soluble in the solvent alone. This is known as *micellar solubilization*, the solubilized substance being termed the *solubilizate*.

Solubilizates are incorporated into the micelle in different ways according to their chemical structure, in particular the presence and disposition of polar and non-polar groups. Saturated hydrocarbons dissolve in the non-polar part of the micelle which in aqueous solutions forms the micellar interior (Fig. 4.34a). Since the M-spacing and thus the volume of the micelle is increased, more amphipath molecules are incorporated into the micellar surface to maintain a suitable packing density. There are therefore larger but fewer micelles and so the I-spacing also increases. Amphiphilic solubilizates, such as *n*-alcohols, form mixed micelles; that is, they are incorporated into the *palisade layer* of the micelle (b), where the molecules are orientated to juxtapose the polar

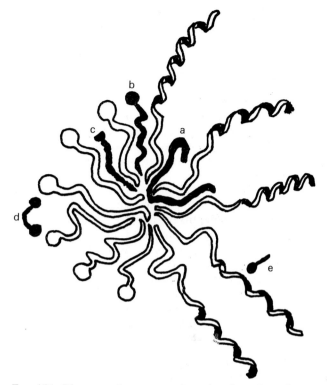

FIG. 4.34. Diagrammatic representation of various sites of solubilization in aqueous solution. Open figures are solubilizer; closed figures are solubilizate. Left: ionic half micelle section; right: nonionic half micelle section.

groups. Weakly polar or polarizable groups such as double bonds enable the solubilizate to be drawn deeper into the palisade layer (c). Incorporation of polar solubilizates tends to result in increased micellar asymmetry with only slight changes in the M and I-spacing. Some water-soluble polar solubilizates are thought to be adsorbed on to the micelle surface (d), but the validity of this has been questioned (Osipow 1962). It appears, however, that complex formation by hydrogen bonding occurs between polyoxyethylene groups and aromatic carboxylic acids such as *p*-hydroxybenzoic acid or phenolic compounds such as chloroxylenol (e).

Micellar solubilization can only occur in the presence of micelles. Often the amphipath forms micelles in the absence of the solubilizate but occasionally aggregation takes place only upon addition of the latter. Thus the addition of an amphiphilic solubilizate to amphipath concentrations below the CMC may reduce the CMC sufficiently for mixed micelles to form: a process known as *co-micellization*. Incorporation of a fourth component to the amphipath-water-solubilizate system may increase the solubility of the solubilizate; for example, octanol forms mixed micelles with sodium 3-hendecanesulphate in water thereby increasing the solubility of a hydrocarbon.

Enhanced solubility of organic compounds may sometimes be achieved by the addition of non-micelle forming forming compounds. Thus sodium acetate or salicylate greatly increases the solubility of theobromine. While such an effect is generally due to complex formation or to decreased hydrophobic bonding, various workers have shown that there is a continuous gradation in solubilizing behaviour between high molecular weight micelle-forming amphipaths and low molecular weight non-micelle-forming amphipaths. The effect of non-micelle-forming amphipaths is known as *hydrotropy* and is due to a 'co-solvent' action, the distinction between hydrotropy and solubilization being rather vague. Even below their CMC, soaps are known to increase the solubility of phenolic compounds.

Factors Affecting Solubilization
Concentration of amphipath. Marked increase in solubility occurs above the CMC, the solubility often being a linear function of the amphipath concentration for dilute solutions (Fig. 4.35). If the amphipath is more concentrated however, the solubility may increase more rapidly, reflecting the changing size and shape of the micelles.

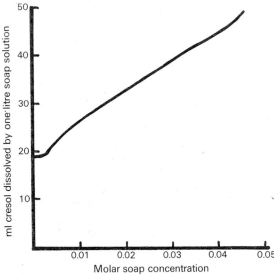

FIG. 4.35. Solubilization of Cresol BP in potassium oleate solution at pH 10.6 and 23°C (soap prepared from Oleic Acid BP).

Nature of the amphipath. For a homologous series of amphipaths, solubilization of hydrocarbons is increased by an increase in alkyl chain length but is decreased by chain branching. The effect of unsaturation in the chain probably depends upon the solubilizate. Enlargement of polyoxyethylene chains of non-ionic compounds appears slightly to reduce their solubilizing power even when calculated on the basis of weight of solubilizate incorporated per unit weight of micelle interior. The type of ionic group also has an effect which is slightly modified by the nature of the counter-ion. However, although McBain and Richards found dodecylamine HCl to be a much better solubilizer than K laurate (C_{12}), data collected by Mulley (1964) suggest that superior solubilizing power is not inherent in any particular class of amphipath. The influence of alkyl chain length upon solubilization of polar compounds is complicated since these solubilizates are incorporated in the palisade layer. Instead of excess solubilizate separating as another phase virtually devoid of amphipath and water, as occurs with hydrocarbons, an excess of alcohols, aldehydes and fatty acids causes separation into two phases each containing a considerable proportion of amphipath. Each of these phases may be isotropic, one containing ordinary micelles and excess water (*L1 phase*) and the other containing inverted micelles and excess amphiphile (*L2 phase*). Alternatively, the two phases may be L1 and liquid crystalline (*LC*) phases. In either case, a turbid emulsion results due to the different refractive index of the phases. L1 and L2 systems separate with amphipaths containing the shorter alkyl chains when increasing chain length results in increasing amount of amphiphile which can be solubilized before separation of an L2 phase. However, solubilization with the longer alkyl chain compounds is limited by the separation of an LC phase at a lower amphiphile concentration than when an L2 phase separates, and this concentration decreases as the amphipath alkyl chain is lengthened.

Nature of the solubilizate. Elworthy et al. (1968) have discussed the effect of the nature of a solubilizate upon the extent of its incorporation into micelles and conclude that generalizations apply only to the simplest compounds. Polarity and polarizability are important, besides molecular geometry. For a homologous series, whether polar or non-polar, an increase in the size of a hydrocarbon group decreases the solubility in a solution of an amphipath of given concentration. Branching of alkyl chains has only a small effect but unsaturation increases the solubility. Cyclization also tends towards enhanced solubility but this remains low for the more rigid polycyclic compounds. Polar compounds are usually more soluble than non-polar ones although octanol is less soluble than octane in a decinormal solution of dodecylamine HCl at 25°C, presumably for reasons discussed in the preceding paragraph. Octanol is, however, more soluble than octane in several other amphipath solutions. The effect of the type of polar group and alkyl chain length upon the system sodium caprylate–water–solubilizate has been illustrated by Mandel! et al. (1967a, b).

Effect of electrolytes. Salts have been shown to enhance the solubility of hydrocarbons in amphipath solutions. Besides promoting the formation of micelles as evidenced by a lowering of the CMC, salts cause an increase in micelle size with a consequent increase in the volume–surface ratio and presumably therefore an increased solubilizing capacity. The solubility of some polar compounds is reduced in the presence of salt and is probably associated with a decreased solubility causing separation of a liquid crystalline phase.

Effect of non-electrolytes. Mention has already been made (p. 57) of the effect of water-soluble substances on the CMC. Similar effects have been noted with regard to the solubilizing power of amphipaths towards hydrocarbons. For example, ethanol suppresses both micelle formation and the heptane and benzene-solubilizing power of cetrimide. Solubilization behaviour is however influenced by the solvent effects of the additive and there will exist a partition of both the hydrocarbon and the polar additive between the micelles and the extramicellar solution. Sometimes the addition of water-soluble compounds enables a given amount of solubilizate to be dissolved using less amphipath: glycerol, sorbitol and sucrose, for example, reduce the amount of non-ionic amphipath required to solubilize vitamin A. The addition of hydrocarbons may also increase the solubility of sparingly soluble compounds. This effect, known as *co-solubilization*, is thought to be due to the increased volume of the micelles upon solubilization of the hydrocarbon. The co-solubilizing action of long-chain alcohols and hydrocarbons has already been mentioned (p. 64). Other polar compounds are also effective co-solubilizers such as long-chain amines or mercaptans.

Effect of temperature. There is little effect upon the solubility of liquid hydrocarbons in dilute solutions of ionic amphipaths although an increase in temperature can markedly increase the solubility of solid solubilizates since the crystal lattice becomes less stable. The solubility of polar solubilizates, however, may increase considerably with temperature particularly when solubility is limited by the separation of a liquid crystalline phase. Increase in temperature may also increase the solubilizing power of non-ionic amphipath solutions but many solubilizates, particularly amphiphilic ones, lower the cloud-point so that the solubility decreases again as higher temperatures are reached (Fig. 4.36).

Effect of pH. Although pH has little effect on the CMC of such compounds as alkyl sulphates, the CMC of fatty acid soaps decreases with a reduction in pH. With the latter compounds a small reduction in pH results in enhanced solubilizing power. When the solubilizate is a weak electrolyte, its degree of ionization is influenced by the prevailing pH. Since the extent of solubilization may frequently be considered in terms of the distribution between the lipophilic interior or palisade layer of the micelle and the extra-micellar aqueous solution (Evans & Dunbar 1965), a shift in pH in the direction which suppresses ionization and makes the solubilizates less hydrophilic will increase the proportion solubilized. Some compounds such as benzoic acid also appear to associate with the polar chains of non-ionic amphipaths by hydrogen bonding. A decrease in pH decreases the ionization of the acid and would increase such binding to the micelle surface. Regardless of the position in the micelle occupied by the benzoic acid, it follows that a decrease in pH results in a decreased extra-micellar concentration for a given total benzoic acid concentration.

Ternary Phase Diagrams

Various physico-chemical characteristics of three component systems at constant temperature and pressure can be mapped out using triangular co-ordinates. The diagrams are constructed using equilateral triangles which have the unique property that the lengths of the three lines radiating from any point within the triangle, parallel to the sides and disposed at an angle of 60° to each other, add up to the length of one side. Similarly the composition fractions of the three components add

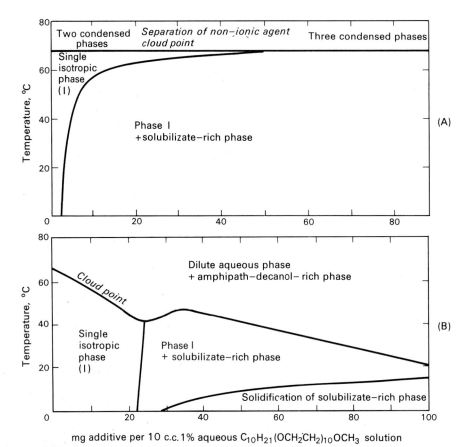

FIG. 4.36. Solubilization and cloud point curves of 1 per cent $C_{10}H_{21}(OCH_2CH_2)_{10}OCH_3$ solution in the presence of A, decane; and B, decanol (after Nakagawa & Tori 1960).

up to the whole system. Thus point A of Fig. 4.37 represents 50 per cent X, 20 per cent Y and 30 per cent Z; point B represents 30 per cent X and 70 per cent Z and point C represents pure component Z.

Line CF contains every possible mixture with components X and Y in the ratio 5:2. Dilution of composition F with component Z causes the resultant composition to pass through A and to reach the corner at C at infinite dilution. Line DE contains every possible mixture with 20 per cent Y, the proportion of X and Y varying according to the position on the line. (See also p. 12.)

Triangular diagrams are constructed as contour maps each contour joining those compositions having some property in common. Thus a phase diagram has contours which circumscribe those compositions exhibiting the same phase type.

A four component system might be represented as a solid figure in the form of a regular

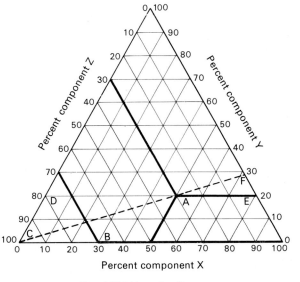

FIG. 4.37. Triangular diagram.

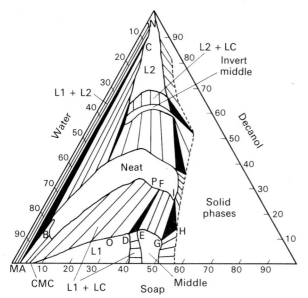

FIG. 4.38. Phase equilibria for the system sodium octanoate–decanol–water at 20°C (slightly modified from Mandell et al. 1967).

tetrahedron or an equilateral triangular prism. Alternatively, the vertical scale of the prism may be used to represent the influence of temperature or of amphiphile chain length upon a three component system.

Fig. 4.38 illustrates the triangular phase diagram. Compositions within the regions denoted by L1 (high proportion of water) and L2 (high proportion of decanol) are isotropic containing micelles and inverted micelles respectively except right in the corners where the soap concentration is below the CMC. The smectic liquid crystalline region is delineated near the centre of the triangle and the two hexagonal mesophases are also shown. Regions between these single phases are composed of a mixture of the relevant phases. Thus at low soap concentrations the mixture separates into two phases (L1 and L2) except when water or decanol is in extreme excess. Mixtures on the *tie-line MN* separate into the two phases whose compositions are *M* and *N*. The proportion of phases of composition *M* and *N* depends on the position of the mixture on the tie-line. Other mixtures separate into L1 and neat phase, L1 and middle phase or L2 and invert middle phase. Thus mixtures lying on the tie-line *OP* separate into two phases of composition *O* and *P*. Between the single liquid crystalline phases are two phase regions, each phase consisting of a different type of liquid crystalline arrangement, for example neat and middle. It will also be noted that there are a number of triangular regions within which the mixture separates into three phases. According to the phase rule these form invariant systems, that is, any mixture within a triangle will separate always into the phases whose compositions are denoted by the corners of that triangle. For a given temperature and pressure, only the relative proportion of the three phases will vary with change in composition of the mixture within the triangle. Thus mixtures within *ABC* separate into L1 + L2 + neat; mixtures within *DEF* separate into L1 + middle + neat and mixtures within *GHI* separate into middle + neat + hydrated solid.

Pharmaceutical Application of Solubilization

Drugs of limited aqueous solubility have been solubilized for both internal and external use. These include oil-soluble vitamins, steroid hormones and antimicrobial agents, the resulting systems being thermodynamically stable.

Solubilization of orally administered drugs results in an improved appearance and may improve an unpleasant taste. It also enables both oil- and water-soluble compounds to be combined in a single phase system as with multivitamin preparations. The amphipath must be non-toxic in the quantities used, have an agreeable taste and odour and be compatible with other ingredients. It should also possess good solubilizing power and stability. Cationic amphipaths are the most toxic but non-ionic compounds generally have a low toxicity and therefore are to be preferred. Because many non-ionic compounds are bitter, careful formulation is required to keep their concentration to a minimum. The monoesters of polyoxyethylene sorbitan or of sucrose are commonly used, often with co-solubilizing agents which may also help to improve the taste.

Solubilization may lead to enhanced absorption and an increased biological activity. It improves the intestinal absorption of vitamin A and the percutaneous absorption of oestrone. Drug absorption from ointment bases and suppositories may also be increased by the presence of an amphipath.

Clear solutions of corticosteroids for ophthalmic use are achieved using non-ionic agents. In order to minimize any irritant effect, low concentrations of amphipath are required, a good solubilizing power being essential.

Amphipaths are more toxic when given parenterally. Ionic compounds readily produce haemolysis and therefore only non-ionic compounds are suitable, such as a polyethylene glycol ether which is used to disperse phytomenadione.

Aqueous concentrates of volatile oils have also

been prepared. Careful formulation is necessary in order to achieve a concentrate which remains clear upon dilution. Soaps are used to solubilize phenolic compounds for use as disinfectants, familiar examples being Lysol and Roxenol. The soap enables the phenol to become readily dispersed throughout systems, such as drains, to which it is added and assists penetration into greasy or coagulated material. While only the phenol in the extramicellar solution is bactericidally active, the micelle acts as a reservoir tending to maintain a constant extramicellar concentration as phenol is used up due to reaction with protein or removal by dirt. The partial phase diagram for a Lysol is given in Fig. 4.39. Line *AF* represents all compositions containing 51 per cent w/w (50 per cent v/v) Cresol. Compositions *B*, *C* and *D* are clear solutions (L2 phase only) whereas *E* is cloudy (L1 + L2). If composition *B* is diluted with water it will remain clear although L1 is eventually produced. It is also apparent that composition *C* contains the minimum of soap that will enable a Lysol to remain clear on dilution. Composition *D*, although clear at first, will pass through the L1 + L2 region upon dilution but will eventually become clear as the single L1 region is reached. This illustrates the use of the ternary diagram which enables the formulator to decide upon a suitable composition. Different soaps and grades of cresol can have a profound effect upon the phase diagram for Lysol. Burt (1965) showed that *p*-cresol with sodium oleate produced a three phase region (L1 + L2 + LC) so that dilution of

such a Lysol always made it pass through a cloudy region.

Disinfectants are also prepared by solubilizing iodine with non-ionic amphipaths. Such a product is called an *iodophore* (meaning iodine carrier) and probably involves a certain degree of complexing between the iodine and the polar groups. The use of an amphipath obviates the necessity of solvents of high glycol content and enables dilution without precipitation of the iodine. Solubilized iodine volatilizes less readily and is less liable to stain fabric or corrode metal. It has however good bactericidal activity and most of the iodine is readily released to the bacterial cell.

Liquid preparations generally require preservation against microbial spoilage. The preservative exerts its effect by dissolution in the aqueous phase. Absorption into micelles reduces its effective concentration and so larger amounts of preservative need to be added to maintain a suitable extramicellar concentration.

The stability of a drug may be enhanced by solubilization. Vitamin A is more resistant to autoxidation in aqueous non-ionic amphipath solutions than in oil. Similarly the oxidation of aliphatic and aromatic aldehydes is less when they are solubilized rather than emulsified. It is probable that the reduced rate of oxidation within micelles is due to dilution of the solubilizate by the amphipath making free-radical propagation more difficult. The catalytic effect of metal ions is also reduced when an aldehyde is solubilized.

Solubilization can also reduce the rate of hydrolysis of drugs such as benzocaine and methantheline bromide. Anionic amphipaths are better than cationic ones in protecting against alkaline hydrolysis since hydroxyl ions are repelled by micelles of the former but attracted by those of the latter. On the other hand, acid hydrolysis may be promoted by anionic compounds which attract hydrogen ions, but some measure of protection may be afforded by the addition of salts whose cations compete with the hydrogen ions at the micelle surface. Non-ionic amphipaths are also capable of reducing hydrolysis rates but if solubilization occurs among the polar groups rather than in the micelle, interior protection from hydroxyl ions is not so marked. The site of the hydrolytic process is in the extra-micellar solution. Increasing the amount of amphipath increases the partition of drug into the micelle thereby reducing the fraction of drug in the aqueous environment with a consequent reduction in the rate of hydrolysis. However, solubilized systems possess a

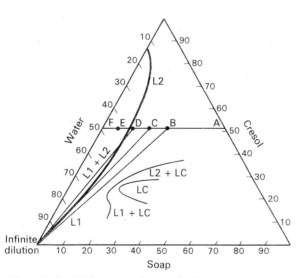

FIG. 4.39. Equilibrium phase diagram for the system potassium oleate–cresol–water at pH 10.7 and 20°C.

large micellar surface area enabling rapid transfer of drug into the hydrolysis-promoting environment. Emulsified oils with a much smaller oil-water interfacial area therefore tend to hydrolyse more slowly.

Further details may be obtained from the reviews by Mulley (1964), Swarbrick (1965) and Elworthy et al. (1968), which also contain good bibliographies.

INSOLUBLE MONOLAYERS

If the non-polar groups of an amphipathic compound are sufficiently large to render it almost completely insoluble, then traces of the compound will usually spread over a water surface to form a monomolecular layer. In such a case the whole of the 'solute' may be said to form the Gibbs excess. As usual, such molecules will have a preferred orientation with the polar groups directed towards the water. Such monolayers may spread not only from liquid amphipaths, or from their solutions in non-aqueous solvents, but also from the solid. Spreading from the solid involves a positive entropy change whereas from the liquid it is negative showing that the monolayer is disorientated relative to the solid but more orientated than in the bulk liquid. Such monolayers behave somewhat like two-dimensional matter in possessing two-dimensional physical states and exhibiting a surface pressure, a surface viscosity and a surface potential. They can form at water–air or organic liquid–air surfaces and also at liquid–liquid interfaces.

Formation of a Monolayer

The liquid or liquids forming the interface must be very carefully purified by redistillation in scrupulously clean apparatus and the trough in which the monolayer is to be spread must also be freed from minute traces of surface-active contaminants. When the water–air or water–oil interface has been formed, residual contamination can be sucked away from the interface through a capillary.

Spreading of the monolayer is generally achieved by preparing a dilute solution of the surfactant using a pure solvent which itself has a positive spreading coefficient. For fatty acids and alcohols at the water–air surface, petroleum spirit (b.pt. 60–80°C) is suitable. An accurately known volume (0.01 to 0.05 cm³) is injected near the surface using a micrometer syringe. The solution floats to the surface, spreads over it and the solvent completely disappears by evaporation and by dissolution in the 'subphase' after a few seconds. Solvent retention at the surface can occur and this

may influence the properties of a monolayer. Such retention is minimized by employing the smallest amount of solvent consistent with complete spreading. If a hydrocarbon is unsuitable as a solvent, a water-soluble alcohol, ethanol or propanol, may be used. Alcohol–water mixtures are used to spread polypeptides, electrolytes being included for protein solutions. The solvent soon disappears from the interface by dissolution in the bulk phase in which it becomes extremely dilute. To ensure that the solute is carried to the surface, the solvent must have a suitable density, or in the case of an oil–water interface, the solution must be injected on a suitable side of it.

Surface Pressure and its Measurement

Since the molecules of the monolayer are confined to an interface, their kinetic motion in the interfacial plane will produce a two dimensional pressure (π) measured in terms of such units as $mN.m^{-1}$. This pressure is augmented by repulsion of ionized groups and opposes the surface tension of the substrate liquid, or the interfacial tension between two immiscible liquids, giving rise to a lower tension (equation 4.24). The surface pressure may therefore be conveniently determined by measuring the reduction in the surface or interfacial tension using a Wilhelmy plate (p. 43).

Just as a change in volume produces a change in three-dimensional pressure, so a change in the area occupied by a monolayer results in a different surface pressure. Measurement of these changes enables π–A plots to be constructed, analogous to P–V plots, A being the average area occupied per molecule or per milligram in the case of proteins.

Knowing the area of the interface and the amount of surfactant injected into it, the area available to each molecule can readily be calculated provided that the molecular weight is known. The surfactant can be injected in small increments and the resulting tension measured each time. A disadvantage of this technique, however, is the necessity to wait many times for the disappearance of solvent from the interface.

Studies at a water–air surface may be facilitated by using a rectangular trough made of Teflon, or of glass rendered hydrophobic by being sprayed with a Teflon aerosol or coated with paraffin wax. The water level may then be made to stand a little above the level of the wall of the trough so that a hydrophobic bar placed across the trough isolates the liquid surfaces on either side of the bar. The Wilhelmy plate dips into the liquid at one end of

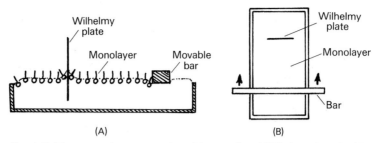

FIG. 4.40. Diagrammatic representation of the trough and Wilhelmy plate; A, side view, B, plan view. (The surfactant molecules are not drawn in proportion).

the trough and the monolayer is spread on the same side of the bar. By moving the bar towards the plate, the area available to each molecule in the monolayer is decreased (Fig. 4.40). The production of non-zero contact angles, particularly with rigid films at high surface pressures, is a source of error.

Direct measurement of the surface pressure can be made using a *film balance* otherwise known as a Langmuir-Adam trough (Fig. 4.41). The Wilhelmy plate is replaced by a 'float' or 'boom', a thin strip of mica rendered hydrophobic in the same manner as the trough. The float lies flat on the water surface and is suspended from a horizontal torsion wire by means of a stiff wire or rigid plastic plate. It extends almost the whole width of the trough, the narrow gaps at the ends being sealed using thin gold or platinum foil or silk treated with petroleum jelly or plastic threads to prevent leakage of the monolayer past the float. Motion of the float is monitored by means of an optical lever. The force exerted on the float by the monolayer can then be determined by the displacement of a reflected light spot, or by the angle of twist to the torsion wire needed to restore the light spot to its null position.

Preliminary cleaning of the water surface is facilitated by the use of movable bars since these can be used to sweep adsorbed contaminants out of the area to be covered by the monolayer. A clean surface can then be demonstrated by reducing the confined surface area when no reduction in surface tension or build-up of surface pressure should be evident. With the film balance it is important to clean the surface on both sides of the float.

When the spread monolayer is highly insoluble, the float of the Langmuir-Adam trough acts as a perfect two-dimensional semi-permeable membrane by allowing free passage only of the substrate liquid. Direct measurements of the surface pressure of soluble monolayers can however be made using a *PLAWM* trough (PLAWM = Pockels-Langmuir-Adam-Wilson-McBain). This is similar to the Langmuir-Adam trough but it is divided into two compartments by a thin highly convoluted rubber membrane under the float. This membrane prevents the seepage of solution to the surface behind the float.

An alternative method of studying soluble monolayers is to follow the changes in tension by means of a strain gauge as a film of solution is stretched between two platinum rings.

Various modifications are necessary for studies

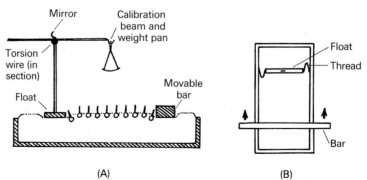

FIG. 4.41. Diagrammatic representation of a film balance; A, side view, B, plan view. (The surfactant molecules are not drawn in proportion).

at the liquid–liquid interface. For example, the trough and barriers may need to be made of a less hydrophobic material than Teflon, such as nylon, while it may be more convenient to use a taut plastic band rather than bars to confine the interfacial film.

Surface Potential and its Measurement

Adsorption of a monolayer of surfactant molecules at a water–air or water–non-polar oil interface changes the potential across the interface due to the separation of charges in or around the polar groups. This potential change (ΔV) is known as the surface or interfacial potential and may be measured by the air-electrode or vibrating plate methods (Alexander & Johnson 1950; Davies & Rideal 1961).

Surface potential measurements can give information relating to the structure of the monolayer. Fluctuations of the potential between different parts of the surface indicate a variation in the packing of the molecules while the actual value of the potential can give information regarding their orientation. The surface potential is analogous to the potential difference between the plates of a parallel-plate capacitor giving the equation:

$$\Delta V = \frac{N.Q.d}{\varepsilon.\varepsilon_o} \text{ volts} \qquad (4.29)$$

where N is the number of charges of magnitude Q coulombs per square metre, d is the distance between the plates, ε is the dielectric constant (relative permittivity) and ε_o is the permittivity of free space ($= 4\pi \times 10^{-7} c^2$ where c is the velocity of light in free space in m.s^{-1}). For a molecule, the product of the charge Q and the separation distance is the dipole moment μ. The distance d is however the separation distance resolved normal to the plane of the monolayer so that if the dipoles make an angle θ to the normal then $Q.d = \mu \cos \theta$. Equation 4.29 then becomes:

$$\Delta V = \frac{N.\mu \cos \theta}{\varepsilon.\varepsilon_o}$$

with N equal to the number of monolayer molecules in each square metre of surface ε generally being taken as unity. Caution must however be exercised in interpreting surface potentials solely in terms of the monolayer structure since the presence of a monolayer can affect the structure of an aqueous substrate adjacent to the monolayer.

Surface Rheology and its Measurement

Two-dimensional distortion and flow of a monolayer is analogous to the behaviour of a bulk phase in three dimensions. A wide range of surface mechanical behaviour can be demonstrated such as viscosity and elasticity in both dilatation and shear. Thus the surface elastic modulus K_s is given by:

$$K_s = -\left(\frac{\Delta A}{A}\right)$$

and its reciprocal is the surface compressional compliance which, for a perfectly elastic film, is also the surface compressibility C_s given by

$$C_s = -\frac{1}{A}\left(\frac{\partial A}{\partial \pi}\right)_T \qquad (4.30)$$

so that $K_s = C_s^{-1}$ which is known as the surface compressional modulus. The compressibility is readily calculated from π–A plots and its value depends upon the state of the film, it being small for closely packed monolayers having the character of a two-dimensional condensed state. The compressibility of a film and its relaxation time are important parameters governing the stability of foams and perhaps some emulsions. The various surface elastic moduli and their interrelationship have been described by Tschoegl (1958).

Resistance to a shear stress in the plane of a monolayer is measured in terms of a surface viscosity (η^s), the unit being a surface Poise ($sP = 1 \text{ mN.s.m}^{-1}$). For a surface,

tangential force per metre $= \eta^s \times$ shear rate

so that η^s has the dimensions MT^{-1} and is related to the three-dimensional shear viscosity (η) by:

$$\frac{\eta}{\eta^s} = \frac{1}{d} \qquad (4.31)$$

d being the film thickness which is of the order of 2 nm for monolayers. Thus a monolayer having a surface viscosity of 10^{-4} sP has a viscosity of about 500 P ($= 50 \text{ N.s.m}^{-2}$) over its thickness. A liquid with such a high viscosity would be termed 'very thick' so that monolayers having surface viscosities of the order of 1 sP or more would generally be regarded as solid.

Surface viscosities can be determined in a number of ways, two-dimensional analogues of tube and Couette viscometers often being employed. The canal method (Fig. 4.42) employs a trough with movable barriers to apply a surface pressure to the film and the pressure difference ($\Delta \pi$) between the ends of the canal can be measured using a film balance.

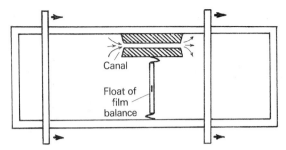

FIG. 4.42. Canal method for measuring the surface viscosity of an insoluble film.

By analogy with the Poiseuille equation

$$\eta^s = \frac{\Delta\pi.W^3}{12\ L(\mathrm{d}A/\mathrm{d}t)} \qquad (4.32)$$

where W and L are the width and length of the canal respectively. Since the flowing film drags some of the underlying water, a correction must be applied so that equation 4.32 becomes

$$\eta^s = \frac{\Delta\pi.W^3}{12\ L(\mathrm{d}A/\mathrm{d}t)} - a.\eta_o$$

where η_o is the 'ordinary' viscosity of the substrate liquid and a depends upon the width and depth of the canal. This method can be used only for insoluble monolayers since partially soluble ones would tend to desorb from the region of high surface pressure and be readsorbed on the other side of the canal.

The drag of the substrate liquid is employed in the so-called 'viscous traction' method. In one variant of this, a petri dish containing the spread film is slowly rotated and a canal between two concentric wire rings suspended at the surface retards the motion of the film. The rings are so fixed that the meniscus between them is slightly concave upwards and talc particles sprinkled on it enable the rate of rotation of the mid-line to be determined. The retardation of the rate of rotation between the rings is a function of the interfacial viscosity, the latter being determined by calibration of the instrument with films of known interfacial viscosity. This method is suitable for both water–air and water–oil interfacial films.

Another method, suitable for liquid–air surfaces, also uses two concentric rings but the inner one is rotated while the liquid is kept stationary. Liquid motion imparted by the rotating ring is kept to a minimum by placing a sheet of mica about 1 mm below the surface. Other techniques that have been used include those which determine the damping of the oscillations of a torsion pendulum.

Creep tests can also be used to study the visco-elastic behaviour of films. This is best achieved by applying a constant torsional stress to a ring or biconical disc suspended in the interface from a torsion wire and observing the displacement with time. The ring or disc must be concentric with the circular dish.

Large increases in surface or interfacial viscosity can result from the formation of mixed monolayers between oil-soluble and water-soluble surfactants, such as between lauryl alcohol and sodium lauryl sulphate or cetyl alcohol and cetrimide. Such monolayers are capable of stabilizing emulsions and foams. The increased surface viscosity resulting from the addition of a little fatty alcohol to an ionic surfactant solution is probably the prime cause of the enhanced foam stability which is obtained (Davies & Rideal 1961).

Structure and State of Monolayers
Just as the bulk state is affected by the three dimensional pressure (P) so changes in surface pressure (π) can alter the state of a monolayer. By the equation analogous to equation 4.31:

$$\frac{P}{\pi} = \frac{1}{d}$$

it follows that if the monolayer thickness is 2 nm, then a surface pressure of $2\ \mathrm{mN.m^{-1}}$ is equivalent to a bulk pressure of $1\ \mathrm{MN.m^{-2}}$ or about ten times atmospheric pressure. Since surface pressures well in excess of $20\ \mathrm{mN.m^{-1}}$ are frequently encountered, it will be appreciated that such monolayers have a strong tendency to maintain their integrity without collapsing and in so doing they exhibit a surface compressibility equivalent to the bulk compressibility of solids or liquids.

The surface pressure of a monolayer is the resultant of three components: that due to kinetic motion (π_k), that due to electrostatic repulsion (π_r) and the opposing effect due to cohesional forces (π_o) which is always negative. Thus:

$$\pi = \pi_k + \pi_r + \pi_o$$

The effect of these pressure components can be seen in Fig. 4.43. Unionized molecules of straight chain fatty acids or alcohols can pack very closely to each other in vertical orientation and cohesion due to van der Waals forces is large. If a large area is available, these form large clusters up to several millimetres in diameter and exert only a very small surface pressure. These clusters behave rather like a two-dimensional liquid with a few 'gaseous' molecules in between. Only when the

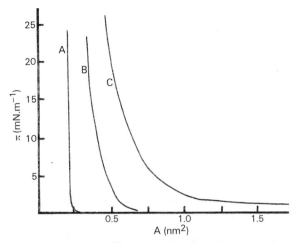

FIG. 4.43. π–A curves illustrating the effect of; A, a straight hydrocarbon chain, octadecanoic acid (stearic); B, a hydrocarbon chain bent by a double bond in the middle, *cis*-9-octadecanoic acid (oleic); C, an ionized polar group, octadecyltrimethylammonium ions on M/2 NaCl.

available area is decreased so that the groups begin to pack tightly does π increase appreciably. Further compression of the monolayers results in large values of π with only a small decrease in A when the compressibility becomes even smaller due to the attainment of a two-dimensional solid state. A little more compression then results in collapse of the film.

A double bond in the hydrocarbon chain particularly with a *cis* configuration prevents close packing of the molecules and reduces interchain cohesion. The monolayer therefore is much more expanded than with saturated-chain acids. Similar behaviour is also observed with other polarizable groups in the hydrocarbon chain such as with hydroxy acids. At large areas both polar groups become anchored to the aqueous substrate so that the molecule occupies a much larger area than when vertically orientated. Appreciable pressures are required to detach the second polar group and to force the molecules into a more or less vertical orientation. This monolayer then has the character of an expanded liquid with the hydrocarbon chains in a more random state than with straight saturated chains and consequently a higher compressibility. Further compression will force the molecules into a closer packing with a smaller compressibility having the character of a condensed film before collapse occurs.

An ionized monolayer, spread on a salt solution in order to reduce its solubility, has an appreciable surface pressure even at very large available areas. Repulsion between the polar groups overcomes the

cohesional forces causing the molecules to fill the surface in a manner anlogous to a gas filling an available space. These monolayers are therefore termed *gaseous*.

Interchain cohesion increases with length of the hydrocarbon chains. Figs 4.44 and 4.45 show the effect of chain length and temperature upon the π–A curves for fatty acids. Fig. 4.44 demonstrates a remarkable similarity to Andrew's P–V curves for a gas above and below the critical temperature suggesting that an increase in interchain cohesion results in a higher critical temperature. The shallow curves on the right hand side of the figure represent highly compressible gaseous films while the steep portions on the left are produced by liquid-like films of low compressibility. For fatty acids below

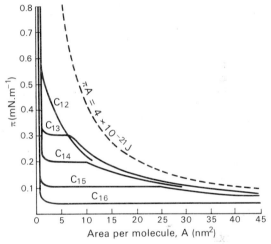

FIG. 4.44. π–A curves for a series of straight chain saturated fatty acids between 12° and 16°C (from Adam 1930).

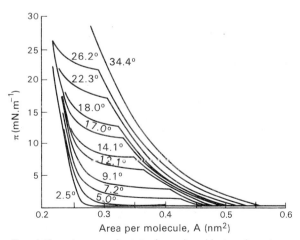

FIG. 4.45. π–A curves for tetradecanoic acid at various temperatures (from Adam 1930).

the critical temperature (in Fig. 4.44 at about 14° with more than 12 C atoms) a horizontal portion represents a first order transition, that is $dA/d\pi$ becomes infinite. Monolayers having a mean area per molecule lying within this transition are composed of discontinuous regions some with coherent molecules, the rest being gaseous. Such a condition leads to surface potentials which fluctuate from one part of the surface to another.

The extreme left hand portion of Fig. 4.44 for the C_{14} acid has been enlarged in Fig. 4.45 which shows the effect of temperature upon the liquid-like state. The steep curves on the right hand side are those for the *liquid-expanded* state whilst on the left hand side the *condensed* state is found. Between these two states is another transition, this time for a second order where $dA/d\pi$ is finite. It is known as a *liquid-intermediate* state and has a higher compressibility than either the liquid-condensed or liquid-expanded states. This transition probably involves the loss of rotational freedom about the long axis of the molecules thereby creating further area for close packing. The sequence of phase changes is summarized in Fig. 4.46. Not all states are given by every compound or at all temperatures. For example, at low temperatures a liquid condensed film may change directly into a gaseous film. Some workers have also distinguished other states such as the *superliquid* which is rheologically liquid but has a compressibility like that of a solid film; cetyl alcohol behaves in this manner.

By analogy with a gas, the simple equation of state for a gaseous film is

$$\pi A = kT \qquad (4.33)$$

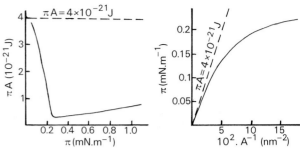

FIG. 4.47. πA–π and π–A^{-1} plots for ethyl hexadecanoate at 16–17°.

where k is the Boltzmann constant, that is the gas constant per molecule (R/N). This assumes that the film pressure has no contribution from cohesional or electrostatic repulsive forces and is due only to kinetic motion so that $\pi = \pi_k$. Thus equation 4.33 is a limiting law and can be represented by a rectangular hyperbola having a value of about 4×10^{-21} J at room temperature (see also Fig. 4.44). Gaseous films tend to approximate to such a curve only at areas per molecule approaching 100 nm² as shown in Fig. 4.47.

This ideal gaseous film equation (4.33) suggests that A becomes vanishingly small as π becomes very large. A better equation of state is obtained by taking into account the effective area (A_o) of the molecule when

$$\pi_k(A - A_o) = kT \qquad (4.34)$$

Films likely to obey equation 4.34 are those which are uncharged $(\pi_r = 0)$ and which have no interchain cohesion $(\pi_o = 0)$. Interchain cohesion is virtually eliminated at an oil–water interface since the oil molecules penetrate between the hydrocarbon chains and satisfy their London attraction forces (Fig. 4.48). This leads to greater surface pressures for a given area per molecule at the oil–water interface. The surface pressures of films of quaternary ammonium ions do however have an

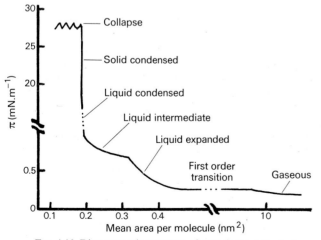

FIG. 4.46. Diagrammatic sequence of monolayer states (values on abscissa represent only the usual order of magnitude).

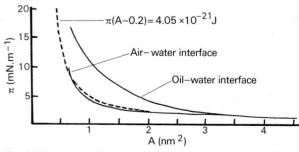

FIG. 4.48. π–A curves for hexadecyltrimethylammonium bromide on salt solution at 20°.

electrostatic repulsion component and the $\pi(A - A_o)$ hyperbola is therefore not coincident with the curve for the oil–water interface. Approximate coincidence with the curve for the air–water surface implies that the cohesive forces and the electrostatic repulsive forces are opposite and of nearly equal magnitude.

Interchain cohesion becomes appreciable in gaseous films under high surface pressure or in liquid-expanded films. For an uncharged film $\pi = \pi_k + \pi_o$ whence $\pi_k = \pi - \pi_o$ and equation 4.34 becomes

$$(\pi - \pi_o)(A - A_o) = kT$$

This equation of state is analogous to the van der Waals equation for real gases and in the case of liquid-expanded films π_o is nearly independent of A.

Since condensed films have nearly linear π–A plots, their equation of state can be written

$$\pi = b - aA$$

where a and b are constant for a given compound and set of physicochemical conditions. Comparison with equation 4.30 shows that aA is the surface compressional modulus (C_s^{-1}).

Extrapolation of a linear plot to zero pressure gives information concerning the packing and orientation of the film molecules. Saturated straight long-chain fatty acids at room temperature show both the liquid and solid condensed states with limiting areas (A_o) per molecules of about 0.24 to 0.26 nm^2 and 0.203 to 0.205 nm^2 respectively. These areas are independent of chain length at a water–air surface (although not at a water–oil interface) and indicate a vertically orientated monolayer. That of the solid condensed state is about 0.02 nm^2 greater than the area of cross-section (0.185 nm^2) in the three-dimensional crystal.

At high surface pressures, many straight-chain compounds have limiting areas of about 0.205 nm^2 Besides the fatty acids, this is found with alcohols, amides and esters where staggering of the polar groups allows the area to be limited only by the interlocked hydrocarbon chains. Since the cross-section of the polar groups is larger than that of the chains, a larger limiting area is often found at low surface pressures; for example, alcohols and esters pack to about 0.22 nm^2 and nitriles to about 0.27 nm^2. However, association between the polar groups by hydrogen bonding, with amides for example, may ensure a low limiting area even at low surface pressures.

For a given surface pressure, the area per molecule of a liquid-condensed film decreases slightly with an increase in chain length due to the increased interchain cohesion. Thus at 5 mN.m^{-1} and 25° a hexadecanoic acid molecule occupies 0.24 nm^2 whereas an eicosanoic acid molecule occupies only 0.23 nm^2. Under these conditions, tetradecanoic acid would form only an expanded film with an area per molecule of 0.37 nm^2.

The effect of an unsaturated bond depends upon the position and configuration. A double bond near the middle of the chain with a *cis* configuration produces too much bending of the chain for a condensed film to form whereas the chain of a *trans* compound is straighter and can produce such a film. Condensed films also form if the double bond is next to a terminal carboxyl group, the liquid condensed phase then having a limiting area of 0.287 nm^2.

Steric hindrance to close packing also results from chain branching. Thus 16-methylheptadecanoic acid forms a much more expanded film than octadecanoic acid although both are saturated C_{18} acids. If the methyl group is near the middle of the chain, the film is even more expanded for a given surface pressure.

Sterols such as cholesterol with a hydroxyl group at the 3 position also form condensed films with a limiting area between 0.37 and 0.42 nm^2 according to the stereochemical configuration of the A and B rings. Such molecules tend to stand nearly upright at a surface, packing closely to form a film of low compressibility. The tilt of the sterol nucleus is affected by the type and position of the polar group. Sometimes the molecules are caused to lie nearly flat at low surface pressures and consequently they possess large limiting areas. Such films have a much greater compressibility than cholesterol.

A liquid condensed film of a straight-chain fatty acid has been shown to have an appreciable compressibility, the area per molecule decreasing from about 0.25 to about 0.205 nm^2 due to a rearrangement of the carboxyl groups. The polar groups of 1–monoglycerides are also closely packed with a limiting area of about 0.263 nm^2 but are not rearranged by compression. Their low compressibility suggests that the molecules are held apart by structure formation between the polar groups. The head groups of p-alkyl-phenols are also closely packed with a limiting area of 0.24 nm^2. Low compressibility in this case suggests that the benzene rings are vertically orientated in a closely packed layer about 0.6 nm thick and that these take up the whole of the compression.

The areas quoted above refer to unionized films

and for fatty acids apply to films spread on dilute HCl or on fresh very pure water. On water, trace contaminants such as polyvalent cations may eliminate the liquid-condensed state causing the solid state to persist down to low film pressures. Alkaline substrates cause ionization and expansion of fatty acid monolayers. Although electrostatic repulsion between ionized carboxyl groups would be expected to have some effect, association of the carboxyl groups with the hydrated cations appears to be the prime cause of the expansion. Liquid-expanded films of octadecanoic acid are produced at pH 13 on solutions of LiOH, NaOH and KOH and it is probable that the size of the hydrated cation *in the surface* increases in the order Li Na K, producing the same order of effect upon expansion of the monolayer. Traces of Ca ions however markedly reduce the expansion effected by mono-valent cations. At pH 8.5, using bicarbonates, compression of the now incompletely ionized monolayer causes monovalent cations to be ejected. These changes in the condition of the monolayer are reflected in the surface potential which becomes considerably reduced by dipolar opposition of the counter-ions.

The conclusion, therefore, is that the state of a given monolayer and its transition from one state to another is influenced by three independent variables. These are the temperature, surface pressure and the extent to which the polar groups interact with the liquid substrate. In the latter case this is affected by the composition of the substrate such as the presence of electrolytes and the prevailing pH. Additional to these factors the configuration and size of the hydrophobic groups influence the cohesive forces and extent of packing of different monolayers.

Mixed Monolayers

While monolayers of water-insoluble amphipaths such as octadecanoic acid tend to be coherent, those composed of less hydrophobic substances tend to be fully solvated, that is, they are penetrated by water to form two-dimensional aqueous solutions. Compression of such monolayers causes the water molecules to be squeezed out at some critical pressure which is less than 0.1 mN.m^{-1} in the case of octadecanoic acid but between 28 and 30 mN.m^{-1} for sodium dodecylsulphate.

Water-soluble surfactants can also penetrate into an insoluble monolayer, the free energy of the penetrant molecules being decreased by dilution in the monolayer. The excess free energy of mixing monolayers of long-chain alcohols with some ionic surfactants has been shown to be a minimum when the monolayer contains equimolecular proportions of the two components. Interchain cohesion and screening of the ionic groups by the intervening alcohol groups are both probably involved in maintaining the integrity of the mixed monolayer.

Molecular association between two components requires a strong interaction between the polar groups but this is accompanied by monolayer penetration only if the soluble molecules have large enough hydrocarbon groups whereby they can form a strong interchain cohesion with the insoluble molecule. Sometimes the association in the monolayer is strong enough for stoichiometric complexes to be distinguished. Thus a cholesterol film on NaCl solution has a limiting area per molecule of about 0.4 nm^2. If the film is expanded and sodium hexadecylsulphate is injected underneath, a very large rise in surface pressure occurs upon recompression with collapse at about 0.6 nm^2 per cholesterol molecule. This indicates that some hexadecylsulphate molecules become squeezed out of the monolayer upon compression but that the remaining molecules strongly adhere in a 1:1 ratio. The surface complex is less stable in the absence of salt. Some hexadecylsulphate also appears to be adsorbed underneath the monolayer and this may enhance the stability of the film.

Similar 1:1 complexes have been found to form between other amphipaths such as between cholesterol and the steroidal saponin digitonin whilst 1:2 or 1:3 complexes have been detected with some other substances. Many other mixed monolayers also have collapse pressures and areas larger than those of the pure insoluble component but not all form stable 'complexes'. Thus molecular association occurs between long-chain alcohols and sodium hexadecylsulphate but a stoichiometric relationship is not found. In such cases the association is strongest when the alcohol possesses a straight hydrocarbon chain.

Surface association is paralleled in bulk solution by the formation of mixed micelles or liquid crystals. A thermolabile complex of cholesterol and digitonin can crystallize from alcohol. Complexing may also affect certain properties in the bulk phase. Thus sodium hexadecylsulphate loses its haemolytic power and is not precipitated by silver nitrate when its solutions contain an equimolar proportion of cholesterol. The extent of molecular association at a water–oil interface is also implicated in the stability of emulsions and may involve multilayer formation.

Monolayer penetration may be accompanied by a change in the physical state of the film. Thus a solid film of ergosterol becomes liquid on injection of saponin or sodium hexadecylsulphate into the substrate whilst a liquid film of cholesterol becomes solid on injection of saponin but remains unchanged with sodium hexadecylsulphate.

If cholesterol is added to a liquid expanded film of a long-chain fatty acid in the molecular proportion of 1:4, the bulky cholesterol molecule restricts the oscillatory motion of the acid molecules causing them to occupy the smaller area of a condensed film. A mixed monolayer of cholesterol and lecithin also occupies a smaller area for a given surface pressure than the sum of the areas of the separate components. Although it has been suggested that the components of the film form molecular complexes, it would seem that the mean molecular area simply reflects the best arrangement of the molecules in accordance with their mutual attractive forces.

Macromolecular Films
Like monolayers of simple molecules, macromolecular films can exist in various physical states ranging from gaseous to solid, compressed films frequently being visco-elastic. They are more expanded at the water–oil interface than at the water–air surface because of reduced intermolecular cohesion due to the penetration of oil molecules between the hydrophobic groups.

Proteins are able to form monomolecular films on water having a thickness of 1 nm or more. This involves the unfolding of the molecule and may result in film formation being irreversible because of the diminution in solubility which accompanies the exposure of hydrophobic side chains. At low surface pressures, protein films occupy an area around $1 \text{ m}^2\text{mg}^{-1}$ with the unfolded molecules lying flat on the surface. Higher pressures cause the hydrophobic side chains to become orientated away from the water and at collapse pressures an insoluble coagulum is produced. Interfacial tensions are a minimum when solutions of proteins such as gelatin are at the isoelectric point because the molecules then have a relatively large intra and inter-molecular cohesion and so are likely to pack better at the surface. This tends to be accompanied by a maximum interfacial viscosity. Greater adsorption on to solids has been noted by a number of workers at or near the isoelectric point.

Many hydrocolloids are adsorbed at solid–water and oil–water interfaces whereby they can stabilize dispersions. The interface between benzene and acacia, sodium alginate or gelatin solutions takes several hours to achieve an equilibrium tension presumably due to multilayer formation. Highly branched stiff-coiled molecules such as acacia form rigid films whereas unbranched chains such as sodium alginate tend to produce liquid films. The properties of these films have an important bearing upon the stability of emulsions. No denaturation of acacia occurs upon adsorption although the first layer appears to be irreversibly adsorbed with the film becoming noticeably rigid within about 20 seconds. The thickness of an acacia multilayer varies with the type of oil. Strong films of potassium arabate about 100 nm thick appear to be formed with aliphatic hydrocarbons whereas weaker thin films form with benzene.

Various statistical mechanical models have been proposed for the conformation of adsorbed macromolecules (Hoeve, DiMarzio & Peyser 1965). It is suggested that the molecule may become anchored at the interface by only a fraction of the groups along its length, the rest of the molecule forming loops into the water. In such an event it is likely that the ends of the molecule are also anchored at equilibrium. The extent of looping into the solvent and the resulting thickness of the adsorbed layer can depend on the solvent. Polymer coils tend to extend in good solvents and would produce thick layers of low density. The density of multilayers probably decreases, that is solvation increases, with distance from the interface.

Biological Membranes
Multimolecular films form the boundary around all living cells and organelles such as mitochondria and chloroplasts. They are composed of lipids and protein molecules held together by hydrophobic and electrostatic interactions to form *lipoprotein*.

The lipids consist of non-ionic amphipaths such as cholesterol and amphoteric amphipaths called *compound lipids*. Compound lipids are long-chain fatty acid esters of alcohols containing other polar groups; for example, a glycerophospholipid is based upon glycerol which contains a phosphoric acid residue and a nitrogenous base this being choline in the case of lecithins (p. 45). Another phospholipid is based upon inositol while the sphingolipids are derived from the unsaturated amino alcohol, sphingosine. Hydrolysis of some compound lipids also yields sugars such as galactose from cerebrosides and sialic acids from gangliosides. Phospholipids predominate in animal cells.

Membranes differ considerably in their lipid and

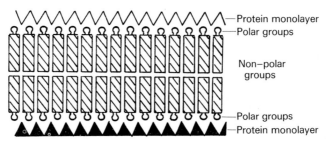

FIG. 4.49. The Danielli-Davson concept of a cell membrane as modified by Robertson (1967).

protein content according to their source and function. Thus myelin membranes contain a dry weight fraction of over 0.7 of lipid whereas rat liver mitochondria membranes contain less than 0.3, proteins making up most of the remaining weight. The proportion of cholesterol in the lipid also varies considerably, constituting about 0.4 of myelin lipid but only 0.06 to 0.14 of mitochondrial lipid and being absent from chloroplast lipid, while bacterial membranes contain little or no cholesterol.

Unlike films formed at an air–water or an oil–water interface, biological membranes are bounded on either side by an essentially aqueous environment. This requires that a multilayer be formed with the hydrophobic groups orientated towards each other inside the membrane, with the more polar groups or molecules exposed on the surface. If the lipids are extracted from erythrocyte membranes and spread as a monolayer upon water they occupy twice the area of the original erythrocyte surface demonstrating that the lipid portion of the membrane is two molecules thick.

Danielli and Davson proposed that cell membranes consist of a biomolecular lipid leaflet bounded on either side with a layer of protein molecules (Fig. 4.49). Electron-microscopic evidence for such a structure in membranes forming the myelin sheath of nerves has been obtained by Robertson (1967) where the bimolecular lipoprotein forms a repeating unit about 7.5 nm thick. However the protein does not appear to be held on the outside of the lipid bilayer merely by coulomb interaction but some portions of the protein molecules must penetrate to the interior where they are held by hydrophobic interactions.

Myelin lipids contain a high proportion of saturated and long-chain fatty acids which favours the formation of a condensed bilayer. Although containing a considerable proportion of polyunsaturated fatty acid esters, human erythrocyte lipids can also form a condensed bilayer within most of the membrane due to the condensing effect of the high proportion (0.42) of cholesterol. Such tightly organized membranes function as permeability barriers. On the other hand, membranes such as those of mitochondria and chloroplasts which are associated with the metabolic activity of the cell, contain lipids which are rich in polyunsaturated or branched-chain fatty acid esters and contain little or no cholesterol. These are unable to form condensed bilayers and are associated with a high proportion of protein. Other, more loosely organized, structures have been proposed for organelle membranes which involve two dimensional arrays of protein interposed by lipid (O'Brien 1967). One such model (Fig. 4.50) consists

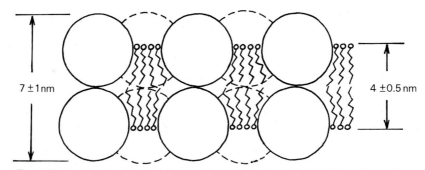

FIG. 4.50. Protein crystal model for membranes showing a double layer of protein molecules (large circles) with liquid bilayer regions filling the pores (after Vanderkoon & Green 1970, 1971).

of a bimolecular array of globular protein having predominantly non-polar amino acids towards the centre of the layer, the cavities between the protein molecules containing the lipid bilayer. It would also appear that some protein molecules extend right across a single membrane and may even extend across two membranes when these are stacked together.

Membranes are not only essential for maintaining the integrity of cells and organelles, but play other vital roles. They are selective to the passage of substances into and out of the cell, ranging from electrolytes to large molecules. 'Active transport' mechanisms are frequently encountered which can be biochemically modified. The difference in permeability of ions together with the Donnan equilibrium gives rise to a *resting* electrical potential which if affected by increasing the permeability of Na^+ during 'stimulation' gives rise to an *action* potential. Many enzymes are bound to membranes which therefore become the sites for certain metabolic pathways such as protein synthesis and respiration. Immunological reactions are also based at the membrane.

The structure and functions of biological membranes have been reviewed by Gross (1971). Their study has been facilitated by the use of artificial membranes. The formation and properties of the latter have been reviewed by Castleden (1969). Chapman (1968) and Sutton (1969) have also written short articles.

LIQUID–SOLID INTERFACE

INTERFACIAL ENERGY, CONTACT ANGLE AND ADHESION

A surface free energy γ_s exists at solid surfaces just as it does at liquid surfaces. If a liquid surface rests at equilibrium on a solid then the surface free energies are related by the equation:

$$\gamma_s = \gamma_{sl} + \gamma_l \cos \theta \qquad (4.35)$$

where γ_{sl} is the *interfacial free energy*, γ_l is the liquid surface energy (numerically the surface tension) and θ, measured within the liquid, is known as the *contact angle* (Fig. 4.51). The surface energies may be considered as surface tensions but surface tensions cannot be directly measured in the case of solids. Strictly, equation 4.35 should be corrected for the equilibrium film pressure π_e of adsorbed vapour on the solid-air surface when:

$$\gamma_s = \gamma_{sl} + \gamma_l \cos \theta + \pi_e$$

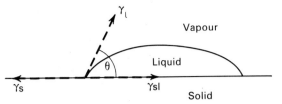

FIG. 4.51. Equilibrium contact angle for a liquid on a solid.

The work of adhesion W_{sl} between the solid and liquid is given by the Dupré equation (see p. 37):

$$W_{sl} = \gamma_s + \gamma_l - \gamma_{sl} \qquad (4.36)$$

and by combining equations 4.35 and 4.36 we have *Young's equation*:

$$W_{sl} = \gamma_l (1 + \cos \theta)$$

Strong adhesion between the solid and liquid produces low contact angles and if the adhesion is equal to, or greater than, the cohesion of the liquid ($2\gamma_l$) a zero contact angle is obtained. This is really only a statement of the obvious since if the molecules of liquid attract those of the solid more strongly than they do each other, then the liquid will spread and completely cover the solid surface.

Since van der Waals forces operate across all solid–liquid interfaces there can never be a contact angle of 180°, that is W_{sl} is never zero. Water on a smooth surface of a *pure* solid paraffin wax gives an angle of about 110° corresponding to $W_{sl} = 48$ mJ.m^{-2}, a figure close to the interfacial tension between paraffins and water (see Table 4.4). Polyethylene and polytetrafluoroethylene give contact angles with water of 94° and 108° respectively at room temperature. If a block of stearic acid is cut, the contact angle will be anywhere between 50° and 105° according to the direction of the cut with respect to the bimolecular layered structure of the crystal.

If the surface is composed of small patches of two different kinds of surface, then the effective contact angle $\bar{\theta}$ is given by the relationship

$$\bar{\theta} = f_1 \cos \theta_1 + (1 - f_1) \cos \theta_2 \qquad (4.37)$$

where f_1 is the fraction of surface having a contact angle of θ_1.

Surface roughness influences the contact angle. If θ on a smooth surface exceeds 90°, roughness increases the contact angle, whereas if θ is less than 90°, a decrease is found. Thus roughened paraffin wax with water can exhibit an apparent contact angle in excess of 130° whilst mica is roughened for use as a Wilhelmy plate to ensure an effective zero angle of contact (see p. 44).

Contact angles are generally affected by motion of the liquid edge on the solid. When the liquid advances over a dry solid surface, the advancing contact angle increases while the receding angle decreases (Fig. 4.52). The reason is that the receding edge is in contact with a more lyophilic surface due either to liquid penetration into the surface or to removal of lyophobic contaminants.

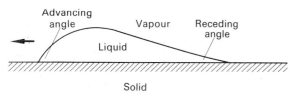

FIG. 4.52. Dynamic contact angles.

ADSORPTION ON TO SOLIDS

Many compounds are adsorbed on to solids from solution. Clay minerals such as kaolin, bentonite and attapulgite and antacid powders such as aluminium or magnesium hydroxides or silicates have been shown to adsorb such drugs as alkaloids, phenothiazine drivatives and the B vitamins. In such cases the rate and even extent of adsorption of drugs from the gastrointestinal tract may be considerably reduced.

Adsorption is often '*physical*' due to van der Waals forces of interaction between the adsorbate and the substrate in which case it is largely reversible by changes in pH or electrolyte concentration, but it may be '*chemical*' which involves a chemical reaction at the substrate surface when desorption may be far less easily accomplished. The extent of adsorption is influenced by the solvent since this too may be adsorbed, the polar/non-polar natures of the solute, solvent and substrate all being involved. The nature of composite and individual isotherms has been discussed by Gregg (1961) and Kipling (1964) while Giles et al. (1960) have classified composite isotherms relating their shape to orientation of the adsorbate and penetration of the adsorbed layer by solvent molecules.

Rowland et al. (1965) have discussed the adsorption of macromolecules at the liquid–solid interface. Natural and synthetic hydrocolloids such as acacia and the cellulose derivatives and amphipaths such as the saponin glycosides of quillaia are adsorbed on to the surface of suspended particles which are not normally wetted by water.

This produces an increase in the hydrophilic character of the solid surface thereby promoting wetting.

PROMOTION OF WETTING

If a non-zero angle of contact exists between a solid and a liquid, a suspension of powdered solid in the liquid will contain a considerable proportion of the powder floating at the surface attached to air bubbles thereby producing an unsightly scum or froth. Homogeneity of the suspension may be difficult or impossible to achieve and shaking may make matters worse. Such a state of affairs may be observed if aspirin or precipitated sulphur is dispersed in water. Wetting of these two solids is accomplished using acacia and the saponins in quillaia extract respectively. There are many wetting agents available, initial selection being determined by the use of the suspension. Gums, cellulose derivatives and non-ionic amphipaths such as the polysorbates are suitable for internal use. For external applications, ionic amphipaths can be used but some gums are precluded on account of their sticky nature. The addition of a wetting agent is essential for the adequate dispersion in water of a number of powders apart from those already quoted, cortisone and the sulphonamides being examples. The foaming and resuspension properties will influence the final choice of wetting agent. A wetting and deflocculating action may frequently go hand in hand since the wetting agent increases the attraction for the liquid dispersion medium and, if ionic, confers repulsive charges on the solid particles.

Young's equation (p. 79) shows that increasing the work of adhesion between the solid and the liquid decreases the contact angle. A similar reduction in contact angle can be achieved without adsorption on the solid if an amphipath is merely adsorbed at the liquid-air surface since the surface tension is thereby reduced. Frequently poor wettability of a powder arises from the porous nature of the particle surface which entraps air: penetration of the pores by the liquid is then required. If r is the effective mean pore radius, then the capillary pressure ΔP is given by the Young-Laplace equation (p. 35) as:

$$\Delta P = \frac{2\gamma_l \cos \theta}{r}$$

This shows that for good pore penetration γ_l should be as large as possible. The better wetting agents therefore act mainly by a specific adsorption on to the solid.

Wetting agents are necessary for fungicide and insecticide sprays since these have to spread over a waxy cuticle or penetrate hairy surfaces of leaves and insects (see below). Some of the best compounds have a high CMC because of their irregular molecular shape and so high monomer concentrations are obtainable giving their solutions exceptionally low surface tensions. One of the better known of these wetting agents is sodium dioctyl-sulphosuccinate. A good wetting action is also necessary for detergent solutions since intimate contact with the cleaned surface is a prerequisite for the removal of dirt.

DETERGENCY

This is the removal of solid particles and greasy films from solid surfaces by means of solutions containing amphipaths. Adsorption of amphipath occurs at both the solid–liquid and oil–liquid interface thereby reducing γ_{sw} and γ_{ow}. Equation 4.38, analogous to equation 4.35, shows that θ must decrease as a result:

$$\gamma_{so} = \gamma_{sw} + \gamma_{ow} \cos \theta \qquad (4.38)$$

thereby causing a greasy dirt to 'roll-up' and to become more readily detached from the solid surface by gentle agitation (Fig. 4.53). These globules then form an emulsion or are solubilized within the micelles. Solubilization probably occurs to a considerable extent with polar dirt. Lawrence (1961) showed that soap is concentrated at the surface of amphiphilic dirt and slowly penetrates

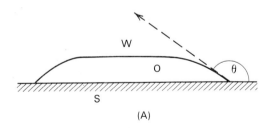

W

O

θ

S

(A)

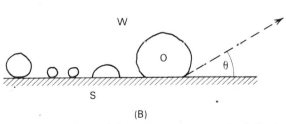

W

O

θ

S

(B)

FIG. 4.53. Illustration of the 'rolling-up' process; A, oil film in the absence of soap; B, globules produced in the presence of soap.

it, forming a liquid crystalline phase. This phase becomes sufficiently mobile to break away upon agitation, when it becomes diluted to form an L1 isotropic phase with or without globules of L2 phase dispersed in it (see p. 64).

Emulsification or solubilization of liquid dirt, or adequate wetting and deflocculation of solid particles is necessary in order to prevent the dirt from becoming redeposited. Emulsification is assisted by a scouring action and by removal of the dirt into the foam while further adhesion is prevented by the adsorption of amphipath on to the cleansed surface. Rinsing involves dilution with water and may enable some deposition of L2 phase. In such cases a preliminary rinse in dilute detergent solution should be undertaken.

Commercial detergent formulations contain a number of additives or 'builders'. A high proportion of a sequestering (chelating) agent such as pyrophosphate is incorporated. This removes polyvalent ions such as calcium present in hard water which might otherwise cause the detergent-dirt mixture to produce an insoluble scum and become redeposited. Much of the solid dirt is also held on to the substrate by adsorbed polyvalent ions. The inclusion of sodium carboxymethylcellulose in the detergent also reduces the risk of redeposition of dirt by forming an hydrated adsorbed layer over the substrate. Liquid detergents also include a hydrotrope (p. 64) in order to increase the surfactant solubility. Since rapid solubilization of fatty dirt requires this to melt, simple surfactant solutions may have an efficient detergent action only at high temperatures. The inclusion of an organic solvent such as xylene, in a solubilized form, enables the detergent to function at lower temperatures.

Dry cleaning may involve the use of detergent solutions containing predominantly an organic solvent and water solubilized within inverted micelles. The water-soluble dirt is solubilized in this case.

WATER-REPELLENCY

Cationic amphipaths are not good wetting agents for many purposes. A dilute solution of cetrimide, for example, can render a clean glass surface hydrophobic by exchange of the cations so that the hydrocarbon chains of the adsorbed monolayer extend outward. A high contact angle can also be obtained by treating such surfaces as glass or steel with a silicone or a methylchlorosilane. Even the single layer of methyl groups in a monolayer of these compounds greatly decreases the adhesion of the surface to water.

Water repellency may be desirable for a number

of reasons. For example, rendering the surface of steam condensers hydrophobic prevents the formation of a continuous film of condensed water which would impede the removal of heat by conduction. A water-repellent surface inside glass vials may also be desirable so that solutions or suspensions can be drained completely from them. Dimethicones are suitable for this purpose.

In mineral flotation the wanted ore is rendered hydrophobic while impurities remain wetted. Small amounts of 'collectors' such as zanthates are added to the slurry. These coat the surface of the ore particles with the alkyl groups on the exterior (provided only a monolayer is adsorbed) so that the air bubbles become attached and float the ore. The ζ-potential (p. 91) of the ore particle should be reduced to zero in order that the work of adhesion W_{sl} should be as low as possible since for hydrophobicity $W_{sl} < 2\gamma_l$.

Woven fabrics may be rendered hydrophobic by coating the fibres with silicone polymers or with cationic amphipaths. The regular small mesh structure of fabrics leads to especially large effective contact angles. If f_1 is the solid fraction of the surface, equation 4.37 reduces to:

$$\cos \bar{\theta} = f_1 \cos \theta - (1 - f_1)$$

since $\theta_2 = 180°$. Thus even if $\theta_1 < 90°$, the average angle $\bar{\theta}$ can be considerably greater than 90°. This is essential for tents and raincoats where the receding contact angle must be greater than 90° for raindrops to 'pearl' off the fabric.

To prevent water penetration through a porous fabric however, θ_1 must exceed 90° (Fig. 4.54). The curvature of the meniscus between the fibres produces a negative capillary pressure which can become very large if the gaps between the fibres are very small. Some microporous plastics are also water-repellent and water-proof wound dressings made from these are required to withstand a hydrostatic head of 50 cm. Such dressings prevent liquid water from penetrating to the wound while allowing the free passage of air and water vapour.

Numerous examples of water-repellency assisted by a broken surface are to be found in nature. The regular structure of the feathers of aquatic birds is one such example where it is essential that the barbules are kept hydrophobic by the secretion from a special oil gland. Some aquatic insects are covered with fine hydrophobic hairs which maintain a thin but permanent film of air around the body. Gaseous exchange occurs across this air film rendering it unnecessary for the insect to replenish its air supply. Many plants also possess highly water-repellent surfaces, due either to a rough waxy cuticle or to a covering of hydrophobic trichomes.

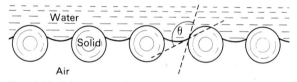

FIG. 4.54. A contact angle greater than 90° makes a fabric water-repellent.

REFERENCES

ABU-HAMDIYYAH, M. (1965) *J. phys. Chem., Ithaca,* **69**, 2720.

ADAM, N. K. (1930) *The Physics and Chemistry of Surfaces,* London: Oxford University Press.

ADAMSON, A. W. (1967) *Physical Chemistry of Surfaces,* 2nd ed., New York: Interscience.

ALEXANDER, A. E. & JOHNSON, P. (1950) *Colloid Science,* London: Oxford University Press.

BALMBRA, R. R., CLUNIE, J. S., CORKILL, J. M. & GOODMAN, J. F. (1962) *Trans. Faraday Soc.* **58**, 1661.

BLANDAMER, M. J. (1970) *Q. Rev. chem. Soc.* **24**, 169.

BURT, B. W. (1965) *J. Soc. cosmet. Chem. Br. Edn.* **16**, 465.

CAMPBELL, J. A., CHRISTIAN, J. E. & EATON, J. R. (1955) *J. Am. pharm. Ass. sci. Edn.* **44**, 501.

CASTLEDEN, J. A. (1969) *J. pharm. Sci.* **58**, 149.

CHAPMAN, D. (1965) *Sci. J., Lond.* **1(8)**, 32.

CHAPMAN, D. (1968) *Sci. J., Lond.* **4(3)**, 55.

CLAYFIELD, E. J. & MATTHEWS, J. B. (1957) *Proc. 2nd Intern. Congr. Surface Activity,* **1**, 172–187, (Ed. Schulman, J. W.) London: Butterworths.

DAVIES, C. M. & LITOVITZ, T. A. (1965) *J. chem. Phys.* **42**, 2563.

DAVIES, J. T. & RIDEAL, E. K. (1961) *Interfacial Phenomena,* New York: Academic Press.

DOUGLAS, H. W. (1950) *J. Sci. Instrum.* **27**, 67.

ELWORTHY. P. H., FLORENCE, A. T. & MACFARLANE, C. B. (1968) *Solubilisation by Surface-Active Agents*, London: Chapman & Hall.

EMERSON, M. F. & HOLTZER, A. (1967) *J. phys. Chem., Ithaca*, **71**, 3320.

ERLANDER, S. R. (1969) *Sci. J., Lond.* **5A(5)**, 60.

EVANS, W. P. & DUNBAR, S. F. (1965) *Surface Activity and the Microbial Cell*, S. C. I. Monograph, **19**, 169.

FERGUSON, A. (1923) *Trans. Faraday Soc.* **19**, 407.

FORDHAM, S. (1948) *Proc. R. Soc.* **A194**, 1.

FOWKES, F. M. (1964) *Ind. Engng Chem. int. Edn.* **56 (12)**, 40.

FOX, H. W. & CHRISMAN, C. H. (1952) *J. phys. Chem., Ithaca*, **56**, 284.

FRANK, H. S. & EVANS, M. W. (1945) *J. chem. Phys.* **13**, 507.

GILES, C. H., MACEWAN, T. H., NAKHWA, S. N. & SMITH, D. (1960) *J. chem. Soc.* 3973.

GREGG, S. J. (1961) *The Surface Chemistry of Solids*, 2nd edn, London: Chapman & Hall.

GROSS, W. (1971) *Angew. Chem. int. Edn.* **10**, 388.

HARKINS, W. D. & BROWN, F. E. (1919) *J. Am. chem. Soc.* **41**, 499.

HARKINS, W. D. & JORDAN, H. F. (1930) *J. Am. chem. Soc.* **52**, 1751.

HOEVE, C. A. J., DIMARZIO, E. A. & PEYSER, P. (1965) *J. chem. Phys.* **42**, 2558.

JORDAN, D. O. & LANE, J. E. (1964) *Aust. J. Chem.* **17**, 7.

KIPLING, J. J. (1964) *Chemy Ind.* 1007.

LAWRENCE, A. S. C. (1961) *Chemy Ind.* 1764.

MANDELL, L. & EKWALL, P. (1967a) Proc. 4th Intern. Congr. Surface Active Substances (Brussels, 1964), pp. 659–671, (Ed. Overbeek, J. Th. G.) New York: Gordon & Breach.

MANDELL, L., FONTELL, K. & EKWALL, P. (1967b) Advances in Chemistry, American Chemical Society Series No. 63, pp. 89–124, Washington D.C.

MCBAIN, J. W., BROCK, G. C., VOLD, R. D. & VOLD, M. J. (1938) *J. Am. chem. Soc.* **60**, 1870.

MOILLIET, J. L., COLLIE, B. & BLACK, W. (1961) *Surface Activity*, 2nd ed., London: Spon.

MULLEY, B. A. (1964) *Advances in Pharmaceutical Sciences*, **1**, 86–194. edit. Bean, H. S., Beckett, A. H. & Carless, J. E., London: Academic Press.

NAKAGAWA, T. & TORI, K. (1960) *Kolloid-Zeitschrift*, **168**, 132.

O'BRIEN, J. S. (1967) *J. theor. Biol.* **15**, 307.

OSIPOW, L. I. (1962) *Surface Chemistry*, New York: Reinhold.

POLAND, D. C. & SCHERAGA, H. A. (1965) *J. phys. Chem., Ithaca*, **69**, 2431.

PORTER, A. W. (1933) *Phil. Mag.*, **15**, 163.

PRESTON, J. (1948) *J. Phys. Coll. Chem.* **52**, 85.

ROBERTSON, J. D. (1967) *Protoplasma* **63**, 218.

ROE, R-J., BACHETTA, V. L. & WONG, P. M. G. (1967) *J. phys. Chem., Ithaca*, **71**, 4190.

ROSEVEAR, F. B. (1968) *J. Soc. cosmet. Chem.* **19**, 581.

ROWLAND, F., BULAS, R., ROTHSTEIN, E. & EIRICH, F. R. (1965) *Ind. Engng Chem. int. Edn.* **57(9)**, 46.

SCHICK, M. J. (1963) *J. phys. Chem., Ithaca*, **67**, 1796.

SHINODA, K. (1954) *J. phys. Chem., Ithaca*, **58**, 1136.

SHOTTON, E. (1955) *J. Pharm. Pharmac.* **7**, 990.

SHOTTON, E. & KALYAN, K. (1960) *J. Pharm. Pharmac.* **12**, 116.

STAUFFER, C. E. (1965) *J. phys. Chem., Ithaca*, **69**, 1933.

SUGDEN, S. (1921) *J. chem. Soc.* **119**, 1483.

SUGDEN, S. (1922) *J. chem. Soc.* **121**, 858.

SUGDEN, S. (1924a) *J. chem. Soc.* **125**, 27.

SUGDEN, S. (1924b) *J. chem. Soc.* **125**, 32.

SUTTON, A. (1969) *New Scient.* **42**, 125.

SWARBRICK, J. (1965) *J. pharm. Sci.* **54**, 1229.

TARTAR, H. V. & WRIGHT, K. A. (1939) *J. Am. chem. Soc.* **61**, 539.

TSCHOEGL, N. W. (1958) *J. Colloid Sci.* **13**, 500.

VANDERKOOI, G. & GREEN, D. E. (1970) *Proc. Nat. Acad. Sci. U.S.* **66**, 615.

VANDERKOOI, G. & GREEN, D. (1971) *New Scient.* **50**, 22.

WARD, A. F. H. & TORDAI, L. (1946a) *Nature, Lond.* **158**, 416.

WARD, A. F. H. & TORDAI, L. (1946b) *Trans. Faraday Soc.* **42**, 413.

WINKEL, D. (1965) *J. phys. Chem., Ithaca* **69**, 348.

ZUIDEMA, H. H. & WATERS, G. W. (1941) *Ind. Engng Chem. analyt. Edn* **13**, 312.

5

Colloidal Systems

Pharmaceutical materials coming under the heading of 'colloids', include a wide range of substances such as suspensions of solids in liquids, emulsified liquids, clays, gels and solutions of soaps and proteins. The feature that is common to such a variety of systems is the fine state of subdivision of the dispersed phase. Early investigations were concerned with preparations such as colloidal suspensions of sulphur and gold and their characteristic properties were correctly thought to be due to the subdivision of the particles which were not in true solution. It is now recognized however, that colloidality is a state of subdivision attainable with almost any material under suitable conditions, e.g. soaps form a colloidal solution in water due to aggregation of soap molecules, but form a non-colloidal solution in alcohol. Some colloidal systems consist of true solutions of very large molecules, e.g. proteins, or colloidal aggregates of small molecules.

It is difficult to give a precise definition of the colloidal state but the following definition is frequently quoted: 'A colloidal system is a two phase system, one phase dispersed as minute particles (*disperse phase*) throughout the other phase (*continuous phase or dispersion medium*).' This, however, ignores such systems as soap films which are of colloidal dimensions as regards film thickness. If the term 'minute particles' is taken to include particles which have at least one dimension lying in the range between 1 nm and 1 μm, the definition can be taken to include fibres and films as well as three dimensional solid and liquid particles. Emulsions and suspensions used in

pharmacy are somewhat coarser than 1 μm but are generally included because their behaviour is similar in many ways to that of true colloids (Hiestand 1964). When the dispersion medium is a liquid the colloidal systems are called *sols*.

The term 'colloid' (from Greek *kolla*, glue) appears to have been applied first by Graham (1851 to 1861) to solutions of proteins such as albumin or gelatin and to naturally occurring gums. He found that crystalline substances could be separated from 'colloids' by placing the mixture inside a bag made of a thin membrane of animal gut and immersing it in water, since the colloids remained inside while simple salts diffused out through the fine pores in the membrane.

The extensive interface between two phases is a predominant feature of colloidal dispersions and it exerts a considerable influence on the physical and chemical properties of the material. In the interior of a solid, the ions, atoms or molecules are attracted equally to their neighbours by electrostatic, covalent bonds or van der Waals forces, respectively, but at the surface unsaturated forces are capable of interacting with forces emanating from molecules of other substances. Thus, finely divided solids can adsorb gas molecules on their surfaces and if the ratio of surface area to weight of solid is large, they will be effective adsorbants. It follows also that colloidal particles close to each other will be mutually attracted but there must be some mechanism responsible for stabilizing the particles, otherwise the colloidal suspension could only exist for a relatively short time before the particles agglomerated.

Before discussing the mechanism of stabilization of colloidal sols, it is convenient to classify colloidal systems into *lyophobic* or *lyophilic* colloids. By definition lyophobic colloids are mere suspensions and not solutions. There is little affinity between the solvent and particle and the system is thermodynamically unstable.

Lyophilic colloids comprise true solutions either of very large molecules or of aggregates (micelles) of smaller molecules that achieve dimensions in the colloidal range. There is strong attraction between the solvent and particle and the solutions are thermodynamically stable. Lyophilic sols differ from solutions of smaller molecules only in the size of the molecules, and many molecules of biological interest fall in this category, e.g. proteins, nucleic acids, starches as well as synthetic polymers. Although it is convenient to designate colloids as lyophilic or lyophobic, it is not possible to draw a sharp line of demarcation between these two groups. For instance, colloidal dispersions of a number of metallic hydroxides, e.g. aluminium hydroxide, possess intermediate properties.

LYOPHOBIC COLLOIDS

Lyophobic colloids can be classified according to the nature of the disperse phase and dispersion medium (Table 5.1).

TABLE 5.1

Dispersed phase	Dispersion medium	Class
Solid	Liquid	Sol
Solid	Gas	Aerosol (smoke)
Liquid	Liquid	Emulsion
Liquid	Gas	Aerosol (fog)
Gas	Liquid	Foam
Gas	Solid	Solid foam (e.g. pumice)

Particles in colloidal solution are subject to the same kind of random thermal motion as are individual molecules, except that their mean displacement per unit time is smaller because of their larger size. The random movement, called Brownian movement, is observed for particles up to about $2 \mu m$, at which level the particles can be observed under an optical microscope. To observe particles small in comparison to the wavelength of light, e.g. $<0.1 \mu m$, the ultramicroscope has been used. The suspension is illuminated by a narrow intense beam of light at right angles to the angle of viewing, when the particles appear as bright dots against a dark background in the same way that dust particles can be seen when a beam of sunlight enters a darkened room.

The beam of light appears as a whitish path as it passes through the suspension. This phenomenon was studied by Tyndall, and bears his name, the Tyndall effect.

The main differences between lyophobic and lyophilic sols are summarized in Table 5.2.

TABLE 5.2

	Lyophobic	Lyophilic
Concentration	Usually very dilute (less than 1 per cent of the disperse phase)	High concentrations are possible
Behaviour towards eloctrolytes	Readily precipitated	Not easily precipitated. High concentration causes 'salting out'
Gel formation	Do not form typical gel, coagulum resulting from precipitation is not easily redispersed	Coagulation gives a gel which is readily redispersed
Behaviour towards lyophobic sols	Sols of opposite charge precipitate each other	Protect lyphobic sols from precipitation
Optical properties	Well defined Tyndall effect	Weak Tyndall effect

PREPARATION OF LYOPHOBIC SOLS

Dispersion methods. Grinding of coarse suspensions in mills known as colloid mills can reduce particles in a liquid phase to $1 \mu m$ and less. Some colloid mills consist of a high speed rotating smooth disc, separated from a stationary disc by about $25 \mu m$ between the two surfaces. Great stresses are developed in the fluid film between the surfaces and these disrupt solid particles present in the gap. Rotor dimensions are such that speeds of between 1500 and 6500 m/min are obtained at the working surfaces. Owing to the unstable nature of the sol, small amounts of lyophilic colloid or other stabilizing agents must be added to prevent agglomeration of the colloidal particles.

Condensation methods. Sols can be prepared from an initially molecular dispersion by controlled growth to colloidal size. The experimental conditions must be carefully controlled to prevent excessive growth and hence precipitation of the particles. During the preparation of sols, van Weimarn found experimentally that small particles are formed by precipitation from either very concentrated or very dilute solutions, while coarse particles formed at intermediate concentrations. In concentrated solution many nuclei are formed simultaneously and growth of these by deposition of solute present above the saturation point is rapid due to close proximity of solute molecules to the nuclei. The result is small colloidal particles of nearly uniform size. In less concentrated solution, the rate of formation of nuclei will be less but solute will still diffuse quite rapidly to the smaller number of nuclei and will produce a coarser sol. In very dilute solutions, the growth process will be slower, although new nuclei will still be forming from the supersaturated solution, and the resulting particles, again colloidal, will be less uniform in size.

Besides these precipitation methods for producing sols, other chemical processes can be used. For example, colloidal ferric hydroxide can be formed by boiling a solution of ferric chloride and allowing the escape of the HCl produced by the hydrolysis:

$$2FeCl_3 \rightleftharpoons 2Fe(OH)_3 + 6HCl$$

Colloidal sulphur sols can be produced by the decomposition of dilute solution of sodium thiosulphate in the presence of acids.

In the preparation of colloidal silicic acid, a solution of sodium silicate is added to excess hydrochloric acid and the sodium chloride removed by dialysis:

$$Na_2SiO_3 + 2HCl \rightarrow H_2SiO_3 + 2NaCl$$

Colloidal sols of the noble metals can be obtained by striking an arc between electrodes of the noble metal, immersed in the dispersion phase. The metal vapour, produced by passing a large current, condenses in the liquid phase, to which may be added traces of electrolyte in order to stabilize the colloidal particle.

Colloidal solution of gold, e.g. Gold (^{198}Au) Injection BP is prepared by reducing a salt of gold-198 with a reducing agent such as dextrose in alkaline solution in the presence of gelatin.

Where a chemical or electrical method may not be applicable, sols may also be prepared by adding a solution of the substance to a second liquid which is a poor solvent for the original solute, e.g. sulphur in ethyl alcohol added to water.

In all these cases, the colloidal particles formed may tend to clump together or flocculate unless additional substances are added to stabilize the sols. The addition may be trace electrolytes or protective colloids. This is discussed later.

PURIFICATION BY DIALYSIS

Low molecular weight impurities, e.g. electrolytes, can be separated from colloidal particles by *dialysis*. The process is most simply carried out by enclosing the solution in a Cellophane sac which is immersed in a large vessel of water. Cellophane tubing, tied off at each end is usually used. The pores in cellophane membranes are sufficiently large for low molecular weight solutes to pass through whilst retaining the larger colloidal particles. Other membranes that are suitable for aqueous sols include parchment, collodian and cellulose acetate. If electrolyte is present in the colloidal sol it diffuses through the pores of the membrane and, by repeatedly changing the water, diffusion will continue until the dialysate remaining is substantially free from electrolyte.

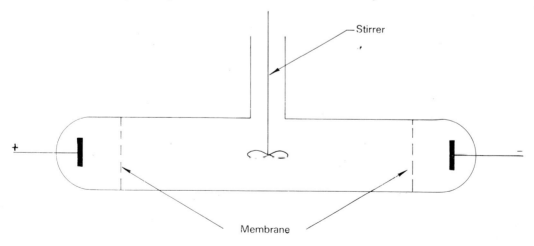

FIG. 5.1. Electrodialysis cell.

This process is relatively slow and the dialysis of electrolytes can be greatly facilitated by the application of a direct current. For this purpose an apparatus illustrated in Fig. 5.1 is used. This technique known as *electrodialysis* is thus a combination of dialysis and electrolysis. The colloid to be purified is introduced into the middle section which is separated from the right and left sections by dialysis membranes. Provision is usually made for circulation of water on both sides of the colloid, and the removal of the electrolyte is achieved by direct current applied by means of electrodes.

Recently electrodialysis has come into prominence in connection with the desalination of water. The success of this operation is due to the development of membranes which will pass only negatively-charged or only positively-charged ions. This enables multi-compartment dialysis cells to be used where the cationic membranes are only permeable to cations and the anionic membrane only permeable to anions. The migration of anions and cations to the relative cell compartment enables deionized water to be collected in the alternate compartments as shown in Fig. 5.2.

A modification of the electrodialysis technique is *electrodecantation* developed by Pauli. The colloid is not stirred and because of its charge will be pulled towards one of the membranes and hence the density near the membrane is increased and the dense solution sinks to the bottom. This provides a method of preparing concentrated colloids as the dense lower layer can be removed and more fresh solution supplied to the cell.

Electrophoresis convection is an extension of this method and is used to fractionate mixtures containing colloids of different mobilities. The component with the highest mobility will reach the membrane first, sink and become concentrated in the bottom of the cell while the less mobile will be enriched in the top of the cell. Suitably designed cells have been used to separate proteins into pure fractions, e.g. γ-globulin.

Dialytic separations may also be effected by *ultrafiltration* (Ferry 1936). This process differs from dialysis only in that the passage of the electrolyte solution through the membrane is accelerated by applying pressure. The membrane needs to be supported on a sintered glass plate to prevent rupture as considerably high positive pressures are required to achieve reasonable rates of filtration. The pore size of the membranes can be increased to some extent by soaking them in solvents that

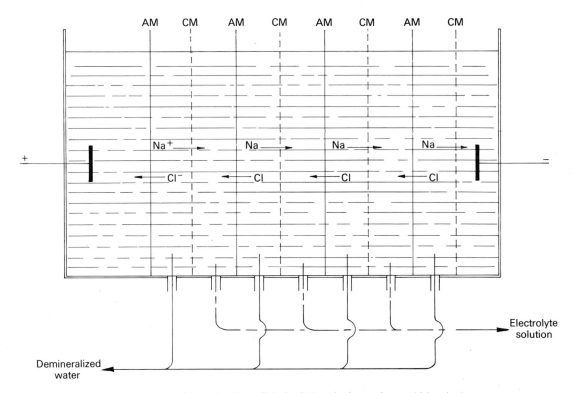

FIG. 5.2. Demineralization of water by electrodialysis; CM, cationic membrane; AM, anionic membrane.

cause swelling, e.g. Cellophane swells in zinc chloride solutions, collodion membranes swell in alcohol. Although there is adequate information in the literature on methods of preparing collodion (nitrocellulose) membranes by controlled evaporation of alcohol–ether solutions, it is difficult to obtain reproducible pore sizes. In practice it is more usual to use commercially available material such as Cellophane which is available in tube or sheet form.

An example of the use of dialysis in pharmacy is the purification of enzymes such as pepsin. The form of pepsin known as 'precipitated pepsin' is prepared by scraping off the mucous membrane of the lining of the stomach of the pig and steeping in diluted hydrochloric acid for some time. The extracted pepsin is then precipitated by adding a saturated solution of sodium chloride, separated by filtration, redissolved in water and dialysed. The sodium chloride and hydrochloric acid pass through the membrane; the pepsin remains in colloidal solution as the dialysate, from which it may be later precipitated by the addition of alcohol.

Fractionation of enzymes by fractional precipitation from solution may be effected by 'salting out' with ammonium sulphate; dialysis or electrodialysis is then used to remove the contaminating electrolyte. Prolonged electrodialysis can sometimes cause inactivation owing to removal of a coenzyme. For instance, malt amylase becomes inactivated in this way and subsequent addition of salts to the deionized material is necessary to restore its activity.

The success of the artificial kidney machine depends on the reduction of blood urea by passage of the patients blood through coils of Cellophane tubing immersed in suitable rinsing fluid. The molecular composition is designed to create a diffusion gradient from blood to rinsing fluid of substances which are present in excess in the blood (e.g. urea) and from the rinsing fluid to blood of substances which are deficient in the body (e.g. bicarbonate), while the concentration of those diffusible substances which are present in normal amounts in the blood is kept unaltered by having them present in the same concentration as in the rinsing fluid. The length of the tubing is about 60 m giving a dialysing surface area of just over 3 m². Other kidney dialysis units utilize sheets of dialysing membranes in place of coils.

Cellophane is an ideal semi-permeable membrane for haemodialysis as its pore size is such that electrolytes, urea and glucose can all pass freely across it, while the larger molecules such as the plasma proteins, lipid fractions and blood cells, cannot pass. The Cellophane tubing does not allow bacteria to pass across it, so that only the inside surface need be sterilized. The method of operation is discussed by Anderson (1964) and shown schematically in Fig. 5.3.

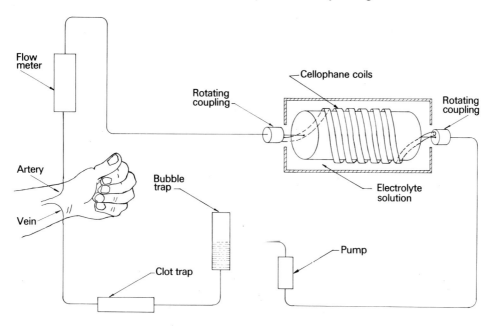

FIG. 5.3..Circuit diagram of artificial kidney (Anderson 1964). The cellophane coils are supported on a drum rotating in the electrolyte solution.

STABILITY OF LYOPHOBIC COLLOIDS

All particles are attracted to one another by van der Waals forces. It is these forces that are primarily responsible for the liquefaction of gases, departure of gases from ideal behaviour, and adsorption of gases on to solids. The origin of the force is electrical and it can be explained easily in qualitative terms. The motion of electrons in their orbitals within the atom gives rise to a fluctuating electromagnetic field which exerts an influence upon the electrons in neighbouring matter, causing a net shift of the centre of positive (nuclear) and negative charges in such a direction that there is attraction between the two separate particles. This force falls off very rapidly with distance and is thus negligible except when the particles are quite close together (e.g. <100 nm). In the absence of repulsive forces between the particles in a colloidal sol they would rapidly aggregate together. The fact that stable lyophobic colloidal sols can be prepared is due to the electrical charges on the particle opposing the van der Waals attraction, and from a quantitative assessment of these opposing forces theories have been proposed notably by Verwey and Overbeek (1948) in Holland and Derjaquin in Russia to explain and predict the stability of lyophobic colloids.

The electrical charge on particles dispersed in a liquid may arise from dissociation of substances

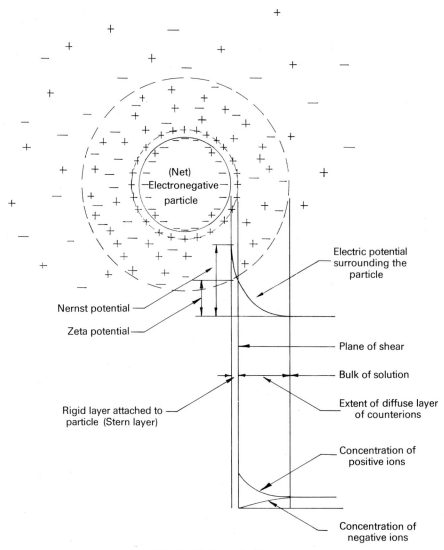

FIG. 5.4. Electrical double layer.

which are an integral part of the crystal lattice of the particle, e.g. sodium ion of Na bentonite clay or Ba^{2+} and SO_4^- ions of barium sulphate. Frequently the change arises from the adsorption of some specific ion with the surface. For example, $Fe(OH)_3$ sols become charged in the presence of excess Fe^{3+} which is adsorbed on the surface.

This fixed layer of charges is called the Stern layer. Ions of opposite charge to those in the Stern layer cluster around the particle, but random thermal motion prevents the existence of a rigid shell of opposite charges. The diagrammatic representation of this electrical double-layer is shown in Fig. 5.4.

The zeta potential, ζ, refers to the electrostatic charge on the particles which causes them to move in an electric field towards a pole of opposite charge. The zeta potential is measured at the surface of shear of the particle and this does not necessarily correspond with the Stern layer. In the absence of hydration the surface potential of the particles should be identical with the zeta potential. Zeta potential can be defined as the work necessary to bring unit charge from infinity to the surface of shear of the particle. The calculation of the decay of electrical potential with distance from the particle is very complex, but it can be solved fairly readily assuming that colloidal particles have an infinite uniform flat surface compared to the reference point where the potential is required. If the surface potential is small it falls to $1/e$ of its initial value (e is the base of natural logs 2.718) in a distance δ given by:

$$\delta^2 = DkT/8\pi^2 ne^2 z^2$$

In water at 25° $\delta^2 \cong 9 \times 10^{-16}/z^2 M$

M = molar concentration of counter ions,
z = valency of counter ions,
k = Boltzmann constant,
D = dielectric constant,
n = number of counter ions per cm^3 of solution,
e = electronic charge.

δ is often called the thickness of the double-layer and is about 1 nm in 0.1 M monovalent electrolyte.

The basic concept underlying the stability of lyophobic colloids is the mutual repulsion due to interacting double layers and the van der Waals force of attraction. For infinitely large flat plates not too close together, the attractive energy V_A between the particles per cm^2, is given by:

$$V_A = A/48\pi d^2$$

where A = van der Waals' constant,
d = distance/2 between the surfaces.

The repulsive energy V_R, arising from the interaction of the double layers was calculated by Verwey and Overbeek (1948) by considering the free energy of the system of the two double layers as a function of their distance of separation. From this knowledge of repulsive and attractive forces, it is possible to construct diagrams showing the interaction energy between a pair of colloidal particles as a function of the separation of their surfaces. In Fig. 5.5 the vertical axis represents the interaction energy, the horizontal axis the distance between two particles. From the summation of the attractive and repulsive forces, a net interaction curve is obtained.

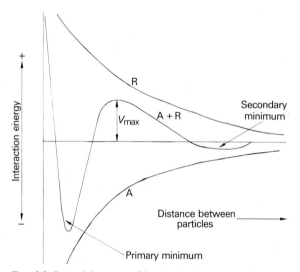

Fig. 5.5. Potential energy of interaction between particles. R, repulsion energy of interaction; A, attractive energy of interaction.

When the particles are far apart, the interaction energy approaches zero, but becomes infinitely large when the particles touch, due to the mutual repulsion of the electrons in the outermost atoms of the particles. For particles to come together at the primary minimum they must surmount the energy barrier of magnitude V_{max}. Particles in the primary minimum will be then irreversibly agglomerated.

As the repulsive forces fall off more rapidly with distance than do the attractive forces, a secondary minimum is produced when the particle surfaces are about 100 nm apart. This weak attraction causes slight flocculation of colloidal particles but the floccules can be redispersed on shaking. Experimental evidence indicates that flocculation in the secondary minimum is restricted to the larger colloidal sizes and is probably unimportant for particles below say 0.1 μm. The rate of coagulation of particles in a sol is obviously a function of the V_{max}. Provided that V_{max} exceeds 20–25 kT, where k is the Boltzmann constant and T the absolute temperature, the particles are unable to gain sufficient energy to surmount the energy barrier and so they remain in a deflocculated condition. Three types of potential energy curve are shown in Fig. 5.6.

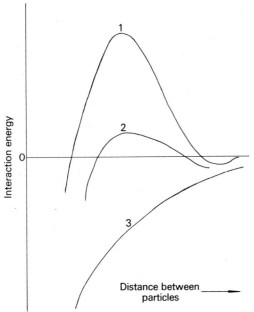

FIG. 5.6. Potential energy curve. 1, stable sol; 2, sol of intermediate stability; 3, spontaneous agglomeration.

Curve 1 has $V_{max} > 25\ kT$ and represents a stable sol. Curve 2 has maximum of only low kT and the particle will agglomerate fairly rapidly due to Brownian movement producing collisions of sufficient energy. Curve 3 represents a sol that will agglomerate instantaneously as no net repulsive forces are operating.

Many attempts have been made to correlate the zeta potential with lyophobic colloid stability; a high zeta potential would give rise to a high V_{max}. The theoretical basis for the potential energy of interaction curves, deduced by Verwey and Overbeek (1948) depends on a knowledge of the potential at the surface of the particle, i.e. at the Stern layer. The zeta potential which is derived from electrokinetic experiments such as electrophoresis (p. 94) is not identical with the surface potential. This is because the method involves the measurement of movement of particle through a liquid and the flow of liquid past the particle does not occur exactly at

the particle–liquid interface but at a plane in the liquid some distance from the true interface. The zeta potential is the potential at this plane and is therefore generally much smaller than the surface potential. However, the zeta potential is readily determined experimentally and in the literature there is evidence that zeta potential can help in predicting whether or not sols will flocculate in the presence of electrolytes. The application to pharmaceutical suspensions is discussed by Nash and Haeger (1966).

SIZE OF COLLOIDAL PARTICLES

ULTRAMICROSCOPE

Light passed in a convergent beam transversely through a sol is scattered and polarized by the dispersed particles and the path of the beam when examined laterally is seen as an illuminated cone. A true solution, examined similarly, appears optically empty, i.e. the Tyndall effect is absent. The ultramicroscope is simply a device for observing the Tyndall effect microscopically. The microscope is perpendicular to the beam of light passing through the sol in a shallow glass cell. The colloidal particles appear as bright spots against a dark background, similar to dust particles seen in a beam of sunlight in a darkened room. The actual shape cannot be seen but from the concentration of the sol and the dimensions of the cell, the number of particles per unit weight of dispersed phase can be calculated and hence the average particle size. The normal optical microscope method will not resolve particles less than wavelength of visible light (0.4–0.8 μm).

ULTRAFILTRATION

Particle size of colloids can be roughly determined by ultrafiltration through membranes of known pore size. Elford (1937) prepared nitrocellulose membranes with graded pore size by controlling the solvent composition in which the nitrocellulose was dissolved; good solvents favour dispersion and give dense membranes of small pore size while poor solvents produce more open membranes. Elford found that the size of large particles passing through the membranes corresponded fairly well with the pore size, but smaller particles (e.g. virus particles) were held back by membranes whose pore size was larger than the particle, probably due to adsorption effects.

ULTRACENTRIFUGE

Colloidal particles cannot be sedimented in the usual laboratory centrifuges because, being small and light, they are kept in random motion by Brownian movement. Centrifugal force of upwards of 400 000 g in the ultracentrifuge originated by Svedburg, is required to produce sedimentation at a reasonable rate. In this instrument the sol is placed in a glass cell in the centrifuge rotor and arranged so that light passing through the cell may be photographed. The centrifuge is rotated at 50 000 rev/min and higher and the rate of sedimentation is derived from the change in light adsorption, or refractive index of the sol during centrifugation. It is possible not only to estimate molecular weight but also to determine the relative homogeneity of the system with respect to molecular weight. The molecular weight of proteins has been calculated from sedimentation velocity, e.g. pepsin 35 500, insulin 41 000, gelatin, 10 000–70 000.

OSMOTIC PRESSURE

The method is based on van't Hoff's law, according to which the osmotic pressure p depends on molar concentration of the solute and on temperature. This is shown in the following equation, where C = concentration (in grams per litre); M = molecular weight and T = absolute temperature:

$$P = \frac{RTC}{M}$$

The equation is valid for very dilute solutions in which the molecules do not interact mutually. However, if association occurs the plot of reduced osmotic pressure, P/C against C will not be linear and it is necessary to extrapolate the curve to infinite dilution to obtain RT/M.

Osmotic pressure is inversely proportional to molecular weight, so that the pressures observed for, say, proteins of molecular weight 50 000 will be very low and special osmometers are employed. The dialysis membranes used for osmometry are permeable to small ions and the distribution of ions across membranes led to discrepancies in the measurement of the molecular weights of polyelectrolytes such as proteins. The protein molecule is a colloidal ion with several charges balanced by normally sized ions. Donnan in 1911 found that the invariably low results for molecular weight obtained from osmotic pressure measurement were due to the unequal distribution of ions across the membrane. He found that by dissolving the protein in electrolyte solution (0.1 M or higher) and using the same salt solution outside the membrane, he was able to swamp out the Donnan effect.

LIGHT SCATTERING

When a light beam is passed through a colloidal solution, the intensity of the scattered beam depends upon the following factors: (1) intensity of the incident beam, (2) wavelength of the incident beam, (3) difference between the refractive index of the particle and the medium, (4) volume of the particles, and (5) the number of particles which scatter the light. In some cases the intensity of light scattered at different angles may differ and can be used to give some indication of the shape of macromolecules. The work of Debye, Doty, Zimm and others (1944 to 1949) led to prediction of equations which correlate the molecular weight M with the intensity of scattered light. This relation, in the case of uncharged species, is expressed by the equation:

$$\frac{HC}{\tau} = \frac{I}{M} + 2BC$$

where τ is the turbidity measured at 90° to the incident beam, C the concentration of solute (grams per litre). M is the molecular weight, B is the interaction constant which, as in osmotic pressure measurements, depends on the degree of non-ideality of the solution. The proportionality constant H is a complicated function of the wavelength of incident light, refractive index and rate of change of refractive index with concentration.

A plot of HC/τ versus C should give a straight line at low concentrations and extrapolation to infinite dilution will give the value of I/M and hence the molecular weight.

ELECTRICAL PROPERTIES OF COLLOIDS

IONIZATION

Soaps in aqueous solution form micelles of colloidal size, in which the molecules are orientated with their hydrocarbon chains forming the interior of the micelle and their polar groups forming the outer layer. Consider a fatty acid soap, $C_nH_{2n+1}COONa$ which ionizes to $C_nH_{2n+1}COO^-Na^+$ in water. The colloidal particle is thus a colloidal anion and the Na^+ ions set free into the aqueous solution form the outer layer of the double layer. Proteins are another group of substances in which the electrical charge arises by ionization. Proteins contain both basic and acidic groups in the molecule and are termed *ampholytes* or *amphoteric electrolytes*. In alkaline solution the acidic group COOH will ionize to COO^- so that the particle carries a negative charge. In acid solution the basic group NH_2 will ionize to NH_3^+ so that the particle now carries a positive charge. At a certain definite pH, the total number of positive charges will equal the total number of negative charges and the net charge will, therefore, be zero. This pH is known as the *isoelectric point*. The protein is probably ionized at the isoelectric point, existing in the *zwitterion* form but the net charge is zero provided no other ions are adsorbed. The electrical state of the protein molecule can thus be depicted as

$$R\underset{COO^-}{\overset{NH_2}{<}} \underset{-OH^-}{\overset{+OH^-}{\rightleftharpoons}} R\underset{COO^-}{\overset{NH_3^+}{<}} \underset{-H^+}{\overset{+H^+}{\rightleftharpoons}} R\underset{COOH}{\overset{NH_3^+}{<}}$$

Negative protein   Isoelectric protein   Positive protein
(zwitterion)

(R denotes the residue of the protein molecule)
(A protein is least soluble at its isoelectric point and is readily precipitated. The protein, insulin, is precipitated from aqueous alcohol by adjusting the solution to the isoelectric point of insulin pH 5 to 6.)

ADSORPTION

The preferential adsorption of an ion by a particle is responsible for the charge on non-ionizing particles, e.g. addition of Fe^{3+} ions to freshly precipitated ferric hydroxide will produce a sol of hydroxide; the Fe^{3+} ions are adsorbed by the particles of ferric hydroxide and the Cl^- ions form the outer shell of the electrical double layer. The spontaneous dispersion of a precipitate on the addition of a small amount of a third substance is known as '*peptization*', a term introduced by Graham. The substance, generally an electrolyte, causing this dispersion is called a '*peptizing agent*'.

The presence of the electrical double layer gives rise to the electrokinetic effects electrophoresis, electroosmosis and streaming potential.

ELECTROPHORESIS

Electrophoresis is the movement of colloidal particles with respect to the liquid when a potential difference is maintained across the sol. The zeta potential can be calculated from the mobility of the particle.

Spherical particles—small compared with the thickness of the double layer. These include protein molecules, fine silver iodide sols, etc. The derivation made by Debye & Hückel was that if the externally applied potential gradient is E and the charge on the particle, Q (coulombs), the particle will experience a force QE tending to accelerate it in the direction of the field. The hydrodynamic resistance to its flow is given by Stokes' Law as $6\pi\eta r v$ where η is viscosity, v the particle velocity and r the particle radius. The particle moves with a constant velocity as the two forces rapidly attain balance. The velocity of the particle in an electric field of 1 eV/cm is given by:

$$v = \frac{QE}{6\pi\eta r}$$

For spherical particles the relation between Q and the zeta potential ζ in a liquid of dielectric constant D is:

$$Q = Dr\zeta$$

so that

$$\zeta = 6\pi\eta v/D$$

If ζ is expressed in millivolts, v in $\mu m/sec$ per V/cm, the equation becomes $\zeta = 21.2v$ for water at 20°.

Particles large compared with the thickness of the double layer. Particles visible under an optical microscope belong to this category. The particle and its double layer are more appropriately treated as a parallel plate condenser. The equation relating zeta potential to its measured mobility becomes:

$$\zeta = 4\pi\eta v/D$$

This is generally referred to as Smoluchowski's equation. For water at 25° this expression is reduced to:

$$\zeta = 12.87 v$$

where ζ is expressed in millivolts and v in $\mu m/sec$ per V/cm.

Experimental methods. The electrophoretic mobility of colloidal particles can be measured from the rate of movement of the boundary of a sol using a simple U tube apparatus shown in Fig. 5.7.

The apparatus is designed so that a sharp boundary is formed between the sol and an electrolyte solution of the same concentration as that in the sol. If the sol is coloured or opaque, e.g. gold sols, emulsions, the position of the boundary can be followed visually. If the sol is colourless, then the boundary has to be observed by measuring the change in refractive index along the column using

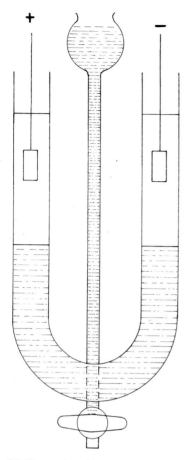

FIG. 5.7. Electrophoresis cell (moving boundary).

where direct observation is made of the movement of the particles. A cylindrical microelectrophoresis cell is shown in Fig. 5.8. At each end of the tube is a porous plug leading to a reversible electrode (Ag–AgCl, Cu–CuSO$_4$, etc.) and a tap is provided for filling and cleaning. For low salt concentrations (below about M/100) platinum electrodes may be used.

The cell is mounted horizontally on the microscope stage and on applying the electrical field (about 10 V/cm) the velocity of the particles is measured by timing their movement across the plane of a calibrated graticule placed in the microscope eye piece. In addition to the electrokinetic potential at the interface between the particles and the liquid, a similar potential usually exists between the walls of the tube and the liquid. Thus the particles are subject to both electrophoretic movement and electroosmotic movement of the liquid near to the walls of the tube. In a closed cell, as shown in the figure, the liquid moving electroosmotically at the wall must return along the centre of the tube. Thus at a certain level in the cell, the two opposing movements cancel each other out and the velocity of the particle in this stationary level will be the true electrophoretic mobility. Bacteria, emulsion droplets, suspensions, etc. have been studied by this method (Alexander & Johnson 1949).

A simplified method for the electrophoresis of lyophilic colloids, e.g. proteins, nucleic acids, is *paper electrophoresis*. A strip of filter paper is moistened with a suitable buffer solution and supported horizontally with its ends dipping into separate reservoirs of buffer. A potential gradient is applied along the paper by electrodes inserted in the reservoirs. A drop of protein solution is spotted on to the paper and a direct current of about 10 mA at 10 V/cm of paper is passed for several hours. The filter paper acts merely as a support for the liquid phase through which the protein mole-

special optical equipment (Schlieren method). This technique is used for the studying of the electrophoretic mobility of components in mixtures, e.g. proteins.

If the colloidal particles are visible under a microscope, an alternative method of electrophoresis is possible. This is microelectrophoresis,

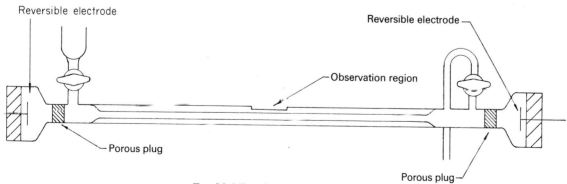

FIG. 5.8. Microelectrophoresis cell.

cules migrate. At the conclusion of the experiment, the paper is removed and the position of the protein is detected by dipping the paper in a dye solution or spraying with a solution, staining the protein but not the paper. A mixture of proteins can be resolved into separate zones if the mobilities of the components are different.

The pH of the buffer solution is important; in alkaline and acid solutions the proteins will migrate in opposite directions, the ions being $RCOO^-$ and RN^+H_3, respectively. If the pH of the buffer solution corresponds to the isoelectric point of the protein, the latter molecule will be present as the zwitterion, $N^+H_3 \ldots COO^-$ and will not migrate. It is, therefore, possible to extend the scope of the method by choice of suitable buffers. Fig. 5.9 shows

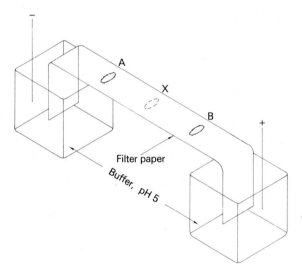

FIG. 5.9. Paper electrophoresis. X, original positions of proteins A and B; A, final position of protein A (I.E.P., pH 4); B, final position of protein B (I.E.P., pH 6).

the appearance of a filter paper strip after electrophoresis of two proteins A and B of isoelectric points pH 4 and 6, respectively when the paper is buffered at pH 5.

ELECTROOSMOSIS

The atmosphere of counter ions around the particles confers a charge on the dispersion medium. The sign of this charge is opposite to that of the particles. Hence, as the particles move towards one pole, the liquid tends to move towards the opposite pole. This phenomenon can be observed if a tube is plugged in the middle with a porous material, e.g. glass powder, with electrodes immersed in dilute buffer solution on either side of the plug. A glass

surface in contact with water bears a negative charge due to the adsorption of OH^-. As the current passes, the liquid will move towards the positive electrode, and this can be best observed if the ends of the tubes are connected to capillary tubes, so that small displacements of the liquid are apparent. Fig. 5.10 shows electroosmotic flow of

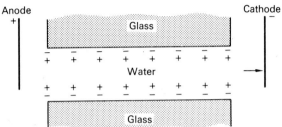

FIG. 5.10. Electroosmosis.

water in a glass capillary tube on application of a potential difference across the ends of the tube.

STREAMING POTENTIAL

This is the converse of electroosmosis. If the electrodes in the electroosmosis apparatus (Fig. 5.10) are replaced by a galvanometer in the circuit, no current would be detected when the liquid is stationary. However, if the liquid is forced through the tube the galvanometer will indicate a current. This streaming potential is due to the displacement of the charges equilibrated in the double layer around the solid. This technique can be used to measure the zeta potential of relatively coarse solids which would sediment rapidly in an electrophoresis cell. The liquid is forced through a plug of the powdered solid at a constant rate and the potential difference across the plug is measured.

PRECIPITATION OF LYOPHOBIC COLLOIDS

The stability of lyophobic colloids depends on the electrical repulsion exerted by the electrical charges on their surfaces. As discussed in a previous section, trace amounts of electrolytes adsorbed on to the colloidal surface may be responsible for the electrical charge and hence stability. However, if excess of electrolyte is added, this may cause reduction in the thickness of the double layer, lowering the zeta potential below the critical value. The reduction of V_{max} (see Fig. 5.5) to a few kT will lead to coagulation in the primary minimum. Ions of charge opposite to that of particles are most effective in coagulating colloids. Furthermore the valency of the ion is important. The coagulating effect of bivalent ions is not just twice that of monovalent ions but the activity increases between ten and a hundred fold on increasing the valency of the acting ion by one. This is known as the Schulz–Hardy rule. Salts of monovalent cations have coagulation values for negative sols around 0.05 mole of cation per litre where the accompanying anion is Cl, SO_4 or NO_3. Acetates and citrate ions tend to be adsorbed even by negatively charged sols and higher concentrations of these salts are required to produce coagulation.

PRECIPITATION OF LYOPHILIC COLLOIDS

The stability of lyophilic colloids depends mainly on interaction of the colloid with the solvent, the so called *solvation*. With water as solvent this interaction is called *hydration*; solvation is a more general term for any liquid. Rubber dissolves in benzene and a stable colloid is formed, as the macromolecules of rubber become solvated by the benzene. There is an enormous variety of electrically charged lyophilic colloids, e.g. proteins, pectins, agar, acacia, alginic acid and their stability in aqueous solution depends to a large extent on hydration and to a lesser extent on electrical charge.

The electrolyte concentrations needed for the precipitation of hydrophilic colloids are many times greater than those needed for coagulation of hydrophobic sols. To precipitate the various proteins of blood plasma not less than 1.3 to 2.5 mole/litre of ammonium sulphate is necessary. The effect of adding electrolytes to a hydrophilic colloid is two-fold: the electrical properties and degree of hydration are both affected. At low concentrations the electrical charge is affected by ions of opposite charge and at high concentrations both charge and hydration are affected, ions having the greatest affinity for water being the most effective in 'dehydrating' the colloid. The precipitation by the action of high concentrations of electrolyte is usually called 'salting out', and the order of effectiveness of various ions for this purpose can be arranged in a series known as the Hofmeister series. The most common ions, arranged in order of decreasing salting out effect for, say, protein solutions, is as follows:

sulphate/2 > acetate > chloride > nitrate > chlorate > bromide > iodide.

For cations, the series is less definite and is as follows:

lithium > sodium > potassium > ammonium > magnesium/2.

Proteins are most readily precipitated if the pH of the solution is adjusted to the isoelectric point where the net charge is zero. The subsequent addition of a dehydrating agent, e.g. alcohol, acetone or electrolyte, will then precipitate the protein. For proteins of similar chemical constitution the salting out concentration of electrolyte decreases as the molecular weights of the proteins increase. Enzymes have been fractionated by repeatedly dissolving and salting out with ammonium sulphate or magnesium sulphate. The purified enzyme is then freed from electrolyte by dialysing against distilled water. Fractionation of human blood plasma into globulins, fibrinogen and thrombin, depends on selective precipitation by organic solvents under conditions of controlled pH, ionic strength and temperature.

STABILIZING EFFECT OF HYDROPHILIC COLLOIDS

When a hydrophilic colloid is added to a hydrophobic sol in sufficient amount, the hydrophobic particles become coated with hydrophilic material and thus acquire the stable properties of a hydrophilic colloid. This protective action of hydrophilic colloids such as gelatin, acacia, cellulose ethers, polyvinylpyrrolidone, etc., has led to the term *protective colloid* to describe this type of colloid. Attempts have been made to express the protective action quantitatively in terms of the amount of colloid needed to protect a gold sol from precipitation, on the addition of sodium chloride. The *gold number* is the weight of protecting substance in milligrams which is just sufficient to prevent the coagulation of 10 ml of red gold sol when 1 ml of 10 per cent sodium chloride is added to it. However, the effectiveness of protective colloids measured in this way must depend on the affinity of the hydrophilic colloid for the gold and will not necessarily correlate with the degree of protection in other systems. The binding of the protective colloid to the hydrophobic surface, may sometimes lead to flocculation, particularly if the two colloids are oppositely charged and are present in approximately equivalent amounts. In such a case, further addition of protective colloid may overcome this difficulty.

In pharmacy, there are numerous examples of protective colloids. Resinous tinctures can be diluted with a dilute solution of tragacanth or acacia to form a colloidal solution, even in the presence of electrolytes. In the absence of these gums, immediate coagulation of the resin occurs. Acacia and sodium carboxymethylcellulose are used to prepare stable emulsions of oil in water. Gelatin and serum albumin are used to stabilize silver oxide in the preparation of silver protein products (Silver Protein and Mild Silver Protein, BPC 1968). On addition to water, a colloidal silver oxide sol is formed which is suitable for application as eye-drops. Gelatin is also used to maintain gold sol in a stable form for injection [Gold (^{198}Au) Injection BP].

GELS

Lyophilic colloids such as gelatin, agar and pectin are soluble in hot water and on cooling give rise to a semi-solid, jelly-like structure termed a gel. The mechanical strength of the gel is due to partial aggregation of the colloidal particles which form an interlaced network with the solvent held within the meshes. The gelation process can be regarded as a half-way stage between a colloidal sol and a completely precipitated sol. Thus electrolytes which promote precipitation of colloidal sols will also promote gelation, whereas peptizing agents will have the opposite effect. For instance, a low concentration of calcium or zinc ions tends to increase the gel strength of the negatively charged bentonite gel, whereas excess will result in precipitation and breakdown of the gel.

PREPARATION OF GELS

Temperature effect. The solubility of most lyophilic colloids, e.g. gelatin, agar, sodium oleate, is reduced on lowering the temperature, so that cooling a concentrated hot sol will often produce a gel. In contrast to this, some materials such as the cellulose ethers owe their water solubility to hydrogen bonding with the water. Raising the temperature of these sols will disrupt the hydrogen bonding and the reduced solubility will cause gelation.

Flocculation with salts and non-solvents. Gelation is produced by adding just sufficient precipitant to produce the gel state but insufficient to bring about complete precipitation. It is necessary to ensure rapid mixing to avoid local high concentrations of precipitant. Solutions of ethyl cellulose, polystyrene, etc., in benzene can be gelled by rapid mixing with suitable amounts of a non-solvent such as petroleum ether.

The addition of salts to hydrophobic sols brings about coagulation, and gelation is rarely observed. However, the addition of suitable proportions of salts to moderately hydrophilic sols such as aluminium hydroxide, ferric hydroxide and bentonite, produces gels. As a general rule, the addition of

about half of the amount of electrolyte needed for complete precipitation, is adequate. With positively charged hydroxide sols, divalent ions such as SO_4^{2-} are more effective than univalent ions such as Cl^-. The gels formed are frequently thixotropic in behaviour.

Such hydrophilic colloids as gelatin, proteins and acacia are only affected by high concentrations of electrolytes, when the effect is to 'salt out' the colloid and gelation does not occur.

Chemical reaction. In the preparation of sols by precipitation from solution, e.g. $Al(OH)_3$ sol prepared by interaction in aqueous solution of an aluminium salt and sodium carbonate, an increased concentration of reactants will produce a gel structure. Silica gel is another example and is produced by the interaction of sodium silicate and acids in aqueous solution.

STRUCTURE OF GELS

Elastic Gels
Gels of agar, pectin and gelatin are elastic, the fibrous molecules being linked at the points of junction by relatively weak bonds such as hydrogen bonds and dipole attraction. If the molecules possess free COOH groups, then additional bonding may take place in the presence of Ca^{2+} when a salt bridge of the type —COO—Ca^{2+}O$^-$OC— is formed between two adjacent strands of the network. The types of links that could be formed are shown below (Alexander & Johnson 1949).

Coulomb forces: $-COO^- \; H_3^+N\,-;$
$\qquad\qquad\qquad -SO_4^- \; Ca^{2+} \; SO_4' -$
$\qquad\qquad\qquad -COO^- \; Ca^{2+} \; OOC' -;$
$\qquad\qquad\qquad NH_3^+ \; SO_4'' \; H_3^+N\,-$

Hydrogen bonding: $-COO^- \; H_2N\,-;$
$\qquad\qquad\qquad\quad -COOH \; H_3^+N\,-$

Dipole forces: $\qquad \overset{\delta^-}{>}\overset{\delta^+}{C=O}$
$\qquad\qquad\qquad\qquad \underset{\delta^-}{O} = \underset{\delta^-}{C} <$

Rigid Gels
In contrast to elastic gels, rigid gels can be formed from macromolecules in which the framework is linked by primary valence bonds. Silica gel is such an example, where silicic acid molecules are held together by –Si–O–Si–O– bonds to give a polymer structure possessing a network of pores, most of which are scarcely larger than a few molecular diameters in width. Because of the resultant large

surface area, silica gel is a useful adsorbent particularly for water vapour and hence its use as a desiccant.

Thixotropic Gels

The bonds between particles in these gels are very weak and can be broken down by shaking or stirring. The resultant sol will revert back to a gel due to the particles colliding and linking together again; Brownian movement being responsible for the particle–particle collisions. This reversible isothermal sol–gel transformation is termed *thixotropy*. It is most likely to occur in colloidal systems with non-spherical particles such as rods or plates which can be easily built up into a scaffold-like structure. Many clay minerals dispersed in water show this effect, due not only to the plate-like structure of the particles, but also due to the faces and the edges of the platelets carrying charges of opposite sign.

Bentonite and acid-washed kaolin platelets have many positively charged edges while all the faces are negatively charged due to disocciation of positive counterions such as Na^+, Ca^{2+}. This results in a face to edge attraction giving a scaffold structure in which solvent is easily enmeshed. Mechanical shearing breaks the structure and liquefies the gels. The effect of adding citrate ions to clay dispersions may be to neutralize the positive charges on the edges of the platelets, thus minimizing the formation of three-dimensional gels. Other examples of thixotropic gels, include aluminium hydroxide in water, many concentrated emulsions, particularly those prepared with emulsifying waxes, and oils gelled with aluminium monostearate.

The different possibilities of gel structure are presented schematically in Fig. 5.11. Evidence for the coherent network structure has been obtained from a number of experiments. For instance, a fluid dispersion of graphite in a non-conducting oil does not conduct electricity until the system is allowed to set to a gel, when it does conduct, indicating that the particles have linked together. Shaking this thixotropic gel will liquefy it when it will act as a non-conductor as before. The open structure of a gel is apparent if one considers the small proportion of solid phase present. For instance, water can be gelled by as little as 0.5 per cent agar, small molecules and ions are free to diffuse in the solvent through the relatively large meshes and it is therefore surprising that the diffusion of low molecular weight substances in gelatin and agar gels is the same as in water, provided no chemical interaction or adsorption occurs. If the concentration of gelling agent is increased the mesh size of the gel is reduced and there will be a limiting concentration that can be used before the diffusing molecule is restricted.

Syneresis

Swollen gels on storage may spontaneously contract with the liberation of dispersion medium e.g. pectin, starch gels. This exudation is probably due to increased particle–particle linkages of the gelling agent resulting in the squeezing out of the enmeshed liquid. This is shown schematically in Fig. 5.12.

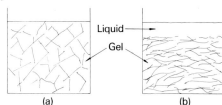

(a)   (b)

FIG. 5.12. Syneresis in gels; A, Original gel; B, Aged gel—increased particle–particle links causing syneris.

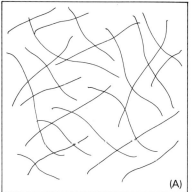 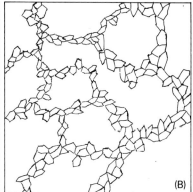 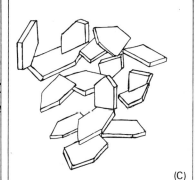

(A)   (B)   (C)

FIG. 5.11. Representation of cell structure; A, Network of macromolecules, e.g. gelatin gel; B, Gel of flocculated solid particles; C, Gel of clay particles (face to edge flocculation), e.g. bentonite.

REFERENCES

ALEXANDER, A. E. & JOHNSON, P. (1949) *Colloid Science*, London: Oxford University.

ANDERSON, J. K. (1964) *Pharm. J.*, 497.

ELFORD, W. J. (1937) *Trans. Faraday Soc.* **33**, 1094.

FERRY, J. D. (1936) *Chem. Rev.* **18**, 373.

HIESTAND, E. N. (1964) *J. pharm. Sci.* **53**, 1.

NASH, R. A. & HAEGER, B. E. (1966) *J. pharm. Sci.*, **55**, 829.

VERWEY, E. J. W. & OVERBEEK, J. T. G. (1948) *Theory of the Stability of Lyophobic Colloids.* Amsterdam: Elsevier.

6

Adsorption

The particles (ions, atoms or molecules) making up a solid are held together by certain forces (electrostatic, valency or van der Waals forces) and each particle in the bulk of the solid is attracted equally by its neighbours, in all directions. At the surface of the solid, the forces are not balanced because the surface particle is not completely surrounded by neighbours. There will be resultant attraction perpendicular to the surface, tending to draw the particles inwards, and they will be at a higher potential energy than those in the bulk of the medium. These surface particles can attract other molecules to them, due to the imbalance of forces giving rise to the phenomenon of *adsorption*. For instance, large quantities of gases such as oxygen or nitrogen are taken up by charcoal cooled in liquid air. The gas is said to be adsorbed on to the surface of the charcoal which may amount to several square metres for each gram of charcoal.

There is a distinction between adsorption, which is a surface process and *absorption* which refers to a uniform distribution of one substance throughout another, e.g. solution of hydrogen in palladium, solution of gases in liquids. It is sometimes difficult to define clearly the interface of highly porous solids and the term *sorption* has been used by workers, notably J. W. McBain, to describe the uptake of gases by porous solids. The substance that is attached to the surface of the solid is called the *adsorbate*. Since adsorption is a surface phenomenon the most effective *adsorbents* are those with high surface areas, e.g. finely divided solids.

TYPES OF ADSORPTION

PHYSICAL ADSORPTION

Physical or van der Waals adsorption is characterized by low heats of adsorption (about 20 to 40kJ per mole of gas) and the forces responsible for this type of adsorption are the same as those that cause liquefaction of gases and deviations of gases from ideal behaviour. Physical adsorption of gases is common at low temperatures when the thermal agitation of the molecules is not sufficient to cause complete evaporation of the adsorbed layer from the surface of the solid. As the temperature is raised, the amount adsorbed becomes progressively less and no detectable adsorption of low boiling point gases, e.g. N_2, O_2 would be detected at room temperature and atmospheric pressure. Adsorption of gases is most marked at temperatures near to their liquefaction temperatures and at partial pressures approaching one. The gas in the adsorbed layer is in equilibrium with the gas molecules in the bulk gas phase, the position of equilibrium depending on: (1) the nature of the adsorbent, (2) the nature of the adsorbate, (3) the surface area of the adsorbate, (4) the temperature, and (5) the pressure of the gas. A decrease in temperature or an increase in pressure increases the amount of adsorption. The relationship between pressure of a gas and amount adsorbed at fixed temperature has been expressed by many equations, one of the earliest of these is the empirical Freundlich isotherm (Fig. 6.1) the equation of which is:

$$x = KP^{1/n}$$

where x = weight of gas adsorbed per unit weight of adsorbent,

P = equilibrium gas pressure, and

K and n = constants depending on the temperature and nature of adsorbent and adsorbate.

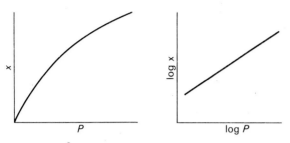

FIG. 6.1. Freundlich adsorption isotherm.

When plotting experimental data, the logarithmic form of the Freundlich equation is more convenient and permits a graphical solution for the constants K and n:

$$\log x = \log K + 1/n \log P.$$

Thus plotting $\log x$ versus $\log P$ gives a straight line of slope $1/n$ and the intercept on the ordinate is $\log K$.

LANGMUIR ADSORPTION ISOTHERM

Whereas the earlier equations were only empirical, a great advance was made by Langmuir in 1916 who derived a theoretical equation for adsorption based on the short range forces that exist between molecules. The equation assumes that:

(1) the layer of gas molecules adsorbed is only one molecule thick,

(2) gas molecules are adsorbed on fixed sites on surface,

(3) the rate of evaporation from the surface is related to the number of filled sites, and

(4) the rate of condensation is proportional to the number of unfilled sites.

At equilibrium at any particular gas pressure, the rate of condensation would equal the rate of evaporation. Thus if θ = fraction of surface covered at a given instance, then $(1 - \theta)$ = fraction of surface not covered by molecules and therefore available for adsorption. The rate of condensation is $K_1(1 - \theta)P$, in which K_1 is a constant and P is the pressure of the gas. Let K_2 represent the rate of evaporation from a completely filled surface so that the rate of evaporation from a partially filled one, will equal $K_2\theta$. At equilibrium the two processes must balance so that:

$$K_1(1 - \theta)P = K_2\theta, \qquad (6.1)$$

or $$\theta = \frac{K_1 P}{K_2 + K_1 P}, \qquad (6.2)$$

and $$\theta = \frac{kP}{1 + kP} \quad \text{where} \quad k = \frac{K_1}{K_2} \qquad (6.3)$$

If x = number of molecules adsorbed at the surface and x_m = number of molecules necessary to fill the surface (i.e. monolayer capacity) then the Langmuir equation becomes:

$$\frac{x}{x_m} = \frac{kP}{1 + kP}, \qquad (6.4)$$

or $$x = \frac{kPx_m}{1 + kP}. \qquad (6.5)$$

Inspection of the adsorption isotherm (Figs. 6.2a and 6.3, Type I) shows that at low pressures, the

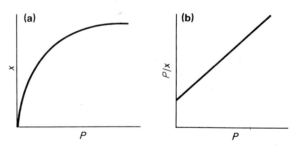

FIG. 6.2. Langmuir adsorption isotherm.

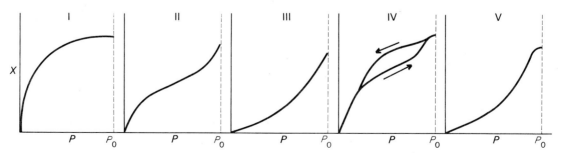

FIG. 6.3. Types I to V adsorption isotherms. (P_o = saturation vapour pressure).

amount adsorbed is proportional to the pressure and at higher pressures the adsorption becomes progressively less and eventually levels off to a constant value, due to all the available sites being filled. This can be inferred from equation (6.5) for when $P \rightarrow \infty$, $x \rightarrow x_m$. At low pressures where $P \rightarrow 0$, $x \rightarrow kPx_m$. The monolayer capacity can be estimated from the value of x where it reaches a limiting value. An alternative method is to plot the Langmuir equation in its linear form:

$$\frac{P}{x} = \frac{1}{kx_m} + \frac{P}{x_m}. \qquad (6.6)$$

Thus a plot of P/x versus P should give a straight line and the monolayer capacity x_m can be calculated from the slope (Fig. 6.2a).

BET ADSORPTION ISOTHERM

Brunaver, Emmett and Teller in 1938 extended Langmuir's ideas to cover adsorption where more than one molecular layer could form. This situation occurred at low temperatures and at pressures approaching saturation pressure when an S-shaped isotherm was obtained (Fig. 6.3, Type II). They assumed that the molecules were adsorbed on to fixed sites and there was no lateral interaction between the molecules. Secondly, that the heat of adsorption of a molecule to any layer other than the first was equal to the heat of condensation. They found that the amount adsorbed per unit weight of adsorbent x, should be related to the pressure P, by the expression:

$$\frac{P}{x(P_0 - P)} = \frac{1}{xc} + \frac{(C-1)P}{x_m CP_0},$$

P being the saturation vapour pressure, x_m the monolayer capacity, c a constant given by $c = e(E_1 - E_2)/RT$, E_1 the heat of adsorption of the first layer, E_2 the latent heat of condensation of the adsorbate, R the gas constant and T the absolute temperature.

This equation has found extensive application in the determination of surface areas of powders by nitrogen adsorption. The monolayer capacity of nitrogen at the temperature of boiling liquid nitrogen is determined and from a knowledge of the cross-sectional area of the nitrogen molecule the surface area is calculated from the equation:

$$S = Nx_m A \times 10^{-16},$$

where S is the surface area (cm^2/g), N is the Avogadro number, x_m is the monolayer capacity (gram moles) and A is the cross-sectional area of the nitrogen molecule (0.162 nm^2). This method is restricted to powders of particle size below a micron in order to obtain measurable amounts of adsorption. To give some idea of the weight of gas adsorbed, 1 m^2 of a monolayer of nitrogen (0.162 nm^2) would weigh only 0.29 mg. Thus on 1 g of a powder made up of equal cubes of edge 1 μm and density 3 the monolayer adsorption would amount to nearly 0.6 mg of nitrogen. Measurements of this magnitude can be made by use of sensitive micro balances (McBain–Bakr balance) or by measuring the volume changes of gas produced by adsorption, using manometric apparatus (Gregg 1961).

A very large number of isotherms have appeared in the literature but the majority can be grouped into the five types of the Brunauer–Emmett–Teller (BET) classification represented in Fig. 6.3. Type II is the one best represented by the BET equation and is usually characteristic of non-porous solids of very fine particle size. Type IV is typical of adsorption of water vapour on gel-like materials such as cellulose, starches and silica gel where the uptake of water vapour with increase in pressure gives an adsorption isotherm which differs from the curve obtained during desorption of the gel. The hysteresis loop so obtained has been explained on the basis of capillary condensation of the liquid within micropores of the gel. Multilayer adsorption occurs as the pressure is increased and, at pressures near to saturation, leads to complete filling of the capillaries. During the filling and emptying of the pores, i.e. during adsorption and desorption, the advancing and receding contact angle between the liquid and solid differ and can account for the difference in vapour pressure for a given amount of vapour adsorbed (Gregg 1961).

In physical adsorption, the shape of the isotherm is determined primarily by the nature of the adsorbent, although different adsorbates which differ in molecular cross-section will also influence it. The equilibrium of gas adsorption is rapidly attained and any delay observed may be due to the time taken for the gas to diffuse to the surface, particularly if the solid has a high internal surface such as charcoal.

Chemisorption

This is chemical combination of the adsorbate at the surface of the adsorbent. It is characterized by a high heat of adsorption (40 to 400 kJ/mole) and unlike physical adsorption it is irreversible. In many cases the chemical adsorption is slow because the molecules have to acquire an energy of interaction before they can react with the adsorbent.

The rate of uptake will then be accelerated by increase of temperature. Examples of chemisorption include tungsten–hydrogen and tungsten–oxygen. The tarnishing of silver on exposure to the atmosphere is a case of chemisorption where gaseous sulphur compounds interact with the silver surface.

ADSORPTION FROM SOLUTION

Solids can also adsorb solutes from solution but the phenomenon is more complicated than adsorption at the gas–solid interface due to competition of the solute and the solvent for the solid–liquid interface. The measured quantity is now the change in the concentration of the solution and is thus only an apparent adsorption, since it is a function of the relative adsorptions of the solute and the solvent. However, in dilute solutions the adsorption of solute follows a similar adsorption pattern to that of gases, so that Freundlich, Langmuir or BET equations can be used to describe the adsorption, the pressure term being replaced by concentration. Langmuir isotherms have been obtained for adsorption of promazine on attapulgite and charcoal (Sorby 1965); strychnine on kaolin, halloysite and attapulgite (Barr & Arnista 1957a, b, c); cetyl-pyridinium bromide on talc and kaolin (Batuyios & Brecht 1957).

The commonest adsorbents used are activated charcoal, bone charcoal, alumina, silica gel, kaolin, kieselguhr and Fuller's earth. The main requirement for an effective adsorbent is a large, accessible surface area attained either by fine subdivision or by an open porous structure. In the use of adsorbents, thorough stirring for a time adequate for the achievement of equilibria is most important. Reference to the Freundlich or Langmuir isotherm shows that adsorption is relatively greater from dilute than from more concentrated solution. In general, high molecular weight solutes are more readily adsorbed than low molecular weight solutes because the van der Waals forces of attraction increase with size of molecule. Thus a number of dyestuffs, e.g. methylene blue, form a complete monomolecular adsorbed layer on powdered graphite even at very low concentrations. As a general rule adsorption is greater from a solvent in which the solute is sparingly soluble. The pH of the medium has a marked effect on the adsorptive capacity of charcoal; positively charged substances, e.g. methylene blue and crystal violet, are most readily adsorbed from alkaline solution; negatively charged substances, e.g. acidic dyes and most coloured impurities encountered in chemical manu-facture, are best adsorbed from alkaline solution; amphoteric solutes such as proteins are best adsorbed in the region of their isoelectric point.

Since an equilibrium exists between the solute in solution and that at the solid surface, a single shaking of the solution with the adsorbent will not remove the entire amount of solute from solution. There may be exceptions to this when the affinity of adsorbent for solute is very high as in the case of methylene blue on charcoal. In many cases it may be necessary to deplete the solution of its solute successively by passing it through a column of the adsorbent when it comes into continuous contact with fresh adsorbent during its travel.

The different affinities exhibited by different substances for adsorbents are responsible for the phenomenon of *selective adsorption*. If charcoal is added to a solution of magenta, the dye is adsorbed and the solution becomes colourless. Addition of saponin to the system restores the colour to the solution because the saponin is more strongly adsorbed than the dye and displaces it from the surface of the adsorbent. Advantage is taken of this principle in the removal of extraneous colouring matter and impurities in preparative work and clarification of pharmaceutical preparations; the substances removed, being complex, are readily adsorbed.

The reverse process of adsorption, *desorption* depends on the same principles. A solvent from which adsorption is poor will normally bring about desorption. Desorption of ionic solutes may also be effected by change in pH. Strongly adsorbed substances such as saponin and other surface active agents may be used to displace adsorbed material.

CHARCOALS

Medicinal Charcoal
This is prepared by carbonizing wood, cellulose residues or coconut shells out of contact with air. The charcoal so obtained may not be a very effective adsorbent and it is 'activated' by heating in steam or carbon dioxide at about 950°C in order to drive out the hydrocarbons adsorbed during the carbonization and probably to increase its surface area. Mineral matter is removed by washing with acids.

Decolorizing Charcoals
Almost any vegetable substance can be destructively distilled to produce a decolorizing char. Some methods are based on carbonizing such materials as sawdust, seaweed, peat, molasses

mixed with a porous substance, e.g. pumice, insoluble salts, etc. This method produces a material similar to bone char in that it has a porous structure as well as considerable mechanical strength. Another method consists of depositing carbon on an inorganic base such as lime, chalk or calcium chloride and after carbonizing the inorganic matter is dissolved out. Sulphuric acid and zinc chloride may also be included to act as activating agents.

Gas Adsorbing Charcoals

The most effective gas adsorbing charcoals are produced by carbonizing dense woods, in particular log wood, lignum vitae and coconut shells. For the adsorption of gases, the charcoals are usually packed in relatively thick beds through which the vapour laden air is passed. High density carbons are necessary to get the maximum volume of charcoal packed into beds or columns and a granular product ensures easy vapour flow.

Standardization of Adsorbents

Standardization of an adsorbent usually involves testing that the adsorbtive capacity does not fall below an acceptable limit. The pharmacopoeial test for the decolorizing power of decolorizing charcoal is based on the partial decolorization of a solution of bromophenol blue which is compared with a standard solution. Charcoal BPC has to comply with a test for adsorption of phenazone from solution and also a test for adsorption of chloroform vapour. These can only be regarded as comparative tests and in practice the only satisfactory standard may be based on determination of adsorption isotherms for the particular solute that is being adsorbed. A charcoal that is effective for gas adsorption is not necessarily the best for adsorbing solute from solution. Some grades of activated charcoals are standardized by titration with methylene blue solutions. A weighed amount of charcoal is dispersed in water and tritrated with a standardized solution of methylene blue. The end point is reached when the supernatant liquid just acquires a blue colour, more easily seen by centrifuging a sample of the suspension or by spotting out on to filter paper. This test can only be used for adsorbents that have extremely high affinity for the solute, otherwise there is no definite end point.

APPLICATIONS OF ADSORPTION

Decolorization

It frequently happens that a chemical is tinted with colouring matter which is not removed in the usual stages of purification involving partition between immiscible solvents, crystallization or precipitation. A colourless solution may be obtained by shaking with about 1 per cent of activated charcoal or animal charcoal, allowing to stand for some time and then filtering.

The process of decolorization should be used with discrimination since charcoal will adsorb, to a greater or lesser extent inorganic and organic compounds. Alkaloids are readily adsorbed by charcoal and decolorization of solutions of these would best be done with a weaker adsorbent such as kieselguhr.

Adsorption of Water Vapour

Alumina and silica gel are powerful adsorbents of water vapour. These desiccants remain as dry powders even on taking up as much as 40 per cent water, and thus possess definite advantages over calcium chloride and phosphorous pentoxide which eventually liquefy on adsorbing water. Refrigerated silica gel has been used as a desiccant in freeze drying where the low temperature increases the efficiency of the adsorption process.

Medicinal Uses

Kaolin, $Al_2(OH)_6SiO_2$, has a sheet-like structure, not unlike that of talc, but one surface of the sheet is formed of aluminium hydroxide residues that are responsible for its capacity to adsorb both basic and acidic intestinal toxins by ion exchange. The reactions take place only at the surface of the kaolin and as a consequence depend on its particle size. However, there is some doubt as to the value of kaolin or charcoal for adsorbing gases, toxins and bacteria from the lower gastrointestinal tract, since passage through the upper tract saturates and deactivates the agent. The effectiveness of these agents may be due to bulk entraining and dispersing bacterial aggregates contributing to beneficial effects in the lower bowel. Activated charcoal is a valuable emergency antidote in poisoning due to alkaloids taken by mouth, but its value is confined to the first phase of therapy when adsorption takes place from the stomach before the alkaloids are absorbed. The simultaneous administration of adsorbents such as magnesium trisilicate, magnesium hydroxide and kaolin with various medicaments may reduce the absorption from the alimentary tract. Cationic medicaments and nitrogeneous bases are likely to be adsorbed by these adsorbents although there is little information on in vivo experiments at the present time. Sorby (1965) studied the effect of attapulgite and charcoal on the absorption of promazine from the gastro-intestinal tract. He found that attapulgite retarded the absorption of promazine but there was little decrease in total availability while charcoal was found to decrease rate and extent of absorption.

Adsorption of Pyrogens

Contamination of injectable fluids by pyrogenic substances causes an undesirable febrile reaction in the patient. While water for injection can be prepared pyrogen-free by taking the proper pre-cautions, this does not overcome the problem of drugs, particularly those prepared from natural sources, that may contain pyrogens. Brindle and Rigby (1946) have reported the effectiveness of activated charcoal for the removal of pyrogen. If the drug is of low molecular weight and present in fairly high concentrations, e.g. injections containing glucose, sodium citrate, calcium gluconate, loss of drug by adsorption is not likely to be significant. However, high molecular weight drugs and in particular nitrogenous bases may be readily lost from solution.

REFERENCES

BARR, M. & ARNISTA, S. A. (1957a) *J. Am. pharm. Ass. (Sci. Edn)* **46**, 486.

BARR, M. & ARNISTA, S. A. (1957b) *J. Am. pharm. Ass. (Sci. Edn)* **46**, 480.

BARR, M. & ARNISTA, S. A. (1957c) *J. Am. pharm. Ass. (Sci. Edn)* **46**, 493.

BATUYIOS, N. A. & BRECHT, E. A. (1957) *J. Am. pharm. Ass. (Sci. Edn)* **46**, 524.

BRINDLE, H. & RIGBY, G. (1946) *J. Pharm. Pharmacol.* **19**, 302.

GREGG, S. J. (1961) *Surface Chemistry of Solids*, 2nd edn London: Chapman & Hall.

SORBY, D. L. (1965) *J. pharm. Sci.* **54**, 677.

7

Ion Exchange and Chromatography

Chromatography is essentially a process for the fractionation of mixtures by continuous partition of the components between two phases, one of which is moving past the other. In principle, there appears to be no restriction on the nature of the mobile and stationary phases nor on the types of equilibria involved in the partition. In practice, the most important applications have involved a liquid mobile phase and a liquid or solid stationary phase.

In adsorption chromatography a solution of the mixture to be fractionated is placed on top of a column of adsorbent and slowly passed through; according to the affinity of the components of the mixture for the adsorbent, they are held in zones at the top of the column. Passage of more solvent through the column, by fractional elution and readsorption, develops the chromatogram by separating the zones of adsorbed material throughout the column, the more strongly adsorbed substances being nearer the top of the column. A developed chromatogram of leaf pigments is illustrated in Fig. 7.1. If the separate zones are readily located by their colour, in ultraviolet light, or by means of a reagent streaked along the extruded column, they are separated by division of the column and eluted with a suitable solvent. As an alternative technique *elution development* is employed, further solvent is passed through the column in order to elute the components successively as shown by suitable chemical or physical tests on the eluate. Where these methods are inapplicable, the eluate is collected in arbitrary fractions and each fraction is examined separately.

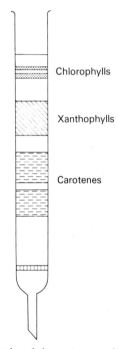

FIG. 7.1. Developed chromatogram of leaf pigments.

In partition chromatography, the column consists of an inert carrier on which is distributed a solvent immiscible with the mobile solvent. Similar principles are exploited in paper chromatography, where selective adsorption on paper or partition between the mobile phase and the water present in paper which has been equilibrated with the saturated vapours of both phases operates to effect the fractionation.

107

Of a number of theoretical treatments of chromatography, the most satisfactory is that of Martin and Synge in which distillation theory is applied to the operation of a column. Although experimental verification of theories of chromatography is available under standard conditions, the optimum conditions for a chromatographic separation are usually worked out empirically.

A useful characteristic of a given set of conditions in a chromatographic system is obtained from the ratio:

$$\frac{\text{Distance moved by solute}}{\text{Distance moved by solvent}} = R_F \text{ or } R$$

The R_F value is of more particular use in partition chromatography, especially on paper, since it is then related to the partition coefficient which remains roughly constant, whereas in adsorption chromatography continuous variation of R is usual. The sequence of the components of a complex mixture is another useful descriptive characteristic since under carefully standardized conditions it is reproducible.

Partition chromatography is suitable for the separation of water-soluble substances while adsorption chromatography finds greater application in the separation of water-insoluble high molecular weight substances.

ADSORPTION CHROMATOGRAPHY

Adsorbents
Among the following commonly used adsorbents of diminishing order of activity: alumina, magnesium oxide, calcium sulphate, calcium oxide, talc, calcium phosphate, calcium carbonate and lactose, together with those whose relative activity has not been thoroughly examined, namely silica, kieselguhr, paper, starch, clays and charcoal, there are enormous variations in adsorptive capacities and specificities which may vary further with the solvents used. A very active alumina is made by heating pure aluminium hydroxide at 380° to 400° for 3 hours or commercial alumina is boiled with successive quantities of water until soluble alkali is removed, then washed with methanol and reactivated by heating at 160° to 200° at 10 mm pressure. In the preliminary selection of an adsorbent, the charge of the mixture placed on the column should be small; in practice, it is frequently possible to fractionate 1 g of a mixture on about 30 g of adsorbent, but the column load influences the degree of fractionation. Chemical changes have

occasionally been observed on very active adsorbents.

Solvents
Fractionation of mixtures of similar substances is often facilitated by elution development with a series of solvents of increasing polarity which exhibit powers of elution in the following ascending order: light petroleum, carbon tetrachloride, cyclohexane, ether, acetone, benzene, esters, chloroform, alcohols, water (at various pH values), pyridine and liquid organic acids. Hydroxylic solvents may cause difficulty because of their solvent action on the adsorbent; thus alumina is appreciably soluble in methanol and in water.

Apparatus and Experimental Methods
The simple device described by Martin is extremely efficient for the preparation of a uniformly packed column. A slurry of adsorbent and solvent of a creamy consistency is poured into the chromatogram tube and thoroughly homogenized by a few rapid strokes of a perforated disc mounted by its centre on a long, thin metal rod. The disc fits the chromatogram tube closely and the diameter of the

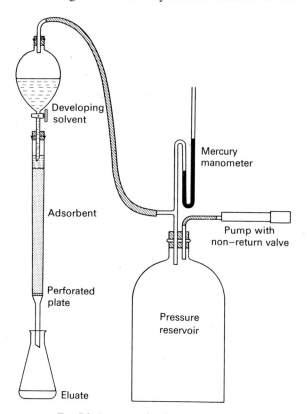

FIG. 7.2. Apparatus for chromatography.

perforations should not be more than about 1.5 mm. The disc is brought to within about 2.5 cm of the bottom of the tube and then moved slowly downwards; this causes the solid to pack beneath it. Rapid homogenizing strokes are followed by slow packing strokes until the whole column is packed. With such columns it is often necessary to accelerate the rate of flow of developing solvent by regulated, positive pressure or suction. A suitable apparatus is illustrated in Fig. 7.2. Even formation of the zones is facilitated by a low rate of flow of developing solvent, uniform pressure and the use of a long column. Unevenness in the development of the zones in large columns is often unavoidable, but is greatly reduced in a multiple column of two or three units with interposed mixing cells. A column built up of filterpaper discs is useful for many purposes.

Location of Zones
For the detection of zones of adsorbed, colourless substances on a column, fluorescence in ultraviolet light, the formation of dark bands on a fluorescent adsorbent or *streak reagents* may be appropriate. Streak reagents are applied with a brush as a longitudinal streak on the extruded column; the zones where a positive reaction is obtained are marked, the surface layer contaminated with the reagent is removed and each zone is separated. Potassium permanganate is a useful streak reagent since it will oxidize many substances and the occurrence of oxidation is made evident by a colour change. The progress of a chromatographic fractionation may frequently be followed by a continuous recording of changes in the physical properties of the issuing eluate; for this purpose changes in conductivity, refractive index and ultra-violet absorbency ratios have been used.

PARTITION CHROMATOGRAPHY

The original partition column, developed by Martin and Synge and intended for the separation of acetylated amino acids, consisted of a column of silica gel on which the stationary phase, water, was distributed; the mobile phase was a water-immiscible solvent saturated with water (chloroform with 1 per cent of *n*-butanol). The individual partition coefficients of the components of the mixture are usually the determining factors in this type of fractionation and under standardized conditions the behaviour of each component of a mixture is summarized in the equation:

$$a = \frac{A_L}{A_S}\left(\frac{1}{R_F} - 1\right)$$

where a = partition coefficient; A_L = cross-sectional area of solvent phase; A_S = cross-sectional area of water phase. Thus components of the mixture that are more soluble in the stationary phase will move slowly down the column. Those components that are very soluble in the moving phase will move more rapidly down the column. Modifications of the stationary and mobile phases and of the support for the stationary phase have led to the application of this technique to a wide range of mixtures.

Types of Partition Column
It appears that to avoid displacement from the support by the mobile phase, the stationary phase must be the more polar. As a consequence, water, buffers or aqueous solutions of acids and bases are most frequently utilized as the stationary phase and a water-immiscible solvent as the mobile phase; other systems, notably reversed-phase systems, are occasionally used. Silica, kieselguhr, starch, powdered cellulose, charcoal and powdered glass are efficient supports for the stationary phase of partition columns. Of these, selected grades of kieselguhr (Hyflo Super Cel and Celite 545) are probably the most generally useful.

Apparatus and Experimental Methods
The apparatus and experimental techniques employed with adsorption columns are used with partition columns. The stationary phase is mixed with the supporting solid by stirring with a rod in a beaker; trituration in a mortar should not be employed. In addition to the methods for the detection of the zones applicable to adsorption columns, suitable indicators may be incorporated in the stationary phase, particularly when mixtures of acids or bases are being examined. Adsorption on the supporting material of a partition column usually leads to a reduction in the operating efficiency of a column.

PAPER CHROMATOGRAPHY

In this process, which was also developed by Martin and Synge, a small spot of solution containing one to several milligrams of a mixture is placed near the top of a strip of filter paper, the end of the paper near the spot is inserted in a trough containing a solvent saturated with water, and the whole is suspended in a suitable chamber whose atmosphere is saturated with the vapours of water and of the solvent. When the solvent has flowed a suitable distance down the paper, the position of the solvent front is marked and the paper is dried. The components of the fractionated mixture are then treated with an appropriate reagent, usually applied by spraying, and finally characterized by comparison of their R_F values with the simultaneously determined values for authentic materials. Caution must be exercised in the characterization of compounds solely on the basis of their R_F values.

In developing a two-dimensional paper chromatogram, the spot of solution is placed near one corner of a square sheet of filter paper and one edge of the sheet is inserted in the solvent trough. After the solvent has flowed nearly to the opposite edge of the sheet, the paper is removed, dried and developed at 90° to the direction of flow of the first solvent with a second solvent in the trough. By using two solvents, the degree of fractionation is greatly enhanced. This is illustrated in Fig. 7.3 for a hypothetical mixture of five components; at stage 2 the components are partially fractionated, and at stage 3 complete fractionation has been effected.

The relative importance of partition and adsorption in effecting fractionation in paper chromatography is doubtful in many cases.

Apparatus and Experimental Methods
Whatman No. 1 filter paper is normally used with solvents usually partially miscible with water and of relatively low volatility, such as *n*-butanol, collidine, lutidine, piperidine, liquefied phenol, although all types of solvent have been used and good results have been obtained with water-miscible solvents.

The scope of this method may be extended by impregnation of the paper with various substances to modify the properties of the stationary phase. The fractionation of water-insoluble substances, e.g. steroids, digitalis glycosides, has been achieved by impregnating filter paper with formamide or glycols and developing with a suitable immiscible solvent.

Among the numerous ingenious modifications of the original experimental techniques, the most important involves development by capillary ascent. For this purpose, the paper strip can be hung from a glass rod fixed in the lid of a tall, glass-stoppered museum jar; the end of the strip adjacent to the spot of the mixture dips into a shallow

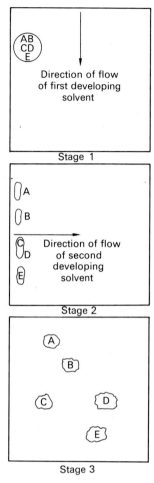

FIG. 7.3. Two-dimensional paper-chromatogram of a hypothetical mixture of A, B, C, D and E.

layer of solvent at the bottom of the jar. The solvent movement is slower than in the descending method and improved resolution of the components is often obtained.

After separation on paper, the components of the original mixture can be eluted without loss and determined quantitatively if a sufficiently sensitive analytical process is known.

Location of Zones
For the detection of colourless substances on a paper chromatogram, a sensitive colour test revealing a number of different substances is most valuable. Ninhydrin is most commonly employed for amino acids; iodine in ethanolic solution or as vapour is useful for most bases, including alkaloids; carbohydrates can be detected by ammoniacal silver nitrate. Certain substances, such as antibiotics

and growth factors, can be detected by their biological effect when the paper is incubated in contact with agar seeded with a selected organism. Radioactive materials can be detected by placing the paper in contact with X-ray film to produce an 'autoradiograph'.

THIN LAYER CHROMATOGRAPHY (TLC)

Instead of using filter paper strips as the supporting media, glass plates are coated with a thin layer of silica gel containing a suitable binding agent. This is achieved by making a slurry of the silica gel with about 13 per cent of plaster of Paris as a binder. This is poured into a spreading device which is drawn across a series of glass plates about 20 cm square. A uniform coating is applied in this way which sets within a few minutes and the plate, after air-drying for about an hour, is heated at 50° overnight. The plates can then be stored over a desiccant until required for use. The sample to be chromatographed is applied in the usual way to one end of the plate and the sample solvent allowed to evaporate. The plate is placed in a glass jar with developing solvent to cover the bottom of the plate to a depth of about 1 cm. The developing solvent ascends by capillarity and the run is usually stopped when the solvent front has moved about three-quarters of the length of the plate. Chloroform, benzene, and mixtures of these with methyl alcohol, are commonly used as developing solvents. For the separation of alkaloids, suitable buffer solutions can be incorporated in the silica gel slurry prior to spreading the plates. The technique is not limited to partition chromatography as it is just as convenient to coat plates with adsorbent powders such as alumina. The advantages of thin layer chromatography over paper chromatography are that separations can be obtained in about 30 minutes, the resolution is often better and a wider range of spray reagents can be used without decomposing the inert support. For instance, corrosive solutions such as hydrochloric or sulphuric acid reagents, unsuitable for use with filter paper, can be used satisfactorily.

GAS CHROMATOGRAPHY (VAPOUR PHASE CHROMATOGRAPHY)

This method was introduced by James and Martin in 1952 for the separation and analysis of volatile materials, i.e. materials that boil below about 300°. The moving phase is an inert gas such as nitrogen and the stationary phase is generally a non-volatile liquid, e.g. silicone oil, mineral oil or polyethyleneglycols mixed with kieselguhr. Kieselguhr is a porous, inert material which holds the stationary phase in the column. A constant flow of nitrogen is passed through the column which is several feet long, and which is maintained at a temperature above the boiling points of the components to be separated (Fig. 7.4). The mixture is injected into the

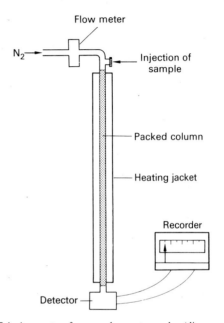

Fig. 7.4. Apparatus for gas chromatography (diagrammatic).

gas stream where it enters the column and immediately vaporizes. The vapour is carried forwards and is distributed between the stationary phase and the moving gas phase (cf. partition chromatography), so that materials which are less volatile and/or more soluble in the stationary phase will tend to move slowly through the column. Different rates of movement of the components will result in their separation. The gas emerging from the end of the column passes through a suitable detector whose function is to produce an electrical current which is proportional to the concentration of vapour present in the carrier gas. A cathetometer is commonly used as a detector. It consists of a thin wire heated by an electric current. The temperature of the wire and hence its resistance varies with the thermal conductivity of the gas surrounding it. The change in electrical resistance can be followed by a suitable potentiometer of the recording type so that the components, as they emerge from the column, are recorded automatically in graphical

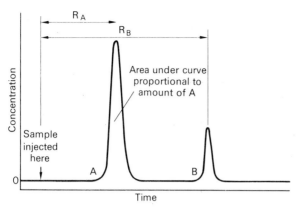

FIG. 7.5. Gas chromatography of mixture of two components, A and B. R_A = Retention time of A. R_B = Retention time of B.

form. Fig. 7.5 represents a result for a mixture of two components A and B.

The time taken for a particular substance to pass through a gas–liquid column operated under standard conditions is a characteristic property of that substance. This *retention time* can be used to aid identification of a substance in the same way that R_F values are used in partition chromatography. The area under the peak is proportional to the amount of substance present so that quantitative analysis is possible from examination of the graph. The advantages of gas chromatography are that separations can be achieved in about 20 minutes and the same column used repeatedly. The method has been used for the identification of components of essential oils, separation of fatty acid esters and hydrocarbons, etc.

APPLICATIONS

A comparison of chromatography with other important general methods for the separation of mixtures, such as distillation, sublimation, fractional crystallization, partition and chemical separations, shows that it possesses two extremely valuable features; it is applicable to small quantities of material and the conditions of operation normally cause no change in the components of the mixture being separated. Its applications to pharmacy are now so extensive that no more than a general indication of its uses can be given.

Pharmaceutical Analysis

Chromatographic methods are of particular value in three types of analytical problem:
(1) Tests for homogeneity of substances liable to contamination with chemically similar substances, such as alkaloids, cardiac glycosides and steroids. Pharmacopoeial test for the absence of related foreign steroids in Betamethasone valerate is performed by paper chromatography.
(2) The identification of pharmaceutical substances and preparations, for example egot alkaloids can be identified by paper chromatography of the amino acids liberated on hydrolysis of the alkaloids.
(3) The determination of the individual components of complex mixtures or of substances in dilute solution. Anthraquinone-containing drugs can be assayed by isolation of the hydroxyanthraquinones on a magnesium oxide–kieselguhr column; these are then eluted and determined spectrophotometrically. Hyoscine and hyoscyamine in solanaceous drugs can be easily determined after separation on a partition column.

Vitamins

Chromatographic methods have been used in the isolation, characterization and determination of many vitamins and allied substances. Vitamin D is separated from other steroids, vitamin A and carotenoids on a column of magnesium oxide and kieselguhr. A method for the determination of the B_{12} vitamins in fermentation liquors and liver extracts involves resolution of the vitamins on paper strips and a microbiological assay.

Antibiotics

Chromatography has been exploited in the isolation of many antibiotics, both on the laboratory and industrial scales. In one method for the assay of penicillins, filter paper is soaked in 30 per cent potassium phosphate buffer of pH 6 to 7 and dried in air; a spot of solution of the mixed sodium salts is then developed on the strip with wet ether and the zones are located by placing the strip on agar inoculated with *Bacillus subtilis*; mixtures of pure penicillins are used as reference standards in the quantitative interpretation of the results.

Radio-isotopes

The absence of radioactive sodium iodate in Sodium Iodide (^{131}I) Injection BP is checked by autoradiograph technique after paper chromatography of the solution. The iodide and iodate ions have different R_F values; all the radioactivity should reside in the iodide ion.

ION EXCHANGE

A substance that can be usefully employed for ion exchange should be insoluble and have the capacity to absorb ions in such a way that they can be reversibly replaced by other ions of the same charge. Thus the reaction can be represented:

$$A^+B^- + C^+D^- \rightleftharpoons A^+D^- + C^+B^-,$$

where A represents a porous insoluble matrix containing the labile ions B^- which are capable of exchanging with anions, in this case, D^- in the surrounding solution. The ions D^- initially distributed throughout the solution must reach the surface of the ion exchange material and then diffuse into the porous matrix so that an equivalent number of B^- ions are released and diffuse out. The exchange proceeds by diffusion throughout the porous material until eventually an equilibrium distribution of B^- and D^- ions is reached. The rate-limiting factor in this exchange reaction is therefore the diffusional process, and this results in the overall rate of reaction being much slower than a chemical reaction in homogeneous solution.

Cation Exchange in Silicates
The natural zeolites were among the first materials to be used for water softening. They are capable of removing unwanted magnesium and calcium ions from hard water and replacing them with sodium ions. The zeolites belong to the class of clay minerals which can be regarded as being built up from an 'aluminosilicate' skeleton together with a sufficient number of cations such as Li^+, Na^+, K^+, Mg^{2+}, Ca^{2+} to neutralize any excess charge on the skeleton. Some or all of these cations are exchangeable for others of equivalent charge provided they can penetrate the pores of the network. The zeolite, analcite $NaAlSiO_6.H_2O$ can be quantitatively converted into $KAlSiO_6.H_2O$ by prolonged leaching with potassium chloride solution. The synthetic aluminosilicates are analogous to the zeolites but their structure consists of irregular pores unlike the perfectly uniform interstices of the zeolite crystals.
Many clay minerals consist of stacks of flat aluminosilicate sheets with the cations attached to the surface of the sheets. The sheet to sheet distance in clays such as mica is about 1 nm so that the exchangeable cations are largely confined to the edges of the sheets. The montmorillonite group of minerals, which includes clays of pharmaceutical importance, e.g. bentonite, attapulgite, has a different layer structure when swells in water due to the penetration of at least two monolayers of water. Swollen sodium bentonite has a multiple sandwich structure with 1 nm layers of water between 1 nm layers of alumino-silicate which enables monovalent and divalent ions to diffuse along the water

filled planes. This accounts for the high exchange capacity of sodium montmorillonites compared with the non-expanding minerals such as illite. The cation exchange capacities of some typical silicates is shown in Table 7.1. Kaolinite

TABLE 7.1

CATION-EXCHANGE CAPACITIES OF SOME TYPICAL SILICATES (AFTER KITCHENER 1957) (mEq/100 g AT pH 7)

Structural type	Mineral	Formula (idealized)	Exchange capacity
Layer lattice (non-expanding)	Kaolinite Illite	$Al_2O_3.2SiO_2.2H_2O$ $(OH)_4K_2(Si_6Al_2)Al_4O_{20}$	3–15 30–40
Layer lattice (expanding)	Mont-morillon-ite	$NaAl_5MgSi_{12}O_{30}(OH)_6$	90–110
Zeolite: open network lattice	Analcite	$NaAlSi_2O_6.H_2O$	588
Amorphous alumino-silicate gel	Synthetic 'Permu-tite'	$Na_2O.Al_2O_2.nSiO_2.H_2O$ $n \approx 5\text{–}6$	150

$Al_2O_32SiO_2.2H_2O$ (natural mineral is kaolin) has a non-expanding lattice and from its structure would appear to have no cations to exchange. However, in practice it takes up 3–15 mEq or even more after prolonged grinding in a mill. This exchange capacity is likely to arise from the broken edges of the silica sheets where the Si–O–Si–O–Si planes are terminated by 5-OH groups. These are only weakly acidic, dissociating as $-S-O^- + H^+$. Additional cation exchange capacity may be due to isomorphous replacement within the sheets, g. Al^{3+} in place of Si^{4+} or Mg^{2+} for Al^{3+} which leaves a net negative charge on the sheet.

Carbonaceous Exchangers
The sulphonation of certain soft coals produces a dark insoluble granular mass with mainly $-SO_3H$ units attached to the aromatic matrix of the coal. These exchangers replace cations by hydrogen ions and are used in the processing of water for chemical plant.

Ion Exchange Resins
The first synthetic ion exchange resins were invented by Adams and Holmes in 1935, whose target was to 'tailor-make' resins for anion and cation exchange. The cation exchange resins were prepared

by condensation of dihydric phenols with formaldehyde so that the OH groups were free and still retained their acidic nature. To introduce stronger acidic groups ($-SO_3H$) the resin was sulphonated after preparation, or phenyl-sulphonic acid was substituted for the phenol in the preparation of the resin. Anion exchange resins were made in a similar way by condensation of amines such as *m*-phenylenediamine with formaldehyde.

Most present day ion exchange resins are prepared by emulsion polymerization techniques which result in well-defined composition of the early condensation resins. An example of this reaction is the polymerization of the unsaturated monomer of the type $CH_2{=}CHX$ which undergoes a chain reaction leading to the structure:

$$-CH_2{-}CH{-}CH_2{-}CH{-}.$$
$$\quad\quad\ \ | \quad\quad\quad\ \ |$$
$$\quad\quad\ \ X \quad\quad\quad\ X$$

This chain polymer is still soluble in certain solvents and in order to produce an insoluble resin it is necessary to incorporate a bifunctional monomer, generally a divinyl compound:

$$CH_2{=}CH{-}R{-}CH{=}CH_2$$

This produces cross linking of the polymer chains and renders the product insoluble. An example of a cation exchange resin prepared by *co-polymerization* is the reaction between styrene $C_6H_5{-}CH{=}CH$ and divinyl benzene $CH_2{=}CH{-}C_6H_4.CH{=}CH_2$. The resultant *co-polymer* is sulphonated with concentrated sulphuric acid.

$$...CH_2{-}CH{-}CH_2{-}CH...$$

$$...CH_2{-}CH{-}CH_2{-}CH{-}CH_2{-}CH...$$

The $-SO_3H$ groups attached to an insoluble polymer matrix are ionizable so that the H^+ is capable of exchanging with other cations in the solution which is in contact with the resin. The polymerization of an emulsion or coarse suspension of the monomer produces a resin in the form of beads of controlled size which are convenient for handling both in the processing operation and in the final usage of the product.

The synthesis of anion exchange resins follows a similar procedure, starting with a cross-linked polystyrene resin and then treating with CH_2ClOCH_3 in the presence of a catalyst (Friedel–Crafts reaction) so that $-CH_2Cl$ groups are attached to the benzene rings in the polymer. A quaternary ammonium resin is then produced by treatment with a tertiary amine:

$$-CH_2Cl + N(CH_3)_3 \longrightarrow -CH_2N(CH_3)_3Cl^-$$

Other resins can be similarly synthesized where the functional groups vary in basic strength; amino groups attached to aromatic nuclei are weak bases but when they are attached to the macromolecular skeleton in the same manner as aliphatic amino groups they give relatively strong bases. Resins containing quaternary ammonium hydroxide functional groups behave as very strong bases.

Cation exchange reactions are reversible and the portion of the equilibrium depends on the proportion of the resin and the electrolyte. When the functional group is $-SO_3H$, the resin RSO_3H is in effect a strong acid and exchange will occur when cations in the ambient solution are combined with the conjugate base of a weak or strong acid, e.g. Cl^- is the conjugate base of the strong acid, HCl, and the following exchange reaction will occur:

$$RSO_3^-H^+ + NaCl \rightleftharpoons RSO_3^-Na^+ + H^+Cl^-$$

Solid resin | Ambient solution | Solid resin | Ambient solution

With the weakly acidic $-COOH$ as the group responsible for the exchange, only cations combined with the conjugate base of a weak acid will undergo exchange:

$$R.COO^-H^+ + CH_3COO^-Na^+$$

Solid resin | Ambient solution

$$\rightleftharpoons R.COO^-Na^+ + CH_3COOH$$

Solid resin | Ambient solution

Phenolic groups are so weakly acidic that exchange occurs only in alkaline solution:

$$ROH + Na^+OH^- \rightleftharpoons RO^-Na^+ + H_2O$$

Solid resin | Ambient solution | Solid resin | Ambient solution

These differences can be exploited for selective exchanges.

The cation taken up by the exchanger can be displaced by washing the resin with mineral acid, whereby the exchanger is converted into its original form and if desired the displaced cation can be recovered.

These synthetic resins are stable in strongly acid or alkaline solutions and can be repeatedly regenerated without decomposition.

Anion exchange reactions with resins containing quaternary ammonium groups $-N^{\pm}$ show reversible anion exchange:

$$RN^+(CH_3)OH + NaCl$$
Solid resin   Ambient solution

$$\rightleftharpoons RN^+(CH_3)Cl^- + NaOH$$
Solid resin   Ambient solution

The resins containing primary, $-NH_2$ or secondary, $=NH$ amino groups do not act as exchangers but can combine with acids as follows:

$$RNH_2 + HCl \rightleftharpoons RNH_3^+Cl^-$$
Solid resin   Ambient solution   Solid resin

The anion fixed by the resin can be displaced by an alkali such as sodium hydroxide. Weak base resins can be regenerated with sodium carbonate.

BEHAVIOUR OF ION EXCHANGERS

No reliable theoretical treatment of ion exchange has yet been developed; an experimental determination of the behaviour of an exchanger is often required. The exchanger is stirred with a series of solutions of the exchanging ion; the equilibrium concentrations in the ambient solution of the two ions undergoing exchange are determined and an *exchange isotherm* summarizing the properties of the exchange can then be plotted.

Exchange Capacity
The capacity of exchangers is usually stated in terms of the uptake of an ion per gram of dry exchanger; the units used for expressing the quantity of the ion are thousandths of its chemical equivalent (mEq). Approximate capacities are given in Table 7.2

Exchange usually takes place fairly rapidly but some aluminosilicates may require 2 to 3 days to attain equilibrium. Within the temperature range at which exchangers are stable, temperature has little effect on the position of equilibrium. It is probable that with many exchangers some surface adsorption and occlusion of solutes occurs simultaneously with exchange.

Exchange equilibria are controlled by a number of factors not directly related to the nature of the

TABLE 7.2

Exchanger	Active groups	Maximum capacity (mEq/M)
	Cationic exchangers	
Zeo-Karb 215* Amberlite IR–1† Wofatit KS‡	$-SO_3H$, $-OH$	2.3–2.5
Zeo-Karb 216* Amberlite IRC–50†	$-COOH$	2.3
Zeo-Karb 225* Amberlite IR–120†	$-SO_3H$	5
Decalso*	Alumino-silicate	0.8
	Anionic exchangers	
De Acidite E* Amberlite IR–4B†	weakly basic groups	4–5
De Acidite FF* Amberlite IRA–400†	Quaternary ammonium groups	2.3

* Permutit Co.
† Resinous Products & Chemical Co.
‡ I.G. Farbenindustrie AG

exchangers. For cations of the same charge, the size of the hydrated ion in solution is the determining factor; for cations of roughly the same size, e.g. Cs^+, Ba^{2+}, La^{3+}, the uptake increases with ionic charge. Correlations of this type have not been detected for anions but the following order of affinity of acids has been found experimentally: $H_3PO_4 > H_2SO_4 > HNO_3 > HCl$; salicylic > citric > acetic > formic > oxalic > benzoic. These differences in the affinities of ions can be exploited for their separation by procedures essentially similar to those employed in chromatography.

Use of Ion Exchangers
Since ion exchange proceeds to a definite equilibrium, a single contact of the ion exchanger with the solution will not give efficient ion exchange. By flowing the solution through a column of ion exchanger, the reaction will go to completion as follows:

e.g.
$$RSO_3^-H^+ + Na^+Cl^- \rightarrow RSO_3^-Na^+ + H^+Cl^-.$$

The apparatus used is essentially similar to that used in chromatography. In a typical exchange of a cation by the hydrogen ion, the cation exchanger, in bead or coarse powder form, is soaked for an hour, with occasional stirring, in 2 volumes of 2 M hydrochloric acid to allow for swelling and to convert the resin into its hydrogen form. It is then transferred to a chromatogram tube of about twice the volume of the resin. To displace air and fine powder, water is passed upwards through the bed of resin until the effluent is free from suspended matter and the excess of supernatant water is drained down to the level of the bed. A volume of 2 M hydrochloric acid equal to the volume of the column of resin is then slowly drained downward through the column; the effluent should be strongly acid. Excess acid is then removed by thorough washing with water. The solution for ion exchange is then passed through the column; if the acidity of the effluent begins to fall before all the solution has passed through, the column is backwashed with water and regenerated by downflow of one resin-column volume of 2 M hydrochloric acid.

APPLICATIONS

Deionization

All the ions can be removed from a solution by using both an anion and a cation exchanger in series or as a mixed bed. For the deionization of water, the mixed bed method is most effective. The bed consists of a mixture of the bead forms of a strong acid exchanger which removes cations (Ca^{2+}, Mg^{2+}) and a strong base exchanger which removes anions (SO_4^{2-}, Cl^-, CO_3^{2-}, HCO_3^-). The electrical resistance of the effluent can be used to assess the quality of the water. Using a mixed bed column, water of specific resistance of 10 MΩ/cm is readily obtained, which is comparable with conductivity water prepared by repeated distillation in a quartz still. For regeneration the two components are separated by back-washing with water; the less dense anion exchanger is then segregated as the upper layer above the denser cation exchanger. The upper and lower layers are separated, regenerated with alkali and acid respectively, rinsed and re-mixed by passing an air stream through the column. By this means, a 2.5-cm column, 1 m high, will yield 22.5 l per hour of water purer with regard to ionic components than distilled water. Purified Water BP may be prepared by ion exchange methods, as an alternative to distillation.

In deionization, by means of a cation and an anion exchanger in series, the effluent from the cation exchanger column is acid:

$$R.SO_3^-H^+ + A^+B^- \rightleftharpoons R.SO_3^-A^+ + H^+B^-$$

| Cation exchanger | Influent solution | Cation exchanger | Effluent solution |

The mixed bed technique does not suffer from this disadvantage and can therefore be used in place of dialysis for the removal of ions from solutions of acid-sensitive colloids. Both methods can be usefully applied to the deionization of an impure solution of any non-electrolyte. Examples of such deionizations are provided by the purification of sucrose, glucose, glycerol, penicillin and enzymes. Iron is removed from lactic acid solutions by passage through a cation exchanger and formaldehyde solutions are deacidified by an anion exchanger.

Exchange of Ionic Constituents

In water softening, calcium and magnesium ions are replaced by sodium ions from a cation exchanger. Potassium salts of penicillins can be converted into sodium salts by cation exchange and streptomycin sulphate is converted into the chloride by anion exchange.

Potassium salts of penicillins can be converted into sodium salts by cation exchange and streptomycin sulphate is converted into the chloride by anion exchange.

Separations of ionic compounds have been achieved by exchangers which take up only one component or group of components of a mixture, e.g. the absorption of basic amino acids in a protein hydrolysate on a carboxyl exchanger, or by chromatographic separation when all the components are absorbed. In the separation of a mixture of amino acids on a sulphonic acid resin, the components of the mixture are absorbed at the top of the column in an order depending on the basic strength of their amino groups; the column is then eluted with a solution of a stronger base and the amino acids pass out of the column in order of their affinities for the resin. Streptomycin can be absorbed on Decalso and, after elution of impurities which are not absorbed, the streptomycin is recovered by washing with sodium chloride solution. Ionic materials can be removed from penicillin solutions by means of columns of anion and cation exchangers in series; the penicillin is not absorbed. Ion exchangers have found extensive applications in the separation of rare earth metals and isotopes.

Recovery Processes

Ion exchangers are extremely useful for the recovery of small quantities of valuable ionic substances from large volumes of solutions containing non-ionic waste products, for example aneurine can be simply recovered from brewery and yeast wastes.

MEDICINAL USES OF ION EXCHANGE RESINS

Prolongation of Drug Action

Ion exchange resins are used to form chemical complexes of acidic and basic drugs which are administered by mouth in order to prolong drug action. Basic drugs such as ephedrine and amphetamine have been combined with cation exchange resins, and to a limited extent acidic drugs, e.g. barbiturate, have been used in combination with anion exchange resins.

The rate of release of the drug from the resin beads depends on the diameter of the beads and the degree of cross linking of the polymer. Both these factors will influence the rate of diffusion of ions through the resin. The acid or basic strength of the resin will also affect the rate of release of basic or acidic drugs in the presence of electrolyte. In the formulation of basic drugs, generally strong acid resins are used, e.g. RSO_3H in order to obtain a reasonably slow rate of release in the acid environment of the stomach. Weak acid types, e.g. $RCOOH$ release the base too rapidly. Amphetamine combined with a cation exchange resin undergoes the following reactions when administered orally:

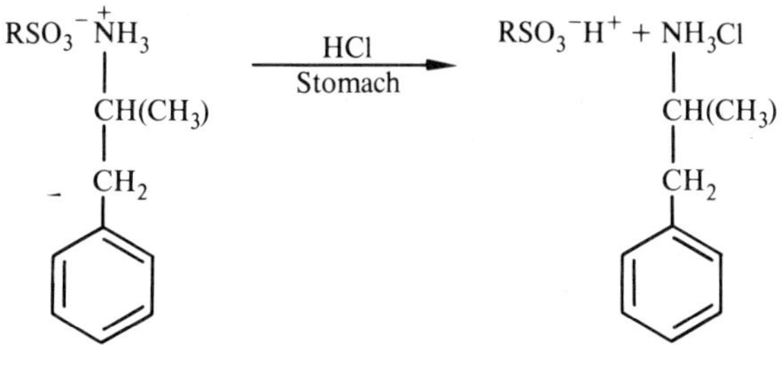

Drug resinate   Amphetamine chloride

Any unchanged drug resin passing from the stomach into the intestine will undergo the following reaction:

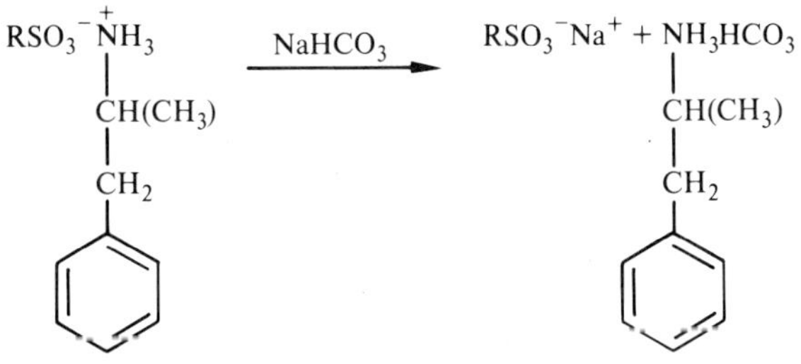

Drug resinate   Amphetamine bicarbonate

The released amphetamine chloride or bicarbonate is then absorbed through the wall of the intestine and the insoluble resin RSO_3Na^+ is excreted. The rate of release of dexamphetamine and ephedrine in vitro has been studied by Chaudry and Saunders (1956).

Resin complexes are also useful in disguising the taste of bitter ionic drugs although in these cases, prolonged action may not be required and a weak acid or basic resin would then be necessary. Ion exchange resins for prolonging drug action are in fine bead form and have a gritty texture when taken by mouth so that it is usual to administer them in tablet form.

Antacids

Weak anion exchange resins have been used as antacids for the relief of symptoms in the treatment of peptic ulcer. The resin combines with the hydrochloric acid in the stomach which is later released in the alkaline conditions of the intestine. The resin is thus excreted unchanged so that there is no ionic disturbance of the ionic content of the body fluids. The reaction can be represented as:

$$\underset{\text{Resin}}{RNH_2} \xrightarrow[\text{Stomach}]{HCl} RNH_3^+Cl^- \xrightarrow[\text{Intestine}]{NaHCO_3}$$

$$\underset{\text{Resin}}{R.NH_2} + NaCl + H_2O + CO_2$$

The resin is usually finely powdered and flavoured to make it palatable.

Control of Electrolyte Balance

Cation exchange resins administered by mouth exchange their cations with those present in the gut and hence effect changes in the electrolyte balance in the plasma. Abnormal physiological conditions in which there is retention of sodium and water, as for instance in cardiac failure, renal disease and toxaemia of pregnancy can be treated by these resins (Payne 1956). The resin is usually the ammonium form, part of which is replaced by the potassium form to prevent undesirable potassium depletion. A side effect of this treatment is the production of acidosis due to the liberation of NH_4^+ ions which on metabolism in the liver produce H^+. It is of course essential that laboratory facilities are available so that a constant check can be kept on the electrolyte balance of the patient being treated by ion exchange resins. An additional hazard of this treatment would be the depletion of essential ions such as Ca^{2+} and Mg^{2+}.

REFERENCES

BUCHI, J. (1956) *J. Pharm. Pharmacol.* **8**, 369.

CHAUDRY, N. C. & SAUNDERS, L. (1956) *J. Pharm. Pharmacol.* **8**, 975.

KITCHENER, J. A. (1957) *Ion Exchange Resins.* London: Methuen.

MARTINDALE, W. (1972) *The Extra Pharmacopoeia*, 26th edn. London: Pharmaceutical Press.

PARTRIDGE, M. W. (1952) *J. Pharm. Pharmacol.* **4**, 217.

PAYNE, W. W. (1956) *J. Pharm. Pharmacol.* **8**, 397.

8

Diffusion

Diffusion is the migration of molecules from a region of high concentration to a region of lower concentration and is a result of the Brownian movement of the solute molecules. The phenomenon of diffusion can be observed if a crystal of copper sulphate is placed in a beaker of water. A saturated solution of copper sulphate forms around the crystal and the coloured zone gradually extends by diffusion until eventually there is a uniform concentration throughout. The migration of solute molecules in the absence of external forces such as movement of the solution by convection gradients is a measure of the escaping tendency of the solute to achieve an equilibrium state. A similar situation arises if a semi-permeable membrane separates two solutions of unequal concentration, when the equilibrium is restored by the diffusion of the solvent molecules through the membrane, i.e. osmosis. Thus, osmosis is concerned with the escaping tendency of solvent molecules, and diffusion with the escaping tendency of the solute. The forces involved in the two processes are equal in magnitude but opposite in direction (Alexander & Johnson 1949)

Fick's First Law of Diffusion
By analogy with the processes involved in heat conduction, this law states that the amount of substance d_m diffusing in the x direction in time dt across an area A is proportional to the concentration gradient dc/dx in the plane of the area:

$$d_m = -DA \frac{dc}{dx} \cdot dt.$$

The proportionality factor D is called the diffusion coefficient. (The negative sign denotes that diffusion takes place in the direction of decreasing concentration.) D is not strictly a constant, since it varies slightly with concentration but it can be regarded as a mean value for the concentration range covered. The dimensions of D are length^2/time.

Fick's Second Law of Diffusion
This is derived from the first law by eliminating the dependent variable m, and expresses the rate of change of concentration at any point:

$$\frac{dc}{dt} = \frac{D d^2 c}{dx^2}.$$

Diffusion and Molecular Properties
The diffusion of colloidal particles is related to the frictional coefficient f, of the particles by Einstein's law of diffusion:

$$Df = kT,$$

where k is the Boltzmann constant and T absolute temperature. For spherical particles the frictional coefficient is given by Stokes' law:

$$f = 6\pi\eta r,$$

where η is the viscosity of the medium and r the radius of the particle.
   Therefore, for spherical particles:

$$D = \frac{kT}{6\pi\eta r} = \frac{RT}{6\pi\eta r N},$$

where R is the gas constant and N the Avogadro number. The effect of temperature and viscosity on diffusion is apparent from this equation as $D \propto (T/\eta)$ for a given solute. For non-spherical molecules the frictional coefficient increases with decreasing symmetry and with particle solvation, e.g. hydration.

MEASUREMENT OF DIFFUSION

Porous Disc Method. A sintered glass disc separates the solvent and solution so that a concentration gradient occurs in the pores of the disc (Fig. 8.1). The liquid in the pores is immobilized

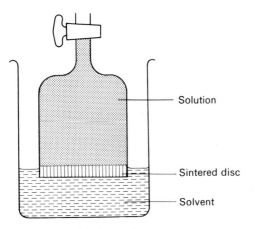

FIG. 8.1. Porous disc apparatus.

and freed from the influence of external disturbance, so that the transport of solute through the pores is due solely to diffusion. Homogeneity of the separate phases is effected by slight convection currents, gentle stirring or rotation of the cell. For small concentration changes Fick's first law can be applied:

$$m = \frac{-DA(C_1 - C_2)}{L}(t_1 - t_2),$$

where m is the amount of solute diffused, C_1 and C_2 are the concentrations of solute on either side of the disc at time t_1 and t_2, A is the cross-section of the pores and L is the effective length of the pores. The quantities A and L are not directly measurable but the ratio A/L can be obtained by calibrating the cell with a solute of known D, e.g. KCl. The method is simple but has the following possible objections: (a) the calibration of the cell with very low molecular weight solutes may not be valid for high molecular weight solutes, especially if molecules of the latter are markedly assymmetric; and (b) entrapped air bubbles in the pores or adsorption of solute would invalidate the results.

Free Boundary Method. An initially sharp boundary is formed between the solvent and solution in a specially constructed diffusion cell. The diffusion is followed by measuring the concentration gradient along the cell by optical methods such as light refraction or light absorption. Very accurate temperature control is essential as convection gradients must be eliminated, since these would disturb the concentration gradient. The change of concentration gradient dc/dt at different times t, is shown in Fig. 8.2. These curves take the shape of Gaussian

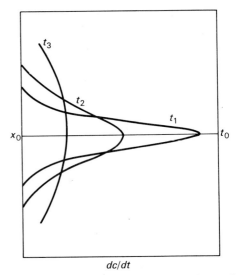

FIG. 8.2. Concentration gradient at different times after formation of sharp boundary ($t_3 > t_2 > t_1$).

distribution curves represented by the equation:

$$\frac{dc}{dt} = \frac{-C_o e^{-x^2/4Dt}}{\sqrt{4\pi Dt}},$$

where C_o is the concentration of solute when $t = 0$. The diffusion coefficient of the sodium dodecylsulphate has been determined by this method (Brudney & Saunders 1955).

Diffusion through gels. The rate of diffusion of low molecular weight solutes through dilute aqueous gels of gelatin and agar is nearly the same as in water alone, provided that chemical interaction and adsorption effects are absent. This is not surprising when one considers that a semi-solid gel of agar could contain as much as 99 per cent water. This water, immobilized by the network structure of the gel, is a continuous phase through which solute can diffuse. As the concentration of gelling substance is increased, the pore size of the gel decreases and the rate of diffusion will fall rapidly when the pore size is comparable with the size of the diffusing molecule. In addition to this sieve-like action of the gel, other factors such as the viscosity of the liquid within the pores will affect the diffusion rate. If the mesh possesses ionizable groups of opposite charge to that of the diffusing particle, adsorption or ion exchange reactions may occur. Agar is an acidic polysaccharide which forms a gel with water at concentrations as low as 0.5 per cent. One-half ester sulphate is present in about 8 to 50 galactose units giving rise to a negatively charged mesh on ionization of the $-O-SO_3H$ groups. These anionic groups will interact with cations such as the basic dyes and quaternary ammonium compounds and retard their diffusion. This can be overcome to some extent by the inclusion of suitable electrolytes in the gel to decrease the ionization of the diffusing molecules. In the case of diffusion through aqueous gelatin gels, the pH of the gel will influence the ionization of the $-NH_2$ and $-COOH$ groups. On the acid side, the isoelectric point, the gel will be positively charged, while on the alkaline side it will be negatively charged (see p. 94).

Let us now consider the diffusion of neutral particles. Fig. 8.3 represents a cylinder of gel in

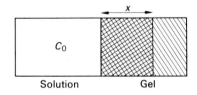

FIG. 8.3. Diffusion of solute from solution into gel.

contact with a solution of concentration C_o. Assuming that the solution is homogeneous and of constant concentration, the relationship between the diffusion coefficient and the concentration of the solute C at a distance x from the gel/solution boundary is given by:

$$C = C_{oe}\left(\frac{-x^2}{4Dt}\right),$$

or

$$1nC = \ln C - \frac{x^2}{4Dt},$$

which may be written with logarithms to the base 10 as:

$$2.301 \times 4D(\log C_o - \log C) = \frac{x^2}{t}.$$

Thus a plot of x^2 against t should be a straight line with a slope of $2.301 \times 4D(\log C_o - C)$ enabling D to be calculated.

Cooper and Woodman (1946) found this equation to apply to the diffusion of crystal violet in agar gels. Sodium chloride was included in the gel to repress the ionization of the dye. The migration of the dye could be followed visually and the coloured edge was matched with a tube containing $1 : 500\,000$ crystal violet ($C = 2 \times 10^{-6}$).

An alternative method of determining D in gels is to dissolve the solute in the gel and follow the rate of diffusion into water in contact with the gel. Nixon, Georgakopoulis and Carless (1967) studied the rate of diffusion of methylene blue from gelatin–glycerin gels using this method.

Cup plate methods of assay of antibiotics are dependent on diffusion through agar gels previously seeded with a test organism. After incubation, the organisms fail to grow where the antibiotic has reached a sufficiently high concentration so that the zone of inhibition can be correlated with antibiotic potency.

Diffusion Through Membranes
Membranes have already been mentioned in connection with dialysis (p. 87) which enables small molecules to be separated from macromolecules. All membranes have a gel-like structure and although the 'pore size' is referred to it should be noted that the pores are not uniform channels but are tortuous, resulting from the random network structure of the gel. The pore size will be affected by the liquid content of the gel, and swelling will result in an increased pore size. Artificial membranes can be prepared from regenerated cellulose (Cellophane), cellulose acetate, etc. (Alexander & Johnson 1949). Natural membranes are usually quite thin, frequently only 10 nm or so in thickness. The permeability of these plays an important part in the rate of absorption of a drug which has to pass through cell membranes to reach its site of action. Permeability can sometimes be explained on the basis of physico-chemical mechanisms (passive transport) but it cannot explain the transport of solutes against a concentration gradient which is mediated through enzymatic action (active transport). This chapter will be concerned only with passive transport and will attempt to indicate the physico-chemical principles that can assist in correlating drug properties with permeability. For instance the relatively rapid passage of a low molecular weight solute across a membrane could be depicted by Fick's first law, although the situation would be complicated for low transport rates by the osmotic flow of water in the opposite direction. Some saline cathartics exert their action

in this way by causing an influx of water into the gastrointestinal tract.

The rates of absorption of orally administered weakly acidic and weakly basic drugs is of particular interest (Brodie 1964). Their absorption can be explained by passive diffusion of the unionized molecular species through the lipoidal membrane of the gastrointestinal tract. The unionized species are generally lipid soluble in contrast to the ionized species which are insoluble in lipid but soluble in water. The proportion of ionized–unionized molecules will thus control the solubility in the lipid, and can be estimated from a knowledge of the pK_a of the drug and the pH of the environment (see p. 23).

A simple model representing the gastrointestinal fluid, the gastrointestinal membrane, and blood as separate compartments is represented in Fig. 8.4. The aqueous phases A (pH 2.0) and C (pH 7.4) represent the alimentary tract and blood compartments respectively. B is the immiscible lipid phase. The driving force, which transports drug from A across the two interfaces will depend on the partition coefficients between A/B and B/C which will be controlled by the pK_a and pH. The ratio of concentration of the drug in the two compartments A and C at equilibrium is given by:

$$\frac{\text{Concentration A}}{\text{Concentration C}} = \frac{1 + 10^{(pK_a - 2)}}{1 + 10^{(pK_a - 7.4)}}$$

$\cdots$ for basic drug,

$$\frac{\text{Concentration A}}{\text{Concentration C}} = \frac{1 + 10^{(2 - pK_a)}}{1 + 10^{(7.4 - pK_a)}}$$

$\cdots$ for acidic drug.

Perrin (1967), using a partitioned cell, studied the rates of transfer of salicylic acid (pK_a 2.96) and amidopyrine(pK_a 5.1) between aqueous buffers (pH 2 and pH 7.4) and an insoluble organic solvent as an in vitro model for a lipoidal membrane. Assuming that the rate of transport followed first

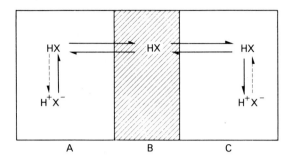

FIG. 8.4. Partition model of acidic drug. A, aqueous phase, pH 2; B, organic phase; C, aqueous phase, pH 7.4 HX, unionized acid; H^+X^-, ionized acid.

order reaction kinetics, the theoretical rates could be correlated with experimental results.

DIFFUSION OF DRUGS FROM DOSAGE FORMS

Sustained release of drugs from tablets has been obtained by incorporating the drug in an insoluble matrix such as plastic resin, wax and fatty alcohol. When brought into contact with the gastrointestinal fluid the drug particles will be slowly leached out as the fluid penetrates the pores of the tablet. Diffusion of the solute through the liquid-filled tortuous paths will play a significant part provided that the tablet retains its framework during the process. Higuchi (1963) suggested that the rate of release of drug from one surface of an insoluble matrix would be governed by the relationship:

$$Q = \left[\frac{D\varepsilon C_s}{\tau} (2A - \varepsilon C_s) t \right]^{1/2},$$

where Q is the amount of drug released per unit area at time t, D is the diffusion coefficient, ε is the porosity of the matrix, C_s is the solubility of the drug, τ is the tortuosity of the matrix and A is the concentration of the drug in the tablet. Desai, Simonelli and Higuchi (1965), discussed the applicability of this equation to the rate of release of sodium salicylate from plastic matrices.

REFERENCES

ALEXANDER, A. E. & JOHNSON, P. (1949) Colloid Science. London: Oxford University Press.

BRODIE, B. (1964) Absorption and Distribution of Drugs (Ed. T. B. Binns). Edinburgh: Livingstone.

BRUDNEY, N. & SAUNDERS, L. (1955) J. Pharm. Pharmacol. 7, 1012.

COOPER, K. E. & WOODMAN, D. (1946) J. Path. Bact. 58, 75.

DESAI, S. J. SIMONELLI, A. P. & HIGUCHI, W. I. (1965) J. Pharm. Sci. 54, 1459.

HIGUCHI, T. (1963) J. Pharm. Sci. 52, 1145.

NIXON, J. R., GEORGAKOPOULIS, P. P. & CARLESS, J. E. (1967) J. Pharm. Pharmacol. 19, 246.

PERRIN, J. (1967) J. Pharm. Pharmacol. 19, 25.

9

Rheology

Rheology is the study of the deformation and flow of matter. A body may deform as a result of a force applied to it and if it is elastic it will return to its original state on removal of the constraining force. As we shall be concerned only with the effects of forces acting uniformly over surfaces, the appropriate measure of these forces is the 'stress', which is a force per unit area. The stress may be applied at right angles or tangentially to the surface and the resulting deformation is known as the 'strain'. The measure of strain is a non-dimensional quantity, a fractional increase or decrease, of length or volume. An ideal elastic body is one in which the strain is directly proportional to the stress and we are able to define a modulus of elasticity which is a ratio of the two parameters. Many materials, however, do not behave in this ideal manner and the deformation may increase with time as long as a stress is applied, or the deformation may not recover completely when the stress is removed. Thus, in characterizing the rheological properties of a body, we are usually concerned with the relations between stress, strain and time.

ELASTIC SOLIDS

Only an elementary treatment will be given in order to introduce the reader to basic concepts. References for further reading are given on p. 139.

MODULUS OF RIGIDITY

Consider a small cube of isotropic material which is subjected to equal forces F applied tangentially over the four faces (Fig. 9.1A) i.e. the cube is subjected to shearing stress (an isotropic material is one in which the physical properties do not depend on direction). The cube is in equilibrium under the action of equal and oppositely opposed couples and we may refer its resulting deformation to the face abcd as a reference plane. The deformed figure has the shape A'B'C'D', abcd. The originally square face ABba has deformed into the rhombus A'B'ba and the amount of deformation can be measured in terms of the angle of shear θ. If L is the length of the side of the cube, the shearing stress $p = F/L^2$ and we can define the 'modulus of rigidity, n, by the equation:

$$n = \frac{p}{\theta}.$$

BULK MODULUS

Consider the cubical body in Fig. 9.1(B) subjected to a uniform hydrostatic pressure, p. If V is the original volume of the body and Δv is the decrease in volume on applying the pressure, then the 'bulk modulus' k is defined by the equation:

$$k = P \left/ \frac{\Delta v}{V} \right. .$$

YOUNG'S MODULUS

If the cube is subjected to a tensile stress (F_2) or a contractile stress (F_1) on two opposite faces (Fig. 9.1C) then Young's modulus, E, is given by:

$$E = p \left/ \frac{\Delta l}{L} \right. ,$$

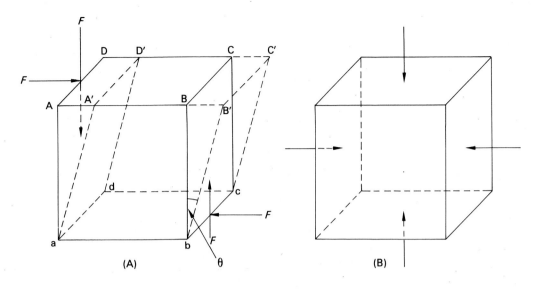

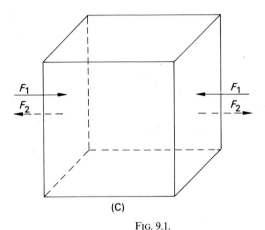

Fig. 9.1.

where Δl = change in length of body in direction of applied stress; L = original length of side of cube.

Young's modulus and the bulk modulus are inter-related by the following equation:

$$E = 3k(1 - 2\sigma),$$

where σ is Poisson's ratio.

This ratio can be defined as the fractional extension at right angles to the applied stress divided by the fractional contraction along the direction of the applied stress. This concept may be visualized if we consider the cube (Fig. 9.1C) subjected to a contractile stress F_1, on the two opposite faces; the remaining faces are unconstrained and we would expect extension of the specimen at right angles to the direction of the force. The quantity

σ is a characteristic of the material and from the equation above cannot be greater than 0.5.

MEASUREMENT OF ELASTICITY

In pharmacy an assessment of the elasticity of gels is important in order to control the quality of gelling agents such as gelatin, agar and pectin. Gelatin gels behave as ideal elastic bodies provided the deformation does not result in the elastic limit being exceeded when irreversible deformation occurs and the gel breaks. Although it is possible to measure the modulus of elasticity of a gel by using cubes of the material and deforming them under a shear stress, it is generally more convenient to use the following methods which have been widely accepted in this country, particularly for gelatin gels.

The Food Industrial Research Association (*F.I.R.A.*) *jelly tester* consists essentially of a small metal vane mounted on a shaft carrying a scale, the whole assembly being rotatable by application of a torque applied by water running at a predetermined rate into a counterpoised bucket connected to the shaft. The vane is inserted into the jelly sample to a definite depth and a torque is applied until the vane has rotated through a definite angle. The weight of water needed to do this is a measure of the jelly strength. A gel box of standard size is used in which the gel is matured under standard conditions; any slight wall effect will give a higher reading for jelly strength, but for comparative work this is not important.

The Bloom Gelometer described in British Standard 757:1959 is the standard instrument for the determination of jelly strength of gelatin. The jelly strength is expressed as a Bloom number which is equivalent to the weight in grams necessary to produce by means of a plunger 12.7 mm in diameter, a 4 mm depression in a jelly of 6.66 per cent w/w, matured at 0°.

The Bloom number has no exact physical significance but is dependent on the average molecular weight of the gelatin. It has been reported by Ellis (1962) that the solubility of glycerin suppositories is influenced by the jelly strength of gelatin and that the solution time of the present BP glycerin suppository is too prolonged, especially if good quality gelatin is used. The specification for BP gelatin is a jelly strength of not less than 150, no upper limit being specified.

An absolute method for the rigidity modulus of gelatin gels has been described by Saunders and Ward (1954). A cylinder of gelatin set in a glass tube is subjected to shearing stresses by applying a known air pressure at one end of the tube. The rigidity of the gel is calculated from the volume displacement which is measured by causing mercury to move along a calibrated capillary tube. The method was used for measuring rigidites of gelatin gels over the range 5×10^3 to 5×10^5 dyne/cm^2 and was suitable for gelatin concentrations up to 10 per cent. Nixon, Georgakopoulas and Carless (1966) using this technique showed that the presence of glycerin up to 40 per cent increased the modulus of rigidity of gelatin gels. No simple relationship was found between Bloom number and rigidity.

FLUIDS

When a shearing stress is applied to a fluid it deforms irreversibly, i.e. it flows. The term strain was used in the previous section to indicate deformation of a solid and in the case of fluids this term is replaced by rate of change of strain or more usually the term 'rate of shear', since the fluid is undergoing flow. Ideal viscous fluids known as Newtonian fluids show a direct relationship between shearing stress and rate of shear, the ratio being known as a coefficient of viscosity. Thus the rate of flow of a Newtonian fluid such as water through a tube is directly proportional to the pressure drop across the tube. Solutions of high molecular weight polymers, emulsions and suspensions show anomalous flow properties and cannot be characterized by a single viscosity value. The term 'apparent viscosity' is sometimes used to indicate that the viscosity determined by a particular viscometer is not an absolute value and in such cases it is important that the exact conditions of the measurement are specified.

VISCOSITY OF FLUIDS

The viscosity of a fluid is the internal resistance or friction involved in the relative motion of one layer of molecules with respect to the next. In order to maintain a constant rate of flow, a shearing stress has to be continually applied. When there are strong attractions between the molecules of a liquid (van der Waals forces, dipole interactions, etc.), the viscosity will be high; when the attractions are weak, the viscosity will be low. In gases, the molecules are in general so far apart that no appreciable intermolecular force exists and the viscosity can be explained by the kinetic theory of gases. Consequently, the viscosity of gases and liquids changes quite differently with alteration of temperature. At high temperatures, the mutual attractions between molecules of a liquid decrease and the viscosity falls, whereas in the case of a gas, the increased kinetic movement of the gas molecules causes an increase in viscosity.

FLOW CHARACTERISTICS OF NEWTONIAN FLUIDS

Consider a fluid flowing smoothly over a horizontal base AB (Fig. 9.2). Every particle of the liquid moves parallel to the surface in the same direction, i.e. it exhibits laminar or streamline flow.

The velocity v at a distance x above the base varies from zero where $x = 0$ to V where $x = h$. The velocity gradient dv/dx is a measure of the laminar flow. Consider a thin stratum of liquid $X_1 Y_1$, $X_2 Y_2$. The more quickly moving liquid above this layer exerts a tangential force tending to accelerate it while the more slowly moving liquid below it will tend to retard it. If the accelerating force from the liquid above $X_2 Y_2$ exactly balances the retarding force from the liquid below $X_1 Y_1$, then the layer $X_1 Y_1 X_2 Y_2$ will move in steady motion. Newton deduced that the tangential force F over the area A was given by:

$$\frac{F}{A} = \eta \frac{dv}{dx}.$$

η is the *coefficient of dynamic viscosity* and has the dimensions of mass × length^{-1} × time^{-1}. The absolute unit is the *poise* (P) (g/cm/sec. In SI Units $1P = 0.1$ Nsm^{-2}). A liquid has a viscosity of 1 P (100 cP) if a steady tangential force of 1 dyne (10 μN) produces a relative velocity of 1 cm/sec between two parallel plates of area 1 cm^2, separated by 1 cm and immersed in the liquid. The kinematic viscosity (v) of a fluid is defined by the equation:

$$v = \frac{\eta}{\rho},$$

where ρ is the density of the fluid. The unit of kinematic viscosity is the *stokes* (S) (For SI Units $1 S = 10^{-4}$ m^2/sec.)

Liquids of equal kinematic viscosities will flow at identical rates through a given tube, when the pressure causing the flow is due solely to the hydrostatic head of the liquid. For any given hydrostatic head, the pressure is proportional to the density. Calculation of the kinematic viscosity is thus readily achieved by comparison with the flow rates of a liquid of known kinematic viscosity, when using a viscometer which is operating under a hydrostatic head. Dynamic viscosities are usually directly measured in other types of viscometers where the flow rate is not dependent on the density of the liquid, e.g. rotational viscometers.

EFFECT OF TEMPERATURE

The dependence of the viscosity of a liquid on temperature is expressed approximately by an equation analogous to the Arrhenius equation of chemical kinetics:

$$\eta = Ae^{E/RT},$$

i.e.
$$\ln \eta = \frac{E}{RT} + \ln A,$$

where A is a constant depending on the molecular weight and molar volume of the liquid, and E is 'activation energy' required to move one molecule past another. As a rough guide the viscosity of many liquids decreases by about 2 per cent for each degree rise in temperature.

Streamline and Turbulent Flow

Fluids flowing relatively slowly on a flat base as in Fig. 9.2, or through pipes, travel in an orderly

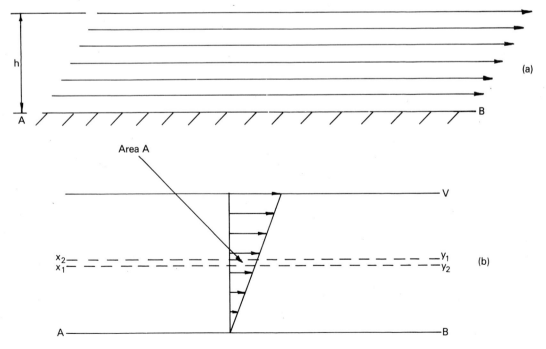

FIG. 9.2. Streamline flow.

manner in what is called streamline flow. The individual particles flow in straight lines parallel to the axis of the tube. Osbourne Reynolds first demonstrated the nature of streamline motion by carefully injecting a fine stream of dye solution into water flowing slowly through a tube. The unbroken filament of dye was carried along the axis of the tube. As the velocity of the fluid was increased, the character of the motion changed and the injected dye was seen to swirl along in the tube becoming thoroughly mixed due to disorderly, turbulent flow of the liquid. By carrying out these experiments over a range of flow rates through smooth tubes, Reynolds was able to show that there was a critical transition velocity V_c, between streamline and turbulent flow given by the following equation:

$$V_c = \frac{Re\,\eta}{\rho D},$$

where ρ = density of liquid,
  D = diameter of tube,
  Re = Reynold's number.

For flow in long smooth tubes, Re was approximately 2000, i.e. $Re < 2000$ results in streamline flow. It should be remembered that the geometry of the entry port leading to the tube can affect the smoothness of flow and this is likely to be most marked when short-capillary tubes are used to study flow rates. It is essential that streamline flow is operating in order to apply Newton's law for the calculation of viscosity. Reynold's number is a dimensionless quantity, i.e. a pure number.

DETERMINATION OF VISCOSITY

Capillary Tube Viscometer
The relationship between the rate of flow of a liquid through a capillary tube, and its viscosity was first given by Poiseuille. The Poiseuille equation for streamline flow is:

$$V = P\pi r^4 t/8l\eta$$

where V = volume of liquid (cm^3) flowing in time
  t (sec),
  P = driving pressure (dynes/cm^2),
  r = radius of capillary (cm),
  l = length of capillary (cm),
  η = coefficient of viscosity (poises).

This equation can be used directly for measuring the viscosity of a liquid, but for accurate measurements it is necessary to apply a correction for the kinetic energy gained by the liquid as it accelerates into the capillary tube from the reservoir. The driving pressure in the Poiseuille equation is that necessary to overcome viscous forces only and any additional force which is used to impart kinetic energy to the liquid must be allowed for. However, the correction term is negligible if the viscometer is designed with a large l/r ratio and the rates of flow are kept extremely low. Inaccuracies will also arise due to errors in measuring l and especially r and in practice the Poiseuille equation is generally used for comparative methods, when the rate of flow of the unknown is compared with the rate of flow of a liquid of known viscosity. If these two liquids have approximately the same flow rates then kinetic energy corrections will be self-cancelling.

The most frequently used capillary tube viscometer is the Ostwald type (Fig. 9.3). This consists

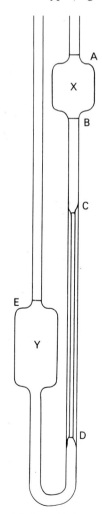

FIG. 9.3. Ostwald viscometer.

of a U-tube bearing two bulbs X and Y and, in one arm, a capillary CD of suitable bore. The tube is placed vertically in a thermostatically controlled bath ($\pm 0.05°$ or better). Sufficient of the liquid whose viscosity (η_1) is to be determined is poured into bulb Y to reach mark E. The liquid is then sucked or blown up to a point 1 cm above A; the time (t_1) for the liquid to fall from A to B is measured with a stop watch. The density of the liquid (ρ_1) is determined. The viscometer is emptied, rinsed out with suitable solvents, dried and the whole operation repeated with a liquid of known viscosity η_2 and density ρ_2. The time of flow is t_2.

From Poiseuille's Law:

$$\eta = \frac{\pi r^4 P t}{8 V l} \qquad (9.1)$$

Where P is due to the force of gravity:

$$P = h\rho g,$$

in which h = height of liquid in area,
ρ = density of liquid,
g = acceleration due to gravity.

As equal volumes of two liquids flow through the same capillary under a driving pressure proportional to density of the fluid:

$$\frac{\eta_1}{\eta_2} = \frac{\rho_1 t_1}{\rho_2 t_2}, \qquad (9.2)$$

and

$$\eta_1 = \frac{\eta_2 \rho_1 t_1}{\rho_2 t_2}. \qquad (9.3)$$

For the measurement of kinematic viscosity the direct comparison with a liquid of known kinematic viscosity simplifies the procedure since:

$$v = \frac{\eta_1}{\rho_1},$$

hence

$$\frac{v_1}{v_2} = \frac{t_1}{t_2}. \qquad (9.4)$$

The kinematic viscosity of a liquid is thus directly proportional to its flow rate.

The rate of flow through a capillary tube depends on r^4, and since Ostwald viscometers can be obtained with r varying from approximately 0.2 to 2 mm, a range of 10^4 in viscosity can be covered. Suitable dimensions for a set of five viscometers of the pattern shown in Fig. 9.3 are given in British Standard 188:1957. The No.0 viscometer can be calibrated with water but the larger sizes require calibration liquids of higher viscosity to ensure streamline flow and also adequate flow times for accurate timing. The Ostwald viscometer is specified for determining the kinematic viscosity of Liquid Paraffin BP.

The measurement of a very viscous liquid in a standard Ostwald viscometer is not convenient due to the difficulty of filling the viscometer with an accurate volume. Drainage errors during the filling procedure may result in overfilling. The suspended level viscometer overcomes this difficulty (Fig. 9.4).

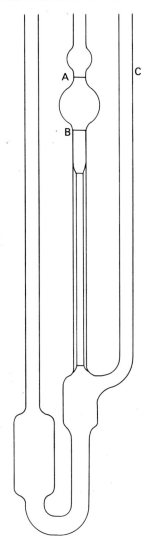

Fig. 9.4. Suspended level viscometer.

The additional side arm C ensures that the exit of the capillary is at atmospheric pressure, so that the total amount of liquid in the viscometer does not require to be fixed. The time of flow of the liquid from A to B is measured and the calculation is as before. This instrument is specified in the BP for determining the viscosity of solutions of methyl cellulose.

Falling Sphere Viscometer

A body falling through a viscous medium attains a constant terminal velocity when the accelerating force (gravity less buoyancy) is equal to the retarding force (viscosity). The retarding force (F) according to Stokes is:

$$F = 6\pi\eta rV \text{ dynes,} \qquad (9.5)$$

for a smooth sphere of radius r cm, moving with a velocity of V cm per sec in a liquid of viscosity η poises. The upthrust on the sphere according to Archimedes' principle is equal to the weight of liquid, density ρ_1 displaced by the sphere, i.e. $4/3\pi r^3\rho_s g$, when ρ_s is the density of the sphere. The net downward force exerted on the liquid is therefore:

$$4/3\pi r^3\rho_s g - 4/3\pi r^3\rho_1 g = 4/3\pi r^3 g(\rho_s-\rho_1). \qquad (9.6)$$

At the terminal velocity, net downward force = net upward force:

$$\therefore \qquad 6\pi\eta rV = 4/3\pi r^3 g(\rho_s-\rho_1), \qquad (9.7)$$

and

$$\eta = \frac{2r^2 g(\rho_s-\rho_1)}{9V}, \qquad (9.8)$$

or

$$\eta = \frac{D^2 g(\rho_s-\rho_1)}{18V}, \qquad (9.9)$$

where D = diameter of sphere.

This equation, known as Stokes' law is only valid for streamline flow of a sphere in an infinite fluid. Streamline flow occurs when Reynolds number (Re) is less than 0.2 where $Re = DV\rho/\eta$.

In the falling sphere viscometer a rust-free ball bearing is timed in falling a measured distance through a cylindrical tube of liquid (Fig. 9.5). For accurate absolute measurements, a correction for the effect of the proximity of the sides of the tube is necessary. The value of η calculated from the equation has to be multiplied by the factor which is approximately $(1+2.1r/R)$ where R is the radius of the tube and where $R > 10r$. The equation in the BP includes this factor calculated for a sphere of 1.55 mm and tube radius of 25 mm. If the instrument is used for relative determinations, corrections for end and wall effects are eliminated.

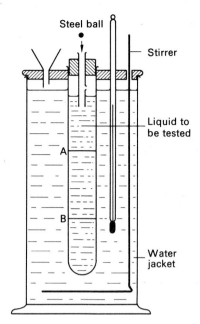

FIG. 9.5. Falling sphere viscometer.

The chief disadvantage of this viscometer is the large volume of sample required, which needs to be clear or translucent.

ROLLING SPHERE VISCOMETER

Whereas the falling sphere viscometer is limited to liquids of high viscosity, the rolling sphere model is capable of covering a range of viscosities from 0.5 to 200 000 P. The instrument consists essentially of a short glass tube of large diameter and a closely fitting ball of either glass or steel (Fig. 9.6). The tube is inclined at a definite angle and the ball is timed between two marks. Unlike the previous viscometer, a large ball falls more slowly than a smaller ball as the liquid has to pass between a smaller gap between the ball and the tube. The Stokes' equation does not apply in these measurements, the viscosity in centipoises is given by the following equation:

$$\eta = t \times (\rho_s-\rho_1)K,$$

where ρ_s = density of ball, ρ_1 = density of liquid, t = time of fall, K = constant for instrument.

The apparatus is calibrated with liquids of known viscosity. The method is capable of high precision provided that adequate temperature control is maintained.

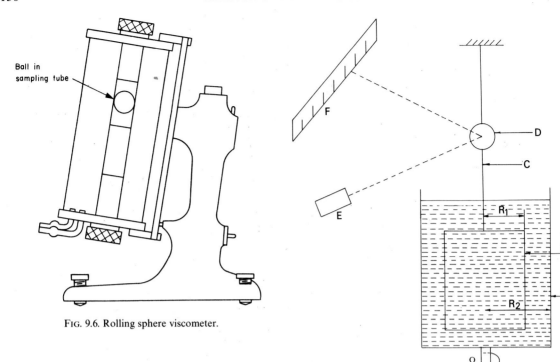

FIG. 9.6. Rolling sphere viscometer.

FIG. 9.7. Concentric cylinder viscometer.

ROTATING CYLINDER VISCOMETER

In this instrument, originally proposed by M. Couette in 1890, the sample fluid fills the annular space between two concentric cylinders, either of which may be rotated by a motor; the other cylinder is suspended elastically so that the torsional couple can be measured. In Fig. 9.7 the inner cylinder B is shown suspended from a torsion wire C and the outer one A is rotated. The liquid rotates in concentric laminar flow and exerts a viscous drag on the inner cylinder, causing a deflection proportional to the viscosity. The angular deflection may be measured by a mirror D attached to the wire, reflecting a light beam on to a horizontal graduated scale F. The rate of shear D at any given radius r is given by:

$$D = \frac{2\Omega}{r^2\left(\dfrac{1}{R_1{}^2} - \dfrac{1}{R_2{}^2}\right)},$$

where R_1 and R_2 are the radii of the inner and outer cylinders respectively.

If the annulus is narrow, an average rate of shear can be used. Many commercial viscometers are calibrated on the basis of the rate of shear at the inner cylinder being operative. The shearing stress exerted on the fluid may be calculated from the dimensions of the instrument and the torsion constant of the wire, or by calibrating the instrument using a liquid of known viscosity. If the rate of shear and the viscosity of the liquid is known, the stress constant for the instrument is readily calculated, since:

Shearing stress $= \eta \times$ rate of shear.

In the design of these viscometers it is desirable that the viscous drag exerted on the two ends of the viscometer is reduced to a minimum. These 'end effects' can be minimized by fitting a stationary guard ring over the upper surface of the inner cylinder or bob, the bottom of which is recessed in order to trap air in the cavity and prevent drag. A deeply recessed upper surface, can be used instead of a guard ring and excess fluid will overflow into this, so that the height of the fluid coincides with the height of the inner cylinder. The Rotovisko viscometer uses this principle.

Examples of commercial rotating cylinder viscometers are the Ferranti Portable, Brookfield and the Rotovisko which will be briefly discussed. For a more detailed description of these and other types, the laboratory manual by van Wazer et al. (1963) should be consulted.

FERRANTI PORTABLE VISCOMETER

This is shown diagrammatically in Fig. 9.8. The rotating outer cylinder is inverted, compared with the conventional Couette type, which permits the determination on bulk fluids into which the cylinder is immersed. The inner cylinder, which is connected to a beryllium copper spring, has its angular displacement indicated by a conventional pointer and scale. The outer cylinder is driven by a synchronous motor with a three- or five-speed gear box giving a range of 1 rev/min up to 300 rev/min. Rates of shear can be varied by speed of rotation and also by choice of inner cylinder. The mean shear rates vary from 930 to 0.15 sec^{-1}. Low shear rates are restricted to liquids of high viscosity and high shear rates to liquids of low viscosity in order to obtain readings on the scale. Size of sample required is usually about 100 ml.

BROOKFIELD SYNCHROLECTRIC VISCOMETER

This viscometer has been in general use in the USA since about 1940. It does not give results in terms of absolute shear rates, but has found widespread use as a comparative instrument. The cylinder that is immersed in the fluid is carried in a rotating spindle driven via a calibrated beryllium copper spring mounted on the motor shaft (Fig. 9.9). The displacement of the spindle due to the viscous drag of the sample is indicated by a pointer attached to the rotating spindle which moves over the scale attached to the motor spindle. Readings are thus complicated by the pointer and scale both revolving,

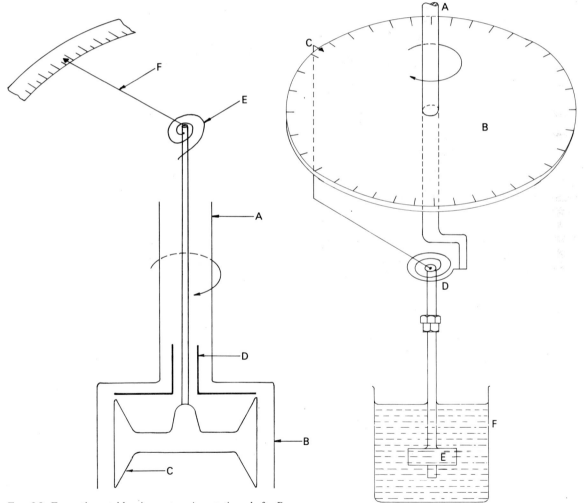

FIG. 9.8. Ferranti portable viscometer. A, rotating shaft; B, detachable outer cylinder; C, detachable inner cylinder; D, guard ring (stationary); E, torque spring; F, viscosity indicating pointer.

FIG. 9.9. Brookfield viscometer. A, driving shaft; B, rotating scale; C, viscosity indicating pointer; D, torque spring; E, interchangeable bob; F, sample.

but it is possible to clamp the pointer to the scale and then to slip the motor in order to take a reading. For this reason, it is not a convenient technique for following viscosity changes while shearing the sample. A wide range of viscosity is covered and very low shear rates are possible. Since the bob operates in an 'infinite sea' of fluid the calibration data are usually expressed in terms of rev/min and Brookfield reading. Although viscosities of Newtonian liquids can be determined, the 'apparent' viscosity of non-Newtonian can only be regarded as comparative measurements.

ROTOVISKO (HAAKE)

This is a very versatile viscometer and will measure viscosities in the range of 5×10^{-3} to 4×10^{7} P. The range of rate of shear is 10^{-2} to 10^{4}/sec. A ten-speed gear box drives the inner cylinder via a flexible cable. As in the Brookfield viscometer, the cylinder is not connected directly to the drive but a torsion spring is interposed between the rotor and the drive shaft. The viscous drag on the rotor causes the spring to twist until its torque is balanced by the viscous drag. The resulting angular displacement of the rotor, relative to the drive shaft, is a measure of the shear stress and is measured by means of a slider arm connected to a potentiometer so that the stress value is read from a galvanometer. A variety of outer and inner cylinders is available in order to cover a wide range of viscosity. A continuous record of stress at a constant rate of shear can be obtained by connecting a recording voltmeter to the output terminals.

CONE AND PLATE VISCOMETER (FERRANTI–SHIRLEY)

Essentially the viscometer consists of a flat plate and a rotating cone with a very obtuse angle (Fig. 9.10). The apex of the cone just touches the plate surface and the fluid sample fills the narrow gap formed by the cone and plate.

The usual cone angles are about 0.3° so that only small samples (0.5 to 1 ml) are required.

The plate is maintained at a constant temperature by circulating water through it and the small volume of sample rapidly reaches an equilibrium temperature.

The rate of shear across the gap for small angles is constant and is given by Ω/ψ; where

Ω = rotation (rad/sec), ψ = cone angle (rad).

The comparison with coaxial viscometers is shown on facing page.

The cone is driven by a variable speed motor through a gear train and a torsion spring is interposed between the driving shaft and the shaft connected to the cone to measure the shearing stress by means of a potentiometer, in a similar way to the Rotovisko instrument. The rate of shear is capable of being varied over a very wide range, e.g. 0 to 18 000 sec^{-1} for a 0.3° cone. The stress is indicated on a galvanometer connected to the potentiometer circuit.

The instrument can be modified to allow the simultaneous recording of shear rate and shearing stress during the constant acceleration of the cone, so that flow curves can be obtained automatically

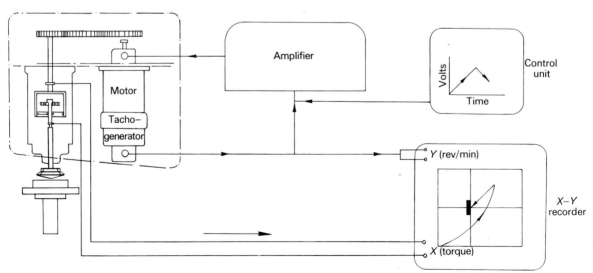

FIG. 9.10. Cone and plate viscometer (Ferranti–Shirley). Schematic diagram of the recording system.

	Co-axial cylinder	Cone plate
G = torque (dyne/cm) Ω = rotation (radian/sec) ψ = cone angle (radians)		
Rate of shear D sec^{-1}	$D_{max} = \dfrac{2}{R_1^2\left(\dfrac{1}{R_1^2} - \dfrac{1}{R_2^2}\right)}$ $D_{min} = \dfrac{2}{R_2^2\left(\dfrac{1}{R_1^2} - \dfrac{1}{R_2^2}\right)}$	$D = \dfrac{\Omega}{\psi}$
S = stress (dynes/cm^2)	$S = \dfrac{\dfrac{1}{R_1^2} - \dfrac{1}{R_2^2}}{4\pi L}$	$S = \dfrac{3G}{2\pi R^3}$

on an X-Y recorder. This is achieved by feeding the torque signal from the potentiometer/torsion spring to the X axis (calibrated in dynes/cm^2) and a voltage proportional to motor speed is fed into the Y axis (calibrated per sec). The control unit permits different rates of acceleration and deceleration of the cone so that rheological properties of fluids that show time-dependent effects, e.g. thixotropy, can be studied. Automatic recording of flow curves is particularly useful when rapid changes of viscosity occur on shearing, as these may be missed when operating the instrument manually. However, a word of caution is necessary as inertial effects of the cone may produce erroneous results, particularly if rapid acceleration–deceleration is applied to liquids of fairly low viscosity. Under these conditions inaccurate hysteresis loops may be obtained with Newtonian liquids.

The advantages of the cone and plate viscometer can be summarized as follows:
(a) Uniform rate of shear across sample.
(b) Sample size 1 ml or less.
(c) Good temperature control.
(d) Easy to clean (the plate is lowered from the cone).
(e) Automatic recording allows flow curves to be obtained quickly and under standardized conditions.

One of the disadvantages of the instrument is that it is unsuitable for coarse suspensions or emulsions, owing to the narrow clearance of cone and plate. Usually suspensions of particles of size not greater than 30 μm can be sheared in the standard cone (0.3°).

Boylan (1966, 1967) has described the use of the Ferranti–Shirley viscometer for measuring the rheological properties of ointment bases.

EXTRUSION VISCOMETER

The F.I.R.A./N.I.R.D. Extruder, manufactured by H. A. Gaydon & Company, Croydon, originally devised by Prentice of the National Institute for Research in Dairying, was used to investigate the consistency of butter. It was found that instrumental readings could be correlated with such subjective qualities as 'spreadability' and 'firmness'. The instrument is equally suitable for assessing the consistency of ointment bases.

The basic principle of the extruder is extremely simple. A sample is removed from the bulk material in a cylindrical borer about 4 cm long and 1.25 cm diameter. The sample is then forced from this cylinder through a circular orifice by a plunger moving at a uniform speed. The thrust required to extrude the material is recorded on a moving chart throughout the test and this chart serves as a permanent record of the firmness of the material. Should any inhomogeneities be present in the sample caused, for example, by the presence of agglomerates of solid particles or air bubbles, the recorded thrust will fluctuate and the nature of the inhomogeneity can often be determined by an examination of the extruded thread of material.

CREEP TESTING

The rheological evaluation of visco-elastic semi-solids (i.e. which possess viscous and elastic properties) can be done by a creep test where a stress is suddenly applied and maintained constant over a period of time. The resultant deformation (strain) of the material with time is known as the 'creep curve'. One type of apparatus used for this measurement consists of two concentric cylinders, the inner cylinder being capable of rotation on application of a torsional couple. The visco-elastic material to be tested fills the annular gap between the two cylinders. To carry out the measurement, a small fixed tangential stress is applied to the material through the inner cylinder and the slow rotation of this cylinder is followed by means of an optical mirror or suitable sensing device (Davies 1969). A typical creep curve is shown in Fig. 9.11 and can be analysed using the theory of linear visco-elasticity. Three separate regions can be identified in this figure: A-B represents an instantaneous elastic component; B-C represents visco-elastic flow; C-D is associated with viscous flow. On removal of the applied stress, the instantaneous elasticity is observed (region D-E) but the material does not completely recover due to some energy

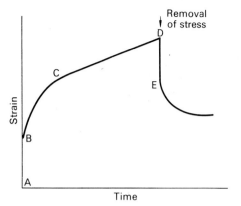

FIG. 9.11. Creep curve of viscoelastic material (constant stress applied).

being dissipated in viscous flow. The visco-elastic properties of ointment bases have been studied by Davies (1969) and by Barry and Grace (1971), the latter workers being interested in the rheology of soft paraffin studied by continuous shear and creep testing. The rheology of pharmaceutical and cosmetic semisolids has been reviewed by Barry (1974).

FLOW PROPERTIES OF NON-NEWTONIAN LIQUID

The viscosity of a Newtonian liquid is completely defined by a single figure, the coefficient of viscosity. This coefficient is the ratio of shearing stress–rate of shear and provided that streamline flow is maintained, it is of course independent of the actual rate of shear. Many colloidal dispersions, suspensions and emulsions cannot be characterized by a viscosity coefficient and it is necessary to determine the relationship between stress and rate of shear over a wide range of shear rate. The resulting plot of stress versus rate of shear is known as a flow curve and examples are shown in Fig. 9.12. Viscometers that are suitable for these determinations are the coaxial and cone-plate viscometers in which the rate of shear can be varied. Fig. 9.12(A) shows the flow curves for two Newtonian liquids of different viscosities.

Pseudoplastic Flow
Solutions of many polymeric substances, e.g. cellulose ethers, tragacanth, alginates, etc., do not show a direct relationship between stress and shear rate

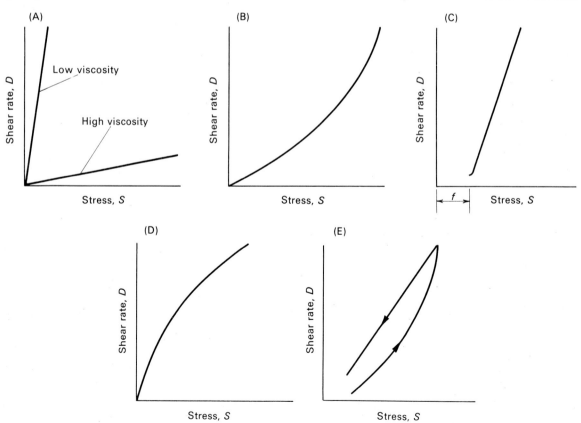

FIG. 9.12. Flow curves of Newtonian and non-Newtonian fluids.

(Fig. 9.12B). At low shear rates the ratio of stress–shear rate (i.e. apparent viscosity) is higher than at the greater shear rates. The flow curve is seen to straighten out at high rates of shear so that the solution reaches a limiting viscosity. This effect is ascribed to molecular interactions resulting in a three-dimensional network structure of solute molecules. For flow to occur this structure must be broken down, and as the rate of shear is increased the molecules will tend to become orientated in the streamlines of the liquid and offer less resistance to flow. Many attempts have been made by rheologists to represent the pseudoplastic curve by equations which have a theoretical basis, but with only limited success. The empirical power law:

$$D^N = \eta' S,$$

has been found to represent the flow curve of some pseudoplastic materials. D is the rate of shear and S the shearing stress. The exponent N is indicative of non-Newtonian flow. If N has a value of unity the equation reduces to the simple Newtonian equation of flow. The greater the values of N above unity the greater the pseudoplastic behaviour of the material. η' is a constant characteristic of the solution and does not have the same physical significance as a coefficient of viscosity. The equation may be written in logarithmic form:

$$\log S = N \log D - \log \eta'.$$

The plot of log S against log D will give a straight line of slope N and intercept of log η' on the log S axis. The advantages of obtaining an equation to fit a flow curve is that the curve may be more conveniently expressed in terms of the parameters N and η' and this simplifies the compilation of data. For instance, these parameters could be obtained for different concentrations of a polymer in solution, and if a correlation between log η' and concentration could be established, the flow properties of a solution of any other concentration could then be calculated. Kabre, De Kay and Banker (1964) applied this approach to the characterization of the viscosity of a number of natural and synthetic gums.

Plastic Flow

Whereas a Newtonian or pseudoplastic liquid will yield under the application of the smallest shearing force, a plastic material fails to flow until a certain shearing stress has been applied. This is typical of concentrated suspensions of solids, ointments and gels and is thought to result from the aggregation of particles forming a continuous but not orientated,

structure throughout the mass. Flow cannot take place until the applied stress exceeds the force of flocculation which causes the particles to adhere together. When flow is initiated the particle layers move relative to the adjacent layers, and the particle contacts are broken but reform again on removal of the stress. Thus the internal structure of the substance is not permanently altered. This behaviour is expressed in Fig. 9.12C. Flow does not commence until the stress reaches the yield value f (dynes/cm^2) above which point the shear rate becomes directly proportional to the shear stress and the reciprocal of the slope of graph gives the plastic viscosity U in poises.

This is expressed by the equation first given by Bingham:

$$U = \frac{S-f}{D}$$

A plastic curve obtained from a coaxial cylinder viscometer is non-linear over the lower portion of the curve and the yield value f is usually obtained by extrapolation.

Dilatancy

If starch is made into a paste with cold water, it can be stirred slowly but tends to solidify if the stirring rate is increased. This effect, common to many concentrated deflocculated suspensions can be explained on the basis of packing characteristics of particles. Deflocculated particles pack into a mass of minimum volume and only a small quantity of liquid is needed to fill the voids between the particles and there is just sufficient to enable the particles to move past each other slowly. When the suspension is sheared rapidly the particles are forced out of their close packing and the void space is increased, i.e. system dilates. There is insufficient liquid to fill the voids completely, the paste appears to 'dry out' and offers considerable resistance to further shearing (Fig. 9.12D). On resting, it liquefies as the particles move back into close packing. Dilatancy is also encountered when a dilute deflocculated suspension settles out on storage. The sediment is dilatant and resists any energetic attempts at stirring or shaking. This effect is known as 'caking' or 'claying' of suspensions and is best avoided by formulating the suspension so that the particles are slightly flocculated.

Thixotropy

The flow curves so far described are not affected by the duration of shearing. However, thixotropic systems undergo gel $\rightleftharpoons$ sol transformation and the equilibrium between proportion of gel to sol is affected not only by the rate of shear, but also by the time for which it is applied. Gel structure is due to particle–particle links and these are broken during shearing, but unlike plastic systems, do not reform instantly on cessation of shear. When determining the flow curve of a thixotropic gel it is usual to take successive readings as the rate of shear is increased in regular increments (up-curve) and then continue the measurements as the rate of shear is decreased (down-curve). The loss in structure due to shearing results in the down-curve being displaced from the up-curve and the resultant hysteresis loop (Fig. 9.12E) can be used as a criterion of thixotropy provided that a standardized programme of shearing is used. Woodman & Marsden (1966) found that the thixotropic properties of an oil-in-water lotion could be characterized more satisfactorily by observing the relaxation of stress during shearing, rather than by hysteresis loop measurement. Boylan (1966, 1967) has reported the thixotropic properties of soft paraffin and some commercial ointments.

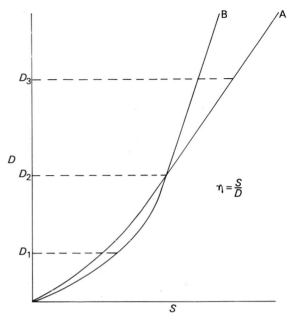

FIG. 9.13. Effect of shear rate on viscosity determination of emulsions A and B.

Selection of Viscometer

Newtonian liquids. For the accurate measurement of liquids of low viscosity, the capillary tube or the Hoeppler viscometer are suitable. These are simple instruments to use and to calibrate. They provide only one shear rate (i.e. single point instrument) and this is adequate as the viscosity of a Newtonian liquid is independent of shear rate.

Non-Newtonian liquids. The majority of emulsions and suspensions are non-Newtonian and, therefore, the limitations of single point measurement should be appreciated. This aspect has been emphasized by Martin, Banker and Chun (1964). Fig. 9.13 shows the flow curves for two emulsions, A and B, where a measurement at shear rate D_1 would indicate that B had a higher viscosity than A, while the opposite result would be obtained at shear rate D_3. At shear rate D_2, the emulsions would apparently have the same viscosity. This shows that even for comparative work single point instruments can be misleading, particularly if no information is available on the type of flow behaviour. Where a simple test for 'viscosity' is required for quality control, it may be sufficient to measure the 'apparent viscosity' at a rate of shear which approximates to the rate of shear to which the product is subjected during usage. Henderson, Meer and Kostenbauder (1961) have calculated the

approximate rates of shear encounted in such operations as milling, pouring from bottles and extrusion from orifices (Table 9.1).

TABLE 9.1

APPROXIMATE RATES OF SHEAR FOR VARIOUS PROCESSES
(after Henderson et al. 1961)

Process	Rate of shear (sec^{-1})
Rubbing on ointment tile	150
Roller mill	1000–12 000
Hypodermic needle	Up to 10 000
Nasal spray (plastic squeeze bottle)	2000
Pouring from bottle	Less than 100

The assessment of thixotropic products requires rotational viscometry in order to plot up and down curves. Lack of reproducibility may be due to lack of standardized pre-treatment of samples before measurements.

A comprehensive treatise on commercial viscometers is given by van Wazer et al. (1963). There is no single viscometer that is likely to be satisfactory for pharmaceutical products that may vary in consistency from water to stiff gels. In selecting a viscometer the following points should be studied:

(a) If low shear rates are required, is the instrument sensitive enough to measure the corresponding stress?

(b) Are the units of rate of shear and shearing stress measured in absolute units or comparative units?

(c) Size of sample available, e.g. a cone and plate may require only a 1 ml sample, while a co-axial viscometer may require several hundred millilitres.

(d) Can the sample be easily maintained at a constant temperature?

(e) Can the instrument be easily cleaned? This is essential when a large number of samples is to be examined.

RHEOLOGY OF SUSPENSIONS

The addition of a disperse phase (solid or liquid) to a liquid increases the viscosity due to the disturbance of the stream lines of the liquid around the particles. Einstein in 1906 to 1911 developed a theoretical expression relating the viscosity of a suspension η, to the volume fraction ϕ of the particles present:

$$\eta = \eta_0(1 + 2.5\phi),$$

where η_0 is the viscosity of the vehicle. This equation is strictly applicable only to very dilute suspensions of rigid spherical particles. In order to extend the equation to higher concentrations, equations of the type:

$$\eta = \eta_0(1 + 2.5\phi + k_1\phi^2 + k_2\phi^3 \ldots),$$

have been developed where k_1 and k_2 are constants for the system.

These equations are of little application to pharmaceutical suspensions as the theoretical treatments have been largely confined to Newtonian flow. The effects of particle shape, particle size distribution and in particular the degree of flocculation of the particles, play a predominant role in determining the flow properties of pharmaceutical suspensions, particularly if the concentration of disperse phase is high. The more uniform the particles, the greater the viscosity of the suspension for a given concentration of solid. Flocculation gives rise to plastic flow properties often combined with thixotropy. If deflocculating agents are added, e.g. surface active agents, peptizing electrolytes, the yield value is reduced or disappears altogether and the flow becomes pseudoplastic, or even Newtonian, depending on the extent of deflocculation. Fig. 9.14 shows the variation of flow properties of suspensions such as kaolin and barium sulphate in water as the concentration is increased. Curve D shows

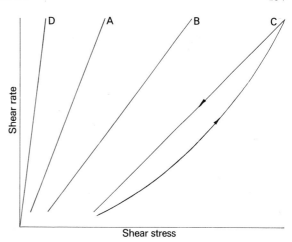

FIG. 9.14. Flow curves of kaolin suspensions in water. A, 20 per cent w/v; B, 30 per cent w/v; C, 40 per cent w/v; D, 40 per cent w/v + 10 per cent sodium citrate.

how the viscosity is reduced in the presence of sodium citrate which deflocculates the suspension.

A similar result is observed with dispersions of zinc oxide in liquid paraffin, where the addition of a little oleic acid produces a similar deflocculation effect.

RHEOLOGY OF EMULSIONS

When droplets of one liquid are emulsified in an immiscible liquid, the viscosity of the emulsion is greater than that of the vehicle, as one would expect from the Einstein equation. This equation is obeyed by very dilute emulsions of small globule size, indicating that the globules are behaving like solid particles. The factors that have been discussed under Rheology of Suspensions apply to emulsions except that the particle shape factor is unlikely to play an important part, since the globules are mainly spherical.

Fig. 9.15 shows the variation of apparent viscosity with volume concentration of disperse phase in a water-in-oil emulsion. The emulsion may invert to an unstable oil-in-water emulsion of low viscosity when the water is increased above a critical amount. The point of inversion depends on the concentration and nature of the emulsifying agent.

The theoretical maximum volume of uniform spheres that can be packed into a given volume is 74 per cent v/v but emulsion droplets are not uniform so that small drops can pack between the larger ones. They can also distort so that emulsions containing as much as 90 per cent v/v internal phase are possible. The viscosity of the internal phase has little or no effect on the viscosity of the

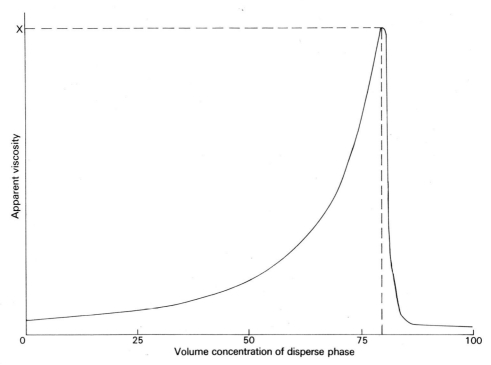

FIG. 9.15. Variation of apparent viscosity with volume concentration (per cent) of water in a water-in-oil emulsion. Maximum viscosity at X—inversion beyond this point.

concentrated emulsions. The important factors influencing the viscosity of emulsions are:

(a) Phase volume ratio.
(b) Viscosity of continuous phase.
(c) Nature and proportion of emulsifying agents.
(d) Globule size and distribution of size.
(e) Aggregation of the globules.

The review by Sherman (1964) should be consulted for detailed information.

Oil-in-water emulsions stabilized by cetyl and stearyl alcohols and water-soluble surface agents have been studied by Axon (1956) who showed that increasing quantities of cetyl alcohol produced an increase in both the yield value and the plastic viscosity of some emulsions. Talman, Davies and Rowan (1967) studied the rheology of similar emulsions and suggested that the large increase in viscosity as the cetostearyl alcohol was increased, was due to the formation of a gel in the aqueous phase due to the interaction of the alcohol with sodium lauryl sulphate. It seems likely that such gel formation would play a dominant role in the viscosity of emulsions containing emulsifying waxes. Barry and Shotton (1967) have studied the thixotropic and visco-elastic properties of the sodium lauryl sulphate–cetyl alcohol–water gel system in the absence of an emulsified phase.

RHEOLOGY OF SUSPENDING AGENTS

The majority of these produce pseudoplastic solutions and have definite advantages over Newtonian liquids such as glycerin or syrups. The high viscosity of pseudoplastics at low rates of shear enables them to stabilize insoluble particles against rapid sedimentation and the shear thinning characteristics enable easy pouring from the bottle. These agents include methyl cellulose, hydroxyethyl cellulose, sodium carboxy cellulose, alginates and clays such as bentonite. Meyer and Cohen (1959) reported that permanent suspensions could be prepared using carboxyvinyl-polymer (Carbopol 934 BF, Goodrich Chemical Co.), which exhibits plastic flow properties. Provided a certain minimum yield value was present, suspensions were observed to be permanent. However, such suspensions should be examined critically since the 'permanency' may be affected by deterioration of suspending efficiency due to chemical deterioration, pH changes, etc. Hiestand (1964) refers to suspending agents that possess yield values, as 'structured vehicles' on account of the structure of the suspending or gelling material. Particles may also remain in suspension due not only to the structure in the vehicle but also to the flocculation of the particles which produces a scaffold structure that extends throughout the suspension. Many long chain polymers induce flocculation of particles due to adsorption of segments of the polymer on to them, the remaining segments being free to project into the vehicle and adsorbing on to adjacent particles. Thus polymer bridge flocculation may be as least as important as the structure of the vehicle itself in preventing suspensions from sedimenting.

Martin et al. (1964) have reviewed the properties of suspending agents and also the effect of processing on the rheology of gums and suspensions.

REFERENCES

AXON, A. (1956) *J. Pharm. Pharmacol.* **8**, 762.

BARRY, B. W. (1974) *Advances in Pharmaceutical Science Vol. 3* (Ed. Beckett, Bean & Carless). London: Academic Press.

BARRY, B. W. & GRACE, A. J. (1971) *J. pharm. Sci.* **60**, 1198.

BARRY, B. W. & SHOTTON, E. (1967) *J. Pharm. Pharmacol.* **19**, 121S.

BOYLAN, J. C. (1966) *J. pharm. Sci.* **55**, 710.

BOYLAN, J. C. (1967) *J. pharm. Sci.* **56**, 1164.

DAVIES, S. S. (1969) *J. pharm. Sci.* **58**, 412.

ELLIS, M. A. (1962) *Pharm. J.* **189**, 177.

HENDERSON, N. L., MEER, P. M. & KOSTENBAUDER, H. B. (1961) *J. pharm. Sci.* **50**, 788.

HIESTAND, E. N. (1964) *J. pharm. Sci.* **53**, 1.

KABRE, S. P., DE KAY, H. G. & BANKER, G. S. (1964) *J. pharm. Sci.* **53**, 492, 495.

MARTIN, A. N., BANKER, G. S. & CHUN, A. H. C. (1964) *Advances in Pharmaceutical Sciences* Vol. 1. (Eds Bean, Beckett & Carless). London: Academic Press.

MEYER, R. J. & COHEN, L. (1959) *J. Soc. cosmet. Chem.* **10**, 143.

NIXON, J. R., GEORGAKOPOULAS, P. P. & CARLESS, J. E. (1966) *J. Pharm. Pharmacol.* **18**, 283.

SAUNDERS, P. R. & WARD, A. G. (1954) *Proc. 2nd Int. Congr. Rheol. p. 284 Oxford.*

SHERMAN, P. (1964) *J. Pharm. Pharmacol.* **16**, 1.

TALMAN, F. A. J., DAVIES, P. J. & ROWAN, E. M. (1967) *J. Pharm. Pharmacol.* **19**, 417.

WOODMAN, M. & MARSDEN, A. (1966) *J. Pharm. Pharmacol.* **18**, 198S.

VAN WAZER, J. R., LYONS, J. W., KIM, K. Y. & COLWELL, R. E. (1963) *Viscosity and Flow Measurement—A Laboratory Handbook of Rheology.* New York: Interscience.

10

Drug Stability

A study of the stability of pharmaceutical products and of stability testing techniques is essential for three main reasons. Firstly it is important from the point of view of the safety of the patient. The present trend in the pharmaceutical industry is towards production of highly specific, chemically complex, potent drugs. It is important, therefore, that the patient receives a uniform dose of drug throughout the whole of the shelf-life of the product. In addition, although a drug may have been shown to be safe for use, this is not necessarily true of the decomposition product(s). It is the duty of the manufacturer to minimize, or if possible prevent, decomposition of the product. This is of particular importance when preparing parenteral solutions, since injection frequently involves a greater risk than other forms of drug administration.

Secondly consideration must be given to the relevant legal requirements concerned with the identity, strength, purity and quality of the drug, and finally such a study is important to prevent the economic repercussions of marketing an unstable product. The sale of such a product is hardly the best advertisement for a manufacturer, and subsequent withdrawal and reformulation of the drug may lead to considerable financial loss.

This chapter concerns the chemical and physical factors causing deterioration of drugs, the application of chemical kinetics to determine the rate of decomposition, and methods of reducing the amount of decomposition. Later sections deal with the use of accelerated storage tests to predict the shelf-life of the product.

CHEMICAL DEGRADATION OF PHARMACEUTICAL PRODUCTS

Pharmaceutical products differ considerably in their composition, so naturally they are subject to different forms of chemical degradation, and in addition there may be several simultaneous decomposition reactions occurring in a product. For example, vitamin A undergoes both isomerization and oxidation, and the alkaloid ergometrine is susceptible to these and also to hydrolysis. Nevertheless, by obtaining information on each isolated degradation process, it is possible to establish reliable methods of reducing, or even eliminating, the causes of instability.

HYDROLYSIS

Hydrolysis is considered to be the major cause of deterioration of drugs, especially for those in aqueous solution. It may be defined as the reaction of a compound with water, and one may distinguish between ionic and molecular forms of hydrolysis. Ionic hydrolysis occurs when the salts of weak acids, e.g. potassium acetate, and bases, e.g. codeine phosphate, interact with water to give alkaline and acidic solutions respectively. As has been discussed in Chapter 2, this is an instantaneous equilibrium process. On the other hand, molecular hydrolysis is a much slower, irreversible process involving cleavage of the drug molecule. This form of hydrolysis is mainly responsible for the decomposition of pharmaceutical products. Esters, e.g. the local anaesthetics amethocaine and benzocaine, and amides, e.g. the sulphonomides, and nitriles, are all substances that are liable to decompose by hydrolysis. The reaction is frequently catalysed by hydrogen (H^+) or hydroxyl (OH^-) ions, and is therefore said to be specific acid- or specific base-catalysed. In many instances, hydrolysis is specifically acid–base catalyzed, and the rate of decomposition is then critically dependent upon the pH of the system. Esters, for example the local anaesthetic procaine, generally exhibit this type of catalysis (Higuchi, Havinga & Busse 1950).

Procaine   p-aminobenzoic acid   Diethylamino ethanol

In many other cases, however, hydrolysis may be catalysed by acidic and basic species other than the hydrogen and hydroxyl ions. According to the Lowry–Brönsted theory, an acid is defined as a species, ionic or molecular, that is capable of donating a proton, while a base is a species capable of accepting a proton. For example, the antibiotic chloramphenicol, as well as exhibiting specific acid–base catalysis, undergoes general acid–base catalyzed hydrolysis (Higuchi, Marcus & Bias 1954). The monohydrogen phosphate ion, mono- and dihydrogen citrate ions, and undissociated acetic acid, all catalyse the reaction:

Chloramphenicol   2-Amino-1-p-nitrophenyl-1,3-propanediol

The drug molecule undergoing hydrolysis may carry a charge or be uncharged. From the preceding discussion, it is evident that a drug may undergo several simultaneous catalytic reactions, all of which are hydrolytic in nature. A prime example of this phenomenon is the decomposition of aspirin into salicylic and acetic acids. Over the pH range of 1 to 12, it has been predicted that six simultaneous reactions occur (Edwards 1950):

(a) Aspirin   Salicylic acid   Acetic acid

(d) [aspirin structure with OCOCH₃ and COO⁻] $\xrightarrow{H^+}$ [salicylic acid structure with OH and COOH] $+$ CH_3COOH

(e) [aspirin structure with OCOCH₃ and COO⁻] $\xrightarrow{H_2O}$ [salicylic acid structure with OH and COOH] $+$ CH_3COO^-

(f) [aspirin structure with OCOCH₃ and COO⁻] $\xrightarrow{OH^-}$ [salicylate structure with OH and COO⁻] $+$ CH_3COO^-

Although hydrolysis will occur principally with drugs in aqueous solution, suspensions and solid dosage forms are also susceptible to hydrolytic attack. Leeson and Mattocks (1958) have shown that moisture is rapidly absorbed on to the surface of aspirin particles causing solution of a portion of the drug in the water layer around the particles. As the aspirin in solution hydrolyses, more of the solid material dissolves and decomposition continues.

OXIDATION

The decomposition of pharmaceutical preparations due to oxidation is nearly as prevalent as that due to hydrolysis. Neoarsphenamine, morphine, adrenaline, fixed oils, fats, oil-soluble and water-soluble vitamins, volatile oils and phenols, are some of the many examples of products that oxidize.

Oxidation of a compound can be defined as the removal of an electropositive atom, radical or electron, or the addition of an electronegative atom or radical. One may make a distinction between those oxidation processes that proceed slowly under the influence of atmospheric oxygen, and those that involve the reversible loss of electrons without the addition of oxygen. The latter type of oxidative change is less frequently encountered than those involving atmospheric oxygen, but is nevertheless important. For example, adrenaline, ferrous salts such as ferrous phosphate, riboflavine, and ascorbic acid are all prone to this form of oxidation. In some instances, it is possible to predict the susceptibility of the compound to oxidation from a knowledge of its standard oxidation–reduction potential, E_o. As has been discussed in Chapter 2, the oxidation–reduction potential, E_h, is related to the proportion of oxidized and reduced forms of the compound and its standard oxidation–reduction potential by the equation:

$$E_h = E_o + \frac{0.0592}{n} \log \frac{[\text{oxidized form}]}{[\text{reduced form}]}, \quad (10.1)$$

where n is the number of electrons transferred per ion. Since E_o is a measure of the oxidizing or reducing tendency of a compound, a compound with a high E_o is more resistant to oxidation than one that has a low E_o value. When two potentially oxidizable compounds are present together, as is the case with many pharmaceutical products, the compound with the lower E_o will be oxidized in preference to that with the higher E_o value. This relationship is utilized in the stabilization of an oxidizable drug by incorporation of a compound of lower E_o value in the formulation. For example, ascorbic acid has been used to protect adrenaline from oxidation in solution. In acid solution (pH range 4 to 7), ascorbic acid undergoes the following reversible oxidation process (von Dolder 1952).

At pH 4.7, the E_o value for ascorbic acid has been found to be $+0.14$ V.

Oxidation of adrenaline results ultimately in the loss of activity of the drug and the production of a red-coloured solution. In acid solution, the first stage of this process involves the formation of adrenaline-o-quinone.

Adrenaline $\xrightarrow[+2H]{-2H}$ Adrenaline-o-quinone

The E_o value for this reversible reaction at pH 4.7 is +0.52 V. Hence, when the two compounds are present in solution at pH 4.7, the ascorbic acid will be oxidized whilst the adrenaline will be protected from attack by oxidizing agents.

Autoxidation is the term applied to those oxidation processes that proceed slowly under the influence of atmospheric oxygen (Ostendorf 1964). Oils and fats containing unsaturated linkages in the molecules are particularly susceptible to autoxidation. Volatile oils, e.g. clove and cinnamon, change colour, consistency and odour. Fixed oils, e.g. the oily injection vehicles ethyl oleate and arachis oil, develop an unpleasant odour and taste, and are said to be 'rancid'. In the majority of cases, the oxidation process is a chain reaction involving the formation of free radicals, and comprises three distinct steps: initiation, propagation and termination.

An organic compound (RH) is converted into an active free radical ($R^\bullet$) during the initiation step as a result of the influence of some factor such as heat, light, presence of trace metals or other free radicals.

$$\cdot RH \longrightarrow R^\bullet + H^\bullet$$

Organic compound   Free radical

The propagation step is the chain reaction during which the free radical absorbs a molecule of oxygen to form a peroxy radical ($ROO^\bullet$). The peroxy radical then abstracts hydrogen from another molecule of RH to form a hydroperoxide (ROOH) and a new free radical $R^\bullet$. $R^\bullet$ will absorb a molecule of oxygen and thus continue the reaction.

$$R^\bullet + O_2 \longrightarrow ROO^\bullet$$
Peroxy radical

$$ROO^\bullet + RH \longrightarrow ROOH + R^\bullet$$
Hydroperoxide

The primary products of autoxidation are the odourless and tasteless hydroperoxides. They, however, break down to yield aldehydes, ketones and short-chain fatty acids that are responsible for the rancid nature of the oil or fat.

In theory, the propagation step can continue until either all of the organic compound, or the oxygen, has been consumed. However, in practice, a termination step intervenes since certain of the free radicals can combine to form inactive products which break the chain reaction.

$$\left. \begin{array}{l} ROO^\bullet + ROO^\bullet \longrightarrow \\ ROO^\bullet + R^\bullet \longrightarrow \\ R^\bullet + R^\bullet \longrightarrow \end{array} \right\} \text{Inactive products}$$

It has been shown, using compounds containing unsaturated linkages, that the initial attack causing formation of a free radical is on the methylene group which is in the α-position to a double bond (Farmer 1942). The complete autoxidation sequence, e.g. for a long-chain unsaturated fatty acid, can be represented thus:

Initiation

$$-\overset{\alpha}{C}H_2-CH=CH-CH_2- \longrightarrow \overset{\bullet}{C}H-CH=CH-CH_2-$$

Propagation

$$-\overset{\bullet}{C}H-CH=CH-CH_2- \longrightarrow -\overset{\overset{OO^\bullet}{|}}{C}H-CH=CH-CH_2-$$

$$-\overset{\overset{OO^\bullet}{|}}{C}H-CH=CH-CH_2- + -CH_2-CH=CH-CH_2- \longrightarrow -\overset{\bullet}{C}H-CH=CH-CH_2-$$

$$-\overset{\overset{OOH}{|}}{C}H-CH=CH-CH_2-$$

Further decomposition to aldehydes, ketones, fatty acids.

Termination

$$-\overset{\overset{OO^\bullet}{|}}{C}H-CH=CH-CH_2- + -\overset{\overset{OO^\bullet}{|}}{C}H-CH=CH-CH_2- \longrightarrow$$

$$-\overset{\bullet}{C}H-CH=CH-CH_2- + -\overset{\bullet}{C}H-CH=CH-CH_2- \longrightarrow \begin{array}{l}\text{Inactive}\\\text{products}\end{array}$$

$$-\overset{\overset{OO^\bullet}{|}}{C}H-CH=CH-CH_2- + -\overset{\bullet}{C}H-CH=CH-CH_2- \longrightarrow$$

If the hydroperoxide content of a compound undergoing oxidation is determined (the 'peroxide value') at various time intervals, the result typically obtained is as shown in Fig. 10.1.

Three distinct stages of oxidation may be identified. Initially, there is an induction period during which oxidation is slow, and the rate at which the chain reaction is terminated is as great

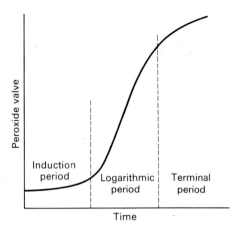

FIG. 10.1. Oxidation rate of an organic compound as shown by peroxide value determination.

as the rate of initiation of the process. There follows a stage where oxidation increases very rapidly at a logarithmic rate. During this period, there are many more free radicals formed than are removed by the termination step. Finally, the rate of oxidation begins to decline. There are fewer and fewer free radicals formed as the chain reaction slows down. It is normally during the latter period that the rancid nature of the oil becomes evident. Several factors can affect the rate of autoxidation as outlined below.

Factors affecting the Rate of Autoxidation
The degree of unsaturation of the organic compound. Highly unsaturated compounds are more susceptible to autoxidation, and therefore oxidize at rates greater than shown by compounds having a lower degree of unsaturation. With compounds containing an unconjugated double bond system, the reactivity of the α-methylene group is enhanced. Consequently, initiation of the process is much easier than is the case when the α-methylene group is flanked by one double bond. For example, linoleic acid

$$[CH_3(CH_2)_4.CH=CHCH_2CH=CH(CH_2)_7COOH]$$

is much more rapidly oxidized on exposure to air than oleic acid

$$[CH_3(CH_2)_7CH=CH(CH_2)_7COOH].$$

The presence of free fatty acids. The presence of a free carboxylic acid group also enhances the reactivity of the organic molecule. Hence free fatty acids oxidize more rapidly than, for example, esters. For instance, methyl linoleate

$$[CH_3(CH_2)_4CH=CHCH_2CH=CH(CH_2)_7COOCH_3]$$

is more stable to air oxidation than linoleic acid. Thus, if unsaturated free fatty acids are produced during oxidation, or are present as impurities in a vitamin, oil or fat, the material becomes more susceptible to autoxidation because of the greater number of free radicals formed from these fatty acids.

Dilution. Dilution of an oxidizable compound with an inert solvent will decrease the rate of oxidation. This follows from the Law of Mass Action (see p. 149). However, a limit will be reached when the concentration of oxidizable material is similar to the concentration of oxygen dissolved in the solvent system. Under these conditions, the proportion of oxidizable material decomposed is very high, although a chain reaction process does not appear to operate. This situation may arise when formulating oily vitamin solutions where the vitamin is present in very low concentrations.

Temperature. The rate of oxidation of an organic compound is increased with increase in the temperature of storage, In addition, the rate at which the hydroperoxides break down into aldehydes, ketones and fatty acids is also accelerated at temperatures in excess of 50°. Thus it is possible for an oxidizable material to have a low peroxide value after storage at an elevated temperature. This, of course, does not signify that there has been a low rate of oxidation, rather that decomposition has advanced to the stage where the secondary products of oxidation predominate.

The presence of pro-oxidants. Pro-oxidants, by definition, accelerate the rate of autoxidation. The hydroperoxides formed during the autoxidation process are themselves pro-oxidants. The addition of hydroperoxides to an oxidizable compound will shorten or even eliminate the induction period.

Heavy metals, e.g. copper and iron, also have a pro-oxidant effect since their variable valency state causes them to act as catalysts for the initiation step. Their mode of action is expressed by the following equations:

$$ROOH + M \longrightarrow RO^{\bullet} + OH^- + M^+$$
$$ROOH + M^+ \longrightarrow ROO^{\bullet} + H^+ + M$$

where M represents the heavy metal.

Heavy metals also influence the propagation and termination steps of the autoxidation process.

The physical state of the oxidizable compound. The oxidation rate of a solid fat is normally very slow in comparison with that occurring in the liquid state. This is primarily due to the fact that there are large quantities of relatively stable, saturated, fatty materials present which act as a diluent for the oxidizable material. In addition, the physical state of the material precludes rapid diffusion of oxygen through the bulk of the material.

When an oxidizable compound, e.g. methyl oleate, is dispersed in water, the rate of oxidation may be profoundly affected, especially if surface-active agents are present to emulsify the system. This phenomenon will be discussed further when dealing with methods of reducing autoxidative degradation of pharmaceutical materials.

ISOMERIZATION

In the present context, isomerization means the conversion of an active drug into a less active, or inactive, isomer having the same structural formula but differing in stereochemical configuration. One may make a distinction between isomerization involving optically active compounds containing one or more asymmetric carbon atoms, and geometrical isomerization. The latter refers to changes in the relative spatial configuration of groupings around a double bond (or bonds) in a molecule.

Optical Isomerization. Optical isomerization as a cause of drug deterioration may be further divided into the processes of racemization and epimerization.

Racemization in solution involves the conversion of an optically active form of a drug into its enantiomorph. The process continues until there are equal concentrations of the two optically active forms present. At this point, the solution no longer rotates the plane of polarized light. Frequently, it is the *laevo*-rotatory form of the drug, e.g. $(-)$-adrenaline, $(-)$-phenylephrine, that has the greater biological activity. When racemization is complete, the drug will still retain a certain degree of potency since 50 per cent of the active form is still present, and the enantiomorph may not be completely inactive. For example, $(-)$-hyoscyamine is readily converted by the action of heat or alkali to atropine which is the racemic mixture of $(+)$ and $(-)$-hyoscyamine. As a mydriatic, $(-)$-hyoscyamine acts with greater intensity than the racemic mixture. The ease with which an optically active compound can racemize depends upon its chemical structure, and especially upon the type of groupings attached to the asymmetric carbon atom. For example, the presence of an aromatic grouping increases the susceptibility of the compound to racemization. The rate of racemization often depends upon such factors as the presence of catalytic hydrogen and hydroxyl ions, heat and light. The racemization of $(-)$-adrenaline is catalysed by hydrogen ions, and hence only becomes a significant factor in the decomposition of the drug at low pH values, i.e. pH 0 to 3 (Schroeter & Higuchi 1958).

Epimerization can occur with a compound having more than one asymmetric carbon atom in the molecule. There is selective racemization of an asymmetric centre that possesses a hydrogen atom and is adjacent to a carbonyl grouping. An equilibrium between the two epimers is attained which does not necessarily correspond to a 50 per cent conversion of the active form of the drug. For this reason, and also because the two epimers do not exhibit equal and opposite optical rotations, the optical activity of the equilibrium system will not be zero, unlike the case of a racemic mixture. For example, upon prolonged storage, solutions containing the alkaloid ergometrine (the 2-amino-1-propanol derivative of D-$(+)$-lysergic acid), as well as decomposing by hydrolysis, undergo isomerization to ergometrinine (Foster, McDonald & Jones 1949).

Ergometrine

The D-$(+)$-lysergic acid portion of the ergometrine molecule contains asymmetric carbon atoms at C_5 and C_8. Epimerization occurs at the C_8 carbon atom to produce the D-$(+)$-isolysergic acid derivative ergometrinine which has little physiological activity.

Geometrical Isomerization. Loss of activity produced by geometrical isomerization is due to the difference in potency exhibited by *cis* and *trans* isomers of some organic compounds. For example, the most active form of the vitamin A molecule has the all-*trans* configuration. However, in

All-*trans* vitamin A

aqueous solution as a component of a multivitamin preparation, in addition to oxidation, vitamin A palmitate isomerizes and forms the 6-mono-*cis* and 2,6-di-*cis* isomers, both of which have much lower potencies (Lehman et al. 1960).

POLYMERIZATION

Degradation of pharmaceutical products by polymerization involves the combination of two or more identical molecules to form a much larger and more complex molecule. Such a reaction is not often the initial cause of drug decomposition, but does occur as a further degradation process of primary decomposition products. Polymerization however, is the prime cause of degradation of the antiseptic formaldehyde. On standing, particularly in the cold, the aldehyde forms paraformaldehyde which is thrown out of solution as a white deposit.

$$HOCH_2[OH + nH]OCH_2[OH + H]OCH_2OH \longrightarrow HOCH_2(OCH_2)_nOCH_2OH$$

Formaldehyde hydrate   Paraformaldehyde

In order to prevent polymerization, 10 to 15 per cent of methyl alcohol is added as a stabilizer.

The straw-coloured solution produced at acid pH values upon autoclaving dextrose injection has been attributed to the polymerization of the major decomposition product 5–hydroxymethylfurfural. Similarly, adrenochrome, the primary oxidation product of adrenaline in acid solution, undergoes further oxidation and is finally converted into black and brown polymeric pigments.

DECARBOXYLATION

As the word implies, decarboxylation is the elimination of carbon dioxide from a compound. This problem is most commonly encountered when parenteral solutions of sodium bicarbonate are autoclaved. In order to minimize the decomposition of sodium bicarbonate, carbon dioxide is passed into the solution for one minute and the containers are sealed so as to be gas-tight prior to autoclaving.

Decarboxylation also occurs when autoclaving the tuberculostatic agent sodium aminosalicylate, and has been identified as a secondary degradation process of procaine. Hydrolysis of procaine yields *p*-aminobenzoic acid which, in weakly acidic solution, decarboxylates slowly with the production of aniline. Aniline darkens on exposure to light, and this could explain the development of colour in old procaine injections.

p-Aminobenzoic acid   Aniline

ABSORPTION OF CARBON DIOXIDE

The absorption of carbon dioxide from the atmosphere by a pharmaceutical product is a more frequent occurrence than the loss of carbon dioxide by decarboxylation. Solutions of potassium hydroxide, sodium hydroxide, calcium hydroxide and lead subacetate become turbid due to the formation of insoluble carbonates. They are therefore stored in well-filled, well-closed, containers. Magnesium oxide and the two volatile nasal decongestants, amphetamine and propylhexedrine, also absorb carbon dioxide from the atmosphere. More important, however, is the effect that carbon dioxide has upon the stability of solutions of the sodium salts of barbiturates. For example, the short-acting intravenous barbiturate sodium hexobarbitone, since it is the salt of a strong base and a weak acid, hydrolyses to give an alkaline solution in water. The solution can absorb carbon dioxide and this results in precipitation of hexobarbitone. This is a serious problem in the preparation of intravenous solutions of soluble barbiturates. They are therefore distributed as sterile powders in ampoules with instructions to dissolve immediately before use in Water for Injections free from carbon dioxide.

PHYSICAL FACTORS INFLUENCING CHEMICAL DEGRADATION

TEMPERATURE

The rates of most chemical reactions increase with rise in temperature. It is, therefore, important to be aware of this when formulating pharmaceutical products for use in tropical areas, or when a product has to be heat sterilized before use. Autoclaving aqueous injections, e.g. dextrose injection, or sterilizing oils, e.g. ethyl oleate, and powders, e.g. sulphanilamide, by dry heat methods can cause decomposition problems when the drug is thermolabile. The observed variation of reaction rate with temperature is an important aspect of the collision theory of chemical raction. According to this theory, a chemical reaction only takes place when molecules collide. The thermal energy of the colliding molecules is converted into energy which is necessary to break chemical bonds and enable the reaction to take place. However, the number of molecular collisions greatly exceeds the number of molecules reacting per second. It has been postulated that reaction only occurs upon collision of molecules possessing a certain minimum amount of energy (the energy of activation). As the temperature of the system is raised, the proportion of molecules having this minimum energy increases. It follows that, at higher temperatures, a greater number of the collisions will result in reaction of the molecules, and it is this that gives rise to the observed greater rate of reaction. The precise relationship between temperature and reaction rate is discussed in the later section dealing with chemical kinetics.

As a result of this phenomenon, it is possible to reduce the rate of decomposition of thermolabile drugs by storing them in a cool place. This technique is particularly useful for biological products such as insulin, oxytocin and vasopressin injections, and also for penicillin and its preparations, which may all be stored in a refrigerator.

There are however, a few instances where low temperature storage may have a tendency to accelerate decomposition. The increased rate of polymerization of formaldehyde at temperatures below 15° has already been mentioned. In certain oxidation processes where the oxygen content of the solution is a critical factor in the reaction, low temperatures can also have an adverse effect on stability. Although a reduction in temperature tends to reduce the rate of oxidation, it also produces an increase in the solubility of oxygen in solution. The increase in oxygen concentration will usually promote the rate of reaction, with the net result that low temperature storage reduces decomposition but not to the extent predicted by application of the rate of reaction–temperature relationship.

MOISTURE

Moisture absorbed on to the surface of a solid drug will often increase the rate of decomposition if it is susceptible to hydrolysis. This is particularly true of aspirin, the penicillins, and other antibiotics such as streptomycin and tetracycline. The presence of moisture may in some instances also increase the rate of oxidation of a susceptible product, since oxygen is dissolved in the water layer surrounding the drug particles. For example, ferrous sulphate crystals are more rapidly oxidized in moist air than in dry surroundings. It is therefore important that such drugs should be stored in as dry a condition as possible. When manufacturing solid dosage preparations from drugs whose chemical stability is affected by moisture, it may be necessary to work in an environment of controlled humidity. This technique has to be used when processing sodium ampicillin and potassium propicillin (Gore & Ashwin 1967). It is equally necessary to ensure that the excipients chosen for the product have moisture contents low enough to prevent transfer of moisture to the active drug.

LIGHT

Numerous references in the pharmaceutical literature refer to the instability of many products when exposed to strong sunlight. Although, in some instances, the instability is due to the heat accompanying the sun's rays, light is a form of energy that can initiate and accelerate decomposition. It is important to distinguish between these heat and light effects in order to determine whether a preparation must be stored below 20°, or protected from light. In the same way that increased temperature can accelerate a thermal reaction, exposure of a light-sensitive drug (photolabile drug) to sunlight supplies sufficient energy of activation to enable decomposition to take place. Only the light radiation absorbed by the drug is effective in producing photochemical reaction. Since a portion, or all, of the light energy may be converted into heat, it should be borne in mind that absorption of light by a compound does not necessarily indicate that a photochemical reaction is proceeding. However, if a photochemical reaction is taking place, the rate will be independent of the temperature of the system.

The relationship between the amount of light absorbed and the amount of reaction taking place was proposed by Einstein in the 'Law of Photochemical Equivalence'. This states that each molecule can only undergo chemical reaction as a direct result of absorption of light, if one quantum of radiant energy causing the reaction is taken up. The unit of radiant energy equivalent to one quantum is called the photon. The energy of the photon is directly proportional to the frequency of the absorbed radiation (inversely proportional to the wavelength). It follows therefore that there is more energy in a photon of short wavelength, than in a photon of light of longer wavelength. For this reason photochemical destruction of pharmaceutical products is usually due to absorption of sunlight of the visible blue and violet and ultraviolet wavelengths (500 to 300 nm). Table 10.1 shows the energy available on absorption per g-mol of substance for different portions of the ultraviolet and visible spectrum.

TABLE 10.1

ENERGY AVAILABLE (kJ/g-mol) AT VARIOUS WAVELENGTHS

Wavelength (nm)	Colour region	Energy (kJ/g-mol)
700	Red	171.6
600	Yellow-orange	200.9
500	Blue-green	238.6
400	Violet	297.2
300	Ultraviolet	357.7

Since there is a relationship between the amount of light energy and the number of molecules undergoing reaction, it follows that a dilute solution of a photolabile drug may be completely inactivated when exposed to light, whereas a more concentrated solution will be only partially destroyed under similar conditions.

Many types of chemical reaction are induced by exposure to light of high energy. For example, amyl nitrite and ethyl nitrite undergo hydrolysis, and many autoxidation processes, e.g. volatile oil oxidation, are initiated. In other cases substances become coloured, e.g. morphine, codeine, and quinine become yellow-brown, while others fade, e.g. the water-soluble dyes indigo carmine and tartrazine incorporated in tablets. There is often a relationship between the structure of the drug and its sensitivity towards light. For example, phenolic substances such as phenol, thymol and salicylates tend to develop colours, while the presence of a conjugated double bond system in the molecule, as in vitamin A and many unsaturated oils, can also induce photolability. Halogenated drugs such as potassium iodide, iophendylate, and the anaesthetics chloroform, tribromomethanol and trichloroethylene are also susceptible to degradation in the presence of light.

Photochemical reactions are rarely simple, since products of reaction are often subsequently involved in thermal reactions, and it is then difficult to distinguish between the primary and secondary processes. For instance, light may initiate the complex autoxidation chain process whose subsequent steps are controlled by factors such as temperature, presence of oxygen, chemical structure of the compound, or the presence of pro-oxidants. Perhaps it is for this reason that, although there are many references to the instability of compounds in the presence of light, relatively few studies have been made of the mechanisms of the decomposition processes. Nevertheless, the photochemical decomposition of cyanocobalamin (vitamin B_{12}) has been well documented. In aqueous solution, in the pH range 3.5 to 6.5, cyanocobalamin is converted to hydroxocobalamin by the action of light. This is a reversible process involving the liberation of the cyanide ion. Hydroxocobalamin is less active than its precursor and is itself susceptible to degradation.

$$\text{Cyanocobalamin} \underset{\text{Dark } CN^-}{\overset{\text{Light } H^+}{\rightleftharpoons}} \text{Hydroxocobalamin} + CN^-$$

Oxidation ↓

Biologically inactive products

Demerre and Wilson (1956) investigated the effect of both intensity and wavelength of light upon the decomposition of the vitamin in neutral solution. They found that exposure to diffuse daylight (intensity about 100 lm/m^2), or daylight of intensity up to about 3000 lm/m^2 produced no noticeable destruction of the solution. When exposed to sunlight at a brightness of about 80 000 lm/m^2, the vitamin lost 10 per cent of its potency for every 30 minutes of direct exposure. Upon exposing the solution to ultraviolet light, a similar amount of decomposition was observed, whereas with light of longer wavelengths (600 to 700 nm) no degradation was evident.

RADIATION

As is discussed in Chapter 28, ionizing radiation can be a useful technique for the sterilization of certain pharmaceutical products, especially those that are thermolabile. Unfortunately, radiation treatment can also produce deleterious changes in the products since the procedure also causes ionization in the irradiated material. The ions formed in the initial stage of the process are subsequently converted into atoms and free radicals which become involved in chemical reactions. In 1960, a preliminary investigation was undertaken to assess the stability of a wide range of pharmaceutical products to γ-irradiation from a ^{60}Co source (A.B.P.I. Report, June 1960, *The Use of Gamma Radiation for the Sterilization of Pharmaceutical Products*). Antibiotics, e.g. polymyxin sulphate and streptomycin sulphate, alkaloids, e.g. atropine sulphate, steroids, e.g. progesterone, sulphonamides and biological products, e.g. insulin and heparin, were all irradiated at dose levels of 2.5 Mrad (sterilizing dose) and also 25 Mrad in order to identify possible decomposition products. The amount of decomposition observed varied from one product to another, and ranged from changes in colour, e.g. with progesterone, to almost complete loss of activity, e.g. insulin injection. The mechanisms of decomposition were not determined for any of the preparations, but it is probable that they differ from those occurring in normal thermal reactions. Irradiation of a drug in aqueous solution produces greater changes than irradiation of the pure material. This is believed to be due to the fact that irradiation of water produces hydrogen peroxide, and free radicals such as $OH^{\bullet}$, $HO_2^{\bullet}$ and $H^{\bullet}$ which have an additional oxidative effect on the drug. Fletcher and Davies (1968) have investigated the stability of 0.5 per cent w/v physostigmine sulphate solutions towards γ-irradiation emitted from a ^{60}Co source. Using dose levels up to 7 Mrad, decomposition was found to be independent of pH in the range 1.5 to 7. This is in contrast to the normal decomposition process which shows a maximum stability in the region of pH 2.2 to 3.0. In addition, the incorporation of 0.5 per cent w/v sodium metabisulphite reduced the amount of decomposition upon irradiation, whereas it had no effect upon the normal decomposition process.

THE APPLICATION OF CHEMICAL KINETICS TO DECOMPOSITION OF PHARMACEUTICAL PRODUCTS

A study of the reaction kinetics of decomposition enables a quantitative assessment to be made of the rate at which the drug is destroyed. In addition, information concerning the number and type of intermediate steps which eventually produce the decomposition products can often be obtained. The application of kinetics also helps us to understand how such factors as concentration of reactants, temperature, composition of solvent system, and the presence of catalysts may affect the rate of reaction.

Chemical kinetic theory is based upon the Law of Mass Action propounded by Guldberg and Waage in 1863. According to this law, the rate of a chemical reaction is proportional to the molar concentrations of the reacting substances each raised to a power equal to the number of g-moles of that substance involved in the reaction. Therefore, for a reaction of the general form:

$$uA + vB + wC \longrightarrow \text{Products}, \quad (10.2)$$

the law may be expressed as:

$$\text{Rate} = k[A]^u[B]^v[C]^w, \quad (10.3)$$

where $[A]$ is the molar concentration of reactant A,
$[B]$ is the molar concentration of reactant B,
$[C]$ is the molar concentration of reactant C,
u, v and w are the numbers of molecules of A, B and C, respectively, involved in the reaction as expressed by equation (10.2),
k is variously known as the rate constant, reaction velocity constant, or specific reaction rate.

DEFINITIONS

Rate of Reaction
The rate (velocity or speed) of a reaction can be expressed either as the decrease in concentration per unit time of any of the reacting substances, or as the increase in concentration per unit time of one of the products. Thus, if the initial concentration of a reactant is a g-mol/litre, and, after time t, x g-mol/litre have reacted, the rate of reaction may be written as either:

$$-\frac{d(a-x)}{dt} \quad \text{or} \quad \frac{dx}{dt}.$$

Molecularity of Reaction
The molecularity of a chemical reaction is equal to the number of molecules or atoms that must collide simultaneously to give the reaction products. If one molecule or atom undergoes change, the reaction is unimolecular. If two molecules or atoms react together, then the process is said to be bimolecular. The stoichiometric equation (10.2) would be trimolecular if u, v and w each had a value of one, since the reaction would depend upon the simultaneous combination of the three molecules A, B and C.

Since molecularity is determined by postulating a mechanism for the reaction, it must be a small number which cannot have fractional or zero values.

Order of Reaction
Since many reactions are complex, experiment often shows that the rate of reaction depends upon

a smaller number of concentration terms than indicated by either the molecularity or the stoichiometric equation for the reaction. Order of reaction expresses the experimentally determined dependence of the rate upon the reactant concentrations. The order of reaction with respect to a single reactant is equal to the power to which the concentration term of the reactant is raised in the experimental rate equation. By way of example, if experiment shows that in equation (10.3), u, v and w have values of 2, 1 and 0, respectively, the reaction is said to be second-order with respect to A, first-order in B, and zero-order in C. In this instance, the experimentally determined rate is only dependent upon the concentrations of reactants A and B. The overall order of reaction is the sum of the powers of the concentration terms affecting the experimentally determined rate. In the above example, the reaction would be third-order overall.

It is evident that, in contrast to molecularity, it is possible for the order of reaction to assume fractional or zero values.

Half-life

The rate of a chemical reaction may also be expressed in terms of the time taken for 50 per cent of the reaction to occur. This time is called the half-life of the reaction, $t_{1/2}$, and depends, in general, upon both the initial concentrations of the reactants and the reaction velocity constant. The exact relationships between these three parameters will be discussed in the following section.

DERIVATION OF THE SIMPLER ORDERS OF REACTION

First-order Reactions

By definition, the rate of a first-order reaction is proportional to the concentration of the reactant. This may be written in the form:

$$\frac{dx}{dt} = k(a-x), \qquad (10.4)$$

where a is the initial reactant concentration,
    x is the amount reacted in time t,
    k is the first-order reaction velocity constant.
Rearrangement of equation (10.4) gives:

$$\frac{dx}{(a-x)} = kdt, \qquad (10.5)$$

and, upon integration of equation (10.5):

$$-\ln(a-x) = kt + \text{integration constant}, \qquad (10.6)$$

when $t = 0$, $x = 0$, and the integration constant =

$-\ln a$. Substituting for the integration constant in equation (10.6) we obtain:

$$k = \frac{1}{t} \ln \frac{a}{(a-x)} \qquad (10.7)$$

It is more convenient to use common logarithms rather than natural logarithms, Hence:

$$k = \frac{2.303}{t} \log \frac{a}{(a-x)} \qquad (10.8)$$

If the change in reactant concentration is followed with respect to time, a plot of the common logarithm of concentration against time will be a straight line whose slope is $-k/2.303$. The first-order reaction velocity constant can then be calculated, and will have dimensions of time^{-1}.

Half-life of a first-order reaction

If the initial reactant concentration is a, at time $t_{1/2}$ the concentration of reactant remaining will be $a/2$. Hence, the first-order kinetic equation becomes:

$$k = \frac{2.303}{t_{1/2}} \log 2 \qquad (10.9)$$

and

$$t_{1/2} = \frac{0.693}{k} \qquad (10.10)$$

Thus, for a first-order reaction, the half-life is independent of the initial reactant concentration, and depends solely upon the reaction velocity constant.

Pseudo-first-order reactions

When defining the order of a chemical reaction, it was stated that the reaction rate often depends upon fewer concentration terms than indicated by the stoichiometric equation for the process. This state of affairs can arise for one or more of the following reasons. Firstly, one or more of the reactants may be present in such large excess that there is no measurable change in its concentration during the course of the reaction. Secondly, if the reaction has several component steps, and if one of these is considerably slower than the rest, it will be the rate-determining step. In this event the kinetics and order of reaction of the process will be those of the rate-determining step. Finally, if one of the reactants is acting as a catalyst in the reaction, its concentration will not change as the reaction proceeds.

A chemical reaction obeys pseudo-first-order kinetics when the rate of the process is proportional to the concentration of only one of the reactants, even though the reaction involves several reactant species. This situation is frequently encountered with drugs that are susceptible to hydrolytic decomposition. Water, although it may participate in the reaction, is in great excess and thus its concentration is essentially constant throughout the process. The hydroxyl and/or hydrogen ions may act as catalysts for the hydrolysis, and thus their concentrations also remain constant. The rate of degradation will then depend solely upon the concentration of the drug.

Procaine hydrochloride undergoes hydrolysis which obeys pseudo-first-order kinetics. A graph of the logarithm of the percentage of the local anaesthetic remaining against time yields a straight line (Fig. 10.2). From the slope of this line, the

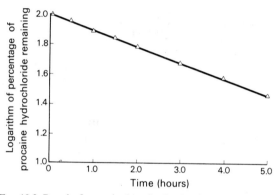

FIG. 10.2. Pseudo-first-order kinetic plot for the decomposition of procaine hydrochloride in ammonium hydroxide–hydrochloric acid buffer, pH 9.7 at 50°. Pseudo-first-order reaction velocity constant $(k) = 0.25$/hour.

reaction velocity constant for the decomposition at 50° in ammonium chloride-hydrochloric acid buffer of pH 9.7 is calculated to be 0.25 hour^{-1}.

Second-order Reactions
The rate of a second-order reaction is proportional to the concentrations of two reacting species. The rate of reaction is given by:

$$\frac{dx}{dt} = k(a-x)(b-x) \qquad (10.11)$$

where a and b are the initial concentrations of reactants A and B. x is the decrease in the concentrations of A and B after time t. Integration of equation (10.11) by the method of partial fractions, and evaluation of the integration constant yields:

$$k = \frac{2.303}{t(a-b)} \log \frac{b(a-x)}{a(b-x)} \qquad (10.12)$$

The value of k may be determined by plotting the function:

$$\frac{1}{(a-b)} \log \frac{b(a-x)}{a(b-x)} \text{ against } t,$$

when the slope of the straight line will be equal to $k/2.303$. The reaction velocity constant for the second-order process will have dimensions of concentration^{-1} time^{-1}.

If the initial concentrations of the reactants are equal, or if the rate of reaction depends upon the square of the concentration of a single reactant, the rate equation takes the form:

$$\frac{dx}{dt} = k(a-x)^2 \qquad (10.13)$$

which upon integration gives:

$$k = \frac{1}{t} \frac{x}{a(a-x)} \qquad (10.14)$$

In this instance, a plot of $x/(a-x)$ against time t, will produce a straight line whose slope is ak.

Anderson and Slade (1966) have shown that the hydrolysis of chlorbutol, in the presence of sodium hydroxide, follows second-order kinetics, since the rate of decomposition depends upon both the concentrations of chlorbutol and hydroxyl ions. The plot for this decomposition process is shown in Fig. 10.3. One molecule of chlorbutol yields three

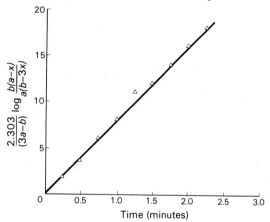

FIG. 10.3. Second-order kinetic plot for the decomposition of chlorbutol in sodium hydroxide at 25° (Anderson & Slade 1966).

chloride ions. In this particular case where there are unequal initial reactant concentrations, to obtain the second-order reaction velocity constant, it is necessary to plot the function:

$$\frac{2.303}{(3a-b)} \log \frac{b(a-x)}{a(b-3x)} \text{ against time.}$$

The slope of the graph will then be equal to k.

Half-life of a second-order reaction

For second-order decompositions that obey equation (10.14), substitution of $a/2$ for x at time $t_{1/2}$ shows that:

$$t_{1/2} = \frac{1}{ka} \qquad (10.15)$$

Hence, it is evident that, unlike first-order reactions, the half-life is dependent upon both the reaction velocity constant and the initial reactant concentration. As the initial concentration increases, the half-life decreases.

For second-order processes where there are unequal initial reactant concentrations, it is not possible to derive a simple relationship between $t_{1/2}$ and initial reactant concentration. However, it is still the case that the half-life decreases with increase in initial reactant concentration.

Zero-order Reactions

Zero-order reaction kinetics are obeyed when the rate of reaction is independent of the concentrations of any of the reactants and does not alter with time. This may be expressed mathematically in the form:

$$\frac{dx}{dt} = k \qquad (10.16)$$

Integrating equation (10.16), we obtain:

$$\int dx = k \int dt \qquad (10.17)$$

Thus $\qquad kt = x + $ integration constant, $\qquad$ (10.18)

when $t = 0$, $x = 0$, and the integration constant $= 0$. Therefore, for a zero-order kinetic process:

$$kt = x \qquad (10.19)$$

A plot of the amount of drug decomposed (or of the amount remaining) against time will yield a straight line whose slope is k. The dimensions of the zero-order reaction velocity constant are concentration time^{-1}.

Half-life of a zero-order reaction

When $t = t_{1/2}$, $x = a/2$, and from equation (10.19)

$$t_{1/2} = \frac{a/2}{k} \qquad (10.20)$$

The half-life is directly proportional to the initial reactant concentration, and inversely proportional to the zero-order reaction velocity constant.

The factor governing the rate of a chemical reaction exhibiting zero-order kinetics might possibly be the concentration of a catalyst, or the amount of light absorbed if the reaction is photochemical. When considering pharmaceutical systems, zero-order processes are most likely to be encountered when investigating the stability of drugs in suspension. For example, let us assume that a sparingly-soluble drug decomposes in aqueous solution according to first-order kinetics. The rate of decomposition will, therefore, be expressed by equation (10.4). In the case of a suspension of the drug, as decomposition proceeds in solution, some of the suspended material will dissolve to maintain the concentration of drug in solution constant. Equation (10.4) must then be modified:

$$\frac{dx}{dt} = ka_s \qquad (10.21)$$

where a_s is the initial drug concentration, and is equal to its solubility in the solvent system.

Under these conditions the rate of decomposition is independent of the drug concentration and hence will obey zero-order kinetics. Kornblum and Zoglio (1967) have shown this to be the case for the hydrolysis of aspirin suspensions in combination with tablet lubricants.

Third-order Reactions

If a reaction appears to obey third-order kinetics, this infers that there is collision of three molecules having sufficient energy to cause reaction. This is an unusual occurrence, and the kinetic equations expressing the rates of reaction are complex and will not be considered further.

COMPLEXITY OF KINETIC RELATIONSHIPS OCCURRING IN SOME PHARMACEUTICAL PRODUCTS

Thus far, an outline has been given of the simple kinetic relationships that may be obeyed in pharmaceutical systems. However, it should be appreciated that certain drugs can exhibit decomposition pathways of considerable kinetic complexity. A brief reference was made earlier to the fact that the overall decomposition reaction may consist of several intermediate steps even incorporating reversible and/or parallel processes. If one of the intermediate steps is slower than the rest, the rate of decomposition will be dependent upon the rate of this step.

As an example of the complexity of some of these processes, the decomposition of the diuretic chlorothiazide will be considered. The final product of decomposition is 4-amino-6-chloro-*m*-benzene

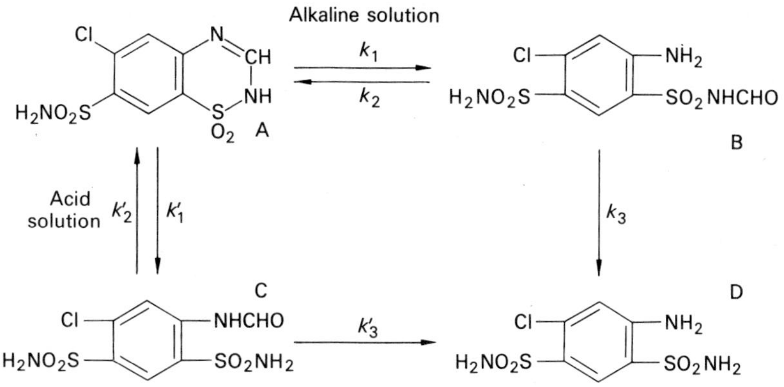

FIG. 10.4. Kinetic processes leading to the decomposition of chlorothiazide (Yamana, Mizukami & Tsuji 1968) k_1, k_1', k_3 and k_3' are the first-order reaction velocity constants for the forward reactions k_2, k_2' are the first-order reaction velocity constants for the reverse reactions. A, Chlorothiazide; B, N-(2-Amino-4-chloro-5-sulphamoyl phenyl sulphonyl) formamide; C, 5-Chloro-2,4-disulphamoyl formanilide; D, 4-Amino-6-chloro-m-benzenedisulphonamide.

disulphonamide. However, this is produced by a series of parallel consecutive first-order reactions as outlined in Fig. 10.4 (Yamana, Mizukami & Tsuji 1968).

THE INFLUENCE OF TEMPERATURE UPON THE RATE OF DECOMPOSITION

As a general rule, the rate of decomposition increases as the temperature is raised. It has long been recognized that the rate of a chemical reaction increases by a factor of between two and three-fold for every 10° rise in temperature in the region of room temperature. By way of example, experiment has shown that the pseudo-first-order reaction velocity constant for the hydrolysis of procaine hydrochloride in pH 9.7 buffer at 40° has a value of 0.11/hour, whilst at 50° the value rises to 0.25/hour.

Arrhenius, in 1889, proposed an equation which related the reaction velocity constant and temperature. The equation was derived from a consideration of the variation of the equilibrium constant of a reversible chemical reaction, K, with temperature, and the relationship between K and the reaction velocity constants of the forward and reverse reactions.

The equation takes the form:

$$\frac{d \ln k}{dT} = \frac{E}{RT^2} \qquad (10.22)$$

where k is the reaction velocity constant,
T is the absolute temperature,
R is the gas constant,
E is the energy of activation which molecules must possess before they will interact.

Integration of equation (10.22) gives:

$$\ln k = \frac{-E}{RT} + \text{integration constant.} \quad (10.23)$$

A more useful form of equation (10.23) is:

$$k = Ae^{-E/RT} \qquad (10.24)$$

where A is a constant which is termed the frequency factor.

The logarithmic form of equation (10.24) can be written:

$$\log k = \log A - \frac{E}{2.303 RT} \qquad (10.25)$$

Thus the common logarithms of the reaction velocity constants at the various temperatures, plotted against the reciprocals of the absolute temperatures will yield a straight line whose slope will be $E/2.303R$.

FACTORS INFLUENCING, AND METHODS OF REDUCING, CHEMICAL DEGRADATION

When the nature of chemical decomposition of a drug has been established, it is possible to develop formulations that minimize the instability by determining those factors that influence the rate of decomposition.

HYDROLYSIS

Adjustment of pH
It will be recalled that when hydrolysis is catalysed by hydrogen and/or hydroxyl ions, the rate of decomposition is critically dependent upon pH.

Often this can be shown by plotting the relationship between the logarithm of the reaction velocity constant for decomposition, and pH. If the reaction exhibits specific acid-base catalysis, a minimum in the curve is observed. For example, Fig. 10.5 shows

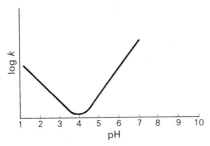

FIG. 10.5. General relationship between $\log k$ and pH for the hydrolytic decomposition of atropine sulphate.

the general form of the curve obtained for the hydrolysis of atropine sulphate. Maximum stability of the drug therefore occurs at pH 3.8. Similarly, a minimum is observed at pH 3.6 for procaine hydrochloride, pH 4.9 for benzocaine, and pH 5 for cinchocaine. It follows that a useful method for reducing hydrolysis of a drug exhibiting specific acid-base catalysis is to adjust the pH to the point corresponding to the minimum in the relationship. In many instances, however, pH affects the solubility and the therapeutic activity of the drug as well as its stability. It is necessary to take all three factors into account when attempting to limit decomposition.

For example, the ophthalmic drugs physostigmine, atropine and pilocarpine are weakly basic in character and show maximum stability in acid solution. Unfortunately, the basic forms of these drugs exhibit the greatest therapeutic activity, probably due to their enhanced lipid solubility in comparison with their salts. Thus neutral solutions of the drugs are more effective than acidic solutions when instilled in the eye. Under alkaline conditions, the drugs precipitate from solution. It is evident that the pH selected in formulating the solutions has to be a compromise. For instance, the basic form of pilocarpine is present to the extent of 99 per cent at pH 9.0, whereas at pH 4.0 (the point of maximum stability) only 0.1 per cent of the drug exists as the base. One successful formulation of pilocarpine eye-drops involves adjusting the pH of the solution to 5.0 with boric acid. A stronger buffer system is not used since, upon instillation into the eye, the pH of the solution is able to rise to that of the tear secretions (pH 7.4) with consequent formation of the more active, basic

form of the drug. Prior to use, storage at pH 5.0 enables a reasonable degree of stabilization to be achieved.

Choice of solvent
Non-aqueous solvents, e.g. alcohol and propylene glycol, have often been used to replace a portion, or all, of the water in a solution in order to reduce hydrolysis of a drug. For example, an elixir of pentobarbitone sodium contains considerable quantities of glycerin and alcohol, while aspirin, which is very unstable in aqueous solution, has been formulated in an alcohol–propylene glycol solvent (Schwartz, Shvemar & Renaldi 1958). The assumption is widespread that replacement of water by a non-aqueous solvent automatically enhances the stability of the product. Although this is true in many instances, there are cases where a non-aqueous solvent may increase the instability of a product. For example, cyclamic acid in aqueous solution hydrolyses at a very slow rate, whereas in alcoholic solution the compound degrades at markedly faster rates (Talmage, Chafetz & Elefant 1968). Only with a knowledge of the chemical kinetics of the process, and the reactant species involved, is it possible to make a valid prediction of the effect that a non-aqueous solvent system will have. It has been shown that the effect depends upon the solubility of the drug in relation to the solubility of its decomposition products, upon the dielectric constant of the solvent system, and upon the chemical nature of the reactant species.

Firstly, let us consider relative solubilities of the drug and the decomposition products in the solvent. In general a reaction will proceed more rapidly if the products of the reaction have a higher affinity for the solvent than the reactants. The quantitative relationship between the reaction velocity constant of the decomposition process and solubility is given by the equation:

$$\log k = \log k_o + \frac{V}{2.303RT}(\Delta\delta_A + \Delta\delta_B - \Delta\delta^*)$$

$$(10.26)$$

where k is the observed reaction velocity constant,

k_o is the reaction velocity constant for the reaction proceeding in an infinitely dilute solution exhibiting ideal behaviour,

V is an approximation for the molar volumes of the reactants A, B and the activated complex formed during the reaction and prior to the formation of the product,

$\Delta\delta_A$, $\Delta\delta_B$ and $\Delta\delta^*$ are mathematical functions that represent the difference in 'polar' characteristics of the solvent and reactant A, reactant B, and the products of the reaction respectively,

R is the gas constant,

T is the absolute temperature.

It follows that if the products of decomposition have polar characteristics similar to that of the solvent (i.e. $\Delta\delta^* \simeq 0$) while the reactants have polar characteristics unlike the solvent (i.e. $\Delta\delta_A$ and $\Delta\delta_B > 0$), then the term $V/2.303RT$ $(\Delta\delta_A + \Delta\delta_B - \Delta\delta^*)$ will have a positive value and the observed reaction velocity will be greater than that occurring in an ideal solution. If, on the other hand, the reactants have similar polar characteristics to the solvent ($\Delta\delta_A$ and $\Delta\delta_B \simeq 0$), and the products have polar characteristics unlike that of the solvent ($\Delta\delta^* > 0$), then the term $V/2.303RT$ $(\Delta\delta_A + \Delta\delta_B - \Delta\delta^*)$ will be negative and the rate of decomposition will be lower in this particular solvent. Generally speaking, highly polar solvents, e.g. water, will accelerate decomposition reactions which form products having greater polar characteristics than the reactants. If the products are less polar than the reactants, the rate of reaction will be slower than expected. When dealing with solvents of low polarity, e.g. alcohol, the reverse argument will apply.

The presence, or absence, of an electrical charge on the drug molecule governs the way in which the dielectric constant of the solvent influences the rate of hydrolytic decomposition. If the process involves a charged drug molecule as well as another ionic species in the system, i.e. H^+ or OH^-, the equation which relates the reaction velocity constant to the dielectric constant of the solvent is:

$$\ln k = \ln k_{D=\infty} - \frac{NZ_A Z_B e^2}{RTr^*} \frac{1}{D} \quad (10.27)$$

where k is the observed reaction velocity constant for the decomposition in a solvent of dielectric constant D,

$k_{D=\infty}$ is the reaction velocity constant for the decomposition in a solvent of infinite dielectric constant,

N is Avagadro's number,

Z_A and Z_B are the charges on the two ionic species,

e is the value of the charge on the electron,

r^* is the distance between the ionic species in the activated complex.

It is evident that by plotting $\ln k$ against $1/D$ a straight line relationship will be obtained. The slope of the line will be negative if the charges Z_A and Z_B are of like sign. Thus, as the dielectric constant of the solvent is decreased, the rate of hydrolytic decomposition will decrease. In this instance, replacement of a portion, or all, of the water (high dielectric constant) with a solvent of lower dielectric constant e.g. alcohol, will decrease the rate of hydrolysis. On the other hand, if the charges Z_A and Z_B are of opposite sign, then the slope of the line will be positive, and decreasing the dielectric constant of the solvent will only serve to increase the rate of decomposition.

If the drug is a dipolar molecule carrying no charge, then the relationship between dielectric constant and the reaction velocity constant is given by:

$$\ln k = \ln k_{D=\infty} + \frac{NZ_A^2 e^2}{2RT}\left(\frac{1}{ra} - \frac{1}{r^*}\right) \cdot \frac{1}{D} \quad (10.28)$$

where Z_A is the charge of the ionic hydrolytic species,

ra is the radius of the ionic species,

r^* is the radius of the activated complex.

As before, upon plotting $\ln k$ against the reciprocal of the dielectric constant, a straight line will be obtained. Since r^* must always be larger than ra, the slope of the line will have a positive value whether the hydrolytic species has a negative or positive charge. In this instance, decreasing the dielectric constant of the solvent system will only increase the rate of decomposition. Marcus and Tarazka (1959) investigated the hydrogen ion-catalysed hydrolysis of chloramphenicol in the presence of high concentrations of perchloric acid and varying proportions of propylene glycol. They found that the rate of hydrolysis of the drug was increased with increasing concentrations of propylene glycol due to the fact that decomposition involved the dipolar chloramphenicol and hydrogen ions.

Production of an Insoluble Drug Form

Hydrolysis only occurs with that portion of a drug which is in aqueous solution. Therefore, if the majority of the drug is present as a suspension with a minimal amount in solution, there will be a reduction in the amount of hydrolysis. The solubility of a drug may sometimes be reduced by adjustment of the pH of the aqueous vehicle. This has been achieved with β-cyclopentyl-propionyl-salicylic acid which hydrolyses in suspension by only 1 per cent a year at pH values less than 3.5 (Garrett 1957). In other instances, solubility may be reduced by a careful selection of the drug vehicle or by producing an insoluble salt of the drug. This latter technique has been successfully used to produce the insoluble procaine salt of benzylpenicillin. Only a small proportion of the salt exists in solution as undissociated procaine penicillin and the penicillin ion (Swintosky et al. 1956).

The Presence of Surface-active Agents

Surface-active agents are widely used in pharmacy as solubilizing and emulsifying agents. Hence it is important to determine the effect they may have upon drug hydrolysis, especially when present in concentrations in excess of their critical micelle concentrations. The presence of surface-active agents can often result in a significant improvement in stability, but this is by no means the general rule. Their effect is dependent upon a variety of factors including the water solubility of the drug, the type, chain length and concentration of the surface-active agent, and the type of hydrolytic species, i.e. H^+ or OH^- ions, present.

Riegelman (1960) investigated solubilized solutions of the relatively water-insoluble drug benzocaine, which is subject to base catalysed hydrolysis. He found that increasing the concentration of the surface-active agent resulted in greater partition of the drug in favour of the micellar pseudophase. With ionic surface-active agents, the rate of hydrolysis steadily decreased as the concentration of the surface-active agent increased. The anionic agents afforded greater protection than the cationic agents, presumably due to the fact that the negatively charged anionic micelles produced a definite barrier to the attack by OH^- ions. The protective effect of non-ionic surface-active agents was not as great as that obtained with the ionic agents. The drug was present in the hydrated palisade layer of the non-ionic micelles, where attack by OH^- ions could take place to a limited extent.

A more complex situation arises when we consider the effect that surface-active agents have upon the hydrolytic decomposition of highly water-soluble drugs. Since these will not be preferentially soluble in the semi-protective environment of the micellar pseudophase, it might be thought that surface-active agents would have little or no effect upon the stability in aqueous solution. In fact, as Nogami et al. (1960, 1962, 1963) have shown, using methantheline bromide, this is only true to a limited extent. The hydrolysis of this cationic, highly water-

soluble, compound is specific acid-base catalysed. Cationic and non-ionic surface-active agents had little effect upon the base-catalysed hydrolysis of the drug, whereas anionic agents produced a high degree of stabilization. This latter phenomenon was attributed to the formation of a water-insoluble complex between the drug and a proportion of the surface-active agent. The complex was preferentially soluble in the micellar pseudophase produced by the remainder of the surface-active agent. The drug was further protected from hydroxyl ion attack because of repulsion of the ions by the negatively charged micelles. When drug hydrolysis was catalysed by H^+ ions, the drug-surface-active agent complex showed increased susceptibility to attack, presumably due to the fact that H^+ ions were attracted to the micelles.

The general conclusions of Nogami and Awazu (1962) and Riegelman (1960) can be seen to be complementary when we consider the stability of solutions of a drug whose solubility in water changes with pH. Nogami and Awazu (1962) examined the stability of aspirin in solutions of non-ionic, cationic and anionic surface-active agents. Unionized aspirin is only sparingly soluble in water, whereas the acetyl salicylate ion is very water-soluble. With change in pH, the composition and hence total water solubility of the drug will change. As mentioned previously, the hydrolysis of aspirin is catalysed by both H^+ and OH^- ions, and six contributory reactions are known to occur

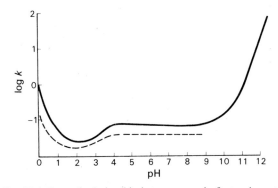

Fig. 10.6. General relationship between pseudo first-order rate constant and pH for aspirin in the presence (broken line) and absence (solid line) of 5 per cent w/v cetylethyldimethylammonium bromide.

over a range of pH. Fig. 10.6 shows the general shape of log k–pH profile for the pseudo-first-order hydrolysis of the drug in the presence and absence of a 5 per cent w/v concentration of the cationic surface-active agent cetylethyldimethylammonium bromide.

In the pH range 1 to 5, Nogami found that the non-ionic, cationic and anionic surface-active agents all reduced the rate of hydrolysis. This can be ascribed to the fact that the drug was present almost entirely in the form of the undissociated species, and therefore was preferentially soluble in the semi-protective micellar pseudophase. Both hydrogen and hydroxyl ion-catalysed attack was inhibited. From pH 5 to 7.5, however, the drug was increasingly in the ionized form, and anionic and non-ionic surface-active agents had little effect on its stability. The cationic agents reduced the rate of hydrolysis because of the formation of a water-insoluble complex with the ionized drug which was preferentially soluble in the micellar pseudophase. Close to pH 1, the drug was undissociated and hydrolysis was due to hydrogen ion-catalysed attack. The rate of decomposition was reduced when using cationic and non-ionic surface-active agents, but was promoted when an anionic agent was utilized. The drug present in the negatively-charged micelles was subjected to increased attack by H^+ ions attracted to the micelles.

The rate of hydrolysis of emulsified systems of a water-insoluble compound has been found to be affected by the ability of the surface-active agent to solubilize the material. Since the bulk of the drug is present in oil globules and is inaccessible to hydrolytic attack, the rate of decomposition is normally slow. However, an investigation of the stability of ethyl benzoate emulsions, using the cationic surface-active agent cetrimide, has shown that increasing the concentration of cetrimide increased the rate of decomposition to a maximum (Mitchell 1962). At this point the quantity of surface-active agent present was sufficient to solubilize all the compound. The observed increase in rate of hydrolysis was due to the increasing proportion of drug in solution (partitioned between the true aqueous phase and the micellar pseudophase) relative to that in the emulsion droplets. As one might expect, upon increasing the surface-active agent concentration beyond the point where complete solubilization was achieved, there was a decrease in the rate of decomposition as more of the material was partitioned in favour of the semi protective micellar pseudophase.

The Presence of a Complexing Agent

The concept of protecting a drug from hydrolysis by the addition of a chemical stabilizer was introduced by Higuchi and Lachman in 1955. They postulated that adding a compound which would form a water-soluble complex with the drug might

in some measure decrease the rate of decomposition. To this end they determined the effect that caffeine has upon base-catalysed hydrolysis of the local anaesthetics benzocaine, procaine and amethocaine. In all cases caffeine was found to decrease the rate of decomposition. As the concentration of caffeine was increased, the degree of stabilization also increased. Higuchi and his co-workers showed that, as more caffeine was added, a greater proportion of the drug existed in the complexed form and was protected from attack by OH^- ions. For example, with benzocaine the complex was found to be of stoichiometric ratio 1:1 viz:

Benzocaine + Caffeine $\rightleftharpoons$

[Benzocaine 1:1 Caffeine].

The observed first-order reaction velocity constant for the system could be represented by the equation:

$$k = k_f F_f + k_c F_c \qquad (10.29)$$

where k is the observed reaction velocity constant for the decomposition of benzocaine in the presence of caffeine,

k_f is the reaction velocity constant for the decomposition of free benzocaine,

k_c is the reaction velocity constant for the decomposition of benzocaine in the caffeine–benzocaine complex,

F_f is the fraction of free benzocaine in solution,

F_c is the fraction of benzocaine in the caffeine–benzocaine complex.

By calculation, it was determined that the rate of decomposition of the local anaesthetic in the complex was insignificantly small (approximately one hundredth of the rate of the free benzocaine), and that for all practical purposes the complexed form does not contribute to the decomposition. Thus:

$$k \simeq k_f F_f \qquad (10.30)$$

The molecular structure and forces involved in the formation of the complex are unknown, and it is surprising that this type of mild molecular action can result in such efficient stabilization. The effect may be due to steric factors, since the relatively large size of the complexing molecule could prevent the approach of OH^- ions to the drug. Alternatively, the presence of the complexing agent may alter the electrical charge distribution over the drug molecule and reduce the tendency for OH^- ions to interact with it. Whatever the exact mechanism of the phenomenon, it has been shown that caffeine will also protect the more complex drug riboflavine in a similar manner. Polyvinylpyrrolidone, desoxycholic acid and 1-ethyltheobromine all have a similar, but less marked, stabilizing effect upon local anaesthetics.

The technique of reducing hydrolysis by addition of a complexing agent has been of practical value in the stabilization of procaine in an injection containing 3.42 per cent w/v of an equimolecular compound of procaine and caffeine in a sodium chloride vehicle.

OXIDATION

The presence of antioxidants
The decomposition of many readily oxidizable materials, e.g. fats, may be reduced by adding a small quantity of a substance that will retard the autoxidation process. Such substances are known as antioxidants, and the ideal antioxidant has the following properties:
(i) Effective in low concentrations.
(ii) Adequately soluble in the oxidizable products.
(iii) Non-toxic and non-irritant at the effective concentration, even after prolonged storage.
(iv) Odourless, tasteless and should not impart colour to the product.
(v) Decomposition products should be non-toxic and non-irritant.
(vi) Stable and effective over a wide range of pH.
(vii) Neutral, and should not react chemically with other constituents present.
(viii) Of low volatility to ensure that loss does not occur during storage.

The term antioxidant embraces several classes of chemically unrelated compounds which may pos-. sess different modes of action. However, it is possible to make a broad distinction between compounds acting as primary antioxidants and those acting as synergists.

Primary antioxidants (antioxygens) act by interfering with the propagation step of the autoxidation process. To maintain the propagation chain process, an $R^\bullet$ or $ROO^\bullet$ free radical is required. The antioxidant molecule (AH) has the ability to react with such radicals, and this results in the formation of free radical $A^\bullet$ which is not sufficiently reactive to sustain the chain process:

$$AH + R^\bullet \longrightarrow RH + A^\bullet$$

Antioxidant　　Free radical

$$AH + ROO^\bullet \longrightarrow ROOH + A^\bullet$$

Subsequently, the antioxidant radical is annihilated by combination with another antioxidant radical or some other free radical:

$$A^\bullet + A^\bullet \longrightarrow AA$$
$$A^\bullet + R^\bullet \longrightarrow AR$$

It follows that for effective stabilization against autoxidation, the A–H chemical bond of the antioxidant should be weaker than the R–H bond of the autoxidizable substance. However, if the bond is too weak, then the antioxidant will be destroyed rapidly by reaction with atmospheric oxygen:

$$AH + O_2 \longrightarrow A^\bullet + HO_2^\bullet$$

It is evident that a primary antioxidant is used up by taking part in the chain process instead of the drug. It only retards the onset of autoxidation of the drug, which proceeds normally when all of the antioxidant has been destroyed. The antioxidant will be rapidly used up if it is added to a product which has already undergone partial oxidation, since there will be many free radicals present. It is therefore important that the antioxidant be added at the earliest possible stage in the preparation of the product. The overall antioxidant effect is to increase the length of the induction period of the autoxidation process. The 'protection factor', defined as the ratio of the length of the induction period in the presence of the antioxidant to that in the absence of any antioxidant, is a measure of the relative efficiency of primary antioxidants in protecting a product. The concentration level at which the antioxidant is incorporated in the product can often be critical. Within a certain range, efficiency increases with concentration until an optimum concentration is reached. In the presence of an excess concentration of antioxidant, there may be a pro-oxidant effect due to the reaction of hydroperoxides with the antioxidant molecules to form free radicals:

$$ROOH + AH \longrightarrow RO^\bullet + A^\bullet + H_2O$$

The classes of primary antioxidants more commonly used to retard autoxidation in pharmaceutical products are outlined below.

Tocopherols. Tocopherols are naturally occurring substances often present in vegetable oils. They are considered to be the major class of natural antioxidants, and are present in optimum concentrations, i.e. in the range 0.01 to 0.1 per cent. Addition of an antioxidant to a vegetable oil already containing tocopherols may accelerate the decomposition. The processes used for refining vegetable oils tend to remove these antioxidants, and subsequent readdition does not usually produce the same level of stabilization. Concentrates of the tocopherols have been added to liquid paraffin to prevent flavours caused by oxidation of the small amounts of aromatic compounds present.

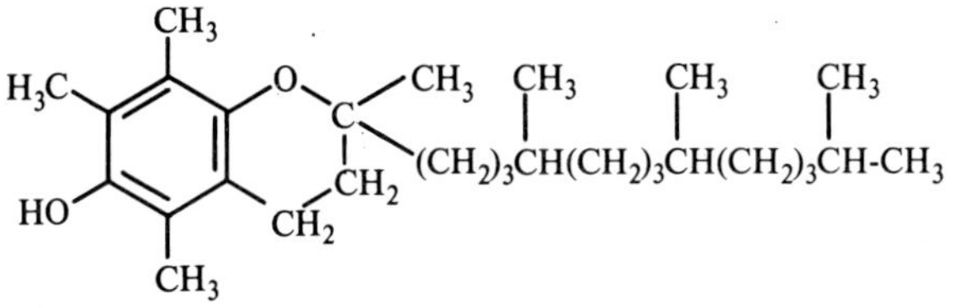

α-Tocopherol

Gallic acid and the gallates. Gallic acid is soluble in water and nearly insoluble in fats. Esterification of the carboxylic acid group with fatty alcohols produces esters which become progressively less soluble in water and more soluble in fats as the molecular weight of the alcohol increases. The gallates are widely used in the preservation of oils, fats, cosmetics and perfumes. The most commonly used esters are propyl, octyl and dodecyl gallates:

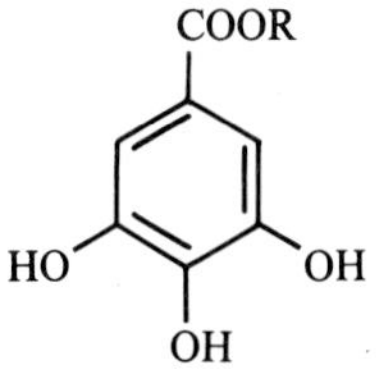

where R = H = gallic acid
R = C_3H_7 = propyl gallate,
R = C_8H_{17} = octyl gallate,
R = $C_{12}H_{25}$ = dodecyl gallate

Rancidity in most oils is prevented by the addition of up to 0.1 per cent of propyl gallate (or higher alkyl gallate). The amount required depends upon the degree of unsaturation of the oil. The addition of 0.002 to 0.01 per cent to ether retards the formation of peroxides, and 0.01 per cent reduces the decomposition of paraldehyde. For essential oils and emulsions, concentrations of 0.2 to 0.5 per cent of propyl gallate may be employed.

The alkyl gallates are effective antioxidants, but discolour in the presence of iron and its salts. The octyl and dodecyl esters are heat-resistant and non-volatile with steam.

Butylated hydroxyanisole. Butylated hydroxy-anisole (BHA) is the monomethyl ether of hydro-quinone containing a tertiary butyl side chain to increase its fat solubility. Chemically, it is a mixture of two isomers. It is most effective in stabilizing animal fats, and its antioxidant activity increases with concentration up to about 0.01 per cent while remaining approximately the same at higher levels.

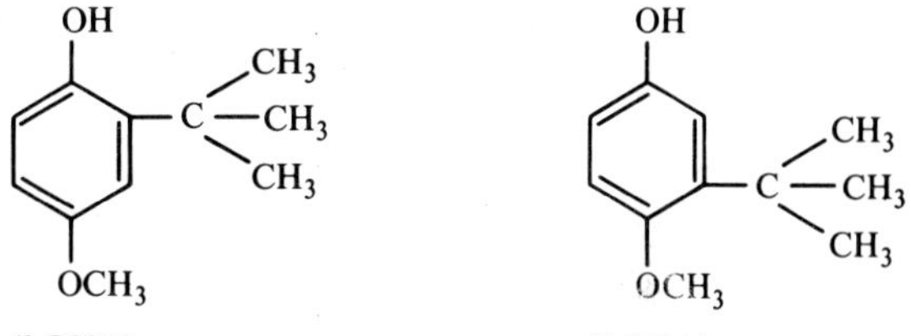

(3-BHA) (2-BHA)

Butylated hydroxyanisole

Butylated hydroxytoluene. The antioxidant properties of butylated hydroxytoluene (BHT) are similar to those of BHA. In pure fats it is less effective than propyl gallate but better than BHA. BHT does not have an optimum concentration; the stability of products to which it is added continues to increase with concentration, although the rate of increase is less at higher levels. The mode of action of primary antioxidants can be clearly seen using BHT as the example:

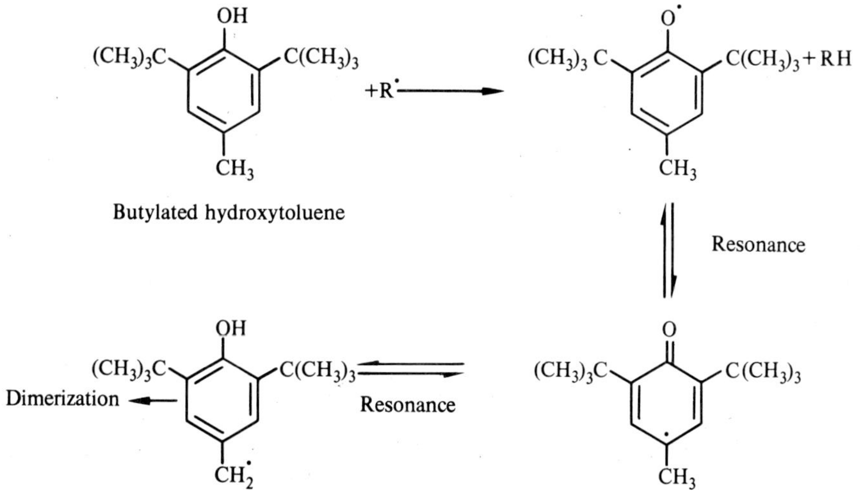

Butylated hydroxytoluene

Nordihydroguaiaretic acid. Nordihydroguaiaretic acid (NDGA) is extracted from a desert plant, and is effective in preventing oxidation in animal fats and fat emulsions. It is much less effective in vegetable oils than animal fats. It has a slightly bitter taste even in low concentrations.

Nordihydroguaiaretic acid

The synergist class of antioxidants have little inherent antioxidant activity. However, when used in conjunction with a primary antioxidant, they have the ability greatly to enhance antioxidant efficiency. Organic and inorganic compounds, containing several hydroxyl and/or carboxylic acid groupings, have been used as synergists, e.g. adipic, tartaric, phosphoric and sulphuric acids, phospholipids, and ascorbic acid. Since they are acidic in character they are sometimes referred to as 'acid-type' antioxidants. Synergists are commonly employed with phenolic antioxidants for the preservation of fats and oils: Table 10.2 shows some of the primary antioxidant–synergist combinations in common use.

TABLE 10.2

SOME COMMONLY USED PRIMARY ANTIOXIDANT–SYNERGIST COMBINATIONS

Primary antioxidant		Synergists
Propyl gallate	+	Citric and phosphoric acids
NDGA and BHA	+	Ascorbic, phosphoric and citric acids
BHA with BHT and NDGA	+	Citric and phosphoric acids, lecithins

The mode of action of synergists is not fully understood, but there are two plausible explanations. Firstly, it is thought that the synergist may provide a supply of hydrogen for regeneration of the inactivated antioxidant radical. Alternatively, it may be that the synergist forms chelates or complexes with the trace quantities of heavy metals that act as pro-oxidants of autoxidation.

Metal complexing agents such as ethylenediaminetetra-acetic acid (EDTA) and *N,N*-di(2-hydroxyethyl)glycine also have a protective effect by removing heavy metal contaminants. EDTA in combination with an antioxidant has been used to retard the coloration of adrenaline solutions.

The Presence of Reducing Agents

In some instances, oxidation of pharmaceutical products may be retarded by the addition of a reducing agent. In contrast to antioxidants, reducing agents are effective against oxidizing agents as well as atmospheric oxygen, and act by being oxidized in preference to the drug they are protecting. The reducing agents most commonly used in pharmacy are the potassium and sodium metabisulphites, bisulphites and sulphites (Schroeter 1961). Sodium metabisulphite is used in aqueous solutions of phenolic drugs such as adrenaline, sodium salicylate, morphine and apomorphine. It is often employed at a concentration of 0.1 per cent, but concentrations in the range 0.01 to 1 per cent have been used. The minimum concentration that gives the desired protective effect should be chosen. Metabisulphites are normally employed in acid solutions, the bisulphites at intermediate pH levels, and the sulphites are the reducing agents of choice where the solution is unbuffered or alkaline in nature. Although widely used, sodium metabisulphite has several disadvantages. It decomposes in air, especially on heating, and an appreciable amount may be lost before it is able to exert its effect when autoclaving an aqueous product. Its reaction with oxygen and oxidizing agents results in a fall in the pH of the preparation. Solutions of sodium metabisulphite may also react with the rubber closures of multidose containers, and this will cause depletion of the reducing agent in solution. Under certain conditions, sodium metabisulphite may react with adrenaline and other derivatives of *ortho*- and *para*-hydroxybenzyl alcohol, with dyes and flavouring agents.

The action of sodium bisulphite is inhibited by mannitol, hydroquine and many phenols. Drugs containing aldehyde and ketone groupings react with bisulphite to give hydroxysulphonic acids. However, bisulphites have been shown to be effective in stabilizing dextrose, streptomycin and dihydrostreptomycin, sulphadiazine, sodium aminosalicylate, morphine and neomycin solutions.

Adjustment of pH

Many of those oxidative decompositions involving a reversible oxidation–reduction process are influenced by the hydrogen ion concentration of the system. For example, this has been shown to be true of the decomposition of aqueous solutions of ephedrine salts, ascorbic acid and riboflavine. It follows that the oxidation–reduction potential, E, and therefore the stability of these preparations will be affected by the pH of the system. In many instances, decreasing the pH (increasing the hydrogen ion concentration) results in an increase in the value of E and hence an increased resistance to oxidation. This technique has been used for stabilizing adrenaline solutions whose pH–E_0' relationship is shown in Fig. 10.7 (E_0' is the standard

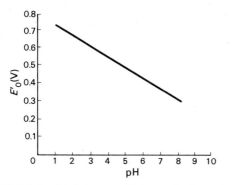

FIG. 10.7. Relationship between oxidation–reduction potential and pH for adrenaline solution.

oxidation–reduction potential at a given pH value). By adjusting the pH of the solution to 4.0, adrenaline has been found to be twice as stable as at pH 6.0.

Removal of Oxygen

By limiting contact of the drug with the atmosphere, those oxidative decompositions dependent upon atmospheric oxygen may often be minimized. In some instances, it is only necessary to store the drug in well-filled, air-tight, containers, e.g. codeine phosphate. More stringent precautions are required for neoarsphenamine, sulpharsphenamine and calciferol which have to be packed in sealed containers under vacuum. With single-dose injections it is often possible to reduce oxidation by displacing the air with an inert gas. Nitrogen is frequently used for this purpose, e.g. injections of ergometrine maleate, chlorpheniramine maleate and chlorpromazine hydrochloride. Carbon dioxide may also be employed, e.g. injection of apormorphine hydrochloride. Since the gas is approximately one and a half times as heavy as air, it has the advantage that it does not escape as easily from the container as nitrogen. Unfortunately, carbon dioxide is appreciably soluble in water, and this often results in a lowering of the pH of the solution.

The Presence of Surface-active Agents

Oxidizable materials, such as oil-soluble vitamins, essential oils and unsaturated oils, have been formulated as solubilized and emulsified products. It is necessary to determine the effects that surface-active agents may have upon the stability of such systems. In general, the rate of autoxidation of a drug in solubilized and emulsified systems is dictated by the concentration of drug in the oil and/or micellar pseudophase. As was pointed out when discussing hydrolysis of drugs in the presence of surface-active agents, the exact effect will depend upon the water solubility of the drug, the type and concentration of the surface-active agent, and the nature of the phase in which the drug is preferentially soluble. For example, the water-insoluble oil methyl linoleate exhibits a low rate of oxidation when dispersed in water, since very little of the material is soluble in the continuous phase. When potassium laurate is added to the system, emulsions are formed. Upon increasing the concentration of the surface-active agent, more of the oil becomes solubilized until ultimately only a homogeneous solution is present.

Carless and Nixon (1960) showed that the rate of oxidation in the emulsified systems was greater than that occurring in dispersions of the oil. As the concentration of the surface-active agent was increased, the rate of oxidation increased until the point was reached where the compound was completely solubilized. Beyond this point, addition of more surface-active agent resulted in a decrease in the rate of decomposition. From these results it appeared that the higher rate of oxidation in emulsified systems was due to the presence of solubilized methyl linoleate. Initiation of the autoxidation process was thought to occur in the micellar pseudophase, and the free radicals were subsequently transferred to the oil droplets where the propagation rate was higher because of the presence of large numbers of oil molecules. The reduced rate of oxidation in completely solubilized systems was attributed to the fact that there were relatively few oil molecules per micelle. Increasing the surface-active agent concentration further only served to increase the proportion of micellar pseudophase and lower the number of methyl linoleate molecules per micelle. Thus there was a greater and increasing probability of termination of the autoxidation process in the micelles. With solubilized systems of linoleic acid, it has been found that maximum stability was achieved when the highest possible concentration of surface-active agent was present (Swarbrick & Rhodes 1965).

Investigation of the autoxidation of the more water-soluble compound benzaldehyde in the presence of potassium laurate or cetomacrogol showed that the initial high rate of oxidation in aqueous dispersion gradually fell with increasing concentration of surface-active agent. This parallelled the gradual transformation from the emulsified to the solubilized state of the material (Carless & Nixon 1957).

The oxidation of benzaldehyde in betaine–water systems was studied by Swarbrick and Carless (1964a, b), who examined decomposition in the isotropic aqueous (L_1) phase, the isotropic 'oily' (L_2) phase, the anisotropic liquid crystalline (L_c) phase, and also the multiphase systems $L_1 + L_2$ (conventional emulsion system), $L_c + L_1$, $L_c + L_2$, and $L_1 + L_2 + L_c$. In the separate phases, the rate of oxidation was found to be in the order $L_2 > L_1 > L_c$, and this phenomenon was though to be due to increasing difficulty with which the propagation could take place in the increasingly structured systems. With multiphase systems, the oxidation rate varied with the proportion and number of phases present. Thus, before making a valid prediction of the influence that a surface-active agent may have upon the stability of such a system, it is necessary to take account of these factors.

PHOTOCHEMICAL DEGRADATION

The photochemical degradation of a sensitive material can be reduced by protecting it from light. This may be achieved by storing the product in a clear glass container, and then either placing it in the dark or enclosing it in an opaque wrapper. Alternatively, light-resistant containers may be used. Since degradation is chiefly due to the absorption of light of shorter wavelength, the British Pharmaceutical Codex defines a light-resistant container as one that does not transmit more than 15 per cent of incident radiation between 290 and 450 nm. The amount of light transmitted through a glass container depends upon the composition and thickness of the glass. The light transmission characteristics of several types of glass container have been reported by Dimbleby (1953), and Fig. 10.8 shows some of the results plotted in terms of percentage transmission per millimetre thickness against wavelength. It can be seen that the yellow-green and amber glasses are satisfactory since they transmit very little light below 400 nm. Medium green containers are less effective, while colourless and blue glass transmit high percentages of the ultraviolet wavelengths. The inspection of solutions for any sign of precipitation or discoloration is difficult in coloured containers, and for this reason many parenteral solutions are packed in clear glass containers and placed in a light-proof enclosure.

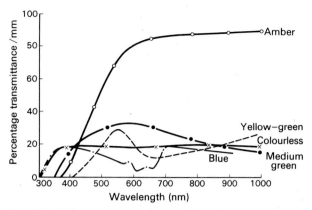

FIG. 10.8. Light transmission characteristics of coloured glass (Dimbleby 1953).

PHYSICAL DEGRADATION OF PHARMACEUTICAL PRODUCTS

Loss of volatile constituents

A wide range of materials, e.g. iodine, camphor, menthol, alcohol and anaesthetic ether, are volatile at ambient temperatures and may be lost from pharmaceutical preparations. Even tablets containing nitroglycerin may lose potency because of volatilization of the drug (Banes 1968). In all cases, deterioration may be prevented by placing such products in well-closed containers. Since the rate of volatilization increases with temperature, volatile substances should also be stored in a cool place.

Loss of Water

Evaporation of water from liquid and semi-solid oil-in-water emulsions may cause cracking of these systems. Loss of water from aqueous solutions will give rise to concentration, and possibly crystallization, of the solute. In addition, some salts, e.g. borax, caffeine, sodium sulphate, quinidine sulphate and sodium carbonate, are efflorescent. The tendency for these materials to lose water will depend upon the humidity and temperature of the environment. The result will be a decrease in weight with a corresponding increase in potency of the materials. Water loss may be prevented by storing the products in well-closed containers.

Absorption of Water

Absorption of moisture from the atmosphere is a common cause of deterioration of a variety of products. For example, glycerin suppositories will absorb moisture and become opaque, while gelatin capsules will soften. Some salts, e.g. calcium chloride, potassium citrate, potassium hydroxide and potassium carbonate, are deliquescent. Their tendency to deliquesce will depend upon the humidity and temperature of the atmosphere. Other materials, such as glycerin, dehydrated alcohol, sulphuric acid and most dry extracts are hygroscopic. Effervescent tablets and granules will react prematurely in a moist atmosphere. Storage of all such materials in well-closed containers will prevent this form of deterioration.

Crystal Growth
The deposition of crystals from aqueous solution occurs when the vehicle becomes supersaturated with respect to the solute. This usually results from a fall in temperature with a consequent decrease in solubility of the solute. A classic example of the phenomenon is often seen with injection of calcium gluconate. Concentrated solutions, containing 10 per cent w/v calcium gluconate, are commonly used. At 20° such solutions are supersaturated and relatively stable provided they are free of suspended particles of solid matter. In order to reduce the risk of crystallization, the *British Pharmacopoeia* allows not more than 5 per cent of the gluconate to be replaced by other harmless calcium salts. Calcium saccharate is usually employed as a stabilizer, although calcium lactobionate has also been used.

In suspensions of finely divided solids, growth of the crystals is also undesirable. There is a tendency for the crystals to bind together to form a hard cake which is difficult to redisperse. Large particles produce a gritty texture which is unacceptable in topical and ophthalmic preparations. When present in suspensions for injection, there is a danger that large crystals may block the hypodermic needle. Higuchi (1958) has discussed the causes of crystal growth in suspensions, and these may be summarized as follows:
(i) Temperature fluctuation; a rise causing increased solubility and a fall causing supersaturation and crystallization.
(ii) The presence of a metastable form of the crystals which has a greater solubility than the stable form. The solution will be supersaturated with respect to the stable form.
(iii) Small crystals have a greater solubility than large crystals so that the solution is supersaturated with respect to the latter.
(iv) Change of crystal structure due to the presence of dispersing solvent.

Prevention, or reduction, of crystal growth may be achieved by avoiding the use of the metastable form of a drug, and by storing in an environment which exhibits the minimum of temperature fluctuation. A narrow size range of crystals should be used, and incorporation of a surface-active agent, which is adsorbed on to the crystal surfaces, also inhibits the rate of deposition of solute molecules. Diffusion of solute molecules to the crystal surfaces may also be hindered by increasing the viscosity of the suspending medium. A stable aqueous suspension of cortisone acetate powder for use as eye drops has been produced by grinding the material with aluminium hydroxide and including methyl cellulose in the suspending medium (Flitcroft & Birchall 1957).

In order to minimize the effect of temperature fluctuations, suspensions should ideally be confined to insoluble solids, or, at least, to solids whose solubility does not increase greatly with rise in temperature.

Polymorphic Changes
As has been discussed in Chapter 3, many substances are known to exist in two or more polymorphic forms. Upon storage in the dry state or in suspension there is the possibility of interconversion of these forms. Since such changes may cause alteration in solubility and possibly crystal growth in aqueous suspension, it is essential that the formulated product should contain a stable crystalline form of the drug.

Colour Changes
A change in colour of a pharmaceutical product is usually just a visual indication that some form of chemical or photochemical decomposition is occurring. It is thus necessary to investigate and remove the cause of chemical instability. Medicines are often coloured for aesthetic reasons, and colour fading is a fairly common source of instability. Certain water-soluble dyes, e.g. indigo carmine, tend to fade rapidly in the presence of reducing substances such as lactose and dextrose (Kuramoto, Lachman & Cooper 1958). The process is also affected by the pH of the solution. Scott, Goudie & Huetteman (1960) showed that non-ionic surface-active agents, e.g. Tween 20 and Myrj 52, also accelerated the fading of indigo carmine, tartrazine and orange G in aqueous solution. They attributed this phenomenon either to an interaction of the dyes with the polyoxyethylene groupings of the surface-active agents, or to the presence of impurities in these materials. Dyes also tend to fade when present in tablets exposed to light. An attempt has been made to reduce the amount of fading by incorporating an ultraviolet light-absorbing compound in the tablet formulation.

Lachman et al. (1962) found that tablets coloured with brilliant blue or tartrazine were more stable when the compound 2,4-dihydroxybenzophenone was present. The problem of colour development in pharmaceutical products is also often encountered. For example, solutions containing physostigmine or adrenaline become red on exposure to air, while apormorphine hydrochloride solutions turn green. Solid dosage forms can also show colour development, e.g. aspirin tablets may become pink, ascorbic acid tablets will gradually age from white to a yellowish-brown colour. The colour stability of ascorbic acid tablets is particularly affected by the presence of lubricants such as magnesium or calcium stearate (Wortz 1967).

STABILITY TESTING

In the past, before a product is marketed, it has been the practice to assess its stability by placing it on storage test. The test, which involves examining for quality and potency at suitable time intervals, is conducted for a period corresponding to the normal time that the product is likely to remain in stock or in use. Since this period can be as long as two years, a storage test of this nature is time-consuming and expensive. It has, therefore, become essential to devise a technique for use during the product development stages that will enable rapid prediction of the long-term stability of a product. It is then possible to identify the most stable and suitable formulation without resorting to the lengthy, conventional, storage testing process. A prediction of the life of the product may be made by accelerating the decomposition process and extrapolating the results to normal storage conditions. Nevertheless, accelerated storage tests cannot be expected to replace the conventional stability testing programme for the product finally marketed, although they do minimize the effort and expense of testing new formulations.

ACCELERATED TESTS FOR CHEMICAL STABILITY

When determining the chemical stability of a pharmaceutical product, it is essential that the assay employed should be sufficiently specific to distinguish between the drug and its decomposition products. This is particularly important where the degradation process involves isomerization. Identification of the product (or products) of decomposition is a more sensitive approach than assaying for the undecomposed drug. However, this can be time-consuming when there are several pathways of decomposition. If data are available on the relative toxicity of the decomposition products, analysis can be restricted to assays for the most toxic product, and for the undecomposed drug.

Acceleration of chemical decomposition is achieved by raising the temperature of the preparations. Application of the principles of chemical kinetics to the results of accelerated storage tests carried out at three or more elevated temperatures enables prediction to be made of the effective life of the preparation at normal temperatures. The order of reaction for the decomposition process is determined by plotting the appropriate function of concentration against time and obtaining a linear relationship. As has been discussed in the section dealing with chemical kinetics, the reaction velocity constant, k, for the decomposition at each of the elevated temperatures can be calculated from the slope of the line. The Arrhenius relationship (equation 10.24) is then employed to determine the reaction velocity constant for the decomposition at room temperature. This is obtained from the linear plot of the logarithms of the determined reaction velocity constants against the reciprocals of absolute temperatures, which is extrapolated to room temperature (25°). The value of k at 25° may then be substituted in the appropriate rate equation, and an estimate obtained of the time during which the product will maintain the required quality or potency (shelf-life). By way of example, the hydrolysis of allopurinol has been found to obey pseudo-first-order kinetics in alkaline solution (Gressel &

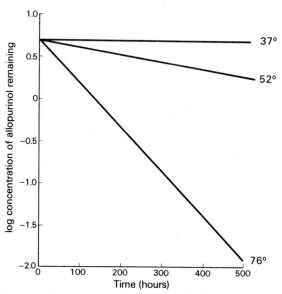

FIG. 10.9. First-order kinetic plot for the decomposition of allopurinol at pH 10.8 (Gressel & Galleli 1968).

Galleli 1968). At pH 10.8, from the slopes of the first-order plots (Fig. 10.9), the reaction velocity constants were calculated to be 1.22×10^{-2}, 1.09×10^{-3} and 1.38×10^{-4}/hour at 76°, 52° and 37° respectively. The Arrhenius plot of these results is shown in Fig. 10.10 and the extrapolated value of k at 25° is estimated to be 2.92×10^{-5}/hour. The potency or quality level below which a product is no longer acceptable will vary from product to product depending upon the form of decomposition. For example, the level is often taken to be 90 per cent of the initial potency of the product. Alternatively, it could be the level at which a toxic breakdown product can no longer be tolerated, or at which a certain degree of odour or colour change is evident. Assuming that the allopurinol preparation is acceptable until the drug content is 90 per cent of the initial concentration, substitution in the first-order rate equation shows that the shelf-life will be 150 days.

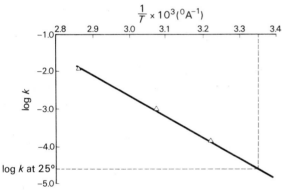

FIG. 10.10. Arrhenius plot for allopurinol decomposition at pH 10.8.

The results of an accelerated test are obtained using comparatively short periods of storage which are known with accuracy. When the bulk or low heat conductivity of the product prevents rapid temperature equilibration with the test environment, the exact times of storage at elevated temperature may be subject to considerable error. There may be a considerable time lag before the product sample reaches the equilibrium storage temperature, and also before it returns to room temperature upon removal from the test environment. These two sources of error do not necessarily cancel each other out. It has been shown (Eriksen, Pauls & Swintosky 1958) that the magnitude of the errors introduced by ignoring heating and cooling times is related to the heating and cooling rate coefficients of the product, the storage time, the

difference between room and storage temperature, and the energy of activation of the decomposition process. With the exception of accelerated stability tests of tablets, powders and other solid dosage forms, the problem is not normally of great significance. Nevertheless, where it is essential to determine accurately the amount of decomposition, rather then obtain an estimate of the change of concentration with time, it is possible to correct for the errors by employing the concept of equilibrium temperature–time equivalents. These are the storage periods corrected for the heating and cooling times encountered in the accelerated storage test. Eriksen et al. (1958) have been able to calculate equilibrium temperature–time equivalents from a knowledge of the order and energy of activation of the chemical decomposition, and the heating and cooling rate coefficients of the product.

Apart from the normal accelerated storage test procedure described, techniques have been devised that enable both the energy of activation and the decomposition reaction velocity constant at room temperature to be determined from a single experiment (Rogers 1963; Eriksen & Stelmach 1965). Such methods involve raising the temperature of a product under test in accordance with a predetermined temperature–time programme. Samples are withdrawn and assayed at suitable time intervals in the usual manner. The programme devised by Rogers (1963) is so arranged that the reciprocal of temperature varies logarithmically with time, i.e.:

$$\frac{1}{T_0} - \frac{1}{T_t} = 2.303b \log(1+t) \qquad (10.31)$$

where T_0 is the initial temperature (°A) of the programme,

T_t is the temperature (°A) of the programme at any time t,

b is the programme constant which enables the length of the experiment and the temperature range to be chosen at will.

Using equation (10.31) in conjunction with the Arrhenius relationship (equation 10.23) and the rate equation for the relevant order of reaction of the decomposition process, the following general equation is obtained:

$$\log f = \log k_0 \quad \log(1 + Eb/R)$$
$$+ (1 + Eb/R) \log(1+t)$$
$$+ \log\left[1 - \left(\frac{k_0}{k_t}\right)^{1+R/Eb}\right] \qquad (10.32)$$

where the function f corresponds to $(c_o - c_t)$ for a zero-order, $(2.303 \log(c_o/c_t))$ for a first-order, and $[(1/c_t) - (1/c_o)]$ for a second-order process.

c_o and c_t are the concentrations initially and at time t respectively,

k_o is the reaction velocity constant at the initial temperature of the programme,

k_t is the reaction velocity constant at time t,

E is the energy of activation of the process,

R is the gas constant.

Although the term $\log[1 - (k_o/k_t)^{1 + R/Eb}]$ varies with time, it rapidly tends to zero as k_t becomes substantially greater than k_o, i.e. at approximately $10°$ above the initial programme temperature. Thus, after this period, a plot of $\log f$ against $\log(1 + t)$ will be a straight line. The slope of the line is $(1 + Eb/R)$, whilst the intercept value at $\log(1 + t) = 0$ is $\log k_o - \log(1 + Eb/R)$. Measurement of these two values enable k_o to be calculated. With a knowledge of k_o and E, substitution into the Arrhenius equation will produce a value for the reaction velocity constant at room temperature.

The programmed temperature rise technique has the advantage that only a single experiment is performed to obtain all the necessary information for the prediction of shelf-life. The fact that a straight line graph is produced provides a check that the correct order of reaction has been assigned to the decomposition process. The temperature–time programme may be chosen according to experimental convenience and selected to fit into the working day. However, since the predicted shelf-life is calculated using the slope and intercept values from the graph, it may be subject to considerable error unless care is taken in the measurement of these quantities. Where the decomposition process exhibits a substantial reverse reaction, it may not be possible to produce a linear equation as easily as has been indicated with the simple rate equations (Carstensen, Koff & Rubin 1968).

Limitations of Accelerated Storage Tests for Chemical Stability

The predicted shelf-life of a preparation will only be valid if the accelerated test is carried out on the final packaged product. This is an essential prerequisite because the pathway or rate of decomposition may depend in some measure upon the container used for storage, e.g. the use of an air-tight container will reduce the rate of oxidation in a drug.

It is not possible to extend the prediction to all climatic conditions, especially those encountered in tropical regions where there are large diurnal variations in temperature. Such conditions have been simulated using temperature cycling ovens which repeatedly cycle the product through a temperature range, e.g. -10 to $37°$. Interpretation of the data in terms of normal storage conditions is very complex.

The accelerated testing technique can only be applied to those forms of decomposition which increase with rise in temperature. Before valid conclusions can be drawn from such tests, it is necessary to determine that the elevated temperatures do not alter the order of chemical reaction from that occurring at room temperature. For example, it is possible for the zero-order decomposition of a drug in suspension to become first-order at higher temperatures because of complete solution of the drug in the vehicle. When the decomposition process is complex, involving a series of simultaneous and/or consecutive reactions each having a characteristic energy of activation, storage of the product at elevated temperatures may produce a change in the relative contributions of the component reactions. This could result in an inaccurate prediction of shelf-life. For example, the fact that determination of peroxide value gives a misleading estimate of the rancidity of an oil stored at high temperature has already been referred to. It is also possible that elevated temperature may induce a decomposition process that is not normally significant at ambient temperatures. This is true of autocatalytic reactions which are accelerated by the products of decomposition.

The shelf-life prediction only applies to the product formulation investigated. One cannot expect the prediction to be valid for different formulations of the same drug.

Although accelerated chemical stability tests are not infallible, if the above limitations are taken into consideration, the prediction of shelf-life may be accepted with confidence. Such tests have a secondary function in that they may be used as a quality control method for the manufactured product. In this way it is possible to ensure that no change has occurred during the manufacturing process that alters the previously obtained stability pattern of the product.

ACCELERATED TESTS FOR PHOTOCHEMICAL STABILITY

Accelerated tests for photochemical stability induce rapid decomposition by means of an intense artificial light source simulating the effects of sunlight and room illumination. Extrapolation of the results obtained to predict the effect of normal storage conditions is often very difficult. Although there is a relationship between reaction rate and intensity of illumination, it is a unique function of the product under test and is not of general application. Thus it is necessary to determine the correlation between normal and accelerated storage conditions for every individual product. The artificial light source used should have a radiant energy distribution similar to that of the sun. It has been found (Lachman, Swartz & Cooper 1960) that daylight fluorescent tubes have the most suitable spectrum. Figure 10.11, shows the spectral energy

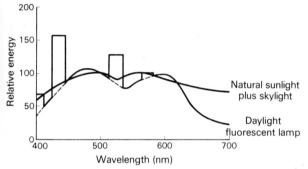

FIG. 10.11. Spectral energy distributions of natural sunlight plus sky light and a daylight fluorescent lamp of equal intensities (Jones & Grimshaw 1963).

distributions for natural sunlight plus daylight and a daylight fluorescent lamp. Correction has been made for the difference in intensity of the two sources. Fluorescent lamps are cool sources of illumination and do not promote thermal reactions in the product under test. Lachman and Cooper (1959) calculated that a bank of eighteen 60-W fluorescent tubes placed at a distance of 1 m from the product sample give a light intensity of about $12\,000\ \mathrm{lm/m^2}$. This is of the order of twenty times the intensity of light found in many storage areas. Such a system has been used in the investigation of the accelerated photodecomposition of dyes incorporated in tablet formulations (Lachman et al. 1960).

As was pointed out, the relationship between the intensity of light and rate of photodegradation is a unique function of the product formulation. In order to determine this relationship, a quantitative method of measuring photochemical decomposition is required. To this end an instrument has been designed which provides radiant energy of the required wavelength and of sufficient intensity to make such studies possible (Price & Osborne 1964). The quantity of light absorbed by the drug sample

is determined by measuring the difference in the intensity and quantity of light incident upon and transmitted by the product. In the future, the use of similar equipment may provide a more rational approach to the design and evaluation of accelerated photochemical stability tests.

ACCELERATED TESTS FOR PHYSICAL STABILITY

As a result of the many and varied causes of physical instability in pharmaceutical products, it is not possible to devise a single universal test that will accelerate the breakdown of all preparations. This is in contrast to accelerated tests for chemical and photochemical stability where exaggerated conditions of heat and light are employed, respectively. It follows that there are as many accelerated physical stability tests as there are types of product. Furthermore, our knowledge of the relationship between physical degradation under a high degree of stress and stability under normal storage conditions is very limited. Generally speaking, one has to be content with applying a high degree of stress and assume that the product is stable on normal storage if it withstands the stress. The discussion of accelerated storage tests for physical stability will be confined to an outline of tests that have been applied to assess stability towards moisture. Some specific test techniques for emulsions and suspensions will also be discussed.

Accelerated Tests for Moisture Absorption

The deterioration of products due to the absorption of moisture is normally accelerated by placing them in an environment of high relative humidity and controlled temperature. In order to obtain as much information as possible, it is preferable to employ a range of humidites. This is achieved by using a number of small cabinets each containing a different saturated salt solution that produces the desired humidity conditions. The final packaged product must be tested in this manner, but it is also useful to apply the test beforehand to the unpackaged material. It is then possible to determine rapidly whether the product is susceptible to moisture, and also whether the final container needs to provide a high degree of protection.

Another approach has been adopted by Carstensen et al. (1966) for the accelerated testing of unpackaged products. They determined the effect of moisture upon the stability of vitamin A acetate tablets by incorporating various quantities of water into the pre-dried granules prior to tabletting. They thus produced tablets having various moisture contents which were stored in well-sealed containers at a series of elevated temperatures.

Accelerated Tests for Emulsion Stability

Elevated temperature storage and centrifugation have both been employed to accelerate the breakdown of emulsions. Storage of an emulsion at a temperature between 45° and 70° is a technique that is often used, since raised temperature causes increased thermal agitation and decreased viscosity of the continuous phase (Levius & Drommond 1953). Both factors facilitate increased frequency of collision of the oil globules and accelerate the tendency for the emulsion to crack (Colburn 1951). If the emulsion withstands such treatment, it is normally correct to assume that it will be stable at normal temperatures. However, the reverse argument does not always apply. There are cases where an emulsion has been found to be perfectly stable under normal conditions even though it cracked during high temperature storage. This phenomenon can be caused by a change in the relative solubility of the emulsifying agent in the two phases at high temperature, and is likely to happen when the emulsifier is a non-ionic surface-active agent. It may also be due to the fact that elevated temperature may accelerate chemical decomposition of one or more of the emulsion constituents and contribute to the deterioration. Both factors can give rise to an inaccurate estimate of the susceptibility of the product to decomposition.

Centrifugation of an emulsion greatly exaggerates the effect of gravity, and therefore predominantly accelerates the rate of creaming. The degree of acceleration of creaming will obviously depend upon the speed of centrifugation. If it is assumed that the rate of creaming is directly proportional to the strength of the gravitational field, it is theoretically possible to establish a direct relationship between speed of centrifuging and normal storage conditions. Indeed, Garret (1962) successfully used an analytical ultracentrifuge, running at speeds up to 60 000 rev/min, to predict the shelf-life of an intravenous oil-in-water emulsion. Unfortunately, it is unlikely that such a simple correlation holds for the majority of highly stable pharmaceutical emulsions. Since centrifugation exaggerates the value of g in Stokes' Equation, the results of the accelerated test can give rise to some misleading conclusions when several emulsion formulations are being compared. For example, it is possible for a stable emulsion, whose disperse and continuous phases have dissimilar densities, to appear inferior to a product that is inherently less stable but which has a smaller difference in density between the two phases.

Accelerated Tests for Suspension Stability

The most common form of physical instability occurring in suspensions is the settling out of the solid phase with the formation of a sediment which is difficult to redisperse on shaking. One might expect centrifugation to be a suitable method for accelerating such a change, but the technique is of little value because the majority of pharmaceutical suspensions are flocculated systems. The centrifugal force is great in comparison with the forces of flocculation, and this will result in destruction of the structure of the suspension. The net effect of such an accelerated test would be to produce a close-packed sediment regardless of the stability of the product. However, low speed centrifugation producing an effect equivalent to about four times that of gravity may be of value in some cases (Jones & Grimshaw 1963).

Crystal growth is also a cause of physical deterioration in some suspensions. Acceleration of crystal growth may be achieved by simulating the temperature fluctuations occurring under normal storage conditions, but at greatly increased frequency. Such a test has more significance than attempting to increase the degree of stress (Carless & Foster 1966). The daily variations of temperature have been reproduced by cycling suspensions between 23° and 33° using a cycling time of 16 minutes. Cycling sulphathiazole suspensions one hundred times produced significant crystal growth with a consequent broadening of the particle size distribution. The degree of acceleration of growth produced by such a test, and its relationship to normal storage conditions, depends upon the particle concentration, the bulk particle solubility, the slope of the solubility curve, the temperature fluctuation range and the frequency of fluctuation. (Varney 1967).

REFERENCES

ANDERSON, R. A. & SLADE, A. H. (1966) *J. Pharm. Pharmacol.* **18**, 640.

BANES, D. (1968) *J. pharm. Sci.* **57**, 893.

CARLESS, J. E. & FOSTER, A. A. (1966) *J. Pharm. Pharmacol.* **18**, 697.

CARLESS, J. E. & NIXON, J. R. (1957) *J. Pharm. Pharmacol.* **9**, 963.

CARLESS, J. E. & NIXON, J. R. (1960) *J. Pharm. Pharmacol.* **12**, 348.

CARSTENSEN, J. T., SERENSON, E., SPERA, C. D. & VANCE, J. J. (1966) *J. pharm. Sci.* **55**, 561.

CARSTENSEN, J. T., KOFF, A. & RUBIN, S. H. (1968) *J. Pharm. Pharmacol.* **20**, 485.

COLBURN, W. J. (1951) *J. Soc. cosmet. Chem.* **2**, 193.

COLES, C. L. J. (1969) *Pharm. J.* **202**, 308.

DEMERRE, L. J. & WILSON, C. (1956) *J. Am. pharm. Ass. (Sci. Edn)* **45**, 129.

DIMBLEBY, V. (1953) *J. Pharm. Pharmacol.* **5**, 969.

EDWARDS, L. J. (1950) *Trans. Faraday Soc.* **46**, 723.

ERIKSEN, S. P., PAULS, J. F. & SWINTOSKY, S. V. (1958) *J. Am. pharm. Ass. (Sci. Edn)* **47**, 697.

ERIKSEN, S. P. & STELMACH, H. (1965) *J. pharm. Sci.* **54**, 1029.

FARMER, E. H. (1942) *Trans. Faraday Soc.* **38**, 340.

FLETCHER, G. & DAVIES, D. J. G. (1968) *J. Pharm. Pharmacol.* **20**, 108S.

FLITCROFT, J. & BIRCHALL, M. E. (1957) *Pharm. J.* **178**, 79.

FOSTER, G. E., MACDONALD, J. & JONES, T. S. G. (1949) *J. Pharm. Pharmacol.* **1**, 802.

GARRET, E. R. (1957) *J. Am. pharm. Ass. (Sci. Edn)* **46**, 584.

GARRET, E. R. (1962) *J. pharm. Sci.* **51**, 35.

GORE, D. N. & ASHWIN, J. (1967) *J. Mond. Pharm.* **10**, 365.

GRESSEL, P. D. & GALLELI, J. F. (1968) *J. pharm. Sci.* **57**, 335.

HIGUCHI, T. (1958) *J. Am. pharm. Ass. (Sci. Edn)* **47**, 657.

HIGUCHI, T. & LACHMAN, L. (1955) *J. Am. pharm. Ass. (Sci. Edn)* **44**, 521.

HIGUCHI, T., HAVINGA, A. & BUSSE, L. W. (1950) *J. Am. pharm. Ass. (Sci. Edn)* **39**, 405.

HIGUCHI, T., MARCUS, A. D. & BIAS, C. T. (1954) *J. Am. pharm. Ass. (Sci. Edn)* **43**, 129.

JONES, W. & GRIMSHAW, J. T. (1963) *Pharm. J.* **191**, 459.

KORNBLUM, S. S. & ZOGLIO, M. A. (1967) *J. pharm. Sci.* **56**, 1569.

KURAMOTO, R., LACHMAN, L. & COOPER, J. (1958) *J. Am. pharm. Ass. (Sci. Edn)* **47**, 175.

LACHMAN, L. & COOPER, J. (1959) *J. Am. pharm. Ass. (Sci. Edn)* **48**, 226.

LACHMAN, L., SWARTZ, C. J. & COOPER, J. (1960) *J. Am. pharm. Ass. (Sci. Edn)* **49**, 213.

LACHMAN, L., URBANYI, T., WEINSTEIN, S., COOPER, J. & SWARTZ, C. J. (1962) *J. pharm. Sci.* **51**, 321.

LEESON, L. G. & MATTOCKS, A. M. (1958) *J. Am. pharm. Ass. (Sci. Edn)* **47**, 329.

LEHMAN, R. W., DIETERLE, J. M., FISHER, W. T. & AMES, S. R. (1960) *J. Am. pharm. Ass. (Sci. Edn)* **49**, 363.

LEVIUS, H. P. & DROMMOND, F. G. (1953) *J. Pharm. Pharmacol.* **5**, 743.

MARCUS, A. D. & TARAZKA, A. J. (1959) *J. Am. pharm. Ass. (Sci. Edn)* **48**, 77.

MITCHELL, A. G. (1962) *J. Pharm. Pharmacol.* **14**, 172.

NOGAMI, H. & AWAZU, S. (1962) *Chem. Pharm. Bull. (Japan)* **10**, 1158.

NOGAMI, H., AWAZU, S. & NAKAJIMA, N. (1962) *Chem. Pharm. Bull. (Japan)* **10**, 503.

NOGAMI, H., AWAZU, S. & IWATSURA, M. (1963) *Chem. Pharm. Bull. (Japan)* **11**, 1251.

NOGAMI, H., AWAZU, S., WATANABE, K. & SATO, K. (1960) *Chem. Pharm. Bull. (Japan)* **8**, 1136.

OSTENDORF, J. P. (1965) *J. Soc. cosmet. Chem.* **16**, 203.

PRICE, J. C. & OSBORNE, G. E. (1964) *J. pharm. Sci.* **53**, 811.

RIEGELMAN, S. (1960) *J. Am. pharm. Ass. (Sci. Edn)* **49**, 339.

ROGERS, A. R. (1963) *J. Pharm. Pharmacol.* **15**, 101T.

SCHOU, S. A. & MARCH, J. (1959) *Archiv. Pharm. og Chemi.* **66**, 231.

SCHROETER, L. C. (1961) *J. pharm. Sci.* **50**, 891.

SCHROETER, L. C. & HIGUCHI, T. (1958) *J. Am. pharm. Ass. (Sci. Edn)* **47**, 426.

SCHWARTZ, T. W., SHVEMAR, N. G. & RENALDI, R. G. (1958) *J. Am. pharm. Ass. (Pract. Edn)* **19**, 40.

SCOTT, M. W., GOUDIE, A. J. & HUETTEMAN, A. J. (1960) *J. Am. pharm. Ass.* (*Sci. Edn*) **49**, 467.

SWARBRICK, J. & CARLESS, J. E. (1964a) *J. Pharm. Pharmacol.* **16**, 596.

SWARBRICK, J. & CARLESS, J. E. (1964b) *J. Pharm. Pharmacol.* **16**, 670.

SWARBRICK, J. & RHODES, C. T. (1965) *J. pharm. Sci.* **54**, 903.

SWINTOSKY, J. V., ROSEN, E., ROBINSON, M. J., CHAMBERLAIN, R. E. & GUARINI, J. R. (1965) *J. Am. pharm. Ass.* (*Sci. Edn*) **45**, 34.

TALMAGE, J. M., CHAFETZ, L. & ELEFANT, M. (1968) *J. pharm. Sci.* **57**, 1073.

VARNEY, G. (1967) *J. Pharm. Pharmacol.* **19**, 19S.

VON DOLDER, R. (1952) *Pharm. Acta Helv.* **27**, 54.

WORTZ, R. B. (1967) *J. pharm. Sci.* **56**, 1169.

YAMANA, T., MIZUKAMI, Y. & TSUJI, A. (1968) *Chem. Pharm. Bull.* (*Japan*) **16**, 396.

Part II
PHARMACEUTICAL OPERATIONS

11

Extraction

The process of solvent extraction is involved in the preparation of most drugs. Synthetic drugs or those produced by fermentation are often purified, or separated from the mother liquor by liquid–liquid extraction. Constituents contained within plant or animal tissues are also extracted by means of solvents, but a preliminary leaching process is usually necessary. Fixed oils may be obtained in this way, but are also removed by direct expression of the tissues, and volatile oils are separated by steam distillation. (See Chapter 14.)

With the advent of numerous synthetic drugs, the demand for drugs of natural origin is diminishing. Some plant and animal products still remain important, however, including alkaloids, glycosides and other sugar derivatives, spices, fixed and volatile oils, proteins and polypeptides. Separation of the active constituents is desirable for the following reasons:

(1) Potency is more readily controlled.
(2) Deterioration, e.g. by enzyme action, is diminished.
(3) Preparations of the drug are more easily formulated, more stable, more palatable and more elegant.
(4) Tabletting of the crude material may not be possible.
(5) Injection of the crude material may be undesirable or dangerous.
(6) Smaller bulk facilitates storage and transport.

Often a single chemical, such as hyoscine or reserpine, is isolated by the extraction process, and is obtained as a crystalline solid. Sometimes, however, the active principle consists of a number of chemical compounds each of which is desired in the final product. The extraction process may then be stopped short of isolating the pure substances and the drug is used as a dry extract, a viscous soft extract, a concentrated infusion or a tincture. These crude extracts are known as galenicals. They were once used much more extensively than they are at present and included also simple infusions and decoctions made by extraction of the raw material with hot or boiling water. They were intended for extemporaneous dispensing and were required to be freshly prepared, because they rapidly produced a deposit due to coagulation of inert colloidal material and readily supported microbial growth because they lacked preservatives. Suitable assays could not be applied to them, and they were therefore usually prepared from materials whose constituents had little pharmacological activity. Galenicals are now rarely made extemporaneously; their preparation is usually time consuming and uneconomical for small quantities, and they also need to be subject to adequate quality control.

LEACHING PROCESSES

The process of leaching has been discussed by Peck (1936). Two main methods are employed, termed *maceration* and *percolation*, both being operated as batch processes. The choice of method depends upon the physical characteristics of the raw material and upon economic considerations and is designated in the monographs of the official preparations. On an industrial scale, however, there is often little difference between the operation of the two methods.

MACERATION

The general process, on a small scale, consists of placing the solid material to be extracted in a closed vessel with the whole of the menstruum, or extraction solvent, and allowing them to stand for seven days, shaking occasionally. The liquid is strained off and the marc, or solid residue, is pressed to remove as much solution as possible. The liquids so obtained are mixed and clarified by subsidence or filtration.

The solids must be in a suitable state of subdivision, either crushed or cut small, or in moderately coarse powder. Fine powders are not used because subsequent clarification would be difficult. Sufficient time is then allowed for the menstruum to penetrate the plant tissues and for the soluble components to diffuse out. Diffusion may be assisted by shaking, or on a large scale by stirring, in order to disperse the concentrated solution which would otherwise accumulate round the particles of solid material. A closed vessel is essential to prevent evaporation and batch variation.

At the end of the maceration process there should be a uniform concentration of active constituents in both the plant debris and in the solution surrounding it. The solution, sometimes called the miscella, is then strained off through cloth or other suitable material and the maximum yield of liquid is obtained by expressing the marc; special presses are used for this purpose. The solution so obtained may be cloudy and may contain small particles of debris, and time must be allowed for any colloidal material to coagulate. Sometimes several weeks are needed for this purpose. Precipitated matter is then removed by filtration through a filter-press or other suitable filter. If filtration is carried out too soon, the initially clear solution will become cloudy again due to further coagulation of colloidal material.

Solutions made by maceration of organized drugs are generally prepared by adding a definite volume of solvent to a definite weight of raw material. Provided that equilibrium has been attained, the potency of the resulting solution will remain the same regardless of the efficiency with which the marc is pressed. These solutions are therefore not adjusted to volume since the potency would then depend on the amount of liquid expressed from the marc. With unorganized drugs such as benzoin, however, the residue cannot be pressed, and so the solution is filtered from the marc and the latter is rinsed by passing more solvent through the filter to produce a definite volume. In the case of Aromatic Cardamom Tincture, other oils are added to the expressed solution and in order that the concentration of these should not vary, the solution is adjusted to volume.

Modifications of the General Process of Maceration
Repeated maceration may be more efficient than a single maceration, since an appreciable amount of active principle may be left behind in the first pressing of the marc. Double maceration is used for concentrated infusions which contain volatile oil, e.g. Concentrated Compound Gentian Infusion. Where the marc cannot be pressed, a process of triple maceration is sometimes employed. The total volume of solvent used is however large and the second and third macerates are usually mixed and evaporated, before adding to the first macerate. This precludes the use of the process for preparations containing volatile ingredients.

In a few cases it is desirable to change the physico-chemical nature of the solvent during a single maceration process. Thus, Opium Tincture is prepared by first pouring boiling water over the sliced opium to disintegrate it. Then, after macerating for 6 hours, 90 per cent alcohol is added to the cold mixture and maceration is continued for a further 24 hours. The addition of the alcohol during the second period of maceration prevents the solution of much of the gummy material in the final tincture.

PERCOLATION

In this process the raw material is packed into a column and the solvent is allowed to percolate through it. Although some materials may be packed into a percolator in the dry state, e.g. Ginger, most drugs require preliminary moistening. The solid material is mixed with sufficient solvent and the moist mass is allowed to stand for 4 hours in a well-closed vessel. This preliminary moistening is important because the dried tissues may swell on contact with the solvent and, if packed in the dry condition, subsequent swelling might reduce the porosity of the material and choke the column. This swelling would be particularly marked with solvents which are mainly aqueous, and the greater the swelling the larger the volume of solvent required for preliminary moistening. Subsequent packing into the percolator is also assisted, since the solvent displaces occluded air and enables the material to be more evenly distributed. If the material is not packed evenly, the percolating solvent will run mainly through the largest channels, resulting in inefficient extraction. Preliminary moistening also makes the fine particles less liable to be washed out of the column during percolation.

After allowing the moist mass to imbibe the liquid, it is packed evenly into the percolator. Fig. 11.1 illustrates a type of percolator used on a commercial scale. The drug is supported on a perforated metal plate covered with sacking or straw. The top of the apparatus is removable for charging the column with raw material and is provided with portholes for inspection and running in of solvent. At the base the outlet is fitted with a tap, and a pipe leads the percolate away for subsequent treatment or to the top of a second percolator in order to use the solvent more efficiently. On a small scale glass percolators can be used and the raw material is supported in a loose plug of tow or other suitable substance which has been previously moistened with solvent. In order to achieve even packing the moist material is introduced layer by layer, each one being lightly tapped with a rod or other suitable implement, to give even compression. The pressure to be exerted depends on the nature of the swollen material and its permeability. To prevent disturbance of the packed solids, a piece of filter paper may be place on top of them and weighted down with sand. If there is a risk of further swelling of the raw material, it is preferable to use a percolator that is slightly conical, as the sloping sides allow better expansion of the bed than would cylindrical columns. The latter have the added disadvantage that solvent often fails to permeate through material near the sides at the bottom.

After packing the column, sufficient menstruum is poured over it to saturate it and when liquid begins to drip from the bottom of the percolator the tap at its base is closed. Enough of the menstruum is then added to maintain a layer above the drug, since the column must not under any circumstances be allowed to become dry, which would produce cracks in the bed. The closed column is then allowed to stand for 24 hours. This period of maceration allows time for complete penetration of the tissues by the solvent and a considerable amount of leaching of the soluble material. It makes for more efficient use of the menstruum than if percolation were allowed to proceed continuously from the start of operations.

After this preliminary *maceration*, the outlet is opened sufficiently to produce a controlled slow rate of *percolation*. The volume of percolate to be collected for a given weight of raw material depends upon the nature of the final product. For some tinctures prepared on a small scale, about three-quarters of the volume of the finished product is collected and the *marc is pressed*, giving about 80 to 90 per cent of the final volume. If no assay is available for the extractive, the mixed products of percolation and expression are made up to volume with more of the menstruum. In some cases additional ingredients e.g. glycerol, are added before the final adjustment is made. In the case of more potent tinctures the percolate is assayed and the calculated amount of menstruum required to give a product of the required strength is added. In this process the assumption is made that the marc will be exhausted of the active principles which are to be extracted and adjustment to volume is therefore justified. The marc is

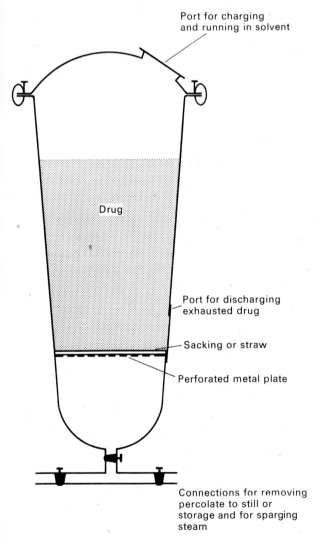

Port for charging and running in solvent

Drug

Port for discharging exhausted drug

Sacking or straw

Perforated metal plate

Connections for removing percolate to still or storage and for sparging steam

FIG. 11.1. Commercial scale percolator (approximately one ton capacity).

pressed only to avoid wastage of solvent. This is in contrast to the maceration process where the liquid expressed from the marc is assumed to be of equal strength with that separated by straining.

Reserved Percolation

Liquid extracts are more concentrated preparations than tinctures, and percolation to exhaustion will produce a preparation that is too dilute. It is therefore necessary to reduce the volume of the percolate by evaporation. In certain instances, e.g. Liquorice Liquid Extract, the whole of the percolate may be concentrated by evaporation, but in others thermolability of the active principle may preclude this. Moreover, evaporation of a dilute alcohol would remove alcohol at a faster rate than water with the result that the concentrated extract would be largely aqueous and probably incapable of retaining the extracted matter in solution.

This is overcome by reserving the first portion of the percolate, which contains the bulk of the active constituents, owing to the preliminary maceration. The rest of the percolate is collected separately, percolation being continued until some simple test shows that no more active principle is being leached out. This second, dilute, percolate is then evaporated by means of, for example, a climbing film evaporator or vacuum still. The percolate is evaporated to the consistency of a soft extract, so that almost all the water is removed. It may then be dissolved in the reserved portion, which is usually strongly alcoholic, without risk of precipitation.

On a commercial scale, percolation and evaporation of the percolate may be carried out simultaneously; sometimes, with simple solvents such as acetone, the condensed vapour from the evaporator may be returned to the top of the percolator to continue the extraction.

CHOICE OF LEACHING PROCESS

Although percolation usually results in a more rapid and complete extraction than does maceration, it is not a suitable process for treating all raw materials. Many tissues are readily compressible when wet, for example, squill and animal tissues, while resinous materials form sticky masses. The permeability of a bed of such material is too low for the percolation process to be practicable. With a few materials (e.g. ground calf's stomach from which rennet is extracted using strong salt solution) the porosity of the bed is increased by mixing the raw material with an inert, relatively coarse substance, which prevents colloids like mucin from blocking the column (Placek, Bavisotto & Jadd 1960). Alternatively, it may be possible to increase the rate of percolation by increasing the pressure gradient through the bed of raw material, but this is not often done because an increased pressure on the bed is likely to compress it and render it less permeable.

Occasionally, a restricted volume of solvent must be used to leach a large amount of raw material, because of the small amount of active principle contained therein. In such a case the proportion of solvent to raw material is too low to permit effective percolation.

Operation of the process of percolation requires skill, care and frequent attention. On the other hand maceration requires little skill and is economical in time; it is efficient for drugs that are easily extracted and in such cases is the method of choice, provided that the product obtained is satisfactory.

Because of the inevitable wastage of rectified spirit, the manufacture of tinctures on a commercial scale frequently departs from the official procedures, and a method is used which combines maceration and percolation techniques. This follows what is called a 'cover and run-down' technique, whereby the raw material is moistened with suitably diluted industrial methylated spirit, packed into a percolator and macerated for a few hours, after which the liquid is run off. The partially extracted material may then be covered with more solvent, macerated as before and a second volume of liquid collected. This process may be repeated several times, but the later, weaker, percolates may be used to start the extraction of a fresh batch of drug. Belladonna, ipecacuanha, senega and squill, may be extracted in this way. Since no preparation for internal use must contain methanol, the percolate is evaporated under reduced pressure until tests show the absence of this toxic substance (Sergeant 1950). After assay for alkaloid or total solid content, the concentrated extract is diluted with water and ethanol to produce a liquid extract or tincture containing the correct concentration of alcohol and active principle. This process cannot be used for materials which contain volatile material or which undergo change during the evaporation stage. Cocillana, for example, would become resinous if evaporated to a soft extract, and it is extracted by reserved percolation, which also retains the characteristic odour of the product.

FACTORS AFFECTING THE EFFICIENCY OF THE LEACHING PROCESS

Pretreatment of the Raw Material and the Mechanism of Leaching

Some preliminary treatment of the raw material is nearly always necessary in order to facilitate extraction of the active principles. Where these are contained in cells near the epidermis, drastic comminution is unnecessary, and bruising or slicing thinly is adequate before maceration. Further treatment could, indeed, lead to an inferior product due to loss of volatile constituents. Occasionally, the raw material needs to be freshly prepared; thus cardamon seed must be freshly removed from the fruit and used immediately after being bruised or coarsely powdered.

Tissues which yield their active principles less readily must be reduced to a powder before extraction and it is very important that this should produce material of the right *particle size*. The smaller this is, the greater will be the surface area exposed to the solvent, and the shorter will be the distance through which this must diffuse to reach the solute and extract it. Increasing the degree of comminution will therefore lead to a faster rate of extraction. The most suitable particle size, however, is not necessarily the smallest, and it will depend on the physical nature of the raw material and of the solvent employed. Hard, woody, materials that are leached by a solvent which causes little swelling of the tissues, can be reduced to a fine powder e.g. ipecacuanha, which is extracted with 80 per cent alcohol. Tissues which swell in the solvent, however, would produce a bed of low permeability if similarly treated. Also, although the cell walls of organized drugs retard the leaching of active constituents, they perform a useful function in preventing the extraction of unwanted high molecular weight constituents. Rupture of a considerable proportion of the cells by reduction to a fine powder may therefore yield an excessive amount of inert material which could hinder subsequent purification of the active principle or render difficult the clarification of a galenical (Bull 1935, 1936). Fine dry grinding may also affect the chemical properties of plant constituents and thereby initiate chemical reactions in which the active principle forms complexes with other cell constituents from which the pure compound becomes difficult to separate (Pirie 1956).

If the cell walls remain intact, diffusion through them may be the rate determining step and this will be in accordance with Fick's first law of diffusion (see Chapter 8). Extraction is not, however, always governed by molecular diffusion since dialysis and slow dissolution may be controlling factors (Karnofsky 1949a). Other factors may also be important; for example, Othmer and co-workers (1955, 1959) demonstrated that, when soybean flakes are shaken with solvent, the oil extraction rate is controlled by capillary action within the broken cells. They showed the dependence of this upon the surface tension, density and viscosity of the solvent. Hydrostatic pressure, particle cohesion and convection currents are also important.

Dean et al. (1953) observe, however, that the rate of leaching finally depends upon the permeability of the cell wall. They suggest that Belladonna and Stramonium Tinctures may be rapidly prepared by passage of the drug suspended in the solvent through a colloid mill followed by clarification in a centrifuge. Another method which, on a small scale, might increase the efficiency of extraction of plant tissue is to subject the macerating material to ultrasonic vibration. Thompson and Sutherland (1955) postulated that this decreased interfacial resistance to mass transfer, increased the interfacial area by reducing particle size, and increased the rate of dispersion of active principle away from the interface into the bulk of the solvent. As has been said above, however, such methods may lead to the extraction of unwanted material.

Since the raw material must form a bed of adequate permeability the *particle size distribution* should be sufficiently narrow to achieve this. A wide distribution would lead to a low porosity, because the smaller particles would tend to fill the voids between the larger particles. For this reason the monographs of the official preparations indicate a suitable degree of comminution and reference should be made to the official classification of powders.

The Nature of the Solvent

The ideal solvent should be selective in dissolving only the wanted constituents, but is rarely if ever met. The commonest solvent, water, is almost non-selective and alcohol is often insufficiently so. In practice dilute alcohols are used for many extractions but in some cases stronger alcohol may be necessary to avoid solution of unwanted substances of high molecular weight, such as gums.

Additional processing is occasionally needed in order to remove undesirable constituents. Thus, before extracting ergot alkaloids with acid alcohol, the powdered ergot must first be defatted with low boiling-point petroleum. In other cases the extract may be defatted. Thus on a small scale, in making Nux Vomica Liquid Extract, a liquid–liquid extraction may be used; the percolate, after concentration, is heated and shaken with hard paraffin, which retains the fat on cooling. Nux Vomica can also be extracted by a 'cover and run-down' process using boiling water. Several of these extractions, each lasting about a day, may be needed to extract an economical amount of alkaloid. The aqueous extract can then be separated from the oil, concentrated by evaporation and re-extracted with strong alcohol to remove unwanted colloidal material. Further evaporation gives a soft extract which, after assay, can be suitably diluted with alcohol to make the tincture.

Aqueous extracts are subject to degradation by enzyme action. This can be inhibited by including alcohol to give a concentration of 25 per cent or more, but the enzyme is not destroyed and care must be taken to avoid subsequent conditions in which the enzyme activity can be restored. Water also supports the life of micro-organisms which may degrade the drug constituents and it is therefore usually necessary to include preservative to prevent this. For most purposes alcohol is used, as it inhibits microbial activity at about the same concentration as is required to inhibit the isolated enzymes. Chloroform Water is used for the cold extraction of liquorice on a small scale, but it is lost when the extract is concentrated by evaporation, and preservation is maintained by addition of alcohol.

It has already been pointed out that some tinctures may need to mature for some time before being finally clarified. Undue deposition of inactive constituents may sometimes be prevented by enhancing the solvent power of the final product, e.g. glycerol is included in Compound Rhubarb Tincture as a solvent for tannins. Alternatively, precipitation of the unwanted material may be ensured by adjustment of the solvent; thus ammonia added to Senega Liquid Extract produces a slight alkalinity which precipitates inert matter and a bright product is obtained after filtration. With liquorice, however, a bright extract of nearly neutral pH can be obtained without the addition of ammonia and so a check for its absence is included in the official monograph. An increase in pH above neutrality considerably enhances the colour intensity and a variable product would be obtained if unspecified amounts of ammonia were present (Oakley & Stuckey 1949). The colour intensity of Liquorice Liquid Extract is also in-

fluenced by its trace metal content (Collett 1950, 1953). The equipment used for making it must therefore be carefully chosen.

If the solvent is to remain in the final product, it must of necessity be non-toxic. A number of liquids which are good solvents for the principles to be extracted may therefore be unsuitable for use. If, however, the solvent is to be removed by evaporation, freedom from toxicity is less important, provided that there is no hazard in its use. It must be completely volatilized during the evaporation process, but its boiling-point should not be so low as to cause difficulties during the leaching process, which might necessitate the use of specially constructed equipment operating under pressure. The solvent should also be plentiful and cheap and have a low specific heat in order to reduce the cost of its removal. Preferably it should also be non-inflammable. It should also have a low viscosity, for this facilitates the leaching of solute from the tissues, the percolation of solvent through the bed of the material and the pressing of the marc and subsequent handling of the solution. Concentration of the solution by evaporation is also influenced by the viscosity, since a high viscosity reduces the rate of heat transfer and increases the risk of overheating thermolabile solutes. A high solution viscosity also restricts the design of suitable evaporators.

For the solvent extraction of oils, such solvents as benzene, light petroleum, or trichloroethylene can be used, while ether is used for the extraction of Male Fern. Where traces of water might interfere with the extraction process, a water-miscible solvent, such as acetone, may be preferred. Acetone is used for the extraction of spices and Ginger Oleoresin. For Capsicum Oleoresin, however, alcohol may be preferred on an industrial scale, since a liquid–liquid extraction may be used later to get rid of water-soluble material. This is an alternative to percolation with acetone and removal of this, followed by cold extraction of the residue with alcohol.

Besides alcohol, hydrocarbons are also used to extract alkaloids. The raw material must, however, first be moistened with water or an alkaline solution to liberate the free alkaloidal base. This technique can be used to obtain reserpine, the moistened rauwolfia powder being extracted with hot benzene in a Soxhlet apparatus (Boehringer et al. 1957). Purification of an alkaloid may be facilitated by such a procedure. The extract as first obtained will consist of a mixture of compounds, often chemically related but of differing pharmacological activity. One or more of the alkaloids will need to be further extracted from this mixture, perhaps by a change of solvent. An alkaloid may be partitioned from solution in a hydrocarbon into acidified water. By careful adjustment of the pH of the aqueous extract, separation of closely related compounds can be achieved by further liquid–liquid extraction. Final purification of alkaloids may also be assisted by careful choice of the acid used to make a crystalline salt (Svoboda & Shahovsky 1953).

Careful selection of solvent may be necessary, not only to achieve a maximum extraction of active principle, but also to prevent undue destruction during the extraction process (Campo & Gramling 1953). Racemization may also be an undesirable result of poor choice of solvent (Carkhuff & Gramling 1952).

Various workers have investigated the effect of adding surfactants to the solvent (Helman 1969). Non-ionic compounds in alcoholic solvents may improve the extraction of alkaloids and, by enhancing the imbibition of solvent by the vegetable tissue, lead to a more rapid extraction with increased selectivity for alkaloid (Butler & Wiese 1953; Srivastava & Chadha 1963). In comparing the different classes of surfactants however, Brochmann-Hanssen (1954) concluded that non-ionic surfactants had little or no effect on the yield of alkaloid. He demonstrated that salts of cationic surfactants gave the best extraction, whereas anionic, compounds were unsuitable due to solubilization and an increased permeability of the cell wall, although an ion exchange mechanism was postulated for cationic surfactants, many alkaloids being combined with cellular constituents such as acids, proteins and cell wall components (Witt, Jirawongse & Youngken 1953). Such adjuvants can only be used where the alkaloids are to be further purified, otherwise they would be present in the final product.

Temperature

The use of elevated temperatures is often precluded by the thermolability or volatility of the active principle, or by an increased extraction of unwanted constituents. For the isolation of a pure thermostable compound, however, raising the temperature of the solvent has the effect of hastening the leaching process, owing to the increased rate of diffusion, stronger convection currents and better solubility of the active principles. An enhanced solvent action is also assisted by loss of the integrity of cell walls and membranes.

Obsolete processes involving the use of hot solvents include the preparation of fresh infusions and decoctions. Fresh infusions were prepared by macerating the drug in a covered vessel for periods ranging from 15 minutes to 2 hours, followed by straining. Generally the water was boiling when first added, but occasionally cold water was used either to prevent too much leaching or to avoid gelatinization of starch. Fresh infusions were not adjusted to volume. Decoctions were prepared by boiling the drug with water, the process being restricted to drugs whose active principles were not volatile in steam. After straining, the volume was adjusted by passing water over the contents of the strainer.

Both maceration and percolation processes are amenable to the use of hot solvent. Maceration is accomplished by heating the drug and solvent in a closed vessel, this modification being known as *digestion*. Hot solvent is sprayed over the bed of raw material in some industrial processes.

Hot water is used for extracting liquorice and cascara, as a precursor to the official processes, but apart from thermolability or volatility of active principle, many drugs are not amenable to such treatment since inert extractive may tend to precipitate for months afterwards. An additional advantage with cascara, however, is that the elevated temperature reduces enzymic degradation (Fairbairn & Simic 1970). Hot extraction is also used for non-official or non-medicinal products: thus quassia is extracted with hot water and buchu with hot alcohol.

Occasionally it is necessary to subject the raw material to the action of hot solvent for an extended period of time, particularly when the solute is not readily soluble, or penetration of cellular tissue is slow. Such cases include the extraction of fixed oils from seeds and of alkaloids by means of such solvents as hydrocarbons, chloroform or methanol, and of ginger oleoresin with acetone.

A small scale extraction apparatus is shown in Fig. 11.2. It consists of a flask, a Soxhlet extractor and a reflux condenser. The raw material is usually placed in a 'thimble' made of filter paper and inserted into the wide central tube of the extractor. Solvent is placed in the flask and boiled, its vapour passing up the large right hand tube into the central space above the drug and thence to the condenser. The condensate then drops back on to the drug, through which it percolates, leaching

vapours encircle the material to be extracted, though the short period of maceration undergone in the Soxhlet apparatus is sacrificed.

A large-scale plant has also been designed based on this principle.

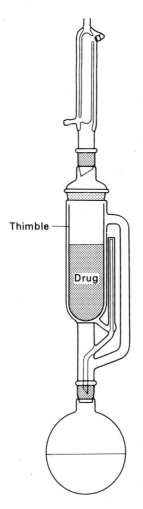

Thimble

Drug

FIG. 11.2. Small-scale extraction apparatus.

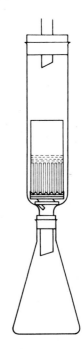

FIG. 11.3. Apparatus for continuous extraction of drugs.

solutes in the process. When sufficient of the solution has collected to raise its level to that of the top of the syphon tube, shown on the right hand side, the whole of the collected percolate syphons over into the flask. The suction effect of the syphoning assists permeation of solvent through the drug. A limited amount of hot solvent is thus made to percolate repeatedly through the raw material, the solutes from which are transferred to the flask.

This principle of continuous hot extraction is sometimes used to extract a drug for the purposes of assay. A simple form of apparatus is described in the British Pharmacopoeia. It is shown in Fig. 11.3 and has the advantage that the hot, rising

Enzyme Activity

Enzyme action may increase solvent penetration of tissues, for example autolysis of lung tissue facilitates the extraction of heparin. Sometimes, fermentation may alter the composition of the soluble constituents, but occasionally the actual yield of an active principle is increased. The sapogenin content of Dioscorea, for example, is increased if the tubers are homogenized with water and allowed to ferment before extraction.

Generally, however, enzyme activity needs to be minimized. The use of strong alcohol and elevated temperatures has been mentioned previously. Protein precipitation may also be used. In the Stoll process for the extraction of Digitalis glycosides, for example, hydrolytic enzymes are inhibited by precipitation with ammonium sulphate added directly to the homogenized tissues. The glycosides can then be extracted by maceration with 70 per cent alcohol with minimum loss.

LIQUID–LIQUID EXTRACTION

Liquid–liquid extraction is used for some commercial scale procedures and is chosen when a pure compound is required. Thus, the production of bacitracin involves partitioning from the bacterial growth medium into butanol (Inskeep et al. 1951). To obtain a satisfactory distribution between solvents it is necessary to select these so that there is as large a difference as possible between the partition coefficients of the various constituents of the crude extract. The distribution between water and an organic solvent will depend on the hydrophilic and hydrophobic groups present in the molecule, and if the hydrophilic groups are ionizable, pH will be an important factor (Newton & Abraham 1950). If the ionization constants of isomers are appreciably different, then separation of these can be achieved (Walker 1950).

The properties of a liquid–liquid interface affect the rate and energy of mass transfer across it. Decreases in interfacial tension in some cases greatly increase liquid–liquid extraction rates (Chu, Taylor & Levy 1950). This may be due to an increase in interfacial area permitted by the lower tension (Garner & Skelland 1956). West et al. (1952) suggest that impurities adsorbed at the interface between immiscible solvents may retard the transfer of solute. This may be overcome by the addition of short-chain (C_6) alcohols which replace the impurities at the interface and destroy the interfacial barriers.

OILS

The method of removal of oils from vegetable and animal tissues depends on the nature of the oil and of the tissues containing the oil. Vegetable fixed oils are removed by *expression* or by *leaching*, whereas animal oils are obtained by a process known as *rendering*. Such oils generally need to be refined. *Steam distillation*, on the other hand, affords a means of obtaining volatile oils in a form which requires little or no further processing. One other process of very limited application is *enfleurage*, used to collect some perfume oils.

VEGETABLE FIXED OILS

Fixed oils are contained in seeds or fruits and, when removed, provide a valuable by-product of protein-rich meal for feeding livestock. The processing of seeds is therefore designed not merely to obtain a good quality oil, but also a useful residue.

Expression

Two main techniques are employed in expression. Hydraulic pressing is a batch process in which the oil is squeezed out by hydraulically exerting pressure on a mass of the material. The other process involves continuous mechanical screw pressing, in which the material is conveyed through a gradually decreasing aperture and the oil is squeezed out by the resulting pressure. In either case, cold or hot expression may be used. Equipment used in these unit operations has been described by Hutchins (1949) and by Dunning (1950, 1956).

The efficiency of pressing is largely determined by pretreatment of the feed material. Seeds may need to be sorted from foreign material, dried and (as for example with peanuts) dehulled by passage through rollers having grooves or cutting edges. Cottonseed also requires delinting. The resulting undamaged seeds are then known as 'meats' and are generally further processed immediately before pressing. Linseed is crushed by passage through rollers; olives are ground to a paste, and peanuts are broken in a hammer mill. Where *cold expression* is necessary in order to preserve the quality of the oil, as with castor and olive oils, the meats are fed directly to the press.

A more complete extraction is, however, achieved by using *hot expression*. The meats, containing a controlled amount of moisture, are first cooked in order to coagulate protein and phosphatides and to rupture the cellular tissue, thereby making the oil more readily available. Most of the moisture is then removed by evaporation and the dried cooked meats are fed to the press while still hot.

Storage of seeds, particularly if they are moist, leads to fermentation. This, together with cooking, tends to increase the fatty acid content of the expressed oil. Hot pressing may also impair the flavour and colour by increasing the amount of aldehydes, ketones and colouring matter, owing to their higher oil solubility at elevated temperatures. The stability of the oil may also be diminished, since the higher temperatures may affect the natural anti-oxidants, initiate autoxidation, or increase the proportion of substances which accelerate fermentation.

The oil that flows from the press will still contain some solids even though the meat has been cooked to coagulate proteins and phospholipids. These solids, known as 'foots', are allowed to settle and are removed by filtration.

Solvent Extraction

In order to achieve an efficient rate of leaching and to minimize the liberation of fines into the miscella, the seeds need to be rolled into flakes of about 0.25 mm thickness. Preliminary cooking before rolling may also be advantageous, for example with soybeans. When seeds are pre-pressed, granulation of the cake may produce a more uniform leaching of the residual oil and enable solvent to be more readily removed from the meal.

Both maceration ('immersion-type') and percolation processes are used; various types of extractors have been described by Karnofsky (1949b). Percolation requires a porous bed and carefully prepared flakes, but has the advantage over immersion-extraction of producing clear miscella by the filtering action of the solids and in permitting adequate drainage of miscella within the flakes. In order to achieve a continuous maceration process, a filtration-extraction technique is commonly employed. Reynolds & Youngs (1964) cite a number of references to the processing of various seeds by this technique. For example, cottonseed flakes are mixed with hexane, agitated, and the oil-laden solvent is removed using a horizontal rotary vacuum filter. The cake may then be washed by more solvent and the washings used to process fresh feed (D'Aquin et al. 1953).

The quality of the oil and the residual cake will depend to a large extent upon the type of solvent chosen. Solvents suitable for glycerides include the straight-chain hydrocarbons. Pentane has too low a boiling-point but hexane can be readily condensed and, being plentiful and cheap, is widely used. Where an elevated temperature is necessary in order to increase oil solubility, heptane may be suitable. Trichlorethylene is also used, but while it is stable and non-inflammable, it has a high specific gravity making it difficult to separate from solids, and it is toxic and may sometimes extract unwanted constituents. Aromatic hydrocarbons are not generally used because they extract too much colour and yield dark oils. Water-miscible solvents such as alcohols and ketones have the disadvantage that traces of water reduce their limited solvent powers for the oil and increase the extraction of water-soluble constituents such as

sugars. Their use does, however, assist in the refining of the oil (Parkin 1950).

Clarification of the miscella, which may contain up to 30 per cent oil is achieved by straining or filtration, or by centrifugation if a finely ground material was extracted by immersion. The solvent may then be removed by passage through a series of evaporators operating at atmospheric or reduced pressure (Hutchins 1968). Removal of the last traces of solvent is achieved by steaming followed by vacuum drying and rapid cooling before contact with air.

Refining

This has been reviewed by Rini (1960). Contaminating components in a crude oil are free fatty acids, phosphatides, colour, moisture and solids. Although olive oil may need little or no refining, most oils require fairly drastic treatment in order to improve their flavour, colour and stability.

While the phosphatides are soluble in dry oil, hydration causes them to precipitate, and they must be removed in order to make the oil palatable. Caustic soda solution may be added in order to neutralize free fatty acids present and to achieve some degree of discoloration. Careful selection of alkali strength, mixing conditions and temperature is very important, since too much caustic soda would saponify an appreciable amount of glyceride. Saponification of the oil can be prevented by employing Clayton's soda ash process which uses a concentrated sodium carbonate solution instead of the caustic soda. The soaps formed from the free fatty acids also entrain phosphatides, proteins, sugars, pigments and resinous substances and are removed by centrifuging, after first dehydrating the oil–soap mixture, followed by careful rehydration just sufficient to cause the soap-stock to break out from the oil without forming an emulsion or entraining too much oil. Although arachis oil may need no further alkali treatment, cotton and linseed oils require further refining with caustic soda in order to remove pigments (Thurman 1949). Bleaching may also be accomplished by treating the hot oil with a suitable adsorbent such as Fuller's earth, kieselguhr or charcoal (Baldwin 1949; Crossley, Davies & Pierce 1962).

An oil processed in the above manner may still not be properly bland and a deodorization process may be necessary. This consists essentially of fractional distillation of the minute amounts of odoriferous materials from the oil with the minimum of injury to the oil itself. Volatile constituents such as peroxides and aldehydes are removed by heating the oil to about 230° in a tank operating at only a few mmHg and injecting steam-free air or oxygen. Rapid cooling before contact with air is necessary in order to prevent deterioration of the oil.

Traces of metallic soaps formed from processing equipment can cause rapid deterioration of oils, but the soaps may be inactivated by residual amounts of phosphatides in the oil. Naturally occurring anti-oxidants include the tocopherols, while the addition of butylated hydroxyanisole and butylated hydroxytoluene is also permitted. Anti-oxidants suitable for highly unsaturated oils are reviewed by Thompson and Sherwin (1966).

ANIMAL OILS

A process called *rendering* is used to separate fat such as lard or tallow from the fatty tissues of animals (Vibrans 1949; Dormitzer 1956). This process consists essentially of freeing the oil by careful heating of the tissue, either under vacuum or by treatment with live steam or warm alkali. The production of fish liver oils also involves such treatment.

A good quality cod liver oil is obtained by 'cooking' the fresh livers with low pressure steam at a temperature not exceeding 85°. After allowing separation to take place, the oil is removed from the water, refined, and chilled to remove high melting point components (*Pharmaceutical Journal* 1970, *205*, 276). The use of high temperatures is desirable since this destroys lipase. Halibut liver oil may be obtained by treatment of the livers with weak alkali. This process may remove some of the natural anti-oxidants from the oil, but the vitamin A stability does not seem to be impaired (Hartman 1950).

VOLATILE OILS

As the name implies, the components of these oils are all sufficiently volatile for a distillation process to be used. Occasionally, while the greater proportion of an oil is volatile, it may be desirable to have much less volatile components present as well, and collection by distillation would yield an inferior product. Such is the case with lemon oil, which is therefore obtained by expression.

A process of *steam distillation* is normally used, the temperature of distillation being close to 100°. The vapour pressure is largely that of the steam, thus enabling the oil to distil at temperatures well below its normal boiling point. *Destructive distillation*, on the other hand involves much higher temperatures. For thermolabile oils steam distillation under reduced pressure may be employed.

Alternatively, a process of limited application known as *enfleurage*, involves the natural volatility of oils at ambient temperatures (Trease & Evans 1966).

Steam Distillation
Prior treatment of the raw material will depend on the accessibility of the steam to the oil containing tissue. Flowers and leaves may be processed whole, whereas woody materials are chipped or cut small and seeds such as caraway are crushed. The distillation is carried out in stills specially constructed for the purpose, the raw material being placed in baskets or trays through which steam is made to pass from underneath. The distillate is collected and the oil separated from the aqueous layer. Some oils such as Turpentine Oil may require to be rectified in order to obtain an oil free from resinous materials. This may be accomplished by further steam distillation.

PROTEINS AND POLYPEPTIDES

Proteins and polypeptides of pharmaceutical importance are derived mainly from animal sources. With a few exceptions, such as gelatin, most are required in a highly purified state. The conversion of skin and bone collagen to gelatin by treatment with lime or dilute acid and its subsequent warm water extraction has been described by Ward & Saunders (1958). The physico-chemical behaviour of gelatin depends largely upon its method of preparation, alkali-precursor gelatin having a much lower isoelectric point than acid-precursor gelatin.

Extraction of other proteins and polypeptides prior to their purification generally involves mincing the animal tissue with a suitable solvent followed by filtration. The choice of solvent depends largely upon the physico-chemical nature of the extractive and the need to reduce the loss of active principle by denaturation or hydrolysis to a minimum. For example, insulin is extracted using cold acid alcohol, the alcohol content, after addition to the minced pancreas, being about 60 per cent. Use of a stronger alcohol would render the insulin insoluble.

Isolation and purification of a particular protein or polypeptide involves adjustment of the physico-chemical conditions of the crude solution in order to precipitate the active principle while keeping impurities in solution. The solubility of a protein depends upon its molecular weight and conformation, the presence of other proteins, the ionic strength, temperature, pH and the proportion of water-miscible non-solvent such as alcohol or acetone which may be present. Further, susceptibility to solvent precipitation is greatest at the isoelectric point, which varies from one protein to another according to the amino acid composition. Careful control of the conditions may therefore be used for the precipitation of proteins. These can then be redissolved in aqueous buffer and reprecipitated to achieve greater purification. By using different solvents at successive stages, a variety of impurities can be removed and finally different protein components themselves can be separated. A good example of this is the fractionation of plasma proteins. Careful adjustment of the ethanol or ether concentration, pH, temperature and ionic strength, enables crude separation into several main fractions, which are then further purified by altering the conditions of precipitation (Nance 1950; Revol 1956). By using aseptic precautions, commercial quantities of purified fibrinogen, thrombin, albumin and various globulin fractions may be obtained in solution, which may be used as such or may be freeze-dried.

The hydration of proteins is also affected by the addition of electrolytes, which compete for the water of hydration. Since the susceptibility to precipitation varies with different proteins, salting out with ammonium sulphate is commonly used. Such a procedure is employed to purify and concentrate the specific tuberculoprotein produced in the culture medium of the tubercle bacillus. The precipitated protein is then separated, dialysed and redissolved in an aqueous solution of suitable pH. Addition of graded amounts of ammonium sulphate to blood plasma can also be used to effect a crude separation of various proteins, particularly the globulin fraction with which antibodies are associated.

The formation of insoluble complexes with heavy metal ions, or with compounds such as Reinecke salt, picric acid, or trichloracetic acid, is also used in the purification of polypeptides. Picrate precipitation, for example, is used in the isolation of insulin, subsequent crystallization being accomplished by the use of zinc chloride. Occasionally, highly specific reactions are possible. Thus correct admixture of a solution of a bacterial toxin with the appropriate antitoxin will precipitate the toxin-antitoxin complex. This affords a highly selective means of purification.

REFERENCES

BALDWIN, A. R. (1949) *J. Am. Oil Chem. Soc.* **26**, 610.

BOEHRINGER, A., BOEHRINGER, E., LIEBRECHT, I. & LIEBRECHT, J. (1957) Brit. Patent 772,122.

BROCHMANN-HANSSEN, E. (1954) *J. Am. pharm. Ass. (Sci. Edn)* **43**, 27.

BULL, A. W. (1935) *Q. Jl Pharm. Pharmacol.* **8**, 378.

BULL, A. W. (1936) *Q. Jl Pharm. Pharmacol.* **9**, 347.

BUTLER, W. J. & WIESE, G. A. (1953) *J. Am. pharm. Ass. (Sci. Edn)* **42**, 382.

CAMPO, J. M. & GRAMLING, L. G. (1953) *J. Am. pharm. Ass. (Sci. Edn)* **42**, 747.

CARKHUFF, E. D. & GRAMLING, L. G. (1952) *J. Am. pharm. Ass. (Sci. Edn)* **41**, 660.

CHU, J. C., TAYLOR, C. C. & LEVY, D. J. (1950) *Ind. Engng Chem.* **42**, 1157.

COLLETT, S. (1950) *Mfg Chem.* **21**, 421.

COLLETT, S. (1953) *Mfg Chem.* **24**, 124.

CROSSLEY, A., DAVIES, A. C. & PIERCE, J. H. (1962) *J. Am. Oil Chem. Soc.* **39**, 165.

D'AQUIN, E. L., VIX, H. L. E., SPADARO, J. J., GRACI, A. V., EAVES, P. H., REUTHER, C. G., MOLAISON, L. J., McCOURTNEY, E. J., CROVETTO, A. J. & GASTROCK, E. A. (1953) *Ind. Engng Chem.* **45**, 247.

DEAN, S. J., BRODIE, D. C., BROCHMANN-HANSSEN, E. & RIEGLEMAN, S. (1953) *J. Am. pharm. Ass. (Sci. Edn)* **42**, 88.

DORMITZER, H. C. (1956) *J. Am. Oil Chem. Soc.* **33**, 471.

DUNNING, J. W. (1950) *J. Am. Oil Chem. Soc.* **27**, 446.

DUNNING, J. W. (1956) *J. Am. Oil Chem. Soc.* **33**, 462.

FAIRBAIRN, J. W. & SIMIC, S. (1970) *J. Pharm. Pharmacol.* **22**, 778.

GARNER, F. H. & SKELLAND, A. H. P. (1956) *Ind. Engng Chem.* **48**, 51.

GRIFFIN, E. L., PHILLIPS, G. W. M., CLAFFEY, J. B., SKALAMERA, J. L. & STROLLE, E. O. (1952) *Ind. Engng Chem.* **44**, 274.

HARTMAN, L. (1950) *J. Am. Oil Chem. Soc.* **27**, 409.

HELMAN, J. (1969) *J. pharm. Sci.* **58**, 1085.

HUTCHINS, R. P. (1949) *J. Am. Oil Chem. Soc.* **26**, 559.

HUTCHINS, R. P. (1968) *J. Am. Oil Chem. Soc.* **45**, 624A.

INSKEEP, G. C., BENNETT, R. E., DUDLEY, J. F. & SHEPARD, M. W. (1951) *Ind. Engng Chem.* **43**, 1488.

JUDAH, M. A., BURDICK, E. M. & CARROLL, R. G. (1954) *Ind. Engng Chem.* **46**, 2262.

KARNOFSKY, G. (1949a) *J. Am. Oil Chem. Soc.* **26**, 564.

KARNOFSKY, G. (1949b) *J. Am. Oil Chem. Soc.* **26**, 570.

NANCE, M. (1950) *J. Pharm. Pharmacol.* **2**, 273.

NEWTON, G. G. F. & ABRAHAM, E. P. (1950) *Biochem. J.* **47**, 257.

OAKLEY, J. H. & STUCKEY, R. E. (1949) *J. Pharm. Pharmacol.* **1**, 714.

OTHMER, D. F. & AGARWAL, J. C. (1955) *Chem. Engng Prog.* **51**, 372.

OTHMER, D. F. & JAATINEN, W. A. (1959) *Ind. Engng Chem.* **51**, 543.

PARKIN, F. P. (1950) *J. Am. Oil Chem. Soc.* **27**, 451.

PECK, W. C. (1936) *Q. Jl Pharm. Pharmacol.* **9**, 401.

PIRIE, N. M. (1956) *Modern Methods of Plant Analysis*, Vol. 1, p. 26. (Eds Paech, K. & Tracey, M. V.) Berlin: Springer-Verlag.

PLACEK, C., BAVISOTTO, V. S. & JADD, E. C. (1960) *Ind. Engng Chem.* **52**, 2.

REVOL, L. A. (1956) *J. Pharm. Pharmacol.* **8**, 84.

REYNOLDS, J. R. & YOUNGS, C. G. (1964) *J. Am. Oil Chem. Soc.* **41**, 63.

RINI, S. J. (1960) *J. Am. Oil Chem. Soc.* **37**, 512.

SERGEANT, G. A. (1950) *J. Pharm. Pharmacol.* **2**, 434.

SRIVASTAVA, G. P. & CHADHA, T. N. (1963) *J. pharm. Sci.* **52**, 299.

SVOBODA, G. H. & SHAHOVSKOY, G. S. (1953) *J. Am. pharm. Ass. (Sci. Edn)* **42**, 729.

THOMPSON, D. & SUTHERLAND, D. G. (1955) *Ind. Engng Chem.* **47**, 1167.

THOMPSON, J. W. & SHERWIN, E. R. (1966) *J. Am. Oil Chem. Soc.* **43**, 683.

THURMAN, B. H. (1949) *J. Am. Oil Chem. Soc.* **26**, 580.

TREASE, G. E. & EVANS, W. C. (1966) *A Textbook of Pharmacology* 9th Edn. London: Bailliere, Tindall & Cassell.

VIBRANS, F. C. (1949) *J. Am. Oil Chem. Soc.* **26**, 575.

WALKER, C. A. (1950) *Ind. Engng Chem.* **42**, 1226.

WARD, A. G. & SAUNDERS, P. R. (1958) *Rheology. Theory and Applications*, Vol. 2, p. 313, (Ed. Eirich, F. R.) New York: Academic Press.

WEST, F. B., HERRMAN, A. J., CHONG, A. T. & THOMAS, L. E. K. (1952) *Ind. Engng Chem.* **44**, 625.

WITT, J. A., JIRAWONGSE, V. & YOUNGKEN, H. W. (1953) *J. Am. pharm. Ass. (Sci. Edn)* **42**, 63.

12

Drying

In the preparation of medicinal chemicals, drying is usually the final stage of processing and is designed to yield a stable homogeneous product which is easy to manipulate in subsequent operations of packing or formulating. In some cases, this involves converting a wet filter cake into a free-flowing solid; in others, such as spray-drying or drum-drying, a solution is both evaporated and dried in a single operation. Vegetable drugs are dried prior to extraction, partly in order to avoid deterioration on storage and transport and partly to facilitate grinding. Drying is also an important stage in some formulating operations, notably during tabletting by 'wet-granulation'. Various methods and equipment are available, the choice being dependent on such factors as:

(a) the heat sensitivity of the product,
(b) its physical characteristics prior to drying,
(c) the nature of the solvent to be removed,
(d) the need for asepsis,
(e) the scale of operating,
(f) available sources of heat.

THEORY

When a material is exposed to air a definite temperature and humidity, it will either gain or lose moisture until an equilibrium is established. The moisture content at equilibrium varies with the nature of the material and with the temperature and humidity of the air. Thus, starch exposed to air at a relative humidity of, say, 60 per cent at room temperature, may contain at equilibrium up to 15 per cent of water. Conversely, a non-porous insoluble solid such as talc has a very low equilibrium moisture content at all temperatures and humidities. It is possible to distinguish progressive stages in the drying of moist material. Consider for example, a slab of material of sufficiently high moisture content so that its surface is wet. In contact with a current of warm air, superficial water diffuses through the surrounding stationary air film and is carried away rapidly by the moving air stream. The rate of evaporation is determined by the temperature and the humidity of the air when the air is moving at constant velocity. Provided that water can move freely from the interior of the slab to the surface to replace that lost by evaporation, the rate of evaporation proceeds at a constant rate as shown by the line AB in Fig. 12.1. At this stage, the rate of drying is controlled by the rate at which the vapour can

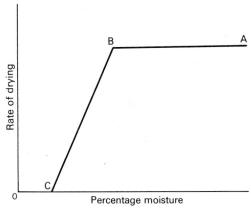

FIG. 12.1. Rate of drying curve

186

diffuse through the surface air film. As drying continues, the surface is no longer completely wetted and the drying rate falls; line BC represents this 'falling-rate period' which will vary according to the thickness of the slab. The limiting factor is now the rate of movement of water from the interior to the surface; water molecules may diffuse through the solid or capillary forces may be responsible for this movement. The point B at which the falling-rate occurs is known as the 'critical moisture content'. As drying proceeds further, the curve eventually approaches zero rate at point C, which corresponds to the water content in equilibrium with the air. Thus, in order to dry a material, two processes are necessary; firstly, heat must be supplied to provide the latent heat of vaporization, and secondly, the liberated vapour must be removed, generally by a moving air stream. The rate of mass transfer of water from the solid to the moving air during the constant-rate period is directly proportional to the difference between the humidity of the air at the liquid surface of the solid and the bulk of the air, and the area of surface exposed to the air. Thus, the rate of mass transfer $= A(H-h)K$, where $A =$ area of interface, $H =$ humidity of saturated air, $h =$ humidity of air stream, $K =$ mass transfer coefficient.

The rate of heat transfer from the air to the wet solid can be expressed as follows:

Rate of heat transfer $= U.A.\Delta t$, where $U =$ overall coefficient of heat transfer, $\Delta t =$ temperature difference between the air and surface of the solid.

Combining these equations for rates of mass transfer and heat transfer, the following expression is obtained:

$$U.A.\Delta t. = A(H-h)K.L$$

where $L =$ latent heat of vaporization, then:

$$H - h = \frac{\Delta t.U}{K.L}$$

During the constant-rate period, the surface of the material resembles a wet bulb hygrometer since heat transferred from the warm air is used to evaporate water at the temperature of the surface of the slab. During the falling-rate period, the amount of heat input is unchanged, but, since the rate of evaporation is less, the temperature at the surface rises and care must be taken with thermolabile materials to avoid decomposition. Air velocity cannot affect the rate of drying in this falling-rate period. During the constant-rate period,

the thickness of the surface air film will influence the rate of diffusion of vapour through it; high air velocities will reduce this film thickness and increase the rate of drying.

EQUIPMENT

All drying processes involve evaporation of the solvent by heat, but the design of equipment varies considerably according to the way in which the heat is applied. For efficient working, it is necessary to establish a balance between (i) removal of solvent vapour from dryer, (ii) evaporation of solvent from the exposed surface, and (iii) diffusion of remaining solvent to the surface. Equipment may be described according to whether it is designed to cope with damp solids or with slurries and solutions.

DAMP SOLIDS

The Tray Dryer
This is essentially a hot air oven in which the material is placed in thin layers in trays. There are many variants of design according to the source of heat used and also as a result of added modifications such as vacuum, forced air circulation and thermostatic control. In small laboratory dryers the material is placed on trays which slide into the drying cabinet while in large installations the interior may be designed for the wheeling in of trolleys containing the trays.

The simplest form of heating places the source of heat (e.g. a steam coil) at floor level and relies on natural convection. Most modern equipment, however, uses fans to provide a forced circulation

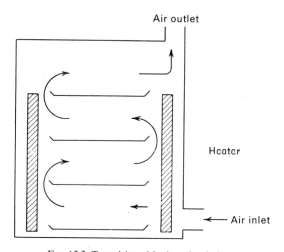

FIG. 12.2. Tray drier with air recirculation.

of air across the trays. In small ovens there may only be provision for a single passage of heated air while in larger units thermal efficiency is improved by recirculation of air which is reheated after its passage over each shelf as shown in Fig. 12.2.

In order to appreciate the relationship between temperature and drying conditions in the dryer under ideal conditions it is necessary to consider some of the basic concepts of humidity, and the terms that are commonly used will first be defined.

Absolute humidity is the weight of water vapour present in unit volume or unit mass of moist air.

Relative humidity is the ratio of the actual vapour pressure to the saturation pressure at the same temperature and usually expressed as a percentage.

Dew point is the temperature at which the saturation vapour pressure equals the actual (partial) pressure of the water vapour in the air.

Wet bulb temperature is the dynamic equilibrium temperature attained by a water surface when exposed to air under adiabatic conditions so that the sensible heat transferred from the gas to the liquid is equal to the latent heat of evaporation of the liquid. The rate at which the temperature is reached depends upon the initial temperatures and the gas flow rate. The wet bulb temperature is the same as the adiabatic saturation temperature.

The relations between absolute humidity and temperature under equilibrium conditions can be seen in Fig. 12.3 which represents a section of a

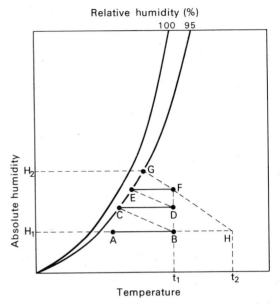

FIG. 12.4. Temperature-humidity relations during recirculation of air in tray drier.

humidity chart. The 100 per cent relative humidity is the 'saturation curve' and represents the humidity–temperature relation for saturated air, and is equivalent to the wet bulb temperature plotted against absolute humidity. The group of lines to the right of this curve are the adiabatic cooling lines. These serve two very useful purposes. Firstly they can be used to determine humidity from a knowledge of wet bulb and dry bulb temperatures. From a point on the saturation curve corresponding to the wet bulb temperature one follows the adiabatic cooling line until the co-ordinate corresponding to the dry bulb temperature is reached, at which point the absolute humidity is read off from the scale on the left. Secondly, the adiabatic cooling lines show the change in humidity in drying under adiabatic conditions. If the humidity of the air in contact with the damp solid is shown by point Z in Fig. 12.3 and this air is then heated to point X the passage of air over the damp solid follows the adiabatic cooling line to meet point Y.

Now consider the humidity chart in relation to the conditions during reheating of the air in a recirculating tray dryer (Fig. 12.2). If air of humidity and temperature at A (Fig. 12.4) is passed over heating coils to a temperature of t_1, the absolute humidity remains constant and the air reaches point B. This air on passing over a tray of moist material will leave at near saturation point, say 95 per cent relative humidity so that the adiabatic

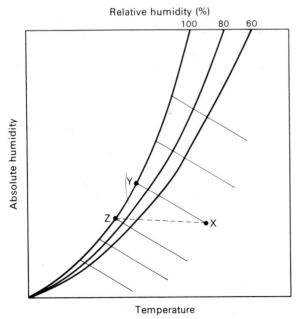

FIG. 12.3. Humidity chart (diagrammatic).

cooling line BC represents the condition of the air during this process. The air is reheated, represented by line CD, and passes over the second tray resulting in a further pick-up of moisture leading to point E. A further cycle of heating and passage leads to point G. The original air humidity H_1 has thus been increased to H_2 after a total of three air circulations. If the dryer operated on a single passage of air, and the same amount of drying was to be achieved, the temperature of the inlet air would need to be raised to t_2. HG is the adiabatic cooling line. The recirculation method thus has two obvious advantages:

(1) Given weight of air takes up more water than is possible in a single pass.

(2) Drying air of lower temperature can be used to obtain the same reduction of moisture.

Vacuum drying may be performed in ovens in which a quantity of material is spread on trays placed on steam-heated shelves in an oven which can be evacuated. The disadvantages are (1) that even though most materials swell and dry as a friable mass, a grinding process is necessary to get a powdered product; (2) the danger of finely powdered material being drawn off by the vacuum pump is considerable, and filters that require frequent cleaning have to be provided; and (3) the material is subjected to heat for the period required to dry the whole. If the shelves of the oven are steam heated, they will be at a temperature of 100° to 110°, or even more, depending on the steam pressure. While the material is wet it will not much exceed the temperature of the boiling point of water at the reduced pressure of the oven, but as the moisture is evaporated and the absorption of heat, as latent heat of vaporization, no longer keeps the temperature down, there will be nothing to prevent the material reaching the same temperature as that of the shelves. This may not matter in some cases, and as a general rule it is less objectionable for the material to reach this temperature when dry. If there is a real objection to the material being so heated, a source of heat of lower temperature must be used. Hot water circulation can be used, but special precautions must be taken to see that the flow of water is arranged evenly through all the shelves of the oven, and that sufficient water is circulated to supply the necessary amount of heat at the lower temperature. As there is very little air present in these ovens, transmission by air convection between the shelf and the product is practically non-existent. Most of the heat passes by direct contact conduction between the tray and the shelf and to a less extent by radiation, although radiation will be small if low temperature heating is used. Early types of vacuum ovens had shelves consisting of a tube bent in the form of a grid; on such a shelf the trays are only in contact along the lines of the pipe, a very small part of their area. Modern ovens have flat steam shelves in which steam is admitted to a space between the upper and lower surfaces of the shelf. The bottom of the tray is in contact with the shelf over its whole surface so that heat transmission by conduction is greatly improved. Trays on such shelves should be carefully handled in order to prevent denting of the under-surface. The degree of 'vacuum' (i.e. the reduction in pressure) is usually shown on a gauge of the Bourdon type graduated in inches of mercury, reading from 0 to 30; a reading of 27 or 28 is quite good for ordinary practice. The 'vacuum' as shown on the gauge is not always strictly accurate; the reading will be affected by the external barometric pressure. When the barometric pressure is high a much better 'vacuum' will be shown on the gauge than when it is low. The actual pressure inside the apparatus is unaffected by external changes in atmospheric pressure and is given by the difference between the external barometric pressure and the reading on the gauge.

The Tunnel Dryer

This is a modification of the tray dryer in which the oven is replaced by a tunnel which receives damp material at one end and discharges the dried product at the other. It may be operated in batches or continuously. One arrangement is that the trays are carried on trucks which move slowly along the tunnel. Another replaces trays by a belt conveyor, either single or multiple. In the latter, partially dried material having completed one circuit spills over the end of the first conveyor on to a second travelling in the opposite direction. In this way, the product may make as many as five successive passages along the tunnel before it is discharged.

The Rotary Dryer

This was originally designed for handling large quantities of chemicals, since it can cope with an input of several tonnes per hour. More recently, small rotary dryers have been introduced for sterile processing. Essentially, the equipment comprises a horizontal tube, slightly inclined, so that material fed in at one end will gradually work its way to the other as the tube slowly rotates. Heating is either applied directly, by a hot air current within the tube, or indirectly via an outer shell containing steam tubes or heated gases. As the tube rotates, the charge is raised by lifting vanes fitted to the walls of the tube, whence it falls into the path of the hot gases, thus producing a tumbling effect. A recent advance in design is the Rotary Louvre Dryer in which hot air is fed into the tube through vents or louvres. In this way, the material to be dried continuously meets fresh streams of air and is maintained as a semi-fluidized bed.

When recovery of the solvent is important, a rotary vacuum dryer may be used. This has a stationary steam-jacketed cylinder fitted with a rotating agitator carrying spiral mixing blades which perform the same function as the lifting vanes of the rotating tube model. Small rotary vacuum dryers have been adopted for aseptic work, such as the removal of solvents from antibiotics. These dryers are of stainless steel and all parts can be sterilized. A further type of rotary vacuum dryer is the Apex 'Rotacone' which is essentially a jacketed double-cone mixer. One of the hollow trunnions on which the dryer is mounted supplies steam or hot water to the jacket while the other acts as a vacuum connection. It is claimed that the continuous tumbling action maintains a uniform temperature in the batch and avoids prolonged contact with the hot surfaces.

Infrared Heating
Infrared rays have been used as a source of heat in drying and evaporating in the pharmaceutical industry. Infrared rays of wavelengths between 2.4 and 3.6 μm can be used for evaporation at temperatures of 55° to 30° or even lower.

The term infrared is misleading as it is possible for all the electromagnetic spectrum to generate heat as its ultimate form of dispersion. By using the middle infrared band, heat is available in useful quantity with the added advantage that infrared rays can (a) pass through certain materials without being absorbed, (b) be reflected 95 to 100 per cent from suitable surfaces, and (c) be absorbed in most industrial products of a heterogeneous nature with generation of heat within the substance. Its properties of absorption and reflection from different substances vary with the wavelength. With any fresh material, tests should be made with different wavelengths to ascertain the temperature which will be generated by adsorption. Sources of heat are used which combine a high proportion of infrared radiation with control over the wavelength of the rays emitted. The most common forms of heat source are specially designed gas burners, electric lamps or electric heating elements.

Kay (1951) describes a dryer which uses 54 bar-type 0.5 kW infrared emitters suspended at equal distances in pairs over the surface of the material and fitted with parabolic reflectors. Provision is made for exhaust connection to the top of the dryer casing, so that water vapour is removed by a gentle flow of air over the material. With such an arrangement sodium bicarbonate, for example, can be heated to 50° at the rate of 750 kg/h, with a consumption of 12 kW. Among the advantages of this type of plant, the author lists (i) ease of control (both of heat and flow of material), (ii) small space requirements, and (iii) suitability for connection to a continuous-flow system in which materials are fed from storage bins dried, cooled, weighed and mixed continuously.

Fowler (1952), gives an account of the pharmaceutical uses of infrared heating and concludes that drying by this method appears to be satisfactory for certain types of pharmaceutical preparations when using a peak wavelength of about 3.9 μm. The method was used successfully, with shorter drying times, for fresh drugs, granular preparations, wet precipitates and lozenges. The author found infrared heating unsuitable for extracts and soft pastille masses. The report suggests that the method does not harm the majority of substances commonly used in tablets and that it appears to offer a means of drying tablet granules quickly.

Fluidized Bed Dryer
Fluidized bed dryers operate by the passage of heated air through a fine mesh which supports the bed of powder. The Aeromatic dryer shown diagrammatically in Fig. 12.5 consists of a conical vessel of either plastic or stainless steel with a perforated bottom, into which the material to be dried is placed. Filtered air, drawn in by the induction fan is heated and filtered and then passes through the powder bed. An air filter above the bed retains any airborne particles. The temperature of drying can be controlled by regulating both the inlet air temperature and the flow rate of air. As the velocity of the air is increased, the pressure drop of the air through the bed becomes at a certain point equal to the net effective weight of the solid per unit area and the bed begins to expand. Further increase beyond this point known as 'onset of fluidization', where the particles are supported by the air, causes rapid expansion of the bed and particles begin to show turbulent motion. The particles are not in direct contact with each other and efficient heat exchange occurs between the particles and the flowing air, the moist air being

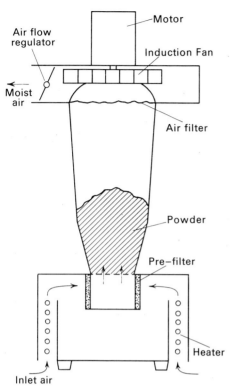

Air flow regulator

Moist air

Motor

Induction Fan

Air filter

Powder

Pre—filter

Heater

Inlet air

FIG. 12.5. Fluidized bed drier.

it forms a thin film which dries rapidly. As the drum slowly rotates, the film approaches a knife which then pares or flakes off the dry solid in the same manner as the doctor blade operates on a rotary filter. Since many solids are extremely adhesive, the correct adjustment of the knife is very important. Different methods are used for applying the liquid to the drum; the original process made use of a shallow pan or trough into which the drum dipped. Alternative arrangements are to splash the liquid on the drum from beneath or to run it on from the top, the latter method giving the thickest layer. Twin drums are sometimes set up in parallel, rotating in opposite directions and with a common feed line but separate knives. A vacuum drum dryer encloses both drums and feed line in a vacuum chamber.

The Spray Dryer

Solutions or slurries may be dried in one operation by spraying into heated air, the very large surface of contact between the drops and the air making possible a very high rate of vaporization. This rapid evaporation keeps the temperature of the droplets low, allowing high air temperatures to be used. The important steps in the spray drying operation are the atomization of the liquid, the drying process and the recovery of the product. Atomization may be achieved by a centrifugal disc atomizer or a pressure type nozzle. The former has the advantage of high capacity and has little tendency to clog. In general, nozzle atomization produces larger particles.

A laboratory model Niro Spray Dryer is shown diagrammatically in Fig. 12.6. Air is drawn through the electric (or gas) heater A by means of a fan B, and is heated to a maximum of 350°. The liquid is fed by gravity to the atomizer D, the disc of which is driven by an air turbine and spins at 35 000 rev/min (max). The sprayed droplets come into contact with the hot air introduced just below the disc at C. The droplets rapidly evaporate as they are carried in the eddy currents in the drying chamber E. The dry powder is separated from the exhaust gas in the cyclone separator F, and is discharged into container G. Inlet and outlet temperatures are controlled by the heater A and also by the valve H which controls the flow rate of air. The evaporative capacity is from 1 to 6.5 litres of water per hour depending on drying temperatures applied. Too high a temperature can result in drying and case hardening of the outer surface of the droplet before the liquid in the interior has evaporated. Under these circumstances, the rapid

carried away rapidly. The drying cycle of tablet granules can be as little as 30 minutes compared with the 24-hour cycle of conventional tray driers. The intense agitation of the granules may cause attrition but the use of suitable binders for making the granules can overcome this. Many organic powders develop electrostatic charges during the fluidization particularly near the end of the drying process so that efficient electrical earthing of the drying chamber and the cloth filters is necessary. Machines are available with capacities from a few kilogrammes to several hundred kilogrammes. The floor space for a given capacity is small compared with a tray dryer.

SLURRIES OR SOLUTIONS

If a solution will not crystallize readily, or if it is desirable to minimize the period of contact with the heating surface, methods are available for converting a slurry or solution into the dry state in a single operation.

The Drum Dryer

This comprises a horizontally mounted steel cylinder heated from within by steam. The liquid to be dried is run on to the hot surface where

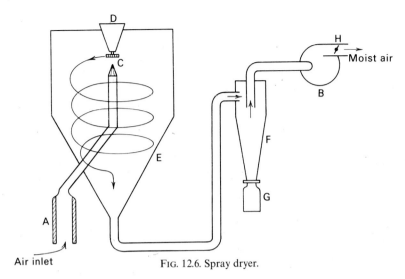

FIG. 12.6. Spray dryer.

heat transfer causes the liquid in the particle interior to vaporize, causing the outer shell to expand forming a hollow sphere. Sometimes the rate of vapour generation is sufficient to disrupt the particle. The particle size of the product depends on the solids content, liquid viscosity, feed rate and disc speed of the atomizer.

Spray dryers can be designed for drying under sterile conditions. Other modifications include operation under closed cycle conditions, which allows feed solvent to be recovered and would also enable drying to proceed under oxygen free conditions.

Riegelman et al. (1950) investigating the characteristics of spray dried powders, found that the rate of solution of boric acid and methyl cellulose powders was substantially increased by the process. Spray drying of sulphur resulted in a free flowing, more easily wetted dispersible powder. Spray dried lactose, because of its good flow properties can be tabletted by direct compression, unlike conventional lactose which requires granulation. However, it suffers the disadvantage of being less pure than crystallized lactose, the impurity 5(hydroxymethyl) 2-furaldehyde causing browning of the tabletted material on storage. Newton (1966) has provided an excellent review wherein the physical characteristics of spray-dried powders are discussed, as well as specific practical consideration for operating spray-dryers.

FREEZE-DRYING

The removal of water vapour from a frozen solution by sublimation forms the basis of freeze-drying. The process of drying from the frozen state is carried out by subjecting the material to be dried to low absolute pressures, after it has been frozen at temperatures below $-40°$. Under these conditions the frozen water will sublime, i.e. pass from the solid to the gaseous state without becoming liquid. The water vapour is removed from the system by condensation in a cold trap maintained at a lower temperature than the frozen material. The principles of the process can be appreciated by referring to the phase diagram of water which shows the relation between the temperature and vapour pressure of ice, water, and water vapour (Fig. 12.7). Vapour, liquid, and solid exist in the

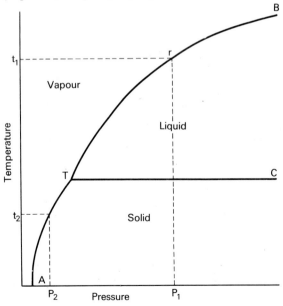

FIG. 12.7. Solid–liquid–vapour equilibria (atmospheric pressure) (not to scale).

areas so indicated in the diagram. TA is the vapour pressure curve of ice. Above TA only water vapour exists, and below TA only ice exists. The line TB is the vapour pressure curve of water. Above this line only water vapour exists, and below this line only liquid water exists. Along TB liquid water and water vapour are in equilibrium. P_1 refers to 760 mmHg when water boils at $100°$ shown as t_1. The line TC represents the effect of pressure on the melting point of ice. Since the line TC slopes slightly to the left it is seen that the melting point is only slightly decreased as the pressure is increased. At point T, solid, liquid and vapour are in equilibrium with one another. This point where three phases are in equilibrium is termed the triple-point. Since the melting point varies very little with pressure, the triple point is very near to the melting point, it being $0.0075°$ and 4.6 mmHg.

The first consideration in freeze-drying any solution is the temperature at which it must be held for sublimation to occur from the solid state. From Fig. 12.7 it can be seen that it is necessary to cool the solution to below the triple-point temperature and to reduce the pressure in the drying chamber to below 4.6 mmHg. Under conditions represented by temperature t_2 where the equilibrium vapour pressure is P_2 then direct change of solid to vapour can occur without conversion to a liquid phase. Freeze-drying will not take place if these equilibrium conditions are maintained, so it is necessary to remove the vapour by a refrigerated condenser operating at a lower temperature than t_2. Alternative methods for removing water vapour include the use of chemical desiccants and mechanical pumping of the vapour. Heat must be supplied to provide the latent heat of evaporation of ice (approximately 2.9 MJ/kg over the range $-30°$ to $0°$).

The principles outlined above have been restricted to the simplest case where ice is sublimed in the absence of any dissolved solid. When a solution of solids is dried, the depression of freezing point of water by the solutes must be considered. It is essential that the temperature is bought below the eutectic point so that no liquid phase is present. Failure to achieve a sufficiently low temperature would result in severe frothing of the product under high vacuum.

Greaves (1946) has emphasized that the rate of drying depends solely on the rate at which heat can be supplied to the material. The factors that limit this rate include (a) maintenance of low condenser temperature, (b) the rate of transfer of heat through the frozen material, (c) the highest 'safe' temperature at which the material can be dried. Since the vaporization of ice can only occur at the surface, it is necessary to expose a large surface area to the source of heat. When large volumes are to be dried, rotation of the vessel during the freezing stage has been used to get a frozen layer around the periphery of the vessel. For efficient vapour flow to the condenser, the freeze-drying apparatus should be designed and operated so that the water vapour is not obstructed by high partial pressure of non-condensable gases (i.e. should be leak free), or by long narrow paths that arise from badly designed manifolds or the use of narrow necked vials.

Greaves (1946) gives the following conditions for the production of dried plasma: condenser temperature $-40°$ (equivalent to v.p. of 0.1 mm); drying temperature of the frozen serum $-21°$ (equivalent to v.p. of 0.7 mm). The pressure difference is 0.6 mm and this results in rapid evaporation. The freeze drying of biological materials has been reviewed by Davies (1968).

It is impossible to remove all trace of moisture under conditions of freeze-drying alone. Lowering the condenser temperature will result in lower moisture content of the sample but there are obvious limits to their values. Under the conditions stated by Greaves, the freeze-dried serum contains a minimum of 5 mg of water per g of dried serum. This is reduced by 3 to 4 days exposure to phosphorous pentoxide.

A freeze-dried powder differs considerably in physical properties from a solid prepared by evaporation of a liquid under reduced pressure or by spray- or roller-drying (p. 191). This is readily seen by comparing samples of human serum dried by different methods. If water is removed by distillation under reduced pressure, there is a general concentration of the solution of the serum solids into a glue-like scale, which ultimately contains from 5 to 10 per cent of moisture. This scale is not completely soluble in water, which indicates some denaturation of the proteins. Spray-dried plasma also shows evidence of slight denaturation; here again the solution passes through similar stages of concentration during evaporation but over a much shorter interval of time. In freeze-drying, evaporation takes place from the solidified solution; no concentration occurs and the evaporated solid occupies practically the same volume as that of the original frozen solution. In these circumstances no denaturation of the plasma proteins occurs. Similar conditions obtain in the freeze-drying of penicillin. The production of freeze-dried material may be considered in three stages: preliminary freezing, vacuum evaporation and heat requirement for evaporation.

Preliminary freezing. Amounts of solution of the material containing a definite quantity are introduced into the final containers. There is a limit to the volume of liquid capable of being satisfactorily freeze-dried in any fixed type of container; beyond a certain limit of depth of liquid to be evaporated the method is unsuitable. The covered containers are first cooled to $2°$ in the cold room and then transferred to the deep freeze cabinet where they are rapidly cooled to $-50°$. The more rapid the rate of freezing the smaller the crystals and the more amorphous and more readily soluble is the final product. The frozen containers are then loaded into the vacuum desiccators.

High-speed vertical spin-freezing. Greaves (1942) introduced this method the drying of serum or plasma. The bottles containing the plasma are spun on their vertical axes at between 750 and 1000 rev/min. The liquid is thereby distributed uniformly inside the bottle round the periphery, leaving a conical air space in the centre reaching to the bottom of the bottle. The liquid after supercooling freezes suddenly in this position, giving small crystals and a very soluble product. If this is done in the vacuum chamber, frothing is avoided and both evaporation and freezing occur. Thus prefreezing is abolished and the freezing becomes the first stage of the drying process.

Vacuum evaporation. The maintenance of the contents in the solid, frozen condition during the application of the vacuum is vitally important. If liquid is formed as a result of partial thawing, a considerable amount of degassing would occur with probable loss of the material, which would froth over the sides of the container. Air is exhausted by double-stage, high-vacuum pumps until a suitable vacuum is obtained (a vacuum of 0.01 mmHg is possible). During evaporation, some water vapour must be carried over into the oil of the pump from which it must be removed either by heating or centrifuging. A condensing coil at the bottom of the chamber is maintained at $-50°$ by means of a special refrigerating plant. When the pressure is sufficiently low, ice evaporates and condenses on the coils. As ice forms on the condenser it acts as an insulator and the heat interchange becomes less efficient.

Heat requirement for evaporation. Latent heat being required for evaporation, the solution would cool still further; a small source of radiant heat is therefore placed in the chamber head and evaporation takes place rapidly with the frozen material remaining at $-20°$ until all the ice has evaporated.

REFERENCES

DAVIES, J. D. (1968) *Process Biochem.* **3**, 11, 48.

FOWLER, H. W. (1952) *J. Pharm. Pharmacol.* **4**, 932.

GREAVES, R. I. N. (1942) *J. Hyg., Camb.* **41**, 489.

GREAVES, R. I. N. (1946) Medical Research Council Spec. Report Series No. **258**. London: HMSO.

KAY, A. W. (1951) *Chem. Trade J. Chem. Engng* **128**, 741.

NEWTON, J. M. (1966) *Manuf. Chem. & Aerosol News* (4) **37**, 33.

RIEGELMAN, S., SWINTOSKY, J. V., HIGUCHI, T., & BUSSE, L. W. (1950) *J. Am. pharm. Ass. (Sci. Edn)* **39**, 444.

13

Evaporation

The vaporization of a portion of solvent from a solution of a solid is termed evaporation. This process is distinguished from distillation in that the volatile component, which is usually water and thus of little value, is not condensed and collected separately. In distillation, the volatile components are required and the term is frequently applied to the separation of components that have different boiling points. Evaporation is employed in the isolation of a non-volatile solute from solution, or for the concentration of such a solution. The term evaporation when used in its widest sense, implies the free escape of vapour from the surface of a liquid below its boiling point. In industrial practice, evaporation is generally carried out at the boiling point of the liquid in order to obtain rapid removal of the vapour. In principle, it is difficult to distinguish between evaporation and drying, although the latter operation is mainly concerned with removal of relatively small amounts of water from a solid, while evaporation is concerned with the removal of large amounts of water or other solvent.

GENERAL PRINCIPLE OF EVAPORATION

Vapour Pressure
Liquids and solids exert a vapour pressure which measures the tendency of the substance to evaporate. The vapour pressure of a liquid increases with rising temperature. In a closed system evaporation of the liquid takes place till an equilibrium is set up between the molecules leaving and molecules re-entering the liquid. The vapour above the liquid is then *saturated* and exerts a *maximum vapour pressure*; before equilibrium is attained, or if insufficient liquid is present to saturate the gas space by evaporation, the vapour is said to be *unsaturated*. The pressure is usually stated in terms of the height of a column of mercury (in cm or mm) which exerts an equivalent pressure.

Boiling Point
The temperature at which the vapour pressure of a liquid is equal to the pressure applied externally is called the boiling point of the liquid. Thus at 100°C the vapour pressure of water is 760 mm and in an atmosphere at this pressure, the water boils. At the boiling point, vapour is formed in the body of the liquid as well as at the surface and drives off the vapour from the surface; below the boiling point, vapour is liberated by diffusion mainly from the surface layers of the liquid.

The boiling point varies with the externally applied pressure; at lower external pressures, there is a reduction in the boiling point and at higher external pressures, an elevation in the boiling point. The following values for boiling points at different pressures illustrate this point: water 100°/760 mm; 0°/4.6 mm; glycerin 290°/760 mm, 130°/1.5 mm; eucalyptol 176°/760 mm, 20°/1.3 mm. An average organic compound may exhibit the following values: 350°/760 mm, 220 to 250°/20 mm; 170 to 200°/0.1 mm, 40 to 60°/0.001 mm. A pressure of 20 mm is attainable on a water pump; 0.1 mm on a good oil pump and 0.001 mm on a mercury diffusion pump backed by an oil pump.

Because of the pressure exerted by the hydrostatic head of liquid, the lower layers boil at a higher temperature than the upper layers so that the average temperature of the boiling liquid is higher than that which would correspond to the external pressure in the vapour space. This effect is significant in large evaporators in which the hydrostatic head may be several feet.

Effect of Dissolved Substances

The vapour pressure of a liquid is lowered when a substance is dissolved in it and consequently the boiling point of the liquid is raised. For dilute solutions of non-volatile solutes equimolecular quantities of different substances dissolved in equal volumes of the same solvent lower the vapour pressure by an equal amount (Raoult's Law). This relationship forms the basis of the ebullioscopic method of molecular weight determination. The effect of volatile solutes is considered under 'Fractional distillation' (p. 210).

Heat Supply and Vapour Removal

In both evaporation and distillation, heat must be supplied to the liquid and the vapour above the liquid surface must be continuously removed. If the vapour space above the liquid is saturated, no evaporation can take place. The vapour from boiling liquids is most conveniently removed by a condenser so that the equilibrium between liquid and vapour is never attained. Evaporation of liquids below their boiling point can be expedited by the passage of a current of air across the surface. In considering the principles of evaporation and distillation, attention must be paid to (a) heat transfer from the heating medium to the liquid and (b) separation of vapour from liquid.

Heat transfer.   The function of an evaporator is to transfer heat to the evaporating liquid so as to provide the latent heat of vaporization. When steam is used as a source of heat there are three obstructions to the transfer of heat from the steam to the substance being heated: (1) the wall of the evaporator, (2) the film of condensed steam on the steam side of the wall; and (3) the liquid film of the substance being heated on the other side of the wall. The significance of these factors will now be discussed in more detail. Consider the simple case of heat transfer to a liquid flowing through a tube which is surrounded by steam; the temperature gradient across a section of the wall is shown diagrammatically in Fig. 13.1. On the steam side, saturated steam at temperature t_1 will condense

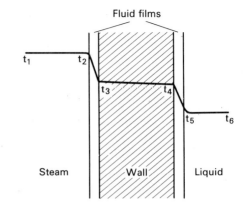

FIG. 13.1. Temperature distribution across the wall of an evaporator.

when it comes into contact with the cooler surface of the wall, resulting in a film of condensate coating the surface. This film offers a considerable resistance to the passage of heat since heat can only be transmitted through this film by conductivity. Most liquids and gases are poor conductors of heat. By calculation from coefficients of conductivity it will be found that a film of water 0.003 inches thick will offer a far greater resistance than a wall of copper 0.125 inches thick. A considerable temperature drop occurs across this film (t_3–t_2). The obstruction caused by the wall itself is proportional to its coefficient of conductivity but for copper, iron and stainless steel the differences are negligible when compared with the film resistances. In practice there are also obstructions due to corrosion, encrustations and deposited solids on the wall of the evaporator. These coatings or scale have a much lower conductivity than the wall itself and in addition their surface roughness will increase the effective thickness of the liquid films in contact with them. The temperature drop across the wall is t_4–t_3 and is seen to be small compared with the drop across the films. Inside the tube, next to the wall, a relatively slow-moving film of liquid will be present even though the liquid towards the centre of the tube may be flowing in a turbulent manner. The thickness of this streamline layer depends on the viscosity and velocity of the fluid and on the surface roughness of the wall. As heat can only be transferred through this film by conduction the temperature drop t_5–t_4 is relatively large. Finally, the heat passes to the bulk of the liquid which reaches an approximately uniform temperature t_6 due to mixing by turbulence.

The amount of heat which must be transmitted through the wall of the vessel varies with the liquid to be evaporated. If the liquid is aqueous with a low solids content then the latent heat of vaporization, 540×4.2 J/g, will be provided by the condensation of an equal weight of steam in the jacket. If benzene is being evaporated, with a boiling point of about $81°$ and a latent heat of vaporization of 90×4.2 J/g, then the condensation of one part of steam will provide the heat to vaporize about six parts of benzene. These comparative figures of course, do not take into account differences in heat transfer across the films of the two liquids. Benzene which has the lower viscosity would have a relatively thin streamline layer in contact with the wall, resulting in better transfer of heat.

The general equation for heat transfer can be expressed as follows:

$$q = UA\Delta t$$

where q is the rate of heat transfer, A is the area of heating surface, Δt is the mean temperature difference between the heating surface and the evaporating liquid, U is the overall heat transfer coefficient. The heat exchange element may be either a jacket, e.g. steam-jacketed pan, or a series of tubes, e.g. calandria unit.

The overall heat transfer coefficient, U, for an evaporator can be regarded as the reciprocal of the sum of the individual thermal resistances. Thermal resistances, like electrical resistances, are additive and the reciprocal of resistance is a measure of conductance. The greatest thermal resistances are those caused by the fluid films next to the wall of the evaporator; the resistance of the metal wall can usually be neglected since this is small in comparison. Thus to obtain high values for the overall heat transfer coefficient, under specified temperature conditions, special attention should be paid to those factors that reduce the thickness of the stagnant film, e.g. use of high liquid velocities. In practice, the overall coefficient may be seriously lowered by the corrosion of the surface or by the deposition of solid material from the evaporating liquid. Another barrier to heat flow may result from the presence of uncondensable gases in the heating steam; air, if present in the steam, will tend to become concentrated next to the wall surface as the steam condenses. Removal of this air by adequate venting is necessary.

Film coefficients. Rate of flow of heat for steady conduction = temperature difference/resistance (cf. flow of electrical current = potential difference/resistance). Flow of heat through a solid can be represented by the equation:

$$\frac{q}{A} = \frac{\Delta t \, k}{L}$$

where q is the rate of heat flow across cross-sectional area A, Δt is the temperature difference across length L and k is the thermal conductivity. For flow of heat through a fluid film, the equation is expressed:

$$\frac{q}{A} = \Delta t \, h$$

where h is the film coefficient. In Fig. 13.1 the overall temperature difference across the wall of the evaporator is $t_6 - t_1$. The total resistance per unit of cross-sectional area is the summation of the fluid film resistances and the wall resistance and equals:

$$\frac{1}{h_1} + \frac{L}{k} + \frac{1}{h_2}$$

where h_1 and h_2 are the film coefficients of the steam film and the liquid film respectively.

The reciprocal of this resistance can be treated as a conductance U so that:

$$\frac{1}{U} = \frac{1}{h_1} + \frac{L}{k} + \frac{1}{h_2}$$

and the rate of heat flow from the steam side to the liquid is:

$$\frac{q}{A} = \frac{t_6 - t_1}{1/U} = (t_6 - t_1) U$$

U is the overall heat transfer coefficient.

In the general equation for heat transfer, q is proportional to Δt. This relationship is valid for the heat transfer to boiling liquids provided that Δt is not increased above a certain upper limit. If the heating surface is very much hotter than the boiling liquid, the increased vaporization will result in the heating surface being insulated by a nearly continuous film of vapour and the rate of heat transfer will be greatly reduced. This effect can be observed when a drop of water is heated on a hot plate. At a temperature of about $110°$ the drop wets the surface and evaporates rapidly. At a temperature of, say, $160°$ the drop dances about on a cushion of steam and evaporates more slowly than at the lower temperature. This effect is likely to be encountered in the evaporation of low boiling point solvents especially if pressure steam is used for heating. Generally, a temperature difference of $20°$

to 30° is ample for rapid evaporation of solutions.

To provide a large heating surface many evaporators are made up of a number of tubes in parallel. The tubes are mounted together to form a unit known as a calandria. The boiling liquid is generally contained within the tubes and the heating steam outside. The rapid evolution of vapour within the tube carries the liquid upwards at high velocity reducing the thickness of the fluid film next to the heating surface and so increasing the amount of heat transferred per unit area of wall surface. Long tube evaporators promote high liquid velocities without the aid of auxiliary pumping equipment.

Separation of liquid and vapour. In small vertical tube evaporators the separation of vapour and liquid usually takes place by gravity since the liquid droplets which are carried some way upwards with the vapour eventually fall back into the boiling liquid. At high vapour velocities and particularly when operating under reduced pressure, fine drops may be carried along by the vapour to the condenser. To prevent this *entrainment*, there are usually special separators through which the vapour must pass. An example is a cyclone separator to which the vapour is introduced tangentially to its periphery causing a circular motion of the vapour. The centrifugal force so produced causes the suspended droplets to be deposited. The separation of vapour from foaming liquids often presents difficulties; loss of product may be serious in spite of the use of entrainment separators. In these instances, the use of long tube evaporators to give high liquid velocities is often effective in breaking up the foam.

SMALL SCALE METHODS

Small quantities of liquids may be evaporated in a shallow porcelain or glass basin. In general, direct heating from a Bunsen flame on a wire gauze should not be employed, since, as the solution becomes more concentrated, its boiling point rises and serious overheating of the solute is likely to occur; removal of the last portions of solvent at a high temperature causes spurting. For aqueous solutions, a water bath or steam bath is used as a source of heat; higher temperatures may be attained on a sand bath or oil bath. The last traces of a solvent may be incompletely volatilized at a temperature well above the boiling point of the solvent owing to the high concentration of the solution. In such cases, evaporation is completed in vacuo. Evaporation of large volumes of liquid or solutions having expensive solvents is effected by distillation at atmospheric pressure or in vacuo.

LARGE SCALE METHODS

Heat Transfer Considerations
When a liquid is heated on a laboratory scale there is no necessity to consider the efficiency of the process as the operation is usually completed quite quickly. On a manufacturing scale however, the problem of scale-up from small scale is very important. In order to make a comparison consider the following cases: (a) 100 ml of water in a hemispherical basin, and (b) 500 litres of water in a hemispherical steam jacketed pan.

As we are more interested in the relative rates of heating and cooling rather than the absolute rates, the calculation can be simplified as follows:

The volume V of a sphere of radius R is proportional to R^3 while the surface area is proportional to R^2. It follows that the ratio of surface to volume for a sphere (or hemisphere) is $1/R$. Considering the 100 and 500 000 ml hemispherical vessels the ratios of the surface to volume are proportional to $1/100^{-3}$ $(1/4.64)$ and $1/500 000^{-3}$ $(1/79.35)$, respectively. As the passage of heat to the liquid must take place through the hemispherical surface of the vessel it can be seen that the larger vessel will only heat up at approximately one-seventeenth the rate of the smaller for the same amount of heat passing per unit area of surface. Evaporation which takes place from the surface of the liquid will also be reduced by the same proportion. This scaling up calculation applies to many of the operations which the pharmacist has to conduct and may be a serious matter if the heat of reaction liberated in a chemical process has to be controlled.

Heating by Steam
Most evaporators use steam as a source of heat. Heating is uniform over the whole wall of the evaporator and the temperatures which are obtainable depend on the pressure. Table 13.1 shows the relative pressure and temperature of steam to the nearest degree Centigrade.

Higher temperatures than those shown in Table 13.1 are obtainable by superheating, but as will be shown, superheating is of little value when steam is required as a source of heat. Superheated steam is used to improve the economy of steam engines, but this is not a matter for consideration here. A slight degree of superheat is of advantage to prevent condensation in the steam lines and is easily

TABLE 13.1

Properties of saturated steam

| Pressure by gauge | | Temperature (°C) |
lb/in²	kg/cm²	
0	0	100
5	0.35	109
10	0.70	116
15	1.05	121
20	1.40	126
30	2.10	134
40	2.80	142
50	3.50	148
75	5.25	160
100	7.00	170
120	8.40	176

obtained by throttling so as to have a pressure in the boiler slightly higher than that of the steam mains.

When steam is used a study of heat transmission is of great importance. Gases and vapours are very bad conductors of heat and give up their heat very slowly. Liquids give up their heat much more quickly.

The specific heat of water is 4.2 kJ kg⁻¹
The latent heat of steam is 2.2 MJ kg⁻¹
The specific heat of steam at constant pressure is 2.0 kJ kg⁻¹

The first two of the above are given up when saturated steam condenses on a surface. The specific heat of the steam must be given up before condensation takes place; this does not take place easily because gases are bad conductors of heat. When steam is superheated the additional heat is in the form of specific heat of the steam as a vapour. Suppose we wish to distil xylene with a boiling point of 136° and we use saturated steam at 30 lb/in² (2.1 kg/cm²) which has been raised by superheating to something above 136°. We shall be able to use only the specific heat of the steam. Steam will come away from the jacket of the still at 136° and very little xylene will be distilled. If we use steam at 100 lb/in² (7.0 kg/cm²), the temperature of which is 170°, in cooling to 136° condensation will take place and we shall be able to use the latent heat in addition to the specific heat given up in cooling from 170° to 136°. The steam trap will void water at 136°, which coming into atmospheric pressure will immediately be cooled at 100° by a part of it flashing into steam, the heat represented by the 36° of temperature difference being converted to latent heat in the steam produced. This loss cannot be avoided.

STEAM TRAPS

Under ideal conditions live steam, i.e. steam that has not been condensed and given up its latent heat, should never leave the jacket or coil of a vessel that is being heated. In order to control the discharge the outlet of the heating element should always be fitted with a steam trap. There are many different types available. An older pattern consists of a bucket which floats until the amount of condensate in the trap swamps it, causing it to sink and open a valve. The condensate is blown out of the trap, emptying the bucket which again floats and closes the valve. This trap has an intermittent or blast discharge (Fig. 13.2). There is no provision

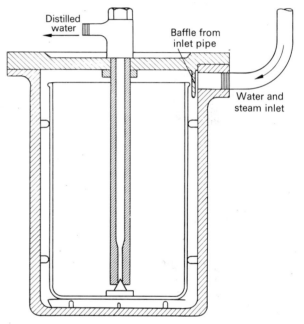

Fig. 13.2. Bucket steam trap (from *The Making of a Chemical*, Lewis & King).

for air to pass this type of trap. A modern type of trap is operated by a thermostatic device depending on the expansion of a liquid sealed in a flexible metal capsule. As this type of trap depends on temperature for opening and closing, both air and water will be voided. A thermostatic trap is shown in Fig. 13.3. A strainer is shown combined with the trap to keep back grit and particles of scale which would get on the valve seat and prevent proper closing. A filter can be used with advantage in conjunction with any form of trap. The trap operates in the following way. A closed vessel, which we will call 'A', made of copper alloy corrugated like a concertina so that it will expand

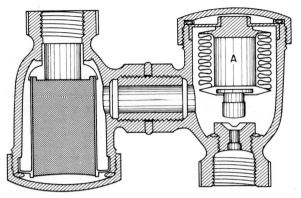

FIG. 13.3. Thermostatic steam trap in section (Spirax Manufacturing Co. Ltd.).

and contract, can be seen in the right-hand half of Fig. 13.3. At the bottom of the element is a valve which is free to enter a valve seat. The part 'A' is held rigidly at the top and is filled with a spirit mixture which usually has a boiling point lower than that of water. When 'A' is heated to the boiling point of water at any pressure a greater pressure will be developed inside than the steam pressure on the outside. The element will then expand and close the valve. As water collects in the trap it cools and the pressure in 'A' is reduced; 'A' contracts, the valve opens, the water is blown out and the cycle is repeated. The temperature at which the trap operates can be arranged by selecting the boiling point of the liquid in 'A' so that condensate can be voided at nearly steam temperature or at considerably below that temperature. The makers will advise on the temperature of discharge and also on the distance between jacket and trap; this distance has an effect on the temperature of the condensate in the trap. These traps have the advantage of being small and easily installed; they do not hold water when not in use so that they can be fixed outdoors without danger of freezing, and since the valve is wide open on starting up, air is easily swept out. Their disadvantage is that the thermostatic element can be damaged by water hammer, and they are therefore unsuitable where there is a large and variable amount of condensate.

The cost of steam on a manufacturing scale is a very important consideration and every effort should be made to conserve heat, not only by the use of efficient traps, but also by lagging pipes, the outside of steam heated vessels, and any part from which heat may be lost. The water voided by the steam traps will be hot. It should be kept free

from contamination and returned to a hot well to be used as boiler feed.

Evaporation at Atmospheric Pressure

Evaporation pans. On a manufacturing scale, aqueous extracts are evaporated in open pans or in vacuum evaporators; the final stage of evaporation from soft extract to dryness is done in vacuum ovens, alcoholic solutions or extracts are evaporated in stills so that the alcohol may be recovered. The still is usually incorporated in the extraction plant. Evaporation in open pans is usually confined to the final stages of the process in the preparation of soft extracts, because: (1) the amount of water to be evaporated is small; (2) it is easy to stir the pan by hand; and (3) it is easy to remove the product. If the extractive is liquid or remains liquid while hot, evaporation in vacuum pans is to be preferred, because the water is removed much more rapidly at a lower temperature, and there is economy of time, heat and labour.

Open evaporating pans are simple in construction. The pan may be made of copper, stainless steel, aluminium, enamelled iron or other metal. They vary in the proportion of depth to diameter, depending on whether they are required simply as heating and mixing vessels or for evaporation. Fig. 13.4 shows sections of two typical pans. The

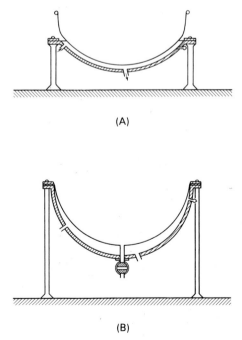

(A)

(B)

FIG. 13.4. Sections of steam-jacketed pans.

shallow pan where the jacket covers only the lower part of the pan, in spite of its limited heating area, will give rapid evaporation by reason of the large surface of the liquid exposed; it also provides for easy stirring in the final stage of the preparation of soft extracts. Shallow copper or stainless steel pans are, for the same capacity, more expensive to construct because the metal of the pan must be thicker than that of a hemispherical pan in order to withstand the steam pressure in the jacket.

Pans up to about 90 litres capacity may be made to tilt on trunnions by the use of a hand lever; above this capacity, the weight of the pan plus contents becomes too great for hand operation and mechanical tilting gear is fitted. In tilting pans the steam inlet and exhaust is made through the hollow trunnions by means of glands. The jacket is cast iron and the pan itself is of stainless steel.

In open evaporating pans, a usual rate of evaporation is about 2 gal/ft^2 (100 l/m^2) of surface per hour with steam at a pressure of 40 lb/in^2 (2.8 kg/cm^2) in the jacket and the liquid in a state of ebullition. This figure is reduced as the liquid becomes concentrated and circulation retarded.

In any room in which open pans are used for evaporation there must be efficient ventilation to remove the vapour. Unless this is done the room quickly becomes filled with a dense fog of condensed vapour and water falls from the roof and runs down the walls. Hoods and electric fans fitted over the pans not only remove the steam and prevent condensation in the room but also accelerate the rate of evaporation by quickly removing saturated air from above the surface of the liquid.

Calandria
In order to get sufficient heating surface, tubes are generally employed, with steam on the outside and the liquid inside. In order still further to increase the capacity, the tubes are multiplied forming a calandria (Fig. 13.5), or are lengthened as in the climbing film type of evaporator (Fig. 13.7). The size and length of the tubes is subject to careful calculation and the form of the heating element is most important. The tubes may be about 1.2 m long and 5 cm in diameter, but the size varies with the nature of the substance to be evaporated. There is a space below, often containing a steam coil to give extra heating capacity, and large enough to afford room for rapid circulation of the liquid; there is a larger space above to allow for spray to separate from the vapour before it leaves the evaporator. The height of the liquid in the evaporator is arranged so that the tubes of the calandria are only partly immersed

and the liquid boils up the tubes, floods over the top and goes down the large central tube, thus ensuring rapid circulation. Fig. 13.6 shows in diagram a type of inclined tube evaporator which has the advantage that by opening the bottom of the inclined calandria the tubes are easily reached for cleaning.

Climbing Film Evaporators
For this type of evaporator numerous advantages are claimed. It differs essentially from the ordinary calandria type in having a small number of long tubes encased in a steam jacket instead of a large number of short ones. The liquor, previously heated, is led through a pipe into a number of tubes fitted into upper and lower tube plates and surrounded by a steam jacket. Steam is admitted to the jacket at the inlet valve causing ebullition to take place inside the tubes and this releases a volume of vapour which must find its way to a region of lower pressure by passing up the tube. As this volume of vapour ascends, it forms itself into a core in the centre of the tube, carrying with it the liquor as a film round the inner surface of the tube, the vapour passing at a higher velocity than the liquor itself. On reaching the top of the tubes, the vapour and liquid pass into a separator, where separation of the concentrated liquor and vapour take place. Advantage is taken of the velocity of the liquid to bring about separation by centrifugal action. The vapour emerging at the outlet may be used to preheat the liquid before admission to the evaporator or may become the source of heat for another effect.

The tubes in a climbing film evaporator are about 6.9 m long with an internal diameter of 5 cm. The vapour and liquor leave the tubes and enter the separator at a speed of about 27 m per sec; it will therefore be seen that the liquor is in contact with the source of heat for such a short time that there is little chance of injury to the product even though a much higher temperature is used than is customary for the same liquor undergoing evaporation in an ordinary type of evaporating pan. All the conditions for good heat transmission are fulfilled. The amount of vapour leaving the evaporator throughout its operation is constant, and this enables the separator to be so designed that entrainment is reduced to a minimum. The high velocity of the liquor reduces scaling in the tubes.

Horizontal Film Evaporators.
The evaporator consists of four or six pairs of horizontal concentric tubes placed one above the

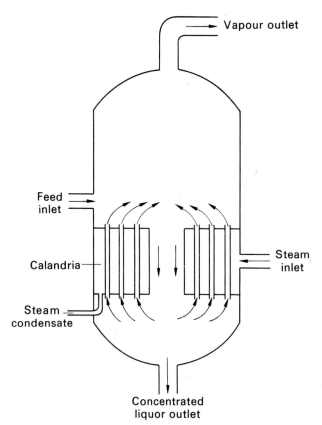

FIG. 13.5. Evaporator with calandria heat exchanger.

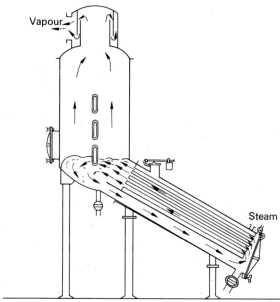

FIG. 13.6. Inclined tube vacuum evaporator.

other, and connected by butt ends so that a horizontal hairpin coil is formed. The liquor passes through the inner tubes, entering at the bottom and passing upwards; the steam enters at the top and passes downwards between the inner and outer tubes of each pair, so that the transference of heat is on the counter-current principle. On leaving the top element, the concentrated liquor and vapour pass into a centrifugal separator from which the liquor is withdrawn by a pump and the vapour passes to a jet condenser and wet pump. Provision is made for preheating the liquor by passing it through a jacketed tube situated below the evaporator tubes. All the parts that come into contact with the liquor are usually made of stainless steel, but in special cases the tubes can be made of glass and the other parts of Keebush, so that all metallic contact is eliminated. Cleaning of the tubes is made easy by the removal of the butt ends which are held in place by means of a stirrup fitted with a single eye-bolt.

The capacity of these evaporators varies greatly, depending on the nature of the liquid, the degree of concentration, the steam pressure and the vacuum. The horizontal tube evaporator described above, working under suitable conditions with a cascara extractive, has a capacity of 135 to 155 l per hr when the feed liquor is concentrated from 5 to 25 per cent. Larger evaporators of this type are available, with capacities of three to four times this amount. The climbing and falling film evaporators have larger capacities, averaging about 450 l per hr, the smallest standard size having a capacity of 225 l per hr when concentrating an aqueous extract of liquorice. The calandria type are made in very large sizes, calandria 4 m in diameter with tubes 1.5 m long being not unusual.

Evaporation under Reduced Pressure

Vacuum evaporation is used wherever possible because there is a saving of time, heat and labour. A factor affecting evaporation is the mean hydraulic depth of the liquid. In big evaporators, and particularly in multiple effect evaporators, the temperature difference between the steam or vapour used for heating and the liquid which is to be evaporated is kept low in order to improve the coefficient of heat transmission. To start and continue ebullition, the heating steam or vapour must be at a higher temperature than the boiling point of the liquid at the pressure at the point where ebullition is to be started. This pressure is increased by the depth of the liquid. To state an extreme case, suppose we have a depth of liquid of

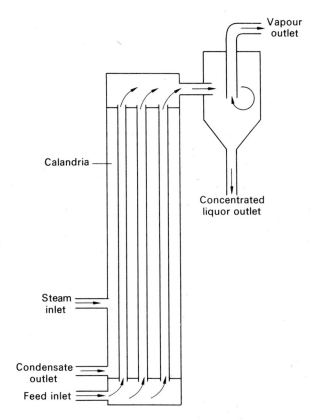

FIG. 13.7. Climbing film evaporator.

(0.7 kg/cm²), having a temperature of 116°, the temperature difference is therefore only 4°, which is hardly enough to allow for the fall in pressure due to condensation across the calandria. If the pressure of the steam were only 5 lb/in² (0.35 kg/cm²) and its temperature therefore only 109°, it would not have a temperature high enough to cause ebullition in the liquid. The above is, of course, an extreme case. Calandria are not made so deep, 4 to 5 ft (1.2 to 1.5 m) being the usual depth, and the temperatures are lower in vacuum evaporators. Nevertheless, the mean hydraulic depth is a factor taken into account in the design of large evaporators. With relatively concentrated solutions, the effect of the solute in raising the boiling point must also be considered.

Widely different types of vacuum evaporators are used in the pharmaceutical industry. The difference is mainly in the method of heat transmission. In evaporation the heat used as latent heat of vaporization is, for all practical purposes, the same in amount whether the liquid is evaporated at reduced pressure or at atmospheric pressure. This heat goes off in the vapour, and it is in an endeavour to save this heat loss that multiple effect evaporators are used. These evaporators are only suitable for very large scale evaporation and are employed in the manufacture of salt, caustic soda and in other continuous processes. Although multiple effect evaporators are not used in the pharmaceutical industry, the principle is of interest and should be understood. If water is evaporated in an open pan, every gram of water evaporated takes away 2.2 kJ as latent heat of vaporization plus that due to the difference between 100° and the atmospheric temperature. In a single effect evaporator, part of this heat may be recovered by using the vapour to preheat the liquid which is

15 ft (4.5 m) in the tubes of a calandria, which will give a pressure at the bottom of the tubes of 7.5 lb/in² (0.525 kg/cm²) over the pressure in the vessel at the surface of the liquid. Under such an additional pressure, if the vessel were at atmospheric pressure and the solution fairly dilute, the liquid at the bottom of the tubes would have a boiling point of about 112°; with steam at 10 lb/in²

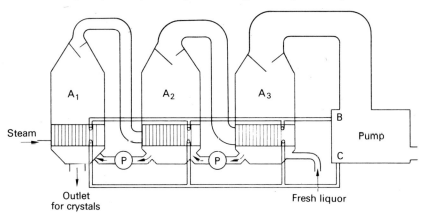

FIG. 13.8. Diagram of triple-effect vacuum evaporator.

to be evaporated. Fig. 13.8 is a simplified diagram illustrating the arrangement of a triple effect evaporator, using vessels heated by calandria. The form of calandria, in the simple type illustrated is that of a drum with vertical tubes, a segment being left at one side as a down-take to ensure circulation. The evaporator A_1 is heated by steam at about 20 lb/in² (1.40 kg/cm²) pressure which enters the calandria. The liquid in the evaporator boils and the vapour is passed over to the calandria of evaporator A_2. The vapour from A_2 is in turn used to heat A_3 and the vapour from A_3 is removed by the pump. It follows that the latent heat of vaporization from A_1 is recovered in A_2 and that from A_2 is recovered in A_3, but after that, unless it can be used to preheat liquor, it is lost through the pump and condenser water. The number of evaporators, or effects as they are called, is limited by the temperature difference over the whole. Suppose steam at a pressure of 20 lb/in² (1.4 kg/cm²) produces a temperature of 126° in the calandria of A_1 and the pump produces a 'vacuum' of 65 cm the liquid in evaporator A_3 will boil at 42°. The total temperature difference will be therefore $126° - 42° = 84°$ to be divided between the three evaporators giving approximately 28° for each.

The liquid in evaporator A_1 will boil at $126° - 28° = 98°$
The liquid in evaporator A_2 will boil at $\;\;98° - 28° = 70°$
The liquid in evaporator A_3 will boil at $\;\;70° - 28° = 42°$

The calandria of A_2 and A_3 are working at pressures lower than atmospheric, and so the condensate must be removed by the pump. If A_3 is made the final evaporator, the liquid can be circulated by the effect of the vacuum. The temperature in A_3 is, however, lower than that in A_1, and it is generally necessary to have the more concentrated liquid, which will have a higher boiling point, in the hottest evaporator, in which case circulation must be induced by means of pumps, indicated at P, between the effects. The pipe indicated diagrammatically at B is for the removal of air from the calandria, and that at C is for the removal of the condensate. It should be noticed that the vapour pipes joining the effects increase in size to allow for the expansion of the vapour with reduced pressure.

This principle of multiple effect evaporation can be applied to other types of evaporators such as the climbing film, but it always involves very large scale evaporation in a continuous process and is unsuitable for small scale pharmaceutical operations.

Wet Vacuum Pumps

Where large volumes of water vapour are to be evacuated, as in the larger types of evaporators, a wet vacuum pump is generally employed. Condensation of the vapour is effected by bringing it into contact with a spray of cold water. The condensed vapour and the water used to condense it together with any air, are all passed out through the pump. As a mixture of air and water is to be evacuated an ordinary type of reciprocating pump is not suitable because the ports and valves would not take away the water quickly enough to prevent a water hammer in the pump.

Entrainment

This term is used to describe the loss of liquid frothing or 'blowing over' during evaporation. In certain kinds of evaporators, some of the liquid undergoing evaporation is usually found in the condensate, which should, of course, theoretically consist only of pure solvent. The condensate obtained in certain types of evaporators during the evaporation of a coloured aqueous extract, such as that of liquorice or cascara, is invariably coloured because particles of the liquid have been carried over mechanically with the aqueous vapour. During rapid boiling, particles of the liquid tend to be projected vertically and are carried away by the vapour. When vacuum evaporation is employed, entrainment is very troublesome because of the high velocity of the expanded vapour. In vacuum evaporators it is usual to design some form of separator to allow the free passage of vapour but obstruct the passage of liquid particles. For a liquid which has any tendency to froth during evaporation in a vacuum, complete separation of liquid particles appears to be impossible and a certain amount of entrainment is inevitable. The object must be to keep this loss as low as possible.

14

Distillation

Distillation is a method of separating substances which differ appreciably in their vapour pressures. It is used in pharmacy either to extract volatile active principles from vegetable drugs or to separate volatile substances from their less volatile impurities; it also provides a method of recovering volatile solvents, notably alcohol, for further use. With the exception of 'destructive distillation', the term is normally applied to liquid–solid systems; the following qualifications are used.

Simple distillation is the process of converting a liquid into its vapour, transferring the vapour to another place, and recovering the liquid by condensing the vapour, usually by leading it into contact with a cold surface. The apparatus used consists essentially of three parts; the *still* in which the volatile material is vaporized; the *condenser* in which the vapours are condensed; and the *receiver* in which the distillate is collected. Simple distillation can produce partial separation of components with different boiling points in a liquid mixture, the more volatile component being obtained in increased concentration in the vapour. The process is generally used for the separation of liquids from non-volatile solids, e.g. preparation of distilled water and recovery of alcohol in the preparation of dry extracts.

Fractional distillation (or rectification) is the process employed to separate miscible volatile liquids having different boiling points. It differs from simple distillation in that partial condensation of the vapour is allowed to occur in a *fractionating column*, through which the vapour must pass before reaching the condenser. This column enables the ascending vapour from the still to come in contact with the condensing vapour returning to the still, and this results in the enrichment of the vapour in the more volatile component.

Steam distillation is used for the distillation of water-immiscible liquids of high boiling points, e.g. turpentine, aniline. By bubbling steam through the liquid, the mixture boils at below the normal boiling point of either component. The distillate consists of the two liquids in the same proportions as in the vapour.

Destructive distillation is the term used to describe the decomposition of a substance, usually a natural product, by heat followed by the condensation and collection of the volatile products of decomposition. It is not a pharmaceutical process but is used in the manufacture of some substances used in medicine, examples being the destructive distillation of wood and of coal to produce tars.

SIMPLE DISTILLATION UNDER ATMOSPHERIC PRESSURE

SMALL SCALE

For simple distillations in the laboratory, a distillation flask with side arm sloping downwards is used. The temperature at which the vapours distil is observed on a thermometer, inserted through a cork, and having its bulb just below the level of the side arm. The flask should be of such a size that it is one-half to two-thirds full of the liquid to be distilled. Bumping, due to superheating, is avoided by adding a small chip of porous pot before distillation; if the distillation is interrupted, a fresh pot chip should be added. Pot should not be added to the superheated liquid, otherwise an instantaneous evolution of a large volume of vapour will occur.

When large quantities of water are to be condensed, a spray or jet condenser is frequently used, which brings the vapour in direct contact with the cooling water. The condenser is used in conjunction with a wet vacuum pump or a barometric leg.

Condensers

A condenser is fundamentally a heat exchanger. Almost every type of condenser embodies a surface which is kept cold by a stream of water on one side, the vapour to be condensed impinging on the other side. A large volume of cooling water is required on account of the latent heat of vaporization, which is evolved on condensing the vapour. In cooling 1 g of water from 100° to 15°, approximately 360 J are evolved; in condensing 1 g of steam to water at 100°, 2.27 kJ are evolved; the latent heats of vaporization of alcohol and ether are 8.48 kJ and 3.78 kJ respectively. For the condensation of liquids which boil at from about 120° to 150°, a stream of cooling water may cause the condenser walls to crack, owing to the high temperature gradient across the walls; stationary water in the jacket is usually used in these cases. For liquids boiling above about 150°, simple air cooling is used.

The main points in condenser construction are as follows:

(1) The condenser must be so constructed as to be easily cleaned.

(2) The cooling surface must be large because the rate of condensation is proportional to the area of condensing surface.

(3) The condensing surface must be a reasonably good conductor of heat because the rate of condensation is proportional to the rate at which the surface conducts away the heat. For this reason, metal, when suitable, is preferable to glass.

(4) The film of condensed liquid is a bad conductor and must be removed quickly in order to avoid serious impairment of the efficiency of the condenser.

(5) The warmer water in contact with the condensing surface must be quickly carried away and its place taken by fresh cold water. The cooling water is arranged to move on the counter-current principle, i.e. its direction of flow is opposite to that of the flow of vapours to be condensed.

In carrying out a distillation on the laboratory scale, the contents of the still are heated gradually and, as the liquid begins to boil, the temperature recorded on the thermometer rises rapidly as the rising ring of condensate ascends the neck of the flask. If the liquid is pure, the temperature recorded when the condensate passes down the side arm remains steady when the uncondensed vapours follow. Heating is then continued at such a rate that a drop of liquid every 1 to 2 sec falls from the condenser. When inflammable liquids are distilled, the distillate is collected in a second distillation flask attached to the condenser; on the side arm of this receiver is attached a length of rubber tubing to lead inflammable vapour on to the floor away from the vicinity of flames.

LARGE SCALE

When it is only necessary to separate a volatile constituent, such as alcohol or acetone from a non-volatile extract, a simple form of still such as that shown in Fig. 14.1 may be used. A still of this

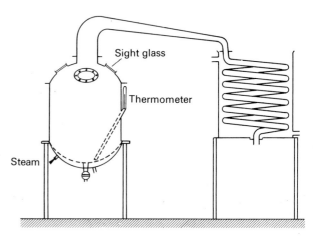

FIG. 14.1. Steam-jacketed still.

kind has a limited heating surface and functions perfectly with volatile solvents, but it is useless for concentrating watery solutions.

Operations which are in frequent or continuous use often have specially designed stills suited to one product or group of products. In pharmacy the best-known example is the continuous water still for producing distilled water for various purposes including Water for Injection.

On a manufacturing scale, distilled water is required in large quantities as a component of many preparations, and for the aqueous extraction of drugs, where the accumulated residues from the use of tap water would be objectionable. The steam condensate from the heating jackets and coils of the plant is quite unsuitable, because it may contain traces of chlorine, derived from the public supply, and will certainly be contaminated with iron from the surfaces of the pipes, etc. The distilled water required should be specially prepared.

The Manesty Automatic Water Still
A steam heated form of this continuous action water still, of the size often used in manufacturing laboratories, is shown in section in Fig. 14.2. Ordinary water from the public supply or condensed steam from the plant enters at the base of the still and surrounds the condenser tubes, which are vertical and open at both ends. As the water rises in the jacket around the condenser tubes, it condenses the steam descending the tubes. By a suitable adjustment of the rate of flow, the condensing water is heated almost to boiling point at the top of the jacket where dissolved gases are released and are allowed to escape into the air. Much of the heated water from the jacket flows to waste, but the remainder passes into the bowl-

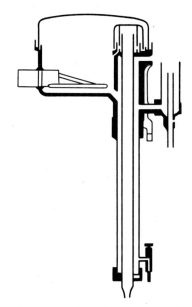

Fig. 14.3. Manesty electrically-heated automatic water still. Internal structure.

shaped still head, where it is boiled by steam circulating under pressure through a copper coil. The steam from the boiling water is unable to escape except through the condenser tubes, the upper ends of which protrude into the still head. The descending steam is condensed into distilled water, which flows from the lower ends of the tubes.

The heat generated by the condensation of the steam is therefore used to preheat the water entering the head, not only driving off dissolved gases but also economizing in the amount of steam used in the coil.

Fig. 14.3 shows a smaller, electrically heated form of the Manesty automatic water still, the principle of which is the same as that of the steam heated type.

SIMPLE DISTILLATION UNDER REDUCED PRESSURE

SMALL SCALE

The effect of pressure on boiling point has already been discussed. From this it is clear that liquids, which are unstable at their boiling point under atmospheric pressure, may be distilled at a much lower temperature under reduced pressure with less likelihood of decomposition. Similar considerations apply in the concentration of solutions of thermolabile substances. Distillation under reduced pressure is very commonly used for the evaporation of the menstruum in the preparation of extracts

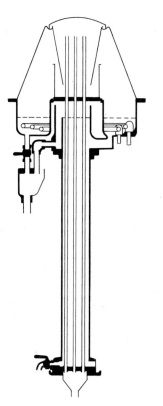

Fig. 14.2. Manesty steam-heated automatic water still. Internal structure.

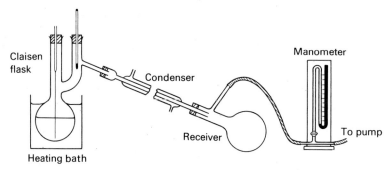

FIG. 14.4. Vacuum distillation apparatus.

(Chapter 13). Evaporative distillation in high vacua is of great importance in the purification of vitamins.

Vacuum distillation is most conveniently carried out in a Claisen flask (Fig. 14.4). The second neck prevents splashing of the violently agitated liquid. Bumping occurs very readily during vacuum distillation, but is easily prevented by means of a stream of air bubbles from a tube drawn out to a very fine capillary dipping in the boiling liquid. The capillary should be sufficiently fine to permit only a slow stream of bubbles to be blown by mouth through a little ether in a test tube. It is usual to use apparatus with interchangeable ground glass joints. Heating with a naked flame requires considerable practice, so it is advisable to use a water bath or oil bath maintained at about 20° higher than the boiling point of the liquid under reduced pressure. In all vacuum distillations, a small pressure gauge (manometer) should be inserted between the pump and the receiver. In carrying out the distillation, heating is not commenced until the required vacuum is attained; evacuation of an apparatus containing hot liquid will almost invariably result in the liquid frothing over into the receiver. Thin walled glass apparatus, such as flat bottomed flasks and conical flasks, should never be used for vacuum distillation.

For the evaporation of extracts under reduced pressure at below 60°, the apparatus shown in Fig. 14.5 is very convenient for laboratory scale work. Two water pumps, one of which is used intermittently, are required. The apparatus is evacuated and a suitable quantity of liquid is allowed to flow into the still by opening screw clip A. Screw clip B is closed and the second pump is turned off. The liquid is heated by means of a water bath to 50° to 60° and the distillate is collected in the Büchner flask. During distillation, screw clip A is adjusted so that the extract enters the still at the same rate as it distils. When the Büchner flask is nearly full, stopcocks C and D are closed, screw clip B is opened and the receiver may be detached and emptied; in the meantime the distillate is collected in E. The receiver is replaced and then evacuated by the second pump, clip B is closed, cock D opened and the distillate from E is run into the Büchner flask by opening C. The whole process is then repeated.

In some instances persistent foaming occurs during vacuum distillation. This may be overcome by adding capryl alcohol to the liquid to be distilled, or by inserting a second air capillary in the thermometer neck of a Claisen flask; the stream of air drawn through breaks the rising foam. Antifoaming still heads have been devised and are very effective for dealing with this problem.

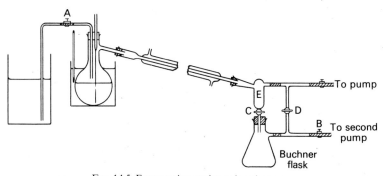

FIG. 14.5. Evaporation under reduced pressure.

LARGE SCALE

Vacuum Stills

These are employed for distilling substances that have a high boiling point at atmospheric pressure, or for substances that are damaged by a high temperature, or for removing the last traces of a volatile solvent. Fig. 14.6 shows the arrangement of a vacuum still. To facilitate the collection and removal of the distillate, without stopping the distillation, two receivers are fitted. By a suitable arrangement of cocks they may be used alternately, the distillate being run off from one while the other is connected to the still under vacuum. Stills vary in design more than any other plant; usually they are specially made to do a particular class of work. A vacuum still with column is shown in Fig. 14.7.

The vacuum used for distilling should be the best possible, especially if fractional distillation is to be done. For pressures of 3 to 5 mmHg with a large vacuum fractionating still, a double-stage dry pump of good capacity, is necessary. To produce pressures of 1 mmHg and less on anything larger than laboratory scale plant requires special design of plant and is only attempted for very special purposes. The wet type of pump and the type of dry pump giving a vacuum of about 68 cm are quite unsuitable for use with vacuum stills, although the dry pump may be used for the removal of the last traces of volatile solvents from non-volatile extracts. It is possible to use more than one oven or evaporator with one pump, provided that the capacity of the pump is big enough, but when working vacuum stills the aim should be to use a separate pump to each still. If two or more stills are working at the same time with only one

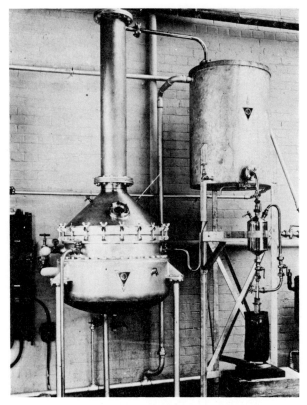

FIG. 14.7. Vacuum still with column.

pump, then the vapour pressure of a substance which is being distilled in one still will probably hinder obtaining a good vacuum in the others. The volume occupied by the vapour of a substance in the high vacuum used in distilling is very great. At a pressure of 5 mmHg the vapour is expanded 152 times. It is important that the swan-neck of the condenser and the fractionating column if present, are of adequate size to prevent back pressure caused by the friction due to the high velocity of the vapour in restricted tubes.

With the high vacuum required for distilling, the prevention of leaks assumes great importance. They frequently arise in the packing of the glands of valves and the bottoms and tops of plug cocks. Leaks in the bottoms of plug cocks can be eliminated by using those specially designed for vacuum work; the bottoms of the cocks are closed and glands are fitted to the spindles. Another common source of leak is in the bottom outlet of the still. This valve or cock fitted to a pipe which must pass through the steam jacket, gets hard wear and strain due to the quick and extreme changes of temperature. If other means such as a dip pipe

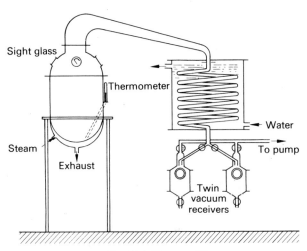

FIG. 14.6. Vacuum still.

can be used for emptying the still, it is a good plan to dispense with this outlet, but very often the final residue is too viscous to be easily removed except through a bottom outlet. It will be found economical to use only the very best quality of valves and cocks on vacuum stills.

FRACTIONAL DISTILLATION

THEORETICAL CONSIDERATIONS AND SMALL SCALE METHODS

Fractional distillation is the process employed to separate miscible volatile liquids having different boiling points. In a mixture of two liquids, each may be regarded as dissolved in the other, and the possibility of separating the two liquids by fractional distillation depends on the effect each has on the vapour pressure of the other.

Vapour Pressure of Miscible Liquids
When the two components of a binary mixture are completely miscible, the vapour pressure of the mixture is a function of the composition as well as the vapour pressures of the two pure components. In an ideal solution where the relation of vapour pressure and composition is given by Raoult's law, the partial vapour pressure of each volatile component is equal to the vapour pressure of the pure component multiplied by its mole fraction.

Thus for a mixture of A and B:

$$P_A = P_A{}^0 X_A$$

$$P_B = P_B{}^0 X_B.$$

Where P_A and P_B are the partial vapour pressures of the components when the mole fractions are X_A and X_B respectively. The vapour pressures of the pure components are $P_A{}^0$ and $P_B{}^0$. The total vapour pressure P of the system is then $P_A + P_B$ (Fig. 14.8).

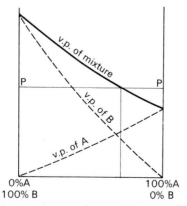

FIG. 14.8. Vapour pressure and composition of miscible liquids.

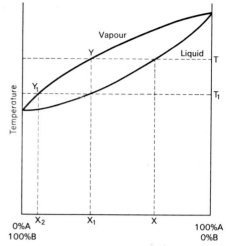

FIG. 14.9. Boiling point and composition of miscible liquids.

Binary mixtures that follow Raoult's law are those where the attraction between A and B molecules is the same as those for the pure components, e.g. benzene/toluene and paraffin mixtures. When the interaction of A and B molecules is less than between the molecules of the pure constituents, the presence of B molecules reduces the A–A interaction and similarly the A molecules reduce the B–B interaction. The partial vapour pressure is now greater than expected from Raoult's ideal solution law and the system is said to exhibit *positive deviation* e.g. benzene/ethyl alcohol, chloroform/ethyl alcohol. *Negative deviation* occurs when the A–B attraction is greater than the A–A or B–B attraction and the vapour pressure is less than expected, e.g. chloroform/acetone.

Referring to the ideal system (Fig. 14.8), the partial vapour pressure of the more volatile constituent B is higher so that the vapour phase will contain more of this component. By removing and condensing this vapour a liquid richer in B is obtained. This aspect is more readily seen from the curves relating to the boiling points of the various compositions rather than the vapour pressures.

BOILING POINT DIAGRAMS AND FRACTIONAL DISTILLATION

The boiling point diagram for an ideal mixture corresponding to Fig. 14.8 is shown in Fig. 14.9. The lower curve shows the manner in which the boiling point of the mixture changes with composition; the upper curve relates the composition of the vapour in equilibrium with the liquid at the same temperature. Hence the boiling point of the mixture X is T. The vapour at T will have a composition fixed by point Y, which corresponds to a mixture richer in B than in A. If this vapour is condensed, a liquid having the same composition (X_1) will be obtained. The boiling point of the mixture X_1 is T_1 and when it is boiled, vapour having the composition Y_1, which yields a liquid X_2 on condensation, is obtained. X_2 is nearly pure B. Hence in this example, extensive fractionation has been achieved by boiling the mixture and condensing the vapour in equilibrium with the liquid and repeating the process with the condensed vapour. The volume of distillate (composition X_2), obtained will be small, since as the vapour is drawn off, the liquid remaining in the still gradually becomes poorer in component B and its boiling point rises. Fractional distillation is based on these principles.

The difference in composition between X and X_2 is equal to that produced in a fractionating column of two theoretical plates. Many laboratory columns bring about separations equivalent to ten or more theoretical plates so that efficient separation of the two components is possible. The change from X to X_1 is the composition difference corresponding to one theoretical plate and under ideal conditions this would occur in simple distillation.

Azeotropic mixtures. An azeotropic mixture or *constant boiling mixture* is one in which the composition of the liquid and the vapour in equilibrium with it is the same. Thus the mixture behaves like a pure liquid in so far as it distils without change in composition or boiling point. Miscible binary liquids form azeotropic mixtures when the vapour pressure curve of the mixture exhibits a maximum or minimum. Such mixtures cannot be separated into their pure components by distillation. It is possible to separate them by distillation only into one component and a constant boiling mixture. Their behaviour on distillation is most easily followed by referring to the boiling point versus composition curves as shown in Fig. 14.10; (A) represents a mixture which possesses a maximum vapour pressure, i.e. low boiling point azeotrope; (B) represents a mixture with a minimum vapour pressure, i.e. high boiling point azeotrope. In this figure the concentration changes arising during distillation using a fractionating column equivalent to two theoretical plates are shown, i.e. X to Z. From (A) it can be seen that repeated fractionation will produce a distillate tending to the composition of the azeotropic mixture represented by point C. The material left in the still will be richer in B than it was originally; eventually pure B will be left after the

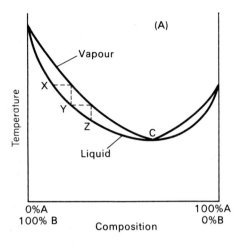

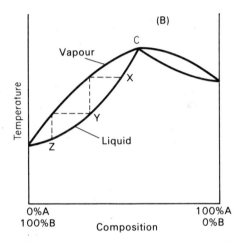

FIG. 14.10. Boiling point composition graphs; A, Minimum boiling azeotrope; B, Maximum boiling azeotrope. C is the composition of the constant boiling mixture.

whole of A has been distilled off in the form of the azeotropic mixture. If the original composition lies to the right of C, then by similar reasoning A will be left in the still. Mixtures of minimum boiling point are more common than mixtures exhibiting a maximum boiling point, e.g. alcohol and water, alcohol and benzene, alcohol and chloroform. Alcohol, boiling point 78.3°, and water boiling point 100° form a mixture of minimum boiling point 78.15°, containing 95.57 per cent w/w alcohol. The composition of mixtures of minimum boiling point varies with pressure as, for example, water and alcohol can be completely separated by distilling at 28° under 7 cm pressure.

On distilling a mixture of maximum boiling point, the distillate will be richer in the component A or B depending on whether the original concentration lies to the right or left of C. Fig. 14.10

(B) shows the original concentration X lying to the left of C and the distillate thus becomes richer in B.

Ternary mixtures. Mixtures of three components, which do not form azeotropes may be separated by fractional distillation in the same way as binary mixtures. Azeotropic ternary mixtures of maximum vapour pressure (minimum boiling point) are important. Water, boiling point 100°, alcohol, boiling point 78.3° and benzene, boiling point 80.2°, form a ternary azeotropic mixture, boiling point 64.85°, containing 18.5 per cent of alcohol, 7.4 per cent of water and 74.1 per cent of benzene; the boiling point of this mixture is lower than the boiling point of any binary mixture of any of the components. Fractionation of this ternary mixture is used on the large scale for the production of absolute alcohol. Absolute alcohol cannot be obtained by normal fractionation of dilute alcohol since a constant boiling mixture of 95.57 per cent w/w is formed. Benzene is added to the alcohol–water azeotrope and when distilled the mixture yields first the ternary water–alcohol–benzene azeotrope, boiling point 65.85°, until all the water is removed from the system. Next a binary alcohol–benzene azeotrope, boiling point 68.2° distils over and finally absolute alcohol, boiling point 78.3°. Trichloroethylene may be used instead of benzene in this process. Solutions in a solvent such as benzene may be dried by azeotropic distillation; benzene forms a constant boiling mixture with water, boiling point 69.3°. All the water present in the benzene is removed when about 10 per cent of the solvent has been distilled.

Fractionating Columns

If a mixture of chloroform, boiling point 61.2° and benzene, boiling point 80.2°, is distilled, the vapours first evolved will be richer in the more volatile component, chloroform; as this is distilled off, the vapours will become gradually richer in benzene, and the temperature of distillation will gradually rise. By changing the receiver when the temperature recorded on the thermometer in the head of the still has risen from 61° to 63°, a *fraction* is obtained which is richer in chloroform than in benzene. Other fractions, which are increasingly rich in benzene, may be collected over the ranges 63° to 68°, 68° to 73°, 73° to 78°, 78° to 80°. Repeated separate distillations of the intermediate fractions, fractions of the same boiling range being combined, will ultimately result in a separation of the liquid into two main fractions, boiling point 61° to 63°

and 78° to 80°, which represent a rough separation of the two constituents of the mixture. This process is very tedious and the same, or a better effect can be achieved in a single distillation through a fractionating column. It should be remembered that complete fractionation by distillation is possible only with liquids which do not form azeotropic mixtures.

A fractionating column, which is inserted between the still and the condenser, acts by bringing about repeated distillations throughout the length of the column. The action of the column is partially to condense the vapours rising from the boiling liquid; this condensate will be richer in the more volatile component than the original liquid and it is vaporized again by the condensation of more ascending vapours; the vapours so produced will be still richer in the more volatile component, and when condensation and vaporization takes place further up the column, further enrichment in the more volatile component will be effected. Under ideal conditions this will result in the lower boiling point component arriving at the top of the column and the higher boiling point component being left at the bottom of the column. Thus a temperature gradient will be established along the column when distillation is in progress, and ultimately the vapour passing out of the column will be very rich in the low boiling point component. This series of events may be easily visualized by considering the action of a bubble-cap column which is used in large scale distillation plant. The column consists of a number of plates mounted above one another, over which flows the condensed liquid (reflux), and through which the ascending vapour is made to bubble. Fig. 14.11 shows three bubble-cap plates in section. If we assume that at each plate, the

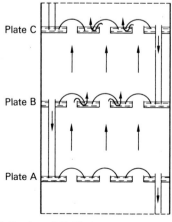

Fig. 14.11. Section of distillation column (bubble-cap type).

vapour and liquid reach equilibrium conditions, i.e. each plate is theoretically perfect, the change in composition of liquid on passing from plate A to plate C will be equivalent to that produced by three theoretical plates. Ascending vapour from the still passes through the bubble-caps on plate A and the vapour rising from it will be richer in the more volatile component. This vapour passes through the liquid on B, condenses, and the heat of condensation partially vaporizes the liquid. The process of condensation and vaporization will be repeated at C and so on, all the way up the column. In this simplified consideration of column action, each bubble-cap plate has the same effect as a separate still. The changes in composition at each plate can be estimated from the boiling point versus composition curves.

Design of fractionating columns. The purpose of a fractionating column is to achieve an extensive liquid–vapour interface so that equilibrium between ascending vapour and reflux can be rapidly attained. In the laboratory, packed columns are frequently used; the packing may consist of single

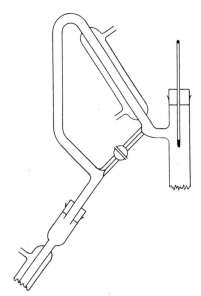

FIG. 14.13. Total condensation variable-take-off still head.

turn helices (spirals) of wire or glass, glass rings, cylindrical glass beads, stainless steel rings, etc. The Vigreux column which in the best types has indentations in the walls, spirally arranged and occupying most of the interior, acts as a packed column. In the Widmer column (Fig. 14.12) fractionation occurs in the central spiral which is kept warm by the vapour around it. Condensed liquid is returned to the still by a trap.

The separation of a mixture in a column depends upon the proportion of vapours traversing the column which are condensed and returned to the still—*the reflux ratio.* A column operating under total reflux will not yield distillate; a state of dynamic equilibrium is reached and a maximum degree of separation of the components is obtained along the length of the column. If the quantity of distillate removed at a time is small, this will minimize disturbance of equilibrium conditions and the concentration gradient along the column will remain resonably stable. For columns operating above about 60°, heat loss should be prevented by insulation, e.g. asbestos cord, silver vacuum jacket. For temperatures above 100° the column is surrounded by a heating jacket which is generally adjusted to the temperature of the vapour that emerges from the top of the column. Heat loss will cause excessive condensation within the column which may result in flooding and also will disturb the steady temperature gradient along the column. Under adiabatic conditions the temperature gradient is determined by the vapour–liquid equilibria

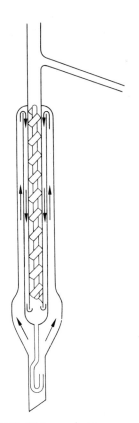

FIG. 14.12. Widmer column.

in the column. For efficient separation it is essential to use a high reflux ratio and collect distillate slowly so that the column is operating under equilibrium conditions. The reflux ratio is conveniently controlled by means of a suitable still head. Fig. 14.13 shows a total condensation variable take-off still head. In operation the vapours are refluxed with the tap closed until equilibrium and the resulting optimum separation are attained; the tap is opened and a small quantity of distillate is taken off; the tap is closed, the column again operated under total reflux and more distillate is then run off. By this means very sharp separations are achieved both at atmospheric and under reduced pressure. Heat input to the still should be controlled—if too little, the packing is insufficiently wetted by reflux and if too much, the vapour velocity may be too great for equilibrium to be attained.

Efficiency of Fractionating Columns

The efficiency of a column is commonly measured by the *height equivalent to a theoretical plate* (HETP). At a theoretically perfect plate, the vapours are brought into equilibrium with the liquid through which they pass; the length of a column required to achieve this is defined as the HETP, and vapour drawn off from the top of such a length of column is in equilibrium with the liquid at the bottom. The HETP value is obtained by analysis of the liquid in the still, the vapour at the head of the column and from data for the composition of liquid and vapour in equilibrium with one another.

Fractional Distillation under Reduced Pressure

Any of the apparatus described for fractionation at atmospheric pressure may be used for fractionation in vacuo. In some instances a short fractionating column is made to fit into the neck of the still. The most convenient receiver for vacuum fractionation is one of the forms of the Perkin triangle (Fig. 14.14). By suitable manipulation of the taps the receiver may be changed without interrupting the distillation. Azeotropic mixtures may be separated by vacuum fractionation. Vacuum fractionation has found extensive application in the separation of the mixed fatty acids derived from oils and fats.

Molecular Distillation

In molecular distillation or evaporative distillation, the pressure of the vapour above the liquid is much lower than the pressure of a saturated vapour in equilibrium with the liquid. The distance between the evaporating surface and the condenser is about equal to the mean free path of the vapour molecules at that very low pressure. Molecules leaving the surface of the liquid are therefore more likely to hit the condenser surface than to collide with other molecules and little or no recondensation at the surface of the liquid takes place. In ordinary distillation at atmospheric pressure and under reduced pressure, conditions approaching equilibrium are maintained and a considerable amount of recondensation (refluxing) occurs. Molecular distillation is usually carried out at 0.001 to 0.00001 mm pressure. There is no well-defined temperature at which distillation commences, unlike ordinary distillation procedures. An extensive review of the principles and techniques has been given by Hickman (1944). This technique has been applied with great success to the purification of vitamin A. For this purpose the fish liver oil is fed continuously as a thin film on to heated discs rotating in a high vacuum.

DISTILLATION IN STEAM

THEORETICAL CONSIDERATIONS AND SMALL SCALE METHODS

Vapour Pressure of Immiscible Liquids

In a pair of immiscible liquids each liquid exerts its own vapour pressure and neither liquid has any appreciable effect on the vapour pressure of the other. The vapour pressure of the mixture at a given temperature is equal to the sum of the vapour pressures of the two pure components at that temperature. Completely immiscible liquids are not known, although the miscibility of mercury and water, for instance, is very low indeed. For practical purposes, the miscibility of many organic liquids, e.g. turpentine or toluene, and water is negligible and calculations of the relative volatilities of such mixtures from their vapour pressures yield approximately correct results.

Distillation of Immiscible Liquids

A mixture of immiscible liquids begins to boil when the sum of their vapour pressures is equal to the atmospheric pressure. Thus in the case of water and a liquid which boils at a much higher temperature than water, the mixture boils below the

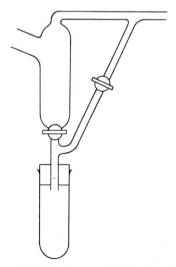

FIG. 14.14. Simple form of Perkin triangle.

boiling point of pure water. The boiling point of turpentine is about 160°, but when it is mixed with water and heated, the mixture boils at about 95.6°. At this temperature the vapour pressure of water is 647 mm and that of turpentine, 113 mm; the sum $647 + 113 = 760$ mm which is the normal atmospheric pressure. From these facts, it will be seen that a high boiling substance may be distilled with water at a temperature much below its boiling point. For substances which are insoluble in water and not decomposed by it, this provides an alternative to distillation under reduced pressure. Certain volatile solids, e.g. camphor, may be distilled in the same way.

For volatile substances which are miscible with water, distillation in steam would involve the same principles as fractional distillation.

The composition of the vapour over a pair of immiscible liquids may be calculated approximately from the vapour pressures and molecular weights of the components. Since in distillation this vapour is condensed, this also represents the composition of the distillate. If the vapour pressures of the two components at the boiling point of the mixture are p_1 and p_2, by Avogadro's hypothesis, the number of molecules present in the vapour is proportional to the vapour pressures, p_1 and p_2. The weights of the components in the vapour will therefore be in the ratio, $p_1 M_1 : p_2 M_2$, where M_1 and M_2 are their respective molecular weights. Hence the proportion by weight, w_1, w_2, of the two components in the distillate is given by the equation:

$$\frac{w_1}{w_2} = \frac{p_1 M_1}{p_2 M_2}$$

For turpentine, which contains a high proportion of pinene, $C_{10}H_{16}$, molecular weight 136, and water, molecular weight 18, the vapour pressures at the boiling point of the mixture, 95.6°, are 113 mm and 647 mm respectively and the distillate will contain turpentine and water in the ratio, $113 \times 136 : 18 \times 647$ or 1.32:1. For camphor, $C_{10}H_{16}O$, molecular weight 152, boiling point at 760 mm 206°, the vapour pressures at the boiling point of the mixture, 99°, are 24.6 mm and 735 mm and the distillate will contain camphor and water in the ratio $24.6 \times 152 : 735 \times 18$ or 1:3.54.

From these calculations, it can be seen that a substance of low volatility can be satisfactorily distilled in steam provided its molecular weight is considerably higher than that of water. Water is particularly suitable for the special case of *codistillation*, termed steam distillation, on account of its

low molecular weight and high boiling point. Other compounds of similar molecular weight to water, e.g. hydrogen sulphide, ammonia, methane, are gases at ordinary temperatures. Liquids other than water have been used for codistillation, e.g. paraffins for the codistillation of indigo. Substances which are only very slowly distilled with steam at about 100° may be distilled with superheated steam.

Small Scale Apparatus

A suitable apparatus for steam distillation on the laboratory scale is shown in Fig. 14.15. The safety tube in the steam generator permits the expulsion of some water if excessive pressure is developed. The distillate separates into two layers, water and the other component; these are separated in a separating funnel. The actual yield is often somewhat greater than the calculated yield since minute particles of the substance are carried over mechanically by the steam.

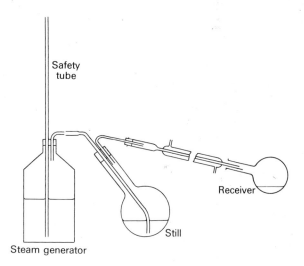

FIG. 14.15. Steam distillation apparatus.

Steam distillation is used for the determination of volatile oils in drugs and, conversely, distillation with toluene is used for the determination of moisture in drugs.

Large Scale Apparatus

Steam distillation is used to extract most of the volatile oils, such as clove, aniseed, eucalyptus, and so on. When the distillation is done in the locality where the material grows, special forms of still are used, often quite primitive, and arranged to meet local conditions. A common form of water still is

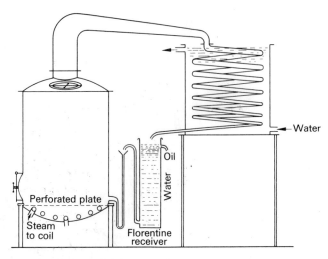

FIG. 14.16. Still for steam distillation of volatile oils.

shown diagrammatically in Fig. 14.16. A still of this kind has a jacket and, in addition, live steam is sometimes injected below the material, which is supported on a perforated false bottom. Means of charging and discharging the still are provided by manholes in the top and side.

Most volatile oils are lighter than water and will separate from the distillate as an upper layer. If a Florentine receiver, shown between the still and condenser in Fig. 14.16, is used the water can be run off from the spout on the left and can be returned to the still, as shown in the diagram, or run to waste. The oil which collects on the surface is run off from the upper spout. Some volatile oils are heavier than water, in which case the operation is reversed. Where the specific gravity of the oil is so near 1.0 that separation does not take place, it may be necessary to collect the whole of the distillate and extract it with a volatile solvent, subsequently distilling off the solvent from the oil.

15

Centrifugation

Centrifuging provides a convenient method of separating either two immiscible liquids or a solid from a liquid; it finds several applications in drug manufacture where it may be used either as a batch process or continuously. Essentially the centrifuge comprises a bowl or 'basket' capable of being rotated at high speed; for small batchwise operations, it is mounted vertically but larger centrifuges designed for continuous working have their axes horizontal. Apart from the angle of mounting, the main difference in design relates to the 'basket' itself. For the separation of crystals from mother liquor, for example, it is perforated and lined with filter cloth. Spinning forces the liquid through the cloth and leaves a cake of crystals on the inner surface of the basket. The alternative design is a non-perforated basket, and this may be used for separating solid–liquid or liquid–liquid systems. With the former, spinning causes the solid to build up on the walls of the bowl while the liquid is removed through an overflow. For the latter, the effect is to create an outer layer of the denser liquid and an inner layer of the lighter; separate overflow points can be arranged so as to remove the components continuously.

Theoretical Considerations
The force acting upon a particle compelled to move in a circular path around an axis is given by the equation:

$$F = MR\omega^2 = \frac{Mv^2}{R} \qquad (15.1)$$

where F is the centrifugal force, M is the mass of the particle, R the radius of curvature, ω the angular velocity and v the peripheral velocity. It can be seen that for any given peripheral velocity, the force varies inversely as the radius of curvature. The equation gives the total centrifugal force due to the mass of the rotating body and has to be taken into account in the design of centrifuges, so that the centrifuge basket is not subjected to excessive strains. In comparing relative performances of centrifuges, it is useful to express the centrifugal force as a relative force. The *relative centrifugal force* (RCF) or centrifugal effect is defined as the ratio of centrifugal force to gravitational force acting upon a given body. Thus:

$$RCF = \frac{F}{Mg} = \frac{R\omega^2}{g} = \frac{v^2}{gR} \qquad (15.2)$$

A more practical form of the equation can be derived in which the centrifugal effect is related to the rate of revolution. Thus,

$$RCF = \frac{R}{g}\left(\frac{2\pi NR}{60}\right)^2 = 11.17 \times 10^{-6}RN^2 \qquad (15.3)$$

where R is in cm and N the velocity in rev/min.

The main method of increasing the RCF is to increase the speed of operation but a limit is set upon the peripheral velocity by the maximum safe strain in the basket wall. Increasing its thickness above a certain amount, in order to get additional strength, does not help because it adds to the weight and increases the strain. For the same peripheral velocity, a larger centrifugal effect is obtained with a smaller basket (see equations 15.1 and 15.2).

The rate of settling, V, of a particle diameter D, at a given distance from the axis of rotation, may be calculated from Stokes's Law (see p. 129) in which g has been substituted by $R\omega^2$.

Thus
$$V = \frac{D^2(\rho_1 - \rho_2)R\omega^2}{18\eta} \qquad (15.4)$$

where ρ_1, and ρ_2 are densities of the solid and liquid respectively; η is the dynamic viscosity of the liquid. When using a continuous type centrifuge of the solid basket type such as the Sharples, the rate of flow of the feed must be considered in relation to the rate of settling of the particle. The simplest form of this type of centrifuge can be considered to be a rotating cylinder through which the feed material is passed. If the liquid lies in such a bowl in a thin layer of thickness S, and is fed continuously at one end and discharged at the other, the time t, during which the liquid is in the bowl is X/Q, where X is the volume of liquid in the bowl at a given time and Q is the rate of flow of liquid through the bowl. If S is small, then the velocity of the particle will be nearly uniform and the distance x settled in time t can be calculated from equation (15.4). Thus:

$$x = \frac{D^2(\rho_1 - \rho_2)R\omega^2}{18\eta}\frac{X}{Q} \qquad (15.5)$$

Particles at a distance less than x from the wall will therefore be removed from the liquid. Thus the rate of flow Q can be calculated in order that particles of the desired size settle out before the liquid leaves the centrifuge. This example only applies to ideal conditions and is given merely as a guide to the correct operation of a continuous centrifuge of the solid basket type.

The critical speed of a centrifuge is that corresponding to the natural period of vibration of the basket. It may be better understood from the following experiment. If a weight is suspended from elastic held in the hand and made to vibrate up and down, it does so at a definite rate, which is the same whatever the amplitude of the vibration. This is the critical speed. If the hand moves up and down slower than this the weight follows, but if the speed of movement is increased the length of the up and down motion of the weight increases, and when the rate approaches that of the natural vibration (or critical speed) of the weight, the motion of the weight becomes so violent that the elastic will be broken. If the speed is increased

so quickly that the critical speed is passed before the weight can build up this violent motion, the motion of the weight will be reduced less and less, and when the motion is very rapid the weight will hardly move at all. In a centrifuge, the basket corresponds to the weight, the buffer bearing to the elastic, the out-of-balance weight to the amplitude of vibration of the hand, and the speed of the machine to the rate of vibration of the hand. A centrifuge has a critical speed of vibration which is slower than the running speed; it is therefore important that the full speed is attained quickly, so that the machine does not run long enough at the critical speed to build up vibration and become dangerous.

Laboratory Equipment

Centrifuges for laboratory use are generally of the horizontal swinging arm type. The glass tubes holding the liquid are supported in metal buckets which are free swinging from the rotor head. When the rotor revolves, the tubes swing out in a horizontal position so that the particles sediment along the length of the tube. If the centrifuge tubes are held at a fixed angle, about 45 to 50° to the vertical axis, both while at rest and while rotating, the sedimenting particles have only a short path to traverse to the sides of the tube. This type of centrifuge is known as the angle centrifuge and is useful for the rapid sedimentation of particles provided that they do not adhere to the sides of the tube. The RCF obtained in small centrifuges of the types mentioned is about 2000 at approximately 5000 rev/min. In making comparisons between centrifuges, it is, of course, important to specify whether the RCF is measured at the free surface of the liquid or at the tip of the tube. High-speed centrifuges (10 000 g can be used to separate bacteria from aqueous fluids. The ultracentrifuge which is capable of causing sedimentation of protein molecules may operate at speeds up to 85 000 rev/min resulting in an RCF of up to 250 000. The size of the rotating head of this type is limited to a few inches in diameter.

High-speed centrifuging is always accompanied by heat generation due to air friction. This can be disregarded for the majority of centrifuging processes but if controlled temperature conditions are required, refrigeration of the centrifuge chamber and operation under vacuum may be necessary.

Zonal Centrifugation

This allows high resolution separation of biological cells and viruses due to the differences in density

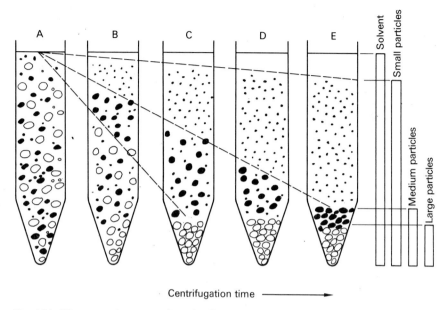

Centrifugation time ⟶

FIG. 15.1. Diagrammatic presentation of sedimentation of particles in conventional centrifuge tube; C, all large particles have sedimented; E, all large and medium particles have sedimented (Anderson 1964).

and size. In an ordinary centrifuge tube, particles in the initially homogeneous suspension settle in the centrifugal field resulting in a distribution of particles of different sizes along the tube (Fig. 15.1). There is no clear-cut separation of particles of different size because the large particles that have settled out will also contain smaller particles that were initially present near the bottom of the tube. Similarly as the intermediate particles sediment they form a layer above the large particles which is contaminated with still smaller particles. By repeated sedimentation fairly clear-cut fractions can be obtained, but generally with considerable loss of material. In zonal centrifugation, the centrifuge tube is filled with a liquid whose density increases towards the bottom and a small sample of particles in suspension is layered over it (Fig. 15.2). This technique gives zones of sedimenting particles, the rate of movement depending on size and density of the particles. Zonal centrifuges are designed to eliminate swinging buckets or centrifuge tubes and provision is made for sedimentation to occur in special rotors. The zones are recovered by displacing them by a denser fluid which is pumped into the outer periphery of the rotor while it is rotating at low speed, the stability of the gradient being maintained by centrifugal force. The effluent is then recovered as a series of discrete samples. This technique has been used to separate glycogen particles present in liver cells and the

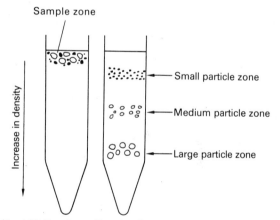

FIG. 15.2. Zonal centrifugation (in conventional centrifuge tube).

separation of virus particles from tissue homogenates.

Supercentrifuge

This consists of a relatively long hollow cylindrical bowl of small diameter suspended from a flexible spindle at the top and guided at the bottom by a loose fitting bushing. The speed of rotation is up to 22 000 rev/min with a standard motor drive or up to 50 000 rev/min with an air turbine. Figure 15.3 shows the supercentrifuge fitted with a bowl for separating two immiscible liquids. The feed is introduced into the bottom of the bowl by gravity feed and the heavier liquid is thrown out against

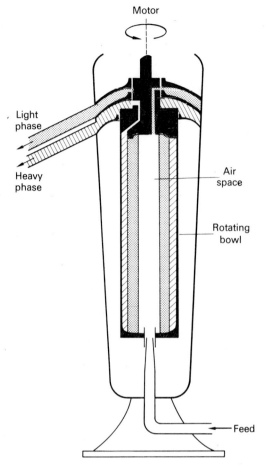

FIG. 15.3. Supercentrifuge fitted with bowl for separation of two immiscible liquids.

the wall, with the lighter liquid forming an inner layer. The separated liquids are taken off from the top of the bowl through separate outlets as shown in Fig. 15.3. For the clarification of liquids the separating bowl is replaced by the clarifier bowl which has one outlet at the top through which the clarified liquid passes, leaving the deposited solids on the wall of the bowl. This centrifuge is limited to the clarification of suspensions of low solid content due to the limited dimensions of the bowl. This restriction does not apply to the separation of liquid–liquid dispersions as there is a continuous take-off of both components.

LARGE SCALE EQUIPMENT

Vertical Centrifuges
With perforated basket. These may be used for separating crystalline drugs, such as aspirin, from their mother liquors. If the basket is mounted above

the driving shaft, the centrifuge is described as 'under-driven'; conversely, if suspended from the shaft, it is 'over-driven'. A common type of centrifuge for the separation of crystals, or a precipitate when the quantity of solid is large in proportion to the total volume of the slurry, is shown in Fig. 15.4. The important part is the 'basket', which may be made of steel, sometimes covered with vulcanite or lead, or of copper, monel or other suitable metal, according to the nature of the material for which it is to be used. It may be plain or perforated.

When a fully loaded basket is rotating at its maximum speed the centrifugal force puts a great strain on the shell. Corrosion and wear can reduce the strength of the shell beyond a safe working limit causing the basket to burst with disastrous results. It is of the greatest importance, therefore, that the basket be well constructed from suitable materials which offer the greatest resistance to corrosion, and it must be examined carefully and frequently. Any bulging of the wall is a sign that it requires immediate attention. Perforated baskets are usually employed. For fine crystals the perforations may be 3 mm in diameter, but for finer grained material which would tend to pass through these holes the basket is lined with a fine-meshed gauze, or with a cloth supported on a coarse gauze. Figure 15.4 shows an electrically under-driven centrifuge with a perforated basket. The whole machine is suspended from flexible joints, two of which can be seen. The lever attached to the side operates the brake which stops the machine when the power is switched off. This type is made with baskets from 90 to 180 cm in diameter. The 90 cm basket has a capacity of 0.085 m^3, runs at 1000 rev/min, and requires about 5 kW for starting and 2 kW for running.

Centrifuges may be driven by belt pulleys and shafting, by water turbines or electric motors operating through a friction clutch. The power required for running is small compared with that required for starting and bringing it up to full speed.

The loading of the material into the basket must be done to give even distribution, as an unbalanced basket running at high speed causes great strain and vibration. After starting, the top speed must be attained quickly, so that the machine quickly passes, and does not run at, the critical speed.

With non-perforated basket. When the deposited solid offers a high resistance to the flow of liquid through it, the non-perforated basket is the method of choice. The suspension is fed continuously into

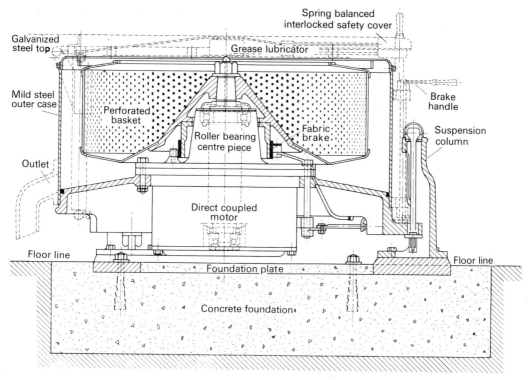

FIG. 15.4. Electrically under-driven centrifuge (Thomas Broadbent & Sons, Ltd.).

the basket and the resulting clarified liquor is removed over a weir or through a skimming tube (Fig. 15.5). The operation is stopped when a suitable depth of solid has been deposited on the walls of the basket. The solids are then scraped off by hand or by a scraper blade. The supercentrifuge discussed previously is also an example of a non-perforated basket centrifuge.

Fig. 15.6 shows a solids ejecting type separator.

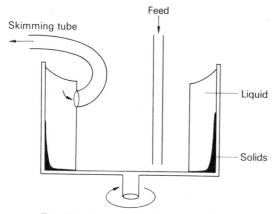

FIG. 15.5. Non-perforated basket centrifuge.

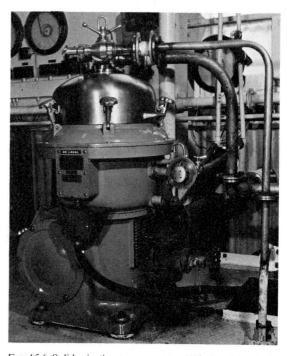

FIG. 15.6. Solids ejecting type separator (Alfa-Laval Co. Ltd.).

The machine runs continuously, the clear liquid being discharged from the spout and the solids collected on the inside of the bowl. The process can be continued until it is necessary to stop to remove the accumulated deposit. Figure 15.7 shows

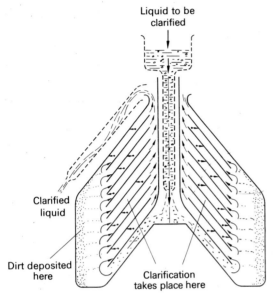

FIG. 15.7. Section of bowl of De Laval clarifier (Alfa-Laval Co. Ltd.).

a section of the bowl used for clarifying in which there are a number of cones separated by narrow spaces. The liquid enters down the centre of the bowl and passes out by ascending the spaces between the cones. The high gravity solids are thrown outwards, travel down the undersides of the cones and the lighter liquid finds its way out over the rim of the bowl. Referring to the diagram it can be seen that the spaces between the cones are very narrow. The impurities therefore have to travel only a very short distance before they are removed from the liquid. This feature allows a slower speed to produce a high degree of clarification. By regulation of the speed it is possible to separate a coarse sediment from a mixture containing a fine powder in suspension.

Horizontal Centrifuges

It has already been pointed out that vertical centrifuges can be designed for the continuous separation of two immiscible liquids. For the continuous removal of solids, however, a horizontal centrifuge is normally employed. The conical centrifuge provides a well-known example. Here the solid–liquid suspension is fed into a horizontally mounted basket through a hollow shaft and the solid is spun to the periphery in the normal way. Inside the basket, there is mounted co-axially a spiral scraper which rotates at a slower speed than the basket itself. As the scraper rotates, it removes most of the solid cake, apart from a slight 'clearance', and forces it along to a point where it first receives a spray of wash liquid and is then dried and discharged. Figure 15.8 illustrates a centrifuge of this type.

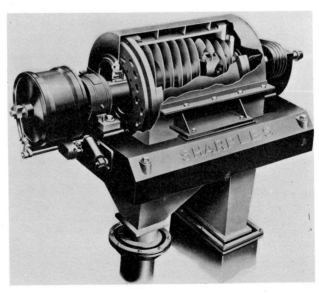

FIG. 15.8. Horizontal centrifuge: the Sharples Super-D-Canter (Sharples Centrifuges, Ltd.).

16

Filtration

This may be defined as a process whereby a solid is separated from a liquid or gas by means of a porous medium which retains the solid but allows the fluid to pass. When solids are present in small proportions the process is usually spoken of as clarification.

Mechanism of Filtration
The retention of particles by a filter can be due to:
(a) Sieving action where the particles are larger than the pores of the filter and the solid is retained at the surface of the filter medium and eventually builds up a thick layer. This is commonly referred to as cake filtration.
(b) Capture of particles in the depth of the filter where the particles retained are always smaller than the average size of the voids in the solid bed through which the fluid flows. This is called depth filtration.

The mechanism of sieving action of a filter is self explanatory but in depth filtration the particles can only be removed by capture at the solid surface by van der Waals forces or by electrical forces, both of which can only operate at short distances from the solid surface. What is the mechanism by which particles in suspension are brought close to the solid surface? For particles less than 1 micron, diffusion plays a major role but for particles larger than say 20 microns, diffusion could be insignificant compared with inertial and gravitational forces. For instance particles may be captured by impact where their trajectories cause them to strike a filter fibre without crossing a fluid strain line or by inertia when their mass is such that they have sufficient inertia

to cross the streamlines and so touch the fibre surface.

In depth filtration, which is used exclusively for the removal of small amounts of contaminants from relatively large volumes of liquid, the filter medium is made up of fibrous or particulate solids arranged in such a manner that the length of travel of the liquid is large in comparison to the size of particles being removed. A special case of depth filtration is the so called sheet filtration where the material to be clarified is passed through a series of pads mounted edgewise to the flow of fluid. The pads commonly consist of a mixture of asbestos fibres embedded in cellulose.

Factors affecting the Rate of Filtration
A typical filter operation is shown in Fig. 16.1.

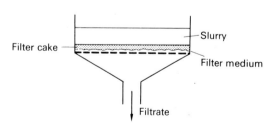

FIG. 16.1. Diagram of a simple filter.

The suspension of solids in liquid, often referred to as the slurry, is poured on to the medium and the formation of a layer of solid (filter cake) is shown. The resistance to flow of liquid thus increases progressively throughout the operation as

223

the cake increases in thickness. The factors affecting rate of filtration are:

(a) The area of filter surface.
(b) The resistance of the filter cake + filter.
(c) The viscosity of the filtrate.
(d) The pressure difference across the filter.

The effects of these variables will now be discussed:

The rate of flow will be greatest at the beginning of the process since the resistance is at a minimum, and will be proportional to the filter area. Once the filter cake forms, its surface acts as the filter medium and solids are continually deposited adding to the thickness of the cake. This cake is composed of a bulky mass of particles and the liquid flows through the interstices. If it is assumed that these interstices correspond to a multiplicity of capillary tubes, the flow of liquids through these may be expressed by Poiseuille's Law as indicated by the equation:

$$V = \frac{P\pi r^4 t}{8\eta l}$$

where V is the volume of liquid of viscosity η flowing through a tube length l, radius r under pressure P, in time t. For a given set of circumstances, V is directly proportional to P, and inversely proportional to l; the length of the pores is unknown but we may assume that it is proportional to the thickness of the cake. The radius r (average) will remain constant for rigid non-compressible cakes. When the solid consists of soft, easily deformable particles, e.g. magnesium hydroxide, increased pressure may cause closer packing of the particles and the resistance to flow is increased. This rate of flow may be only slightly increased, or even decreased, by an increase in pressure. The flow rate is inversely proportional to the viscosity of the filtrate. Viscosity is reduced by a rise in temperature and the filtration of viscous oils, syrups, etc., is often expedited by filtering while hot.

An extension of the Poiseuille equation to make it applicable to porous bed, based on a capillary type structure leads to the Kozeny-Carmen equation which is the most widely used filtration equation:

$$Q = \frac{AP\varepsilon^3}{\eta S^2 K L (1-\varepsilon)^2}$$

where Q is the rate of flow, A the cross sectional area of bed, P the pressure drop across bed, ε the porosity of bed, S the specific surface of bed, L the depth of bed and K the Kozeny Constant,

usually taken as 5. The effect of compressibility of the cake on flow rate can be appreciated from this equation since the flow rate is proportional to $\varepsilon^3/(1-\varepsilon)^2$. A 10 per cent change in porosity can produce almost a three fold change in Q.

In ordinary gravity filtration, P will be due to the head of liquid above the filter. P may be increased by positive pressure or by applying a vacuum to the receiving vessel. In vacuum filtration the greatest vacuum that can be applied will be equal to the vapour pressure of the filtrate. Vacuum filtration is undesirable for very volatile liquids owing to the loss of vapour into the vacuum system. By application of direct pressure to the liquid, the maximum pressure is determined solely by the construction of the apparatus. Another advantage of positive pressure filtration is the ease of filtration of liquids which foam under reduced pressure.

Filter Media

The selection of a suitable filter medium depends upon the purpose of filtration and the quantity to be filtered. In general, it is desirable that a medium should:

(a) be inert, e.g. no chemical interaction and little physical change such as shrinking of solution in the fluid,
(b) allow the maximum passage of liquid while retaining the solid,
(c) sufficient mechanical strength to withstand filtration pressure,
(d) adsorb negligible amounts of dissolved material.

Filter Aids

When clarifying liquids containing slimy compressible materials, e.g. colloidal sludges, the filter medium is soon clogged and it may be necessary to incorporate a material known as a filter aid. This functions by building up a porous rigid structure which can retain the solid particles and allow the fluid to pass through. A filter aid thus tends to counteract unfavourable characteristics of badly filtering material. In practice, a filter aid may be used in two ways:

(a) adding to the suspension and the mixture handled in the usual way, or
(b) making a suspension of the filter aid in a suitable liquid and then filtering so that the filter medium receives a precoat of filter aid.

The important characteristics of filter aids is that they should be chemically inert, of low specific gravity, porous rather than dense and preferably recoverable. Examples include kieselguhr, talc, charcoal, asbestos, paper pulp, bentonite, Fuller's earth. Materials such as activated charcoals will adsorb to a greater or lesser extent inorganic and organic compounds from solution. Alkaloids are very readily adsorbed by charcoal, and a filter aid such as kieselguhr is preferable for the clarification of alkaloidal solutions.

Pretreatment of Materials

Some materials which are practically non-filterable may be modified by suitable pretreatment.

Heat treatment. The collection of materials precipitated from solution may be facilitated if the precipitate is made up of coarse particles. Precipitation from concentrated solutions at a raised temperature results in coarser particles than from dilute cold solutions. Unwanted proteins in aqueous vegetable drug extracts may be removed by heating the solution and the coagulated protein then filtered off. Waxes which soften when warm are not easily filtered unless they are chilled to make the particles more rigid.

Filter aids. These may be added to suspensions to render the filter cake more open and less compressible so that the flow through the filter is not blocked. Their use in the clarification of turbid liquids has been discussed previously.

Removal of tannins. When the turbidity of alcoholic preparations is due to the tannin content it may be removed by the addition of gelatin or isinglass which combine with the tannin to form an insoluble complex and this can be filtered off.

pH *effects.* A protein in solution is least soluble at its isoelectric point and is easily precipitated in a filterable form.

METHODS

In pharmaceutical operations filtration is used chiefly as a method of separating and rejecting small amounts of extraneous matter (including bacteria) from relatively large volumes of liquid. This contrasts with chemical processes where the objective is usually to isolate a crystalline precipitate and to discard the filtrate. This distinction affects both the design of the equipment and the choice of filtering medium.

Filter Funnels

These can be fitted with either paper, sintered glass, sintered metal or asbestos according to the type of filtration required.

The most commonly employed filtering medium on the small scale is filter paper, which consists of spongy, absorbent paper ('bibulous' paper) that has not been 'dressed' or glazed.

Filter papers differ considerably in porosity and texture. The porosity is usually tested by precipitating barium sulphate from a solution of barium chloride and filtering off the precipitate, afterwards washing it on the filter paper. A fair quality paper should be capable of preventing the passage of this salt. Papers of finer texture are tested in a similar manner by suspensions of the oxides of antimony and tin. Filter paper is purified commercially by frequent washing with hydrochloric and hydrofluoric acids, and further washing to remove the acids. Poor quality paper sometimes gives a distinct reaction for chloride. The amount of ash left on ignition of the paper is of importance in gravimetric analysis, but not as important in pharmaceutical operations, where the chief qualities required are freedom from soluble impurity together with rapid filtration.

Funnels for taking filter paper may be of glass or porcelain, the latter being usually modified to take a flat disc of paper supported on a perforated plate. These are known as Büchner or Hirsch funnels and the supporting plate permits the paper to withstand the strain of vacuum filtration.

Büchner and similar funnels (Fig. 16.2) are employed in conjunction with a pressure flask of stout glass (Fig. 16.3) the funnel passing through a rubber bung in the mouth of the flask and the outlet on the left being connected to the pump. If for any reason the water pressure falls, the pressure in the flask may be momentarily less than that within the pump itself, so that water in the pump may be

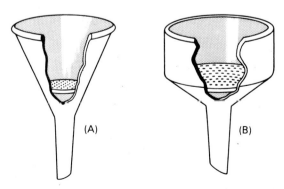

FIG. 16.2. (A), Büchner funnel; (B), Hirsh funnel.

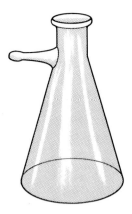

Fig. 16.3. Pressure flask.

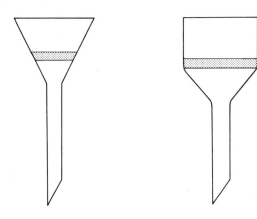

Fig. 16.4. Sintered glass filters.

drawn via the connecting tube into the flask and contaminate the filtered liquid that it contains. The same may occur if the tap is turned off at the conclusion of the process before the flask is disconnected from the pump. To obviate the risk of 'back-suction', a second pressure flask is interposed between the pump and the receiver through the rubber bung of which passes a glass tube, reaching to the bottom of the flask. This tube is connected directly to the pump and the outlet of the interposed flask is connected to the outlet of the receiver, any water sucked back from the pump will be caught in the intermediate flask instead of passing into the receiver.

Hot filtration is sometimes necessary, particularly for syrups or oils which are viscous at room temperature. For this purpose a conical glass funnel may be surrounded by a water-jacket or heating coil.

Sintered Glass Filters
These consist of a filtering medium composed of particles of Jena or Pyrex glass powdered and sifted to produce granules of uniform size which are moulded together into the form of flat or convex plates.* The plates may be fused into glass apparatus of any required shape (Fig. 16.4) which may then be used in the manner of Büchner funnels for filtration under reduced pressure, or, in the case of the coarser grades as ordinary funnels. The porosity of the filter depends upon the size of the granules used in its preparation, and is indicated

by a number. The number is preceded by a letter which indicates the kind of glass employed and the letter is preceded by a number which represents the size and shape of the apparatus into which the plate is fused. Sintered glass filters are useful for filtering such liquids as parenteral injections, official solutions of potent substances, and solutions of salts used in dispensing. For use in the preparation of injections, eye-lotions, etc., they may be sterilized in an autoclave. For the filtration of viscous liquids, such as glycerins, syrups, etc., it may be necessary to surround the filter by a lead tube through which hot water or steam is passed. The filters are also useful for filtering substances such as corrosive liquids and oxidizing agents. In dealing with a large volume of liquid it is useful to employ a coarse grade to remove most of the suspended matter and afterwards to filter through a finer grade. Sintered glass filters may be cleaned by scrubbing gently with a soft brush and sending a stream of water through in the reverse direction, or by chemical means.

Seitz Filters
For use with small quantities of liquids the form shown in Fig. 16.5 is probably the most successful. In this case an asbestos filter sheet is supported by a burnished stainless steel disc which is perforated and lies between the upper and lower parts of the glass funnel. In use the pad is placed on the disc and acts as a gasket between the glass flanges of the funnel. The glass parts are held by two chromium plated metal clamping rings which are drawn together by screws with milled heads.

If desired the apparatus may be used in conjunction with a sterilizing grade of asbestos filter sheet. After assembly the whole apparatus is wrapped and autoclaved and its stem fitted aseptically into

---

* The term 'sintered' is applied to these filters on account of the similarity in appearance and other physical properties which they bear to siliceous sinter. 'Sinter' is a German name for a porous mineral precipitated in crystalline form from mineral waters; there are vaious kinds of sinter, such as calcareous sinter (a variety of calcium carbonate), pearl sinter or florite, etc.

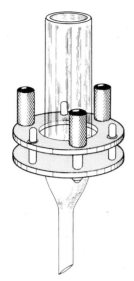

FIG. 16.5. Filter holder for clarification and sterilization.

a sterile filter flask. The liquid comes only into contact with Pyrex glass and a disc of stainless steel so that there is no risk of contamination by toxic metals. The apparatus is easily cleaned and sterilized and is simple in operation.

Membrane Filters

These are thin porous membranes produced from cellulose esters or similar polymeric materials. The pores are uniform in size and pass directly through the entire thickness of the membrane and are virtually non-connecting. The filtration action is mainly sieve-like and the particles are retained on the surface. The membranes are produced in more than 20 distinct pore sizes from 0.01 μm to about 14 μm, in discs ranging from approximately 1.5 to 30 cm in diameter. The porosity or pore volume is estimated as 80 per cent of the total filter volume and this results in flow rates about 40 times faster than with conventional filter media such as sintered glass or unglazed porcelain with the same particle size retention properties. In operation the membranes need to be clamped on a porous grid such as sintered glass or stainless steel mesh and special holders are commercially available for this purpose. Because of the small pore size, the filters are invariably operated under pressure, either positive or negative. Due to the absence of fibres or particles in the membrane, these filters are particularly useful for the preparation of 'particulate free' solutions for parenteral or ophthalmic use.

Cellulose ester membranes are suitable for aqueous solution of drugs, dilute acids, alkalies, aliphatic and aromatic hydrocarbons or non-polar liquids. They are not suitable for use with ketones, esters, ether–alcohols or strong acids and alkalis, in which case they can be replaced by Nylon or Teflon membranes. A wide range of different membrane materials is available and the technical information of the manufacturer should be consulted. The major producers of membrane filters are Millipore Filter Corporation, Sartorius, and Gelman.

For filtration on a factory scale, disc filters are available up to 29.3 cm diameter and are mounted in a filter holder as shown in Fig. 16.6. For the production of very large volumes of filtrate multiplate units are available which may contain up to 60 disc filters, all acting in parallel (Fig. 16.7). The assembly consists of a bell housing containing a vertical stack of perforated screen filter support plates between which the individual filters are clamped under pressure. Whatever type of disc filter unit is used it is always necessary to ensure that the liquid is being pumped under steady pressure since pressure fluctuations may rupture the membrane. A more obvious disadvantage of membrane filters is their brittleness when dry thus making handling difficult. This can be overcome by the

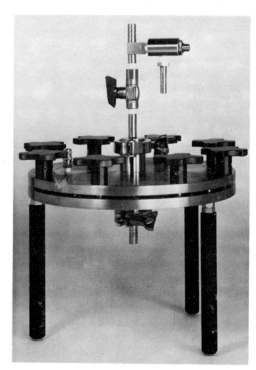

FIG. 16.6. Millipore filter holder (293 mm) (Millipore (UK) Ltd.).

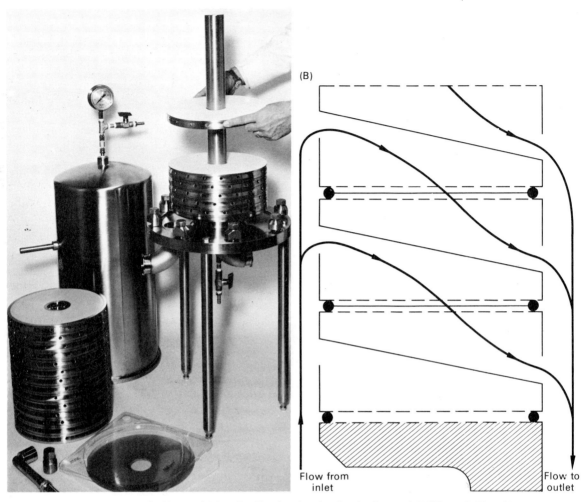

FIG. 16.7. Assembly of the multiplate disc filter housing showing the flow path (Millipore (UK) Ltd.).

use of filters in cartridge form. One commercial product has the membrane material held between two sheets of meshed synthetic fabric which is supported on a hollow tube of polypropylene suitably perforated for the flow of liquid through it.

Membrane filters by virtue of their sieve-like action tend to become clogged by particulate matter and their useful life can be extended by the use of a prefilter such as a depth filter. This type of filter can remove large quantities of contaminant from the fluid and prevent the membrane filter from becoming clogged prematurely. Filter cartridges are available which combine prefilter and membrane filter in the same unit. The advantage of the cartridge type unit is that 'in line' continuous filtration can be carried out which reduces handling of the solutions and thus minimizes the chance of contamination. A series of 'in line' filters shown in

Fig. 16.8 illustrates a possible combination of filters suitable for the production of a pharmaceutical product sterilized by filtration.

Glass-fibre paper. Glass fibres are straight and have uniform cross section; they do not swell and are available in well defined ranges of diameter. 'Paper' manufactured from these fibres is available in a range of pore sizes, the finer pore sizes being produced from fibres of smaller diameter. The advantages claimed for these filters is that the retention efficiency and flow rates are greater than for membrane filters. The mechanism of filtration is not a surface sieving action but is due to trapping of particles in the depths of the filter. For this reason it is not possible to give a significant value for pore size of these filters as the retention property of fibrous filters is dependent upon flow rate, fluid

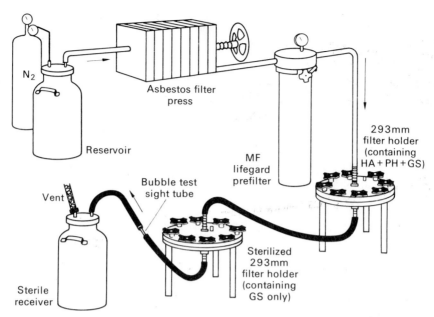

FIG. 16.8. A typical train of filters used to produce a pharmaceutical product such as a vaccine. Mean pore size of filters: prefilter 0.5 μm; HA 0.45 μm PH 0.3 μm; GS 0.22 μm (Millipore (UK) Ltd.).

viscosity, type and concentration of the contaminant, together with the complexity of the spatial arrangement of the fibres. Efficiency of particulate contamination can only be realistically determined by direct measurement. It should be noted that the filtration efficiency of fibrous filters increases during their life and can be explained by the increase in surface area brought about by the deposited contaminant. At the same time the resistance to flow of fluids increases with volume of flow through the filter and the useful life of the filter may be relatively short if clogging of the pores occurs. The filtration performance of glass-fibre paper in terms of flow rates during the building up of retained solids would appear to be much better than membrane filters or cellulose filter paper which tend to clog (Fig. 16.9).

The Filter Press
This is widely used in industry since it is compact and economical, and can be adapted to most filterable materials either for clarification or for the removal of a solid phase as a filter cake. Filter presses vary in design and in materials of construction but the basic principle is the same throughout. A series of square filter units are mounted on bars and are held in position between a fixed head and a moving head. The filter cloth is supported on the

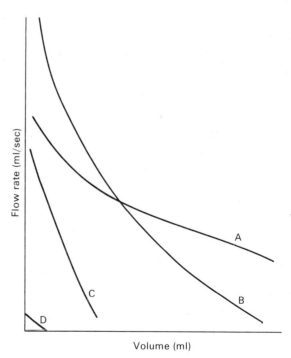

FIG. 16.9. Comparison of filtration performance of glass fibre paper, cellulose paper and cellulose acetate membranes. Data for filtration of river water (suspended solids 7 ppm). A, Whatman glass fibre (GF/B); B, Whatman glass fibre (GF/A); C, Cellulose ester membrane (1.2 μm); D, Whatman paper (42) (from Whatman Technical Information B71/2).

two faces of each plate which are compressed together by means of a thrust screw applied to the moving head so as to make a hermetic seal. These plates are arranged alternately with the filter cloth clamped between them. The feed channel is through one corner of the frame, the slurry entering the space formed by the frame. The plates have ribbed surfaces of such a form that the filter cloth will not be forced to the bottom of the ribs by the pressure used, thus leaving channels for the filtrate to reach the exit ports. Filtration can be continued until the filter cake fills the compartment or until the build-up reduces the efficiency of filtration. Delivery from the press may be either separately from each plate or united into a common channel. As a general rule it is advisable to have a tap on each plate, giving control over each filter unit, then if a filter cloth fails, that unit can be cut off avoiding the necessity of stopping filtration to open the press and find the fault. If it is necessary to force the filtrate to a higher level than the outlet of the press, a combined outlet gives the means of doing so, the pressure being supplied by the filter pump. It is an advantage in such a case to fit a short length of glass tubing into the outflow, so that the condition of the filtrate can be observed.

Washing the filter cake free from mother liquor is not done by passing the wash water through the same channels as for filtration, since the water would take the easiest path and pass through the cake in the region of the outlet port, but with the filtrate outlet of the washing plate closed so that the water passes through the inlet port on the washing plate and then through the whole thickness of the cake to the grooves of the filter plate.

When the runnings from the press are free from the impurity of the mother liquor the cakes are removed and dried. When the deposit is of no value it is usual to add kieselguhr or some other filter aid to the first portion of the liquor. This forms a coating on the filter cloth, giving a better filtering surface, and when cloth is used without filter paper it enables the deposit to be easily scraped off when the press is opened for cleaning.

Fig. 16.10 illustrates a type of filter press that is used in pharmaceutical production departments. The plates and frames are usually make of aluminium alloy and lacquered for protection against weak corrosive chemicals and steam sterilization. A wide range of filter media is available including filter sheets, woven fabrics (Nylon, Terylene etc.), diatomaceous earth and platics. Synthetic fabrics have greater chemical resistance than wool or cotton which are affected by alkali and acid

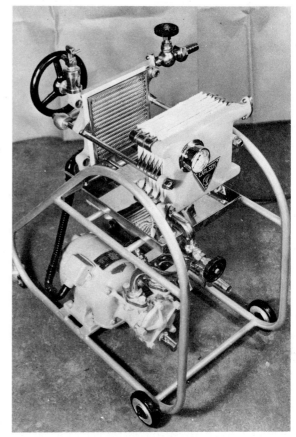

FIG. 16.10. A modern filter-press: the Carlson Pilot Princess. (Floor model, with pump unit).

respectively. Filter sheets composed of a blend of asbestos and cellulose are capable of retaining bacteria so that sterile filtrates can be obtained provided that the whole filter press and filter medium have been previously sterilized. This is usually done by passing steam through the assembled unit.

The manner of feeding the liquid to the press is of great importance. It must be supplied under pressure, which must be as steady as possible, any surging caused by the pump will tend to drive sediment through the filtering medium. As the solids are deposited the resistance to the passage of the liquid becomes greater and increased pressure must be applied until either the space in the press is filled with solid or the resistance has reached the maximum pressure for which the press is constructed. Presses will generally work up to a pressure of 75 to 100 lb/in^2 (0.525 to 7.0 kg/cm^2). The rate of filtration can be increased in some cases by increasing the pressure, but very often the use of too high a pressure will result in the deposition of a compact cake, which will quickly slow the rate of filtration. Lower pressures and a smaller feed often result in a more open cake and an increased amount of liquid filtered over a longer period.

The output of filter presses varies with the size and number of the plates, the nature of the solid to be collected, the viscosity and temperature of the liquid and the pressure applied. Relative rates for different sizes of presses for the same liquid can be calculated from the area of their filtering surfaces.

The main features of the filter press may be summarized as follows:

Advantages. (i) It is simple in construction, can be made from a variety of materials, and has no moving parts. (ii) It is compact, i.e. provides a large filter area in a small floor space. (iii) It is flexible and can be adjusted easily to different batch sizes. (iv) It has low maintenance costs. (v) It produces a dry cake in slab form.

Disadvantages. (i) Operating costs are high (preparing plates and discharging cake). (ii) Washing is not very efficient. (iii) Frequent dismantling increases wear and tear of filtering media.

The Metafilter

For some manufacturing processes the filter presses just described are frequently not convenient, because presses are generally adapted to filter large volumes and work continuously on one particular product. When it is necessary to change from one preparation to another and the batches are moderate in size, the volume of the residual liquor which is finally left in the pump and press may be large in proportion to the batch. In such cases some other form of filter is more advantageous. A useful form of clarifying filter which can be built up in units adapted to the size of the batch is the Metafilter. The permanent filter support is made up of rings on a grooved column. The rings, Fig. 16.11, are 22 mm in external diameter and have raised portions, shown shaded. The height of these raised portions may be made to vary from 0.025 to 0.2 mm, to suit requirements. The raised parts are only on one side of the rings, so that when the rings are threaded on the column, as shown in Fig. 16.12, channels are formed between the raised parts of one ring and the flat side of the next. The columns of rings are used as units to build up a filter in which they are the permanent base on which a filter bed of kieselguhr, charcoal, decolorizing carbon or other filter aid is deposited.

These pressure filters may also be fitted with a steam jacket for the filtration of very viscous liquids such as syrups or oils which can be rendered less viscous by warming.

This type of filter can easily be cleaned by back-flushing with water or steam, which because of the shape of the pores in the rings, will wash away the filter bed completely.

Drum Filter

The modern drum filter (Fig. 16.13) is a metal cylinder mounted horizontally, the curved surface being a perforated plate supporting a filter cloth. Internally, it is divided into several segments in which a vacuum is created independently as they enter the slurry and is discontinued when they are no longer immersed. The speed of rotation varies

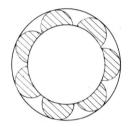

Fig. 16.11. Rings used a metafilter (Metafiltration Co. Ltd.).

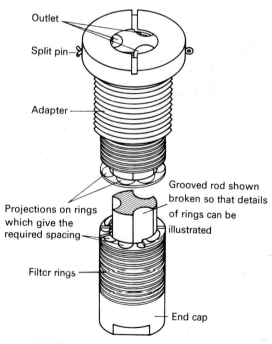

Fig. 16.12. Assembly of rings on column for metafilter (Metafiltration Co. Ltd.).

with the material to be filtered, but is usually less than 1 rev/min. As the segment leaves the slurry, the filter cake on its surface may be washed with a water spray and consolidated by means of a 'cake compressor'. It is then removed either by a doctor knife or a string discharge. The latter is particularly useful for products which yield a firm cake. Some rotary filters include a hot air drying zone and are capable of producing a cake with less than 1 per cent moisture.

AIR FILTRATION

Filtration is an important part of the system of air conditioning which is a normal feature of the pharmaceutical factory. Its purpose may be to produce either a dust free atmosphere where products can be handled under clean working conditions, or a sterile atmosphere for aseptic processes (Sykes & Carter 1953). (See also Chapter 31.)

Air filters must be of open construction to ensure high flow rates and thus the openings are large compared with the size of particles that are filtered out. The removal of a particle is due to a chance collision with the filter material rather than by any positive sieving action. The most important factors governing the removal of particles are impingement forces at high velocities and diffusion at low velocities. Small particles striking any surface will tend to adhere because of van der Waals forces, and if electrical charges are present the forces of adhesion may be increased.

Impingement. This can occur when the particles follow the streamlines of air close to the individual fibres of the filter, allowing the particle to come into contact with the fibre. The air streamlines bend round the fibre and small particles in the outer streamlines will miss the fibre. Larger particles, however, especially at high velocities, will not follow the curve of the streamline around the fibre but will continue on a straight course and collide with the fibre. This inertial effect is effective for particles of 5 μm upwards especially at high velocities of air flow (Stairmand 1950).

Diffusion. Inertial effects for particles less than 1 μm are unimportant. Filtration of these particles is, however, effective at low flow rates, and may be

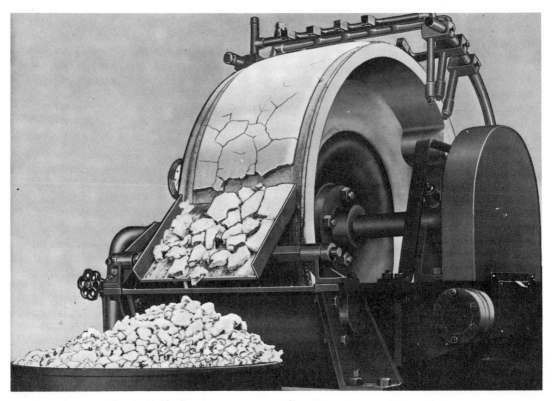

FIG. 16.13. The Paxman rotary vacuum filter (Davey, Paxman & Co. Ltd.).

explained on the basis of increased Brownian movement resulting in increased particle–fibre collisions. The efficiency of an air filter may be at a minimum when flow rates are too fast for diffusional movements to be effective and too slow for impingement.

Methods

Two general methods are available, the first being based on the use of oiled metal plates or mesh, and the second ('dry-type') on fibrous or granular material such as cotton wool, slag wool or glass wool. A third method, although sometimes described as filtration, actually involves the separation of solid particles by electrostatic precipitation.

Oil or viscous filters are designed so that the air passes over a large area of oil-coated metal either in the form of corrugated plates or wire mesh. Larger models have a rotary metal screen which passes through an oil trough. Dry filters comprise frames packed with asbestos, glass wool, slag wool, or various mixtures of these. Normally, they are discarded at the end of their time cycle, but some can be cleaned for re-use.

The electrostatic method is more expensive than the foregoing but is extremely efficient. Incoming air passes through an electric field of high potential gradient thus causing dust particles to become ionized. A series of wires carry a potential of about 12 kV and a corresponding series of 'Collector' plates are at about 7 kV. The charged particles are thus attracted to and held by the 'Collector' plates of opposite charge; these are periodically cleaned by spraying with water. An efficiency of 98 per cent against dust has been claimed for this method.

The correct working of an air filter may be checked photometrically by passing filtered and unfiltered air simultaneously through standard areas of chemical filter paper. The relative discoloration is a measure of efficiency. Bacteria-proof filters are checked by using a standard 'infected' air and testing by slit sampler and after filtration.

REFERENCES

DICKEY, G. D. (1961) *Filtration*. New York: Reinhold.

GREEN, H. L. & LANE, W. R. (1957) *Particulate Clouds: Dusts, Smokes and Mists*. London: Spon.

STAIRMAND, G. J. (1950) *Trans. Inst. Chem. Engs* **28**, 130.

SYKES, G. & CARTER, D. V. (1953) *J. Pharm. Pharmacol.* **5**, 945.

WYLIE, D. M. (1959) *Fundamentals of Filtration*. Journal of Cosmetic Chemists Congress Proceedings. Cosmetic Science.

17

Comminution, Sizing and Handling of Powders

SIZE REDUCTION

Size reduction or comminution is the process of reducing substances to small particles, an operation that has to be applied in greater or lesser degree to most drugs for the sake of easy administration and so that they present a large surface to the action of a solvent, thus aiding solution in the case of chemical substances and, in the case of crude drugs, allowing rapid penetration of the liquid used to extract their active constituents.

It is an important preliminary stage in the preparation of compressed tablets, where granular material has to be prepared for the tabletting process. Relatively few drugs can be compressed alone into satisfactory tablets; in general other ingredients have to be added—excipients, disintegrants, diluents and lubricants—and their particle size characteristics have a major influence on the properties of the finished tablets. Comminution is very relevant to the preparation of pharmaceutical dispersions, pastes and fluids, where properties such as consistency, tendency to sediment, appearance and general storage characteristics again depend on the particle size of the solid ingredients.

For sustained release preparations such as testosterone and oestrone, the drug must be within a particular size range if its effects are to be prolonged over a period and if it is not to be excreted too rapidly from the body.

Finally, the reduction of materials to a fine state of subdivision is an essential preliminary to the preparation of pharmaceutical capsules, insufflations (i.e. preparations inhaled directly into the lungs), suppositories, pessaries and ointments, where the requirement is that the solid constituents should be impalpable, i.e. less than about 60 μm in diameter.

GENERAL PRINCIPLES

The main object in most size reduction operations is to obtain a product smaller than a certain specified size. Drugs which are to be dispensed in some vehicle for oral or parenteral administration must be in the form of a very fine powder (usually less than 20 μm). Where a coarse product is required, e.g. vegetable drugs in a form suitable for extraction, a minimum proportion of fine particles is usually required. The type of size reduction apparatus plays an important part in this respect.

Machinery used for size reduction may be divided into three classes, depending on the size of the product required. Coarse crushers usually accomplish breaking by the application of a continuous pressure, and they yield a product generally greater than 1000 μm in diameter.

Intermediate machines employ blow or impact methods and produce powders in which the majority of particles are between about 100 μm and 1000 μm in diameter.

Finally there are the machines which employ grinding or abrasion methods and which are used for preparing the finest powders down to 1 μm diameter or below. No sharp dividing line can be drawn between the three classes of machines, but for pharmacists generally the intermediate and fine machines are of greater interest than the crushers.

Mechanism of Size Reduction

The mechanisms involved in size reduction are very complex (Bickle 1961) and, as they vary with the nature of the material, no comprehensive treatment is generally available. Theory is of limited use in the choice and operation of machines, and art and experience are still required in order to produce a desired result, since some drugs require individual treatment.

When a solid particle is struck, or is loaded with a force greater than its breaking strength, it generally breaks to form a few relatively large particles and a number of fine particles, but relatively few particles of intermediate size. Increasing the energy of the blow usually increases the number of both large and small particles and decreases the size of the former, but not of the latter. This indicates that the size and number of the large particles is determined by the energy and nature of the breaking process, but that of the smaller particles by the internal structure, nature and presence of fissures in the material concerned.

The energy supplied during comminution is distributed in elastic and plastic deformation of particles, in lattice rearrangements within crystals, and in the increased energy of the material associated with the new surfaces that have been formed. These are produced by fractures which occur along lines of weakness in the material and which open up under pressure or impact, but a very large proportion of the energy supplied is dissipated in the form of heat without achieving any useful result. It has been estimated that in most machines less than 2 per cent of the energy actually supplied is used for producing new surfaces, the rest going in overcoming friction and inertia of the machine parts, in friction between particles and deformation of particles without breaking them.

Many attempts have been made to develop equations for the useful work required to effect a given size reduction (Dobie 1952; Carey & Stairmand 1952). Rittinger's Law assumes that the energy consumed is proportional to the fresh surface produced. Kick's Law assumes that the energy required for the sub-division of a definite amount of material is the same for the same fractional reduction in size of the individual particles. Thus, if 1.5 kW is required to crush a given weight of a substance from 2 cm to 1 cm pieces, the energy required will be the same for crushing 1 cm to 0.5 cm or 0.5 cm to 0.25 cm pieces. For crushing large particles this appears to give better results than Rittinger's Law, which can be applied more satisfactorily to fine grinding.

A law combining both the above is due to Bond and can be expressed by:

$$E = E_i \left(\frac{100}{L_2}\right)^{1/2} \left(1 - \left(\frac{L_2}{L_1}\right)^{1/2}\right)$$

where L_1 is the initial diameter of the material in microns, L_2 is the final diameter of the material in microns, and E_i is the so-called work index, i.e. the amount of energy required to reduce unit mass of the material from a very large size down to a size of 100 μm. Work indices for many drugs and excipients are now available.

Size Distribution during Comminution

At all stages during a comminution process there will be a size distribution of particles; no machine can produce a completely uniformly sized product though some, which combine comminution with classification, very nearly do so. Fig. 17.1 shows schematically the change in particles size distribution which occurs as comminution proceeds (Herdan et al. 1960).

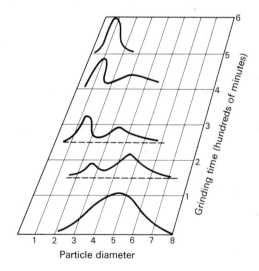

FIG. 17.1. Frequency distribution during milling.

At the start, when particles of many sizes are present, the distribution curve is rather flat and bell shaped, but in a short while a secondary peak develops and gradually moves to the left. At the same time its height rises indicating increasing production of small sized particles. The height of the secondary peak continues to rise at the expense of the primary, while its width decreases. The final stage is represented by the topmost curve.

By taking samples from a machine after different

periods of comminution, and plotting the histograms, it is possible to establish the most satisfactory and economical milling conditions.

COMMINUTION MACHINERY

Five main types of equipment are in regular use for size reduction of drugs and other pharmaceutical materials and they may be summarized briefly as (Cremer & Davies 1957; Neuman & Axon 1961):
hand operated or mechanical pestles and mortars,
impact or hammer mills,
pin mills,
ball mills and vibration mills, and
micronizers.

In addition there are the techniques of spray and freeze-drying, crystallization and precipitation, which are being increasingly used for producing drugs in a fine state of division without grinding.

Mortar and Pestle Types

The hand mortar and pestle has for centuries been the standard equipment for achieving size reduction, and is still very widely used for small scale purposes. Its mechanical counterparts are the end runner mill (Fig. 17.2) and the edge runner mill.

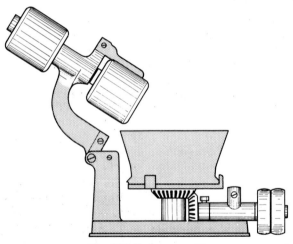

FIG. 17.2. End runner mill.

The end runner mill consists of a weighted pestle mounted eccentrically in a ceramic, granite or metal mortar, which is rotated by a motor. The pestle rotates by friction and is free to rise and fall in the mortar so that its grinding action involves both impact and shear, the material being crushed and rubbed between it and the rotating mortar. Spring loaded scrapers ensure that material is constantly returned to the grinding area and at the end of the

operation the pestle can be swung clear of the mortar to facilitate emptying and cleaning.

The edge runner mill consists of one or two heavy steel or granite rollers mounted on a horizontal shaft and turned round a .central vertical shaft on a bed of steel or granite. The stones may vary from 0.5 to 2.5 m in diameter, the larger size weighing up to about 6 tonnes. The material to be ground is kept in the path of the runners by scrapers. The reduction is partly due to crushing by the weight of the stones, but more to friction between the surfaces of contact between the runners and the bed stone. Although edge runner mills are gradually being replaced by more sophisticated machines they are still used, particularly for reducing extremely tough and fibrous materials—roots and barks—to the form of powder.

Impact and Hammer Mills

There are numerous commercially available types of impact mills, all working at high speed. The material is fed into the body of the machine and ground between rapidly rotating fixed or swinging blades and the corrugated mill casing. It passes out through screens round the circumference of the mill chamber. The Apex Comminuting Mill is an example of this type of machine. Basically it consists of a stainless steel grinding chamber (Fig. 17.3) the lower part of which holds interchangeable screens. A rotor carrying a series of blades is fitted to a shaft passing· through the chamber and, like the screens, the blades are interchangeable. For pulverizing, a hammer blade is used, while for cutting or dicing, a blade with a concave edge is the most effective. The Type 1141 blade has a hammer face on one side and a cutting edge on the other. A number of other types of dual faced blades and hammers have been developed, each having a special usefulness for certain operations or products.

The material to be processed is led via a feed pan to a throat or chute, the design of which may be modified to suit the physical nature of the product concerned. Pulverized material falls through the screen and is collected in drums or other suitable receivers. The speed of the mill may be adjusted, usually between 1000 and 5000 rev per min, and when temperature control is important, as for example when dealing with thermolabile drugs, the grinding chamber may be water-jacketed. For aseptic processing, a model is available which can be dismantled easily for cleaning and sterilizing. The Apex Mill and Fitz Mill (Fig. 17.4) are suitable for producing coarse to ultrafine powder (> 1 μm diameter) from such varied materials as drugs,

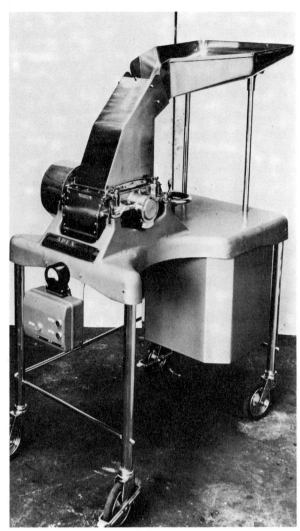

FIG. 17.3. Apex comminuting mill (Apex Construction Ltd.).

down to fine powder by the series of impacts as it passes outwards between the revolving and stationary pins. The maximum pulley speeds of the 'Reddrop-Periflo' Mill are 1450 on the smaller and 1000 rev per min on the larger sizes. The top cover is removable for cleaning and for changing the discs, which can be supplied in different forms to suit different materials. Discharge is from the bottom of the casing which is connected to a bag, or by a sleeve to a box. Two or three filter sleeves are fitted to the openings in the top cover, to allow the escape of air which is drawn in by the centrifugal action. These mills are adapted for the fine grinding of substances with low melting points, such as resin, soap, sugar, etc. The mill described is the smallest size and has an output of up to 100 kg per hr, with a power consumption of 1.5 kW. Larger sizes are made with outputs up to 6 tonnes per hr and power consumptions of 30 kW.

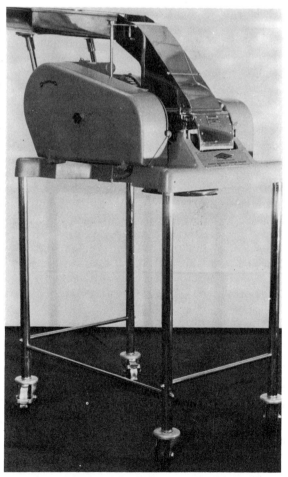

roots, herbs, glands, livers, soaps, etc. They can also be used for size enlargement or granulation of powders as a preliminary to tabletting (see Chapter 19).

Pin Mills

These rely on the high speed rotation of a series of pins located on a plate which revolves against a similar plate leaving a small clearance for the passage of the drug being comminuted. Typical is the 'Reddrop-Periflo' Mill.

The upper disc is fitted to the cover while the lower disc rotates, driven by a vertical spindle and gearing. The material is fed in through the centre of the upper disc and is thrown outwards by the centrifugal force of the rotating disc and broken

FIG. 17.4. Manesty Fitzmill comminuting machine (Manesty Machines Ltd.).

Ball Mills

In ball mills the material is ground by the impact and friction of a large number of balls in a rotating vessel. Different models vary greatly in size and form. They produce fine powders; the fineness depending on a number of operating variables such as the speed of the mill, the size, nature, path and load of the balls and the charge of material being handled. A great deal of work has been done on all these aspects over the last few years (Hukki 1959; Riley 1965). Steel balls are often the most efficient, but they may produce deterioration or contamination of certain acidic products and porcelain, flint, steel, nylon or rubber balls can be employed instead: mills can be of steel or porcelain or may be rubber-lined. There are considerable variations in the recommendations for ball load. With steel balls, a load of about 33 per cent of the mill volume is often used, but for porcelain or nylon balls it may be as high as 55 per cent. Overloading causes the mill to 'choke'.

The mill speed should usually be between about 50 and 65 per cent of the critical centrifugal speed, i.e. the speed at which the balls stick to the inner walls of the rotating vessel. This ensures that their motion is that of cascading, i.e. slipping smoothly over each other, rather than being thrown—cataracting—or sliding en masse round the walls of the vessel. Generally, the balls should be as small as practicable, consistent with the size of the feed and the arrangements available for straining them from the product; commonly they are 12 mm or less in diameter and spherical in shape, though for some purposes 'cylpebs' (cylindrical pebbles) are preferred. There appear to be no particular advantages in using balls of mixed sizes, though it has been claimed that they sometimes help to maintain the charge mobility in the mill.

A modification to the conventional ball mill is the Hardinge mill. This has a conical centre section and as the charge rotates, differential centrifugal forces cause the finer particles to move to the discharge end. In this way, the mill operates simultaneously for size reduction and classification. It may be connected also to an air classifier in which a stream of air is passed through the mill, the fines being transported upwards and recovered in a cyclone separator. The principle of closed circuit grinding, thus outlined, is widely used in the pharmaceutical industry, and has the advantages of accelerating the grinding process by continuously removing the fines which otherwise tend to cushion the larger particles, eliminating problems of dust and overheating, and producing a closely graded product free from oversized and undersized material.

Vibration Mills

Vibration mills are similar to ball mills in that particles of the material are crushed between porcelain or metal balls and the mill body. Here, however, the energy is supplied by vibrating the mill body. The mill is supported on a spring base and is subjected to forced vibrations induced either by rotating out of balance weights or by electromagnetic means.

Laboratory models are usually restricted to one frequency and amplitude of vibration. Fig. 17.5 shows details of the GEC VM25 electromagnetic vibration mill which has been successfully employed on a semi-production scale. Drugs and excipients are readily ground to less than 5 μm diameter, the grinding time being considerably less than is required in normal ball milling. As a result the efficiency of the comminution process in vibration milling is a good deal greater than it is in ball milling (Rose & Sullivan 1961).

Micronizing

The process of micronizing or jet milling is now frequently employed in the pharmaceutical industry and involves grinding particles upon themselves (Dotson 1962).

Coarse particles are fed into a flat cylindrical grinding chamber of highly resistant stainless or alloy steel; air, or superheated steam at high pressure, is then injected through the jets spaced round the periphery of the chamber, causing the material to circulate at high speed. The violent impacts, which occur rupture the particles and, as a result of the centrifugal motion, classification takes place into different sizes. The larger particles move to the outer grinding zone and the finer ones towards the centre of the chamber, being eventually expelled in the exhaust gas, from which they are recovered with a cyclone collector, which may or may not be an integral part of the equipment.

Commercial micronizers range in size from about 5 cm to 1 m in diameter and have throughputs of up to 2000 kg per hr depending on their size, the characteristics of the product and the size range required. When operated at relatively low jet pressures, e.g. 20 to 40 lb per in² (1.4 to 2.8 kg/cm²) their main action is in breaking up aggregates of particles without rupturing the individual crystals and at these pressures therefore, there is little change in the surface area of the powder as measured for example, by nitrogen adsorption. But

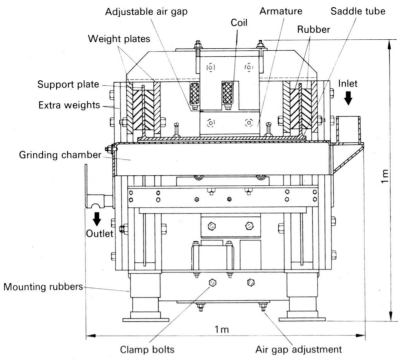

Adjustable air gap · Armature · Saddle tube · Coil · Rubber · Weight plates · Support plate · Extra weights · Inlet · Grinding chamber · Outlet · Mounting rubbers · Clamp bolts · Air gap adjustment · 1 m

FIG. 17.5. Vibration mill.

at higher pressures, 60 to 80 lb per in² (4.2 to 5.6 kg/cm²), the individual crystals are ruptured and there is a large increase in surface area. On the whole, micronized drugs are smoother and less irregular in shape than those which have been ground by other methods; particles become increasingly spherical in shape as the period of micronizing is increased.

The mills described in the above section are only a selection of the available types. All have their particular advantages and no one mill will do all that is required in pharmaceutical practice.

The art of milling requires much experience to be able to select the right kind and size of mill to give the required result. While flour milling has been reduced to a practically automatic process, drug milling cannot be done in this way, since each different material has its own distinctive properties and requires special treatment. A powdered drug produced in a ball mill differs from that produced in a micronizer even though both powders may be screened to the same fineness, the difference being due to the shape of the particles, their roughness and their internal pore structure. A fibrous material ground in an Apex mill will give a much more fluffy powder than the same material ground in a ball mill. Substances of a resinous or oily nature should not be subjected to heavy pressures or much

heat, as a pasty mass may result; they are better treated in a micronizer or hammer mill, than in a heavy edge runner mill. Much heat is produced in the grinding process and this is particularly noticeable in high speed mills. When a current of air passes through the mill, as in closed circuit grinding, the material often loses considerably in weight due to the evaporation of moisture. Powders that have lost weight in this way usually tend to regain it on storage.

In the *British Pharmacopoeia*, the degree of comminution of materials varies according to the purpose for which they are required, from crushed, e.g. gentian for the preparation of tincture, to very fine, e.g. calomel in injections of mercurous chloride.

Particle size characteristics, particularly in the case of sparingly soluble drugs, have a profound influence on their rate of absorption in the stomach or gastrointestinal tract, and hence on their efficiency when administered orally. Penicillin in a medium of aluminium monostearate plus arachis oil, appears to be most effective when 90 per cent of the particles are smaller than 5 μm. The relatively insoluble sulphonamides attain their maximum antibacterial activity at crystal sizes of about 1 μm or below (Neuman & Axon 1961). For insufflations the drug should usually be smaller than about 5 μm.

For the preparation of extracts of vegetable drugs, the grade varies from coarse to fine powder, the components of compound powders are all finely powdered and in the preparation of tinctures, bruised to moderately coarse powders are used. Powders used for extraction by percolation should not contain a large proportion of fines, as this would result in uneven extraction of the material. Coarse and moderately coarse powders, with a minimum of fine powder are most easily obtained by using a high speed impact mill. Materials such as cascara, liquorice, belladonna leaf and root, and ginger are all easily broken down in such mills. When fine powders are required, many drugs can still be broken down in high speed impact mills by fitting finer screens; the finer the screen the slower the process becomes, and with very tough materials the process is very slow.

Fine powders of tough or fibrous materials such as nux vomica or ipecacuanha are often produced in two stages, a preliminary treatment in an Apex mill and a final grinding to the required grade in a ball mill or edge runner mill. Substances which are hygroscopic such as potassium carbonate, or very poisonous such as triturations of the alkaloids, are most easily prepared in closed porcelain ball mills. The fineness of grinding of some drugs produces changes in their properties. For example, the viscosity of mucilage of tragacanth prepared from No. 60 powder will be greater than that prepared from No. 120 powder, both powders having been prepared from the same sample of gum. Tragacanth should therefore never be ground to a finer powder than is necessary. The industrial grades of acacia which sometimes tend to give ropy solutions are often improved by fine grinding. Powders used as absorbents have that property enhanced by fine grinding. Spontaneous combustion sometimes occurs in finely powdered resins and hard soap since the greatly increased surface area accelerates oxidation and produces heat. In the case of soap, it can generally be traced to the quality of the olive oil used in its manufacture, unrefined oil often being the cause.

The colour of powders is affected by the degree of comminution and also by the proportion of particles which are finer than the designated grade. As previously stated, there is a difference between powders of the same grade produced in different mills. Powders produced in ball mills and particularly in edge runner mills usually contain a high proportion of fines which tend to cause a 'white' powder to appear 'whiter' and affects the tint of a coloured powder.

OTHER TECHNIQUES FOR PRODUCING FINE PARTICLES

Mention will be made elsewhere in this book of certain other techniques for producing materials in the form of fine particles, but for completeness it will be convenient to give brief details of them here also, since they are widely employed in industry in the preparation and purification of drugs and other pharmaceutical powders.

Precipitation

Precipitation occurs when solutions of materials which react chemically are mixed to form a product which is but sparingly soluble in the liquid, and therefore deposits out. Precipitation is a convenient method for producing solids in a very fine state of subdivision down to 0.1 μm in diameter. It is also widely used as a method of purifying powders since the required product and its impurities will generally be soluble to different extents in the liquid medium that has been employed. Examples of pharmaceutical substances commonly prepared by precipitation are calcium and magnesium carbonates made by treating the respective chlorides with sodium carbonate solution, ammoniated mercury made by adding a solution of mercuric chloride to a solution of ammonia, and yellow mercuric oxide made by adding a warm solution of mercuric chloride to a solution of sodium hydroxide.

Hot, concentrated solutions usually produce heavy, coarse precipitates which can be fairly readily freed from contaminating salts by washing. But the precipitates from cold dilute solutions are usually much finer and it may be difficult to free them from impurities adsorbed on to their very large surface area. In many cases the order of mixing the solutions can influence the type of precipitate obtained. For example, when a solution of an iron salt is poured into an excess of a solution of sodium carbonate, iron carbonate $Fe_2(CO_3)_3$ is produced, but if the procedure is reversed the product will also contain basic salts such as $Fe(HCO_3)_3$, $Fe(OH)(CO_3)_2$, etc., which may be difficult to remove.

Crystallization

Crystallization differs from precipitation in that the product deposits from a supersaturated solution, rather than from a liquid in which it is insoluble. The basic steps in crystallization are first to achieve a supersaturated solution, then to provide nuclei on to which the material can deposit in the form of microcrystals, a few hundredths or even thousandths of a micron in size, and finally to allow these microcrystals to grow up to normal crystal dimensions so that they settle to the bottom of the containing vessel and can be separated from the supernatant liquid. Crystals will only grow if the solution is supersaturated and the rate of growth is proportional to the degree of super-saturation (Dunning 1961; Dunning & Albon 1959).

The shapes and sizes of the crystals formed are markedly dependent on the conditions under which the crystallization is carried out. For example, griseofulvin crystallized from acetone has a different form from the same drug crystallized from benzene or chloroform. A derivative of an organic acid used in an insufflation has large needle shaped crystals when precipitated from hot alcohol and cubic crystals when precipitated from acetone–alcohol mixtures. Crystallization, like precipitation, is also widely used as a method for removing impurities from pharmaceutical products before they are incorporated in capsule or tablet formulations. The need for lengthy grinding in machines can often be avoided by correctly choosing the conditions of the crystallization itself to produce the drug directly in the state of fineness that is required.

Crystallization equipment is most readily classified according to the method employed for producing the supersaturated solution. Supersaturation can be achieved by cooling, by evaporation of the solvent, by a combination of cooling and evaporation and by salting out, i.e. adding another solute to the solution to reduce the solubility of the substance in question. Equipment in commercial use includes tank crystallizers, agitated batch crystallizers, the Svenson Walker Crystallizer, the Krystal and other vacuum crystallizers and details of their design and operation will be found in textbooks of chemical engineering (Badger & Banchero 1955).

SIEVING AND SIFTING

A feature of the modern pharmaceutical industry is the increased use that is being made of materials in a fine state of subdivision. Numerous methods have been developed for sifting powders and determining their particle size. Of these sieving is undoubtedly the most common, being applicable to practically all powders from about 40 μm upwards.

SIEVING

In the U.K., the British Standard Sieve is extensively used both for scientific work on powders and for separating them into fractions on a commercial scale. In Europe the German DIN (Deutsche Industrienormen) is widely used. But different standards are used for German, American and other sieves. To state that a sieve has a certain mesh is meaningless unless the diameter of the wire constituting the mesh is also specified. This will determine the size of the opening. Clearly the opening will always be smaller than the measurement suggested in the 'mesh designation'.

TABLE 7.1

WIRE MESH SIEVES

Sieve Number	Preferred Average Wire Diameter	Tolerance for Average Aperture Size	Approximate Sieving Area
mm	mm	mm	per cent
3.35	1.25	0.10	53
2.00	0.90	0.060	48
1.70	0.80	0.051	46
1.18	0.63	0.035	43
μm	μm	μm	
710	450	28	37
600	400	24	36
500	315	20	38
425	280	17	36
355	224	14	38
250	160	13	37
180	125	11	35
150	100	9.4	36
125	90	8.1	34
106	71	7.4	36
90	63	6.6	35
75	50	6.1	36
53	36	4.8	35

TABLE 7.2

PERFORATED PLATE TEST SIEVE

Sieve Number	Preferred Plate Thickness	Minimum Width of Bridge	Tolerance on Nominal Aperture Size	Sieving Area
mm	mm	mm	mm	per cent
6.70	1.0	1.3	6.70	47

To obtain reproducible results in a particle size analysis it is necessary to adhere closely to the detailed procedure given in British Standards 410 (1969). The powder under test is passed through a number of sieves of increasingly smaller mesh size and the weight remaining on each sieve is measured. The method of shaking the sieves is important; for rapid sieving it is usual to use a mechanical shaker that imparts gyratory and vibratory movement to spread the material over the whole of the mesh. Errors can arise if the sieves are overloaded or if insufficient time is allowed for the particles to pass through (Heywood 1963).

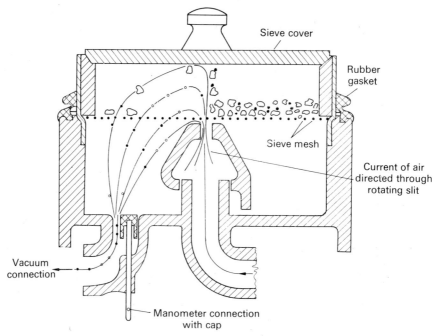

FIG. 17.6. Alpine airjet sieve.

The Alpine Airjet Sieve

In recent years the Alpine Airjet sieve has been developed to extend the range of conventional sieves which tend to block at particle sizes below about 80 μm. The action of the sieve depends on a jet of air instead of mechanical vibration. Its purpose is to fluidize the powder, thereby preventing blocking of the mesh and at the same time cushioning the particles from impact with the mesh which, in the case of soft powders, artificially produces fines.

The apparatus shown in Fig. 17.6 consists essentially of a metal housing into which the sieve mesh is fitted. Powder is placed on the mesh which is then covered by a close fitting lid and is fluidized by an upward jet of air directed on to its lower surface through a rotating slit. A vacuum is simultaneously created in the interior of the housing so that the undersized powder is sucked through the sieve into a paper filter from which it can be recovered if required.

Having checked that the upper edge of the rotating slit is level with the upper edge of the housing, the finest sieve is fitted into the machine and the plastic sealing ring drawn downwards until an airtight seal is obtained.

About 10 g of the material under examination is carefully weighed, and spread on to the sieve, and the cover placed in position. The slit is set into rotation and the suction adjusted until the manometer reads 200 mm. Sieving is continued for 2 minutes, the residual powder is weighed, transferred to the next sized mesh with a fine brush and the process continued until the sieve anlysis is complete.

Airjet sieving has a number of advantages over the more conventional method. It is rapid, produces closer and more reproducible size cuts, is not subject to the clogging which occurs in hand or vibration sieving at small sizes in particular, and probably gives a truer result since there is less tendency for fines to be formed as a result of the sieving itself. Against these advantages, however, must be set the fact that Airjet sieves have a relatively small capacity which makes them unsuitable for handling large quantities of powders. They are thus primarily used for determining the particle size range of a powder rather than for classifying it.

CLASSIFIERS AND SIFTERS

Most commercial classifiers and sifters are based on the principle of sieving (Cremer & Davies 1957). Thus in the Pascall Turbine Sifter there is a cylindrical screen which is divided into two or three compartments, in each of which there is a turbine beater, which drives an air current through the screen and carries the fine powder with it. This is drawn off from the base of the machine, the air is recirculated and the coarse material is discharged from a spout at the side. Brush sifters employ brushes to separate the fine and coarse particles on the sieve mesh and are useful for greasy or sticky powder such as waxes and soaps. One design has three circular brushes mounted on a triangular structure. The sieves are mounted on a delivery funnel of stainless steel or enamel and the whole unit (Fig. 17.7) is supported on a wheeled trolley for ease of movement.

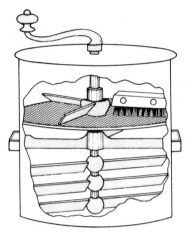

Fig. 17.7. Brush sifter.

In recent years there has been an increasing demand for pharmaceutical powders like griseofulvin, and aspirin in an extremely fine state of subdivision, i.e. less than 10 μm and this has necessitated the use of what are essentially centrifugal classifiers. One example is the Cutrock classifier (Goodridge, Badzoick & Hawksley 1962). It consists of three rotating discs mounted in a cylindrical chamber. The drug flows from a buffer along a vibrating feeder and is drawn into the classifier by a stream of air passing along an axial inlet. It then flows radically outwards between discs.

The rotation of the discs causes the air stream to spin with the result that the larger particles circulate in an annular gap between the edge of the discs and the casing of the chamber, while the smaller ones are expelled through the exit and can be collected in a bag. By appropriately choosing the speed of operation of the machine, it is possible to collect only the particles smaller than a particular size and return the rest for further grinding until they meet the specification that has been set.

For larger scale classification the Alpine Mikroplex and the Hosokawa types are useful. These again employ the centrifugal principle and have rotating blades which can be set at different angles to achieve separations ranging from 3 up to about 50 μm diameter. Depending on the material being handled and the particle size of the fraction to be collected, the outputs from these machines are between about 50 and 5000 kg per hr.

DETERMINATION OF PARTICLE SIZE

There are a number of methods available for measuring the sizes of particles in a powder (Edmundson 1967) and in principle all would yield the same result if the particles were uniform in size, spherical, smooth and non-porous and of equal density. In fact, however, real powders contain particles of a range of sizes, shapes, densities and porosities and the value obtained thus depends to a considerable extent on the method of measurement and on the conventions used for defining particle size. The particle size may be defined in terms of the dimensions and shape of the particle, e.g. a mean diameter based on direct observation, or one may refer to a mean diameter calculated from the volume of the particle or its surface area (Heywood 1963). Particles having similar shapes may be compared for size by microscopic examination or sieving; particles with similar hydrodynamic properties by sedimentation or elutriation and particles with similar porosities and surface characteristics by gas permeability or gas adsorption. The size ranges covered by some of these different methods are indicated in Table 17.3.

TABLE 17.3

Method	Useful range
Sieving	Above 33 μm
Optical microscopy	0.2 to 100 μm
Electron microscopy	0.005 to 1 μm
Sedimentation and elutriation	2 to 50 μm
Gas permeability	5 to 100 μm
Gas adsorption	0.005 to 20 μm
Coulter counters	1 to 100 μm

MICROSCOPY

A representative portion of the powder is placed in a glass slide and viewed through a microscope. The images are compared with reference circles of known size inscribed on a graticule and in this way

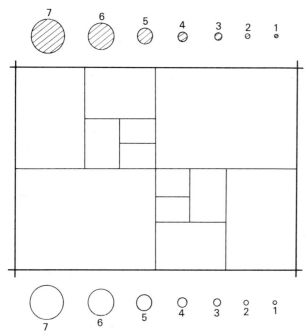

FIG. 17.8. Diagrammatic standard graticule (approximately to scale).

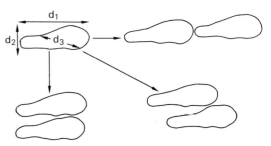

FIG. 17.9. Beam splitting device.

applied to the beam splitting device to get the two images into edge to edge contact.

SEDIMENTATION METHODS

These are based on the measurement of the rate at which particles of the powder settle out from a liquid in which they have been dispersed. The technique is widely employed and can be extended down to sizes of about 0.5 μm under special circumstances by using a centrifuge to accelerate the settlement.

the relative number of particles of each size present in the sample may be determined. In most powders the frequency of occurrence of particles increases rapidly as their size diminishes and it is therefore necessary to measure large numbers of particles— 200 to 300—to ensure a representative count. The actual procedure to be adopted has now been standardized and is described in British Standards, the standard graticule being illustrated in Fig. 17.8.

The percentage by weight of particles in each size range, i.e. between consecutively numbered circles on the graticule, is denoted q_r, thus

$$q_r = 100 N_r d_r^3 / \sum (N_r d_r^3)$$

where N_r is the number of particles of this size per unit area of the graticule, d_r is their mean diameter and the symbol $\sum$ denotes the summation of all the products of $(N_r d_r^3)$.

In cases where the powder contains particles of irregular, non-spherical shape, double image microscopy is useful. The microscope is fitted with a beam splitting device (Timbrell 1959), which is situated between the objective lens and the eyepiece. This forms two identical images of any particular particle which is in the field of view. The images are brought into edge to edge contact along different diameters, as illustrated in Fig. 17.9 and the length of each diameter $d_1 d_2 d_3$ is obtained in turn by reading off the shear that has been

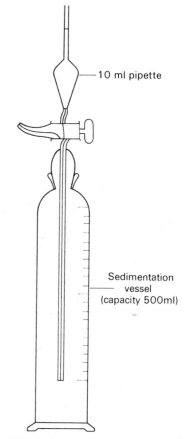

— 10 ml pipette

Sedimentation vessel (capacity 500ml)

FIG. 17.10. Andreasen apparatus.

In the incremental method (British Standards 1963) the powder is suitably dispersed in the liquid contained in a tall vessel, as shown in Fig. 17.10. Ten ml samples are withdrawn at redetermined times from a known depth below the surface and the weight of powder present in each sample is determined either by evaporating the liquid and weighing the residue, or by some suitable assay method.

In order to calculate the range of particle sizes present in each sample, use is made of Stokes's Law. This applies strictly only to dilute dispersions where the concentration of solid is less than 2 per cent (w/w).

This can be written as

$$V = \frac{h}{t} = \frac{d^2(\rho - \rho')g}{18\eta}$$

where V is the velocity of fall of a particle, h is the depth in cm below the surface from which the sample is withdrawn after t s, d is the diameter of the particle in cm, ρ is the density of the material in g per ml, ρ' is the density of the liquid in g per ml, g is the gravitational constant 981 cm s^{-2}, η is the viscosity of the liquid in poises.

Knowing all the terms in this equation, d, the diameter of the largest particles present at the depth h cm after t s, can be calculated and this sets the upper limit of size in each 10-ml sample of liquid that has been withdrawn.

For the calculation it is convenient to write

$$d = 175 \sqrt{\frac{h\eta}{(\rho_1 - \rho_2)t}} \ \mu m,$$

where η and t are now expressed in centipoises and minutes, respectively.

The cumulative percentage W of material smaller than size d is given by:

$$W = \frac{w \times V}{w_s \times V_\rho} \times 100$$

where w is the weight of the solid in the withdrawn sample, V is the total volume of the sedimentation vessel (usually about 1 litre), w_s is the weight of the withdrawn sample (usually about 10 g), V_ρ is the volume of the pipette in ml, and is plotted against particle size to give a cumulative distribution curve in the usual way.

The cumulative method of sedimentation analysis is carried out with a sedimentation balance (Stairmand 1947).

As before, the powder is uniformly dispersed in a liquid but now a continuous record is kept of the weight that settles on a balance pan which is immersed in the liquid column. For the purpose of computation:

$$W = w - \frac{dw}{d \ln t}$$

where w is the weight of particles that settle in time t seconds, and W is the fraction by weight of particles greater than a particular diameter in microns, which is calculated by Stokes' Law from a knowledge of the height of the suspension above the balance pan, the density of the particles and the density and viscosity of the medium. For accurate results it is necessary to observe a number of precautions when using a sedimentation balance. These include ensuring its freedom from vibration, accurate temperature control to eliminate convection currents and the employment only of dilute suspensions less than about 2 per cent w/w.

GAS PERMEABILITY

The gas permeability of a powder provides a measure of its surface area and if it is assumed that the particles are all of equal size and spherical in shape, then their mean diameter can be evaluated.

In the Lea and Nurse method (Orr & Dallavalle 1959), dry air is forced at constant pressure through a bed of the powder under investigation. In the Rigden method, which has been adapted from it, air is allowed to escape from a reservoir through the powder bed and the time for the pressure to fall from one specified level to another is measured.

The Rigden apparatus is shown schematically in Fig. 17.11. The two ends of the cell E containing the powder are connected to the two ends of a U tube containing a non-volatile oil. The equilibrium level of the oil is at C. The oil is sucked into one arm Y of the manometer by means of the bulb F and as it returns to the equilibrium level, it forces air through the powder bed. The time taken for a given volume of oil to travel between the starting line to mark A or B on the manometer is measured and the specific surface is calculated from the Kozeny equation. This can be written:

$$S = \left[\frac{\varepsilon^3}{(1-\varepsilon)^2} \frac{A}{5\eta L} \frac{\beta\rho g}{V} \ln\left(\frac{h_2}{h_1}\right) \frac{t}{d^2} \right]^{1/3}$$

where S is the specific surface in cm^{2}g^{-1}, ε is the porosity, A is the cross-sectional area of the powder bed, η is the gas viscosity in poises, L is the length of the powder bed, β is the atmospheric pressure in cm of liquid of density ρ g cm^{-3}, g is

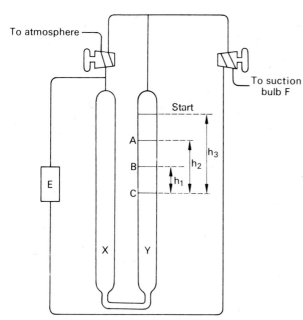

FIG. 17.11. Rigden apparatus (schematic).

the gravitational constant in cm s^{-2}, V is the volume of the reservoir, h_2 is the final reservoir pressure in cm of liquid, h_1 is the initial reservoir pressure in cm of liquid, d is the density of the powder sample in g cm^{-3}, t is the time in s for the air pressure to fall from h_1 to h_2.

For a given apparatus and porosity the equation reduces to:

$$S = \frac{K}{d} \sqrt{t},$$

where K is a constant.

A convenient, semi-automatic piece of equipment employing the same principle, is the Fisher sub-sieve sizer in which air at a constant pressure is forced through the powder bed. The pressure drop is read off from a water manometer and by means of a calculator chart is converted into an average value of particle size.

GAS ADSORPTION

The amount of gas that will be adsorbed by a powder also provides a means of determining its total surface area, and this type of measurement is conveniently carried out with the Perkin-Elmer Shell Sorptometer (Fig. 17.12). Basically the apparatus consists of two valves for controlling the flow of nitrogen and helium gas.

These flow through a cold trap then through the

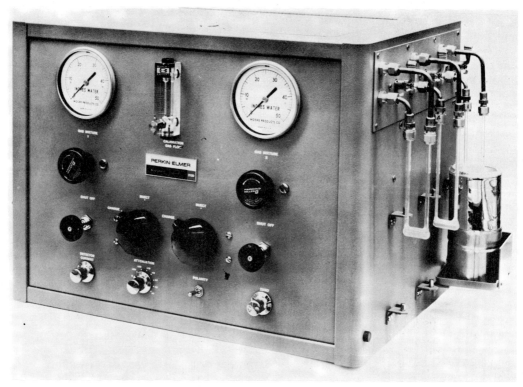

FIG. 17.12. Perkin Elmer sorptometer.

reference arm of a detector unit, then through an adsorption tube containing a known weight of the sample which has previously been freed from adsorbed gas by subjecting it to a high vacuum, and finally through the measuring arm of the detector. The amount of nitrogen adsorbed by the powder at a series of different partial pressures of nitrogen is obtained by continually measuring the thermal conductivity of the emergent gas stream, and the surface area per g of the sample, is then obtained from the BET equation.

COULTER COUNTER

This apparatus is coming increasingly into use in pharmacy for determining the particle size of powders (Edmundson 1967) and depends on the ability to prepare a suspension of the sample free from floccules or aggregates. The suspension is made up in a suitable electrolyte solution, e.g. NaCl, and is then drawn through a small orifice, having an electrode on each side, Fig. 17.13. As each

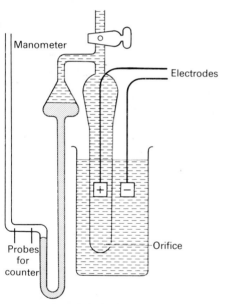

FIG. 17.13. Coulter counter.

particle passes through, it displaces its own volume of electrolyte within the orifice and momentarily increases its electrical resistance. The resulting voltage pulses are proportional to the particle volume; they are amplified, scaled and counted and yield a particle size distribution curve extending, under ideal circumstances, down to about 0.2 μm. On the whole the results agree fairly well with

those obtained by sedimentation. But on occasions there can be considerable discrepancies with the microscopic results. This is probably due to the difficulty encounted in some cases in achieving complete dispersion of the particles.

PARTICLE SHAPE

Even to describe a moderately irregularly shaped body in exact mathematical terms is a matter of great complexity and in practice it is more usual to simplify the procedure by assuming that all particles can be considered as ellipsoids, whose axes are a_1, a_2 and a_3 such that $a_1 > a_2 > a_3$. The ratio a_1/a_2 is defined as the elongation ratio and a_2/a_3 as the flatness ratio. If a_1 is similar to a_2 and $a_2 \gg a_3$, the elongation ratio is about unity, the flatness ratio is large and the particle is described as disc shaped. If $a_1 \gg a_2$ and a_2 is similar to a_3, the elongation ratio is large, the flatness ratio is about unity and the particle is described as acicular (needle-shaped). If $a_1 \gg a_2 \gg a_3$, then both the flatness and the elongation ratios are large and the particle is described as ribbon shaped (Neumann 1967).

A more refined way of defining shape (Heywood 1963) is to include in these ratios a term which also takes into account the geometrical form, e.g. a prism, ellipsoid, tetrahedron, to which the particle most closely approximates, but even this procedure breaks down in the case of complex shaped particles, for example, those containing bends, re-entrant angles or cavities.

In order to specify the 'shape' of a powder, it is necessary to examine a large and representative number of particles, usually under the microscope, and calculate an average value for the elongation and flatness ratios. Alternatively, the shape may be defined simply as the ratio of the average particle diameter, as determined in some direct way, like sieving or microscopy, to the average particle diameter determined in an indirect way like sedimentation or gas permeability. Each pair of methods will give rise to a different shape factor.

The shape of particles is often affected by the method employed for preparing them. Spray dried products, for example, tend to be spherical in shape, as do micronized products. The angularity of products seems to increase with the type of mill used for reducing them to powder form in the order micronizer, ball mill, pin mill, hammer mill (Rose 1961).

As in the case of particle sizes, the shapes of particles have an important influence on certain of their properties which are relevant in pharmaceutical practice. In the dry state, irregular particles tend to be less free flowing than spherical particles, but may be able to pack together more closely giving a higher bulk density. The rheological properties of pharmaceutical suspensions are also affected by the shapes of the particles that they contain.

HANDLING PROPERTIES

SLIDING AND FLOW

With the increasing employment of materials in powder form, not only in pharmacy, but also in many other branches of technology, it has become necessary to examine what, for a better term, may be designated the handling properties of powders. This means the way in which powders slide in pipes or chutes, pack down when stored in silos, flow from hoppers and form into heaps when tipped or dumped. Pharmacists have long recognized that some powders are inherently more cohesive than others, that fine grade griseofulvin, for example, is less free flowing than spray dried lactose, so that it cannot be sieved through a 30 μm sieve even when its individual particles, as measured by gas adsorption or sedimentation, may be as small as 5 μm.

If one separates a powder or granular mass into its different sizes and then measures the rate at which these flow through a particular size of orifice, one finds that a graph can be plotted between flow rate and particle size, as shown schematically in Fig. 17.14.

There are two regions where the orifice blocks,

one where the particle diameter exceeds about one fifth of the diameter of the orifice, the other at the very small particle size, below about 100 μm. Here they form into a dome over the orifice, rather like bricks over a doorway.

This sort of behaviour is characteristic of virtually all materials, though the position and height of the maximum in the curve, and the position where blocking occurs, vary from one material to another, being dependent on such properties as the density, shape, roughness of the particles concerned.

It is convenient to label material that will pass through an orifice as free flowing, but material which will not, even though its particles are very much smaller than the orifice, as cohesive. A number of techniques is available for studying powders in both the free flowing and in the cohesive size range.

Methods for Free Flowing Powders and Granules
(a) The angle of friction α may be defined as the angle to which a particular surface must be elevated from the horizontal before the powder begins to slide upon it. It is measured conveniently by placing the material on a chute, which is pivoted at one end and raised at the other by means of a screw. Clearly the value obtained for α will depend on the roughness of the surface. But it also depends on the thickness of the powder bed. In general, the thicker the bed and the more it has been packed down during preparation the greater the value of α (Jones & Pilpel 1966).

(b) The so-called angle of repose of a powder θ, is the angle of elevation to the horizontal at which the powder commences to slide upon itself. Numerous methods have been devised for measuring it (Pilpel 1965; Neumann 1967). Thus the powder may be allowed to flow out of a funnel to form a conical heap and θ calculated from the base radius r and hypotenuse h of the cone by substituting into the expression: $\cos \theta = r/h$.

Alternatively, the cone may be formed by placing an open ended cylinder on a base of the same radius, filling it with powder and then raising it slowly to leave a conical heap behind. Both these methods yield a so-called three dimensional angle of repose. The two dimensional angle of repose can be obtained with similar equipment to that used for the angle of friction, but noting this time the angle of elevation when the surface layer of powder begins to slide on the rest of the bed. For this purpose it is clearly necessary to use a chute with a rough surface to prevent the whole powder bed sliding off it.

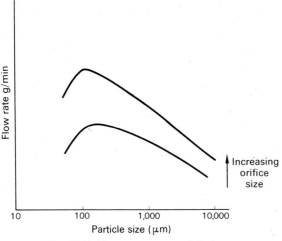

FIG. 17.14. Flow rate versus particle size.

The angle of repose varies within about $\pm 2°$ depending on the experimental method employed; other factors affecting its value are the size of the particles in the powder, their shape and roughness. The angle decreases fairly regularly with particle size in the range 200 to 2000 μm and can be expressed by:

$$\theta = AD_p^{-1} + B$$

where A and B are constants for any particular material and D_p is the particle size concerned.

The presence of fines, additives and moisture can produce considerable changes in the value of the angle of repose and for this reason its measurement is usefully employed as a means of monitoring the quality of powders being produced in batch or in continuous processes. For example, if one observes an increase in the angle of repose, the powder may have become damp or may now contain an increased proportion of fine sizes.

(c) The most direct method for free flowing powders is simply to measure the rate at which they emerge through the orifice of a suitable container or hopper. A large number of investigations of this type have been reported (Pilpel 1965; Neumann 1967). One rather unexpected finding is that whereas the rate of flow of a liquid through an orifice is directly proportional to the head of liquid, in the case of a powder, the head height has practically no effect on the rate. This arises in part because of the complex movement of the powder in the immediate vicinity of the orifice, as shown in Fig. 17.15.

Outside the trumpet-shaped region above the hole, denoted E, the powder is at rest. In region A the particles are sliding rapidly over region B, which in turn is sliding slowly over region E. Particles from A and B slide into C down slopes which are inclined to the horizontal at angles greater than the angle of repose and then move rapidly downwards and inwards into D. Once in D they accelerate and emerge in a stream which is noticeably narrower than the orifice. This phenomenon is referred to as the vena contracta.

The most important single factor controlling the rate at which a powder emerges from a circular horizontal orifice appears to be the orifice diameter D_0 and one can therefore write:

$$W \propto D_0^n$$

where W is the flow rate in g/s, D_0 is the orifice diameter in cm and n is a numerical term, which for many materials lies between 2.5 and 3.2. Other factors controlling the flow rate include the particle

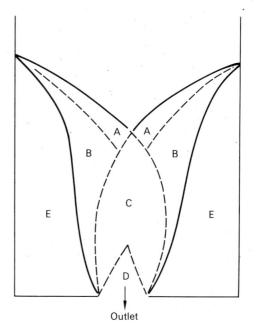

FIG. 17.15. Flow contours in a hopper (schematic).

shape, size, density and roughness and the geometry of the containing vessel. The equation:

$$D_0 = A\left(\frac{4W}{60\pi\rho\sqrt{g}}\right)^{1/n}$$

where A and $1/n$ are functions of these factors and g is the acceleration due to gravity, has been successfully used for predicting the flow rate of different materials, not only when they have been sieved into close size cuts, but also when they contain a range of sizes in the free flowing region. In this case one employs a geometrical mean particle diameter for the purpose of evaluating the terms A and $1/n$ (Jones & Pilpel 1966). Some typical figures illustrating the agreement between flow rates as measured and those predicted from the equation are shown in Table 17.4.

TABLE 17.4

TERNARY MIXTURES OF MAGNESIA GRANULES

Mixture per cent w/w size (cm)			Orifice D_0 cm	Flow rate (g/min) Calcu- lated	Observed	Error (per cent)
0.056	0.025	0.009				
10	20	70	0.90	586	678– 684	− 14
60	20	20	1.35	1750	1930–2015	− 9
60	20	20	0.74	363	372– 387	− 2
0.056	0.025	0.005				
10	10	80	0.90	394	356– 387	+ 2
50	40	10	1.35	1763	1968–2040	− 10
50	40	10	0.74	368	350– 361	+ 3

Methods for Cohesive Powders

The problem of expressing in quantitative terms the handling properties of non-free flowing materials is more difficult and has recently been reviewed in detail (Pilpel 1971). One earlier technique (Hawksley 1947) is to mix into the powder coarser particles of sand until the mixture just starts to flow through a particular size hole and use the amount of sand required as a measure of the cohesiveness of the powder but the method is not very sensitive.

The split plate method (Dawes 1952) involves dredging the powder to form a loose bed on a split, roughened flat surface, one half of which runs on ball bearings. On slowly tilting, the bed separates and if one knows the cross-sectional area of the bed A and the mass of it in the half that has separated, m, then the Tensile Strength is given by:

$$T = \frac{mg \sin \beta}{A} \text{ dyn cm}^{-2}$$

β being the angle of tilt that has caused the bed to separate.

From both the theoretical and the practical point of view, probably the most satisfactory method for measuring the cohesiveness of fine pharmaceutical powders is the shear box method (Jenike 1961; Ashton, Cheng & Farley 1965). The apparatus Fig. 17.16 consists of a cylindrical brass cell which is divided horizontally into a base section, a centre section and a moulding ring, the three being aligned and held in position while filling with powder by means of three vertical pins.

The base section can be moved along steel rails by a motor-driven shaft at a constant speed of 1.25 mm per min and this causes the centre section of the cell to bear against a device which records the shear stress.

Having filled the cell with powder and established the number of twists that must be applied to the lid correctly to consolidate the specimen, the tests consist of applying various normal loads to the lid and measuring the shear stress needed to split the bed horizontally. The results are plotted as shown in Fig. 17.17 to give a series of yield loci, each appropriate to the value of the bulk density achieved during the initial consolidation of the

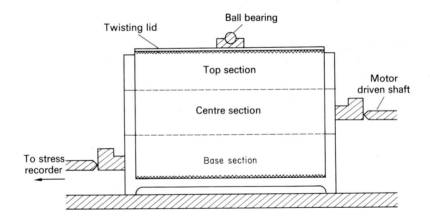

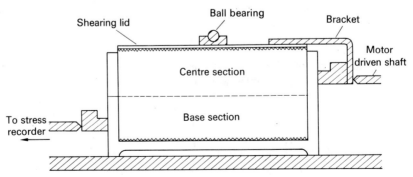

FIG. 17.16. Jenike shear cell, Schematic arrangements for consolidation and shearing respectively.

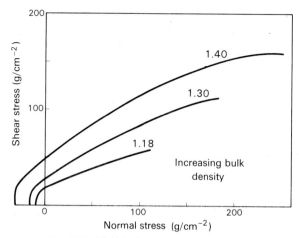

FIG. 17.17. Yield loci at different bulk densities.

specimen. The slope of the yield locus is the internal angle of friction of the powder and its intercept on the ordinate is its cohesiveness.

Data of this type are useful for predicting the way in which pharmaceutical powders are likely to behave during manufacture and during such processing operations as transportation, sieving, granulation, storage and tabletting. A highly cohesive powder tends to compact on storage, flow with difficulty and thus cause blocking of pipes and orifices. It tends to be difficult to sieve into fine fractions as it balls up on the sieve mesh. It may also prove difficult to mix in the dry state with excipients and other ingredients as the first stage in compressing into tablets or filling capsules.

MIXING OF POWDERS AND PARTICULATE SOLIDS

Because of its antiquity and apparent simplicity, it was for a long time assumed that the subject of mixing and blending powders did not require scientific study. But in the last few decades serious limitations in the empirical approach have become apparent as a result of the increased speed of industrial operations and the increased degree of automation in many pharmaceutical firms (Valentine 1965).

Mixing is one of the commonest pharmaceutical operations and occurs in the preparation of many types of formulations. The simplest examples are compounded powders administered as such, e.g. ipecacuanha and opium powder. These may contain natural drugs and medicinal chemicals in varying proportions according to their respective potencies. Mixing is also an intermediate stage in most tablet making processes.

The ease with which different substances will blend to a reasonably homogeneous whole varies considerably, being dependent on various physical properties of the individual components and on their relative proportions. Obviously it is easier to mix equal weights of two powders of similar fineness and density than to incorporate a small proportion of a fine powder in a large mass of a coarse, denser material. Apart from density and particle size, the stickiness of the additive is also important and it may require prolonged mixing effectively to distribute lubricants, wetting agents, etc., into tablet granules.

Mixing is sometimes achieved by feeding two or more materials simultaneously to a mill, if both require grinding. In other cases mixing is accomplished by kneading, and the equipment modified accordingly. In pharmaceutical operations, mixing is usually a batchwise process, although a batch may be as large as 1 tonne. Equipment for continuous mixing is available from the food and other industries, but has only recently been used in pharmacy.

The simplest mixing machines are adapted from the old manual method of heaping materials on the ground and then repeatedly cutting and piling them. One method suitable for materials the granular or crystalline structure of which might be damaged by more vigorous agitation is the tumbling barrel.

It comprises a box or drum in which the powders are mixed by slow rotation. A very simple method of mixing is to place the drum on rollers so that the ingredients within perpetually cascade over one another. Large bulks of mixed powders and powdered drugs, e.g. nux vomica, jalap, etc., which need to be sampled for assay and adjustment of strength, must be thoroughly mixed if the samples taken are to be representative. For quantities of powder of 500 kg or more mixing drums of the type illustrated in Fig. 17.18 are used.

A more efficient design is that of the double cone blender, which is a shallow drum with conical ends which is rotated so that the powder flows from one cone to the other. A further advance on this design in the Y cone blender in which one end is conical, while the other consists of two cylindrical 'legs'. As the blender rotates, the moving mass of powder is continually divided and recombined while entering and leaving the 'legs'. Conical blenders are made in stainless steel or in transparent plastic, the smaller models take a charge of about 20 kg and rotate at 35 rev per min and the larger ones a charge of about 1 tonne, rotating at about 15 rev per min.

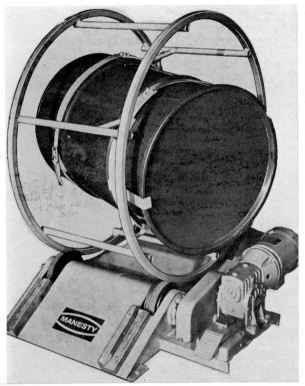

FIG. 17.18. Drum-mixer (Manesty Machines Ltd.).

fitted at the bottom with a distributor, through which compressed air is introduced (Anon 1966). Air emerging from the distributor at a speed of several hundred m per s, causes the powder or granules to spiral upwards. Considerable turbulence occurs in the outer region of each spiral and this is responsible for the mixing action.

Air mixers are fabricated in capacities up to about 50 m^3 and achieve their action in a matter of a few minutes, in comparison with up to several hours in more conventional machines. On the other hand such mixers are not very suitable for sticky or cohesive powders, for very dense substances or for mixtures which contain ingredients having substantially different densities, which cause them to segregate.

Ideally, perfect mixing could be said to have occurred when each particle of one material was lying as nearly adjacent as possible to a particle of another material. But in practice a convenient definition of the degree of mixing of a powder is its standard deviation σ. For a mixture of two components this can be defined by:

$$\sigma = \sqrt{\frac{xy}{N}}$$

where x and y are the proportions of the minor and major constituents and N is the number of particles in the sample taken. Mixing of pharmaceutical powders should be continued until the amount of the active drug that is required in a dose is within ± 3 SD of that found by assay in a representative number of sample doses. To achieve this it is clearly necessary to make N large by milling the ingredients to a sufficient degree of fineness (Train 1960).

For quite a range of pharmaceutical products, particularly those containing cohesive ingredients which tend to ball up into aggregates or ingredients which, as a result of their differing flow properties, tend to segregate or demix, agitation mixers are generally more satisfactory than tumbling mixers.

They consist essentially of a stationary shell with a horizontal or vertical agitator moving inside it. The agitator may take the form of blades, paddles, or a screw. Detailed descriptions of the various types will be found in the Chemical Engineers Handbook.

The preliminary mixing of stiff pastes, such as toothpastes requires slow speed mixers which must be very robust to overcome the friction due to the viscosity of the mixture. The mixer in Fig. 17.19 is a typical example, where two 'Z' blades of polished steel revolve in opposite directions and at different speeds to each other resulting in efficient kneading of the paste.

A recent development in powder mixing is the employment of compressed air or fluidization. The substances to be mixed are introduced through a weight or volume dosimeter into a conical vessel,

GRANULATION OF POWDERS

In pharmaceutical practice two main methods are used for preparing tablets from powders which, in their original state, are neither free flowing nor compressible. These are slugging and wet granulation. Quite recently fluidized bed methods have also been described. (See also Chapter 19.)

Slugging involves strongly compressing the powder between rollers and then breaking it up. The resulting granules are fed into a tabletting machine and because of the double compression to which they have been subjected, now produce satisfactory tablets.

Wet granulation can be done in several ways (Rumpf 1962). The drug, binder, excipients, etc., are mixed together with sufficient water to produce a

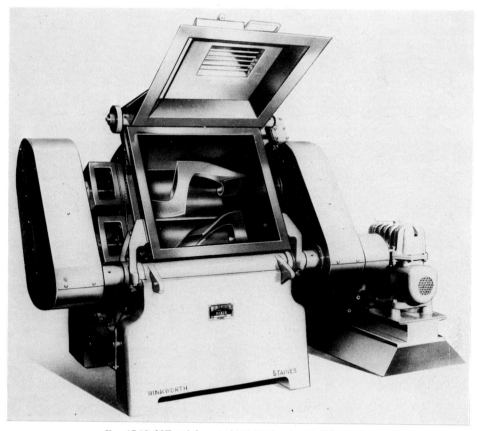

FIG. 17.19. 29Z stainless steel 'Z' blade mixer (162 l capacity).

dough and this is then pressed through a sieve mesh, either mechanically, or by hand. Alternatively, the dough may be extruded through a multiple spout extruder or 'mincing' machine. After drying, the granules are lightly shaken on a B.S. No. 22 sieve, to free them from adhering fine material that may still be present. The Apex and similar mills, e.g. the Fitz mill, which have already been described in connection with comminution of solids, can also be applied to the granulation of powders by feeding in the materials as a dough and using a slow operating speed and a coarse grade of mesh during the breaking process.

Another method of granulation by spray drying is to form the powder into a slurry with water and then spray it downwards against a rising current of hot air in the form of fine droplets. The water evaporates and one is left with rounded, light and porous granules which, when made in this way, generally flow freely. They have a minimal tendency to block the hopper or clog the dies of multi-punch tablet making machines (Raff, Robinson & Svedres 1961).

Recently a bowl method has been developed for granulating pharmaceutical powders which, though still in the development stage, has commercial potentialities. The materials to be granulated are placed in a large copper or stainless steel bowl, which is mounted on the shaft of a driving motor and tilted at an angle of about 30° to the horizontal. They are made to tumble by revolving the bowl at a speed of about 30 rev per min at the same time spraying in a fine mist of water, or a dilute solution of a suitable binder, such as polyvinyl pyrrolidone or gum. As the powder becomes moist, the particles start to agglomerate and by correctly choosing the speed of rotation, the amount of liquid, and the processing time, they can be made to grow up to any desired size. (In some cases, tumbling of the powder needs to be assisted by fitting shallow baffles in the interior of the bowl.) A stream of warm air is then directed into the bowl, which dries off the granules and the final drying is done by spreading them on flat trays in an oven and heating at about 80°.

Granules prepared by this method are generally

smoother and more uniformly spherical than those obtained by the other methods that have already been described.

It is appropriate to conclude this chapter by referring briefly to one or two other aspects of powder science that are relevant in the practice of pharmacy, in the context of the handling properties of powders.

TRANSPORT

The transport of materials in bulk by pneumatic methods, employing air slides and pipelines, is coming into increasing use because of its obvious advantages over the conventional method of carrying in sacks, cartons, or other containers. Losses due to spillages or torn containers are reduced, contamination and dust formation are minimized and savings can be achieved by reduced labour costs and the lower freight rates that apply to the transport of materials in bulk.

An air slide consists of a chute with a porous metal base through which air is passed at about 1 lb/in² (0.07 kg/cm²) and 5 ft (1.5 m)/min. This partly fluidizes a fine powder, reducing its angle of friction very nearly to zero so that it can flow down the slide even when this is almost horizontal. In this way, the powder can be transported a long distance horizontally.

In a pneumatic pipeline system on the other hand, a high velocity stream of air is passed through the conveying line and the powdered materials are fed into it from storage hoppers or from mechanical conveyors, being delivered into the appropriate receptacles which are vented to the atmosphere through suitable dust filtration equipment.

For the design and satisfactory operation of pneumatic conveying systems, it is necessary to know a good deal about such properties of a powder as its density, particle size distribution, cohesiveness, angles of friction and repose, and fluidization characteristics. The same properties are clearly of relevance to the pharmacist in the formulation of powdered insufflations, where the patient has to·inhale a fine powder directly into the lungs.

DUST CONTROL

The control of dust is an important aspect of modern pharmaceutical practice, not only for the purpose of maintaining the sterility of products, but also for preventing the loss and widespread dissemination into the air of powdered drugs, which might have an adverse effect on the health of factory workers and other members of the community. Dust is a potential hazard as a source of explosions and fires and in reports from the Chief Inspector of Factories, starch and dextrin dusts, in particular, have been mentioned as dangerous in this respect.

The main methods used for controlling dust in the pharmaceutical industry are filtration, inertial separation and electrostatic precipitation (Green & Lane 1957; Hammond 1958).

In filtration, air which contains dust is sucked or blown through some suitable material whose pores are sufficiently small to retain the particles of solid. Materials used for the purpose include paper, felt, wool, cotton wool and nylon. Filters often take the form of pads or panels fitted to the walls and windows of buildings. But there is also a large variety of filter bags, stockings and cabinets, etc., which can be attached to particular machines where dust is being produced, thereby preventing it from escaping into the atmosphere.

Intertial separators are exemplified by cyclones, in which air is caused to spiral through a cone-shaped vessel. Due to centrifugal force, any particles of dust that it contains are thrown outwards to the walls of the cyclone and then slide down to a hopper from which they can be subsequently withdrawn.

Cyclones are particularly suitable for attaching to machines in which large amounts of dust are being produced; they form an integral part of the design of certain mills and mixers.

Finally, electrostatic precipitators consist of a number of earthed tubes, between which are stretched fine metal wires charged to several thousands of volts d.c. The high potential difference between the tubes and the wires ionizes any particles of dust that are being carried by air streaming over the precipitator and the dust is deposited on metal plates from which it is collected periodically.

REFERENCES

Anon (1966) *Br. chem. Engng* **11**, 725.

Ashton, M. D., Cheng, D. C. & Farley, R. (1965) *Rheol. acta* **4**, 206.

Badger, W. L. & Banchero, J. T. (1955) *Introduction to Chemical Engineering*. London: McGraw Hill.

Bickle, W. H. (1961) *Society of Chemical Industry Monograph*, No. 14, London.

British Standards (1963) 3406, Parts 2 and 4.

British Standards (1969) 410.

CAREY, W. F. & STAIRMAND, C. J. (1953) *Recent Developments in Mineral Dressing* 117. London: Institute of Mining & Metallurgy.

CREMER, H. W. & DAVIES, T. (eds) (1957) *Chemical Engineering Practice*, Vols 1–9. London: Butterworths.

DAWES, J. G. (1952) *Safety in Mines*, Research Establishment Report, No. 36.

DOBIE, W. B. (1952) *Recent Developments in Mineral Dressing*. London: Institute of Mining & Metallurgy.

DOTSON, J. M. (1962) *Ind. Engng Chem.* **54**, 62.

DUNNING, W. J. (1961) *Society of Chemical Industry Monograph*, No. 14, 29. London.

EDMUNDSON, I. C. (1967) *Advances in Pharmaceutical Sciences*, Vol. 2 (Ed. by Beckett, Bean & Carless) 95. London: Academic Press.

GOODRIDGE, A. M., BADZOICK, S. & HAWKSLEY, P. G. W. (1962) *J. sci. Instrum.* **39**, 12.

GREEN, H. L. & LANE, W. R. (1957) *Particulate Clouds Dusts Mists and Smokes*. London: E. & F. N. Spon.

HAMMOND, R. (1958) *Separation and Purification of Materials*. London: Heywood.

HAWKSLEY, P. G. W. (1947) *Institute of Fuel, Conference on Pulverized Coal*, p. 656. London.

HERDAN, G. et al. (1960) *Small Particle Statistics*. London: Butterworths.

HEYWOOD, H. (1963) *J. Pharm. Pharmacol.* **15**, 56T.

HUKKI, R. T. (1959) *Br. chem. Engng* **4**, 446.

JENIKE, A. W. (1961) *Bulletin*, No. 108. Engineering Experimental Station University of Utah. U.S.A.

JONES, T. M. & PILPEL, N. (1966) *J. Pharm. Pharmacol.* **18**, 429, 182S.

NEUMAN, A. C. C. & AXON, A. (1961) *Society of Chemical Industry Monograph*, No. 14, 291.

NEUMANN, B. (1967) *Advances in Pharmaceutical Sciences*, Vol. 2 (Ed. Beckett, Bean & Carless). London: Academic Press.

ORR, C. & DALLAVALLE, J. M. (1959) *Fine Particle Measurement*. London: Macmillan.

PILPEL, N. (1965) *Chem. Proc. Engng* **46**, 167.

PILPEL, N. (1971) *Advances in Pharmaceutical Sciences*, Vol. 3 (Ed. Bean, Beckett & Carless). London: Academic Press.

RAFF, A. M., ROBINSON, M. J. & SVEDRES, E. V. (1961) *J. Am. pharm. Ass.* **50**, 76.

RILEY, R. V. (1965) *Chem. Process Engng* **46**, 189.

ROSE, H. E. (1961) *Society of Chemical Industry Monograph*, No. 14, 130.

ROSE, H. E. & SULLIVAN, R. M. E. (1961) *Vibration Mills and Vibration Milling*. London: Constable.

RUMPF, H. (1962) *Agglomeration*. London: Interscience.

STAIRMAND, C. J. (1947) *Suppl. Trans. Inst. Chem. Engs* **25**, 131.

TIMBRELL, V. (1959) *Lab. Pract.* **8**, 33.

TRAIN, D. (1960) *Pharmac. J.* 6th August, 129.

18

Emulsions

An emulsion has been defined by Becher (1965) as 'a heterogeneous system, consisting of at least one immiscible liquid dispersed in another in the form of droplets whose diameters, in general, exceed 0.1 μm. Such systems possess a minimal stability, which may be accentuated by such additives as surface-active agents, finely-divided solids, etc.' The liquid droplets, generally known as the *emulsion globules*, form the *disperse phase* (or *internal phase* while the liquid in which they are dispersed is known as the *continuous phase* (or *external phase*). If oil globules are dispersed in water, the system is called an *oil-in-water* emulsion (o/w type); conversely, the dispersion of water in oil produces a *water-in-oil* (w/o) emulsion. The ratio of internal phase volume to the *total* volume is known is known as the *phase volume* or the *phase volume ratio*.

It is not necessary to have an oil or indeed water to form an emulsion. When a coacervate (Kruyt 1949) first separates it does so in the form of colloid-rich globules. Conversely, both phases may be non-aqueous. Occasionally, a *multiple emulsion* can be formed as when minute oil globules are dispersed in the water globules of a w/o emulsion: this might then be described as an o/w/o emulsion.

Globule sizes can vary enormously but are generally in the range 0.25–25 μm diameter. Emulsions with predominantly large globules are sometimes referred to as *coarse emulsions* while those with globules of mean diameter below about 5 μm are considered to be *fine emulsions*. Even finer emulsions can sometimes be formed with globule diameters as small as 10 nm; these are known as *microemulsions*. Unlike ordinary emulsions which are generally 'milky', microemulsions may be transparent having globules only a little larger than micelles.

Except with some microemulsions, emulsification is generally not spontaneous and certainly not in the thermodynamic sense, and energy must be supplied in order to increase the interfacial area between the phases. Considering a 1 cm diameter globule of liquid paraffin in water with an interfacial energy (γ_{ow}) of 55 mJ.m^{-2}, the interfacial energy is:

interfacial area × energy per unit area

$$= \pi d^2 \gamma_{ow} = (3.1416(10^{-2})^2)55 = 0.017 \text{ mJ}$$

If this globule is broken into globules of 10 μm diameter then:

$$\frac{\text{volume of original globule}}{\text{volume of emulsion globule}} = \frac{d_1{}^3}{d_2{}^3} = 10^9 \text{ globules}$$

and the interfacial energy is then:

$$10^9(\pi d_2{}^2)\gamma_{ow} = 10^9(3.1416(10^{-5})^2)55 = 17.28 \text{ mJ}$$

requiring an energy input of $17.28 - 0.017 = 17.26$ mJ. Reduction of globule size to 1 μm diameter would have required an energy input of 172.8 mJ or almost 330 mJ for each ml of liquid paraffin emulsified. Much less expenditure of energy is required if the interfacial energy is decreased by the addition of surface-active agents to, say, 1 mJ.m^{-2} when only $330/55 = 6$ mJ would be needed for each ml of oil in order to make a fine emulsion (assuming, highly unrealistically, 100 per cent efficiency of the mechanical process!).

The mechanical disruption of the disperse phase may be achieved by shaking or stirring if γ_{ow} is very small, otherwise some kind of machine is required. Non-vigorous agitation generally leads to polydisperse globules with a wide range of sizes, so that the emulsion frequently needs further and more vigorous treatment in a homogenizer. Homogenization can be achieved by forcing the crude emulsion through a narrow orifice under high pressure, which produces extremely large shearing forces causing the globules to be strung out into high speed liquid jets which are ruptured into minute globules by the action of the interfacial tension on the perturbations. Colloid mills are also used. Alternatively, a fine emulsion can be achieved by means of an ultrasonic dispersator. Propellor mixers and shrouded turbines are favourite instruments on a small scale while the pestle and mortar may suffice for extemporaneous dispensing. Some emulsifying equipment is described at the end of this chapter.

Since there is a positive interfacial tension between the internal and external phases, emulsions are thermodynamically unstable. Collision of unprotected globules will very probably result in their coalescence, thereby producing a rapid coarsening of the emulsion. This process is known as *breaking* or *cracking*. It follows that some barrier to coalescence is needed and this is achieved by the use of *emulsifying agents* otherwise known as *emulgents*.

EMULSIFYING AGENTS

There are basically three classes of these:
1. *amphipaths* such as soaps, long-chain amines and alcohols,
2. *hydrophilic colloids* such as acacia, sodium alginate, gelatin and methylcellulose, and
3. *finely-divided solids* such as magnesium and aluminium hydroxide and bentonite.
All are surface-active in that they tend to congregate at an oil–water interface, but a marked lowering of γ_{ow} is found mainly with amphipaths whereas hydrophilic colloids generally produce only a moderate lowering. The mechanism of adsorption of the latter has been discussed in Chapter 4 while that of fine particles is dealt with here.

The surface-activity and emulsifying power of single oil and water-soluble surfactants and blends of these have been classified semi-empirically by

Griffin (1949, 1954) in terms of the *hydrophile–lipophile balance* (HLB). This has been discussed by Becher (1965) and by Sherman (1968). HLB numbers may be determined experimentally or calculated in a manner similar to the parachor (see Chapter 4), and afford a means of blending surfactants so as to achieve a desired type of emulsion.

Oil soluble amphipaths have low HLB values whereas water-soluble ones have high values. Thus sorbitan mono-oleate has a value of 4.3 while polyoxyethylene sorbitan mono-oleate has a value between 10 and 15 depending upon the length of the oxyethylene chain. Blending of these amphipaths gives an HLB of intermediate value. For an o/w emulsion, an HLB value within the approximate range 8–18 is required, while within the range 3–6 a w/o emulsion would be produced. The HLB value of an individual surfactant is correlated with its dielectric constant and, for o/w emulsions, the more polar the oil, the more polar must be the emulgent. This means that the more polar oils need emulgent blends of higher HLB value. In connection with this, it is worth noting that the spreading coefficients of an oil on aqueous solutions of various surfactants, or of water on solutions in oil, have been correlated with the HLB value.

PREPARATION AND PROPERTIES OF EMULSIONS

In the labelling of medicines the term 'emulsion' is generally restricted to o/w emulsions intended for oral use, but it does in fact cover all aspects of the dispersion of one immiscible liquid in another and so includes creams and some lotions, liniments and applications.

o/w Emulsions containing amphipaths
Reference was made in Chapter 4 to the work of Schulman and Cockbain who demonstrated that molecular association between an oil-soluble and a water-soluble surfactant was necessary for good emulsion stability and that stability of the film is a prerequisite for emulsion stability. These workers concluded that this stability was conferred by a charged liquid-condensed monolayer at the oil globule–water interface. Since strength and compactness of the interfacial film seemed important, 'complex' formation was considered necessary (Chapter 4). This condition is achieved using mixtures of the anionic surfactant sodium lauryl sulphate with cetostearyl alcohol (as in Aqueous Cream) or of cationic cetrimide with cetostearyl

alcohol (as in Cetrimide Cream). Since the Helmholtz double layer thickness is less than 10 nm in water, oil globules carrying an appreciable ζ-potential have an appreciable potential energy barrier to surmount before they can approach close enough to coalesce (see Chapter 5). It is possible however for these globules to flocculate in the secondary minimum and this is commonly observed especially in concentrated emulsions such as many creams. Stabilization due to the electrical charge is supplemented by the Marangoni–Gibbs effect since close approach of two potentially colliding globules causes deformation of the opposing faces due to the resistance to ejection of the intervening medium. The resulting *localized* increase in interfacial area causes depletion in monolayer packing with a concomitant increase in interfacial tension so that the distorted faces act like stretched membranes. The tension gradient which is produced then rapidly brings monolayer molecules from behind the globules ·to fill the weakened gaps and these molecules drag water with them thus opposing further thinning of the aqueous lamella between the globules. Delay in adsorption of more amphipath from the water allows time for elastic rebound and the globules will then have survived their encounter (Fig. 18.1).

A liquid-condensed monolayer is not necessarily a prerequisite for good emulsion stability since dilute monolayers of sodium oleate with oleic acid have been shown to be effective. Nor is it necessary to use an ionic amphipath since equally good emulsions can be obtained using the non-ionic surfactant cetomacrogol 1000 with cetostearyl alcohol (as in Cetomacrogol Cream). Globules of such an emulsion may still acquire an appreciable ζ-potential, presumably by adsorption of contaminant ions and friction with the aqueous medium. However, entropic stabilization appears to be more important with non-ionics (Elworthy & Florence 1969).

The three creams mentioned above may be prepared in two slightly different ways. Commonly the water-soluble and oil-soluble amphipaths are dissolved in their respective phases with the aid of gentle heat, the two phases are mixed at about 60–70° and then stirred gently till cool or passed, with cooling, through an emulsifier. Alternatively an *emulsifying wax* is used which consists of the two amphipaths intimately mixed by melting and dissolution. This 'wax' is melted, dissolved in the warm oil phase and mixed with the warm aqueous phase. Emulsification is then achieved as before

since the water-soluble component rapidly partitions out of the oil.

The consistency of the product and its appearance may be influenced by the method of preparation. Since the concentration of water-soluble surfactant is in excess of the CMC, some of the cetostearyl alcohol partitions into the aqueous phase to form mixed micelles. Low concentrations of the alcohols give fluid emulsions but concentrations near or above the saturation concentration

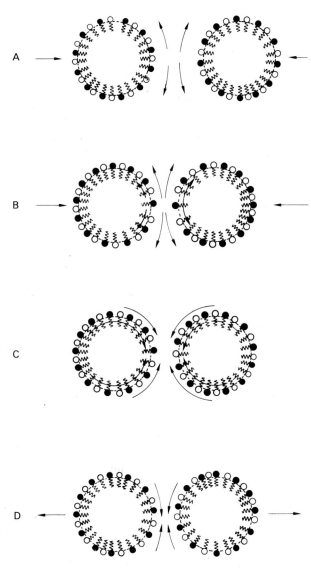

FIG. 18.1. Elastic collision of mixed amphipath stabilized oil globules in water (letters indicate time sequence in the Marangoni-Gibbs effect).

in the oil produce semi-solid creams, i.e. they possess a yield stress (see Chapter 9) and will not flow under their own weight. This *bodying* action as it is called is due to gelation of the aqueous phase, probably as the result of the formation of liquid crystalline structures (Lachampt 1970) (see Chapter 4). The visco-elastic gel network which forms when the emulsion is first cooled is partially disrupted when sheared, resulting in a reduced yield stress. However there may be some thixotropic recovery.

Evidence so far accumulated suggests that, for a given amount of oil-soluble component, ionic water-soluble surfactants produce stiffer creams than an equal molar concentration of a non-ionic one. The consistency however depends largely on the rate of cooling of the cream during manufacture and on the mechanical dispersion process since this affects the degree of partitioning of the oil-soluble component before the structures are 'frozen' in position. It is possible that ionic surfactants behave rather differently from non-ionic ones. Structure build-up is rapid with the former and occurs during the cooling process whereas structural changes occur over a period of several hours in cooled non-ionic creams (Barry & Saunders 1971c). In order to obtain a cream with a smooth texture, the oil and water-soluble components should be readily capable of forming a ternary liquid crystal phase, otherwise granular textured creams may be produced containing waxy particles in the aqueous phase. These latter probably arise due to mechanical separation from the oil by the action of the homogenizer and may result when a low concentration of water-soluble component is used in conjunction with a fatty acid instead of an alcohol. Using cetrimide or ceto-macrogol 1000, the optimal chain length of saturated fatty alcohols for a bodying action is C_{14} and C_{16} or a mixture of C_{16} and C_{18}, but a marked visco-elasticity has been noted using shorter chain alcohols.

Unsaturated alcohols such as oleyl alcohol, have no bodying action but do permit the production of stable creams. Increasing the volume of oil (producing a larger phase volume) has the effect of increasing the viscosity of the emulsion. This effect is supplemented by raising the proportion of oil-soluble component.

Details concerning the bodying action of mixed emulsifiers may be found by reference to the work of Barry, and Talman and their coworkers (cited in Barry & Saunders 1970, 1971a,b,c; Talman & Rowan 1970a,b).

Stable emulsions may be produced in which the oil and water-soluble components are not chemically distinct. Soaps such as Soft Soap used in Turpentine Liniment partially hydrolyse so that co-adsorption of ionized and unionized molecules at the o/w interface produces a complex film. The soap may also be formed in situ (*nascent soap* method) as when aqueous ammonia is added to oleic acid–paraffin oil in the preparation of Ammonia Liniment BPC 1949.

w/o Emulsions containing amphipaths
Schulman and Cockbain concluded that loss of charge together with rigidity in an interfacial monolayer leads to the formation of an emulsion where the globules are formed from the aqueous phase. Since an interfacial monolayer has two sides, one attracted strongly to the water and the other held by the oil, two different tensions, in effect, are operating and the film will *tend* to curve towards the side of greatest tension. Thus a reduction in water attracting power, for example by reducing ionization, may have the effect of causing an o/w emulsion to change or *invert* to a w/o emulsion. A similar effect might be expected if the film becomes more bulky on the oil side as when the carboxyl groups of two fatty acids are joined by a divalent cation leaving the two hydrocarbon chains free to move on the oil side (Fig. 18.2). Thus, shaking the o/w Ammonia Liniment with a little magnesium chloride causes complete inversion to a w/o emulsion. During shaking the least abundant phase would tend to be broken up but in the absence of the magnesium the aqueous phase globules readily coalesce so that the stable oil globules accumulate. Upon shaking the liniment with the magnesium salt, it is the turn of the oil globules to become unstable while the stabilized water globules accumulate.

A similar process occurs during the preparation of White Liniment. An o/w emulsion of turpentine oil is made using ammonium oleate (formed in situ) and this is then inverted upon shaking it with ammonium chloride dissolved in the rest of the water. Both w/o emulsions mentioned here contain emulgents whose water solubilities are low. In the first place, addition of the magnesium salt would cause precipitation of a magnesium oleate gel, while in the second ammonium chloride has a salting-out effect also potentially leading to a gel. Whether the film surrounding the water globules is a monolayer is obviously questionable since a gelatinous multilayer might well produce a suitable mechanical barrier. However, a surfactant mixture, such as

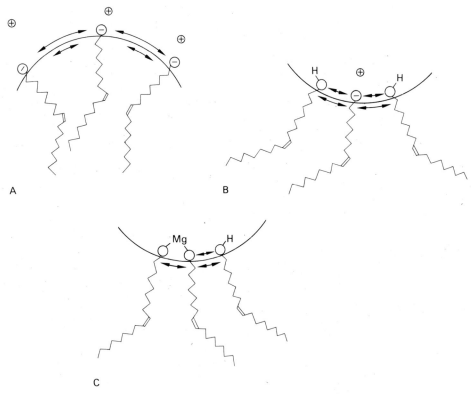

Fig. 18.2. Influence of hydrophilic and lipophilic groups on interfacial curvature. A, sodium oleate. Tension low on water side due to repulsion of ionized groups and ion-dipole interaction. Result o/w. B, sodium oleate plus oleic acid. Entropic repulsion on oil side predominates since ionization on water side reduced. Result w/o. C, magnesium oleate plus oleic acid. Charge neutralization and strong linking of polar groups. Result w/o.

lecithin–cholesterol in a ratio below 8:1, can form monolayer stabilized w/o emulsions. Close approach of two water globules leads to the formation of a lipid bilayer which, however, retains some oil and complete thinning of the oil lamella with consequent coalescence of the globules is resisted.

Water globules have been demonstrated to possess charges, the effect of which is long ranging due to the low permittivity of the intervening oil. In such instances, the Helmholtz double layer thickness can exceed 1 μm producing a considerable energy barrier with respect to infinite separation of the globules. The globules are, however, not separated by vast distances so that geometric distribution of the globules necessarily means that part of the barrier is already surmounted and the net repulsion is considerably reduced.

Hydrophobic soaps produced by reaction between divalent and trivalent cations and fatty acids are nearly always formed in situ. Such is the case with Zinc Cream and Oily Calamine Lotion, both of which contain calcium oleate formed by the interaction of calcium hydroxide solution and oleic acid. They will also contain traces of zinc oleate from the zinc oxide and calamine respectively. Emulsions prepared using these soaps alone tend to break readily, therefore in each case woolfat is added to enhance the stability. This contains long-chain alcohols and hydroxysterols such as cholesterol which on their own tend to produce w/o emulsions but may be used to stabilize both w/o and o/w emulsions. By contrast, it should be noted that Calamine Cream is an o/w emulsion utilizing sodium lauryl sulphate, the corresponding divalent salts of which are much more soluble in water than those of fatty acids.

Multiple emulsions
These may form when a system does not strongly favour one particular emulsion type or when three phases are present. Certain aspects of their formation have been discussed by Mulley and Marland (1970).

Emulsions containing hydrophilic colloids

Macromolecular films at the oil–water interface have been described in Chapter 4. Since the emulgents used are non-toxic and hydrophilic they are commonly employed in the preparation of o/w emulsions for oral use. A mechanically strong gel barrier forms around the outside of the oil globules while a considerable viscosity is imparted to the intervening aqueous phase thereby reducing the probability and energy of encounter between oil globules. The mechanical strength of the gel barrier largely determines the stability of the emulsion and this may be enhanced by ensuring physicochemical conditions for least solubility of the emulgent. Thus pH control may be important as demonstrated by the fact that gelatin is most effective at its isoelectric point. The rate of coalescence of oil globules protected by anionic hydrocolloids such as carboxymethylcellulose is reduced at low pH where the interfacial film strengths are high even though the aqueous solution viscosities are reduced.

Since the interfacial energy of macromolecular film-stabilized emulsions is generally fairly high, perhaps in excess of 20 mJ.m^{-2}, considerable energy needs to be expended in order to achieve a fine emulsion. Generally, the oil is dispersed in an aqueous solution of the hydrocolloid by means of a homogenizer or other suitable mechanical mixer which does not incorporate much air. For very small quantities of acacia stabilized emulsions, a pestle and mortar technique may be used where the oil–water–gum proportions are initially carefully controlled so that the relative viscosities of the two phases allow adequate shearing of the interface. This is further described in Chapter 24.

Since globule size reduction involves an increase in interfacial area, more hydrocolloid needs to be adsorbed. If there is an excess of hydrocolloid, coverage of the extra area need not be at the expense of the thickness of the interfacial film. In the presence of very thick films (of the order of 100 nm) such as occur in acacia stabilized liquid paraffin emulsions, the effective phase volume increases as the emulsion is made finer, resulting in an increased viscosity of the emulsion (Shotton & White 1963). Low viscosity grades of cellulose derivatives are desirable in order that these may be present in suitable concentration to produce a good coverage of the globules without increasing the viscosity of the external phase too much.

Emulsions containing solids

The extent of adsorption of solids, such as gelatinous precipitates, at an o/w interface depends very largely upon their physical state. Energy conditions for adsorption are illustrated in Fig. 18.3, Liquid Paraffin and Magnesium Hydroxide Emulsion BPC being an example of C. This is also illustrated in Fig. 4.54 where a necessary condition is a non-zero angle of contact (θ) such that $|\cos\theta| < 1$. In order to achieve this, the solid may be modified by the controlled addition of amphipaths or by reaction with a component of the oil in situ. The most stable emulsions are obtained when $\cos\theta \approx 0$.

An extremely rigid interfacial film of closely packed particles can be produced by capillary forces as illustrated in Fig. 18.4 the effect being enhanced with most particles by the irregularity of their surface. The phase having the greatest affinity

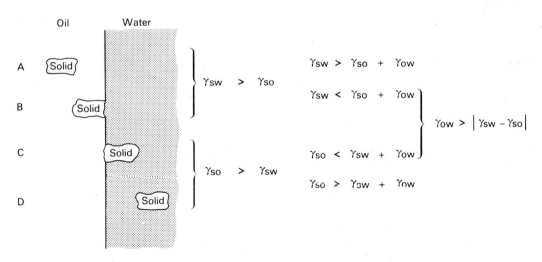

FIG. 18.3. Interfacial energy considerations for adsorption of solids at oil-water interfaces.

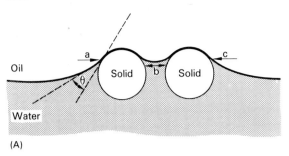

(A)

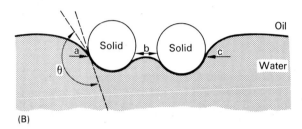

(B)

FIG. 18.4. Capillary forces cause similar particles to be drawn together so that they cohere strongly. The closer the particles, the more curved is the meniscus at b and the lower the pressure there compared with that at a and c. A, solid preferentially wetted by water; $\theta < 90°$: result o/w B, solid preferentially wetted by oil; $\theta > 90°$ result w/o.

for the solid forms the external phase. Thus magnesium and aluminium hydroxides may be employed, where appropriate, in o/w emulsions for oral use, whereas bentonite can be used in both o/w and w/o emulsions for external application.

These emulsions tend to be rather coarse but their stability can often be enhanced by the addition of other surface-active materials and these, together with the preparative technique, may influence the emulsion type. Thus a bentonite stabilized cream incorporating Self-emulsifying Monostearin would be o/w whereas that made with calcium oleate might well be w/o.

It is probable that many w/o emulsions, whose stability is commonly attributed to monolayers, are actually stabilized by fine particles, probably with monolayers filling the gaps, and a similar mechanism might be postulated for some o/w emulsions where gelatinous structures are known to exist in the aqueous phase (Sanders 1970; Davis 1971). A necessary criterion is that the solid particles shall be much smaller than the globules which they are to protect. Since their desorption involves, at least temporarily, an increase in interfacial energy, these emulsions can be very stable. This stability may be enhanced if the particles carry a charge, resulting in globules having a high ζ-potential.

SPONTANEOUS EMULSIFICATION AND MICROEMULSIONS

If some non-equilibrated oil and water phases are brought together, an emulsion may form near the interface without mechanical agitation. One of three mechanisms may be involved. Firstly, contact of an oily solution of a fatty acid with aqueous alkali may lead to interfacial turbulence owing to local variations in lowering of γ_{ow}. Secondly, the diffusion of oil-soluble acid or alcohol into the aqueous surfactant may carry oil which then becomes stranded as the environment becomes predominantly aqueous. At the same time, water diffused into the alcohol laden oil becomes stranded as the alcohol passes out into the aqueous phase. The result is an o/w and a w/o emulsion on either side of the original interface. Emulsions formed spontaneously in this way are not thermodynamically stable.

The third mechanism leads to the formation of transparent or faintly turbid o/w or w/o *microemulsions* with globule diameters in the range 8 to 80 nm; less than one order of magnitude larger than micelles. Low molecular weight hydrocarbons have been microemulsified probably due to the formation of an interfacial duplex film of low tension which is opposed by an imbalance of forces on either side of the film, tending to produce a negative interfacial tension. A non-negative tension is then restored by the spontaneous curvature of the interface (Prince 1967). Such emulsions are therefore unique in being thermodynamically stable.

STABILITY OF EMULSIONS

Since pharmaceutical emulsions have a positive interfacial energy they are thermodynamically unstable in the sense that breaking is the spontaneous process whereby globules coalesce to form larger globules and eventually separate completely into another layer with a minimum interfacial area. The rate of coarsening of an emulsion depends upon the effectiveness of the interfacial barrier to coalescence and upon the frequency and duration of globule encounter. The latter is increased if the globules collect into a smaller volume owing to a difference in density of the internal and external phases. This phenomenon is known as *creaming* by analogy with the concentration of oil globules at the top of a bottle of milk. By similar analogy, it will be appreciated that the process of creaming can be readily reversed by agitation whereas breaking cannot so easily be reversed.

Creaming should be minimized or eliminated

since it *tends* to reduce the stability and elegance of an emulsion. Obviously, if an emulsion possesses a yield stress, the globules will be kept from moving by the structure of the external phase. In the absence of a yield stress, the Stokes equation points to the ways in which creaming may be controlled:

$$v = \frac{d_{st}^2 \Delta \rho g}{18 \eta}$$

This shows that in a gravitational field of acceleration g, the velocity v of a globule can be reduced by decreasing its effective size (d_{st}) and difference in density from the external phase ($\Delta \rho$) and by increasing the viscosity (η) of the external phase. Reducing the effective globule size means not only that the individual globules should be as small as possible but that they should be kept from flocculating by means of a suitably high ζ-potential. It is not usual to reduce $\Delta \rho$ but this could be done by adjusting the oil density using a mixture of a light and a heavy oil such as a paraffin or vegetable oil and a brominated oil. The viscosity of the external phase may be increased by incorporating more bodying agent, such as a long-chain acid or alcohol in amphipath stabilized emulsions. The emulsifying waxes have a *self-bodying* action, that is, the consistency of a cream may be controlled entirely by the proportion of 'wax' added. Thus Emulsifying Wax BP is used in both Benzyl Benzoate Application and in Aqueous Cream but whereas the former contains only about 2 per cent 'wax' and is fluid and prone to creaming, the latter uses 9 per cent and is semi-solid.. Emulsions intended for oral use may include hydrocolloid thickening agent such as tragacanth or a small quantity of high molecular weight methylcellulose. Alternatively, sodium alginate may be thickened by the addition of traces of a calcium salt.

Phase volume may influence emulsion stability. Obviously if the internal phase volume is large, the mean distance between globules will be small. A large phase volume may involve considerable flocculation of globules and flattening of the regions of contact which will increase the chances of coalescence. The proportion of oil to water may occasionally decide whether an o/w or a w/o emulsion is obtained but with those emulgents where this is so the preparative technique may be the overriding factor. Sometimes it pays to prepare one type of emulsion, say a fine o/w emulsion, and then to *invert* this to w/o by the addition of more oil or by cooling. In this way, smaller water globules may be obtained than would otherwise be possible. White Liniment affords an example where the preparative technique involves inversion, in this instance due to an alteration in the nature of the emulgent.

Occasionally, however, only incomplete emulsification may be achieved. This might be due to a poor technique or to some unsuspected change in the quality of an ingredient. Instead of obtaining a white emulsion, an unsightly, immiscible, coarse mixture of o/w and w/o emulsions is obtained. It may be possible to break the emulsion by heating and then to make another attempt at emulsification, perhaps using another instrument, but usually it is best to start again. An example where difficulty might be encountered is in the preparation of Turpentine Liniment. If the soft soap is dispersed in the oil and this is then shaken vigorously with the water, an o/w emulsion may not be made successfully. However, o/w emulsification is readily produced with only a few shakes if about a one minute interval is allowed between each shake. This allows time for redistribution of the ionized soap and free fatty acid between the oil, the water and the interface and results in a very thick stable o/w emulsion. Slight changes in pH may also lead to emulsion instability. With soft soap, this might result from the absorption of carbon dioxide.

Breaking of an emulsion during storage may be due to a number of interacting factors. Temperature fluctuations should be avoided. Elevated temperatures may lead to the emulsifier favouring a different emulsion type since changes in the interfacial film often become pronounced above 40°. With o/w emulsions particularly, warm conditions enhance evaporation and chemical degradation processes such as oxidation of oils. The use of well-closed containers is therefore essential. The stability of most emulsions is also diminished by cooling to near or below 0°. Besides alteration of the emulgent properties, formation of ice crystals ruptures the interfacial film, thereby breaking o/w emulsions. In order to counteract loss of water from o/w dermatological creams, a humectant is frequently added. This is commonly glycerin or sorbitol. In sufficient amounts these compounds reduce the evaporation rate from the container and the skin, but the concentration is limited by their tendency to dry the skin.

Another source of instability is the growth of microorganisms. o/w Emulsions prepared with materials of natural origin such as gums, carbohydrates and proteins are particularly prone to such spoilage, fungi, yeasts and bacteria all being implicated. Synthetic compounds such as cellulose and sorbitan derivatives are therefore to be preferred. Preservation requires the addition of one or more compatible, water-soluble, non-toxic compounds which have a long-lasting, wide spectrum of activity against microorganisms even in low concentration. Usually they should be undetectable by the senses. For oral use, benzoic acid is commonly employed, which may be supplemented with chloroform as in Liquid Paraffin Emulsion. Esters of *p*-hydroxybenzoic acid are used for both oral and topical use. Sometimes, the emulgent itself has a preservative action as in Cetrimide Cream but in others a compound such as chlorocresol is a suitable additive. Since microbes grow in the aqueous phase, a sufficient preservative concentration must be found here and partitioning into the oil must be allowed for (Bean, Konning & Malcolm 1969). Further aspects of preservation are discussed in Chapter 36.

Instability of an emulsion is not associated merely with flocculation, creaming or breaking. Emulsions used as bases must not impair the activity of the medicament. Generally, an ionic emulgent will be incompatible with medicaments whose active ion is of opposite charge such as sodium lauryl sulphate with neomycin sulphate. Ionic incompatibility is not always obvious as for example the incompatibility of hexachlorophene with quaternary ammonium surfactants due to the anionic character of the phenolic group. Nonionic emulgents may be used when ionic reactions are at risk but even these are not immune from incompatibility due for example, to their micellar adsorption of phenolic compounds. Incompatibilities are not always visible although emulsion breaking may ensue. Sometimes a colour change may be seen as when proflavine hemisulphate is incorporated in an anionic base, but discoloration may develop only slowly as when hydrocortisone is incorporated in a cream stabilized with a triethanolamine soap. It is important to choose a base which is chemically unreactive and which gives the medicament the desired degree of skin penetration and release to the body tissues.

Another form of instability has been observed when the medicament is *suspended* in an emulsion. Liquid Paraffin and Phenolphthalein Emulsion requires the phenolphthalein to be very finely dispersed otherwise it settles out and cannot easily be redispersed upon shaking.

Occasionally, emulsions are deliberately made with an inherent instability. An o/w barrier cream may be used which liberates a film of oil when applied to the skin. Sometimes, emulsion breaking is an essential part of a manufacturing process such as the separation of woolfat from wool scouring wastes. Yet another application is the formation of foams from emulsified aerosol propellants which vaporize on release from the container.

Reference should be made to the review by Garrett (1965) for further details.

GLOBULE SIZE

Microemulsions having globule diameters below about 50 nm are transparent, while those with larger globules are decidedly turbid. If the globules are above about 100 nm extremely white emulsions are produced but as the diameters increase much above 10 μm a greyish or cream colour is developed. The whiteness of fine emulsions is due to the reflections and refractions at the many interfaces. If, however, the two phases have the same refractive index, a *transparent* emulsion is produced except when they differ in optical dispersive power and then a highly coloured *chromatic* emulsion results.

Globule size may be represented by any of the equivalent spherical diameters, the mean size generally being weighted by number. Although some size distributions may be approximately Gaussian, they are usually skewed but often capable of normalization by a logarithmic transformation in which case the distribution parameters are simply related by the equations of Hatch and Choate. Various other, largely empirical, distribution functions have also been proposed.

Size distribution is influenced by: (*a*) method of preparation of the emulsion, (*b*) temperature during mixing, (*c*) viscosity, (*d*) type of oil and its phase volume and (*e*) type and concentration of emulgent. Size reduction involves an increased interfacial area and interaction between globules resulting in appreciably higher viscosities only with the more concentrated emulsions (phase volume greater than 0.5). A more uniform size distribution also affords more resistance to flow. Thus concentrated emulsions having the same mean globule size may differ considerably in viscosity if they have different standard deviations. Reference has already been made to the increase in viscosity upon homogenizing emulsions stabilized by thick hydrocolloid films.

Size reduction may also lead to enhanced flocculation. This also increases emulsion viscosity. In the event of flocculation, care has to be taken in interpreting size parameters especially if nonmicroscopic methods of analysis are used.

Coarsening of an emulsion tends to follow first order kinetics and is observed as an increase in mean globule size. This may be accompanied by a broadening of the size distribution but sometimes a more nearly monodisperse system of large globules results.

Sherman (1964), Becher (1965) and Hamill and Petersen (1966) have reviewed the literature concerning the influence of globule size while Sherman (1968) has discussed its determination.

TESTING OF EMULSION TYPE

Several methods are available for testing emulsion type. The *dilution* method involves placing a little of the emulsion in water. If the emulsion readily disperses it is o/w, otherwise a w/o type is indicated. Thick o/w creams may require slight agitation but usually emulsion type is readily observed especially as lumps of o/w cream appear dull in water whereas w/o creams are shiny and usually float to the top.

The *dye solubilization* method involves dusting a small amount of a water-soluble dye, such as methylene blue, on the surface. Rapid dye diffusion indicates that water is the external phase. It is often useful to supplement this by dusting an oil-soluble dye such as scarlet red on another part of the emulsion surface. Dye diffusion then indicates contact with oil as in the case of w/o emulsions, but for this test to be valid the top surface of the emulsion should first be removed otherwise coloration may merely indicate a thin oil film on top of an o/w emulsion due to contamination from manufacturing equipment. Alternatively, it might indicate an unstable o/w emulsion.

Electrical conductivity is another method relying on the poor conductivity of oils compared with aqueous solutions. The conductivity may be measured by standard low frequency a.c. methods, and it will be low where oil is the continuous phase as in w/o emulsions. Ionic emulgents used for the production of the latter give higher conductivities than non-ionic emulgents.

If a drop of emulsion is placed on filter paper, the external phase will tend to spread quickly if it is aqueous. The *filter paper wetting* method however, is useless for thick o/w creams or for emulsions of water in thin oils which themselves spread.

The tests mentioned above may be applied rapidly but the results must be interpreted with caution. They will, for instance, not indicate whether a multiple emulsion has been produced. This must be resolved by *microscopy*.

EMULSIONS IN PHARMACY

Emulsions may be administered orally, rectally, parenterally and topically. Occasionally a medicament forms all or most of one phase but generally, emulsions serve merely as carriers.

Oil-in-water emulsions are used for oral administration serving to mask the unpleasant taste of water-insoluble liquids such as liquid paraffin. Fine emulsification may enhance the absorption of lipid-soluble medicaments such as oil-soluble vitamins but these must use an absorbable oil as carrier: liquid paraffin would hinder their absorption. It should be noted that liquid paraffin emulsions should not be too fine since fine globules of paraffin can be absorbed. Hydrocolloids or non-ionic amphipaths such as polyoxyethylene sorbitan esters are employed for oral use.

Emulsions used as enemas are also of the o/w type but may use soaps. The incorporation of a surfactant in suppositories has been reported to influence drug absorption either by increasing its rate or by prolonging it. The choice of surfactants for parenteral use is very limited and has already been discussed in Chapter 4. Phytomenadione Injection may be in the form of a fine o/w emulsion.

By far the greatest use of emulsions is in dermatology. Oil-in-water creams and lotions form the washable variety whereas w/o creams may be used to act as barriers to aqueous solutions. Topical applications are common in the cosmetic field while in the medical treatment of diseased skin, emulsions are often used as carriers for a drug. Generally only a superficial drug action is required and undue penetration of the skin may need to be avoided as in the case of corticosteroid creams. Percutaneous absorption is mainly a function of the drug itself and not of the vehicle containing it. Where penetration does occur, the hair follicles, sweat ducts and stratum corneum may all be implicated, absorption being greatest for those substances which have both a water and lipid solubility with the hydrophile–lipophile balance in favour of lipid. Since drug action requires partitioning out of the emulsion base, a base having a poor solvent action for the drug should be used. Percutaneous absorption is greatly affected by the condition of the skin such as its relative hydration and greasiness. It may be modified by vasodilation and by the accumulation of sweat during the use of occlusion dressings which involve covering the treatment area with a plastic film. Water-in-oil bases also may inhibit evaporation of sweat, reduce heat radiation and increase skin temperature.

The skin is a natural barrier with a pH between 5 and 6. Ideally, therefore, cream bases should have a neutral or slightly acid pH. Buffered Cream BPC is one such o/w emulsion, this being similar to Aqueous Cream BP having the pH adjusted to about 6 with sodium phosphate and citric acid. The electrolyte content of the aqueous phase of a cream may be an important consideration when treating hypersensitive skins.

de Kay (1962) and Becher (1965) have surveyed much of the literature relating to the topical use of emulsions.

EMULSIFYING EQUIPMENT

A wide variety of machines is available for finely dispersing the internal phase of an emulsion.

Among factors which influence the suitability of a particular machine are (i) the amount of emulsion to be processed, (ii) the flow characteristics, (iii) the need to blend ingredients such as powders, (iv) the temperatures involved and (v) the desired rate of cooling if elevated temperatures are used.

Large and small batches may often be made conveniently by using propeller-mixers operating in suitable mixing vessels, the latter being steam-jacketed if initial heating is required. If a thick emulsion or cream is produced, the propeller-stirrer can be replaced by a gate-stirrer assisted by scraper arms. Fluid emulsions may also be prepared by means of a shrouded turbine such as a Silverson mixer-emusifier. Models are available for batch processing quantities from a few ml up to several

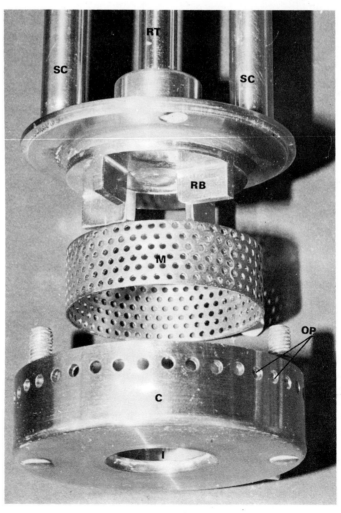

FIG. 18.5. Exploded head of a Silverson mixer-emulsifier.

thousand litres while continuous processing can be achieved by incorporation into a pipe-line. Fig. 18.5 shows the components of the working head of a large laboratory scale model. The columns SC support the head in which turbine blades RB are driven. These are powered by a motor above the supporting columns which act via the drive RT. Centrifugal forces expel the contents of the head through the mesh M and on to the cover C when large shearing and impaction forces produce a fine emulsion which emerges from the openings OP. Circulation of material through the head is maintained by the suction produced in the inlet I at the bottom of the head.

Homogenization can also be obtained by forcing the crude mix through a small annulus so that a high velocity jet is made to impinge on an impact ring set at right angles to the flow. One such instrument, the A.P.V. Gaulin homogenizer, uses a high pressure pump and the shearing action is divided between two independently adjustable stages (Fig. 18.6). Ormerod Q.P. homogenizers work on the same principle, the hand-operated model being commonly used for dispensing purposes. The plate jet, illustrated in Fig. 18.7, is fitted into a reciprocating piston which is filled with the crude mix (held in the bowl) upon its downward stroke. The upward stroke causes expulsion via the shearing and impaction surfaces, the valve loading being controlled by rotation of the drip-cup.

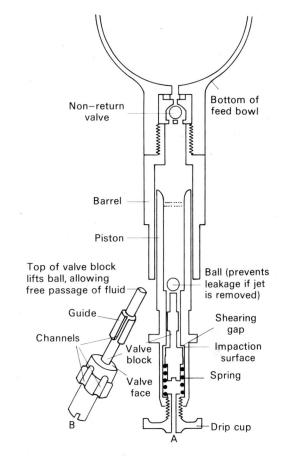

FIG. 18.7. The Q.P. laboratory emulsifier. A, emulsifier in section B, components of the plate jet (Omerod Engineers Ltd.).

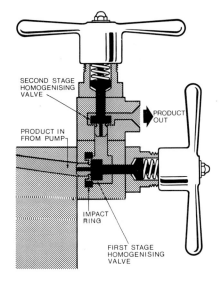

FIG. 18.6. The A.P.V. Gaulin two stage homogenizing valve (A.P.V. Co. Ltd.).

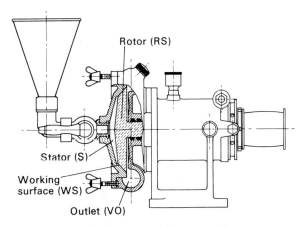

FIG. 18.8. Premier colloid mill in section.

A Premier colloid mill is shown in section in Fig. 18.8, side and top loading models being obtainable.

The rotor RS runs at several thousand rev/min with its working surface WS in close proximity to the stator S, the gap being adjustable from about 50 μm upward. Crude mix is fed via the funnel on to the centre of the rotor and is flung outwards via the shearing surfaces to be discharged at VO.

Cavitation effects the break up of liquid in ultrasonic equipment. In the Rapisonic Homogenizer, a portable machine made by Ultrasonic

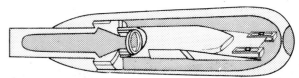

FIG. 18.9. Interior of the Rapisonic homogenizer.

Ltd., crude mix is sucked into one end of a long U-tube and ejected at the other end over a blade which vibrates at its natural frequency of about 30 kHz. The emulsifier head is illustrated in Fig. 18.9.

REFERENCES

BARRY, B. W. & SAUNDERS, G. M. (1970) *J. Colloid Interface Sci.* **34**, 300.

BARRY, B. W. & SAUNDERS, G. M. (1971a) *J. Colloid Interface Sci.* **35**, 689.

BARRY, B. W. & SAUNDERS, G. M. (1971b) *J. Colloid Interface Sci.* **36**, 130.

BARRY, B. W. & SAUNDERS, G. M. (1971c) *J. Pharm. Pharmacol.* **23**, 2405.

BEAN, H. S., KONNING, G. H. & MALCOLM, S. A. (1969) *J. Pharm. Pharmacol.* **21**, 173S.

BECHER, P. (1965) *Emulsions: Theory and Practice*, 2nd edn, New York: Reinhold.

DAVIS, S. S. (1971) *J. Pharm. Pharmacol.* **23**, 161S.

ELWORTHY, P. H. & FLORENCE, A. T. (1969) *J. Pharm. Pharmacol.* **21**, 70S.

GARRETT, E. R. (1965) *J. pharm. Sci.* **54**, 1557.

GRIFFIN, W. C. (1949) *J. Soc. Cosmet. Chem.* **1**, 311.

GRIFFIN, W. C. (1954) *J. Soc. Cosmet. Chem.* **5**, 249.

HAMILL, R. D. & PETERSEN, R. V. (1966) *J. pharm. Sci.* **55**, 1268.

DE KAY, H. G. (1962) *Am. Perfumer & Cosmetics* **77(10)**, 109.

KRUYT (1949) (Ed.) *Colloid Science*, London, Vol. II, 232, Elsevier.

LACHAMPT, F. (1970) *Am. Perfumer & Cosmetics*, **85(1)**, 27.

MULLEY, B. A. & MARLAND, J. S. (1970) *J. Pharm. Pharmacol.* **22**, 243.

PRINCE, L. M. (1967) *J. Colloid Interface Sci.* **23**, 165.

SANDERS, P. A. (1970) *J. Soc. Cosmet. Chem.* **21**, 377.

SHERMAN, P. (1964) *J. Pharm. Pharmacol.* **16**, 1.

SHERMAN, P. (1968) *Emulsion Science*. London: Academic Press.

SHOTTON E. & WHITE, R. F. (1963) *Rheology of Emulsions* (ed. Sherman, P.). Oxford: Pergamon Press.

TALMAN, F. A. J. & ROWAN, E. M. (1970a) *J. Pharm. Pharmacol.* **22**, 417.

TALMAN, F. A. J. & ROWAN, E. M. (1970b) *J. Pharm. Pharmacol.* **22**, 535.

19

Tablets and Capsules

Solid medicaments may be administered orally as powders, pills, cachets, capsules or tablets. As these contain a quantity of drug which is given as a single unit they are known collectively as solid unit-dose forms even in the case of sustained action preparations which, technically, contain the equivalent of several normal doses of drug. The stringent formulation requirements of modern medicaments, the many advantages of tablet and capsule medication, coupled with expanding health services and the concomitant need for large-scale economic manufacture, have lead to a steady decline in the prescribing of powders and pills. A few medicaments such as the salts of para-aminosalicylic acid are administered as cachets and the production of these dose-forms is described elsewhere in this volume. Tablets and capsules, on the other hand, currently account for well over half the total number and cost of all National Health prescriptions issued in the U.K.

TABLETS

Tablets are solid masses made by the compaction of suitably prepared medicament (granules) by means of a tablet machine. Although it is possible to manufacture tablets in a wide range of shapes, official tablets are defined as circular discs with either flat or convex faces. The *British Pharmacopoeia* 1973 includes monographs for over three hundred tablets.

Advantages of Tablet Medication
When correctly formulated and manufactured, tablets provide an accurate, stable dose of drug with the necessary physical and chemical properties for the required duration and intensity of therapeutic action. Modern methods are capable of large scale economic production with a high degree of tablet uniformity both within and between batches. Suitable formulations provide sustained release characteristics and coatings can be applied to improve palatability or reduce the incidence of gastric irritation. Of all dose forms, the tablet presents the medicament in the highest practicable state of compaction. This permits the use of light weight, low cost containers for packaging, while emergency supplies of the drug can be conveniently carried by the patient.

Disadvantages of Tablet Medication
Some patients, particularly children and the seriously ill, may experience difficulty in swallowing tablets. If the tablet is too large, reformulation as two smaller units each containing half the required dose may minimize the problem in some cases. Occasionally a particular property of a medicine, such as the demulcent action of a linctus, cannot effectively be obtained with a tablet. Absorbents are available which allow the production of tablets containing a small amount of liquid, but it is usually more satisfactory to formulate as a soft capsule.

Types and Uses of Tablets
To secure rapid release of drug the majority of tablets are required to break down (disintegrate) rapidly in the stomach, but there are a number of exceptions to this general rule. If the drug is inactivated at low pH, causes gastric irritation, or

269

is intended to exert its effect on the lower part of the gut, an enteric coating is applied to ensure that disintegration does not take place in the stomach but readily occurs in the small intestine. Examples are enteric coated tablets containing erythromycin or the alkali metal halides. Only part of the medicament in a sustained action tablet is released in the stomach to obtain prompt therapeutic action while the remainder is released at a controlled rate as the tablet progresses along the gastrointestinal tract. As an alternative to enteric coating for the minimization of gastric irritation, the drug e.g. aspirin, may be formulated as a soluble tablet to be dissolved in water prior to administration; an effervescent base, as in Effervescent Potassium Tablets BPC, improves palatability. If the preferred site of absorption is the oral mucosa the tablet is directed to be dissolved in the mouth (isoprenaline), under the tongue (ethisterone) or chewed (phenolphthalein). For lozenges slow solution in the mouth, rather than disintegration, is required.

A number of preparations, not intended for oral administration, are also prepared by compression, examples being Mouth-wash Solution Tablets BPC, Testosterone Implants BP and Acetarsol Pessaries BPC. Solution tablets are dissolved in water and the solutions applied to mucous surfaces or externally. A distinctive shape and colour is used for solution tablets that contain a poison.

GRANULATION

THE TABLET COMPRESSION CYCLE

Further processing, that is, granulation, is usually required before a drug can be tabletted. To a large extent the requisite physical properties of the granules are determined by the design of the tablet machine and the nature of the compaction process. Details of machine design are given later, but a brief discussion of the compression cycle, specifically that of the single punch tablet press, is relevant at this point to a proper understanding of the objectives to be attained by granulation.

Granules flow from the hopper (Fig. 19.1) into a feedshoe which oscillates over the die to promote uniform flow of material into the die-cavity. For a given granule the *volume* of the cavity, which is adjustable, governs the weight of the tablet. At the end of the filling stage the toe of the feedshoe is deflected so that it smooths the surface of the granules in the die and cannot foul the top punch as it is lowered to compact the granules. The penetration of the top punch into the cavity can be adjusted to regulate the degree of compaction, that is the tablet hardness. The top punch is then quickly raised and, after a short delay, the bottom punch moves upwards to eject the tablet. Finally, the bottom punch drops to the filling position and the ejected tablet is pushed towards the collection chute by the toe of the feedshoe as it moves forward to commence the filling cycle of the next tablet.

ESSENTIAL GRANULE PROPERTIES

From the foregoing it should be clear that for the successful production of tablets the granules must fulfil a number of requirements. With both single punch and rotary tablet presses only about a fifth of a second or less is available for filling the die-cavity. Rapid, reproducible, flow of granules is essential if the tablet weight is to remain constant throughout the batch. Furthermore, particles of

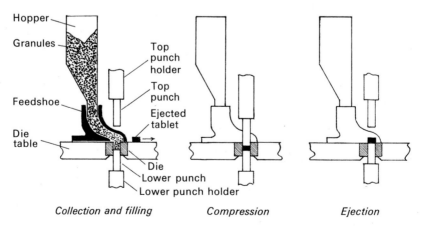

Collection and filling   Compression   Ejection

FIG. 19.1. The compression cycle for a single punch tablet machine.

different size or density must not separate in the hopper as a result of machine vibration if both tablet weight and composition are to be maintained. Granules of uniform size minimize difficulties due to separation, but yield tablets with an inelegant pitted surface. A broader size distribution, with a proportion of fines to fill the inter-granule spaces, avoids the latter problem. The conflicting requirements for ˙tablet uniformity and finish must be carefully balanced by rigid control of the granulation process.

During compaction inter-granule bonds must be formed to allow the production of a tablet which combines the required disintegration characteristics with sufficient firmness to withstand damage due to packaging, transport and other hazards. The volume of the granules may be several times that of the tablet into which they are compacted. The reduction in volume is due to removal of air and this must readily escape for the proper development of the inter-particle bonds. Compaction also forces the tablet material into very close contact with the wall of the die. Excessive die-bore wear and damage to the edges of the tablet result if the die-wall friction is not reduced, usually by the addition of a lubricant to the granules.

In addition to the above it is, of course, essential that the medicament in a tablet is stable and released at the required rate. Primarily these are matters of correct formulation and processing.

GRANULATION PROCESSES

Three processes namely, moist granulation, preliminary compression or slugging and dry granulation are in common use and are described in the *British Pharmaceutical Codex*, 1973.

Moist Granulation
This is still the most widely used of the three processes. The mixed, powdered, tablet constituents are converted to a moist cohering mass by the incorporation of granulating fluid. Granules formed by passing the moist mass through a screen are dried, rescreened to break down agglomerates and blended with other tablet adjuvants such as lubricant and disintegrant. Although the majority of drugs are available as powders suitable for direct use in the moist granulation process, in a few cases the particle size of the powder affects the eventual compression characteristics of the granules. Smith (1950), for instance, reports that a powder finer than 80 mesh should be used for the production of tablets containing either phenacetin or phenobarbitone. Often the dose of the drug is very small

and an inert diluent (bulking excipient) should be added before granulation to give, as a minimum, a 50 mg tablet. Some diluents will absorb small quantities of liquids (absorbent excipients); others may be used in the dry granulation process (see Table 19.1). Although the inertness of diluents is generally assumed, there have been reports of their adverse effect on product performance. Stephenson

TABLE 19.1

SOME DILUENTS USED IN TABLETTING

Diluent	Use and comments
Calcium Phosphate BPC	Absorbent diluent. Increases granule density but some grades are abrasive.
Calcium Hydrogen Phosphate USP	Used for direct compression formulations.
Colloidal silica	Small proportion used as an absorbent diluent or to improve granule flow by glidant action.
Anhydrous Dextrose BP	Absorbs moisture at high relative humidity—see BPC.
Dextrose (spray dried)	Useful for direct compression formulations but absorbs moisture at high relative humidity.
Lactose BP	Inert, tasteless, odorless, inexpensive and gives granules by moist granulation which have good tabletting properties. Incompatable with primary amines (Duvall et al. 1965).
Lactose (spray dried)	Used for direct compression formulations but tablets may assume a brown tinge on storage (Brownley & Lachman 1963). Is also incompatable with primary amines.
Lactose (anhydrous)	Used for direct compression formulations. Care should be taken to prevent moisture uptake. Is also incompatible with primary amines.
Mannitol BP	Dissolves readily and has a 'cooling' effect in the mouth.
Microcrystalline cellulose	Mainly used for direct compression formulations; has some lubricant and disintegrant effect and may improve the behaviour of granules made by other methods.
Sodium Chloride BP	Oral tablets containing this substance must be dissolved in water before administration to avoid gastric irritation—see BP. Usually reserved for the formulation of solution tablets. To avoid binding during compression, dry thoroughly and compress while still warm.
Starch BP	Small proportion of dried starch may be used as an absorbent excipient but its main use is as a disintegrant.

and Humphreys-Jones (1951) examined a number of formulations for glyceryl trinitrate tablets and demonstrated the superior stability of preparations using a lactose base. Richman et al. (1965) noted that microcrystalline cellulose permits dry granulation of this drug and yields a more stable product than that obtained with a lactose–sucrose diluent. A carbonyl-amine reaction causes darkening of tablets containing lactose or other reducing sugars together with a primary amine (Duvall et al. 1965). The BPC 1968 states that calcium phosphate may interfere with the absorption of calciferol.

Mixing. To ensure batch uniformity it is essential that the dry powders are thoroughly mixed before moistening. It must be stressed that mixing problems are particularly acute where one or more of the constituents forms only a small proportion of the tablet weight. Such minor components should, if possible, be dissolved in the granulating fluid or other suitable solvent and incorporated during the moistening stage. This method is included in the *British Pharmacopoeia* 1973 monograph on tablets and was specified for Soluble Paediatric Atropine Sulphate Tablets BPC 1968. Train (1960) pointed out that solute migration during the drying stage, analogous to separation on a chromatographic column, will lead to unequal distribution of solute within the granule mass, that is, to virtual demixing and this may be difficult to rectify in subsequent processing. With soluble dyes the effect is visually apparent in the uneven coloration of the dried granules and the mottled appearance of the finished tablet. Jaffe and Lippmann (1964) studied the migration of F.D. & C. Blue No. 1 dye in lactose and noted that tragacanth, acacia and talc tended to 'fix' the dye so reducing its migration. The problem may be circumvented by the use of lake dyes, that is, soluble dyes bonded to an inert base. Lake dyes usually exhibit greater stability to light than the corresponding soluble colorant and are now much used, particularly for tablet coating.

A further mixing difficulty may arise if the drug is physically adsorbed on to the surface of the granules and these have a broad size distribution. A large fraction of the drug will be adsorbed on the fines since these make a disproportionately large contribution to the total granule surface. Should separation of fines occur this again is equivalent to demixing. The deliberate removal of fines to improve the tabletting properties of the granules is particularly suspect in these circumstances as this could lead to the production of low potency tablets. Where solvent dispersion of the minor components is not feasible a concentrated triturate may be prepared and subsequently diluted, in steps, with the remainder of the tablet ingredients. This should improve mixing, as comparable quantities of materials are blended at each stage of the process.

Batches up to a few hundred grams may be mixed in a mortar. Larger quantities of powders require power driven mixers, e.g., Y-cone, Roto-cube, or ribbon blenders. The transference of large quantities of material from the mixing to the moistening equipment may be obviated by the use of trough or change-pan mixers (Fig. 19.2) which are capable of performing both operations. The change-pan mixer is so called because the mixing blades and pan are detachable. Only one drive unit is required to service a number of blades and pans in which separate products may be prepared according to the needs of production. In this way the mixer is utilized more efficiently, transport of granules for further processing is facilitated and cleansing of the blades and pan simplified.

Moistening. This involves the gradual addition of granulating fluid to the dry mixed powders. A pestle and mortar is suitable for small batches, but power

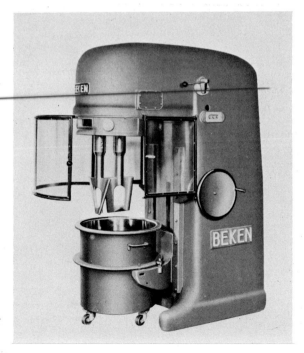

Fig. 19.2. The Beken change pan mixer with working capacity of about 0.1 m^3. The machine is shown with the pan lowered and the guard open (Beken Engineering Ltd.).

driven equipment such as the trough or change-pan mixer is essential for thorough blending action on a larger scale. Initially most of the fluid is held by capillary forces at the points where particles are in contact (Fig. 19.3, Stage 1). Further liquid builds up a continuous film on the external surfaces of the particles and at this second stage the powder is obviously damp and is very coherent. A quite small addition of fluid is now sufficient to produce a film of such thickness that the inter-particle friction is lowered to an extent that close packing of the particles can take place. At this third stage of moistening, air in the voids is displaced by fluid and a wet paste, technically a very concentrated suspension, is formed. This can however be produced once the second stage of granulation has been reached, by prolonged or more efficient blending, without the further addition of granulating fluid, owing to more uniform distribution of existing moistening medium and the mechanical removal of air from the mass. For production of tablet granules the volume of granulating fluid, mixing time and efficiency must be adjusted to give a second stage mass which just coheres when lightly compressed in the hand. Often, this condition may be anticipated by observing the behaviour of the mass which breaks away from the walls of the mixer, while the powder shows obvious signs of aggregation as a result of the greater cohesiveness of the particles.

In some cases moistening may be carried out with a solvent which causes partial dissolution of one or more components. With suitable materials the finished granules retain their structure, as the individual particles have been cemented together with solute deposited by the removal of solvent on drying. Reversion to the original powdered state will occur if substances of low natural cohesiveness are solvent granulated and a binding or adhesive granulating agent is required in these circumstances. The adhesive may be added as a solution or mixed with the tablet ingredients as a dry powder for subsequent activation by moistening with solvent. The latter method is sometimes less effective, as many binders are hydrophilic colloids requiring for complete hydration more solvent and mixing time than is normally used at the moistening stage. Table 19.2 lists some of the more commonly used binders. Ethyl alcohol, isopropyl alcohol, acetone, and chlorinated hydrocarbons are useful moistening agents for water-sensitive drugs; a solvent soluble adhesive may be needed to obtain firm granules. Due to their high cost, the use of anhydrous solvents is usually restricted to those situations where other methods are not feasible. Attention must be given to fire and toxicity hazards and efficient vapour extraction is mandatory.

The most suitable granulating fluid, the volume to be used and the optimum operating conditions are best selected by the production of trial batches of granules. In the early stages of developing a suitable process, when even an approximate value for the volume of granulating fluid is not known, the time taken for moistening may be unduly protracted. Significant amounts of solvent may be lost by evaporation in these circumstances and should be allowed for in subsequent trials. Clearly, the volume of fluid must be sufficient to produce a second stage moistened powder mass and at the same time add sufficient binder to ensure the production of suitable granules. Powdery granules which do not compress well are obtained if the adhesive is too 'weak', is employed in too low a concentration, or if the volume of granulating fluid is inadequate. The converse conditions lead to hard granules which produce excessive amounts of fines when dry-screened. Symptoms of over-moistening are clogging of the screen and agglomeration of the wet granules. Scale-up calculations based on

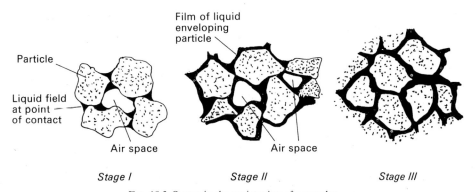

FIG. 19.3. Stages in the moistening of a powder.

TABLE 19.2

ADHESIVE GRANULATING AGENTS

Material	Concentration in the granulating fluid % w/v	Concentration in the dried granules % w/v	Uses and comments
Acacia	5–15	1–5	Use high quality gum to avoid the darkening of white tablets. Clarify the solution. Excess gives very hard granules.
Ethylcellulose	2–5	0.5–3	Soluble in water or alcohol, the latter being used for water-sensitive drugs. Is relatively expensive.
Gelatin	5–20	1–3	Dissolve in hot water and use warm, as the cold solution gels. Produces hard tablets which dissolve slowly—useful for lozenges.
Liquid glucose	10–30	5–20	Strong adhesive action. Tablets may soften under humid conditions.
Methylcellulose	2–10	0.5–3	Use low viscosity grades. May prolong disintegration time.
Polyethylene glycol (Macrogol)	Solvent activated	2–15	Use grades with molecular weight in excess of 5000. Soluble in water and some anhydrous solvents. Has some lubricant action and helps to counteract effects due to the hydrophobic nature of some materials.
Polyvinyl pyrrolidone (P.V.P.)	2–10	0.5–3	See ethylcellulose.
Sodium alginate	2–10	0.5–3	See methylcellulose.
Sodium carboxymethylcellulose	2–10	0.5–3	See methylcellulose.
Starch	5–15	1–5	Mucilage prepared with boiling water and used as warm as possible, as the mucilage gels on cooling. Efficient blending action is essential.
Sucrose	10–50	5–30	Strong adhesive, but tablets tend to harden on storage.
Tragacanth	0.5–2	up to 0.5	Not generally used as an adhesive but is added to lozenges for its demulcent effect. Often solvent activated.

data obtained from small trial batches often overestimate the concentration and volume of granulating fluid on account of the higher blending efficiency of equipment used for large scale manufacture. Finally, granules must be evaluated on a press of the type used for production as their performance may to some degree be affected by mechanical features such as the method for filling the die-cavity, speed of operation and compaction conditions.

Wet screening. Granules will not readily flow into a cavity with which they are comparable in size due to crowding at the entrance of that cavity. On the other hand very fine granules often exhibit poor flow characteristics. Both conditions lead to excessive weight variation in the manufactured tablets. In addition, tablets which are too thin relative to their diameter are prone to breakage when handled. For these reasons the screens used for granulation and the die size for compression are selected (Table 19.3) according to the final tablet weight. The Table must be regarded as a guide only since, for example, a smaller die size may be required if the material to be tabletted is unusually dense, while screens somewhat larger or smaller than those recommended may give granules with better characteristics.

Small batches of moistened mass may be screened by hand, the material being lightly rubbed, rather than forced, through the screen. Too vigorous manipulation at this stage is equivalent to highly efficient blending which, as already explained, may result in the formation of a third stage pasty mass and consequent difficulties due to screen clogging. Hand screening is tedious for more than a few kilograms of moist material, power driven equipment such as the Apex comminutor or the Fitz mill

TABLE 19.3

A GUIDE TO THE SIEVE NUMBER, PUNCH SIZE AND MAXIMUM
PUNCH LOAD FOR THE PRODUCTION OF TABLETS

Tablet weight (mg)	Sieve number[1] for		Punch diameter (mm)	Maximum punch load[2]	
	wet screening	dry screening		Flat or normal concave or flat (kg)	Deep concave or flat bevelled edge (kg)
50	16	20	5–6.5	2000	1300
100	16	20	7	3000	1500
150	12	16	8	3800	1800
200	12	16	8.5	4800	2000
300	10	12	10.5	6500	2500
500	10	10	12	8800	3500
1000	8	8	16	15300	6500

[1] Meshes per inch (2.54 cm).

[2] Applies to special steels used for tabletting punches; for other materials refer to the manufacturer.

being employed for larger batches. The oscillating granulator (Fig. 19.4) also finds considerable industrial use. The base of the hopper is closed by a semi-cylindrical interchangeable screen just above which a rotor oscillates about a horizontal axis. Blades parallel with the axis and integral with the rotor push the moist mass through the screen on to a receiver below. In a recent study Fonner et al. (1966) found that this type of granulator gave smoother, more nearly spherical granules of a starch–lactose formulation than either hand screening or three other commonly used power-driven granulating machines.

Drying. The drying temperature for granules is usually about 60° but may be lower if thermolabile substances are involved. With tray dryers, air exchange is essential to prevent saturation of the oven atmosphere with solvent vapour. By spreading the granules as thin layers on the trays and raking these layers over from time to time, agglomeration of granules and migration of solutes is minimized and even drying of the granules promoted. If different products are to be dried in the oven at the same time care must be taken to avoid cross-contamination. Up to 24 h may be required for the drying of large batches of granules.

The fluid-bed dryer (Fig. 19.5) is now widely used in the pharmaceutical industry because the drying time is only 20 to 30 min, irrespective of batch size which may be 60 kg or more. The amount of granulated solvent to be evaporated decreases as drying proceeds; thus the temperature of the air leaving the fluidized bed rises until it is constant and approximates to that of the input air stream. With experience the effluent air temperature provides a convenient means of establishing the optimum drying time. If drying is prolonged beyond this point attrition of the granules leads to an increase in the proportion of fines. The overdried granules have inferior compressing characteristics and consequently difficulties are encountered in the production of the tablets. On large scale equipment an automatic timer is provided to shut off the heaters and air flow at the end of the pre-determined drying time. Generally, less fluid is needed for granules which are to be dried in fluidbed equipment as the amount of granulating fluid suitable for tray-dried granules gives a moist mass which is too dense and cohesive for correct fluidization of the bed. On the other hand, undermoistening should be avoided as fines may clog the output air filters and impede the air flow.

Dry-screening. This breaks down agglomerates and reduces them to a size compatible with the tablet diameter. Too vigorous dry-screening causes granule structure to be lost with the production of excessive quantities of fines. Although a proportion of these is required to fill the voids between larger granules, so giving a smooth tablet surface, and excess causes trouble at the compression stage.

Other methods of moist granulation. The conventional process has a wide range of application but is time consuming and involves a large number of separate operations. Alternative methods of moist granulation have been developed whereby granule manufacture can be carried out as a single integrated process. Fluid-bed granulation (and drying) stems from the work of Wurster (1959, 1960) who had earlier patented a fluid-bed method for tablet coating. One equipment in current use for moist granulation has a downwards directed atomizer placed centrally above the fluidization chamber. Correct circulation of material is brought about by the special shape of the perforated base and the progressive expansion of the upper part of the chamber. The powders are mixed, granulated by the spray of warm granulating solution and dried while in a fluidized state. Lubricant, disintegrant and any other necessary tablet adjuvants are then added and blended by a further short period of fluidization.

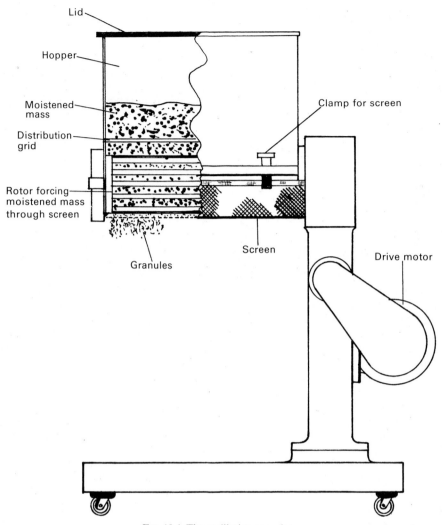

Lid

Hopper

Moistened mass

Distribution grid

Rotor forcing moistened mass through screen

Granules

Clamp for screen

Screen

Drive motor

FIG. 19.4. The oscillating granulator.

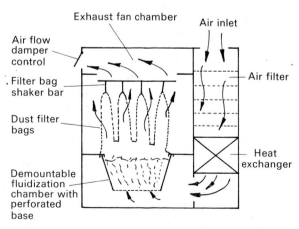

Exhaust fan chamber

Air inlet

Air flow damper control

Filter bag shaker bar

Dust filter bags

Demountable fluidization chamber with perforated base

Air filter

Heat exchanger

FIG. 19.5. The fluid-bed drier.

Granule size is controlled by the volume, temperature and rate of addition of granulating fluid together with the air flow-rate, which determines the expansion and circulation of the bed. Normally, these parameters are automatically controlled by presetting a programming device on the basis of data obtained from previous development batches. A granulator capable of processing up to 60 kg of material in under 2 hr with only minimum supervision, is shown in Fig. 19.6. Other methods for moist granulation are discussed in Chapter 17. The foregoing methods all show a considerable saving in time and labour costs as compared with the conventional method: the granules often possess superior flow properties due to their greater smoothness and sphericity.

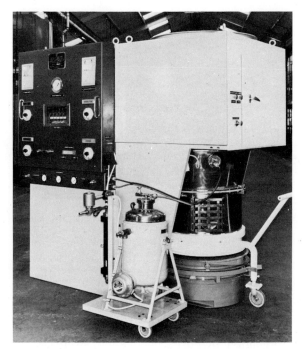

FIG. 19.6. The Calmic fluid-bed granulator. The programming panel may be seen top left. This controls application of granulating agent from the pressure vessel (centre bottom) to the material in the fluidizing chamber.

Preliminary Compression or Slugging

This method is used where the tablet ingredients react chemically when moistened, degrade in the presence of water or when heated, or yield granules with poor flow or compression properties when made by other granulation techniques.

Heavy-duty tablet presses are employed for the compression of the dry, mixed powders. As these rarely flow well, vibratory feed devices may be attached to the hopper while die-cavity filling is facilitated by the use of large (2–5 cm) punches and slow speed operation of the press. Flat faced punches are necessary as the high compaction pressures employed for slugging would splay the edges of a concave faced punch: the clearance between the punch and die-wall is also larger than that used for ordinary tablets to allow rapid escape of air entrapped in the powders. The compaction pressure must be high enough to ensure that the rough tablets (slugs) give material with a granular structure when forced through a screen. It is usually advantageous to add some lubricant and disintegrant prior to slugging, further quantities of these being added to the granules before final compression. Talc is frequently employed as lubricant, since

powder flow rather than die-wall friction is usually the major problem in the preliminary compression stage. Adhesive-containing granules, prepared by moist granulation, tend to retain their structure for long periods in contact with aqueous media. The absence of adhesives from tablets prepared by slugging however usually results in good disintegration.

Paediatric Ampicillin Tablets BPC and the official soluble analgesic tablets containing aspirin may be prepared from granules made by preliminary compression.

Dry Granulation

This is the simplest of the three granulation techniques. The material to be tabletted is screened if necessary, mixed with any additional adjuvants and is then ready for compression. Tablets made in this way are said to have been prepared by direct compression.

Formerly, the alkali metal and ammonium halides, hexamine and potassium chlorate were the only commonly used medicinal substances which could be dry granulated. More recently the list has been extended by the commercial production of suitably granular forms of Dried Yeast, Dry Cascara Extract, Aspirin, some ferrous salts and a few other substances. Provided an increase in the tablet weight can be tolerated, the addition of spray-dried lactose or anhydrous lactose to the medicament, together with lubricant and disintegrant, will often yield granules which may be directly compressed. As Lactose BP does not promote free powder flow, act as a dry binder or possess good compaction properties it would appear that these characteristics reside in the spherical shape of the spray-dried sugar. The applications of this material to tabletting technology have been reviewed by Gunsel and Lachman (1963). Tablets containing spray-dried lactose may assume a brown tinge on storage due, it has been suggested, to the presence in the sugar of 5-hydroxymethyl-furfural (Brownley & Lachman 1963). This darkening should be distinguished from that resulting from the reaction of primary amines and lactose. Other excipients which may be used in direct compression formulae are listed in Table 19.1. Of these, microcrystalline cellulose is of particular interest since, as reported by Reier and Shangraw (1966), this material also possesses marked lubricating and disintegrating properties.

In those cases where one or more ingredients are present in low concentration, efficient mixing may be more difficult with dry than with moist granulation. The problem has a two-fold origin. Firstly, solvent dispersion cannot be used and, secondly, fine powders are essential to secure efficient mixing—but fine powders lack the good flow and compaction characteristics essential to tablet manufacture. The magnitude of the problem may be appreciated by applying the methods described by Train (1960) to the example of 50 mg tablets containing 1 per cent by weight of drug. If the density of the material from which the tablet is formed is 1.5 g.cm^{-3} the particle size should not exceed 20 microns and at least 10^7 particles per tablet are necessary to ensure that 99.7 per cent of the tablets in the batch comply with a ± 10 per cent tolerance in the content of the drug.

Dry granulation is the most economical of the three granulation processes in terms of time, labour and equipment. The availability of the drug for absorption should be good due to the absence of adhesive granulating agents while the elimination of drying and moistening stages obviates many of the stability problems associated with the moist granulation process. Against these advantages must be set the relatively high cost of some diluents used in direct compression formulae and the restricted range of materials manufactured in a suitable granular form. It seems likely however that the more widespread adoption of devices for promoting uniform die-filling with difficult materials will reduce the cost and extend the applicability of the dry granulation process.

FLAVOURS, LUBRICANTS AND DISINTEGRANTS

When moist granulation is employed, these adjuvants are normally added to the dry, screened granules, but the incorporation of internal lubricant or a proportion of disintegrant prior to moistening, as described below, are exceptions. For slugging and dry granulation the addition of these adjuvants has been discussed in the relevant sections.

Flavours
Essential oils are included in a few official tablets. They may be mixed with a small quantity of fines or absorbent excipient and the triturate thoroughly blended with the rest of the granules. Dissolution in a volatile solvent aids dispersion if the volume of flavouring agent is small or, alternatively, the solution may be directly sprayed on to the granules. In both cases solvent must be completely removed before compaction. For non-official tablets a wide range of flavours in powder form is available.

Flavours may not, of course, be added prior to an operation involving the use of heat.

Lubricants
These may promote granule flow (glidants), minimize die-wall friction (die-wall lubricants) or prevent the adhesion of granules to the punch faces (anti-adherents). Talc, for example, is a good glidant but is inferior to magnesium stearate as a die-wall lubricant. In addition to their mode of action, lubricants may also be classified according to the way in which they are added to the granules. External lubricants are incorporated immediately before compression and function by coating the granule surface while internal lubricants are mixed with the dry powders prior to moistening with granulating fluid. Granules prepared in this manner are described as self-lubricating. One step in the moist granulation process can be eliminated by the use of an internal lubricant in conjunction with polyethylene glycol as the binding agent. In suitable cases the water solubility of the glycol permits the formulation of tablets with good disintegration properties. Commonly used lubricants are listed in Table 19.4.

Disintegrants
These assist the disintegration of the tablet by swelling (bursters), by improving the penetration of aqueous liquids (Table 19.5), or by the liberation of gas from an effervescent base. For a number of medicaments, disintegration of the tablet is improved if part of the disintegrant is added to the powders prior to moistening; the disintegrant within the granules assists the disruption of these in contact with aqueous media. Powdered disintegrants e.g., starch, methylcellulose, etc., are normally employed in proportions which significantly increase the fines content of the granules and in unfavourable circumstances this can give rise to compression difficulties. Additionally, premature disintegretation of the tablet may occur in the mouth if excessive amounts of disintegrant are employed and, apart from difficulty in swallowing the powdery mass, any unpleasant taste due to the medicament may prove objectionable. In a few cases an effervescent base is used to promote disintegration. This consists of citric or tartaric acid together with sodium bicarbonate, potassium bicarbonate or calcium carbonate. These react in contact with water to liberate carbon dioxide which disrupts the tablet. A slight trace of moisture is sufficient to initiate the reaction which produces

further water and is thus potentially self-perpetuating. For stability, very dry materials, rigorous exclusion of moisture during manufacture and efficient sealing of the packages are essential—the use of *anhydrous* citric acid in official preparations of this type should be noted.

TABLE 19.4

LUBRICANTS USED IN TABLETTING

Material	Type	Concentration in the granules per cent w/w	Uses and comments
Boric acid	E, L	1–5	Toxic orally, reserve for solution-tablets.
Colloidal silica	E, G	0.1–0.5	Promotes granule flow but has little effect on die-wall friction.
Hydrogenated vegetable oils	I, L	1–5	May prolong disintegration time. 'Hard' grades must be used to avoid punch face adhesion.
Magnesium stearate	E, L	0.1–1	Use minimum effective amount as excess may impede granule flow, reduce tablet hardness, or prolong disintegration. Some grades are slightly 'alkaline'—this causes discoloration of aminophylline tablets (Castello & Mattocks 1962) and promotes the hydrolysis of aspirin (Ribeiro et al. 1955; Kornblum & Zoglio 1967).
Polyethylene glycol	I, L	2–15	Use grades with molecular weight in excess of 5000. Soluble in water and some anhydrous solvents. Has some lubricant action, helps to counteract effects due to the hydrophobic nature of some materials, but main use is as a binder.
Stearic acid	E, L / I, L	0.1–1 / 0.2–2	Use finely powdered grade. Effect on tablet hardness and disintegration not so marked as with the magnesium salt.
Talc	E, G	1–5	Promotes granule flow and inhibits punch face adhesion but is much less effective than the stearates as a die-wall lubricant. Low quality grades may be abrasive causing punch and die wear.

E —External lubricant
I —Internal lubricant
L —Lubricates die-wall
G —Glidant

TABLE 19.5

DISINTEGRANTS USED IN TABLETTING

Material	Concentration in the granules per cent w/w	Uses and comments
Alginic acid	2–10	Burster which may prove better than starch for 'difficult' materials (Berry & Ridout 1950). May be incorporated prior to moistening to improve disintegration. If added to the dry granules, avoid finely powdered grades as these form a coherent gel on the tablet surface and may prolong disintegration time.
Magnesium aluminium silicate	1–10	Burster; Veegum is one variety.
Methylcellulose	2–10	Burster. Use medium viscosity grade in a not too fine powder.
Microcrystalline cellulose	1–10	Has some lubricant properties, higher concentrations used as dry-binding diluent
Sodium lauryl sulphate	0.1–0.5	Wetting agent which improves penetration of the tablet pore system by aqueous liquids. Will counteract the water-repellent effect of, for example, phenothiazine and the stearate lubricants. May minimize the increase in disintegration time which often occurs as tablets age.
Starch	2–10	Burster. Potato and maize starch are usually considered superior to the other varieties. Part may be incorporated prior to moistening.

THE COMPRESSING WEIGHT

This is the weight of granules which must be fed into the die-cavity to give a tablet containing the nominal amount of drug. The most direct method is to assay the granules and from the result calculate the compressing weight. Alternatively, this may be derived from data obtained during the manufacture of the granules and allows production of tablets to proceed without the delay due to the time taken to assay the granules. Whichever method is used, the finished tablets must be examined for medicament content, weight uniformity etc. as discussed later.

Dry granulation. The compressing weight is the sum of the weights of the individual ingredients in each tablet:

Codeine Phosphate	20.00 mg
Stearic acid, in fine powder	0.06 mg
Potato Starch	0.60 mg
Spray dried lactose	39.34 mg
Compressing weight	60.00 mg

As given, this formula would not be adopted for the commercial production of large batches, due to the possible darkening of the spray-dried lactose. It is suitable for the extemporaneous preparation of small batches. If a specified number of tablets must be supplied, an allowance must be made for losses incurred when adjusting the machine for correct tablet weight and hardness.

Preliminary compression. Here, an allowance must be made for losses which occur when slugging and rescreening. Consider typical production data for 100 000 Soluble Aspirin Tablets BP:

	per tablet	for 100 000 tablets
Aspirin, in fine powder	300 mg	31.00 kg
Anhydrous Citric Acid	30 mg	3.10 kg
Calcium Carbonate	100 mg	10.33 kg
Saccharin Sodium	3 mg	0.31 kg
Talc	4 mg	0.41 kg
Theoretical weight of ingredients	437 mg	45.15 kg
Weight of granules after slugging and rescreening		44.30 kg
Weight of talc added prior to final compression		0.80 kg
Total weight of granules for final compression		45.10 kg

Actual number of tablets which may be prepared from the slugged and rescreened material is:

$$\frac{44\,300}{0.437} = 101\,373$$

Compressing weight

$$= \frac{\text{Total weight of granules for compression}}{\text{Number of tablets}}$$

$$= \frac{45\,100}{101\,373} = 0.445 \text{ g}$$

Talc, rather than magnesium stearate, is used to avoid hydrolysis of aspirin and to improve powder flow. Disintegrant is not required as an effervescent base and finely powdered aspirin ensures rapid dissolution when the tablet is placed in water.

The use of anhydrous citric acid avoids premature reaction of the ingredients.

Moist granulation. When calculating the compressing weight of granules prepared by this process it cannot be assumed that the starting materials are perfectly dry or that all moistening solvent is removed by drying. By keeping a record of the weight of the product at each stage of the granulating process calculation of the compressing weight is feasible. The following data might be typical for the manufacture of, say, about 200 000 tablets each containing 0.5 g of medicament:

Medicament	101.0 kg
Adhesive granulating fluid	10.6 kg
Theoretical weight of mass	111.6 kg
Actual weight of moist granules	111.1 kg
Weight of granules after drying	104.6 kg
Weight of granules after screening	104.3 kg

Formula of granules for compression:

Screened granules	104.3 kg
Disintegrant	8.0 kg
Lubricant	0.5 kg
Weight of granules for tabletting	112.8 kg

Number of tablets which could be produced from 101 kg of medicament is:

$$\frac{101\,000}{0.5} = 202\,000$$

Weight of moist mass per tablet:

$$\frac{111\,600}{202\,000} = 0.5525 \text{ g}$$

Number of tablets that may be prepared from the actual weight of moist granules:

$$\frac{111\,100}{0.5525} = 201\,095$$

After drying 104.6 kg of material contains the medicament present in 111.1 kg of moist granules and 104.3 kg of dried material is available for tabletting after screening. The number of tablets that may be produced from the screened granules is:

$$\frac{201\,086 \times 104.3}{104.6} = 200\,518$$

The final compressing weight after addition of disintegrant and lubricant is:

$$\frac{112\,800}{200\,518} = 0.5625 \text{ g}$$

In the previous two examples large quantities of materials are being handled and losses can be kept to a minimum. Much greater losses are incurred when the moist granulation technique is applied to small batches; moistened mass which cannot be recovered from the granulating screen and tablets lost when adjusting the tablet press may represent a large proportion of the total batch. A loss of up to 10 per cent is possible in these circumstances and should be allowed for when calculating the weights of materials required to produce the batch.

PRODUCTION OF TABLETS

THE SINGLE PUNCH TABLET MACHINE

Assembly

Clean the punches and die, set the machine by hand to the filling position, insert the bottom punch in its holder (Fig. 19.7), making sure that the locking notch faces the locking bolt, and lightly secure in position. Carefully fit the die, check that the die-face is flush with the table and then securely tighten the locking bolt. The top punch may now be fitted, lightly secured, and this operation followed by the assembly of the feedshoe but not the connecting rod. Fill the feedshoe with granules, adjust the weight regulating collar so that the punch face is 0.5 to 1 cm below the die table and then fill the cavity with granules. Carefully lower the top punch into the die-cavity and at the same time adjust the hardness control such that the machine drive cannot be turned by hand past the compression position; maintain the load on the punches while their locking bolts are finally tightened. This procedure ensures that the punches are firmly locked in their holders and cannot work loose during tablet manufacture. Finally, reduce the compression control and eject the compact.

Adjustments

Tablet weight. For the filling and compression stages the lifting block pulls down the weight-regulating collar and holds it in contact with the main frame of the machine. The position of the bottom punch face in the bore determines the volume of the die-cavity and hence the tablet weight. For preliminary weight adjustment the collar is adjusted on its thread so that a weighed quantity of granules just fills the cavity. Final weight adjustment is made with the press running normally, as die filling is affected by the dynamic flow properties of the granules under operating conditions.

Ejection. After the compression stage the lifting block moves to its top position and raises the lower punch assembly by engagement with the ejection regulating collar. This is set to bring the punch face flush with the upper surface of the die. Too low a setting will cause part of the tablet to be sliced off as the feedshoe moves forward, while the punch will foul the base of the shoe if the setting is too high. The feedshoe is fabricated from a soft metal to minimize damage in the event of machine malfunction. A locking device is provided to make sure that the regulating collars cannot move during machine operation.

Tablet hardness. The top punch is locked in a holder which moves in a guide to ensure accurate registration of the punch and die-bore. During operation of the press an eccentric cam imparts a vertical movement to the punch holder. Since the amplitude of the upper punch stroke and the centre of rotation of the cam drive are fixed by the machine design, die penetration is controlled by an adjustment which, effectively, alters the distance between the centre of rotation of the cam drive and the face of the upper punch at the bottom of its stroke. If this distance is increased the punch penetrates further into the die-cavity; thus, for a given fill, the granules are more highly consolidated and a harder tablet is formed. The mechanisms used to adjust tablet hardness vary considerably and are best understood by examination of actual equipment. One method is shown in Fig. 19.7; as the holder is moved down the adjusting thread punch penetration is increased.

Feedshoe movement. A rod connects the shoe to its actuating mechanism, transverse oscillation of the feedshoe relative to the die-cavity being controlled by the length of the rod. This should be adjusted to ensure that the cavity is uniformly filled with granules, the top punch does not foul the shoe and the ejected tablet is pushed well away from the vicinity of the die. Once correctly adjusted, little further attention is required for successive production runs.

Operation

Once the machine has been assembled, trial tablets may be made with the feedshoe and the press operated by hand. When soft tablets of the correct weight have been obtained by adjustment of the appropriate controls, the feedshoe operating rod is connected and further tablets produced by hand.

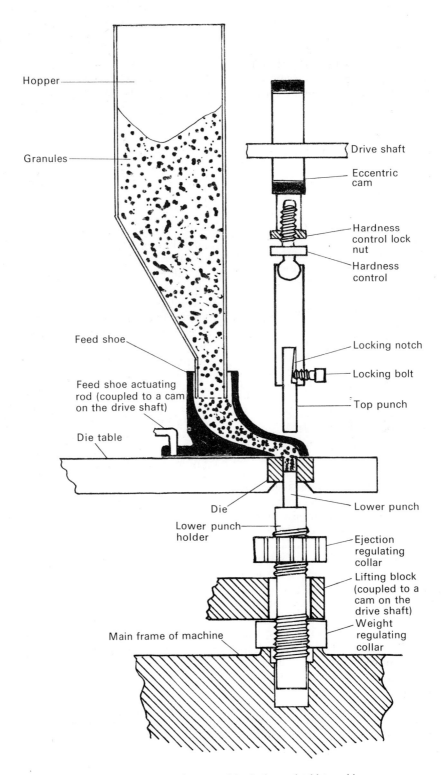

FIG. 19.7. Main operating parts of the single punch tablet machine.

If these are still rather soft, but otherwise satisfactory, power drive may be applied. Make any final adjustments to the controls bearing in mind that the press will 'settle down' after 20 to 30 tablets have been made. The production of soft tablets during the preliminary stages of adjusting the machine is necessary to obviate jamming due to the more efficient filling of the die under power drive.

The optimum tablet hardness depends on the material to be compacted and the ultimate use of the tablets. Uncoated tablets must be hard enough to withstand handling and yet not so hard that the disintegration time is unduly prolonged. Firmer tablets are required to resist the abrasion normal to the film or pan coating processes, but cores for compression coating must be somewhat soft to allow further consolidation when the coating is applied. A crushing test is used to ensure compliance with predetermined specifications for tablet hardness.

There is, obviously, a limit to the compaction force which may be safely developed by a given model of tablet press. Some are fitted with an adjustable overload release whereby the weight regulating collar rests on a spring loaded stop which is deflected downwards should the preselected compacting force be exceeded. In this way jamming and machine damage is avoided. The medium duty press shown in Fig. 19.8 is provided with means for varying the production rate from 40 to 90 tablets a minute and overload release for loads up to 4 tons (4000 kg).

It is essential that precautions are taken to preclude accidental connection of the power supply during assembly and initial adjustment of the press. As large compaction forces are developed, even by hand tablet machines, it should not be necessary to emphasize that the hands must be kept clear of the compressing area during production. On some presses an interlocking switch isolates the power supply until the moving parts are enclosed by a safety screen. The machine must never be operated so that the punch faces come into contact: if it is to be left for a short period the die-cavity must be filled with granules. Finally, the feedshoe connecting rod must be removed and the shoe deflected away from the die area, if it becomes necessary to operate the press in the reverse direction.

THE ROTARY TABLET MACHINE

The most important factor limiting the production capacity of a tablet press is the rate at which the die-cavity can be filled with granules. For the single punch machine the limit is probably of the order

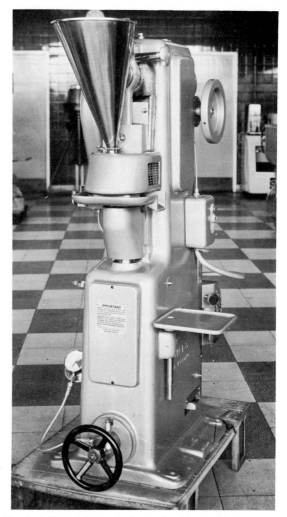

FIG. 19.8. Power-driven single punch tablet machine. The top punch and the bottom punch holder are enclosed by a safety screen. The value at which overload occurs is indicated by the gauge bottom left.

of 8000 tablets/hr but by mounting the punches and dies in a rotating holder (turret) which passes them in sequence through the filling, compression and ejection stages much larger outputs are possible. This is the principle of the rotary tablet machine (Fig. 19.9).

The top and bottom punches move freely in guides bored in the upper and lower sections of the turret (Fig. 19.10) while the centre section forms the die-table. Cam tracks govern the positions of the punches by engaging with the head or the under surface of the 'mushroom' head of the punch. The die-cavity is over-filled with granules as it passes below a flat feedframe (Fig. 19.11) fed from a hopper. Tablet weight is regulated

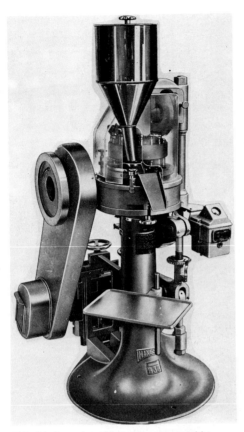

FIG. 19.9. Medium duty 16-station rotary tablet press. The upper turret and punches are visible beneath the plastic dust screen (Manesty Machines Ltd.).

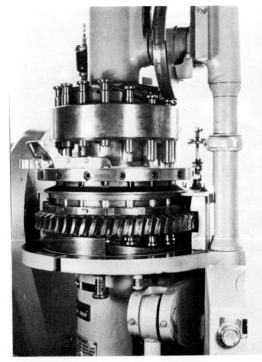

FIG. 19.10. 16-station rotary tablet press. The perspex screens and hopper and lower guard have been removed to show the upper and lower turrets and die table. The upper and lower cam tracks and the upper pressure roller are also visible.

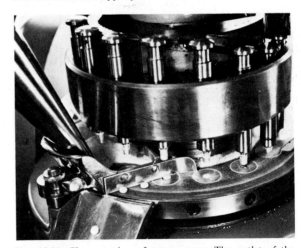

FIG. 19.11. Close-up view of rotary press. The outlet of the hopper may be seen (left) feeding granules into the feed frame. Ejected tablets are being directed towards the collection chute bolted to the end of the feed frame. The upper cam track for lifting the top punch clear of the feed frame is also visible.

by an adjustable section of the lower cam track which, towards the end of the filling period, causes the bottom punch to rise slightly. The excess granules are removed by a scraper bar and retained in the feed frame. The method gives a more consistent die fill than would be obtained by setting the bottom punch at the correct level for the whole of the filling period. Weight adjustment is followed by a slight but sudden drop in the bottom punch level both to remove air by tamping action and lower the level of the granules in the die. This facilitates subsequent compaction and at the same time obviates spillage from the die-cavity due to the centrifugal forces developed by the rotating turret.

At the start of the compression stage the top punch is rapidly lowered to penetrate the die-cavity and then both punches pass between pressure rollers which 'squeeze' the punches towards one another. The position of the upper roller is fixed and it is the adjustable lower roller that controls the separation of the punch faces at the point of maximum compression, that is, the tablet hardness. The lower roller is fitted with adjustable overload protection. Following compression, the top punch is raised rapidly to clear the feed frame and allow the tablet to be ejected as the lower punch rides up the lower cam track which may be adjusted to set the correct height of the punch for tablet ejection. The lower punch is then pulled down for the filling stage on the next revolution of the turret. A scraper bar directs the ejected tablet towards the collection chute. Any granules which have seeped out of the feed frame are carried round on the die-table and returned to the frame behind the scraper bar. With 16 punch and die positions (16 station machines) the output is of the order of 50 000 tablets/hr. Double rotary machines produce two tablets per revolution of the turret; outputs in excess of half a million tablets/hr may be obtained with 69-station double rotary machines (Fig. 19.12).

It is inherent in the processing of particulate solids that dust will be liberated into the environment, a problem which is particularly acute with rotary tablet machines. With highly potent medicaments toxicity hazards must be considered, while inter-product contamination is an ever present problem in all tablet production processes. Modern rotary machines are provided with clear plastic covers over the the moving parts and dust extrac-

tion. In difficult cases the only complete solution may be the provision of individual dust-extracted cubicles for each machine. Finally, as discussed earlier, it should be remembered that granules which 'run' well on a single punch machine may need reformulation for good performance on a rotary machine (and vice versa) due to differences in the modes of die feed and compression.

DEVELOPMENTS IN THE DESIGN OF ROTARY TABLET MACHINES

Granule Flow
The flow of granules into the feed frame is controlled by the height of the hopper outlet above the die-table. A number of materials flow erratically or may even block the hopper outlet. Vibratory devices for attachment to the hopper offer a partial solution to these problems but where a very high flowrate is required—this may be as much as 2 kg/min for ultra high-speed presses producing half a million tablets/hr—more positive feeding is essential. The Stokes metering hopper minimizes blocking by allowing the granules to flow down a wide straight section at the base of the hopper on

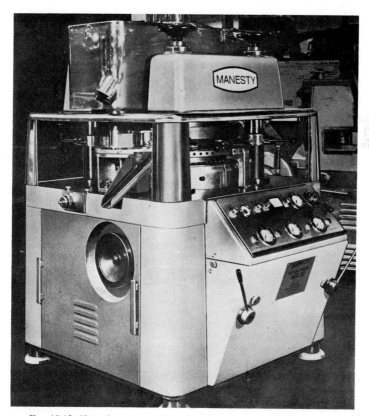

FIG. 19.12. 69-station rotary tablet machine (Manesty Machines Ltd.).

to an inclined plate which in turn directs the granules on to a metering wheel. The form of the latter i.e. perforated disc, mesh or paddle, its rotational speed and the height of the baffle above the wheel, control the flowrate of the granules out of the hopper and into the feed frame.

Die Filling

Even flow of granules from the feed frame into the die-cavity is essential if tablets of uniform weight are to be produced. Even at low operating speeds filling of the die with 'difficult' materials may be erratic with conventional feed frames. A number of devices have been designed to give 'forced', 'assisted' or 'induced' feed of granules into the cavity. The Manesty Rotaflow feeder employs contrarotating vaned rotors in an enclosed feed frame to assist granules into the dies. Some removal of air and slight compaction of the granules in the die-cavity is obtained by the use of this feeder which is so designed that excess granules are automatically returned to the die-feed area. Gold et al. (1968) have reported that with a normal 16-station press the coefficient of weight variation for 500 mg tablets was 0.7 to 2.4 per cent when a granule with good flow properties was used and 3.4 to 3.9 per cent for a poor granule. Using an ultra high speed machine with induced die-feed they found that the coefficient of variation fell to 2 per cent or less irrespective of the type of granule, in spite of a lower tablet weight of 200 mg and a rate of production (3000 to 4000 tablets/min) at least five times that attained with the conventional machine.

Removal of Air

The time taken for compression may not be sufficient for the complete removal of air from the granules in the die-cavity. The air which remains hinders inter-granule bonding and may result in capping, lamination and other difficulties. Many rotary presses are now fitted with precompression rollers for light compaction of the granules ahead of the main compressing position. In this way most of the air is removed from the granule bed which is partially compacted before final compression takes place.

The introduction of devices for improving granule flow, die-filling and the removal of air has made feasible the ultra high-speed production of tablets. These devices will, undoubtedly, find wide application in the direct compression of a wider range of substances than has hitherto been possible with conventional tablet machines.

Multilayer Tablets

One further development, not directly concerned with overcoming flow and compaction problems, has been the introduction of equipment for making multi-layer and compression coated tablets. The latter are discussed in the section on coating techniques. Layer presses are used where chemically incompatible materials, or those which separate in a mixed granulation, must be presented in the same tablet. For sustained action products each layer may be formulated for different release characteristics. The presses employ three filling and compression stages round the turret and as each layer is filled into the die-cavity in sequence the granules are lightly compressed to remove air. When the final layer has been deposited the whole is compressed into a firm tablet in the normal way. Since each layer is thinner than in normal tabletting, fine granules (16 mesh or smaller) must be employed. Excessive fines and lubricants must be avoided to promote good inter-layer adhesion. A sampling device is provided so that the weight of each layer may be checked without stopping the machine. For the successful production of multilayer tablets the granules must not be too dense and should compact to less than half their original volume, otherwise the depth of fill is unmanageably small and difficult to control.

PUNCHES AND DIES

These are usually fabricated from special steels, the working surface being accurately machined and highly polished to ensure proper mechanical operation and well finished tablets. For single punch machines the punches are held, firmly seated in their holders, by wedge action of the locking notches against the tips of the locking bolts; notches or circumferential channels serve the same purpose for the dies. For the manufacture of specially shaped products, such as pessaries, registration of the upper punch and the die must be exact. In the case of rotary tablet machines a key inserted in the guide prevents free rotation of the upper punch. The clearance between the upper punch and die-bore is normally 0.0013–0.004 cm (0.5–1.5 thousandsth of an inch) but for slugging this is increased to 0.008 cm to allow rapid escape of air from the granules. Fines seeping downwards between the lower punch and die-bore would become highly compacted and impede free punch movement but for a slight reduction in the shank diameter some 0.5 cm below the punch face.

In most English speaking countries and some others, punch diameters were, until recently, quoted as multiples of a thirty-second of an inch, but metric sizes have been adopted by the *British Pharmacopoeia* 1973 and *British Pharmaceutical Codex* 1973. The majority of tablets are produced with flat, flat bevelled edge or normal concave punches (Fig. 19.13) but where tablets are to be pan or film coated deep concave punches must be used to facilitate the coating process. Punch faces may be embossed so that tablets with engraved letters or other devices are produced. Diametrical scoring permits more ready subdivision of the tablet by the patient should this be required. The load which may safely be applied to punches is limited by the material from which they are fabricated and by the type of punch face. A load of 8×10^7 kg/m^2 (50 tons/in^2) is permissible for flat or normal concave steel punches but must be reduced to half this figure, or less, depending on the punch diameter and face contour where the edge of the punch face is very thin as is the case with deep concave, bevelled edge and ball punches. This is because the lateral forces developed during compression would splay the thin weak edges of these types of punches. The maximum loads quoted in Table 19.3 are average figures for the special steels used in punch manu-

facture; where other materials are employed the manufacturer of the punches should be consulted.

Punches and dies (tooling) must be stored, lightly oiled, in containers which prevent accidental contact. The ease of manufacture and the final appearance of the tablet depend on unblemished, highly polished working surfaces; punch edges must be sharp and free from burrs. As compaction usually occurs in the middle section of the die-bore, wear 'rings' are formed at this point and hinder tablet ejection. Inversion of the die for alternate tablet batches minimizes ringing and extends the life of the die. Tapered dies may facilitate the compaction of 'difficult' materials, as the progressive increase in clearance (about 0.004 cm in the centre to 0.008 cm at the die-face) permits more ready escape of air and gradual reduction of die-wall friction as ejection proceeds. Tungsten carbide inserts, having greater resistance to wear are particularly useful for the compaction of abrasive materials. Non-metallic tooling may be required for the compaction of corrosive substances. Agate may be employed for this purpose, for instance in the production of tablets containing mercury salts. All stations of a rotary machine must produce tablets of uniform weight and hardness. Maintenance must, therefore,

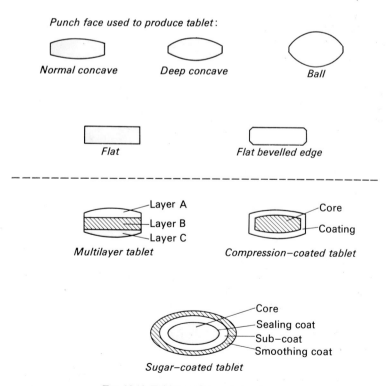

FIG. 19.13. Tablet profiles and structures.

ensure that all punches in a given upper or lower set are of identical length as the weight, hardness and ejection controls are common to all stations of a rotary.

The comprehensive range of tooling required for even a modest tablet manufacturing department represents a large capital investment which rapidly depreciates in the absence of proper maintenance. Additionally, the inferior tablets produced by defective punches and dies do little to enhance the reputation of the manufacturer. Swartz et al. (1962) and Swartz and Anschel (1968) indicate that extended life and improvements in the quality of the tooling supplied by the manufacturer are positive advantages which may be expected from a well organized punch and die quality control programme.

TABLETTING PROBLEMS

Tablets may exhibit a number of defects which are immediately apparent or, as is often the case with capping, appear only after storage. It is important therefore that the appropriate tests be applied at the start of and during a production run in order that remedial action may be promptly taken.

Binding in the Die
When this occurs ejection of the tablet is difficult and is often accompanied by a characteristic 'grunting' noise; the tablet edges are rough or scored. The problem results from those conditions which give rise to high die-wall friction namely, poor lubrication, underdried granules and a dirty or blemished die. Poor lubrication includes inefficient blending of the lubricant with the granules as well as the wrong quantity or choice of this adjuvant. An alternative source of trouble is too large a clearance between the lower punch and the die-bore as a result of excessive wear. Fines seep downwards through the gap and compact to form a tough film which hinders free movement of the punch.

Picking and Sticking
Here the problem is caused by adhesion of material to the punch faces. If localized, portions of the tablet surface are seen to be missing; this is called picking. The tablet has a dull rough appearance when 'sticking' occurs due to adhesion of the tablet to the whole punch face. In either case, if not corrected, the defect worsens progressively and a layer of compacted granules builds up on the punch face. This, effectively, is equivalent to an increase in punch length that causes high compaction pressure and eventual jamming of the press if not promptly rectified. The fault can usually be traced to under-dried granules, poorly maintained punch faces or the use of a lubricant lacking in anti-adherent properties.

Capping and Lamination
These faults can often be traced to inadequate removal of air from the granules in the die-cavity before and during compression. The entrapped air interferes with granule bonding while its subsequent expansion at the ejection stage detaches the top, the 'cap', of the tablet. In other cases the tablet splits into a number of layers (laminates). Excessive fines, incorrectly prepared or overdried granules or too small a top punch/die-bore clearance all hinder escape of air from the die cavity and may be the cause of capping or lamination.

A second cause of the problem is associated with undue elastic compression of the tablet due to the use of too high a pressure at the compaction stage. During ejection, elastic recovery of that part of the tablet protruding from the die gives rise to both lateral and longitudinal forces (Fig. 19.21) which rupture the intergranule bonds and the tablet then caps or laminates. Finally, on occasion, these faults may be traced to distortion of the tablet during ejection from a 'ringed' die or to the use of burred punches.

Excessive Weight Variation
This problem is associated with poor granule flow and separation of granule constituents. Thus granules which are under-dried, too large (see wet-screening, p. 274), too fine or contain a large proportion of fines, are incorrectly lubricated or comprise elements with widely differing densities or sizes, may all be suspected as possible causes of excessive weight variation. If the fault occurs with a rotary machine and granule flow appears to be satisfactory, then it is worth considering the possibility that one or more punches are of different length to the others due, for example, to inadvertent mixing of bottom punch sets. Occasionally, 'difficult' granules are produced in spite of care in processing and tablets of more uniform weight and improved appearance may be obtained at a slower machine speed that allows more time for die-cavity filling.

Fissured or Pitted Surface
If this is not due to sticking or picking the most likely cause is the presence of granules which are uniform in size and lack the fines necessary to fill

the voids. Generally, the problem may be cured by the use of granules with a broader size distribution but care must be taken to see that this does not lead to other problems such as capping or lack of uniformity in the tablet weight.

Soft Tablets

Apart from the use of too low a compaction pressure this problem usually arises when granules have been inadequately dried or the intergranule bonds have been weakened either by traces of air in the granule bed (insufficient to cause capping) or by excessive proportions of fatty lubricant such as magnesium stearate.

Protracted Disintegration

In this case the tablet either rapidly breaks down to form large particles that persist for a long period, or fine particles are produced, but the overall disintegration time is excessive. The fault can usually be traced to:

(i) an adhesive granulating agent which is too 'strong'.

(ii) conditions that inhibit the penetration of water; high degree of compaction, hydrophobic tablet ingredients, excessive quantities of fatty lubricant or gelling of the granulating agent, or

(iii) inefficient bursting action resulting from the use of the wrong type of disintegrating agent, or insufficient of it.

If the granules are intrinsically hydrophobic or have become so due to the unavoidable use of a fatty lubricant, small amounts of surfactant may be included in the tablet formulation to facilitate penetration by aqueous fluids. Alternatively, a hard polyethylene glycol may be employed to provide 'soluble' points in the tablet structure. In suitable cases more efficient bursting action is obtained if part of the disintegrant is incorporated prior to the moistening or preliminary compression stages of granulation. Finally, as discussed later, it should be noted that too *low* a degree of compression may lead to a long disintegration time.

Mottled Tablets

These may be produced if the granule size distribution is discontinuous; the finer particles provide a background of slightly different hue which shows up the larger granules in the tablet surface. The effect is more marked with coloured tablets and is particularly noticeable if dye migration has occurred. If the problem arises when the tablets are stored, instability of one or more ingredients should be suspected.

Variation of Medicament Content

Standards will eventually be set for the drug content of individual tablets. If the content shows excessive variation and those factors contributing to weight variation can be eliminated as a cause, the most likely sources of trouble are migration of solute, physical adsorption with separation at some stage of the production process and inefficient mixing.

Drug Instability

This topic is discussed in detail elsewhere in this volume. The majority of air-dry drugs and tablet excipients contain water and this is also deliberately added, and may not be completely removed, in the moist granulation process. Moisture content must be controlled not only for purely technical reasons associated with the physical processes of tablet production, but also to ensure drug stability. The subject was reviewed by Griffiths (1969).

TABLET COATING

Tablet coatings perform one or more of the following functions. They may: *mask* the taste of unpalatable drugs, *protect* the drug from deterioration due to light, oxygen or moisture, *separate* incompatible ingredients, *control* the release of medicament in the gastrointestinal tract, and *provide* an elegant or distinctive finish to the tablet.

The materials used for coating may largely comprise sucrose (sugar coating), water-soluble film-forming polymers (film coating) or substances which are soluble in the intestinal secretions but not in those of the stomach (enteric coating). These types of coating can all be applied by the pan or fluid-bed processes; the compression coating technique is suitable for sugar and enteric coatings, but not for film coating.

PAN COATING

In this process the tablets are tumbled in a bowl or pan which rotates about an axis inclined about 30° to the horizontal (Fig. 19.14). With the correct pan load a three dimensional circulation is established and sufficient coating solution is added to wet the tablet surfaces. Internal baffles (Sutaria 1968) or hand manipulation of the wetted tablets ensures that the solution is evenly distributed and a satisfactory tumbling action maintained while the coating is dried by a stream of warmed air. Small amounts of dusting powder may be applied to reduce tackiness and cohesion of the tablets during the drying stage. The volume of coating solution

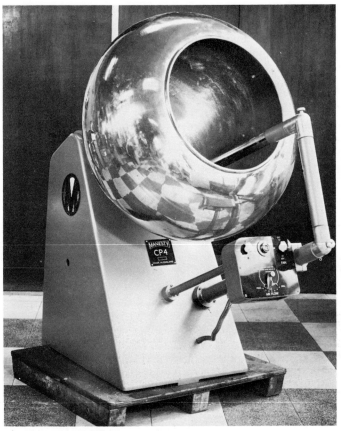

FIG. 19.14. Production model pan coating machine. The diameter of the
bowl is about 1 m (Manesty Machines Ltd.).

for each application is critical; inadequate wetting leads to irregular coating, whereas with too large a volume the tablets agglomerate and do not tumble well. The cycle of alternate wetting and drying is continued to build up a coating of the required properties. Initially, the tablets are subject to considerable abrasive action and for this reason should be more highly compressed than the corresponding uncoated tablets.

Sugar Coatings
This traditional coating imparts a smooth, rounded, elegant appearance to the tablet. Stephenson and Smith (1951) have given a detailed discussion on the composition of sugar coatings.

Sealing.   After all dust has been removed from the the tablets a dextrin, gelatin or acacia coat may be applied to ensure good coating adhesion. Where protection against the effects of water in subsequent coating solutions is required a 30 to 50 per cent solution of shellac in alcohol or other suitable

solvent is employed for sealing, care being taken to avoid over generous application as this leads to a prolongation of the disintegration time.

Subcoating.   To minimize the amount of material which must be used to round the tablet edges the cores are made on deep concave punches. The subcoat is built up in successive layers by wetting the tablets with an adhesive solution, dusting with filler and then thoroughly drying, as retained moisture may cause later cracking of the coat or deterioration of the core. The subcoating solution is usually an aqueous solution of sucrose to which is added acacia, gelatin or both, to impart adhesive properties. Talc and precipitated calcium carbonate are widely used in the subcoating filler together with some sucrose and a small proportion of acacia. A small proportion of inert filler, e.g., talc, may be added to the subcoating solution, which, if it contains gelatin, should be used warm to avoid gelling. Too heavy an application of filler must be avoided as the excess forms 'granules' with the coating solution and these interfere with the formation of a smooth subcoat. This stage of the process is continued until the tablets have a rounded appearance and the edges are well covered. When complete, the tablets are removed from the pan and thoroughly dried.

Smoothing and polishing. The application of a smoothing solution (60 per cent sucrose in water is satisfactory) causes limited wetting of the subcoat, which has been hardened by drying, so that it is smoothed out by the tumbling action. Soluble dye or a lake colour may be added to the smoothing solution if a coloured coating is required. As soon as the coat has become comparatively smooth the volume of smoothing solution per application should be reduced and the tablets dried without the aid of heat. In the final stages, tumbling is limited by 'inching' rather than rotating the bowl so that the coating is not scratched or otherwise damaged. At this stage the tablets will have a perfectly smooth but matt appearance and are thoroughly dried before polishing in a pan specially set aside for the job and coated with a beeswax–carnauba wax or similar waxy mixture.

Film Coating

Sugar coating doubles the weight and increases the size of a tablet and this is obviously undesirable if the tablet, in the uncoated state, is already large. Film coating provides an alternative means of masking the taste of the medicament and providing protection against adverse climatic conditions without significantly altering the tablet weight or size. The obvious advantages of excluding water from the coating process may be secured with film-forming polymers, such as ethylcellulose, polyvinylpyrrolidone or hydroxymethyl propyl cellulose, that are soluble in both water and anhydrous organic solvents. Some 3 to 10 per cent of the foregoing materials can be dissolved in an acetone–alcohol mixture together with 5 to 10 per cent of diethyl phthalate or other plasticizer to produce a film coating solution which may be applied by the pan technique. The plasticizer stops the film becoming brittle with age. Methylene chloride is often added to the solvent to reduce fire hazards, while undue absorption of expensive film forming agent is prevented by the prior application of a shellac sealing coat to the core tablets.

Enteric Coating

Tablets are enteric coated if the medicament is decomposed in the acid secretions of the stomach,

if it causes gastric irritation, or if it is intended to exert its main effect only on the intestine. Some official tablets coated in this way include those containing biscodyl, bismuth and emetine iodide, and erythromycin. Enteric coatings resist the acid conditions of the stomach but readily dissolve in the more nearly neutral fluids of the small intestine. They are also used in the formulation of sustained action preparations as the release of medicament is delayed by the time taken for the tablet to pass from the mouth to the intestine.

Formalized gelatin, keratin, salol, shellac, sandarac, stearic acid and cetyl alcohol have all been used to produce enteric coatings but are either difficult to apply or erratic in their action. The compositions of the fluids in the gastrointestinal tract are not constant but vary with time and from person to person. It is clearly important that the enteric action shall largely be independent of such variations in compositions. Cellulose acetate phthalate is widely used for enteric coating and was reported by Antonides and DeKay (1953) to be the only cellulose derivative of the fourteen evaluated that was satisfactory for this purpose. Only one of the phthalic acid carboxyl groups is attached to the cellulose, the other being free for reaction. The polymer dissolves in a variety of solvents, gives water-soluble salts with a number of bases and forms coatings which are insoluble in, but slightly permeable to, water (Malm et al. 1951). An important feature is the solubility of cellulose acetate phthalate films in buffers having a pH as low as 5.8; thus the requirements for enteric action are a medium with a pH higher than this value which can contribute ions to the coating to form a soluble salt. Such conditions are found in the intestine but not in the stomach.

In addition to 5 to 15 per cent of cellulose acetate phthalate the enteric coating solution may contain a plasticizer such as castor oil or butyl stearate together with a soluble or a lake dye if a coloured finish is required. The materials are dissolved or dispersed in a volatile solvent comprising alcohol, acetone, and, to reduce flammability, methylene chloride.

Automated Pan Coating

Successful use of the pan coating technique depends, in large measure, on the skill of the operator: it is also time consuming. Due to their higher volatility the solvents used for film coating permit rapid drying of tablets after each addition of the coating solution. As with moist granulation, spraying rather than pouring the coating solution is a more controllable technique that relies less on the operator's skills and which is more readily adapted to automatic control. In the case of enteric coated tablets, performance is determined by the thinnest part of the film and for reproducible characteristics between and within batches the coating must be of known uniform thickness. According to Lachman and Cooper (1963), enteric coatings complying with the foregoing criteria may be obtained by means of an automated film coating process. The tablets are tumbled in a baffled pan and a solution of cellulose acetate phthalate together with fillers in suspension is sprayed on to the tablets in repetitive 'bursts' alternating with longer drying periods. The spray gun for applying the coating solution and the hot or cold air flow for removing solvent are controlled by a punched tape programming device. The coating time for an 85 kilogram batch of tablets (90 minutes) is half that required by the corresponding manual procedure, and the weight of the coating is reduced and is more uniform.

Fully automated equipment for pan coating is now commercially available. Provision is made for programmed control of the coating composition, spray application and drying air-flow at each stage of the process. The different paths taken by tablets in a pear-shaped bowl leads to a lack of uniformity in the thickness of coating applied to tablets within the batch. This problem is avoided in the Manesty Autocota by the adoption of a cylindrical coating vessel rotating about a horizontal rather than inclined axis.

FLUID-BED COATING

Wurster (1959) first described the application of sugar or film coatings to tablets suspended in an air stream. In that equipment the coating solution is introduced into the fluidizing airstream at the base of a tall vertical tube in which tablets circulate as they are coated. Evaporated solvent and air are removed at the top of the chamber. The fluid-bed moist granulation equipment described earlier has now been modified by the makers for fluid-bed coating. As the tablets circulate in the air stream they are subjected to considerable abrasive action and for this reason they are compressed with extra firmness on punches which give a well rounded profile.

COMPRESSION COATING

As noted earlier it is desirable on occasion to separate tablet ingredients to avoid incompatabilities, to facilitate manufacture or to produce a sustained action product. Layer tablets provide an acceptable means for ingredient separation but the protective effect of the coat enveloping the tablet is lacking. It is not an easy matter to ensure a sugar coat of the same thickness for all tablets in a batch by pan coating and although reasonable variation in coat thickness and weight is not significant in plain sugar coating such variation cannot be tolerated if the coat contains a potent medicament. The idea of applying granular coating materials to a preformed core was conceived by Noyes in 1896 but could not be commercially exploited until the problem of core centration and the automatic rejection of coreless tablets had been solved. The expected advantages of a compression coating process are:

(i) core tablets are not subjected to abrasive action and need not be especially hard,
(ii) the process is 'anhydrous' and sealing coats are not required,
(iii) the disintegration time of a coated tablet can be comparable with that of the uncoated variety, due to the above,
(iv) good control of coating weight can be obtained,
(v) chemically incompatible ingredients may be separated,
(vi) the core and coat may be formulated for different properties e.g., for a sustained action tablet the coating would provide the prompt dose and the core the sustaining dose,
(vii) the process is continuous, completely mechanized and removes much of the element of skill from tablet coating.

Compression Coating Machines

The essential stages of coating by compression are (Fig. 19.15), deposition of the bottom fill of coating granules, transfer and centration of the core tablet, deposition of the side and top fill and finally compression to bond the coat to the core. The machine described by Whitehouse (1954), the Kilian Prescoter, used preformed cores which were fed into holes on the periphery of a transfer disc and deposited on the lower fill of coating granules as the lower punch dropped in readiness for the top fill. The core was centred by a light tap of the top punch, the top fill deposited and the coating bonded to the core by compression. The force developed during compaction in the presence of a core was sufficient to cause slight deflection of the overload release but failed to do so in the absence of a core. A switch connected to the overload release provided an electrical signal which, when fed to a memory unit, actuated a gate on the

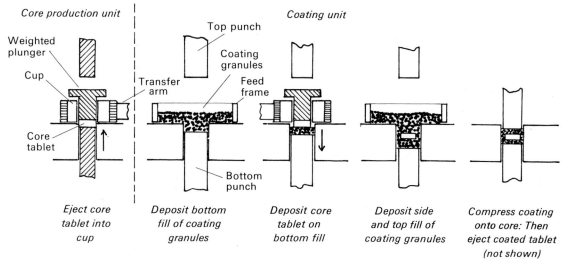

Core production unit | Coating unit

Weighted plunger
Cup
Core tablet
Transfer arm
Top punch
Coating granules
Feed frame
Bottom punch

Eject core tablet into cup | Deposit bottom fill of coating granules | Deposit core tablet on bottom fill | Deposit side and top fill of coating granules | Compress coating onto core: Then eject coated tablet (not shown)

FIG. 19.15. The compression coating of tablets.

collection chute such that coreless tablets were rejected.

The Manesty Drycota (Fig. 19.16) comprises two rotary presses coupled by a transfer unit (Fig.

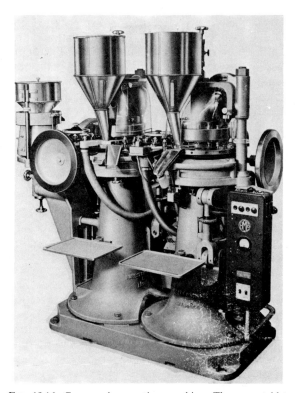

FIG. 19.16. Compression coating machine. The core tablet formed by the left hand unit is carried by the central transfer unit to the coating press or the right.

19.17). The spring-loaded arms of the transfer unit engage with small collars on the upper turret to ensure accurate ejection of the core tablet into a cup fitted with a free sliding weighted plunger. Next, the cup passes over a 'bridge' where dust is removed to avoid contamination of the coating granules and then engages with the collar on the upper turret of the coating press. As the bottom punch drops, the tablet is pushed out of the cup on to the centre of the bottom fill of coating granules by the action of the weighted plunger. The cavity is then filled with granules for the sides and top of the coating, which are bonded to the core by compression. As the cups pass round the transfer unit the plungers are examined by feelers which operate microswitches. If a cup fails to pick up or deposit a core at the appropriate stage in the cycle the signal from the microswitches initiates action for the rejection of coreless tablets.

Requirements for Core Tablets and Coating Granules

Core tablets should be prepared from rather large granules and should be lightly compressed. The surface of a soft tablet made from large granules is somewhat porous and provides a good 'key' for adhesion of the coating. There is a second reason for light compression of the core tablet. Residual stresses in a tablet are not instantaneously relieved when that tablet is ejected from the die. Large residual stresses induced by a high degree of compression may be sufficient to split the coating some time after manufacture has been completed.

The gap between the core and die-wall should

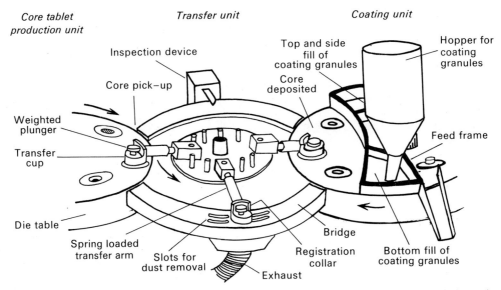

FIG. 19.17. Essential features of transfer mechanism of a compression coating machine (for clarity, only the die tables of the core and coating units and three transfer arms are shown).

be at least 0.13 cm to facilitate uniform deposition of coating granules round the edges of the core tablet and hence to ensure adequate coating strength. For these reasons too, the granule size should not exceed a quarter of the edge coating thickness. On the other hand, excessive amounts of fines or fatty lubricants should be avoided, as these lead to poor coating strength and poor adhesion to the core.

Performance

Provided the requirements for edge thickness are met, the weight of the coating is maintained with considerable precision and may be varied over a wide range. It may be noted that the official test for weight variation applies to compression coated tablets but not to those having a film or conventional sugar coat. Centrifugal and tangential forces due to turret rotation may slant the bottom fill of coating granules and displace the core from its central position. Lachman et al. (1966) concluded that coating granules which gave minimum weight variation also tended to give less core displacement. Coatings may be formulated for a wide range of properties but of these, enteric coatings are of particular interest. Blubaugh et al. (1958) have described the preparation of coating granules containing triethanolamine cellulose acetate phthalate which, when applied by compression, produce a coating with enteric properties. In a more recent paper Srinivas et al. (1966) have reported on the use of a number of carboxylated polymers for the production of entire coating granules.

THE QUALITY CONTROL OF TABLETS

Formerly, tablets were considered satisfactory if they were elegant and firm enough to withstand handling without damage. The realization that such criteria were inadequate for the scientific control of tablet quality led to the inclusion of suitable standards and tests in all national pharmacopoeias. Although corresponding procedures differ in detail or emphasis they serve an identical purpose which may, in general, be understood by a consideration of the requirements of the *British Pharmacopoeia 1973*. These:

define and describe compressed and moulded tablets, chocolate basis and tablet coatings,

restrict flavouring agents and coatings to those products for which specific permission is given for their use in the monograph,

standardize uniformity of tablet diameter and weight, content of medicament and disintegration time, and

prescribe storage and labelling requirements,

and are intended to ensure, not only a fully potent product, but also uniformity in the physical characters of official tablets regardless of source. The latter is essential as the patient quickly perceives, and is concerned about, differences in the appearances of nominally identical tablets.

UNIFORMITY OF DIAMETER

The standard specifies the punch diameter to be employed for a given tablet and the permitted tolerance on the specified size, thus securing dimensional uniformity between tablets of the same kind from different manufacturers. The standards apply only to uncoated and compression coated tablets. They make allowance for the manufacturing tolerances in die fabrication and for tool wear by allowing a deviation about the stated diameter. Generally, the manufacturing tolerance is proportionately less for large than for small dies and the deviation is reduced from ± 5 per cent to ± 3 per cent for diameters in excess of 12.5 mm.

TESTS FOR UNIFORMITY OF WEIGHT AND FOR MEDICAMENT CONTENT

The combined effect of these tests is to ensure that all tablets in a batch are, within reasonable limits, of the same potency. A perfect manufacturing procedure would yield a batch of tablets having identical weight and medicament content; in practice the values of these parameters for individual tablets deviate about the mean values for the whole batch. Such deviations will be of acceptable magnitude if correctly formulated and prepared granules are compressed on properly maintained equipment but will be larger, and probably unacceptable, if the converse conditions apply.

Ideally, the quality of a batch of tablets would be assessed by determining the potency of each tablet in a truly representative sample. The analysis of a large number of tablets by conventional means would be both costly and time-consuming while automated techniques for the analysis of the majority of drugs have still to be dveloped. At the present time therefore the reasonable assumption is made that the variation of the weight of individual tablets is a valid indication of the corresponding variation in the drug content.

Test for Uniformity of Weight

This test does not apply to sugar or enteric coated tablets. The weight of each tablet and the average weight of all tablets in the sample are determined. The standard, summarized in Table 19.6, limits the number of tablets in the sample which may deviate from the average weight by more than specified amounts. Rogers (1956), on the basis of production data then available, showed that the coefficient of variation of tablet weight was reasonably constant for tablets weighing more than 0.2 to 0.3 g but rose steeply for smaller tablets; a similar observation

has been made by Smith et al. (1963). This is not unexpected as there is greater practical difficulty in ensuring the flow, die-filling and air release characteristics necessary for low weight variation, with the finer granules which must be used for the production of small tablets. This factor is recognized by making the weight variation tolerances wider for small than for large tablets.

Twenty tablets represent a very small fraction of a manufacturing batch that will generally exceed 10 000, and may be as large as 1 000 000. If the tablet weights in a batch of, say, 0.3 g tablets are normally distributed and 10 per cent deviate from the average weight by more than 5 per cent, then 0.1 per cent of the tablets in that batch could be expected to deviate by more than 10 per cent from the average weight. Smith (1955) has calculated that there is a 67 per cent probability that the examination of a sample of twenty tablets by the official method would lead to the acceptance of such a batch. With a rotary machine, if the weight variation derives from a few punches of significantly different length from the others in the set, the foregoing calculations that are based on an assumed normal distribution do not apply. Nevertheless, the unsatisfactory nature of a batch of tablets produced under these conditions should be relaxed as indicated in Table 19.7. This table may

TABLE 19.6

SUMMARY OF THE BP 1973 TEST FOR THE UNIFORMITY OF TABLET WEIGHT

Number of tablets in sample	Average weight of tablets in sample	Percentage deviation about average weight	
20	80 mg or less	± 10.0	± 15.0
	More than 80 mg, less than 250 mg	± 7.5	± 12.5
	250 mg or more	± 5.0	± 10.0
	Number of tablets in the sample that may deviate by more than the above percentages	Not more than two	None
10	80 mg or less	± 10.0	± 15.0
	More than 80 mg, less than 250 mg	± 7.5	± 12.5
	250 mg or more	± 5.0	± 10.0
	Number of tablet in the sample that may deviate by more than the above percentages	Not more than one	None

intended to detect abnormal weight variation. While the stringency of the official test could be improved, for instance, by specifying narrower weight tolerances, it is important to remember that the discrimination level must provide a reasonable balance between the risks to the patient arising from over or under dosage and the performance that can reasonably be expected with the currently available manufacturing methods. Although the manufacturer must ensure that the completed batches of tablets comply with official requirements, samples would be examined during production as an extra check on quality and for the early detection and rectification of any faults which may develop.

Content of Medicament

The standards are framed to take into account processing difficulties, variations in the purity of the drug, accuracy of the assay methods and the size of the sample relative to that of the typical manufacturing batch. The stated limits for drug content given in the individual monographs apply to the examination of a sample of 20 tablets; where less than this number is available the sample must comprise at least 5 tablets and the limits are relaxed as indicated in Table 19.7. This table may

TABLE 19.7

BP 1973 STANDARD FOR THE CONTENT OF MEDICAMENT
IN TABLETS

Sample size	Instruction	Weight of drug in each tablet		
		0.12 g or less	More than 0.12 g Less than 0.30 g	0.3 g or more
15	Subtract from lower limit	0.2	0.2	0.1
	Add to upper limit	0.3	0.3	0.2
10	Subtract from lower limit	0.7	0.5	0.2
	Add to upper limit	0.8	0.6	0.4
5	Subtract from lower limit	1.6	1.2	0.8
	Add to upper limit	1.8	1.5	1.0

Allowances to be made when examining samples containing less than 20 tablets where the monograph limits for content of medicament between 90 and 110 per cent.

be used directly where the limits specified in the monograph are *between* 90 and 110 per cent. Thus, for a sample of 20 Promazine Tablets each containing 25 mg of Promazine Hydrochloride the monograph limits are 92.5 to 107.5 per cent of the nominal content of drug and would be widened in the case of a sample of 5 tablets to 90.9 to 109.3 per cent. To comply with official requirements

the tablets must therefore contain between 22.73 and 27.33 mg of drug.

Where the monograph limits fall outside the 90 to 110 per cent range the *Pharmacopoeia* directs that proportionately larger allowances should be made for samples of less than 20 tablets. A method for the calculation has been suggested by Hadgraft (1945).

It is now recognized that although a *sample* of tablets may comply with given standards for drug content, this may not be so for *individual* tablets within that sample. From theoretical considerations, Train (1960) concluded that if 20 tablets are examined and as a whole comply with ± 10 per cent limits, a variation as large as ± 40 per cent might be expected if each tablet was separately assayed. This variation could be due to solute migration and adsorption, granule separation and other effects. As discussed earlier, such variation is more likely to occur where the weight of the medicament is only a small proportion of the total tablet weight. Even a reduction in the proportion of medicament from 90 per cent to 23 per cent doubled the standard deviation of drug content for the tablets examined by Smith et al. (1963). On the other hand, Robinson et al. (1968) failed to detect a deviation greater than ± 15 per cent when examining over 1000 imipramine and desipramine tablets and capsules. In a number of cases the United States *Pharmacopoeia* includes a standard for the drug content of individual tablets; Feldman (1969) has indicated that the number of products affected by this standard will be increased in the future. The BP 1973 requires that, for tablets and capsules described in its monographs, no gross deviation from the stated amount of medicament is permissible when each dose unit is individually assayed. The term 'gross deviation' is not defined. If a formal standard for drug content per tablet is included in future editions of the *Pharmacopoeia*, automated analytical techniques of sufficient rapidity, sensitivity, accuracy and precision will be required. It is evident from the review by Kuzel et al. (1969) that considerable progress has been made in the field of automated analysis since 1960 when Stephenson concluded that for Digoxin Tablets the methods of mixing were probably superior to the then available assay methods.

TEST FOR DISINTEGRATION

Methods

Features common to the tests described in the literature are: an aqueous disintegration medium, agitation of the tablet or medium to simulate peristalsis and means for recognizing the end point, that is, complete disintegration. The many proposed methods may be classified into three types: (i) The tablet, supported on a frame, is immersed in water and the time determined for a weighted wire to pass through the tablet (Berry 1939). The method was abandoned because it gave anomalous results if the tablet disintegrated into large particles or yielded a hard core (Berry & Smith 1944). This stricture on the method might not be so relevant at the present time when, for efficient drug release, it is considered desirable that a tablet should disintegrate completely into very fine particles. (ii) A tube filled with water except for a small headspace and containing the tablet, is rotated end over end (Berry & Smith 1944; Mapstone 1952). (iii) A wire mesh cage (Hoyle 1946) or a tube closed by a wire mesh at the lower end (Prance et al. 1946) is moved up and down in the disintegration medium so that the tablets are constantly agitated. Disintegration is complete when all particles from the disintegrated tablet pass freely through the mesh.

The reader is referred to the BP 1973 for details of the official apparatus which, essentially, is that described by Prance and coworkers. Tablets may fail the test because, for instance, they form a gummy mass in contact with water or a resistant core is left after the rest of the tablet has disintegrated. If tablets fail the test for any reason, it may be repeated with a guided disc (Fig. 19.18)

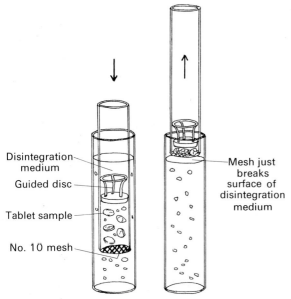

FIG. 19.18. Essential features of apparatus for the BP 1968 disintegration test showing guide disc in use.

Disintegration medium

Guided disc

Tablet sample

No. 10 mesh

Mesh just breaks surface of disintegration medium

placed in the disintegration tube above the tablet sample. The light percussive action of the disc as it rises and falls in the tube assists the breakdown of the tablets.

Requirements

Uncoated and compression coated tablets. The general requirement is that these shall disintegrate within 15 min. There are a number of exceptions. Tablets which are to be dissolved in water prior to administration e.g., Sodium Citrate, Soluble Aspirin, must disintegrate within 3 min. Calcium Lactate Tablets harden on storage and 30 min is allowed for these. The same period is specified for Thyroid Tablets and Prepared Digitalis Tablets as these form a gummy mass which is not easily persuaded through the mesh even with the aid of a guided disc. The test does not apply to products which should dissolve slowly in the mouth, e.g. lozenges, Compound Sodium Bicarbonate Tablets, Glyceryl Trinitrate Tablets, or to those which must be masticated, e.g. Phenolphthalein, Aluminium Hydroxide, or to Effervescent Potassium Tablets BPC. The official apparatus is not used for the latter; they are required to disolve completely within 3 min when placed in water at 20°.

Sugar and film coated tablets. As these coatings may increase the distintegration time, 1 h is allowed. One exception is Quinalbarbitone Tablets which must be sugar coated to mask the bitter taste of the drug. This hypnotic acts very promptly and therefore the tablets are required to disintegrate within 15 min.

Enteric coated tablets. The official apparatus is used but the test is carried out in two stages. It is first ascertained that the coating should not rupture in the stomach by subjecting the tablets to the action of 0.6 per cent v/v hydrochloric acid solution for 3 hr. If the coating is intact at the end of this period the tablets are washed to remove adherent acid and must then disintegrate within 1 hr when a pH 6.8 buffer is used as the disintegrating medium. Except in the case of achlorhydric patients the pH of the stomach is normally very low but the composition of its secretions varies considerably between individuals, in any one individual throughout the day and from day to day. Similar variations are found in the contents of the duodenum and small intestine which are often not as rich in enzymes or bile salts or of as high a pH as was implied by the composition of the alkaline pancreatin solution specified by the BP 1963 for the second part of the test. A number of enteric coatings used in the past depended on enzyme action or a rather high pH and proved erratic in their action. The test solutions prescribed by the BP 1968 have been adopted with a view to the elimination of such coatings.

Comments on the Test

The choice of water as the disintegrating medium is open to criticism. Among others Abbott et al. (1959) observed that the addition of mucoid substances to the test solution had a marked effect on disintegration time, which was often doubled and on occasion increased by a factor of 16. However, as Hartley (1950) has commented, the selection of 15 min for the disintegration time of uncoated tablets is, itself, somewhat arbitrary and may be quite unrelated to the rate at which the drug is absorbed. Generally, prompt action is required but the optional coating of, for example, Benzylpenicillin Tablets leads to the anomalous situation that the permitted maximum disintegration time may be 15 or 60 min depending on whether uncoated or coated tablets have been supplied to the patient. Benzylpenicillin Tablets (Ashby et al. 1954), those of Quinalbarbitone and a number of others (Howard 1951) can be sugar coated without extending the disintegration time beyond 15 min. The coating methods used for these tablets could, presumably, be more widely employed with the consequent potential advantage of more prompt therapeutic action. It is well known that although a tablet may comply with official requirements, the particles freely passing the mesh of the disintegration tube may remain intact for periods in excess of 15 min. Furthermore a number of factors, such as the physical state of the medicament used to produce the tablet, may have a marked effect on therapeutic response. For these reasons it is probably the dissolution rather than the disintegration behaviour which should be tested.

COLOUR

Rolfe (1956) has argued the case for and against the addition of colourants to tablets. Such arguments were, presumably, involved in the decision to remove all former restrictions, in the BP 1968, but the BPC 1973 still prohibits the use of colours except for specific tablets and those which are enteric or compression coated. The colour to be employed for a given tablet is not stated in either book of standards. Even if the proportion of a named colourant were to be specified for a given tablet, considerable difficulties would still arise when attempting to standardize the final shade and depth of colour as these are markedly affected by processing conditions. The problem is obviously more acute if the same product is to be produced by a number of manufacturers.

HARDNESS

Although there is no official test for tablet hardness this property must be controlled during production to ensure that the product is firm enough to withstand handling without breaking, chipping or crumbling, and yet not so hard that the disintegration time is unduly prolonged. Most testers apply a load to the edges of the tablet across a diameter. The load is gradually increased until the tablet fractures, the value of the load at this point (the crushing force) giving a measure of the hardness of the tablet. In the Monsanto Hardness Tester (Fig. 19.19) the tablet is held between a fixed and a moving jaw. The force applied to the edge of the tablet is gradually increased by turning the compression screw. The body of the instrument carries an adjustable scale which can be set to zero against an index mark fixed to the compression plunger when the tablet is lightly held between the jaws. With the Strong Cobb tester the load is

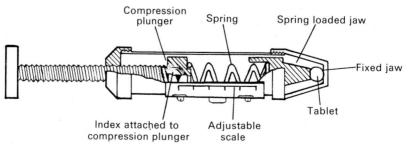

FIG. 19.19. The Monsanto tablet hardness tester.

applied pneumatically, while a pliers mechanism is employed in the Pfizer tester. To minimize errors due to the small force required to hold the tablet in position at the start of the test and the rate at which the load is applied, the mean of several hardness determinations should be used. For tablets of fixed dimensions in an experimental series the method provides comparative estimates of hardness. On the other hand, the optimum hardness for a given tablet in the manufacturing situation can only be set by experience extending over a number of batches. A tablet which was 'soft' and just handleable would give a reading of 1 to 2 kilograms on the Monsanto tester; for highly compacted tablets the reading would be 6 kilograms or more. The performance of a number of commercially available hardness testers has been reviewed by Brook and Marshall (1968) and by Ritschel et al. (1969).

Tablets are usually subjected to a second type of test which, essentially, measures the surface hardness. The Vickers test measures the size of the indentation produced on the tablet surface by a specially shaped loaded point. More usually the tablets are tumbled in a controlled manner and the change in the average weight of the tablets determined after a specified length of treatment. Such a test provides an indication of the likely edge damage that would occur when the tablets are handled during packaging and dispensing. The equipment designed by Webster and Van Abbe (1955) uses a vertical jogging action, whereas in the Roche Friabilator the tablets drop through a fixed distance during each revolution of a horizontally disposed plastic drum. The permissible loss in weight is obviously set by production experience, but with the Friabilator is usually in the range 1 to 5 per cent for 10 min treatment. Incipient capping and lamination usually show up on a tumbling test.

THEORETICAL STUDIES IN TABLETTING TECHNOLOGY

Although a great deal of information on the practical aspects of tabletting had appeared in the literature prior to 1952, very few papers had been concerned with theoretical studies. In that year, however, Higuchi and his associates (1952, 1953, 1954) published the first in a series of papers relating to the physics of tablet compression. Subsequently, as may be seen from the extensive bibliographies of Evans and Train (1963, 1964),

many workers have reported the results of studies in this field.

THE COMPACTION PROCESS

Both tablet machines and ram presses have been used to investigate the compaction behaviour of pharmaceutical substances. Pressures in the range 300 to 3000 kg/cm^2 are usual for tablet machines, but the upper limit may be higher for mechanical or hydraulic ram presses. The use of flat-faced punches simplifies subsequent treatment of the data. Where the time taken for compression is short, as with the tablet machine, transducers must be used to convert the compaction forces, punch displacements, etc. into electrical signals which can be recorded, usually by an ultraviolet oscillograph. The necessary instrumentation has been described by Higuchi et al. (1952, 1954a), Shotton and Ganderton (1960a), Shotton et al. (1963), Goodhart et al. (1968) and by other workers. Fig. 19.20 shows typical results that are obtained using an instrumented tablet machine.

The downwards thrust of the top punch in the die-bore during compaction causes movement of material relative to the wall of the die. The movement is resisted by frictional effects, in part within the bed of material but mainly between that material and the die-wall. As a result, the maximum force transmitted to the lower punch (F_b) is less than the maximum force (F_a) applied by the top punch to the contents of the die-cavity by an amount F_d, that is, the force 'lost' to the die-wall. As compaction also squeezes the compacting material into close contact with the wall of the die this latter experiences a maximum radial force F_r. Even when the top punch has been removed from the die, residual stresses within the tablet give rise to a load normal to the die-wall and therefore an ejection force, maximum value F_e, must be applied to the compact by the lower punch to overcome friction and initiate ejection. The extent to which the material in the die has been compacted may be evaluated from the relative volume (V_r), relative density (ρ_r) or porosity (ε) of the tablet. By loading the edges of the tablet across a diameter the minimum crushing force (F_c), just sufficient to rupture the tablet, may be found. If, as is often the case, the tablet dimensions are maintained in an experimental series, F_c provides a comparative measure of tablet hardness. The foregoing parameters, together with a number of others commonly used in tabletting theory, are defined in Table 19.8.

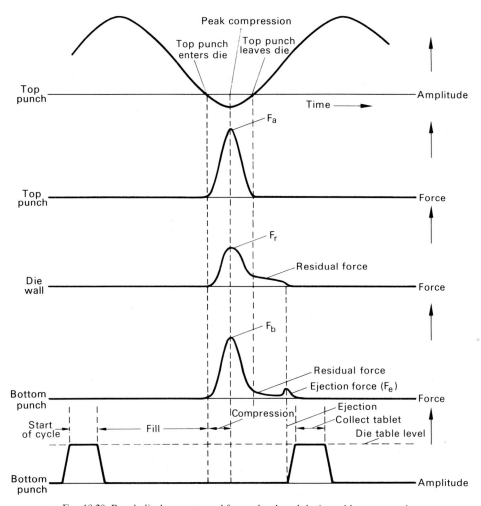

FIG. 19.20. Punch displacements and forces developed during tablet compression.

By finding the values of the parameters described in the previous paragraph at a number of pre-selected maximum upper punch pressures the compaction behaviour of a substance may be studied. Higuchi et al. (1953) determined these values for sulphathiazole compacts made in a ram press. In each case the upper punch pressure (P_a) was raised to its preselected maximum value over a period of 20 to 60 s. Whereas the logarithm of the disintegration time was found to be proportional to P_a, the crushing force (F_c) was linearly related to $\log P_a$. Thus, the compaction pressure had a much greater effect on the disintegration time than on hardness as is shown in Table 19.9. The porosity of the tablets progressively decreased as the pressure was increased but the specific area rose to a maximum at about 1600

kg/cm² and subsequently decreased. This was attributed to fragmentation of granules during the initial stages of compaction followed by bonding of the freshly formed surfaces at higher pressures. Further studies with aspirin, lactose and sulphadiazine (Higuchi et al. 1954b) gave results qualitatively similar to those obtained with sulphathiazole.

Train (1956) compacted alternate layers of normal and coloured magnesium carbonate. When the die-wall was lubricated with graphite the layers compressed evenly, whereas, in the absence of the lubricant, the layers curved downwards from the wall of the die towards the centre of the compact indicating that friction had restricted movement of the particles near the die-wall. Due to intense local shear action a hard 'skin' of distorted strongly bonded particles was formed where the compact

TABLE 19.8

DEFINITIONS OF SOME PARAMETERS USED IN TABLETTING THEORY

Symbol	Definition	Derivation
A	Area of tablet in contact with die-wall	$\pi D L$
A_p	Area of punch face	$\pi D^2/4$
D	Diameter of punch face	
F_a	Maximum upper punch force applied to compact	
F_b	Maximum force transmitted to lower punch by compact	
F_c	Crushing force applied across a diameter to edges of compact, just sufficient to cause rupture	
F_d	Force lost to the die-wall	$F_a - F_b$
F_e	Maximum force applied by lower punch to initiate ejection	
F_r	Maximum radial force at die-wall during compaction	
F_r'	Force normal to die-wall during ejection	
k_d	Die-wall coefficient of friction during compaction	
k_e	Die-wall coefficient of friction during ejection	
L	Observed length of compact	
L_o	Length compact would assume if compressed to zero porosity	$W/A_p \rho_o$
P_a	Maximum upper punch pressure	F_a/A_p
P_b	Maximum lower punch pressure	F_b/A_p
P_m	Mean compaction pressure	$(P_a + P_b)/2$
P_r	Maximum radial pressure during compaction	F_r/A
P_r'	Radial pressure during ejection of compact	F_r'/A
R	Punch force ratio	F_b/F_a
T	Transmission ratio	P_r/P_a
V	Observed volume of tablet	$A_p L$
V_o	Volume compact would assume if compressed to zero porosity	W/ρ_o
V_r	Relative volume of compact	V/V_o
W	Weight of tablet	
ε	Porosity—ratio of void to total volume	$(V - V_o)/V$, $1 - \rho_r$
ρ	Observed density of compact	W/V
ρ_o	True density of material used in compaction study	
ρ_r	Relative density of tablet	ρ/ρ_o, $1/V_r$

It is assumed that the punches are flat faced and circular in section.

TABLE 19.9

THE EFFECT OF COMPACTION PRESSURE ON THE PROPERTIES OF SULPHATHIAZOLE COMPACTS

Compaction pressure (P_a) kg/cm^2	Specific surface area m^2/g	Porosity (ε) per cent	Crushing force (F_c) kg*	Disintegration time s
319	0.25	30	2.9	50
638	0.75	23	5.8	150
957	0.85	17	8.8	285
1276	0.95	15	10.2	560
1595	1.00	11	11.0	1180
1914	0.90	10	12.4	3000
2552	0.70	9	13.1	15000
3828	0.45	5	16.1	—
5104	0.30	4	16.8	—

* Strong-Cobb units $\times 0.73$—see Brook & Marshall (1968).

limited by the available space in the die-cavity. Thereafter, the slope increased abruptly and during the second stage the load was supported by temporary structures of compacting material. At still higher pressures the structures collapsed and the material failed by crushing and plastic flow (third stage) until, in the fourth stage, there was sufficient rebonding of the freshly created surfaces to give a compact with enough strength to involve the normal compression characteristics of solid magnesium carbonate in any further reduction of volume. The data of Higuchi et al. (1953, 1954b) and Shotton and Ganderton (1960a), when plotted in the form used by Train, show that the third and fourth stages of compaction also occur with aspirin, lactose, sulphadiazine, sulphathiazole and sodium chloride. In the cases of the first four substances the abrupt changes in the slope of the $\log P_a/V_r$ plot occur at approximately the same compaction pressures as the maxima in the specific surface area curves. This would be expected if, as Train suggested, fragmentation and rebonding are competitive processes with the latter predominating in the fourth stage of compaction.

TABLET HARDNESS

Effect of Compaction Pressure
The behaviour of granules during compaction, the extent to which they bond together and the strength of the intergranule bonds relative to the strength of the granules determine tablet hardness. Strickland et al. (1956), who used activated carbon to delineate the granule boundaries, found that the carbon did not penetrate the interior of the granules even though these were laterally deformed by compaction. Shotton and Ganderton (1960b)

had been in contact with the die. This 'skin' is often formed on tablets and provides resistance to abrasive damage. The degree of compaction was assessed by measuring the thickness of the layers in each region and was found to be higher in a peripheral ring near the top punch and in a lower central region (Fig. 19.21). The latter may explain why the 'core', often seen towards the end of a disintegration test, breaks down more slowly than the rest of the tablet. A plot of V_r as a function of $\log P_a$ was not a smooth curve but showed several abrupt changes of slope (Fig. 19.22). The initial decrease in V_r was due to closer packing of the magnesium carbonate but this was eventually

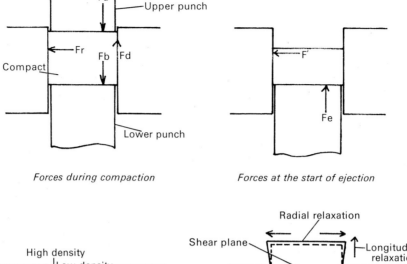

FIG. 19.21. Physical conditions during tabletting.

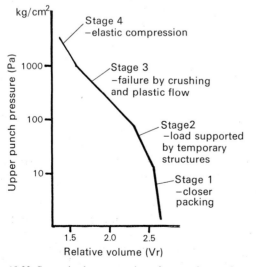

FIG. 19.22. Stages in the compaction of magnesium carbonate.

applied a vividly coloured sucrose coating to preformed spherical granules of that material. The coating remained intact and the granules largely retained their shape at low compaction pressure but as this was increased the granules distorted progressively until, at the highest compaction pressures, the coating had ruptured to such an extent that it appeared as coloured fragments against the white underlying sucrose. The strength of the intergranule bonds formed by light compression was less than that of the granules with the result that the tablets failed along, rather than across, the granule boundaries when submitted to a crushing force. When this was applied to the more heavily compressed tablets the bond strength was large enough to permit the development of faults within the granules which spread across the boundaries and led to failure of the tablet. The rebonding of surfaces formed by fragmentation, rather than granule interlocking, was apparently the more important factor determining the hardness of these tablets.

Effect of Materials Used and Tablet Dimensions
For given compaction conditions the intergranule bond strength is highly dependent on the nature of the base material. Strong bonds offer resistance to the propagation of faults across the grain boundary in which case, according to Orewan (1949) and others, the strength of the compact formed at a particular compaction pressure should be greater with fine than with coarse granules. This effect was noted with sodium chloride and hexamine compacts (Shotton & Ganderton 1961). Aspirin granules, however, formed weak bonds and softer tablets and, since fault propagation was not involved, granule size had little effect on tablet hardness. Coating sodium chloride and hexamine granules with stearic acid to weaken the intergranule bonds, reduced the hardness of the compacts, and abolished the particle-size effect observed with hexamine, but in the case of sodium chloride the hardest tablets were formed by the coarsest granules. Shotton and Ganderton suggested that the particle to particle contact pressure was greater in coarse sodium chloride grains than in fine ones since, for a given weight of that substance, fewer contacts were available to support the applied load. The higher contact pressure with the coarsest granules allowed penetration of the stearic acid film, the formation of strong bonds and, consequently, the production of the hardest tablets.

The majority of tabletting studies have used a constant die size for an experimental series and the thickness of the tablet, over a range of compaction pressures, has been maintained at a particular value by varying the compressing weight of the base material. Rees and Shotton (1969) reported preliminary studies on the effect of tablet dimension on the crushing strength. For sodium chloride their data indicated a relation of the form:

$$\frac{F_c V_r}{D L_o} = k_c P_m + C_c \qquad (19.1)$$

where D is the tablet diameter, L_o the length the compact would assume if compressed to zero porosity and k_c and C_c are constants.

CAPPING AND LAMINATION

Granule Bonding and Relaxation Stresses
Occasionally, at the start of a disintegration test, small radiating cracks appear on the upper face of the tablet and small bubbles of air are released. If air does not freely escape from the granules in the die-cavity, for example, where the fines content is high, the force created by the expansion of entrapped air may be sufficient to disrupt the bonds between the 'cap' and the rest of the tablet when the top punch is removed at the initiation of the ejection stage although, as will be seen later, capping and lamination can occur under conditions which preclude the implication of air as the causative agent. It is well known that too high a compaction pressure may lead to capping and lamination and has been shown to occur, for example, with hexamine (Shotton & Ganderton 1961) and sodium chloride (Rees & Shotton 1969).

In 1956, Train pointed out that on removal of the compacting force the elastic recovery of the dense peripheral ring (Fig. 19.20) would be larger than that of the adjacent, less dense, part of the tablet. The differential stress in this region is aggravated by both longitudinal and radial relaxation of that part of the tablet extruded from the die during the initial stages of ejection (Fig. 19.20). Both effects would increase the tendency to capping and lamination. It may be noted that the increase in tablet dimensions that is due to elastic recovery is usually sufficient to prevent re-insertion of the tablet into the die from which it has just been ejected. Clearly, the strength of the granule bonding may be critical in determining whether the tablet will cap or laminate. According to Shotton and Ganderton (1961) the bonds in sodium chloride compacts were strong enough to support relaxation without laminar failure although this can occur if extreme compaction pressures have been employed (Rees & Shotton 1969). The weaker bonds in aspirin compacts allowed the relaxation stresses to be dissipated by bond weakening and partial separation of the granules within the tablet. Undoubtedly, some loss of hardness must have occurred but the bonding was still sufficient to give a firm tablet. Hexamine tablets capped and laminated by fault propagation across the granule boundaries. This was not due to entrapped air as compacts prepared in vacuo behaved in a similar manner. Coating the hexamine granules with stearic acid eliminated the fault entirely and this was attributed to the bond weakening effect of the fatty acid which permitted dissipation of the relaxation stresses by the mechanism postulated for aspirin.

Residual Die-wall Pressure
Practical experience has shown that some tablets do not cap or laminate immediately, but may do

so on storage. Higuchi et al. (1965) studied the decay of die-wall pressure for a number of materials. In addition to an immediate elastic recovery in the die there was also a residual die-wall pressure (Table 19.10) which decayed slowly over a period of a minute or more, during which time the tablet 'flowed' in a direction opposite to that in which the compacting pressure had been applied. Addition of lubricant lowered the residual die-wall pressure due, presumably, to the 'softer' nature of the tablets (see the values for crushing strength) and to reduced die-wall friction. The fact that a radial pressure persisted at the end of the decay period showed that there was an elastic deformation which could only be relaxed by ejection of the tablet from the die. Internal strains within the tablet might also provide a further source of stress energy which could be dissipated at any time during the life of the tablet. For single punch and rotary tablet machines, upper punch pressure release and ejection take only a fraction of a second. Even if a tablet with a tendency to cap survived the rapid elastic recovery stage on extrusion from the die, the subsequent slower relaxation may cause capping when the tablets are handled and packed. Incipient capping and lamination of this type is usually apparent if a few tablets are shaken in the cupped hands, dropped on to a hard surface or subjected to a friability test.

HARDNESS OF MATERIALS AND TABLET PROPERTIES

Prior to compression, a granule porosity exceeding 60 per cent would not be unusual. As shown in Table 19.9, porosity is reduced to about 20 per cent with light compression and decreases to 5 per cent or less at much higher compaction pressures. The reduction in porosity is due to granule fragmentation giving smaller particles which may be more closely packed, and plastic deformation which allows the granules to 'flow' into the void spaces. The contribution of each process depends on the hardness of the substance being compressed. If it were possible to compress a liquid in a tablet machine P_a, P_b and P_r would be equal i.e., the transmission ratio would be unity. Rubber and silicone putty show 'liquid' behaviour and are used for die-wall pressure calibration. For other materials the transmission ratio will be less than unity. When sodium bicarbonate or sulphathiazole were compressed, Nelson (1955) observed that about a third of the upper punch pressure was transmitted to the die-wall. Windheuser et al. (1963) distinguished three distinct stages in the development of die-wall pressure with increasing values of upper punch pressure. The initial steep rise of P_r was due to the reduction of void space by the removal of air. This was followed by a less rapid rise in P_r during which granule fragmentation and consolidation took place. In the third stage, P_r increased more rapidly than in the second stage and represented the compression of an essentially void-free material, the 'yield value' of which was estimated by extrapolating the third portion of the curve to the abscissa (Fig. 19.23). Generally, the first ascending

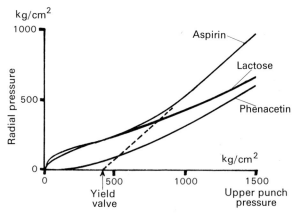

FIG. 19.23. Radial pressure as a function of upper punch pressure (after Windhesuer et al. 1963).

portion of the curve was steeper, the second stage more extended and the yield value higher for the harder materials examined. The reduced hardness of potassium chloride and sulphathiazole tablets containing magnesium stearate (Tables 19.10 and 19.11) was reflected in the smaller yield value obtained when that lubricant was employed. For phenacetin and acetanilide a measurable radial pressure could not be obtained until a significant upper punch pressure had been applied: the second stage was virtually absent. These materials produced poor tablets due to the fact that the crystals were plate-like and tended to compact into layers with poor interlayer bonding. Although there were considerable experimental difficulties, Ridgeway et al. (1969a) obtained values for Young's modulus and the surface hardness for a number of pharmaceutical materials; these values were then related (Ridgeway et al. 1969b) to the transmission ratio and to the surface hardness of the compact. The results of these studies (together with data from other sources) are summarized in Table 19.10 where it will be seen that, as anticipated, the transmission ratio was large for soft materials such as aspirin, and vice versa. Overall, the data in the table generally support the view that the hardness of a

TABLE 19.10

THE RELATION OF THE HARDNESS OF SOME PHARMACEUTICAL SUBSTANCES TO THEIR TABLETTING BEHAVIOUR

Substance	Hardness		Compaction behaviour			Properties of compacts prepared at 1000 kg/cm^2	
	Young's modulus (kg/mm^2)	Vickers surface hardness (kg/mm^2)	Transmission ratio: T	Yield value (kg/cm^2)	Die-wall coefficient: of friction K_d	Vickers surface hardness (kg/mm^2)	Crushing strength: F_c (kg)
Aspirin	9	8.7	0.67	410	0.17	11.6	3.6
Urea		9.1	0.60			8.6	
Hexamine	90	13.3	0.56		0.31	12.8	5.4
Salicylamide	130	15.1	0.50				
Potassium chloride		17.7	0.45	440		16.1	
Sodium chloride	190	21.2	0.40	640	0.40	27.4	9.1
Sucrose	220	63.6	0.33	700			2.8
Reference	(1)		(2)	(3)	(4)	(2)	(5)

Substance	Lubricant	per cent	Transmission ratio T	Properties of compacts prepared at 1290 kg/cm^2		
				Residual die-wall pressure (kg/cm^2)		Crushing strength: F_c
				Initial	Equilibrium	(kg)
Aspirin	—		0.73	36	23	9.4
Sodium chloride	—		0.59	307	200	>19.0
Sucrose	—		0.49	141	119	8.0
Potassium chloride	—		0.71	301	149	14.6
Potassium chloride	Magnesium	2	0.80	178	118	7.3
Potassium chloride	stearate	5	0.84	135	92	7.3
Reference	(6)					

References: (1) Ridgeway et al. (1969a) (2) Ridgeway et al. (1969b)
(3) Windheuser et al. (1963) (4) Lewis & Shotton (1965a)
(5) Shotton & Lewis (1964) (6) Higuchi et al. (1965)

substance is an important factor determining its behaviour both during and after compression.

LUBRICATION

Lubricants are used to improve granule flow (glidants), minimize die-wall friction (die-wall lubricants) and prevent adhesion of the granules to the punch faces (anti-adherents). The extent to which they possess these properties varies; talc is a better glidant than magnesium stearate but is an inferior die-wall lubricant. Excessive proportions of the stearate may actually impede granule flow.

Glidants

The effect of a glidant on the flow properties of a granule may be assessed by measuring the angle of repose, flow-rate through an orifice or by the other methods outlined in Chapter 17. A number of mechanisms have been proposed to account for glidant action. The flow properties of smooth, nearly spherical particles are known to be better than those of more irregular shape: it has been suggested that glidant may fill surface depressions and thereby reduce roughness. If the coefficient of friction of the glidant is less than that of the granules then inter-particle friction may be lowered. Alternatively, the glidant may physically separate the solid particles so that inter-molecular attractive and capillary adhesion forces are reduced. The latter derive from the thin film of moisture normally present on solid surfaces. A proportion of fines will often improve granule flow, presumably by a combination of the foregoing effects although, as discussed earlier, an excess of fines often has an adverse effect on tabletting properties. Some materials acquire a frictional electrostatic charge when handled. The mutual repulsion of particles due to this effect is sufficient to impede proper die-filling during the production of hexoestrol implants. Although the solution to this specific problem resides in recrystallization from a suitable solvent, glidant action may in some cases be

TABLE 19.11

THE EFFECT OF LUBRICANTS ON TABLETTING PROPERTIES

Substance	Lubricant	per cent	Force lost to die-wall: F_d (kg)	Punch force ratio: R	Die-wall coeffi-cient of friction K_d	Ejection force: F_e (kg)	Crushing force: F_c (kg)	Relative density: ρ_r	Ref.
Aspirin	—		438	0.71	0.17	60	3.6	0.975	
Hexamine	—		392	0.74	0.31	144	5.4	0.987	
Hexamine granules	—		392	0.74	0.31	156	14.6	0.965	
Sodium chloride	—		362	0.75	0.40	165	9.1	0.895	
Sucrose	—		Could not be measured—the machine				2.8		
Sucrose granules	—		jammed during the preparation of				2.8		1
			compacts						and
Aspirin	Magnesium stearate	2	129	0.91	0.051	62	2.7	0.982	2
Hexamine	Magnesium stearate	2	90	0.94	0.051	59	1.3	0.995	
Hexamine granules	Magnesium stearate	2	174	0.87	0.093	145	10.5	0.985	
Sodium chloride	Magnesium stearate	2	90	0.94	0.045	26	2.6	0.940	
Sucrose	Magnesium stearate	2	90	0.94		26	1.4	0.890	
Sucrose granules	Magnesium stearate	2	90	0.94		48	4.0	0.860	
Sucrose granules	—		682	0.55		371			
Sucrose granules	Stearic acid	2	78	0.94		22			
Sucrose granules	Magnesium stearate	2	104	0.93		50			3
Sucrose granules	Talc	2	664	0.59		353			
Sulphathiazole granules	—		367	0.69		100	18.3		
Sulphathiazole granules	Magnesium stearate	0.1	105	0.90		20	17.5		
Sulphathiazole granules	Magnesium stearate	0.2	86	0.92		15	17.2		
Sulphathiazole granules	Magnesium stearate	0.4	74	0.93		14	16.1		
Sulphathiazole granules	Magnesium stearate	0.6	65	0.94		11	15.1		
Sulphathiazole granules	Magnesium stearate	1	72	0.93		10	13.9		
Sulphathiazole granules	Magnesium stearate	2	51	0.95		8	11.0		4
Sulphathiazole granules	Stearic acid	0.2	266	0.77		72	17.2		
Sulphathiazole granules	Stearic acid	0.4	187	0.83		50	16.8		
Sulphathiazole granules	Stearic acid	0.6	156	0.85		43	16.4		
Sulphathiazole granules	Stearic acid	1	124	0.88		35	15.9		
Sulphathiazole granules	Stearic acid	2	102	0.90		30	15.3		

(1) Shotton & Lewis (1964)—mean compaction pressure 1000 kg/cm^2
(2) Lewis & Shotton (1965a)—mean compaction pressure 1000 kg/cm^2
(3) Lewis & Shotton (1965b)—mean compaction pressure 1033 kg/cm^2
(4) Strickland et al. (1956)—mean compaction pressure 1390 kg/cm^2
Data is quantitatively comparable within, but not between groups due to different operating conditions.

attributed to the reduction of electrostatic charges. A detailed review of glidant action is given by Jones (1969).

TABLE 19.12

EFFECT OF LUBRICANTS ON THE DISINTEGRATION TIME OF SODIUM BICARBONATE TABLETS COMPACTED AT APPROXIMATELY 1300 kg/cm2

Lubricant concentration per cent	Disintegration time (s) Stearic acid	Magnesium stearate
0	200	200
0.25	370	1500
0.50	520	2000
0.75	680	2200
1.00	900	2300
2.00	1400	2900
4.00	2500	3800

From Strickland et al. (1956).

Die-wall Lubricants

The effects of die-wall lubricants on tabletting behaviour may be seen by inspection of Tables 19.10, 19.11 and 19.12. They reduce the force lost to the die-wall, the ejection force, the crushing strength and the residual die-wall pressure. The relative density, punch force ratio, transmission ratio and disintegration time are increased. In part, the lubricant effect appears to reside in the formation of a tough film on the die-wall. If a die 'conditioned' by the production of tablets from lubricated granules is subsequently used to compact unlubricated granules, easy tablet ejection persists for a short period. Strickland et al. (1956) expressed the view that the reduction of force lost to the die-wall as a result of lubrication (ΔF_d) may be related to the fractional coverage of the die-wall–compact interface. At low concentrations (c) of lubricants they reported an apparent agreement with a Langmuir-type adsorption equation i.e.

$$\Delta F_d = c/(k+c) \qquad (19.2)$$

Materials used as lubricants must shear readily even when highly compressed. In this connection it may be noted that the slip and orientation of layers within the crystal lattice, on which the action of laminar lubricants such as talc depends, are inhibited by large applied loads and degree of compaction. Under these conditions the shear strength of talc is high (Train & Hersey 1960) which undoubtedly accounts for the poor die-wall lubricant action of that substance.

Compression and ejection processes involve movement of material relative to the die-bore surface. The frictional force (F) resisting motion of one surface over another is proportional to the load (L) applied normally to those surfaces, that is:

$$F = kL + C \qquad (19.3)$$

where k is the coefficient of friction applicable to the particular conditions. For consolidation of granules the maximum force resisting further reduction in the length of the compact is related to F_d and the normal load is the die-wall force (F_r). During ejection the resistance to motion of the compact is related to the ejection force (F_e) whilst F_r', the radial force operating as ejection takes place, constitutes the normal load. As $F_r = P_r A$ and $F_r' = P_r' A$, by analogy with equation (19.3):

$$F_d = k_m P_r A + C_m \qquad (19.4)$$

$$F_e = k_n P_r' A + C_n \qquad (19.5)$$

If it is assumed that P_r and P_r' are proportional to a generalized compaction pressure (P) the appropriate substitution in equations (19.4) and (19.5) yields expressions with a common factor (PA), which implies that F_e and F_d are linearly related. This has been confirmed by, for instance, Train (1956), Lewis & Shotton (1965a) and by other workers. Clearly, this is a simplification of a very complex process and could not be expected to apply directly to all materials and compaction conditions. Train's data for the ejection of magnesium carbonate compacts was best represented by a power law, but Lewis & Shotton used linear expressions.

$$F_d = k_d P_m A + C_d \qquad (19.6)$$

$$F_e = k_e P_m A + C_e \qquad (19.7)$$

to describe the compression and ejection of aspirin, hexamine, sodium chloride and sucrose compacts.

In these equations k_d and k_e were coefficients which depended on the frictional conditions at the die-wall. They found that whereas the values of k_d (Table 19.11) were different for each of the unlubricated substances, they assumed (except in the case of hexamine granules) a virtually identical and lower value when 2 per cent magnesium stearate was added to the base materials. The values of k_e showed a similar but less marked trend. In these circumstances the lubricant governed the frictional characteristics of the die-wall–compact interface regardless of the properties of the material being compacted or ejected. The absolute magnitudes of P_r and P_r' are determined by the transmission ratio (T) and this would not be identical for all lubricated substances which explains why these produced different values of F_d and F_e at a given mean compaction pressure.

In common with the investigations described above, most compaction studies have employed a constant compact diameter and thickness in an experimental series. Sometimes, when tabletting 'difficult' granulations, it is found that there is an optimum die-size which minimizes e.g., F_d, F_e, capping, lamination, etc. The effect of thickness and diameter on tabletting properties is therefore of considerable technical interest. From Table 19.8 it can be seen that:

$$\frac{P_r}{P_a} = T \quad \text{and} \quad \frac{F_a}{A_p} = P_a$$

and substituting these in equation (19.4) and rearranging, then:

$$\frac{F_d}{A} = \frac{k_1 F_a}{A_p} + C_1 \qquad (19.8)$$

Also, if the assumption is made that P_r' is proportional to P_a:

$$\frac{F_e}{A} = \frac{k_2 F_a}{A_p} + C_2 \qquad (19.9)$$

Equations (19.8) and (19.9) fitted the results of Rees and Shotton (1969) for the compaction of sodium chloride. As these workers pointed out, these equations are not applicable when the length of the compact is sufficient to prevent proper consolidation of granules near the bottom punch—a condition which should rarely be encountered in normal pharmaceutical tabletting operations. Further studies will be necessary to show whether the expressions are valid for a wider range of materials.

It is implicit in the reduction of residual die-wall pressure and improvement of transmission ratio

(Table 19.10) by die-wall lubricants that they facilitate the movement of material in the die-cavity both during and after compression. The more ready elimination of voids is reflected in the higher relative density of the compacts (Table 19.11). Die-wall lubricants are not, however, without adverse effects on other tablet properties such as disintegration time (Table 19.12). Also, as has been noted earlier, they may reduce the strength of the bonds between particles in a tablet. While this has the beneficial effect of reducing capping and lamination in the case of hexamine, with other substances an undesirable reduction in tablet hardness may occur. Clean surfaces are known to produce the strongest bonds but, as hard tablets can be prepared with lubricated granules, it seems reasonable to suppose that enough of the clean surface produced by fragmentation during compression remains uncontaminated by lubricant and capable of forming strong bonds. If this is so, lubricants should affect the hardness of tablets produced from crystals more than those produced from granules. This is because the crystals, being harder than granules, would tend to fragment to a lesser extent under pressure. In confirmation of this, Shotton and Lewis (1964) found that the strength of hexamine and sucrose tablets prepared from crystalline material was reduced by 76 per cent and 50 per cent respectively by the addition of 2 per cent magnesium stearate. The corresponding reduction in hardness was 28.1 per cent and 18.4 per cent respectively for tablets formed from granulated hexamine and sucrose.

DISINTEGRATION

In the context of tablet technology, disintegration implies penetration of the tablet by an aqueous liquid, disruption of internal bonds and the subsequent breakdown of the tablet. It is reasonable to suppose that rapid penetration of liquid is an essential requirement for rapid disintegration of conveniently formulated tablets.

Theory
A pressure differential P is required to cause liquid of viscosity η to flow with a velocity dL/dt in a horizontal pore of hydraulic radius m at a time t when the meniscus has moved a distance L along the pore.

$$\frac{dL}{dt} = \frac{Pm^2}{k_o \eta L} \qquad (19.10)$$

Here, k_o, a pore shape factor and m, the hydraulic radius, are used because the pore in a compact has

an irregularly shaped rather than a circular cross-section. In all other respects the equation is of the same form as that used to describe the flow of liquids in circular pipes. The pressure differential derives from the drop in pressure across a meniscus:

$$P = \frac{\gamma \cos \theta}{m} \qquad (19.11)$$

where γ is the surface tension of the liquid and θ the contact angle with the pore wall (cf. the corresponding expression for a liquid meniscus in a capillary of circular section). From the foregoing:

$$\frac{dL}{dt} = \frac{m\gamma \cos \theta}{k_o \eta L} \qquad (19.12)$$

If $L = 0$ when $t = 0$ on integration

$$L^2 = \frac{2m\gamma \cos \theta}{k_o \eta} t \qquad (19.13)$$

If the pore is part of a network that is uniform throughout the compact, for penetration into one face of that compact, the volume of liquid in the pores (V) is proportional to L and at any time t:

$$V^2 = kt \qquad (19.14)$$

k being a coefficient representing the properties of the liquid and of the pore network within the compact.

Effect of Granule Properties
For a compact of given porosity the void space may comprise a few large diameter pores or many fine ones. Fine pores are most likely to be formed from soft friable granules that readily fragment into much smaller particles during compression. In these circumstances the size of the pores should be largely independent of the size of the granules used to prepare the compact. Conversely, hard granules do not collapse to the same extent during compaction and thus the pore network will be coarser and dependent on the original granule size. According to equation (19.13), such a network would be more readily penetrated by liquids than that resulting from the compaction of soft materials. Ganderton and Selkirk (1969) made granules from lactose and sucrose by massing with water and found that the hardness and bulk density increased with the amount of water used for granulation. They suggested that this was due to a reduction in intragranule pore volume. Sucrose granules, which were harder and less friable than those prepared with lactose, gave compacts with a coarser pore structure that was more readily penetrated by liquid.

Initially, the imbibition rate for all compacts conformed to equation (19.14), but on many occasions slowed down or stopped abruptly before the theoretical volume of liquid had been absorbed. This was more frequently observed with sucrose compacts, particularly in those circumstances where the porosity was high and the largest, hardest, granules had been used. These conditions were essential for the effect to occur with lactose compacts. It was postulated that compacts showing this type of behaviour had a broad and perhaps discontinuous distribution of pore sizes. Rapid penetration of the wider pores isolated some regions of the compact, occluded air prevented subsequent penetration of the isolated regions and, as a result, a lower than theoretical degree of saturation was attained. By compressing the compacts to a lower porosity the size and lack of uniformity in size distribution was reduced and higher fractional saturation obtained.

In the foregoing experiments liquid penetrated one face of the compact. However, complete immersion of the tablet during disintegration exposes the whole surface to penetrant liquid. In this situation the geometry of the system demands a reduction in the total pore cross-sectional area available for flow as liquid approaches the centre of the tablet. Furthermore, as the pore entrances on all surfaces of the tablet will be sealed by liquid, air entrapment will occur. Liquid will penetrate until the increase in the pressure of the occluded air is equal to the capillary pressure. A larger fraction of the total pore length will be penetrated with fine rather than coarse pores, but this need not necessarily imply good disintegration characteristics. It is quite possible that the back pressure of the occluded air as it compresses in the pore and the decreasing area available for flow could act in concert with the normally operative viscous forces so that the *rate* of penetration was too low for a short disintegration time.

Effects of Die-wall Lubricants

Some medicaments e.g., phenothiazine, and most die-wall lubricants are hydrophobic and impart this property to the pore walls in the tablet. The resultant increase in the contact angle reduces the value of $\cos \theta$ in equation (19.13) and therefore the pore is less readily penetrated by an aqueous liquid. This is reflected in the longer disintegration time which is found when, for instance, the stearate lubricants are used (see Table 19.12). For magnesium carbonate compacts there was a rough proportionality between the concentration of

magnesium stearate and the time taken for the uptake of a given amount of water (Ganderton 1969). This time was extended, other conditions being constant, by increasing the efficiency of the process whereby the lubricant was blended with the granules. When 1 per cent of magnesium stearate was incorporated during the moist granulation stage penetration of water was completely inhibited: the pores were so well coated that the contact angle was greater than 90° and probably approached that of the solid lubricant. As the cosine of an angle greater than 90° is negative, V^2 in equation (19.14) is also negative and penetration cannot occur. Where such a situation arises in tablet manufacture, due either to the intrinsic water repellency of the medicament or the lubricant, a water soluble surfactant may be added to the granules to reduce the contact angle. Surfactants also facilitate the displacement of air from blind pores in a tablet under the conditions of a dissolution test. Studies by Wurster and Seitz (1960) with benzoic acid compacts into which 1 mm diameter artificial holes had been formed by drilling, demonstrated that the total pore surface was not available for attack by simple aqueous dissolution fluids, due to occluded air. This effect was abolished when air was removed from the pores by vacuum treatment or by addition of a surfactant to the dissolution medium.

Mode of Disintegrant Action

Starch has been used for many decades as a disintegrating agent. Since instrumented tablet machines were not available to Berry and Ridout (1950) they used the compression ratio, that is the ratio of the weight of a tablet to its thickness, as a measure of the degree of compaction in their studies. The disintegration time of tablets containing 15 per cent of starch, dry mixed with phenacetin granules, fell linearly from 15 min at a compression ratio of 0.57, to 6 min as that ratio was raised to 0.7; further compaction to 0.75 brought about a steep rise in disintegration time to 24 min. They argued that the disintegrating action of starch was due to swelling and that this would be most efficient when the granules were in close contact with the starch grains in a tablet of low porosity. At still lower porosities (higher compression ratios) imbibition of water was restricted by the small pore size. Similar effects have been noted by Higuchi et al. (1954b) with sulphadiazine tablets. Berry and Ridout compared the effect of starch added as described above with that of alginic acid incorporated during the moist granulation stage. This latter substance also swells in contact with aqueous liquids, but, since it was part of the granule structure, disintegration occurred by erosion and breakdown of the granules into the original particles from which they had been prepared. A low disintegration time of approximately 3 min was maintained up to a compression ratio of 0.65 but then, as with starch, further compaction caused a marked increase in the time taken for the tablet to disintegrate. Burlinson (1950) observed that there was little to choose between aliginic acid and starch if part of the latter was incorporated into the granules during moist granulation of the medicaments.

The assumption that starch facilitates tablet disintegration by swelling action (bursting) is based on the known increase in the dimensions of starch grains exposed to aqueous fluids. Patel and Hopponen (1966) found a 70 per cent increase in volume, but Ingram and Lowenthal (1968) quote a lower figure which, they suggest, is not sufficient to account for the disintegrant action of starch. The latter workers suggest that the irreversible swelling of damaged starch grains is much greater but could not establish a correlation between the degree of damage and the tablet disintegration time. As an alternative to the 'swelling' theory it has been argued that starch may derive its disintegrant properties from capillary action in the intergranule pore system. It is possible that it may also prevent the complete collapse of the pore system during compaction or provide a secondary pore surface of low contact angle against aqueous media.

It seems likely that the disintegration time of tablets is determined by the complex interaction of a wide variety of factors. The rate at which liquid penetrates a tablet, the nature and method of incorporation of lubricants, the action of disintegrants, the degree of compaction and the reduction of inter-particle bond strength in the presence of water, are all clearly of major importance. In practice, granules often contain hydrophilic colloids which, apart from their effect on the surface tension, viscosity and contact angle of the penetrant liquid, may dissolve or gel and this may have a profound effect on the rate at which a tablet disintegrates. Finally, some tablets disintegrate by continuous erosion of an outer wetted layer in which case the complete rapid saturation of the pore system by aqueous media may not be an essential initial step in the disintegration process.

CAPSULES

A capsule consists of a dose of drug enclosed in a water-soluble shell or envelope. Although capsules are predominantly used for oral medication, suppositories, consisting of the drug and a suitable dispersion medium enclosed in a flexible gelatin shell, are available (Senior 1969). There are two types of capsule, the hard variety which is intended for the administration of particulate solids and the soft or flexible capsule used for powders, non-aqueous liquids or pastes. As the shell takes several minutes to dissolve, the taste of unpalatable drugs is effectively masked. Officially, capsules may be spherical (perles), ovoid or cylindrical with hemispherical ends—only the last of these descriptions applies to hard capsules. The shell may include an antimicrobial preservative, can be coloured as an aid to identification and may be rendered opaque by dyes or fillers if the drug e.g., some vitamins and Chlorodiazepoxide, is photosensitive. For official preparations, diluents may not be added to the medicament unless this is specifically permitted in the relevant monograph: a similar restriction also applies to the use of coloured shells for capsules described in the Codex. It is possible to coat capsules with cellulose acetate phthalate or a mixture of stearic acid and butyl stearate if enteric action is required, but it is more usual in these circumstances to formulate if possible as an enteric coated tablet.

SOFT CAPSULES

Formerly, these were extemporaneously prepared by filling and sealing shells which had been made by dipping metal formers or 'olives' into a molten aqueous base containing glycerin and gelatin (glycogelatin). The glycerin ensures that a flexible shell is obtained. The first step in mechanizing the production of soft capsules was the development of a process whereby a sheet of glycogelatin was covered with a measured amount of anhydrous fluid drug. A second sheet was then placed over the drug and the 'sandwich' compressed between plates into which had been set hollow elliptical or hemispherical dies. The pressure forced the glycogelatin sheets and the drug into the dies and formed individual capsules by sealing and cutting at the rims. The capsules were then separated from the residual glycogelatin matrix, washed in solvent to remove traces of oil used as a release agent and dried to give a tough though flexible shell. The process was used until recently but could not complete with the rotary die machine (Figs 19.24 and 19.25) in terms of economic, continuous, high speed production. In this machine the dies are set in a pair of contra-rotating cylinders. Two continuous glycogelatin ribbons, previously warmed

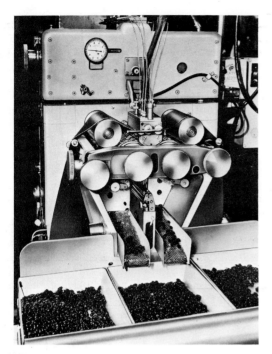

FIG. 19.24. The rotary die soft capsule filling machine (R. P. Scherer Ltd.).

as a soft capsule. Vegetable oils, Liquid Paraffin and Soft Paraffin are used when necessary to dilute or suspend the drug. Vegetable oils are specified for the dilution of the oil-soluble vitamins, as the paraffins are known to interfere with the absorption of these medicaments from the gut. As noted in the BPC 1968, drugs containing water or other gelatin solvent cannot be filled into soft capsules due to the resultant pitting, softening and eventual breakdown of the shell; the water should be removed and the residue mixed with an oil prior to encapsulation. Conversely, anhydrous but hygroscopic liquids may withdraw water from the shell which then hardens and has reduced solubility. Glycogelatin softens markedly as the temperature is raised and it is usual to increase the proportion of gelatin for capsules used for tropical climates. Due to changes in the equilibrium moisture content of the shell, the flexibility of soft capsules varies with ambient humidity. They are hard and inflexible

by the filling wedge to make them plastic, are fed between the cylinders. At the moment when opposing dies converge, a measured fill of drug is forced between the ribbons by a metering pump and simultaneously the edges of the dies seal and cut out a complete capsule. These are separated from the matrix, washed in solvent and dried (*Pharmaceutical Journal*, 1960). It is claimed that the fill of drug per capsule can be maintained to within 1 per cent of the mean fill for the batch.

Depending on machine capacity and capsule size, production rates in excess of 30 000 capsules/h are possible while production lines are available for the formation of the ribbons, sealing of the capsules and their subsequent washing and drying as a continuous integrated process. Rotary die machines have also been developed whereby powders, as such, may be directly encapsulated in a flexible gelatin shell. The ribbon is made to conform to the contour of the die by application of reduced pressure, a 'plug' of powder is forced between the ribbons and the capsules sealed, washed, and dried as described above. Capsules of some tetracycline antibiotics are made by this method.

Virtually any non-aqueous liquid drug or a powdered solid formed into a suspension of suitable consistency by the addition of oil, may be presented

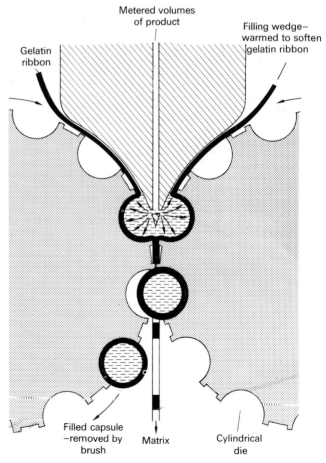

FIG. 19.25. Method for filling and sealing soft gelatin capsules in a rotary die machine (diagrammatic).

at 20 per cent, taut but flexible at 50 per cent, and soft and flaccid at 80 per cent relative humidity. In the latter condition the relatively high moisture content of the shell may encourage the diffusion of any water-soluble substance from the fill into the shell and as a result there may be unwanted reactions between the constituents or changes in the appearance and solubility of the shell.

According to Notton (1956) the oxygen permeability also increases with the moisture content of the glycogelatin envelope. It will be noted that the official storage requirements for both varieties of capsule are framed to prevent moisture uptake and other forms of deterioration as well as crushing and breakage. Sufficient preservative must be used to ensure effective antimicrobial action even where the moisture content of the envelope is high. Additionally, the possibility that preservative may partition between the shell and the capsule content can not be ignored. Studies by Patterson and Lerrigo (1947) showed that beta-naphthol, used extensively at that time as a mould inhibitor, partitioned to such an extent that after approximately 18 months storage the amount of preservative in the capsule contents was more than twice that in the shell. It is unlikely, however, that partitioning would be a serious problem with the ionized antimicrobials, such as potassium sorbate, that are now employed as preservatives for capsule shells.

HARD CAPSULES

These are made by filling the drug as powder, granules or pellets into a preformed cylindrical shell or body, the contents being retained by a shorter shell or cap fitted over the body. Wood (1965) has reported that on occasion the cap may disengage from the body during the act of swallowing. This, clearly, is undesirable, and may be avoided by securing the shell components with a narrow sealing strip. Hard capsules provide an alternative to powders, cachets and tablets for the administration of solid medicaments. They are at least as durable as tablets and correct formulation permits the rapid release and absorption of drug in the gastrointestinal tract.

Hard capsule shells are made by dipping moulds into a gelatin solution, the film on the mould dried, the shell cut to length and then stripped from the mould (*Pharmaceutical Journal*, 1965 & 1966). The shells are made in a range of 8 sizes to accommodate 50 to 1000 mg doses of drug but for veterinary preparations three larger shells are available for 5 to 30 g doses. Particularly where high-speed filling equipment is used there must be no difficulty in removing and replacing the cap, yet the junction of this with the body must form an efficient seal. The necessarily small tolerances on the dimensions of the cap and body are achieved by rigid control of all stages of the manufacturing process. Peck et al. (1964) have described a device utilizing the absorption of β-radiation from a chlorine-36 source for the control of shell thickness.

A description of the small scale filling of hard capsules is given in Chapter 24. For large scale production the capsules are sorted and positioned body downwards and sucked into holes in upper and lower rings which, when separated, retain the cap and body respectively (Fig. 19.26). The lower ring is then presented to a head which fills the body with medicament composition, as either a powder or a lightly compacted pellet. Subsequently the rings are recombined, the body pushed into the

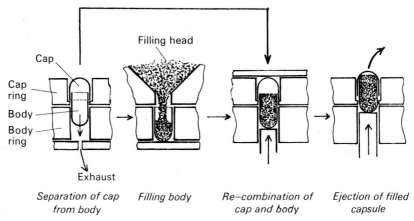

FIG. 19.26. Stages in the filling of hard capsules.

cap, the capsule ejected and any dust adhering to the outer capsule surface removed. In semi-automatice equipment the rings are separated, transferred to the filling head and recombined by hand, but with fully automatic machines these operations are accomplished by mechanical means.

In common with many other pharmaceutical materials such as bacitracin, magnesium trisilicate and starch (Strickland 1962), the moisture uptake–ambient humidity curve for gelatin exhibits marked hysteresis (Strickland & Moss 1962). Thus, the moisture content of the shell, normally 9 to 12 per cent, is determined by both its previous history and the ambient humidity; it may vary between 4 and 16 per cent under extreme conditions. Strickland and Moss concluded that the diffusion of moisture into the capsule contents occurs mainly through the shell surface with only a small contribution due to the junction between the body and cap. Moisture will be absorbed from the environment via the capsule wall if the medicament is more hygroscopic than the shell and for this reason such substances should not be dispensed in capsules. The preparation of the drug and its subsequent filling into the body poses many of the problems which have already been discussed in the context of tabletting, for instance, care must be taken to ensure the efficient mixing of minor constituents with other drugs or diluents. The weight of drug in both tablets and capsules is governed by the volume available for filling and the bulk density of the drug formulation under production conditions, while for low weight variation the powder must flow in a reproducible manner. Unlike the die-cavity of the tablet machine, the volume of the capsule body cannot be adjusted to accommodate a given weight of powder and therefore, with hard capsules, the bulk density of the powder must be adjusted by the addition of an inert diluent such as lactose. Care is necessary in the selection of the diluent as, apart from its effect on powder flow properties there is some evidence, at least in the case of Chloramphenicol Capsules (Withey & Mainville 1969), that high concentrations of lactose may interfere with drug dissolution. In addition to diluent, a lubricant such as magnesium stearate (about 0.5 per cent) may be added for correct operation of the mechanism in the filling head and up to 5 per cent talc may be added to improve the flow properties of the powder. Reier et al. (1968) have reported on preliminary studies to elucidate the effect of medicament type, production rate, capsule size, presence or absence of talc, particle size, specific volume and powder flow on

the semi-automatic filling of hard capsules. These studies showed that, for a given capsule size and production rate, the filling weight was largely determined by the specific volume of the powder, while the action of talc in reducing weight variation was attributed to more reproducible, rather than more rapid, flow of the powder. Computer analysis of the data gave equations for filling weight and filling weight variation which included all possible interactions of the factors listed above, except that terms for medicament type and particle size were not required as their effect was reflected in the flow properties of the powder and these were adequately defined by the flowability and specific volume. As the capsule size is set by the specific volume of the powder, only that parameter and the flowability need be measured, using a small sample, to predict the performance of a given filling composition. Thus, production difficulties may be anticipated and corrected prior to filling trials with large and potentially expensive batches of medicament. Reier and co-workers found excellent agreement between the predicted and observed behaviour of a number of model filling compositions.

QUALITY CONTROL OF CAPSULES

The reasons for controlling the disintegration time, weight variation and medicament content of tablets also apply to capsules and have been discussed in considerable detail earlier in this chapter.

Disintegration
The tablet disintegration apparatus of the *Pharmacopoeia* is specified for the test but the guided disc may not be used. With capsules, it is clearly necessary to distinguish, during the course of the test, between particles of shell and drug; the BP 1973 requires that no portion of *drug* shall remain after 15 min which does not freely pass the 10 mesh screen at the base of the disintegration tube. Aguiar et al. (1968) found that hard capsules containing chloramphenicol disrupted sufficiently to release the drug after a few minutes immersion in simulated gastric fluid, but several hours were required for complete solution of the shell. These authors emphasized that both rapid deaggregation (disintegration of powder aggregates into primary particles) and rapid dissolution were necessary conditions for good biological availability of the drug.

Uniformity of Filling Weight
This cannot be determined by simply weighing the filled capsules as there will be a variation in the

weights of the individual shells. For this reason the weight of the content of an individual capsule is defined as the difference in weight of the intact dose unit and the empty shell. Removal of dry particulate solid from the capsule merely involves detaching the cap or slitting the shell (Method A) but oily contents are squeezed out of the split shell and the remainder removed by washing in solvent (Method B). In all other respects the principle of the test is the same as that applied to tablets: Table 19.13 summarizes official requirements. Only one set of tolerances is specified when Method B is used to determine the weight of the capsule contents as this method applies to soft capsules and it is not usual to fill these with less than about 0.3 g of material.

Content of Medicament
A sample from the bulked contents of the capsules used in the test for weight uniformity is assayed and the dose of medicament per capsule calculated. This must comply with the limits set out in the relevant monograph which is framed to take into account such factors as drug purity, assay accuracy, assay precision and manufacturing difficulties. The general requirement that the drug content of individual dose units shall not show a gross deviation from that stated or prescribed also applies to capsules.

The available literature, see for example Aguiar et al. (1968), Robinson et al. (1968) and Stock (1962), suggests that, provided the capsule contents are correctly formulated and the manufacturing process adequately controlled, there should be few instances where difficulties will be encounted in the large scale production of capsules complying with official requirements.

TABLE 19.13

SUMMARY OF THE BP 1973 TEST FOR UNIFORMITY OF FILLING WEIGHT OF CAPSULES

Method	Applicable to	Sample size	Average weight of contents	Deviation per cent about the average weight	Maximum number of capsules which may exceed the stated weight range
A	Capsules containing particulate solids	20	0.12 g or less More than 0.12 g	±10 ±20 ± 7.5 ±15	Two None Two None
B	Flexible capsules containing oily filling	10	Not stated —see text	± 7.5 ±15	One None

REFERENCES

ABBOTT, D. D., PACKMAN, E. W., REES, E. W. & HARRISSON, J. W. E. (1959) *J. Am. pharm. Ass. (Sci. Edn)* **48**, 19.

AGUIAR, A. J., WHEELER, L. M., FUSARI, S. & ZELMER, J. E. (1968) *J. pharm. Sci.* **57**, 1844.

ANTONIDES, H. J. & DeKAY, G. H. (1953) *Drug Standards* **21**, 205.

ASHBY, F. W., MUGGLETON, P. W., TAYLOR, F. & WOODWARD, W. A. (1954) *J. Pharm. Pharmacol.* **6**, 1048.

BERRY, H. (1939) *Quart. J. Pharm.* **12**, 501.

BERRY, H. & RIDOUT, C. W. (1950) *J. Pharm. Pharmacol.* **2**, 619.

BERRY, H. & SMITH, A. N. (1944) *Quart. J. Pharm.* **17**, 248.

BLUBAUGH, F. C., ZAPAPAS, J. R. & SPARKS, M. C. (1958) *J. Am. pharm. Ass. (Sci. Edn)* **47**, 857.

BROOK, D. B. & MARSHALL, K. (1968) *J. pharm. Sci.* **57**, 481.

BROWNLEY, C. A. & LACHMAN, L. (1963) *J. pharm. Sci.* **52**, 86.

BURLINSON, H. (1950) *J. Pharm. Pharmacol.* **2**, 638.

CASTELLO, R. A. & MATTOCKS, A. M. (1962) *J. pharm. Sci.* **51**, 106.

DUVALL, R. N., KOSHY, K. T. & PYLES, J. W. (1965) *J. pharm. Sci.* **54**, 607.

EVANS, A. J. & TRAIN, D. (1963) *Bibliography of the Tabletting of Pharmaceutical Substances.* London: Pharmaceutical Press.

EVANS, A. J. & TRAIN, D. (1964) *Supplement to Bibliography of the Tabletting of Pharmaceutical Substances.* London: Pharmaceutical Press.

FELDMAN, E. G. (1969) *J. Pharm. Pharmacol.* **21**, 134.

FONNER, D. E., BANKER, G. S. & SWARBRICK, J. (1966) *J. pharm. Sci.* **55**, 181.

GANDERTON, D. (1969) *J. Pharm. Pharmacol.* **21**, 9S.

GANDERTON, D. & SELKIRK, A. B. (1969) Symposium on Powders, Society of Cosmetic Chemists of Great Britain, Dublin.

GOLD, G., DUVALL, R. N., PALERMO, B. T. & SLATER, J. G. (1968) *J. pharm. Sci.* **57**, 2153.

GOODHART, F. W., MAYORGA, G., MILLS, N. & NINGER, F. C. (1968) *J. pharm. Sci.* **57**, 1770.

GRIFFITHS, R. V. (1969) *Manufacturing Chemist and Aerosol News* **40**, 29.

GUNSEL, W. C. & LACHMAN, L. (1963) *J. pharm. Sci.* **52**, 178.

HADGRAFT, J. W. (1945) *Pharmaceut. J.* **154**, 183.

HARTLEY, F. (1950) *J. Pharm. Pharmacol.* **2**, 628.

HIGUCHI, T., ARNOLD, R. D., TUCKER, S. J. & BUSSE, L. W. (1952) *J. Am. pharm. Ass. (Sci. Edn)* **41**, 93.

HIGUCHI, T., RAO, A. N., BUSSE, L. W. & SWINTOSKY, J. V. (1953) *J. Am. pharm. Ass. (Sci. Edn)* **42**, 194.

HIGUCHI, T., NELSON, E. & BUSSE, L. W. (1954a) *J. Am. pharm. Ass. (Sci. Edn)* **43**, 344.

HIGUCHI, T., ELOWE, L. N. & BUSSE, L. W. (1954b) *J. Am. pharm. Ass. (Sci. Edn)* **43**, 685.

HIGUCHI, T., SHIMAMOTO, T., ERIKSEN, S. P. & YASHIKI, T. (1965) *J. pharm. Sci.* **54**, 111.

HOWARD, W. R. (1951) *J. Pharm. Pharmacol.* **3**, 777.

HOYLE, H. (1946) *Quart. J. Pharm.* **19**, 279.

INGRAM, J. T. & LOWENTHAL, W. (1968) *J. pharm. Sci.* **57**, 393.

JAFFE, J. & LIPPMANN, I. (1964) *J. pharm. Sci.* **53**, 441.

JONES, T. M. (1969) Symposium on Powders, Society of Cosmetic Chemists of Great Britain, Dublin, 1969.

KORNBLUM, S. S. & ZOGLIO, M. A. (1967) *J. pharm. Sci.* **56**, 1569.

KUZEL, N. R., ROUDEBUSH, H. E. & STEVENSON, C. E. (1969) *J. pharm. Sci.* **58**, 381.

LACHMAN, L. & COOPER, J. (1963) *J. pharm. Sci.* **52**, 490.

LACHMAN, L., SYLWESTROWICZ, H. D. & SPEISER, P. P. (1966) *J. pharm. Sci.* **55**, 958.

LEWIS, C. J. & SHOTTON, E. (1965a) *J. Pharm. Pharmacol.* **17**, 71S.

LEWIS, C. J. & SHOTTON, E. (1965b) *J. Pharm. Pharmacol.* **17**, 82S.

MALM, C. J., EMERSON, J. & HIATT, G. D. (1951) *J. Am. pharm. Ass. (Sci. Edn)* **40**, 520.

MAPSTONE, T. J. (1952) *Pharmaceut. J.* **168**, 291.

NELSON, E. (1955) *J. Am. pharm. Ass. (Sci. Edn)* **44**, 494.

NOTTON, H. E. F. (1956) *Pharmaceut. J.* **177**, 69.

OREWAN, E. (1949) *Rec. Prog. Phys.* **12**, 185.

PATEL, N. R. & HOPPONEN, R. E. (1966) *J. pharm. Sci.* **55**, 1065.

PATTERSON, S. J. & LERRIGO, A. F. (1947) *Quart. J. Pharm.* **20**, 83.

PECK, E. G., CHRISTIAN, J. E. & BANKER, G. S. (1964) *J. pharm. Sci.* **53**, 607.

PHARMACEUTICAL JOURNAL (1960) **185**, 372.

PHARMACEUTICAL JOURNAL (1965) **194**, 475.

PHARMACEUTICAL JOURNAL (1966) **197**, 169.

PRANCE, H. P., STEPHENSON, D. & TAYLOR, A. (1946) *Quart. J. Pharm.* **19**, 286.

REES, J. E. & SHOTTON, E. (1969) *J. Pharm. Pharmacol.* **21**, 731.

REIER, G. E. & SHANGRAW, R. F. (1966) *J. pharm. Sci.* **55**, 510.

REIER, G. E., COHN, R., ROCK, S. & WAGENBLAST, F. (1968) *J. pharm. Sci.* **57**, 660.

RIBEIRO, D., STEVENSON, D., SAMYN, J., MILSOVICH, G. & MATTOCKS, A. M. (1955) *J. Am. pharm. Ass. (Sci. Edn)* **44**, 226.

RICHMAN, M. D., FOX, C. D. & SHANGRAW, R. F. (1965) *J. pharm. Sci.* **54**, 447.

RIDGEWAY, K., SHOTTON, E. & GLASBY, J. (1969a) *J. Pharm. Pharmacol.* **21**, 19S.

RIDGEWAY, K., GLASBY, J. & ROSSER, P. H. (1969b) *J. Pharm. Pharmacol.* **21**, 24S.

RITSCHEL, W. A., SKINNER, F. S. & SCHLUMPF, R. (1969) *Pharm. acta helv.* **44**, 547.

ROBINSON, M. J., GRASS, G. M. & LANTZ, R. J. (1968) *J. pharm. Sci.* **57**, 1979.

ROGERS, A. R. (1956) *J. Pharm. Pharmacol.* **8**, 1103.

ROLFE, H. G. (1956) *Pharmaceut. J.* **176**, 178.

SENIOR, N. (1969) *Pharmaceut. J.* **203**, 703.

SHOTTON, E. & GANDERTON, D. (1960a) *J. Pharm. Pharmacol.* **12**, 87T.

SHOTTON, E. & GANDERTON, D. (1960b) *J. Pharm. Pharmacol.* **12**, 93T.

SHOTTON, E. & GANDERTON, D. (1961) *J. Pharm. Pharmacol.* **13**, 144T.

SHOTTON, E., DEER, J. J. & GANDERTON, D. (1963) *J. Pharm. Pharmacol.* **15**, 106T.

SHOTTON, E. & LEWIS, C. J. (1964) *J. Pharm. Pharmacol.* **16**, 111T.

SMITH, A. N. (1950) *J. Pharm. Pharmacol.* **2**, 627.

SMITH, C. D., MICHAELS, T. P., CHERTKOFF, M. J. & SINOTTE, L. P. (1963) *J. pharm. Sci.* **52**, 1183.

SMITH, K. L. (1955) *J. Pharm. Pharmacol.* **7**, 875.

SRINIVAS, R., DEKAY, H. G. & BANKER, G. S. (1966) *J. pharm. Sci.* **55**, 335.

STEPHENSON, D. (1960) *Pharmaceut. J.* **185**, 137.

STEPHENSON, D. & HUMPHREYS-JONES, J. F. (1951) *J. Pharm. Pharmacol.* **3**, 767.

STEPHENSON, D. & SMITH, D. S. (1951) *J. Pharm. Pharmacol.* **3**, 547.

STOCK, F. E. H. (1962) *Pharmaceut. J.* **188**, 453.

STRICKLAND, W. A. (1962) *J. pharm. Sci.* **51**, 310.

STRICKLAND, W. A., NELSON, E., BUSSE, L. W. & HIGUCHI, T. (1956) *J. Am. pharm. Ass. (Sci. Edn)* **45**, 51.

STRICKLAND, W. A. & MOSS, M. (1962) *J. pharm. Sci.* **51**, 1002.

SUTARIA, R. H. (1968) *Manufacturing Chemist and Aerosol News* **39**, 37.

SWARTZ, C. J., WEINSTEIN, S., WINDHEUSER, J. & COOPER, J. (1962) *J. pharm. Sci.* **51**, 1181.

SWARTZ, C. J. & ANSCHEL, J. (1968) *J. pharm. Sci.* **57**, 1779.

TRAIN, D. (1956) *J. Pharm. Pharmacol.* **8**, 745.

TRAIN, D. (1960) *Pharmaceut. J.* **185**, 129.

TRAIN, D. & HERSEY, J. A. (1960) *J. Pharm. Pharmacol.* **12**, 97T.

WEBSTER, A. R. & VAN ABBÉ, N. J. (1955) *J. Pharm. Pharmacol.* **7**, 882.

WHITEHOUSE, R. C. (1954) *Pharmaceut. J.* **172**, 85.

WINDHEUSER, J., MISRA, J., ERICKSEN, S. P. & HIGUCHI, T. (1963) *J. pharm. Sci.* **52**, 767.

WITHEY, R. J. & MAINVILLE, C. A. (1969) *J. pharm. Sci.* **58**, 1120.

WOOD, J. H. (1965) *J. pharm. Sci.* **54**, 1207.

WURSTER, D. E. (1959) *J. Am. pharm. Ass. (Sci. Edn)* **48**, 451.

WURSTER, D. E. (1960) *J. Am. pharm. Ass. (Sci. Edn)* **49**, 82.

WURSTER, D. E. & SEITZ, J. A. (1960) *J. Am. pharm. Ass. (Sci. Edn)* **49**, 335.

Part III
DISPENSING

20

Pharmacopoeias, Formularies and Medicines Legislation

The word, pharmacopoeia, is derived from the Greek *pharmakon*, a drug, and *poieo*, I make. Literally, it is a list of medicinal substances, crude drugs and formulae for making preparations from them. Such a list is compiled by recognized authorities, usually appointed by the government of each country. Most of the principal countries of the world have their national pharmacopoeias.

THE BRITISH PHARMACOPOEIA

The *British Pharmacopoeia* came into existence in 1864 replacing the more parochial publications that were then in use. Earlier, pharmacopoeias had been published in London, Edinburgh and Dublin, each containing preparations bearing the same name but differing in strength. There was obviously a need for a single national authority and the Medical Act of 1858 gave the General Council of Medical Education and Registration the responsibility of publishing the *British Pharmacopoeia*. This responsibility was reiterated in the Medical Act of 1956, Section 47 of which states:

'The General Council shall, at such intervals as they may determine, cause to be published under their direction new editions of the British Pharmacopoeia, containing such descriptions of and standards for, and such notes and other matter relating to medicines, preparations, materials and articles, used in the practice of medicine, surgery, or midwifery, as the Council may direct.'

A review of the arrangements for preparing the pharmacopoeia by a sub-committee of the Committee of Civil Research in 1926 led to the recommendation that the General Medical Council should appoint a Pharmacopoeia Commission, entrusted with the detailed work of new editions.

The *British Pharmacopoeia* 1932 was published under these arrangements and subsequent editions have been similarly prepared. Under the Medicines Act 1968, the responsibility for preparing the pharmacopoeia was transferred to the Medicines Commission and under Section 4 of the Act, the *British Pharmacopoeia* Commission was reconstituted by the Health Ministers on the recommendation of the Medicines Commission.

The *British Pharmacopoeia* is the source of official standards for drugs in the United Kingdom and other parts of the Commonwealth. Important though it undoubtedly is as the primary authority for drug standards, it has ceased to have its former significance for practising pharmacists. Generations of pharmaceutical students were brought up to regard the pharmacopoeia as the main source of all their pharmaceutical knowledge. Today most of the drugs and preparations described in the *British Pharmacopoeia* are proprietary products of the pharmaceutical industry and the pharmacopoeia provides information on the standards and methods of anlysis to be employed. The pharmaceutical student has much less occasion in practice today to consult the pharmacopoeia but should nevertheless become thoroughly familiar with its scope, particularly in those aspects where it lays down official methods to be employed, for example, in the preparation of injections.

THE INTERNATIONAL PHARMACOPOEIA

The concept of a single national pharmacopoeia, however, has to some extent outlived its usefulness.

This has arisen not only from the need for a wider international authority but also from the changes that have taken place in the practice of pharmacy and the preparation of medicines. Attempts were made to establish international uniformity of terminology and standardization as long ago as 1874 but it was not until 1906 that an 'International Agreement respecting the Unification of Formulae for Potent Drugs and Preparations' was achieved. Attempts were made to publish an International Pharmacopoeia under the Health Organization of the League of Nations and subsequently under the World Health Organization, and Volume 1 was eventually issued in 1951. The second edition was published in 1967 under the title, *Specifications for the Quality Control of Pharmaceutical Preparations*—a further indication of the changed function of pharmacopoeias and the emphasis placed on the provision of standards of purity.

THE EUROPEAN PHARMACOPOEIA

While the *International Pharmacopoeia* has undoubtedly had a unifying influence it has not replaced the national pharmacopoeias of each country. Under the auspices of the Council of Europe, it has been considered necessary to prepare a European Pharmacopoeia. The participating countries are Belgium, France, the Federal Republic of Germany, Italy, Luxembourg, the Netherlands, Switzerland and the United Kingdom. The *European Pharmacopoeia* takes precedence over the national pharmacopoeias of the participating countries for those substances covered by its monographs.

The future of the *British Pharmacopoeia* in the light of the publication of the European Pharmacopoeia and the Medicines Act, 1968 has been discussed by Hersant (1969) who has suggested that the importance of the *British Pharmacopoeia* may be undermined in the future. However, since publication of a monograph in the *European Pharmacopoeia* can only result from the unanimous agreement of the representatives of the participating countries, this is likely to be a slow process. Hersant has suggested that the function of the *British Pharmacopoeia* in the future will be primarily concerned with the early publication of specifications for new drugs.

THE BRITISH PHARMACEUTICAL CODEX

To a greater degree, similar considerations may influence the scope and function of the companion volume to the *British Pharmacopoeia*, the *British Pharmaceutical Codex*. This publication, originally described as 'An Imperial Dispensatory for the use of Medical Practitioners and Pharmacists', is published by the direction of the Council of the Pharmaceutical Society of Great Britain. The *British Pharmaceutical Codex* differs in several important respects from the pharmacopoeia. It comprises many more drugs and preparations; some may be included in advance of the pharmacopoeia and ultimately acquire official status, others may formerly have been official and are retained in the Codex because they are still used to an appreciable extent. For such preparations the Codex provides standards and tests similar to those in the pharmacopoeial monographs and it should be noted that, like the *British Pharmacopoeia*, it has been accepted as the presumptive standard for legal purposes in Great Britain. It has, for example, been used to decide, in Courts of Law, on the quality of a drug demanded in accordance with the Food and Drugs Act 1938.

In addition to drug standards, the *British Pharmaceutical Codex* since 1923 has been the source of standards for surgical dressings. Furthermore, it provides information on the actions and uses of drugs, their undesirable effects, precautions and the treatment of poisoning. To the practising pharmacist, the codex is useful not only as a source of information on drugs but also because it contains the formulae of most of the preparations still extemporaneously prepared in pharmacy, notably liquid preparations for oral administration, sterile eye drops and eye lotions, ointments and creams, together with recommended methods for dispensing them.

THE BRITISH NATIONAL FORMULARY

For the day-to-day purposes of the prescribing doctor and pharmacist, there is an obvious need for a ready and convenient source of essential information on the drugs and preparations commonly in use. This need is answered by the British National Formulary, a publication produced jointly by the Pharmaceutical Society of Great Britain and the British Medical Association. It is prepared by a Joint Formulary Committee, drawn from the two professions and on which the Department of Health and Social Security is also represented. At the inception of the National Health Service, the Minister of Health, as he was then designated, signified his willingness to accept the Formulary as the standard prescribers' formulary for the Service.

The British National Formulary is not a book of standards and differs in this respect from the *British Pharmacopoeia* and the *British Pharmaceutical Codex.* By close liaison between the authorities responsible for publishing the three books, many preparations from the Pharmacopoeia and the Codex are included in the Formulary. Such is the pace of therapeutic innovation nowadays, however, that the Formulary often has to include new drugs before thay have achieved the status of inclusion in either the Pharmacopoeia or the Codex.

The pharmaceutical student will find much useful information in the British National Formulary. The Classified Formulary section, in which the preparations are listed according to their pharmaceutical form, provides the practising pharmacist with the formulae of commonly dispensed medicines and other details of practical importance. The Classified Notes for Prescribers are arranged according to a pharmacological classification and are primarily intended for the prescribing doctor. The pharmaceutical student, however, will find in them much useful information on the actions, uses and doses of drugs. In addition, the Formulary contains sections dealing with such subjects as dependence on drugs and adverse reactions to drugs.

THE EXTRA PHARMACOPOEIA

The vast number of drugs and proprietary medicines in use today is such that therapeutic information and its retrieval is one of the major problems of the pharmacist, whatever his field of practice. The *Extra Pharmacopoeia* (*Martindale*), published by the Pharmaceutical Society, is a useful reference book, containing information not only on official preparations but also proprietary products and preparations in foreign pharmacopoeias. Many of the leading drug manufacturers produce technical literature which provides another source of information and the filing of such material so that it can be readily retrieved is very well worth the trouble. Under the Medicines Act, each product marketed commercially must be described in a Data Sheet, conforming to the requirements of the Licensing Authority. The data sheets of the leading manufacturers are published annually in a bound volume by the Association of the British Pharmaceutical Industry (ABPI).

MEDICINES LEGISLATION

In recent years, it has become apparent that the introduction of new drugs into medicine is not adequately safeguarded even by the stringent controls applied through pharmacopoeial and other monographs. Before a drug achieves the distinction of being included in the Pharmacopoeia or Codex, it is usually developed in the commercial research laboratories of the pharmaceutical industry, and released for commercial distribution if it passes the requisite tests for toxicity and clinical efficacy. Much effort is put into the investigations required by the pharmaceutical manufacturer to ensure that the products released are safe for the purpose intended. However, there is always an element of risk with any drug developed and experience has shown that there is a need for the central supervision of the testing of new drugs by an independent authority.

The reports of fetal abnormalities following the administration of thalidomide to pregnant women during 1960 and 1961 gave rise to much public concern and a Joint Sub-Committee of the Standing Medical Advisory Committee was set up to advise the Minister of what further steps were considered desirable to ensure the safety of drugs. The Joint Sub-Committee rejected as neither desirable nor practicable the suggestion that responsibility for testing new drugs should be transferred to a central authority. However, it recommended that there should be an expert body to review evidence and offer advice on the toxicity of new drugs.

The Committee on Safety of Drugs was appointed in June 1963 under the Chairmanship of Sir Derrick Dunlop and subsequently of Sir Eric Scowen. The terms of reference of the Committee were as follows:

(i) To invite from the manufacturer or other person developing or proposing to market a drug in the United Kingdom any reports they may think fit on the toxicity tests carried out on it; to consider whether any further tests should be made, and whether the drug should be submitted to clinical trial, and to convey their advice to those who submitted reports.

(ii) To obtain reports of clinical trials of drugs submitted thereto.

(iii) Taking into account the safety and efficacy of each drug and the purposes for which it is to be used, to consider whether it may be released for marketing with or without precautions or restrictions on its use and to convey their advice to those who submitted reports.

(iv) To give to manufacturers and others concerned any general advice they may think fit on the matters referred to in paragraphs (i) and (iii).

(v) To assemble and assess reports about adverse

effects of drugs in use and prepare information thereon which may be brought to the notice of doctors and others concerned.

(vi) To advise the appointing Ministers on any of the above matters. ·

Three sub-committees of the Committee on Drug Safety were established to deal with: (1) toxicity, (2) clinical trials and therapeutic efficacy, and (3) adverse reactions. The Committee started to assess reports on toxicity and clinical trials on 1 January 1964 and both the Association of British Pharmaceutical Industry and the Proprietary Association of Great Britain agreed not to submit a new drug for clinical trial or to market a new drug after that date against the advice of the Committee. The Committee on Drug Safety, therefore, possessed no legal sanctions but operated by the consent and agreement of the medical profession and the main bodies representing commercial interests in pharmacy.

Despite its lack of legal powers, its authority and influence effectively prevented the marketing of drugs which had not passed through the recognized procedure.

There are therefore a number of different bodies responsible for publishing standards for drugs, concerned with drug safety and issuing information about the use of drugs. Clearly there was a need for the work of all these disparate bodies to be co-ordinated centrally and controlled in the public interest. Such co-ordination was established in the Medicines Act 1968 which made new provision for the safety, quality and efficacy of medicinal products for human and veterinary use. the circumstances in which they are sold and supplied, their labelling and description and their sales promotion.

This comprehensive legislation was foreshadowed by a White Paper (Cmnd 3395) published in 1967 and it was also influenced by the recommendations made in the report of the Committee on the Relationship of the Pharmaceutical Industry with the National Health Service (Cmnd 3410). The Act provided for the appointment of a Medicines Commission to advise the Health Ministers on the administration of the Act.

As has been said, among its many functions, the Medicines Commission became responsible for advising the Health Ministers on the preparation of the *British Pharmacopoeia*. The Act also empowers the Secretary of State to assume responsibility for any other compendia giving standards for, or information about substances and articles used in human or veterinary medicine. The publication of the *British Pharmaceutical Codex* is authorized by the Council of the Pharmaceutical Society of Great Britain, and the *British National Formulary* is authorized by the British Medical Association in accordance with the Pharmaceutical Society. It has now been agreed that the *British Pharmacopoeia* will in future be the sole source of official standards for medicinal preparations (including surgical dressings). The *British Pharmaceutical Codex* 1973 is the last edition of that book in which standards are provided. The status of the *British National Formulary* remains unchanged at the time of going to press.

Under the Medicines Act 1968, the Safety of Drugs Committee was reconstituted as a statutory body under the new title of the Safety of Medicines Committee. The Medicines Act also introduced a system of licensing of pharmaceutical preparations and medicines. Before a new drug can be submitted to clinical trial it must first be approved by the Safety of Medicines Committee and granted a Clinical Trial Certificate. Before it is released for commercial distribution, the new drug preparation must further be granted a Product Licence. The grant of clinical trial certificates and product licences is made only after the manufacturer has disclosed, in confidence, to the Safety of Medicines Committee full information on the chemistry, pharmacy, standards, toxicity and stability data of the new preparation.

The Medicines Act 1968 also provided for the setting up of a Medicines Inspectorate. This has the responsibility of inspecting and approving premises in which medicines are manufactured and stored. Each manufacturer is required under the Medicines Act to obtain a licence for his premises and the grant of a licence is subject to a satisfactory report by the Medicines Inspectorate.

The Medicines Act thus covers many aspects of the practice of pharmacy, including requirements for standards of hygiene in places where medicines are manufactured, transported, stored and supplied. It is also concerned with the laws governing the sale of poisons and the retail sale of medicinal preparations. The Medicines Act has had a profound effect on the practice of pharmacy which will continue to be felt in the coming years.

REFERENCE

HERSANT, E. F. (1969) *Pharmac. J.* **203**, 239.

21

Weights and Measures

For many years, three systems of weights and measures were in use in pharmacy: the metric system, the avoirdupois system and the apothecary system. A Committee on Weights and Measures Legislation was appointed by the President of the Board of Trade in 1948 'to review the existing Weights and Measures Legislation and other legislation containing provisions affecting Weights and Measures and the administration thereof and to make recommendations'. The Committee, in a report published in 1951, recommended that the apothecary system should be abolished and that the metric system should be adopted in its place. It recommended further that steps should be taken in concert with the Commonwealth and the USA to abolish the imperial system of measurement in favour of the complete adoption of the metric system over a period of about 20 years.

While the complete adoption of the metric system of weights and measures for the purposes of trade has not yet been accepted, steps have now been taken to abolish the use of apothecary and imperial systems for all dealings in drugs and medicines. Since 31 March, 1969, pharmacists have been required to carry out all dispensing in the metric system. The apothecary and imperial weights and measures became illegal as far as pharmacy is concerned.

The first steps to change over to the metric system appeared in the British Pharmacopoeia and British Pharmaceutical Codex published in 1963. In these editions, the strengths of all single-dose forms of drug presentation (tablets, capsules and injections) were given only in metric quantities.

In order to carry this change into effect, the Weights and Measures (Equivalents for dealings with drugs) Regulations 1964 (S.1 1964 No. 81) stipulated the strength in metric units which *must* be dispensed or supplied when a strength in apothecary units is stated on the prescription or order.

The British Pharmaceutical Codex 1968 and the British National Formulary 1968 extended the use of the metric system to all other liquid forms of drug presentation and the schedule of metric equivalents to be used in place of apothecary and imperial quantities was further extended by the Weights and Measures (Equivalents for Dealing with Drugs) Regulations 1970 (S.I. 1970 No. 1897). The complete adoption of the metric system in pharmacy has therefore been achieved.

While pharmacists are required to use the metric system for dispensing prescriptions, doctors have not been compelled to use the metric system in writing them. There are still in circulation older prescriptions written by medical practitioners before 1969 and a few prescriptions continue to be written in the older system of weights and measures even today. The pharmacist is required to interpret these prescriptions in the metric system, even though they are written in the avoirdupois or apothecary systems. In converting prescriptions from the older systems, the metric equivalents sets out in the Weights and Measures (Equivalent for dealings with drugs) Regulations 1970 (S.I. 1970 No. 1897) must be used. Appendix 32 of the British Pharmaceutical Codex, 1973 gives information on weights and measures.

THE METRIC SYSTEM

The use of the metric system of weights and measures was legalized in this country as long ago as 1897 by the Weights and Measures (Metric System) Act.

The international metre was formerly defined as the distance measured at $0°C$ between two marks on a platinum–iridium bar. This standard was derived from a previous standard which was said to be the one ten-millionth part of the earth's quadrant from the North Pole to the Equator.

For exact measurement it has become necessary to devise a physical means of defining the metre. At the International Metric Convention it was agreed that the metre could be defined in terms of the wavelength of a certain radiation. The radiation chosen was that from krypton-86 and the orange-red line was the chosen emission. Metric length measurements are now derived from the definition of the metre which is equal to 1.65076373×10^6 ^{86}Kr, where $^{86}Kr = 6.0578021 \times 10^7$ metre is the wavelength in vacuo of the orange-red radiation corresponding to the transition between two specific energy levels of the krypton-86 atom.

LENGTH

Basic unit = 1 metre (m)
1 decimetre (dm) = $\frac{1}{10}$th part of 1 metre (10^{-1} m)
1 centimetre (cm) = $\frac{1}{100}$th part of 1 metre (10^{-2} m)
1 millimetre (mm) = $\frac{1}{1000}$th part of 1 metre (10^{-3} m)
1 micrometre (μm) = 1 micron (μm) = $\frac{1}{1000}$th part of 1 millimetre (10^{-6} m)
1 nanometre (nm) = 1 millimicron (mμm) = $\frac{1}{1000}$th part of 1 micron (10^{-9} m)
The terms micron and millimicron according to a resolution of the Thirteenth General Conference of Weights and Measures (1967), should no longer be used.

MASS

The international kilogram is the weight in vacuo of a platinum-iridium cylinder preserved at the International Bureau of Weights and Measures at Sèvres and known as the international prototype kilogram.
Basic unit = 1 kilogram (kg)
1 gram (g) = $\frac{1}{1000}$th part of 1 kilogram (10^{-3} kg)
1 milligram (mg) = $\frac{1}{1000}$th part of 1 gram (10^{-6} kg)
1 microgram (μg) = $\frac{1}{1000}$th part of 1 milligram (10^{-9} kg)

The gramme was formerly spelt thus instead of gram to avoid confusion with grain in prescription writing, and gramme was abbreviated to G not gr or g to avoid confusion with the abbreviation for grain in the apothecary system. However, the symbol g is now the recognized contraction for gram in international practice, and is normally used in prescription writing, although older prescribers may adhere to the use of G.

The British Pharmacopoeia recommends that microgram should not be abbreviated in prescription writing. Where an abbreviation is necessary, mcg should be used. The terms μg and μ should not be used in prescription writing or recording the dosage of drugs.

CAPACITY

The litre (l) is now a special name for the volume occupied by a cube with sides of 1 decimetre. The 1901 definition of the litre under which it was found by later experiment to be 1.000028 dm^3 has been abrogated. The term litre is no longer associated with the results of measurements of volumes to high precision but has been retained for use in medicine.
Basic Unit = 1 litre (l)
1 millilitre (ml) = $\frac{1}{1000}$th part of 1 litre (10^{-3} l)

The millilitre is thus now equal to 1 cubic centimetre (cc). The term mil is sometimes used as an abbreviation for millilitre in writing prescriptions.

LIQUID MEASURES

Conversion to the metric system for single-dose forms of drug presentation (e.g. tablets, capsules, injections) produced few complications. More difficulty was encountered in introducing the metric system for all the liquid oral forms of drug presentation e.g. mixtures, elixirs, linctuses, etc.

For many years such preparations were prescribed in teaspoonful and tablespoonful doses in order to provide a measure which the patient could use conveniently in his own home. There is an enormous variation in the capacity of domestic teaspoons and tablespoons and while such a variation in the dose volume was not important with traditional medicines having little or no therapeutic activity, more accurate measurement of the dose volume is necessary for the administration of modern potent drugs.

Liquid medicines in the metric system have been formulated to a dose volume of either 5 ml or 10 ml and the patient is instructed to take either one or two 5 ml dose volumes. For this purpose a standard 5 ml medicine spoon has been produced (B.S. 3221/4) and the instructions given to the patient are to take one 5 ml spoonful or two 5 ml spoonfuls.

These matters are dealt with more fully in the chapters on liquid preparations. The pharmacist has a clear responsibility to ensure that each time a medicine is dispensed the patient fully understands the dose and frequency of administration.

REFERENCES

British Standard 1922: 1953. Dispensing Measures for Pharmaceutical Purposes (Metric Units).

British Standard 3221/4 (revised) (1969). Metric Medicine Spoons.

British Standard 1679/6. Metric Dispensing Bottles.

British Standard 1679/7. Metric Ribbed Oval Bottles.

CAPPER, K. R. (1960) *Pharm. J.* **185**, 229.

A.B.P.I. Committee's Report (1952) *Pharm. J.* **168**, 284.

Report of the Committee on Weights and Measures Legislation (1951) Cmd. 8219. London: HMSO.

Weights and Measures Regulations, S.I. 1965 No. 320. London: HMSO.

Weights and Measures. (Equivalents for dealing in drugs) Regulations (1970 No. 1897). London: HMSO.

22

Pharmaceutical Calculations

The adoption of the metric system has simplified many of the calculations necessary in the practice of pharmacy, especially of the amounts needed to prepare percentage solutions.

PERCENTAGE SOLUTIONS

The *British Pharmacopoeia* defines four different types of percentage solutions, according to the circumstances:

Per cent w/w (percentage weight in weight) expresses the number of grams of active substance in 100 g of product.

Per cent w/v (percentage weight in volume) expresses the number of grams of active substance in 100 ml of product.

Per cent v/w (percentage volume in weight) expresses the number of millilitres of active substance in 100 g of product.

Per cent v/v (percentage volume in volume) expresses the number of millilitres of active substance in 100 ml of product.

In the case of a liquid dissolved in a liquid the strength is expressed as a percentage volume in volume. For example, a 1 per cent v/v solution of rosemary oil in alcohol consists of 1 ml rosemary oil in sufficient alcohol to produce 100 ml.

In the case of a solid dissolved in a liquid, the strength is expressed as a percentage weight in volume. Thus a 1 per cent w/v solution of morphine sulphate in water contains 1 g morphine sulphate in sufficient water to produce 100 ml. An injection containing 1 per cent w/v of active substance contains 10 mg in 1 ml.

It should be noted that no account is taken of the density of the solvent in calculating per cent w/v solutions. Thus a 5 per cent w/v solution of phenol in water contains 5 g in 100 ml of solution. Similarly, a 5 per cent w/v solution in glycerin contains 5 g phenol in sufficient glycerin to produce 100 ml of solution.

EXPRESSION OF STRENGTHS OF INTRAVENOUS FLUIDS

Developments in biochemical techniques have led to the expression of the electrolyte content of body fluids in terms of millimoles (mmol) or milli-equivalents (mEq) of ions per litre. It is logical, therefore, to express in similar terms the strength of intravenous infusion solutions intended to correct the balance of electrolytes in body fluids. The mole is now the basic international unit for specifying the amount of an element, compound or ion. It is defined by the *British Pharmaceutical Codex* (Appendix 31, 1973) as 'the basic unit of amount of substance of a specified chemical formula, containing the same number of formula units (atoms, molecules, ions, electrons, quanta or other entities) as there are in 12 g of the pure nuclide ^{12}C'. A millimole is one thousandth of this amount. In the case of ions, therefore, a millimole is the sum of the atomic weights in the ion, expressed as milligrams. The milliequivalent of an ion may be defined either as one-thousandth of the gram-equivalent weight of that ion, or as the ionic weight (the sum of the atomic weights in the ion) in milligrams divided by the valency of the ion. The milliequivalent is therefore the millimole divided by the valency of the ion.

The total ionic concentration of plasma is from 300 to 320 millimoles per litre, and the principal ions present are sodium, potassium, magnesium, calcium, chloride, bicarbonate and phosphate. Most of these are contained in the intravenous fluids of the *British Pharmacopoeia, British Pharmaceutical Codex* or *British National Formulary.*

A Table in Appendix 31 of the *British Pharmaceutical Codex* (1973) gives the values of the millimoles and milliequivalents of the principal ions and the weights of various salts containing one millimole or one milliequivalent of these ions.

A further Table in Appendix 31 gives the concentration of ions, in terms of millimoles per litre, in various commonly used intravenous fluids.

Conversion of percentage strength to millimoles per litre:

Let C = percentage w/v strength of salt
W = milligrams of salt containing 1 millimole of the specified ion

100 millilitres of solution contain C grams of salt
1 litre of solution contains $10 \times C$ grams of salt = 10 000 C milligrams

$$\therefore \text{Millimoles per litre} = \frac{10\,000\,\text{C}}{\text{W}}$$

This equation may be used to calculate the number of millimoles per litre from the percentage strength of a salt containing the specified ion. The number of milliequivalents per litre may be obtained by multiplying by the valency of the ion. Thus the numbers of millimoles and milliequivalents of a univalent ion such as sodium are identical whereas the number of millimoles of a divalent ion such as calcium is half the number of milliequivalents.

Example: How many millimoles per litre of bicarbonate ion are contained in a solution of sodium bicarbonate 8.4 per cent w/v?

C = 8.4 per cent w/v

W = 84 milligrams

$$\text{Millimoles per litre} = \frac{10\,000 \times 8.4}{84}$$

$$= \frac{84\,000}{84} = 1000$$

An 8.4 per cent w/v solution of sodium bicarbonate contains 1000 millimoles of bicarbonate per litre.

Conversion of millimoles per litre to percentage strength:

Let M = millimoles of specified ion per litre
W = milligrams of salt containing 1 millimole of specified ion

1 litre contains M millimoles of specified ion
= $M \times W$ milligrams of salt
= $\dfrac{M \times W}{1000}$ grams of salt

$$\therefore 100 \text{ millilitres contain } \frac{M \times W}{10\,000} \text{ grams of salt}$$

$$\text{Percentage strength w/v} = \frac{M \times W}{10\,000}$$

Example: What is the percentage strength w/v, of a solution of potassium chloride containing 20 millimoles of potassium per litre?

M = 20

W = 74.5

$$\text{Percentage strength w/v} = \frac{20 \times 74.5}{10\,000}$$

$$= 0.149$$

Approximately 20 millimoles per litre of potassium are contained in a 0.15 per cent w/v solution of potassium chloride.

OSMOLARITY AND OSMOLALITY

The osmotic activity of a solution may be stated in terms of the milliosmol, which is an expression of the osmotic activity of 1 millimole. The term *osmolarity* is used to express the strength in milliosmols per litre and indicates the total ionic concentration of the solution. Biochemical data often refer to the *osmolality* of body fluids and this is the total ionic concentration per 1000 g water. Since most body fluids are of low concentration, the density is small and there is little numerical difference between the osmolarity and osmolality.

The osmolality of blood serum is approximately 300 mmol and this can be used as a useful factor in adjusting an injection to isotonicity.

Example: How much sodium chloride is needed to adjust to isotonicity a solution containing 20 mmol of calcium per litre (as calcium chloride)?

20 mmol of calcium are provided by 60 milliosmols of calcium and chloride per litre

$\therefore\ 300 - 60 = 240$ milliosmols are to be provided by sodium chloride to give an isotonic solution.

The formula of the solution is therefore:

Calcium chloride ($CaCl_2, 2H_2O$):
$$60 \text{ milliosmols} = 20 \text{ mmol Ca}^{2+}$$
$$= 20 \times 147 = 2.94 \text{ g}$$

Sodium chloride:
$$240 \text{ milliosmols} = 120 \text{ mmol Na}^+$$
$$= 120 \times 58.5 = 7.02 \text{ g}$$

Water for Injection to 1000 ml.

SOLUTIONS FOR PERITONEAL DIALYSIS AND HAEMODIALYSIS

Solutions used for peritoneal dialysis or haemodialysis are required to contain a mixture of anions and cations in approximately physiological concentrations. The bicarbonate present in blood plasma may be replaced by lactate or acetate ions in dialysis solutions in order to overcome some of the problems of formulation, particularly when concentrated solutions are required.

Example: Calculate the quantities of salts required for the preparation of 1 litre of a peritoneal dialysis solution in which the ionic concentration is as follows:

Sodium 130 mmol
Acetate 35 mmol
Chloride 100 (approx) mmol
Calcium 1.5 mmol
Magnesium 0.75 mmol

Since the acetate ions will be contributed by sodium acetate, 35 mmol of sodium will be obtained from this source. The remainder of the sodium (130–35) = 95 mmol will be contributed by sodium chloride.

Quantities required:

Sodium chloride 95 mmol

Sodium acetate 35 mmol

Calcium chloride 1.5 mmol

Magnesium chloride 0.75 mmol

Sodium chloride
$$95 \text{ mmol} = \frac{95 \times 58.44}{1000} = 5.56 \text{ g}$$

Sodium acetate ($CH_3CO_2Na, 3H_2O$)
$$35 \text{ mmol} = \frac{35 \times 136.1}{1000} = 4.76 \text{ g}$$

Calcium chloride ($CaCl_2, 2H_2O$)
$$1.5 \text{ mmol} = \frac{147 \times 1.5}{1000} = 0.220 \text{ g}$$

Magnesium chloride ($MgCl_2, 6H_2O$)
$$0.75 \text{ mmol} = \frac{203.3 \times 0.75}{1000} = 0.15 \text{ g}$$

The chloride content is contributed by the sodium chloride (95 mmol), calcium chloride (1.5 mmol) and magnesium chloride (0.75 mmol), i.e. a total content of 99.5 mmol of chloride. In addition, solutions for peritoneal dialysis are rendered slightly hypertonic by the inclusion of glucose. The concentration of glucose varies between 1.4 per cent and 7 per cent depending upon the rate at which it is required to remove water in the dialysis procedure. A typical formula for peritoneal dialysis solution is as follows:

Sodium chloride 5.56 g
Sodium acetate 4.76 g
Calcium chloride 0.33 g
Magnesium chloride 0.15 g
Glucose (anhydrous) 17 g
Water for Injection to 1 litre

Solutions for haemodialysis have a similar composition but are prepared in concentrated form and are diluted at the time of use in the artificial kidney machine. In addition they may contain a small concentration of potassium (up to 4 mmol per litre) since they are used over longer periods of time than peritoneal dialysis solutions and a dangerous hypokalaemia might be produced by potassium-free dialysis solutions. The concentration of glucose in haemodialysis solutions is usually one-tenth the concentration in peritoneal dialysis solutions.

Example: Calculate the quantities required for 1 litre of a 40× concentrated haemodialysis solution so that the final dilution contains 0.2 per cent glucose and the following ionic concentrations:

Sodium 130 mmol
Acetate 35 mmol
Chloride 100 mmol (approx)
Calcium 1.5 mmol
Magnesium 0.75 mmol
Potassium 1.3 mmol

Quantities required:

Sodium chloride

$$95 \text{ mmol} \times 40 = \frac{95 \times 58.44 \times 40}{1000}$$
$$= 222.4 \text{ g}$$

Sodium acetate

$$35 \text{ mmol} \times 40 = \frac{35 \times 136.1 \times 40}{1000}$$
$$= 190.4 \text{ g}$$

Calcium chloride ($CaCl_2$, $2H_2O$)

$$1.5 \text{ mmol} \times 40 = \frac{147 \times 1.5 \times 40}{1000}$$
$$= 8.8 \text{ g}$$

Magnesium chloride

$$0.75 \text{ mmol} \times 40 = \frac{203.3 \times 0.75 \times 40}{1000}$$
$$= 6.0 \text{ g}$$

Potassium chloride

$$1.3 \text{ mmol} \times 40 = \frac{74.56 \times 1.3 \times 40}{1000}$$
$$= 3.88 \text{ g}$$

Glucose monohydrate
$$0.2 \text{ per cent} \times 40 = 8 \text{ per cent}$$
$$= 80 \text{ g}$$

The formula of the $40\times$ concentrated haemo-dialysis solution, therefore, is as follows:

Sodium chloride 222.4 g
Sodium acetate 190.4 g
Calcium chloride 8.8 g
Magnesium chloride 6.0 g
Potassium chloride 3.88 g
Glucose monohydrate 80.0 g
Purified Water to 1 litre

REFERENCES

HADGRAFT, J. W. (1960) Preparations for water and electrolyte balance. *Pharm. J.* **184**, 277.

OWEN, J. A., EDWARDS, R. D. & COLLAR, B. A. W. (1970) *The Mole in Medicine*. Edinburgh and London: E. & S. Livingstone.

23

Prescriptions

Dispensing is that part of the practice of pharmacy in which the pharmacist or a pharmacy technician under his supervision interprets the doctor's requirements for the drug treatment of his patient. This usually takes the form of interpreting a written prescription but may, on occasion, involve taking instructions given by word of mouth or by telephone. Whenever the doctor does not state his requirements in a written form in the first instance, he should be asked to confirm his instructions in writing at a later stage. However the pharmacist receives the doctor's intentions, it is essential that every precaution is taken to eliminate mistakes, which may arise either in writing the prescription or in its interpretation, since it is at this stage that the patient is given a preparation which he will take in accordance with the directions stated by the pharmacist. It may often be necessary for the pharmacist to emphasize special instructions regarding the administration of the preparation in order to reinforce any directions that the doctor may have given to the patient. He should also be ready to advise the patient about other self-prescribed medication, for example, patients receiving anticoagulant therapy should be warned against taking preparations containing aspirin.

Modern drug treatment uses preparations that are frequently prepared by the manufacturer and which require no further manipulation in the pharmacy. Most modern drugs are available in tablets, capsules or injections which are supplied by the pharmaceutical industry. The process of dispensing has, therefore, become very much simplified, and whereas the pharmacist was formerly required to carry out manipulative processes in the preparation of medicines, he is less frequently called upon to do so nowadays. While the process of dispensing has been simplified, the nature of the drugs used has become considerably more sophisticated, and the potential for serious mistakes to occur in drug administration has become greater.

The development of new and potent drugs makes it even more important for the pharmacist to take the utmost care in the interpretation of prescriptions and to examine each prescription very carefully in order to avoid possible errors of interpretation which may arise because of inadequately or poorly written prescriptions. No preparation should be supplied to the patient until the pharmacist is fully satisfied that he has interpreted the doctor's intentions correctly.

The main procedures involved in dispensing are discussed here, and while they may not often be used in the general practice of pharmacy, it is essential for students to become thoroughly familiar with the principles underlying the procedures in order to develop the correct approach to dispensing. It is also of practical importance to those who will ultimately find themselves working in a hospital pharmacy where the opportunities for carrying out dispensing techniques arise more frequently and to those who wish to make a career in the pharmaceutical industry, since no new pharmaceutical preparations can be developed without, in the initial stages, using some of the basic procedures of dispensing that have been developed over the years.

An increasingly disturbing feature of modern life

is the abuse of drugs, particularly those acting on the central nervous system. The illicit use of such preparations has led to the forging of prescriptions, and it is part of the responsibility of the pharmacist to detect prescriptions which have been forged or altered by the patient. Prescription forms issued by the Ministry of Health, known as FC10 forms, have been stolen and used for writing forged prescriptions. Prescriptions legitimately written by a doctor may have the quantity of the preparation subsequently increased by the patient in order to obtain a larger quantity than that prescribed. Items not prescribed by the doctor may be inserted by the patient in forged handwriting. Wherever there is any doubt about such a prescription, it is the responsibility of the pharmacist to refer it back to the prescriber for confirmation. Particular care should be taken with prescriptions calling for drugs scheduled under the Misuse of Drugs Act (1971) or in the Fourth Schedule of the Pharmacy and Poisons Act (1933).

THE FORM OF THE PRESCRIPTION

Traditionally a prescription consisted of the following four parts.
1. The *superscription*, which is simply represented by the sign R. It has been stated that this sign was originally employed as the sign of Jupiter in the days when medicine was thought to be under astrological influence but there is considerable doubt as to the validity of such a contention. It is now used as an abbreviation of the Latin word *recipe*, take. Similarly, French prescriptions have the superscription P, an abbreviation of *prenez*.
2. The *inscription*, which is the general body of the prescription; it comprises a list of the ingredients and the quantity of each to be used or supplied.
3. The *subscription*, or directions to the dispenser.
4. The *signature*, or the directions to the patient as to how the medicine is to be used, including, in the case of internal medicines, the size and frequency of the dose.

THE LANGUAGE OF PRESCRIPTION WRITING

Alongside the simplification of dispensing there has been a parallel simplification in the language of prescription writing. Nowadays, prescriptions are frequently written in English and medical students are taught to write prescriptions in English. There are, however, a number of Latin terms and phrases which have been traditionally used and which continue to find a place in prescription writing. Pharmaceutical students must familiarize themselves with the more commonly used Latin terms

and abbreviations since they may encounter these in the course of their professional work, particularly in prescriptions written some years ago.

While the British and United States *Pharmacopoeias* have adopted the use of English, the International and European *Pharmacopoeias* continue to use Latin nomenclature for the preparations included. The arguments which have been advanced for the continued use of Latin are as follows:
1. It is understood by pharmacists in all countries.
2. Pharmaceutical Latin names are very similar in all countries. In the case of potent substances, the Latin names in the various *Pharmacopoeias* are often identical.
3. Abbreviated Latin forms a handy shorthand for the busy practitioner.
4. It may be advisable that the patient should not learn the nature of the remedies prescribed for him.

These arguments become increasingly less valid as each year passes and English is likely to become universally used for prescription writing in this country.

DISPENSING ROUTINE

A strict routine is necessary in dispensing in order to ensure safety, speed and neatness. The following general rules apply whether the prescription involves extemporaneous preparation of the medicine or simply the issue of a manufactured product of the pharmaceutical industry.

When receiving a prescription to dispense, the following routine should be followed:
1. Read it carefully. Do not express doubt about it either to the patient or his messenger in terms which question the wisdom of the prescriber. However, it may be necessary, on occasions, to question the patient in order to determine the true intentions of the prescriber. Never feel reticent about asking the advice of a colleague. If for any reason (e.g. the preparation is not in stock) you are unable to dispense the prescription, return it to the patient and advise him how he may best obtain his medicine with the least delay.

Dispense a prescription as soon as possible after it is received. If it involves time in preparation or other prescriptions are awaiting your attention, give the patient a realistic time when he will be able to collect his medicine.
2. Note the dose. If the prescription is for an infant or child, note the age of the patient. Never proceed with the dispensing if you are doubtful about the dose. An easy and interesting method of acquiring

a sound knowledge of posology is to look up the doses of any new drug you encounter in the course of dispensing. Even though the prescription may be for a standard routine dose, you will often find that drugs are given in other less commonly used doses for special purposes.

If you consider the dose to be dangerous or unusual, do not hesitate to consult the prescriber. If this is not possible and you feel confident there has been an error, dispense the normal dose (i.e. within the limits given in the *British Pharmacopoeia, British Pharmaceutical Codex* or *British National Formulary*). This course of action should only be taken in exceptional circumstances. Doses that are underlined, expressed in words as well as figures or individually initialled by the prescriber should be dispensed as written.

Particular attention should be paid to prescriptions for children. The age of the child should be stated on the prescription and this should be noted and taken into account in determining the appropriateness of the dose.

3. If the prescription is a private one, copy it in the prescription book or file. Give it a number and make sure the patient's name and address are recorded.

4. Private prescriptions should be priced according to a definite system which should always be used.

5. Mark the prescription with a rubber stamp to indicate that it has been dispensed. The number assigned to a private prescription should be written in the vacant space of the prescription stamp.

6. Write the label before dispensing the prescription. This is a procedure which serves to prevent the dispensing of an excessive dose since it draws attention not merely to the strength of the preparation to be supplied but also to the actual amount that the patient is to take at a time. As stated above, especial care should be taken in labelling medicines intended for children or infants.

The label should be typewritten if possible but if handwritten it must be neat and legible. Write the patient's name on the lower right-hand corner of the label or in the appropriate space if one is provided.

Nomen proprium labelling is an old Latin instruction which literally means the proper name of the preparation. It is now usually abbreviated to N.P. and means that the name and strength of the preparation should be written on the label.

N.P. labelling is now common practice and National Health prescription forms (FC10) have the letters N.P. printed in a box. If the doctor has not cancelled the letters it means that he intends

the name and strength of the preparation to be written on the label. In general practice pharmacy, the name of the preparation as written on the prescription is used on the label, e.g. if the doctor uses a proprietary name on the prescription, this is the preparation supplied and this is the name which should be used on the label. In hospital pharmacy, there is often a general policy that only official names should be used, where available, even though the prescription involves the supply of a proprietary product.

However, care should be taken in the use of official names in circumstances where the biological availability of the drug differs with different manufacturers. This is of especial importance in the case of digoxin tablets and in such instances the brand name of the preparation supplied or the manufacturer's name should be stated on the label of the dispensed medicine.

The practice of disclosing the name and strength on the label of a dispensed medicine has been adopted by the medical and pharmaceutical professions in recent years in the interests of safety. It should, however, be remembered that such disclosure is not always desirable and should only be made if the prescription indicates that it is the doctor's intention. Disclosure of the names of drugs to patients can in some circumstances cause unnecessary anxiety and distress. Caution should also be exercised in accepting the evidence of the nature of a preparation from the labelled name since patients not infrequently transfer drug preparations from one container to another.

Labels on dispensed medicines customarily carry a warning that they should be kept in a safe place out of the reach of young children. They should also carry any other special storage instructions and an expiry date where appropriate.

7. Use a new, clean container for each occasion on which a prescription is dispensed. This rule should also be followed when stocks of drugs are issued for use in hospital wards.

When dispensing:

(i) Have the prescription always before you. If it is necessary to go to a distant part of the dispensary, take the prescription with you since it will serve as a constant reminder of the name and strength of the preparation required and help to avoid mistakes.

(ii) If the preparation of the medicine involves weighing, test the dispensing scales before beginning to weigh the ingredients.

(iii) Replace containers of stock preparations or drugs in their proper position after use.

(iv) Keep the label uppermost when weighing solid ingredients (especially potent drugs such as morphine hydrochloride) to serve as a constant reminder that the correct drug is being used.

(v) When pouring or measuring liquid ingredients, keep the label uppermost to prevent surplus liquid running down the outside of the bottle and staining the label.

(vi) Care must be taken to keep dispensing scales clean and powder should be transferred from the stock container using a clean spatula. Particular attention should be paid to cleaning the scale pan immediately after use.

(vii) Medicines which are to be used externally (e.g. lotions, liniments, etc.) should be supplied in bottles which are vertically fluted or ribbed so as to be distinguishable by touch. Some proprietary preparations for external use are supplied in plastic containers. These are satisfactory provided they are clearly distinguishable from containers normally used for dispensing medicines to be taken internally.

Medicines to be used externally must be labelled in red or against a red background,

> For External Use Only

(viii) Before the medicine is handed to the patient, again check that the correct preparation in the correct strength has been supplied and the correct directions have been stated on the label. Accuracy in dispensing is dependent on self discipline.

HOSPITAL PRESCRIPTIONS

The principles underlying the dispensing of prescriptions for out-patients in hospital are essentially the same as those in general practice pharmacy. The main difference in the form of the prescription in hospitals is that generally the length of time of the treatment is specified rather than the actual quantity of the medicine to be supplied.

In hospitals there may also be an agreement between the pharmacist and the medical staff regarding the supply of proprietary brands of drugs. Despite the use of different proprietary names, it may have been agreed that one particular make of a drug is to be supplied unless the prescriber indicates that the proprietary brand specified is needed.

The supply of drugs to in-patients in hospitals has taken different forms and given rise to new approaches to dispensing. Traditionally prescriptions have been written on in-patient sheets which are sent to the pharmacy for dispensing. The medicines are either dispensed for the individual treatment of the patient or, in the case of commonly used preparations, a stock bottle is issued from which the nursing staff can take the individual doses for each of the patients requiring that particular preparation. The nursing routine for drug administration varies in different hospitals, but in some, the prescriptions were formerly transcribed on to a Drug Treatment Sheet by the nursing staff, and the ward medicine round conducted from this record.

Although this practice has been largely abandoned, retrospective surveys by Vere (1965) and Hill and Wigmore (1967) showed that when the details of drugs administered (including dose, time of administration, etc.) were checked against the original prescriptions, the frequency with which errors occurred was as high as 18 per cent. Many of these were minor in character (e.g. wrong time of administration) but, nevertheless, a system which involves such a high level of error is undesirable.

In some hospitals, particularly in Scotland, it has been found that more effective control by the pharmacist can be achieved and the errors reduced by a system of ward stocks and the utilization of a specially designed prescription sheet which also incorporates a record of drug administration. An integral feature of this system is that the pharmacist regularly visits the wards, inspects the prescriptions, discusses any problems with the medical and nursing staff and issues instructions to the pharmacy department to ensure that the wards are carrying adequate stocks to meet the demands of the prescriptions. Close pharmaceutical control is necessary if the ward stocks of drugs are not allowed to grow to unmanageable proportions and a regular turnover of the stock is to be maintained. The advantages claimed for such a system is that it brings the pharmacist into active contact with the treatment of the patient on the ward and offers him a better opportunity of influencing decisions on prescribing.

An alternative approach is to reduce the level of stocks of drugs on the wards to a minimum. The whole of the drug treatment sheets for the ward are brought to the pharmacy at pre-arranged times and the drugs are issued for each individual patient at weekly intervals. The drugs are kept separately, in individual trays reserved solely for each patient. The trays are stored in a specially designed medicine trolley which can be wheeled to each patient's bedside in turn during a medicine round. This system can also be operated in association with a specially designed prescription and drug administration sheet. The advantage of the ward trolley system is that it ensures that the pharmacist sees every prescription in its original form and there is no reason why it cannot be operated in association with regular ward visits by the pharmacist. There is a trend in the USA towards the issue of medicines in unit doses (i.e. one dose at a time) and this could follow as a logical development of the ward trolley system.

Small hospitals in remote rural areas may not have the services of a full time pharmacist. Such institutions present special problems for the issue and administration of medicines. The introduction, development and evaluation of a system for prescribing, administration and distribution of drugs in small hospitals was the subject of a special investigation carried out by Shirley Ellis (1972).

Economy in the Use of Drugs in Hospitals
The pharmacist has an important part to play in helping to secure the economic use of drugs in hospital practice. In association with the treasurer, he can prepare quarterly analyses of the money spent on drugs, breaking down the expenditure into different pharmacological groups, e.g. antibiotics, corticosteroids, etc. By this means, the medical staff can be constantly reminded of the level of expenditure and their attention drawn to particular items on which large sums of money have been spent. Hospital regions or areas also have pharmaceutical advisory committees, which not only ensure economic purchasing by arranging contracts but can also issue information on the cost of drugs for circulation to the medical and nursing staff. Apart from his daily contact with doctors, the pharmacist is also able to influence prescribing by participating in a pharmaceutical sub-committee of the medical advisory committee of his hospital.

REFERENCES

VERE, D. W. (1968) *Lancet* **1**, 370.

HILL, P. A. & WIGMORE, H. W. (1967) *Lancet* **1**, 671.

CROOKS, J., CLARKE, C. G., CAIE, H. B. & MANSON, W. B. (1965) *Lancet* **1**, 373.

ELLIS, S. (1972) Control of drugs in small hospitals. The West Cornwall system. King's Fund Hospital Centre Paper.

24

Oral Preparations

Drugs may be administered by a variety of routes but oral administration is adopted wherever possible. It is the safest, easiest and most economical route of drug administration. There are, however, limitations to the use of the oral route. It is obviously unsatisfactory for substances such as insulin and adrenaline which are inactivated or destroyed by the secretions of the gastrointestinal tract. Other substances, although not destroyed, may not be adequately absorbed from the alimentary tract and if required to produce a systematic effect must be administered by other routes. Such drugs may nevertheless be given by mouth to obtain a localized action in the large intestine and bowel. For example, neomycin and the less soluble sulphonamides are administered orally in the treatment of gastrointestinal infections or to reduce the bacterial flora prior to surgery of the bowel.

Another limitation to oral administration is the fact that some drugs irritate the gastric or intestinal mucosa, but this may be minimized by giving the drug after food. Enteric coating may be applied to tablets or capsules to prevent gastric irritation and some drugs, e.g. phenylbutazone and indomethacin, may be administered rectally as an alternative to the oral route.

SOLID PREPARATIONS

For oral administration there is a choice between solid and liquid medicines. Solid forms of drug presentation include powders, cachets, tablets and capsules.

The most commonly used oral preparations, nowadays, are tablets and capsules. Generally speaking, they are more stable and less prone to microbiological contamination than extemporaneously dispensed liquid medicines. However, liquid preparations have advantages for administering drugs to children and patients who have difficulty in swallowing solid preparations.

POWDERS

Drugs administered in powdered form are immediately available for absorption. However, the absorption of substances which are only poorly soluble may be affected by the particle size of the drug. The clinical aspects of the fineness of particles in pharmaceutical practice were discussed by Lees (1963). He gave a number of examples of drugs, of which the gastrointestinal absorption is affected by particle size, including the corticosteroids, sulphonamides and griseofulvin. The absorbability of the latter drug is directly related to the logarithm of the specific surface. The efficacy of other drugs acting locally in the gut may be enhanced by reduction of particle size. In veterinary medicine, the anthelmintic activity of phenothiazine has been shown to be related to particle size.

Dispensing of Powders

Powders may be ordered to be individually wrapped in single doses or in bulk. Individually wrapped powders are used for potent drugs and wherever it is necessary to ensure accurate measurement of the dose. They may be either simple (containing only one active ingredient) or compound (containing more than one active ingredient). Individually wrapped powders provide a useful method of drug presentation if the required dose is not available as a standard tablet or capsule.

Powders are administered by placing the contents of one powder paper on the tongue and swallowing with a drink of water. For administration to children, powders are sometimes mixed with jam, treacle or honey. If the drug is likely to be adversely affected by acids, the responsible person should be warned against the use of jam.

Simple Individually Wrapped Powders
Powders are wrapped in white glazed paper, cut to a suitable size, depending upon the bulk of powder contained in a single dose. Machine or guillotine-cut paper is preferable.

Select a number of papers corresponding to the number of powders ordered and of a suitable size. Turn up one of the longer edges of each paper about half an inch and place the papers in a convenient position on the dispensing bench so that each slightly overlaps the next.

Weigh out the total quantity of powdered drug to be dispensed and replace the bottle. If the drug is caked or lumpy, reduce it to a powder by grinding in a mortar. When six or more powders are to be sent, it is advisable to weigh a total quantity corresponding to one more than is required, because during the weighing there may be slight losses due to powder adhering to the knife or scale pan. Place the total quantity of powder on a large sheet of paper and weigh from this. The latter procedure prevents too many or too few powders being sent and is a check on the weighing.

Wrap the powders so that they are of a size that will fit loosely in the box (a white glazed, slide or hinge-lid box is generally used). Bend the far border over until it is about half an inch from the near border (Fig. 24.1). Turn the margin upwards with the thumb and bend over to form a flap. Fold the flap loosely over on itself to an extent which makes the packet slightly narrower than the interior of the box. Hold the packet over the drawer section of the box and turn the ends down lightly over the ends of the drawer so as to form a slight crease that will act as a guide to the length of the finished powder. Bend each end in turn sharply over a powder knife, holding the knife about 3 mm inwards from the creases made by the ends of the box. Finally, place the folded packet on a sheet of white paper, cover it with another sheet of paper and pass a knife over the upper sheet. This last procedure distributes the

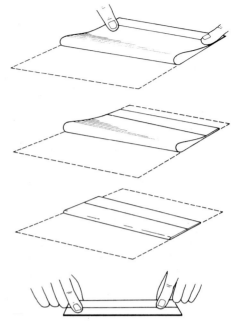

FIG. 24. 1. Wrapping a powder.

powder evenly within the packet and prevents the escape of powder through the folds.

When all the powders have been wrapped, arrange them in pairs, flaps to flaps and encircle the stack with an elastic band before placing them in the box.

Crystalline substances or substances in large or small lumps must be reduced to a fine powder to facilitate administration and hasten solution after administration.

Potent crystalline substances should be powdered in a glass mortar, preferably placed on a black surface. Wedgewood ware or composition mortars are liable to absorb potent drugs to some extent. Iodine is absorbed by composition mortars and stains them badly.

Hygroscopic substances must be powdered and weighed as rapidly as possible, avoiding undue exposure to moisture.

Powders of hygroscopic substances should be doubly wrapped, the inner wrap consisting of waxed paper to protect the powder from moisture.

Volatile substances must also be doubly wrapped in the same manner.

Triturations
A trituration is the term applied to a mixture or dilution of a potent substance with an inert one. Small quantities of finely powdered solids may be mixed on a sheet of white paper by means of a

powder knife or spatula. A mortar should be used when the quantities are too large to be conveniently dealt with on paper. The invariable rule is to add a little of the substance present in greater amount to the whole of the substance present in lesser amount (usually the more potent substance), and mix intimately; the remainder of the substance present in greater amount is then introduced into the mixture in very small quantities at first, but gradually increasing the quantities, until the whole has been added. It is impossible to ensure intimate dispersion of one powder in another by mixing the two substances all at once.

Powders weighing less than 100 mg must be made up to 100 mg by adding an appropriate quantity of lactose.

Consider the following prescription:

R Cortisone acetate 15 mg
 Send 10 powders
Total quantity of cortisone acetate = 10×15 = 150 mg
Add 850 mg of lactose = 1 g total.
 Weight 10×100 mg powders

Small doses of potent substances must not be weighed on ordinary dispensing scales.

Substances having a maximal dose of less than 60 mg should be regarded as potent substances. *These should be weighed either on a chemical balance or upon a delicate pair of dispensing scales specially reserved for the purpose.* In no case should a quantity less than 50 mg be actually weighed. It may happen, of course, that a quantity of potent substance less than 50 mg in weight is to be dispensed and the required amount should be obtained by the method described below.

The general procedure is as follows:

Weigh 100 mg; gradually incorporate a convenient weighed quantity of lactose with this; then weigh a portion of the mixture that will contain the desired weight of the potent substance.

Examples

(1) R Prednisone 8 mg
 Send 4 powders
Method. Weigh 100 mg of prednisone; mix on paper with 900 mg of lactose = 1 g total. 320 mg of this mixture will contain 32 mg of prednisone. Mix this quantity with 80 mg of lactose and divide into 4 powders each weighing 100 mg.

(2) R Pentobarbitone sodium 15 mg
 Send 2 powders
Method. Total required = $2 \times 15 = 30$ mg. Weigh 60 mg of pentobarbitone sodium; mix on paper with 60 mg of lactose = 120 mg total. 60 mg of this mixture will contain 30 mg of pentobarbitone sodium. Mix this quantity with 140 mg of lactose and divide into 2 powders each weighing 100 mg.

Compound Powders in Doses

These are powders containing more than one active ingredient. Small quantities may be mixed on paper by means of a spatula or with a pestle and mortar. Any ingredients that are not finely sub-divided should be reduced to powder form separately before being mixed.

In mixing compound powders it is essential to follow the general rule of gradually incorporating the ingredient present in greatest amount with the whole of the ingredient present in least amount, any other ingredients then being introduced in turn a little at a time. When using a pestle and mortar for mixing, trituration should be light; heavy trituration or grinding tends to make powders denser and less diffusible in fluids. Only hard, crystalline substances require heavy grinding. Caution should be exercised in handling mixtures of oxidizing and reducing agents in a mortar and pestle as an explosion may occur. If it is necessary to mix such substances, they should be powdered separately and then mixed very lightly on paper.

Sifting. Compound powders containing vegetable substances often require sifting to break up small masses of cohering particles. A no. 44 or no. 60 sieve should be chosen and the mixed powder brushed through or rubbed through with a spatula. Various mixers and sifters are obtainable for small quantities.

After sifting, all powders must again be lightly mixed, as there is sometimes a tendency for the ingredients to be separated by the sieve.

Fractional quantities. In some cases it may happen that after all the ingredients have been mixed an awkward fraction is obtained when the total weight is divided by the number of powders to be sent. This difficulty is easily overcome by adding a small quantity of lactose to bring the weight of each powder to a convenient figure. If the total weight of the ingredients is 3.7 g and this is to be divided into 10 powders, it would be advisable to incorporate 0.3 g of lactose (= 4 g total) and divide into 10×0.4 g powders.

Lactose intolerance. It should be noted that there is a rare condition in children which makes them intolerant to lactose. In such cases, an alternative inert diluent must be used (e.g. starch powder).

Powders in Bulk

Sometimes, when the dose is not critical, powders may be ordered in bulk. Often powders of this kind are for use as antacids, e.g. Magnesium Trisilicate Powder, Compound BPC. The quantities are usually so large that it is necessary to use a mortar in mixing, even though the ingredients may be already in fine powder. They should be sent out in *perfectly dry*, wide mouthed, glass bottles with plastic screw caps or other suitable closure. If any of the ingredients are deliquescent or volatile, an airtight container should be used.

CACHETS

Powders can be enclosed in small containers made of rice flour and water, known as cachets. They are available in various sizes holding from 0.2 to 1.5 g of powder. Such preparations have advantages for the administration of nauseating drugs given in large doses. The cachet prevents the patient from tasting the powder and a larger dose can be enclosed in a cachet than in a tablet or a capsule. Sodium aminosalicylate, which is given in a dose of 12 g daily in the treatment of tuberculosis, is commonly prescribed in cachets.

Before administration, a cachet should be immersed in water for a few seconds and then placed on the tongue and swallowed with a draught of water. In this way the outer shell of the cachet is softened, but it retains the enclosed powders long enough for the whole to be swallowed without permitting the powder to come into contact with the palate. After being swallowed, the cachet disintegrates and the powder is liberated.

There are two kinds of cachet; 'wet seal' cachets which are sealed by moistening the edges with water, and 'dry seal' cachets which, as the name implies, require no moisture for sealing.

Wet seal cachets. A wet seal cachet is composed of two similar concave halves, having flat edges (see Fig. 24.2). The weighed powder is deposited into one half, the edges of the other half are moistened with water, inverted over the first half and the flat edges pressed together so that they adhere and enclose the powder.

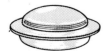 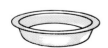

FIG. 24.2. Cachets.

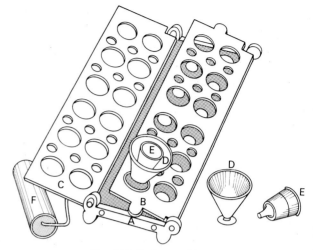

FIG. 24.3. Cachet machine.

Wet seal cachet machine. This consists of three metal plates (Fig. 24.3), the two outermost plates being attached by hinges to the centre one. The halves of the cachets in which the powder is to be inserted are placed in holes in the centre plate, A, where they fit loosely. One of the other plates, B, is then swung over and placed on top of the cachets. This second plate also has holes, which are congruent with the holes in the first plate, and its object is to protect the edges of the cachets while they are being filled. A funnel, D, of the correct size, supplied with the machine, is next placed in each hole of the second plate in turn, and the powder introduced. The powder is pressed down with a small wooden plunger or metal thimble, E, also supplied with the machine.

When the lower halves have been filled, the second plate is folded back. The top halves of the cachets are then placed in the holes of the third plate, C, on the opposite side of the centre plate. The holes in C are somewhat smaller than those of the centre plate, so that the tops of the cachets fit tightly. The edges of the top halves are then moistened with a roller, F, the plate is swung over and pressed down firmly on the centre plate. The top halves of the cachets are thus brought exactly over the lower halves and the edges made to adhere. The upper plate is now lifted, when it brings with it the completed cachets. The finished cachets are finally pushed out gently and boxed.

The amount of moisture used is very important and somewhat difficult to judge correctly. Too much causes the edges to crinkle and become discoloured; too little may produce an imperfect seal and allow the powder to escape at some point on the circumference, or cause the two halves to fall apart completely after the patient has received the cachets.

Dry seal cachets. Dry seal cachets consist of two halves, the upper half fitting over the lower half like the lid on a box (Fig. 24.4). The backs of both

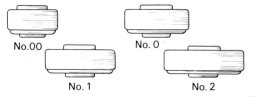

FIG. 24.4. Dry-closing (Secca) cachets.

lower and upper halves have small projections which fit into the holes of the plates of the machine. Since the projections are the same size on all the sizes of cachets, only one machine is required for the whole range of sizes. The lower halves are fitted into the lower plate (Fig. 24.5) of the machine and filled. The upper halves are fitted into the upper plate, D, which is pressed down on the lower one, when the upper halves or 'lids' fit exactly over the lower halves. These cachets are much more substantial than the ordinary type, and there is no likelihood of the powder escaping. They can be prepared more quickly and are more hygienic.

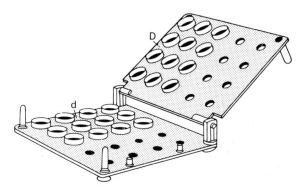

FIG. 24.5. Dry-closing machine (cacheteur Secca).

Dispensing cachets. Cachets are dispensed in boxes or tins in which they are packed on their edges or lying flat. Some manufactured cachets are packed in plastic sleeves, each holding a day's treatment. Cachets should be labelled with directions for administration, e.g. 'Immerse in water for a few seconds and then swallow with water'.

Automatic and semi-automatic cachet machines. The widespread use of cachets for the administra-

tion of sodium aminosalicylate has stimulated the industrial production of cachets in this country. Both dry and wet seal cachets may be filled and sealed by automatic (machine-fed) or semi-automatic (hand-fed) machines. Fig. 24.6 shows an automatic machine in which the adjustable four-punch dosing mechanism delivers a plug of compressed powder to the lower half of the cachet and to this the upper half (automatically moistened if wet sealed) is applied. To achieve consistent dosage from such machines it is essential that the bulk density, particle size and flow characteristics of the powder or blend of powders is accurately controlled.

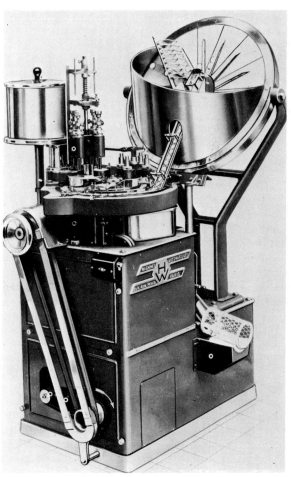

FIG. 24.6. Automatic cachet machine (Smith & Nephew Ltd.).

CAPSULES

Capsules consist of a medicament enclosed in a shell of gelatin; methylcellulose has been used but is no longer recognized by the *British Pharmacopoeia* as a shell material. The shell is soluble in water at 37° and after the capsule has been swallowed, it dissolves and releases the medicament allowing it to be absorbed. However, the mucilaginous coating which forms around the drug as the capsule dissolves may delay absorption, so that its onset of action may be delayed. With very soluble drugs this may not be an important factor, but is more important when the drug is only very sparingly soluble.

The manufacture of hard gelatin and flexible gelatin capsules is described in Chapter 19. Small quantities of hard gelatin capsules may be extemporaneously dispensed by hand-filling.

Hard Capsules

Hard gelatin capsules are available in a range of sizes to hold varying doses of powdered drugs. They are formed of two cylindrical halves, one slightly larger but shorter in length than the other. The medicament is inserted in the longer narrower half, then the other half is fitted over the open end as a cap, held in place by moistening the edges.

Hand filling hard capsules. The smallest size capsule should be selected that will hold the quantity of medicament prescribed.

The lower halves of the capsules may be supported in the holes of a suppository mould or in a block of wood in which holes of a suitable size have been bored. The powders are prepared in the usual way and are poured into each capsule. This operation is facilitated by the use of a small glass or aluminium funnel and a thin wooden plunger that will pass down the stem of the funnel and prevent it from becoming clogged with powder. The outer edges of the lower halves of the capsules are then moistened with water, using a camel hair brush, and finally the caps are pressed on. This forms a seal which prevents the powder from leaking out of the capsules.

Enteric Coated Capsules

Enteric coating is applied to gelatin capsules when they are intended to pass through the stomach and release their contents in the small intestine. A 10 per cent solution of cellacephate (cellulose acetate phthalate) in acetone may be used for this purpose. The capsules are dipped in the solution, removed by means of tweezers and allowed to dry on a sieve. It is usually necessary to apply three coats.

Containers for capsules. Capsules are dispensed in small glass screw-cap tablet bottles or in suitable plastic containers. They should be protected from moisture.

Small scale manufacture of capsules. In hospital practice a hand-operated capsule filling machine may be found useful for the preparation of capsules, particularly special formulations required in the clinical trial of new drugs. The Tevopharm machine (see Fig. 24.7) is suitable for such purposes, and is essentially a device for locating the capsules into two plates which can be brought together to effect closure. Plates are available to accommodate the different sizes of empty capsules and each plate holds 60 capsules. A sorting device is used to drop the capsules, bottom downwards into the holes in the filling plates. The capsules are pushed firmly into the holes and the lower plate is then fixed by the screw on the front. The upper plate is removed, taking with it the tops of the capsules. The lower halves of the capsules are then pushed flush with the lower plate and are gravity filled with the powdered drug. If the dose required cannot be obtained by filling one of the standard capsule sizes, a triturate in lactose must be prepared. After filling the capsules, the top plate is replaced and the lever at the side of the machine operated to engage the rods under the base plate, pushing the bottoms of the capsules upwards at the same time as pressure is applied at the top to force the two halves of the capsules together. The bottom plate is again fixed and the top plate is removed bringing away the filled capsules.

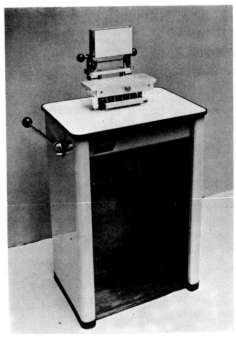

FIG. 24.7. Tevopharm capsule filling machine (Anglo-Continental Machines Ltd.).

LIQUID PREPARATIONS

Drugs administered in aqueous solution or suspension are presented to the gastrointestinal mucosa in a form that is immediately available for absorption. Liquid medicines are, however, generally less stable than solid forms of drug presentation, although, non-aqueous vehicles may be used for drugs which deteriorate in the presence of moisture. Nauseous drugs and those which are irritant to the gastric mucosa are usually unsuitable for presentation in liquid formulations unless well diluted.

MIXTURES

Mixtures are liquid medicines which the patient divides into doses; he may, or may not be directed to dilute each dose before taking. *A draught* is a liquid medicine consisting of one dose only. *A linctus* is a preparation intended for the treatment of a cough and is rendered viscous by the inclusion of glycerin or syrup; it should be administered undiluted in order to obtain the lubricant effect of the vehicle.

The *British Pharmaceutical Codex* 1973 gives the following metric dose volumes for liquid preparations: for linctuses and elixirs, 5 ml; for adult mixtures, 10 ml, or multiples thereof; and for draughts, 50 ml.

Metric medicine bottles. Mixtures are dispensed in clear glass bottles which comply with British Standard No. 1679/6. The following range of sizes of metric bottles are available: 50, 100, 150, 200, 300 and 500 ml.

If the mixture consists of a simple solution in water, it can be adjusted to volume in a measure before being transferred to the bottle. If the mixture contains an insoluble powder or is viscous, the bottle should be calibrated to the correct volume and the final adjustment to volume made in the bottle. This procedure enables the whole of the insoluble powder or a viscous liquid to be transferred to the final container.

Labelling. The dose should be stated in terms of the metric medicine spoon (B.S. 3221/4). This has a capacity of 5 ml and in the case of medicines having a 5 ml dose-volume the label should read, 'One 5-ml spoonful to be taken . . .'. In the case of medicines having larger dose volumes, the dose should be stated in units of the 5 ml medicine spoon, e.g. for a 10 ml dose volume, the label should read, 'Two 5-ml spoonfuls . . .'.

For the medicines which are still prescribed in the apothecary system of weights and measures, the prescription must be transcribed into the metric system (see below) and the doses stated in terms of the metric medicine spoon. The use of domestic teaspoons and tablespoons should be abandoned for measuring medicines.

A plastic medicine spoon should be supplied with each bottle of mixture dispensed.

Mixtures containing an insoluble deposit should always be labelled with the direction, 'Shake the Bottle'.

The *British Pharmaceutical Codex* 1973 gives the following directions for labelling mixtures issued on a medical prescription or for an individual patient:
(1) The prescriber's directions
(2) Any special storage conditions
(3) For suspensions, a direction to shake the bottle
(4) A date after which the mixture should not be used if a recommendation is made by the manufacturer, or if a mixture is diluted before issue.

The requirement to state a date after which the mixture should not be used applies to mixtures containing unstable ingredients. For example, elixir of phenoxymethylpenicillin prepared from granules which have been ready made by an industrial manufacturer. The granules are stable if stored in a cool place, but once the elixir has been prepared by the addition of water, it must be stored in a cool place and used within 7 days.

Tap water is bacteriologically controlled and is free from pathogenic organisms. Purified water, on storage, can become heavily contaminated with microorganisms. Purified water prepared in a deionizer is particularly liable to be contaminated if the water is allowed to stagnate in the resin bed. Purified water, prepared by distillation, should not be stored in large volume tanks or containers which permit it to become contaminated. Polythene tubes and containers may become contaminated and form a reservoir of infection which will proliferate and build up a heavy infection in stored water.

Medicinal waters. Medicinal waters such as peppermint water and cinnamon water are used as flavouring agents and carminatives. Chloroform water is used for its sweet taste and also possesses excellent preservative properties (see Chapter 36).

Infusions. Fresh infusions are no longer used. They are now prepared by diluting concentrated infusions which are 10 times the strength of the original infusions (see Chapter 11).

Suspending Agents

Many insoluble substances, when shaken up, will remain suspended sufficiently long for a dose to be measured without the use of a suspending agent, but others will not and these require the use of a suspending agent. When no suspending agent is ordered by the prescriber, the pharmacist must use his judgement as to whether it is necessary to include one.

The following are the most commonly used suspending agents:

Compound Tragacanth Powder, BP. This is a mixture of powdered tragacanth, powdered acacia, starch and sucrose. It is used in quantities of 25 to 200 mg for each 10 ml of mixture. It is only in exceptional cases that more than 100 mg for each 10 ml is required.

The powder is mixed in a mortar with the substance to be suspended, and the vehicle added gradually with trituration.

Tragacanth Mucilage, BPC. This is employed in quantities up to 1 ml for each 10 ml of mixture, depending on the weight of insoluble matter to be suspended.

Sodium Carboxymethylcellulose BPC. This is available in various viscosity grades, depending upon the degree of polymerization. A medium viscosity grade is preferable for suspending powders in mixtures and is used in a concentration of 0.25 to 1 per cent. It is incorporated in the same manner as compound tragacanth powder.

Powdered tragacanth. This is less satisfactory as a suspending agent since it is liable to coagulate into unmanageable lumps unless it is mixed very intimately with an insoluble powder before addition of the vehicle. If it is prescribed in combination with an alcoholic liquid, tragacanth can be made into a mucilage by adding it to the alcoholic liquid in a dry bottle, adding a large quantity of the aqueous vehicle all at once and shaking vigorously.

Liquids in Mixtures

Measurement of volume. The errors involved in measuring volumes of liquids are discussed by Capper and Dare in their report, *Dispensing Tolerances in Liquid Medicines* (1957). Government stamped metric measures complying with British Standard 1922: 1953 should be used for dispensing purposes.

Measures are graduated to contain and not to deliver. Consequently after the volume of a liquid has been measured, the measure should be rinsed out with some of the vehicle and the rinsings added to the mixture before adjusting to volume. To measure volume correctly, the bottom of the meniscus should be in line with the graduation on the measure and this should be aligned with the sighting mark on the back of the measure.

If a viscous liquid is to be incorporated in a mixture, it should be measured, and then diluted in the measure with some of the vehicle, and mixed with a glass rod before transferring it from the measure. The measure should be finally rinsed with some more of the vehicle. However, glycerin or syrup if combined with an insoluble substance, should not be too much diluted in the measure; if added to the powder in a mortar, they assist in producing a paste free from lumps and this can then be diluted with the vehicle to produce a uniform suspension.

Volatile liquids, such as compound spirit of orange, should always be added last to avoid loss of the volatile ingredients.

Soluble Solids in Mixtures

If there is sufficient water present to dissolve the substance completely, a solution can be prepared in a measure with the aid of a stirring rod. The solution should be filtered through sintered glass and the filter washed through with more of the water before making up to volume.

Large crystals such as those of ferrous sulphate should be powdered and dissolved in a mortar. Scale preparations, such as iron and ammonium citrate, dissolve more readily if they are added to water in a measure, small portions at a time with constant stirring.

Stock solutions. For convenience in dispensing, solutions of stable soluble salts may be kept ready prepared. However, solutions of some salts may become heavily contaminated with bacteria and fungi if stored for more than a few days.

The use of heat. Some substances dissolve only slowly and the rate of solution may be increased by the use of hot water. Care must be taken to ensure that there is sufficient water present in the mixture to keep the substance permanently in solution; and solution should be allowed to cool to room temperature before the final adjustment to volume. If the substance is present in excess of its solubility, the excess will crystallize out when the solution cools and probably form a mass of crystals at the bottom of the bottle. The method for dealing with substances present in excess of their solubility is described below.

Hot water should not be used for substances decomposed at only moderate temperatures e.g. bicarbonates. It should also not be used if volatile ingredients are present.

Substances present in excess of their solubility. The substance is powdered as finely as possible in a mortar and triturated with some of the cold vehicle. The suspension is then transferred to a previously calibrated bottle and the mortar rinsed with further quantities of the cold vehicle, the rinsings being added to the contents of the bottle. The mixture is labelled 'Shake the Bottle'.

Small doses of potent substances. The smallest quantity which can be weighed on a dispensing balance is 50 mg and it may sometimes be necessary to make a liquid triturate in order to obtain the required quantity.

Example
    Hyoscine hydrobromide 0.5 mg
    Chloroform water to 5 ml
    Send 100 ml

Hyoscine hydrobromide is freely soluble in water. The required quantity is $0.5 \times 20 = 10$ mg. Weigh 50 mg; dissolve in 100 ml of chloroform water. Take 20 ml of this solution and dilute with chloroform water to 100 ml.

Insoluble Solids
Diffusible insoluble substances. The general procedure is to reduce the substance to a fine powder in a mortar. The powder is then triturated to a smooth cream with a small amount of the vehicle and this is then diluted by gradually adding about two-thirds of the vehicle required. The suspension is then transferred to a measure or calibrated bottle and the mixture is made up to volume with the remainder of the vehicle, washing out the mortar with successive small portions and adding to the bulk of the preparation. If syrup or glycerin is present in the mixture, it is diluted with a small portion of the vehicle and used to form the primary smooth cream.

This method can be applied to mixtures containing vegetable powders and diffusible solid drugs such as magnesium carbonate, magnesium trisilicate, light kaolin, etc.

Soluble substances with insoluble solids. The soluble substance can sometimes be mixed with the insoluble powder in a mortar before adding the vehicle. However it is usually preferable to dissolve the soluble ingredient separately and use the solution to triturate the insoluble powder in a mortar.

Indiffusible solids. Substances which do not remain in suspension sufficiently long for a dose to be measured accurately must be suspended by means of a suspending agent (see p. 342). Substances which require the use of a suspending agent include the sulphonamides (e.g. sulphadimidine and succinylsulphathiazole), aspirin and phenacetin. Corticosteroids such as hydrocortisone acetate may sometimes be prescribed as suspensions for administration to children but it is preferable for potent substances such as these to be supplied where possible in tablet form, with instructions that they be crushed and mixed with honey or syrup before administration.

The general procedure for indiffusible solids is to reduce the substance to a fine powder in a mortar, triturate with the suspending agent (usually compound tragacanth powder or sodium carboxymethylcellulose) and form a smooth cream with a small portion of the vehicle. The remainder of the vehicle is then added gradually.

DISPENSING IN THE METRIC SYSTEM

As noted above, the liquid medicines in the *British Pharmaceutical Codex* and *British National Formulary* are formulated to a dose of 5 ml or a multiple thereof. When a fractional dose is prescribed, the pharmacist is directed to dilute the medicine with the appropriate vehicle so that the patient is able to measure a full medicine spoonful. Consider the following prescription:

    ℞ Tetracycline mixture
        2.5 ml four times daily
        Send 50 ml

This is dispensed as follows:
    Tetracycline mixture 2.5 ml
    Syrup to 5 ml
    Send 100 ml and label, 'One 5-ml spoonful to be taken four times daily'.

The appropriate diluents for use in each case are stated in the monographs of the *British Pharmaceutical Codex*. Care should be taken to note those preparations which must not be diluted (e.g. Nystatin Mixture). Diluted preparations have only a limited stability and must not be used more than 14 days after the date of preparation. The above mixture therefore should also be labelled 'Do not use after (date)'.

INTERPRETATION OF PRESCRIPTIONS WRITTEN IN
APOTHECARY SYSTEM

In order to effect the changeover to dispensing in the metric system, the Weights and Measures (Equivalents for Dealing with Drugs) Regulations, 1968 include six tables specifying how to convert a prescription from the apothecary system into the metric system. A useful series of articles dealing with the changeover to metric dispensing appeared in the *Pharmaceutical Journal*, February, 1969, and a review of the problems involved was given by Thornton Jones (1969).

EMULSIONS

The theory of emulsions has been described in Chapter 18. In physical chemistry an emulsion is described as a system in which one immiscible liquid is dispersed in another, but in pharmacy the term is restricted to oil-in-water preparations for internal administration. An emulsion is a particularly convenient form in which to administer oily substances such as liquid paraffin and fixed oils. The oil is dispersed in a continuous surrounding aqueous medium in which flavouring agents may be incorporated to mask the nauseous properties of the oil and improve the palatability of the preparation. This chapter deals with the extemporaneous preparation of small volumes of emulsions. Equipment for the large scale production of emulsions is described in Chapter 18.

Small quantities of emulsions may be prepared either in a small emulsifying machine or by the mortar and pestle method. Many machines advertized for cream making can be used for the extemporaneous preparation of emulsions and the results are superior to those produced by the mortar and pestle method. The use of a machine enables a wider range of emulgents to be employed and smaller proportions of emulgents are required.

Hand Emulsifying Machines
The oil, water and mucilage are shaken together to form a coarse emulsion which is poured into the bowl of the machine and pumped by a lever movement of the handle through a fine orifice at high pressure. This gives the shearing effect which produces a fine emulsion.

Mortar and Pestle Method
The most commonly used emulgent for preparing oil-in-water emulsions in powdered acacia, which can be used for fixed oils, volatile oils, oleo-resins and liquid paraffin. Emulsions may be prepared by hand in a mortar and pestle either by a *dry gum method* or a *wet gum method*.

The dry gum method. A primary emulsion is prepared by mixing the oil, water and gum in the proportions indicated below. When the primary emulsion has been formed it may be diluted with more of the external aqueous phase.

To obtain a good primary emulsion, oil, water and gum must be mixed in the following proportions, depending on the nature of the oil:

Fixed oil	4	Volatile oil	2
Water	2	Water	2
Gum	1	Gum	1

It will be observed that the proportion of gum is twice as great in an emulsion of a volatile oil as in one containing a fixed oil. The ratio of water to gum in the primary emulsion is always 2:1.

In preparing an emulsion by hand, an ample sized mortar should be selected with a corresponding pestle with a broad, flat head to provide the maximum amount of shear in use.

Example:
  Olive oil 50 ml
  Powdered acacia, a sufficient quantity
  Chloroform water to 250 ml
  Method: Place in the mortar 12.5 g of powdered acacia; measure 50 ml of olive oil and pour it on to the gum in the mortar, allowing time for the measure to drain. Triturate the oil and gum together to obtain even dispersion of the gum (prolonged trituration is undesrable since it will result in the particles of gum becoming surrounded by oil and they will not readily be hydrated by water). Using a *clean* measure, add 25 ml of chloroform water, *all at once*, and triturate vigorously, working in one direction only and using a whipping action.

As the primary emulsion forms, the preparation changes to a white homogeneous paste and the motion of the pestle produces a crackling sound. The trituration should be continued until a stable primary emulsion has formed. The remaining chloroform water should then be added, in small quantities at first but in increasing quantities as the preparation becomes dilute. Finally, transfer the emulsion to a measure, rinse the mortar with more chloroform water and adjust to volume.

A simple emulsion such as this should be white in appearance and when a few drops are diluted in a large volume of water there should be no visible oil globules on the surface. Emulsions should not cream for several hours and the oily layer should be easily diffused again by shaking.

Failure to obtain a satisfactory preparation may be due to one or more of the following causes: (i) the use of a mortar which is too small or which is too conical; (ii) the use of a narrow-headed pestle which fails to shear the oil into globules; (iii) measuring the oil in a wet measure; (iv) measuring the water in an oily measure; (v) using an old sample of gum, which has acquired an acid reaction; (vi) bad manipulation; (vii) using incorrect proportions of oil, water and gum; and (viii) diluting the primary emulsion before it is completely formed.

The wet gum method. The proportions of oil water and gum used in the wet gum method are the same as those used for the dry gum method. Only the procedure is different.

Example:
  Cottonseed oil 50 ml
  Powdered acacia, a sufficient quantity
  Chloroform water to 250 ml
Method: Weigh 12.5 of powdered acacia and transfer to a suitable sized mortar. Add 25 ml of chloroform water and triturate until the gum has dissolved to form a mucilage. Add the cottonseed oil, drop by drop with constant trituration using a whipping motion. As the oil is added, the liquid in the mortar may acquire a ropy appearance and the oil may not be readily absorbed. When this occurs, add a few drops of chloroform water and triturate the mixture until it becomes homogeneous. Continue to add the oil so log as it is taken up homogeneously, adding a few drops of chloroform water if the preparation shows any tendency to become ropy.

When all the oil has been added, continue triturating until a stable primary emulsion has been obtained. Finally, dilute the primary emulsion with chloroform water, transfer to a measure, rinsing the mortar with further quantities of chloroform water, and adjust to volume.

The wet gum method is more time consuming than the dry gum method. The mucilage should be freshly prepared, since on storage it may become acid in reaction, lose viscosity and render emulsification impossible.

EMULSIFYING AGENTS

Powdered Tragacanth
This is inferior to acacia as an emulgent and its emulsifying properties depend mainly upon the viscosity it imparts to the continuous phase. Tragacanth emulsions are coarser than acacia emulsions and do not have their white colour. The main use of tragacanth in emulsions is as an ancillary emulgent in association with acacia. A mixture of tragacanth, 1 part, with acacia, 15 parts, may be used in place of powdered acacia in the extemporaneous preparation of emulsions.

Methylcellulose, BPC
This is a methyl ether of cellulose and is available in various viscosity grades which are denoted by a number following the name. The lower viscosity grades are used as emulsifying agents, methylcellulose 20 being the most commonly used member of the series for this purpose. The suffix '20' indicates the approximate viscosity in centistokes of a 2.0 per cent w/v solution in water at 20°.

A mucilage of methylcellulose may be prepared by adding the solid to about one-third the required amount of boiling water stirring constantly and adding the remainder of the water, preferably in the form of ice, when the powder is thoroughly hydrated. The mucilage can be used to make emulsions extemporaneously by the wet gum method but better results are obtained if a mechanical stirrer is used.

Methylcellulose 20 is used as the emulgent in Liquid Paraffin Emulsion, BPC.

Agar
This was formerly used extensively (in association with acacia and tragacanth) for the emulsification of liquid paraffin. It was included for its supposed therapeutic action but was present in too small a quantity to be effective. The *British National Formulary* allows Liquid Paraffin Emulsion to be supplied when Liquid Paraffin and Agar Emulsion is prescribed.

Casein
This is the protein which emulsifies fat in milk. Soluble casein or similar products obtained from milk protein may be used as emulgents in the proportion of 12 g of casein for 100 ml of fixed oil. The oil is added to the casein in a mortar and triturated to form a paste and the water is then added gradually with continuous trituration. Emulsions containing casein are particularly liable to microbiological contamination and a preservative should be included. Chloroform, 1:500, may be used for this purpose.

Gelatin Solution
This is an effective emulsifying agent when used on a large scale. A solution containing 120 g of gelatin

with 200 g of potassium carbonate in 5 l of water will emulsify 120 l of liquid paraffin.

SUBSTANCES REQUIRING SPECIAL TREATMENT

Male fern extract. Add it to its own weight of acacia and triturate thoroughly; then add twice the same amount of water with constant trituration. Take care that the extract does not come into contact with water until it is intimately mixed with gum. Otherwise, the emulsion will contain unsightly black particles.

Paraldehyde. This is now usually given by intramuscular injection but may occasionally be administered orally as a draught. One gram of paraldehyde disolves in 9 ml of water and it need only be emulsified if present in excess of its solubility. An emulsion can be prepared by adding the paraldehyde to compound powder of tragacanth (100 mg for each 25 ml of paraldehyde) in a dry bottle, shaking gently to disperse the powder and then adding twice the volume of water and shaking vigorously. The remainder of the water can then be added gradually, shaking after each addition.

REFERENCES

LEES, K. A. (1963) Fine particles in pharmaceutical practice. *J. Pharm. Pharmacol.* **15**, 43T.

Pharm. J. (1969) Changeover to metric **202**, 114, 145, 167.

THORNTON JONES, A. D. (1969) Changeover to the metric system. *Pharm. J.* **202**, 221.

25

Rectal Administration

Drugs are introduced into the rectum in either solid or liquid preparations (suppositories and enemas).

SUPPOSITORIES

Suppositories are solid, uniformly medicated, conical or torpedo shaped for rectal administration. They melt at slightly below body temperature so that after insertion, the mass melts and the medicament is liberated in contact with the rectal mucosa.

Drugs may be administered in suppositories for a local effect in the rectum or so that they may be absorbed and exert a systemic effect. Local anaesthetics, astringent drugs (e.g. hamamelis) and cortiscosteroids are administered in suppositories for the treatment of haemorrhoids. Drugs which are liable to cause gastric irritation may be given rectally in the form of suppositories as an alternative to oral administration. For example, phenylbutazone and indomethacin are sometimes administered rectally for this reason.

Suppository Bases
Medicated suppositories are most commonly prepared in a fatty base which melts below 37°. Water soluble bases may also occasionally be used.

Theobroma Oil. This is a solid fat at ordinary temperatures but melts between 29° and 34°; consequently it is fluid at body temperature. Its specific gravity (0.990 to 0.998) is very near to that of water.

Witepsol bases. These are processed neutral fatty substances, consisting of the triglycerides of saturated fatty acids with varying proportions of partial glycerides. Witepsol H 15 is recommended for large scale production, whereas W 45 is more suitable for small scale dispensing. The melting point of the two substances is the same (33.5° to 35.5°) but Witepsol W 45 solidifies at 29° to 32° whereas H 15 solidifies at 32.5° to 34.5°.

Witepsol and similar proprietary suppository bases have the advantage that lubrication of the mould is unnecessary and they are unaffected by heat whereas theobroma oil requires lubrication and is converted by only a slight excess of heat to an isomorph with a lower melting point. The partial glycerides present in Witepsol bases act as water-in-oil emulsifying agents and enable appreciable quantities of aqueous solutions to be incorporated.

The *British Pharmaceutical Codex*, 1973, states that when theobroma oil is specified as a suppository base it may be replaced by 'any other suitable basis, such as Fractionated Palm Kernel Oil or other suitable hydrogenated vegetable oil, provided that the melting point of the suppositories is not more than 37°'.

Suppositories prepared with Witepsol bases should not be ice-cooled since they are liable to become brittle and fracture if cooled too rapidly.

Glycogelatin base. Suppositories may also be prepared with Glycerol Suppository mass of the *British Pharmacopoeia*. Its use, however, is limited because the gelatin it contains is incompatible with a large number of substances, the laxative action of the suppository base tends to promote expulsion of the medicament. The glycogelatin base can be used by itself as a laxative.

Water soluble bases. Water soluble suppositories may also be prepared with macrogol bases. These are polymers of ethylene glycol which range from mobile liquids to hard waxy solids. Suitable combinations for use as suppository bases have been proposed, such as the following:

Polyethylene glycol 6000 40
Polyethylene glycol 15400 30
Polyethylene glycol   400 30

Suppositories may be prepared by either the fusion method or by cold compression.

The Fusion Method

In this method the medicament is intimately mixed with a melted base and the mixture poured into moulds to solidify.

The mould. Suppository moulds are usually made of an alloy of gun metal type. They have either six or twelve wells into which the melted mass is poured and are divided longitudinally, so that when unscrewed, the two halves of each well can be separated (see Fig. 25.1).

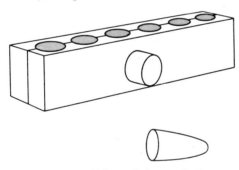

FIG. 25.1. Mould for conical suppositories.

Suppository moulds are made with a nominal capacity of 1 or 2 g. The capacity of a new mould should be ascertained exactly before it is used. The capacity of a mould for theobroma oil is determined by pouring an excess of melted theobroma oil into the holes, cutting of the excess with a sharp knife while the mass is still rather soft, allowing to solidify, removing the suppositories and weighing. A note should be made of the actual capacity of the mould for future reference.

Lubricant. Moulds that are to be used for the preparation of theobroma oil suppositories must be lubricated before pouring in the mass. This is done with a small camel hair brush or on a piece of cotton wool. The latter is better, since it is less likely to leave an excess of lubricant, but care must be taken that no strands of cotton are left adhering to the mould.

The following lubricant may be used:

Soft soap 10 g
Glycerin 10 g
Alcohol (90 per cent) 50 ml

Calculating the quantities. When making suppositories, it is necessary to prepare for a slight excess owing to unavoidable losses during pouring. It is usually necessary to make for eight if six are required and for fourteen if twelve are required.

In determining the amount of theobroma oil required, allowance must be made for the displacement of the theobroma oil by the medicament. This will depend upon the density of the medicament compared with that of theobroma oil. For example, if the medicament has twice the density of theobroma oil, it will displace half the volume of an equal weight of theobroma oil. The density of the medicament compared with theobroma oil is known as its displacement value. The total weight of the medicament is divided by its displacement value and this amount is deducted from the nominal amount of theobroma oil required.

Example:

Ŗ Tannic acid 0.2 g
Theobroma oil q.s.
Send 6 suppositories

Make for 8 suppositories (each 1 g)
Total quantity of tannic acid required
$$= 8 \times 0.2 = 1.6 \text{ g}$$
Displacement value of tannic acid
$$= 1.6$$
Quantity of theobroma oil required
$$= 8 - \tfrac{1.6}{1.6} \text{ g}$$
$$= 7 \text{ g}$$

The *British Pharmaceutical Codex* gives the displacement values of a number of substances commonly prescribed in suppositories.

Making suppositories with theobroma oil. (1) Lubricate the mould and invert it to drain off excess of lubricant.
(2) Cool the lubricated mould over ice to allow it to contract fully before the mass is poured in.
(3) Weigh the theobroma oil (previously shredded by means of a grater) and place in a small porcelain dish over a water bath. The water in the water bath must be hot but not boiling and the heat must be removed before the dish is placed on the bath. Remove the dish from the water bath as soon as the mass is molten.

(4) Weigh the medicament and powder it finely. Place it on a slightly warm porcelain slab.

(5) Pour about half the melted theobroma oil on to the medicament and mix by means of a spatula. Scrape the mixture back into the dish and mix with the remainder of the melted theobroma oil, stirring with the spatula.

(6) When the mixture in the dish has cooled sufficiently to start to thicken and flows sluggishly, pour the mixture into the holes in the mould, filling each to overflowing, and stirring the contents of the dish continuously between pouring. Care must be taken to ensure that the mass is not too warm before pouring as there is a danger that the medicament will form a sediment at the tip of the suppository. Because theobroma oil contracts as it solidifies, it is necessary to fill the mould to overflowing.

(7) Place the mould on ice (or in a cold place) and when the surplus material has attained the consistence of butter, remove it cleanly with a sharp knife.

(8) When the suppositories have completely set hard (usually after about half an hour), open the mould and eject the suppositories by slight pressure on the broad ends.

(9) Remove any surplus lubricant from the surface of the suppositories by rolling them on filter paper.

The main disadvantage of theobroma oil as a suppository base is its tendency to be converted by heat to a polymorphic form which has a lower melting point. It is for this reason that care must be taken not to overheat the suppositories during preparation. The melting point of theobroma oil is lowered by some substances (e.g. chloral hydrate, phenol and volatile oils) and the *British Pharmaceutical Codex* allows the addition of beeswax to suppositories containing such substances provided that the melting point is not above 37°. Beeswax may also be added to suppositories intended for use in tropical or subtropical climates.

Making suppositories with Witepsol base. The procedure is the same as for theobroma oil suppositories with the following exceptions: (1) the mould must not be lubricated; (2) the suppositories must not be cooled rapidly on ice as they are liable to fracture; and (3) there is less need to avoid overheating the mass since the melting point is unaffected by heat.

THE COLD COMPRESSION METHOD

This method is used for the large scale production of suppositories. Theobroma oil or Witepsol base may be used but some manufacturers may modify the base by the inclusion of wool fat, or castor oil and beeswax.

The medicament and the base are intimately mixed and placed in a hollow cylinder. The mass is extruded from this by means of a piston, actuated either by hand or mechanically, through small holes that communicate with the pointed ends of conical cavities based in a metal cap fixed at the end of the cylinder. The cavities are filled by pressure with the mass, which is prevented from escaping by a movable end plate. When the end plate is removed the suppositories are ejected by further extrusion.

GLYCOGELATIN SUPPOSITORIES

The *British Pharmacopoeia* includes a formula for Glycerol Suppositories, containing gelatin, glycerin and purified water.

The gelatin is soaked in purified water for about 5 min until softened. The surplus water is then drained off and the glycerin added. The mixture is heated over a water-bath until the gelatin has dissolved and the contents of the dish have been evaporated to the required weight, which corresponds to 70 per cent w/w of glycerin.

This liquid mass is poured into moulds having a capacity of 1 g (infants), 2 g (children) or 4 g (adults) as may be required.

The gelatin should either be powdered, granulated or cut into small pieces before soaking in water. If sheet gelatin is used, the hard outer portions of the sheets should be removed. During evaporation the liquid mass should be only gently stirred to avoid introducing air bubbles into the finished suppositories. Any skin that may form on the surface should be removed before pouring.

Lubricant. Lubricate the mould with arachis or almond oil applied on cotton wool, and invert the mould so that any excess of lubricant may drain out.

Calculating the quantities. Glycogelatin mass is denser than theobroma oil and a 1 g mould will hold 1.2 g of glycerin suppositories mass. This fact must be borne in mind when calculating the quantities and an excess must also be prepared to allow for losses during pouring.

Making suppositories with glycogelatin base. The displacement values of substances in glycogelatin base are half the values in a theobroma oil base.

The medicament is added directly to the mass in

the dish and mixed by gentle stirring. When pouring the suppositories, each hole of the mould must be filled just to the top. It is unnecessary to fill to overflowing as the contraction on cooling is inappreciable and it is difficult to remove any excess neatly by cutting.

Dispensing Suppositories

Suppositories should be supplied in boxes lined with waxed paper or in containers made of plastic. If they contain volatile ingredients, each suppository should be separately wrapped in metal foil.

PESSARIES

Because their pharmaceutical form is similar to that of suppositories, it is appropriate here to mention the dispensing of pessaries. These are solid preparations, suitably shaped for vaginal insertion, containing medicaments intended to have a local action on the vaginal mucosa. Pessaries may be prepared either by moulding as described for suppositories or by compression in the same way that solution tablets are manufactured (see Chapter 19). Compressed pessaries are usually prepared in special punches and dies to produce an almond or diamond-shaped product, convenient for vaginal administration. Moulded pessaries are usually prepared in 4 or 8 g moulds depending upon the bulk of the ingredients. The basis may be either glycogelatin or a hydrogenated vegetable oil such as is used for suppositories.

Pessaries are dispensed in boxes lined with waxed paper or in suitable plastic containers. Many proprietary pessaries prepared by compression are strip-packed in metal or plastic coated metal foil.

ENEMAS

An enema is a solution or fluid suspension for rectal administration. There are two types: evacuant enemas and retention enemas. The volume given varies according to the type of enema. Retention enemas do not normally exceed 100 ml in volume; evacuant enemas may be as much as 2 l. Large volume enemas should be warmed to body temperature before administration.

Evacuant Enemas

A typical evacuant enema is:
    Soft soap 25 g
    Water to 500 ml
This is a simple solution which may be supplied in a plain screw-capped bottle.

Starch mucilage may be used as an emollient and suspending agent for insoluble solids in enemas. Sodium carboxymethylcellulose may be used for the same purposes.

Retention Enemas

Rectal injections may be given as basal anaesthetics before surgical operations. For example, thiopentone sodium is given in a dose of 40 mg per kg body weight (maximum 2 g). The thiopentone sodium is dissolved in 30 ml of purified water. It must be freshly prepared.

Paraldehyde is occasionally given rectally as a 10 per cent solution in sodium chloride solution (0.9 per cent).

Disposable Enemas

In recent years enemas have become available in disposable plastic bags. They include evacuant enemas such as magnesium sulphate solution and retention enemas of prednisolone. The latter are convenient for the steroid treatment of ulcerative colitis.

REFERENCES

SOULSBY, J. & HOPKINS, S. J. (1956) *Pharm. J.* **176**, 157.
SETRIKAR, I. & FANTELLI, S. (1962) *J. pharm. Sci.* **51**, 566.
BRYAN, G. (1964) *M. and B. pharm. Bull.* **13**, 33.

26

External Preparations

LIQUID PREPARATIONS

Liquid preparations for external application can be classified as follows:

(a) *For application to the skin:* applications, liniments, lotions, and paints.

(b) *For application to the ear:* ear drops.

(c) *For application to the mouth and throat:* gargles and mouth-washes.

(d) *For application to the naso-pharynx:* nasal drops, spray solutions, and inhalations.

Preparations for use in the eye are dealt with in Chapter 27.

APPLICATIONS

Applications are liquid or viscous preparations intended for application to the skin. They often contain parasiticides and are intended for only a limited number of applications (e.g. Dicophane Application, BPC). Compound application of Calamine, BPC, is really an oily lotion since it consists of calamine dispersed in a water-in-oil emulsion. Applications should be dispensed in fluted bottles so as to be distinguishable by touch and should be labelled 'For external use only'. The closure of the bottle should be of plastic screw-cap type.

LINIMENTS

Liniments are liquid preparations for external use and may be applied with or without friction. For the relief of pain, they may be applied on warmed flannel or lint, or may be painted on to the skin by means of a soft brush. As stimulants, liniments may be massaged into the skin with considerable friction. They should not be applied to areas in which the skin is broken.

Liniments may be: alcoholic solutions (e.g. Aconite Liniment, BPC); oily solutions (e.g. Methyl Salicylate Liniment, BPC); or emulsions (e.g. Turpentine Liniment, BP). They should be dispensed in coloured, fluted bottles and labelled 'For external use only'.

LOTIONS

Lotions are aqueous solutions or suspensions intended for application to the skin surface. If they contain insoluble solids in suspension, they are sometimes referred to as 'shake lotions'. On application to the skin, the water evaporates leaving a residue of the medicament on the skin surface. The evaporation causes cooling and lotions are applied to acutely inflamed areas. The cooling effect may be enhanced by the inclusion of alcohol. Glycerin may be included to promote adherence of the residual powder on the skin surface. Suspending agents such as sodium carboxymethylcellulose or bentonite may be present to assist the dispersion of insoluble powders in shake lotions (e.g. Calamine Lotion, BP).

Lotions may also take the form of dilute emulsions, usually of the oil-in-water type and containing emulsifying wax. They should contain a preservative to inhibit the growth of micro-organisms. When purified water is used for the preparation of lotions, it should be freshly boiled and cooled before use.

Lotions should be dispensed in fluted bottles,

closed with a plastic screw-cap. They should be labelled 'For external use only'.

PAINTS

Paints are another group of liquid preparations for external application, usually for circumscribed areas. They may be aqueous or alcoholic solutions and sometimes are prepared with a collodion basis to form a film on the skin. Compound Tincture of Benzoin BPC is also used as a basis for paints for the same reason (e.g. Compound Podophyllin Paint, BPC).

Paints should be dispensed in coloured fluted bottles, preferably closed by means of glass stoppers.

EAR DROPS

Ear drops are often aqueous (sometimes glycerin or alcoholic) solutions dispensed in small quantities (10 or 25 ml) and intended for instillation into the ear. Hydrogen peroxide ear drops (5-volume) and phenol ear drops (6 per cent w/w) are typical examples. It should be noted that glycerin phenol (16 per cent w/w) becomes caustic if diluted with water. When prescribed in ear drops, glycerin phenol must be diluted with glycerin.

Ear drops should be dispensed in coloured, fluted bottles with a dropper and plastic screw-cap closure.

GARGLES

Gargles are aqueous solutions, intended to be used after dilution with warm water. They are intended to bring the medicament into contact with the mucous surface of the throat, but it is now generally recognized that antiseptic substances exert little effect when used in this manner. Gargles may be useful in giving symptomatic relief and may have some analgesic effect. Gargles are usually clear solutions but occasionally aspirin, in the form of a suspension may be used as a gargle and afterwards swallowed.

Gargles should be dispensed in clear, fluted glass bottles closed with a plastic screw-cap. If they are to be swallowed after use, they should be dispensed in clear, plain glass bottles in the same way as mixtures.

MOUTH-WASHES

Mouth-washes are similar to gargles but are intended to wash out the mouth. They may be of value for local hygiene of the mouth but antiseptic substances used in this way are unlikely to be effective.

Mouth-washes should be dispensed in clear, fluted bottles.

NASAL DROPS

Nasal drops are aqueous solutions for instillation into the nostrils. They may contain vasoconstrictor drugs to relieve nasal congestion and are often preserved with chlorbutol (0.5 per cent) or other suitable antiseptic substance. Formerly, oily solutions were commonly used as nasal drops but the oil may retard the ciliary action of the mucosa or, if drops of oil enter the trachea, may even cause lipoid pneumonia. For this reason, oily solutions are no longer recommended.

Nasal drops are dispensed in small quantities (10 or 25 ml) in fluted, coloured glass bottles fitted with a plastic screw-cap and dropper. Proprietary nasal sprays are supplied in plastic, squeeze-type containers. The prolonged use of vasoconstrictor drugs in the nose may damage the nasal mucosa.

SPRAY SOLUTIONS

Spray solutions are aqueous, alcoholic or glycerin solutions intended to be applied to the membrane of the throat or nose by means of an atomizer. Oily solutions were formerly used for this purpose but are no longer used for the same reasons that oily nasal drops have been discontinued.

The type of atomizer used depends upon the viscosity of the spray solutions; the more viscous the solution the more powerful the atomizer needed. When dispensing a spray solution, the patient should be asked whether he possesses a suitable spray. If not, an appropriate one should be supplied and its use explained.

The drugs most commonly dispensed as spray solutions are adrenaline and isoprenaline, which which are both used for the relief of asthma. The use of spray solutions for this purpose has been superseded to a large extent, by the introduction of metered aerosols (see Chapter 37). Metered aerosols have the advantage of producing a more accurately controlled dose of the drug in particulate form. The particle size can be controlled to ensure that the drug penetrates the bronchial tree. Such preparations are not without risk and adverse reactions, including fatalities, have followed the too frequent use of such preparations. It is advisable to warn patients that they should follow very carefully the medical directions in the use of these preparations and should resist any temptation to use them more frequently.

Ergotamine tartrate is also sometimes administered by inhalation from a metered aerosol for the relief of attacks of migraine.

Inhalations are solutions or suspensions of volatile, aromatic or antiseptic substances, the vapour of which is inhaled from the surface of hot water. The directions are usually to the effect that one teaspoonful of the liquid is to be poured on to about one pint of hot, but not boiling, water and the vapour inhaled. Inhalations are useful for the relief of nasal congestion and it is probable that the steam contributes mainly to the effectiveness of these preparations.

Inhalations often consist of alcoholic solutions of substances such as menthol, volatile oils or benzoin (e.g. Benzoin Inhalation, BPC). Occasionally, volatile oils are ordered with water as the vehicle, and in these circumstances the oil is triturated with a small amount of light magnesium carbonate in a mortar and the water added gradually, the suspension being finally rinsed into the bottle and made up to volume with more of the water (e.g. Menthol and Eucalyptus Inhalation, BPC). The object of the light magnesium carbonate is to ensure even dispersion of the volatile oil throughout the vehicle and such inhalations should be labelled with directions to shake the bottle before use. Inhalations should be dispensed in fluted bottles of clear glass.

SOLID PREPARATIONS

The solid or semi-solid preparations for external application are ointments, creams, pastes, poultices, and dusting powders.

Ointments are greasy, semi-solid preparations for application to the skin. They are often anhydrous and contain the medicament either dissolved or dispersed in the vehicle. Substances which are dispersed should be in the form of a fine powder and in some cases, notably the corticosteroids, the solid should be in the form of a micronized powder.

The bases that are used mainly in the preparation of ointments may be classified into hydrocarbon bases, absorption bases, emulsifying bases, and water soluble bases.

Hydrocarbon bases. These may consist of soft paraffin or a mixture of soft paraffin with hard paraffin and liquid paraffin to produce a suitable consistency. Paraffins are inert substances, chiefly saturated, which are unlikely to react with the medicament and do not develop rancidity on storage.

Paraffin Ointment BP is a mixture of white beeswax, hard paraffin, cetostearyl alcohol and white soft paraffin. The *British Pharmacopoeia* directs that when paraffin ointment is used in a white ointment, it should be prepared with white soft paraffin and when used in a coloured ointment, it should be prepared with yellow soft paraffin. The cetostearyl alcohol is included in paraffin ointment in order to improve its spreading properties on the skin. Paraffin ointment is stiffer in consistency than soft paraffin.

The paraffin bases form a greasy film on the skin surface which remains unabsorbed. They reduce the rate of moisture loss from the skin surface and, in dry scaly conditions of the skin, may improve the hydration of the horny layer.

Absorption bases. Absorption bases contain a water-in-oil emulsifying agent, usually in the form of wool fat or one of its derivatives. Simple ointment BP is a mixture of wool fat, hard paraffin cetostearyl alcohol and white or yellow soft paraffin, depending upon whether it is used in a white or coloured ointment. Simple Ointment will absorb about 15 per cent of its weight of water, forming a water-in-oil emulsion.

Wool Alcohols Ointment, BP contains wool alcohols, hard paraffin, liquid paraffin and white or yellow soft paraffin depending upon whether it is used in a white or coloured ointment. Wool alcohols ointment will absorb an equal weight of water. Wool alcohols is liable to oxidize on storage and when preparing ointment of wool alcohols, the outer film of oxidized material should be removed since the emulsifying properties are reduced on oxidation.

Absorption bases such as simple ointment and wool alcohols ointment form a greasy film on the skin surface which modifies the rate of moisture loss in the same way as the hydrocarbon bases. The wool fat or wool alcohols may also assist in hydrating the horny layer by forming a water-in-oil emulsion on the skin surface, thus prolonging the time during which the moisture may be absorbed by the keratin layer.

Although not included in the *British Pharmacopoeia* or *British Pharmaceutical Codex* hydrogenated lanolin is sometimes used in preference to wool fat, since it is a more elegant product and more consistent in its performance. However, wool fat and related products are now less favoured in dermatological vehicles, since some individuals are sensitive to them.

Emulsifying bases. These bases contain oil-in-water emulsifying agents which render them readily miscible with water or 'self-emulsifying'. Depending upon the nature of the emulsifying agent present, emulsifying bases can be classified into three main groups: anionic emulsifying bases, cationic emulsifying bases, and non-ionic emulsifying bases.

Anionic emulsifying bases contain an anionic emulsifying agent and are exemplified by Emulsifying Ointment, BP. This consists of a mixture of emulsifying wax, white soft paraffin and liquid paraffin. Emulsifying wax is a mixture of cetostearyl alcohol and sodium lauryl sulphate which is incompatible with cationic organic medicaments and the salts of barium and heavy metals.

Cationic emulsifying bases are exemplified by Cetrimide Emulsifying Ointment, BP. This consists of a mixture of cetrimide, cetostearyl alcohol, white soft paraffin and liquid paraffin. Cetrimide Emulsifying Wax BPC is a mixture of cetrimide and cetostearyl alcohol which is compatible with cationic medicaments.

Non-ionic emulsifying ointments are exemplified by Cetomacrogol Emulsifying Ointment, BPC. This consists of a mixture of cetomacrogol emulsifying wax, white soft paraffin and liquid paraffin. Cetomacrogol Emulsifying Wax BP is a mixture of cetostearyl alcohol and cetomacrogol 1000 which is compatible with cationic medicaments and fairly high concentrations of electrolytes. Cetomacrogol is a polyethylene glycol ether of cetostearyl alcohol and is incompatible with phenolic compounds.

Because of their surface active properties, emulsifying bases may facilitate contact between the medicament and the skin surface. They are also readily washed off the skin and are used when this property is desired, e.g. on scalp areas.

Water soluble bases. Water soluble bases consist of mixtures of macrogols (polyethylene glycols). These are polymers of ethylene glycol which range from mobile liquids to hard waxes, depending upon the number of ethylene oxide units in the polymer. Macrogol 300 BP contains five or six ethylene oxide units and has a molecular weight of 285 to 325. Macrogol 4000 BP contains 69 to 84 ethylene oxide units and has a molecular weight of 3100 to 3700.

Macrogol Ointment, BPC is a mixture of liquid and hard macrogols which has a consistency similar to that of soft paraffin and is completely soluble in water. Macrogol bases are used for local anaesthetics such as lignocaine and are useful when easy washing from the skin surface is desired, but they reduce the activity of phenolic antiseptics.

Preparation of Ointments
Trituration. When the quantity of ointment is not more than about 50 g, a white porcelain or marble ointment slab (about 30 cm square) should be used in conjunction with a flexible steel spatula.

A steel spatula should not be used when there is a possibility that the medicament may react with the metal, e.g. mercury compounds, tannic acid, salicylic acid and iodine. Stainless steel spatulas are suitable for most substances or a flexible vulcanite spatula may be used.

The whole of the medicament is first intimately mixed with a little of the base, and then the remainder of the base incorporated gradually, the spatula being held flat and worked with a side-to-side motion rather than a rotary one. When the medicament is rather gritty or contains large aggregated lumps (e.g. zinc oxide, calamine or mercuric oxide) it should be levigated on the slab with a few drops of liquid paraffin before incorporation into a paraffin base.

Twin roller mills are available for the preparation of small quantities of ointment by hand. The degree of fineness is determined by the setting of the variable roller. Larger, triple-roll mills, motor driven, capable of handling larger quantities of ointments and having an output up to 5 to 7 kg per h, are also available.

Crystalline, water soluble substances (e.g. resorcinol), present in small quantities, may be dissolved in a little water before incorporation in the basis. It should be noted that soft paraffin is capable of absorbing up to 10 per cent of its weight of water and wool fat will absorb nearly twice its weight of water.

Fusion. Ointments containing ingredients which are quite solid at room temperature (hard paraffin, beeswax, emulsifying wax, wool alcohols) are prepared by melting the ingredients in a porcelain dish over a water bath. The usual method is to melt the substance with the highest melting point first and add the other ingredients of the basis in order of their melting points.

When an insoluble substance is to be incorporated into such a base containing an oil, it is advisable to levigate the solid with the oil in a hot mortar and then to add to it, with constant trituration, the previously melted mixture of the other ingredients. For small quantities of ointment, a heated slab may be used.

If no oil is present, the solid medicament must be finely powdered and sifted into the melted base through fine muslin or a No. 60 mesh sieve, after the base has been removed from the water bath and has just begun to thicken. The mixture is then stirred until cold.

Water soluble bases containing liquid and hard macrogols are also prepared by fusion, using a minimum amount of heat and stirring until cold.

CREAMS

The term 'cream' in pharmacy and medicine is applied to viscous emulsions of semi-solid consistency intended for application to the skin or mucous membrane. They may be of the water-in-oil (oily creams) or oil-in-water (aqueous creams) type.

Preparation of Creams

Microbiological contamination is liable to occur, particularly in aqueous creams, which should always contain an added preservative. In the presence of an oily phase and emulsifying agents, the activity of preservatives may be reduced and if there is heavy contamination, the preservative may not be capable of preventing bacterial growth. Special care should be taken to avoid contamination of creams with *Pseudomonas aeruginosa*, which is commonly found as a contaminant of purified water. Apparatus used in the preparation of creams should be thoroughly cleansed and rinsed with freshly boiled and cooled purified water before use. Purified water must be freshly boiled and cooled before incorporation into creams and hygienic precautions should be taken both during the preparation of a cream and when filling into containers.

Containers. Creams should be dispensed in well-closed containers to prevent evaporation of the aqueous phase. Collapsible metal or plastic containers are preferable, but if a pot with a screw-cap is used, care should be taken to ensure that the liner of the screw-cap is of plastics or is plastic-coated. Bonded cork liners are particularly to be avoided. Creams should be stored in a cool place.

Oily Creams

Oily creams contain a water-in-oil emulsifying agent (see Chapter 18) which may be wool fat, wool alcohols, a fatty acid ester of sorbitan or the salt of a fatty acid and a divalent metal (e.g. calcium).

Oily Cream, BP. Oily Cream, BP, consists of a mixture of equal parts of wool alcohols ointment and purified water.

Method. Melt the ointment of wool alcohols over a water bath. Warm the purified water, freshly boiled and cooled, to about 50° and mix with the melted ointment of wool alcohols. Stir constantly until cold, preferably by means of a mechanical stirrer.

Oily Cream, BP is incompatible with phenolic substances and with ichthammol. It is liable to separate on standing, particularly at summer temperatures. The water is usually readily reincorporated by stirring. For a discussion of the use of wool alcohols see Clark and Kitchen (1960).

Zinc Cream, BP. Zinc Cream BP consists of zinc oxide suspended in a water-in-oil emulsion of arachis oil. The emulsifying agent is calcium oleate and wool fat.

Method. Mix the zinc oxide with the calcium hydroxide and triturate with the oleic acid and arachis oil. Incorporate the wool fat and gradually add sufficient purified water to produce the required weight, stirring vigorously during this addition.

Aqueous Creams

Aqueous creams contain an oil-in-water emulsifying agent (see Chapter 18) which may be one of the emulsifying waxes (see p. 258), and alkali salt of a fatty acid, self emulsifying monostearin or a polyethylene glycol derivative of a sorbitan fatty acid ester.

Aqueous Cream, BP. Aqueous Cream, BP, consists of a mixture of 30 per cent of emulsifying ointment with purified water preserved with chlorocresol.

Method. Boil and cool sufficient purified water. Measure the quantity required and dissolve the chlorocresol with the aid of gentle heat. Add the solution to the emulsifying ointment, previously melted over a water bath. Stir gently until cold.

Hydrocortisone Cream, BPC.

Method: Boil and cool sufficient purified water and measure the quantity required. Dissolve the chlorocresol with the aid of gentle heat; melt the cetomacrogol emulsifying ointment over a water bath; add the chlorocresol solution warmed to the same temperature and stir the mixture until cold. Incorporate the required amount of hydrocortisone acetate in the cream by trituration on a clean ointment slab using a spatula.

Note: Special care should be taken to avoid introducing heavy contamination during preparation, and creams containing coricosteroids are best dispensed in collapsible metal or plastics tubes so that they do not become contaminated during use.

Dimethicone Cream, BPC.

Method: Melt the cetostearyl alcohol with the dimethicone 350 and the liquid paraffin over a water bath. Boil and cool sufficient purified water and measure the required quantity. Dissolve the chlorocresol and cetrimide with the aid of gentle heat. Add the solution to the oily phase at the same temperature and stir mechanically until cold.

Note: Dimethicone 350 is a silicone fluid which is water repellant. Dimethicone cream is used as a protective barrier around colostomies and to prevent bedsores and napkin rash. It is vital, therefore, that is should not be contaminated with microorganisms.

PASTES

Pastes are stiffer preparations than ointments and contain a high proportion of powder dispersed in a fatty basis. They were originally formulated on the principle that the high content of powder would absorb exudate but it is unlikely that a powder which has been preferentially wetted with oil will be capable of absorbing an aqueous fluid. Because of their very stiff consistency, pastes are useful for applying active medicaments (e.g. dithranol and coal tar) to circumscribed areas of the skin since they tend to localize the effect of the active ingredient.

Pastes are usually applied liberally by means of a wooden spatula or palette knife. Zinc and Salicylic Acid Paste, BP (Lassar's paste) is the most commonly used preparation of this type. Medicaments incorporated in zinc and salicylic acid paste are less active than when included in ointments. Higher concentrations of substances such as dithranol may therefore be tolerated if they are combined in zinc and salicylic acid paste. The following example illustrates this:

R∕ Dithranol 0.1 g

  Zinc and salicylic acid paste to 100 g

Method: This preparation is best prepared on a heated ointment slab. Triturate the dithranol with a small quantity of the zinc and salicylic acid paste until it is smooth and completely dispersed. Gradually incorporate the remainder of the zinc and salicylic acid paste, with constant trituration to ensure uniform dispersion of the dithranol. The preparation should be carefully inspected to ensure that no discrete agglomerates of dithranol are present.

POULTICES

A poultice is a viscous, pasty preparation for external use, usually employed with the object of reducing inflammation and allaying pain. The two most commonly used preparations of this type are Kaolin Poultice, BPC and Magnesium Sulphate Paste, BPC.

In the preparation of Kaolin Poultice, BP, heavy kaolin is first sifted and dried at 100° to remove moisture. It is then mixed with boric acid and glycerin and the mixture heated to 120° for 1 h with occasional stirring. After cooling, thymol, methylsalicylate and peppermint oil are added and the mass thoroughly mixed.

Heavy kaolin is liable to be contaminated with bacterial spores (e.g. *Clostridium tetani*) and the heating procedure is necessary to kill these. The temperature is limited to 120° to prevent decomposition of the glycerin.

Kaolin Poultice is stored in well closed containers to prevent loss of volatile ingredients and absorption of moisture from the atmosphere by glycerin.

In the preparation of Magnesium Sulphate Paste, BPC, the dried magnesium sulphate must first be heated at 130° or 150° for an appropriate length of time to ensure that the dried powder contains at least 85 per cent of magnesium sulphate. This is necessary to ensure that the product complies with the standard and does not form a granular crystalline preparation on storage.

DUSTING POWDERS

Dusting powders are mixtures of fine powders which are applied to the skin folds to prevent friction. They may contain talc, zinc oxide, starch and kaolin. Powders such as talc and kaolin, which may be contaminated with bacterial spores, should be sterilized by heating at 160° for 1 h before incorporation into a dusting powder. Talc is included for its lubricant properties whereas starch and zinc oxide absorb moisture. Boric acid should no longer be used in dusting powders since it has been found that it may be absorbed in toxic amounts through abraded skin.

Dusting powders are prepared by the same technique as those described for powders (see p. 337). After mixing, they should be passed through a No. 44 mesh sieve or finer; any powder that will not pass the sieve must be further ground until it will. After sifting, the whole must be again lightly mixed.

REFERENCES

CLARK, E. W. & KITCHEN, G. F. (1960) *J. Pharm. Pharmacol.* **12**, 227.

DODD, M. C., HARTMAN, F. W. & WARD, W. C. (1946) *J. Am. pharm. Ass. (Sci. Edn)* **35**, 33.

EBLING, F. J. (1961) *J. Pharm. Pharmacol.* **13**, 23T.

HADGRAFT, J. W. (1954) *J. Pharm. Pharmacol.* **6**, 816.

HADGRAFT, J. W. (1961) *J. Pharm. Pharmacol.* **13**, 43T.

HADGRAFT, J. W. (1967) *J. mond Pharm.* **3**, 309.

27

Preparations for the Eye

Drugs may be applied to the eye in the form of drops, ointments or lotions. They may also be injected into various regions of the eye. The *British Pharmaceutical Codex* defines the following ophthalmic injections:

Subconjunctival injections—aqueous solutions or suspensions which are injected under the conjunctiva. The volume injected by this route is limited to 1 ml and consequently the amount of soluble drug administered is restricted to the amount which dissolves in that volume.

Intracameral injections—aqueous solutions which are injected into the anterior chamber of the eye during surgery to increase the volume of the chamber, to produce miosis and for zonulysis. Antibiotics are usually satisfactorily administered by subconjunctival injection and rarely need intracameral injection.

Intravitreous injections—used to increase the volume of the vitreous chamber. Reconstituted dried vitreous fluid is used for this purpose and a suitable grade of sterilized silicone oil may also be used.

Retrobulbar injections—aqueous solutions used to produce anaesthesia of the globe and akinesia of the extraocular muscles.

Ophthalmic injections must be sterile and are prepared under the same conditions and by the same methods as other parenteral preparations (see Chapter 31). Solutions used during surgery must also be sterile and contain no preservative. They must therefore be presented in single-use containers and any solution remaining at the end of an operation must be discarded.

EYE DROPS

Eye drops are sterile aqueous or oily solutions or suspensions intended for instillation into the conjunctival sac. They may contain antimicrobial substances such as antibiotics, anti-inflammatory agents such as the corticosteroids, miotic drugs such as physostigmine sulphate or mydriatic drugs such as atropine sulphate. Oily eye drops are nowadays seldom used but may, nevertheless, occasionally be requested. They are usually prepared with sterile castor oil and alkaloids incorporated in such a vehicle must be used in the form of the base; e.g. oily eye drops of pilocarpine consist of pilocarpine base dissolved in sterile castor oil.

STERILITY OF EYE DROPS

Until the Supplement 1966 to the *British Pharmaceutical Codex* 1963, there was no official requirement that eye drops should be sterile. They had previously been regarded as extemporaneously prepared preparations and, although precautions were taken to avoid contamination during preparation, they were not subjected to a final sterilizing process. It became evident, particularly in hospital practice, that contaminated solutions could cause serious infections of the eye and various organisms were incriminated including *Pseudomonas aeruginosa*, *Staphylococcus aureus* and *Proteus vulgaris*. Of these, *Pseudomonas aeruginosa* has given rise to the most concern. It is widely distributed and is a commonly found contaminant of distilled water.

It has simple nutritional requirements and is resistant to the action of many antimicrobial agents and antibiotics. Moreover, it can cause serious infections leading to the loss of an eye.

The intact eye has its own defences against infection. The corneal epithelium provides an effective barrier against infection and the tears contain lysozyme which has a powerful antimicrobial action. However, if the eye is damaged, infection can pass into the non-vascular, underlying stroma which provides a good culture medium in which the organisms can proliferate. The cornea may become ulcerated and loss of sight ensue. It is particularly important, therefore, to ensure the sterility of solutions which may be used in damaged eyes. Fluorescein eye drops, for example, are used as a diagnostic agent to detect foreign bodies and corneal abrasions. In such circumstances, the need for sterility is vital and it is better that such preparations should be used from single-dose containers.

STERILIZATION OF EYE DROPS

The problems of sterilizing eye drops are essentially the same as those involved in the preparation of parenteral solutions (see Chapter 31). Many of the drugs used in ophthalmology are affected by heat and the amount of heat applied in the sterilization procedure has to take account of the stability of the drug. The *British Pharmaceutical Codex* recommends the three following general methods:

1. The medicament is dissolved in the aqueous vehicle containing one of the prescribed antimicrobial substances, the solution is clarified by filtration, transferred to the final containers, which are then closed to exclude microorganisms, and sterilized by autoclaving.
2. The medicament is dissolved in the aqueous vehicle containing one of the prescribed antimicrobial substances, the solution is sterilized by filtration and transferred, by means of an aseptic technique to sterile containers, which are then closed so as to exclude microorganisms.
3. The medicament is dissolved in the aqueous vehicle containing one of the prescribed antimicrobial substances, the solution is clarified by filtration, transferred to the final containers which are then closed so as to exclude microorganisms and sterilized by maintaining at 98° to 100° for 30 min.

The *British Pharmaceutical Codex* permits eye drops to be prepared by any other method provided that the product is identical in appearance, quality and composition with one prepared by the appropriate method described in the individual monograph. Exposure to ionizing radiations is not a permitted method but it may be used provided that the product is sterile and has not undergone chemical degradation so that it fails to comply with the required standards. It should be pointed out, however, that the effect of ionizing radiations on drugs and bactericides has not yet been fully investigated and unusual pathways of degradation may be involved. Trigger and Caldwell (1968) have reported that both sodium sulphacetamide eye drops and fluorescein eye drops darken in colour on exposure to a dose of 2.5 Mrad but this colour change was not associated with any other measurable change in assay, ultraviolet absorption or chromatography. There was also no detectable increase in the irritancy of the eye drops according to the Draize test. The same authors also reported that atropine eye drops and eye ointment bases could be sterilized by exposure to ionizing radiations.

BACTERICIDES IN EYE DROPS

In order to prevent the growth of microorganisms, accidentally introduced during use, eye drops which are dispensed in multi-dose containers must contain a suitable preservative. The preservation of ophthalmic preparations has been reviewed by Brown and Norton (1965). These authors state that there is no ideal preservative for eye drops available at present. The properties of an ideal preservative are:

1. It should be rapidly effective against a wide range of organisms, particularly *Pseudomonas aeruginosa*.
2. It should be non-irritant to the eye, non-toxic, and should not cause pain or stinging.
3. It should be compatible with the medicaments used in eye preparations.
4. It should be compatible with eye drop containers and closures.
5. It should be stable at the temperatures used for sterilization of eye drops.

The *British Pharmaceutical Codex* permits the use of three antimicrobial agents as preservatives in eye drops namely: (a) phenylmercuric nitrate or acetate (0.002 per cent); (b) benzalkonium chloride (0.01 per cent); or (c) chlorhexidine acetate (0.01 per cent). Phenylmercuric salts are unsuitable for use in eye drops which are used over long periods of time (e.g. pilocarpine and physostigmine) since there is a possibility that with prolonged use they may cause deposition of minute traces of mercury in the lens. While this condition appears to be symptomless, it is nevertheless undesirable. Benzalkonium chloride is unsuitable for use in eye drops containing local anaesthetics because the latter abolish the blink reflex and the benzalkonium chloride, because of its detergent action, removes the protective oily layer from the precorneal film. If the blink reflex is normal, the meibomian oily layer is rapidly restored.

Apart from the above considerations, the selection of the preservative to be used in eye drops depends upon its compatibility with the medicament. The preservatives used in the eye drops of the *British Pharmaceutical Codex* are given in Table 27.1.

TABLE 27.1

Medicament	Preservative
Amethocaine hydrochloride	PMA or PMN 0.002 per cent
Atropine sulphate	PMA or PMN 0.002 per cent or BC 0.02 per cent
Carbachol	BC 0.02 per cent
Chloramphenicol	PMN or PMA 0.002 per cent
Cocaine hydrochloride	PMN or PMA 0.002 per cent or CA 0.01 per cent
Cocaine hydrochloride and Homatropine hydrobromide	CA 0.01 per cent
Fluorescein	PMN or PMA 0.002 per cent
Homatropine hydrobromide	BC 0.02 per cent or CA 0.01 per cent
Hyoscine hydrobromide	BC 0.02 per cent or CA 0.01 per cent
Lachesine chloride	PMN or PMA 0.002 per cent
Neomycin sulphate	PMN or PMA 0.002 per cent
Phenylephrine hydrochloride	BC 0.04 per cent
Physostigmine sulphate	BC 0.02 per cent
Pilocarpine hydrochloride	BC 0.02 per cent
Prednisolone sodium phosphate	BC 0.04 per cent
Sulphacetamide sodium	PMN or PMA 0.002 per cent

BC = Benzalkonium chloride, CA = Chlorhexidine acetate, PMN = Phenylmercuric nitrate, PMA = Phenylmercuric acetate.

HYDROGEN ION CONCENTRATION

The lacrimal secretion has a pH value between 7.2 and 7.4 and has a high buffering capacity. Consequently, the eye can tolerate solutions having a wide range of pH values from 3.5 to 10 provided they are not strongly buffered since the tears will rapidly restore the normal pH value of the eye.

Most drugs used in the eye are the salts of weak organic bases (e.g. alkaloids) and are stable at acid pH values. The degree of ionization is affected by the pH value and as this approaches neutrality, the concentration of the unionized organic base is increased. The free base is lipid soluble and will penetrate the cornea more readily than the ionized form of the drug. The therapeutic activity of eye drops may therefore be affected by the pH value but, for reasons of stability, this must usually be kept low.

TONICITY

It was formerly thought that, for reasons of comfort on instillation, eye drops should be made isotonic with the lacrimal secretion. However, it has been established that the eye can tolerate a range of tonicity from 0.5 to 2 per cent sodium chloride before discomfort is experienced. It is often the nature of the medicament itself which causes pain or stinging on instillation. Amethocaine hydrochloride, for example, has surface active properties which cause pain when solutions are instilled into the eye and for this reason concentrations above 1 per cent should not be used. There is now no general requirement in the *British Pharmaceutical Codex* for eye drops to be made isotonic.

VISCOSITY

Attempts have been made to prolong the contact time of the drug in the eye by increasing the viscosity of the vehicle. For this purpose, methylcellulose has been incorporated into eye drops but it is unlikely that the increase in viscosity has any material effect on the efficacy or duration of action of the medicament.

Hypromellose Eye Drops BPC, contain hydroxypropylmethylcellulose which has been selected for the purpose because it produces clearer solutions than methylcellulose. Hypromellose eye drops are intended for use as a substitute for tears in eye conditions in which the lachrymal secretion is deficient. They may also be used as a contact lens solution but may need diluting when used for this purpose. Hypromellose eye drops cannot be used as a general vehicle for eye drops since incompatibilities may arise between the medicament and the bactericide or the hydroxypropylmethylcellulose. Solutions containing cellulose derivatives are coagulated on heat sterilization but will usually go back into solution if shaken while cooling. However, there is usually some reduction in viscosity.

EYE DROP CONTAINERS

For use in hospital practice during and after surgery on the eye, eye drops should be dispensed in single-dose containers. Eye drops which are used in damaged eyes (e.g. fluorescein) should be similarly dispensed. In such a container, there is no necessity for eye drops to contain a bactericide and it should be remembered that solutions used during surgery must not contain any added antimicrobial substance.

Multi-dose containers. For domiciliary use and for intact eyes in hospital practice, eye drops are dispensed in multi-dose containers. The conventional type of eye drop bottle is made of glass and is closed by a screw-cap through which the eye dropper and teat are inserted. The *British Pharmaceutical Codex* specifies that such containers should comply with British Standard 1679: Part 5: 1965. This requires that the bottle is amber coloured, vertically ribbed and made of neutral glass or soda glass which has been surface treated to limit the amount of alkali released into aqueous solutions. The surface treated bottles are known as 'one trip' bottles and should not be autoclaved more than once. Glass droppers are made of neutral glass and the rubber teats must be capable of withstanding autoclaving on one occasion and must not release alkali or other impurities during use. The caps into which the teats are inserted may be made of aluminium or a suitable plastic.

Natural rubber teats not infrequently give rise to difficulty. Certain batches may not withstand autoclaving on a single occasion, while others may be incompatible with the bactericide. On autoclaving in the presence of benzalkonium chloride, they may produce a cloudy solution possibly due to the leaching out of stearates from the rubber. Silicone rubber teats are less likely to absorb the bactericide from solution (see below). Unfortunately, they are considerably more expensive than natural rubber teats and allow considerable loss of water vapour on storage.

Eye drops may also be dispensed with an ordinary screw-cap closure and the sterile dropper provided separately in a suitable pack to maintain sterility. This method of presentation may be adopted to overcome the difficulty of incompatibility between the bactericide and the rubber closure, in which case the rubber liner of the screw-cap must be protected by a disc of ethylene terephthalate ('Melinex'). This method presents practical difficulties since ethylene terephthalate is available only in sheet form and the discs must be hand-cut. Eye drops may also be dispensed in this manner in hospital practice so that a supply of wrapped sterile droppers may be issued with them and a new sterile dropper used every time the drops are applied to the eye in order to minimize the risk of infection.

Aluminium or other metal screw-caps are unsuitable if a phenylmercuric salt is used as the bactericide because of the possibility of chemical interaction.

The *British Pharmaceutical Codex* also permits the use of 'suitable plastics containers' for eye drops. Such containers must be compatible with the preparation and not release undesirable materials (e.g. plasticizers), into the solution. Containers made of nylon have been used for eye drops and are generally satisfactory, but elderly patients may have difficulty in using them to instil the drops into the eye. They are used for some proprietary presentations of eye drops.

PREPARATION OF EYE DROPS

An account of the small scale preparation of eye drops has been given by Smith (1967). The general precautions with regard to cleanliness of apparatus, working environment etc. are the same as those for parenteral solutions.

Containers

Glass containers must be thoroughly cleansed by rinsing in detergent solution and purified water. Rubber teats must also be cleansed by boiling in water and detergent followed by rinsing in purified water. They are then impregnated with the bactericide to be used by autoclaving in a closed container in a solution containing twice the concentration of bactericide used in the eye drops and storing them in this solution for 7 days before use. It is preferable to have a stock of rubber teats all ready for use stored in closed screw-cap jars containing each of the bactericides used in the *British Pharmaceutical Codex*.

The absorption of bactericides from the solution varies with the quality of the rubber. Natural rubber teats absorb all these bactericides readily from aqueous solution. Silicone rubber teats do not absorb appreciable amounts of chlorhexidine acetate and benzalkonium chloride but readily absorb phenylmercuric salts. As mentioned above, benzalkonium chloride may extract stearates from certain grades of natural rubber teats.

Most eye drops are simple solutions in water which should be clarified by filtration before filling into the containers. The *British Pharmaceutical*

Codex limits the volume to be supplied in each container to 10 ml so that the eye drops are not in use over too long a period of time.

Sterilization

The sterilization procedures are the same as those applied to parenteral solutions, which should prove no problem in a well-equipped hospital pharmacy. In general practice pharmacy, it may be necessary to obtain a small, electrically heated autoclave especially for the extemporaneous preparation of eye drops. A suitable autoclave is obtainable from Jacob White and Co. Ltd and is illustrated in Fig. 27.1.

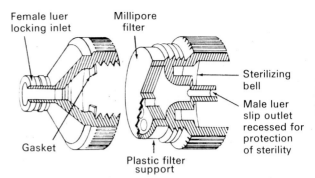

FIG. 27.2. Swinnex-25 filtration unit (Millipore).

after clarification is sucked up into a syringe (preferably a sterile plastics disposable syringe). The plastic bag holding the Swinnex unit is opened by means of sterile scissors and, with aseptic precautions, the unit is attached to the syringe and a sterile needle is fixed to the other end of the unit. The solution is then forced through the membrane filter into a previously sterilized eye drop bottle by pushing down the plunger of the syringe. The closure is immediately placed on the bottle. It is essential that all operations are carried out as rapidly as possible to minimize the risks of contamination.

Labelling

Eye drops which are not issued to the user (i.e. purchased from a pharmaceutical manufacturer) should state: (1) the concentration of the active ingredient, and (2) the name and concentration of the antimicrobial substance used in the eye drops.

It is customary in hospital practice for this information also to be stated on eye drops issued to patients for domiciliary use.

Eye drops which are not extemporaneously dispensed should have a readily breakable seal over the closure to indicate that the container has not been opened. In hospital practice, this usually takes the form of a Viscose ring.

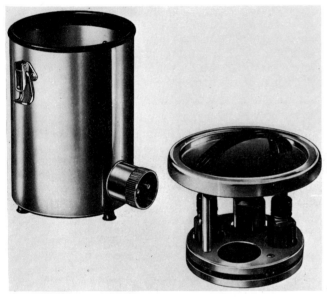

FIG. 27.1. Electrically heated autoclave for small scale preparation of eye drops.

Sterilization by filtration may also be a problem in general practice pharmacy, particularly for the extemporaneous preparation of sodium sulphacetamide eye drops. The small scale preparation of eye drops by filtration has been outlined by Smith (1967) who describes different kinds of modified syringes which can be used to sterilize small volumes of aqueous solutions. The most satisfactory is probably the Swinnex filter unit (Fig. 27.2) which is available pre-sterilized from Millipore U.K. Ltd. Swinnex filter units are available in two sizes (filter diameters 13 or 25 mm) and the membrane filters in two porosities (0.45 and 0.22 μm). The smaller diameter filter is usually adequate for eye drops and it is safer to use the lower porosity membrane, although filtration may be slower.

Using a pre-sterilized Swinnex unit, the solution

EYE LOTIONS

The *British Pharmaceutical Codex* defines eye lotions as either (1) sterile aqueous solutions containing no bactericide for first-aid purposes over a maximum period of 24 h, or (2) aqueous solutions containing a bactericide for intermittent domiciliary administration for up to 7 days. They therefore have only a limited use nowadays, but may nevertheless occasionally be prescribed. Sodium bicarbonate eye lotion is used for the emergency treatment of acid burns of the eye and is known as 'Factory Eye Drops No. 2'. Sodium chloride eye lotion is an isotonic solution which is occasionally used for irrigating the eye. Both these preparations are prepared by conventional sterilization procedures.

Occasionally, a prescription for the older type of eye lotion may be received. This consisted of a solution which the patient was directed to dilute with an equal volume of water for use in an eye bath. When such preparations are prescribed nowadays, they should be issued as sterile solutions even though the patient cannot maintain the sterility of the preparation during use. An example of this type of eye lotion is given by the following prescription:

R Boric acid 2 per cent
   Zinc sulphate 0.4 per cent
   Purified water to 100
   Send 200 ml
   Label: Use with equal volume of warm water in an eye bath

The zinc sulphate and the boric acid are dissolved in purified water, the solution is clarified by filtration and transferred to a fluted bottle, closed with a screw-cap and sterilized by heating in an autoclave.

The patient should be instructed to avoid contamination of the solution during use as far as possible (see also below).

Containers for Eye Lotions

Eye lotions are dispensed in coloured fluted bottles closed with a screw-cap. It is important to ensure that the liner of the screw-cap is not made of cork since this may be a source of microbial contamination. Rubber or plastics liners are suitable and the screw-cap may be either of metal or plastics. Uncoloured or non-fluted bottles may be used if a suitable coloured, fluted bottle is not available.

Labelling

In addition to the words 'For external use only', eye lotions which are used for first-aid purposes (e.g. sodium bicarbonate eye lotion) should be labelled to indicate that the preparation should be used on one occasion only, e.g. with the words 'Discard any lotion remaining after use when the seal is first broken'.

Eye lotions which are issued for domiciliary purposes should be labelled to indicate that they are not to be used more than 24 h (or 7 days if a bactericide is added) after first opening the container, e.g. with the words 'Discard any lotion remaining 24 hours after the container has been first opened'.

EYE OINTMENTS

Eye ointments are required by the *British Pharmacopoeia* to be sterile and as their preparation involves aseptic handling using a previously sterilized medicament, they are seldom dispensed extemporaneously.

Eye ointment basis of the *British Pharmacopoeia* consists of a mixture of 80 per cent of yellow soft paraffin with 10 per cent of liquid paraffin and 10 per cent of wool fat. It is prepared by melting the constituents together, filtering through a coarse filter paper in a heated funnel and sterilizing at 150° for 1 h. It is stored in containers sealed so as to exclude microorganisms before use.

Preparation of Eye Ointment

The *British Pharmaceutical Codex* describes two alternative procedures for the preparation of eye ointments. Aseptic precautions must be observed throughout.

Water-soluble medicaments. Medicaments which are readily soluble in water are dissolved in the minimum quantity of purified water. The solution is sterilized by heating in an autoclave or by filtration and the sterile solution incorporated into the melted, previously sterilized basis by stirring until cold and observing aseptic precautions. The preparation is then transferred to previously sterilized eye ointment tubes which are immediately closed so as to exclude microorganisms. Many medicaments used in eye ointments are thermolabile and in these circumstances filtration is used for sterilization.

Insoluble medicaments. In this method, it is essential to use a previously sterilized sample of the medicament. Observing aseptic precautions, the medicament is finely powdered and triturated with a small quantity of the melted, previously sterilized basis. The mixture is then incorporated with the remainder of the melted basis and the eye ointment transferred to sterile eye ointment tubes which are sealed immediately so as to exclude microorganisms. It is essential that an insoluble medicament should be finely powdered so as to exclude the possibility of a large particle of the drug being introduced into the eye.

Containers for Eye Ointments

Eye ointments should be packed in collapsible metal or plastics tubes or in single-dose containers. Plastics tubes are used for some proprietary formulations of eye ointments but there are no standard empty containers of this type available for dispensing purposes.

Collapsible metal tubes should as far as possible be freed from dust and metal particles before use. This is probably the best achieved by blowing the tubes out with a powerful jet of filtered, dust-free air. Washing the tubes is less effective and often adds more particles than it removes. It has been found that, with present methods of manufacture, it is impossible to produce collapsible metal tubes which are completely particle-free and all the particles may not be removed by cleansing. The particles are not removed until they undergo the shearing action of the ointment as it is expressed from the tubes. Following reports of the occurrence of metal particles in eye ointments, a British Standard was devised to limit the particles present in tubes used for eye ointments. Metal tubes used for dispensing eye ointments must comply with the requirements of British Standard 4230: 1967.

Certain proprietary formulations of eye ointments are available in single-dose containers. These take the form of an elongated, flexible gelatin capsule with one end constricted, and are opened by cutting off the constricted end with sterile scissors.

The container of eye ointments, which are not extemporaneously dispensed, should be enclosed in a readily breakable sealed package to indicate that it has not previously been opened. This can take the form of a sealed paper or plastic envelope or a sealed carton.

Labelling
The *British Pharmaceutical Codex* requires that the label on the tube or outer sealed envelope (except one issued on prescription) should state that the contents are sterile provided that the container has not been opened.

REFERENCES

BROWN, M. R. W. & NORTON, D. A. (1965) *J. Soc. Cosm. Chem.* **16**, 369–387.

SMITH, G. (1967) *Pharm. J.* **198**, 55–61.

TRIGGER, D. J. & CALDWELL, A. D. S. (1968) *J. Hosp. Pharm.* **25**, 259–265.

British Standard 4230 (1967).

Part IV

RADIOACTIVITY

28

Radioisotopes

RADIOACTIVITY AND RADIONUCLIDES: ELEMENTS OF NUCLEAR PHYSICS

DEFINITIONS

The atomic number (Z) is the number of protons in the nucleus.

A nucleon is a heavy nuclear particle of any type (proton or neutron).

The mass number (A) is the total number of nucleons in a nucleus.

A nuclide is a nuclear species characterized by the magnitudes of its atomic and mass numbers. Nuclides may be stable or unstable and unstable nuclides are radioactive (radionuclides). The correct convention for the representation of nuclides is: ^A_Z chemical symbol. However the atomic number is implicit in the chemical symbol and is usually omitted. When speaking of a nuclide the mass number follows the name of the element e.g. ^{226}Ra is described in speech as radium-226.

^1H, ^2H, ^{12}C, ^{23}Na are stable nuclides.

^3H, ^{14}C, ^{22}Na, ^{24}Na are radionuclides.

An isotope is one of a series of nuclides with the same atomic number, e.g. ^1H, ^2H, ^3H are isotopes of hydrogen of which only ^3H (tritium) is radioactive; ^{10}C, ^{11}C, ^{12}C, ^{13}C, ^{14}C are isotopes of carbon of which ^{10}C, ^{11}C and ^{14}C are radioactive.

The electronvolt (eV) is the unit of energy used for radiations and 1 eV is the energy acquired by an electron when accelerated through a potential difference of 1 V. This amount of energy is very small, so the energies of particles are usually given in terms of MeV or KeV:

$$1 \text{ MeV} = 10^3 \text{ KeV} = 10^6 \text{ eV} = 1.60 \times 10^{-6} \text{ erg}.$$

The atomic mass unit (a.m.u.) is the unit of physical atomic weights and 1 a.m.u. is one-twelfth of the mass of the carbon-12 atom:

$$1 \text{ a.m.u.} = 1.66035 \times 10^{-24} \text{ g}.$$

All matter has an energy equivalent (given by the Einstein equation $E = mc^2$). Thus:

$$1 \text{ g of matter (at rest)} \equiv 5.61 \times 10^{26} \text{ MeV},$$

$$1 \text{ a.m.u.} \equiv 931 \text{ MeV}$$

GENERAL REVIEW OF NUCLEAR STRUCTURE

Elementary Particles
A large number of these particles exist and the properties of those which are of interest here are given in Table 28.1. These particles may exist in the nucleus or be emitted from it.

A Picture of the Nucleus
The charge is positive and dependent on the atomic number.

Size. The nuclear radius is the distance from the centre of the nucleus over which the intranuclear forces are effective and is of the order of 1 to 9 × 10^{-13} cm, about one 10000th of the atomic radius.

Mass. Most of the mass of the atom is concentrated in the nucleus which thus has a 'density', a concept of doubtful validity in this context, of about 10^{14} g per cm^3.

TABLE 28.1

THE PROPERTIES OF SOME ELEMENTARY PARTICLES

Particle	Symbol	Charge	Rest mass (a.m.u.)	Stability
Proton	p	$+1$	1.00759	Stable
Neutron	n	0	1.00898	Unstable
Negatron	e^- β^- (from the nucleus)	-1	0.00055	Stable
Positron	β^+	$+1$	0.00055	Unstable
Neutrino Antineutrino	v	0	$<1 \times 10^{-6}$	Stable

Nuclear Stability

A convenient analogy has been drawn between the nucleus and a drop of liquid, the nucleons being envisaged as being in a state of continual motion, as are the molecules in a liquid. Thus the energy of the individual nucleons is changing continually. In a stable nucleus the energy distribution is such that none of the nucleons acquires sufficient energy to undergo transformation or to escape from the nucleus. However with radionuclides this energy barrier is overcome and the energy distribution of the nucleons determines whether a particular nucleus will undergo transformation or not and, within limits, the way in which the transformation will occur. To extend the analogy, it is a common experience, e.g. with mercury, that small drops of a liquid are stable and coherent when subjected to mechanical shock, whereas large drops tend to be unstable and break up. This latter type of situation occurs with very large nuclei, all of which are unstable above atomic number 82 and many of these emit α-particles.

The intranuclear forces are very short range, exchange type forces which are attractive and virtually independent of the charge on a nucleon, i.e. they are similar for n–n, n–p and p–p interactions. Although the electrostatic repulsion in the p–p interaction is outweighed by the total effect of the attractive forces, the repulsive effect is not lost and becomes increasingly important as the number of protons increases. To maintain stability extra neutrons are required so that the total attractive nuclear force is increased and repulsions are overcome.

Fig. 28.1 shows the relationship between the numbers of neutrons and protons for maximum stability. Stable nuclides have a neutron–proton ratio of 1.0 at low atomic numbers, e.g. $^{6}_{3}\text{Li}$, $^{12}_{6}\text{C}$,

$^{20}_{10}\text{Ne}$, and the ratio tends to about 1.5 at high atomic numbers, e.g. $^{55}_{25}\text{Mn}$, 1.20; $^{89}_{39}\text{Y}$, 1.28; $^{127}_{55}\text{I}$, 1.4; $^{181}_{73}\text{Ta}$, 1.47; $^{208}_{82}\text{Pb}$, 1.54. Nuclides with a sufficient neutron excess or deficiency are unstable (radioactive) and generally the greater the excess or deficiency the greater the instability. The degree of instability is reflected in the rate of decay, e.g. for fluorine, stable mass number 19, the relative rates of decay of its four radioactive isotopes ^{17}F, ^{18}F, ^{20}F, ^{21}F are respectively 92, 1, 547 and 1250. Decay always produces a change which results in a nuclear configuration of greater stability.

Binding energy. The binding energy is the energy which binds the individual nucleons in a coherent unit and may be calculated as the energy change resulting from combining the individual particles comprising an atom.

If ΔE = binding energy
M_a = exact mass of the atom in a.m.u.
M_p = mass of a separate proton
M_e = mass of a separate electron
M_n = mass of a separate neutron

then,

$$\Delta E = 931 \left[M_a - Z(M_p + M_e) - M_n(A-Z) \right] \text{ MeV.}$$

Since the mass of an atom is always less than the sum of its constituent particles (the difference is the *mass defect*) ΔE is negative. The relationship between the average binding energy per nucleon ($\Delta E/A$) and the mass number is given in Fig. 28.2 which shows that the binding energy is the source of the energy released in atomic fission, in which a large nucleus splits into two smaller ones, and in the atomic fusion reaction, in which deuterium

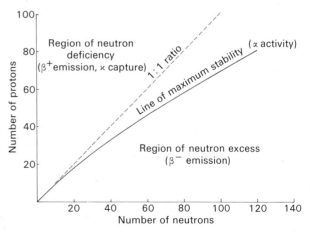

FIG. 28.1. The relationship between the numbers of neutrons and protons for nuclear stability.

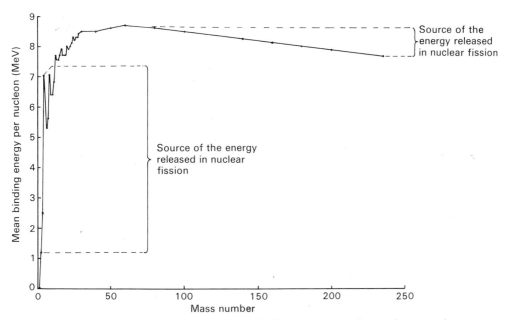

FIG. 28.2. The relationship between the mean binding energy per nucleon and mass number.

is converted into helium. Clearly the latter process is inherently a much greater source of energy than the former.

RADIOACTIVITY

Definition
Radioactivity is the spontaneous transformation of one nucleus into another and is accompanied by the emission of characteristic particles (negatrons, positrons, α-particles, neutrons) or electromagnetic radiation.

The process is completely random and is unaffected by external conditions of temperature, pressure, etc., since the energy which can be applied to the nucleus from outside is very small relative to that required to produce nuclear transformations.

Radioactive Decay
In any given population of nuclei there is a finite probability that a given nucleus will disintegrate in a given time. The probability of decay in unit time is the *decay constant* (λ).

If there are N_0 radioactive atoms present initially and dN of these decay in a time dt then:

$$dN/dt = -\lambda N_0. \qquad (28.1)$$

The function dN/dt is the rate of decay, observed as nuclear disintegrations, and is referred to as the *activity* and measured in disintegrations per second (dps) or disintegrations per minute (dpm).

Integrating equation (28.1) gives:

$$N_t = N_0 e^{-\lambda t} \qquad (28.2)$$

where N_t is the number of atoms present at time t and e is the base of natural logarithms.

Half-life. The half-life ($t_{1/2}$) is the time taken for the activity to decay to one half of its initial value.

If $N_t/N_0 = 0.5$ then, from equation (28.2)

$$e^{-\lambda t} = 0.5 \qquad (28.3)$$

and

$$t = \log_e 2/\lambda = 0.693/\lambda = t_{1/2}. \qquad (28.4)$$

Equation (28.2) is a first order exponential function so that if the logarithm of the activity is plotted against time a straight line results with a slope of $-\lambda$. This is illustrated in Fig. 28.3 which also shows the half-life relationship.

Both λ and $t_{1/2}$ are constants which characterize the rate of decay, but $t_{1/2}$ is the more convenient for general use. If $t_{1/2}$ is known the activity of a sample at any time after initial calibration may be calculated. If the initial activity is I_0 then after one half-life ($1 \times t_{1/2}$) the residual activity (I) is $I_0/2$; after $2 \times t_{1/2}$, $I = I_0/4 = I_0/2^2$; after $3 \times t_{1/2}$, $I = I_0/8 = I_0/2^3$; after $m \times t_{1/2}$, $I = I_0/2^m$. For example, (a) for ^{32}P, $t_{1/2} = 14.3$ days and exactly 3 weeks after calibration the activity is $I_0/2^{(21/14.3)} = 0.3613 I_0$,

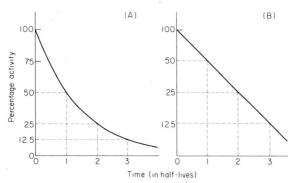

FIG. 28.3. The decay of activity with time; A, arithmetic scale; B, semi-logarithmic scale.

(b) for ^{24}Na, $t_{1/2} = 15.0$ h and exactly 3 weeks after calibration the activity is $I_o/2^{(504/15)} = 7.7 \times 10^{-11} I_o$. Thus if a reasonable excess of activity was present initially the ^{32}P material would still be usable after 3 weeks, whereas there is no possibility of continuing to use a sample of ^{24}Na after the same elapsed time. This is obviously important in the planning of experiments and the maintenance of stocks.

The determination of residual activity after a period of decay may be done graphically (Fig. 28.4) if precise results are not required, but direct calculation or reference to prepared tables (e.g. Table 28.2) is essential for accuracy.

Radioactive equilibria. The situation in which a radionuclide decays to give a radioactive daughter nuclide, which itself decays in turn occurs frequently, e.g. in the natural radioactive series. Taking the simplest case of the daughter decaying to a stable nuclide, the basic rate equation for the daughter is:

$$dN_D/dt = \lambda_P N_P - \lambda_D N_D \quad (28.5)$$

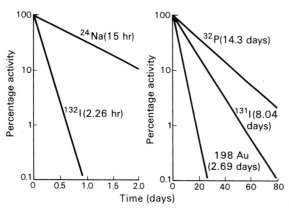

FIG. 28.4. Decay curves, with half-lives, of some common radionuclides.

where N_P, N_D are the numbers of parent and daughter atoms and λ_P, λ_D are their respective decay constants. Thus the net rate of change of the number of daughter atoms is the difference between the rate of production from the parent and the rate of decay of the daughter.

Integrating equation (28.5), assuming the case of a pure parent in which there are no daughter atoms at zero time, gives:

$$N_D = \frac{\lambda_P (N_P)_o}{\lambda_D - \lambda_P} (e^{-\lambda_P t} - e^{-\lambda_D t}) \quad (28.6)$$

where $(N_P)_o$ is the number of parent atoms at zero time and t is the elapsed time. If I_P, I_D are the respective activities, equation (28.6) may be written:

$$I_D = \frac{\lambda_D (I_P)_o}{\lambda_D - \lambda_P} (e^{-\lambda_P t} - e^{\lambda_D t}) \quad (28.7)$$

or

$$I_D = \frac{T_P (I_P)_o}{T_P - T_D} (e^{-\lambda_P t} - e^{-\lambda_D t}) \quad (28.8)$$

where T_P, T_D are the half-lives of parent and daughter. If $T_P \gg T_D$ the term $e^{-\lambda_D t}$ approaches zero with increasing time much more rapidly than does $e^{-\lambda_P t}$, so that the relative amounts of parent and daughter activity reach an approximately constant value. Since $(I_P)_o e^{-\lambda_P t} = I_P$ and assuming the condition that $e^{-\lambda_D t} = 0$, this limiting condition is represented by the equation:

$$\frac{I_D}{I_P} = \frac{\lambda_D}{\lambda_D - \lambda_P} = \frac{T_P}{T_P - T_D} \quad (28.9)$$

which gives the relative activities of daughter and parent at the steady state, when the daughter is said to be in 'equilibrium' with the parent. Following attainment of equilibrium the total activity and the activities of the parent and daughter nuclides decay with the half-life of the parent.

If the half-life of the parent is very long, so that its decay is negligible the condition is known as *secular equilibrium* and this occurs with the natural radioactive series. When parent decay is appreciable the condition is known as *transient equilibrium*. The latter condition occurs in the series

$$^{132}\text{Te} \xrightarrow[\beta^-, \gamma]{78 \text{ h}} {}^{132}\text{I} \xrightarrow[\beta^-, \gamma]{2.3 \text{ h}} {}^{132}\text{Xe},$$

represented graphically in Fig. 28.5. This situation is utilized to store radionuclides of short half-life which otherwise could not be used, since their activity would decay virtually to zero during the time of processing and delivery. Thus ^{132}I is stored

TABLE 28.2

THE RESIDUAL ACTIVITIES OF RADIONUCLIDES AS A FUNCTION OF DECAY TIME

Decay time (half-lives)	0.00	0.02	0.04	0.06	0.08	0.10	0.12	0.14	0.16	0.18
0.0	1.000	0.986	0.973	0.959	0.946	0.933	0.920	0.908	0.895	0.883
0.2	0.871	0.859	0.847	0.835	0.824	0.812	0.801	0.790	0.779	0.768
0.4	0.758	0.747	0.737	0.727	0.717	0.707	0.697	0.688	0.678	0.669
0.6	0.660	0.651	0.642	0.633	0.624	0.616	0.607	0.599	0.591	0.582
0.8	0.574	0.566	0.559	0.551	0.543	0.536	0.529	0.521	0.514	0.507
1.0	0.500	0.493	0.486	0.480	0.473	0.467	0.460	0.454	0.448	0.441
1.2	0.435	0.429	0.423	0.418	0.412	0.406	0.401	0.395	0.390	0.384
1.4	0.379	0.374	0.369	0.364	0.359	0.354	0.349	0.344	0.339	0.335

	.0.00	0.05	0.10	0.15	0.20	0.25	0.30	0.35	0.40	0.45
1.5	0.354	0.342	0.330	0.319	0.308	0.297	0.287	0.277	0.268	0.259
2.0	0.250	0.242	0.233	0.225	0.218	0.210	0.203	0.196	0.190	0.183
2.5	0.177	0.171	0.165	0.159	0.154	0.149	0.144	0.139	0.134	0.129
3.0	0.125	0.121	0.117	0.113	0.109	0.105	0.102	0.098	0.095	0.092
3.5	0.0884	0.0854	0.0825	0.0797	0.0770	0.0743	0.0718	0.0693	0.0670	0.0647
4.0	0.0625	—	0.0583	—	0.0544	—	0.0508	—	0.0474	—
4.5	0.0442	—	0.0412	—	0.0385	—	0.0359	—	0.0335	—

The table gives the fraction of the initial activity present after decay. For example to determine the activity of a source of ^{32}P ($t_{1/2}$, 14.3 day), initial activity 3.1 mCi, after 10 days 6 h.

$$10 \text{ days } 6 \text{ h} = 10.25 \text{ days} = \frac{10.25}{14.3} \text{ half-lives} = 0.717 \text{ half-lives}.$$

From the table the residual activity after 0.7 half-lives is 0.616 and that after 0.72 half-lives is 0.607.
Interpolating, after 0.717 half-lives the residual activity is 0.615.
Therefore the activity of the source is 3.1×0.615 mCi = 1.91 mCi.
(Reproduced by permission of the Radiochemical Centre, Amersham.)

in the form of an equilibrium mixture of $^{132}Te + $ ^{132}I adsorbed on an alumina column and the ^{132}I is eluted with a mixture of 0.01 mol/l NH_4OH plus 0.01 mol/l $Na_2S_2O_3$ as required. Fig. 28.5 shows that, following elution, a further slightly smaller amount of ^{132}I can be eluted after approximately 12 h and this process may be repeated until the ^{132}Te activity has decayed to too low a level, usually 14 days. Similar procedures are used to supply ^{113m}In (half-life 99.5 min), ^{87m}Sr (2.8 h) and ^{99m}Tc (6 h). A ^{99m}Tc radionuclide generator is illustrated in Fig. 28.6.

Determination of half-lives. If measurable decay occurs in a reasonable time the half-life may be determined by measuring the activity of a sample at intervals over a period. For accuracy the period of observation should extend over about 5 half-lives and there should be no appreciable decay during the time required to make each measurement. The slope of the best straight line which fits the data (the logarithm of the activity against time) is calculated to give the value of the decay constant, from which the half-life can be calculated using

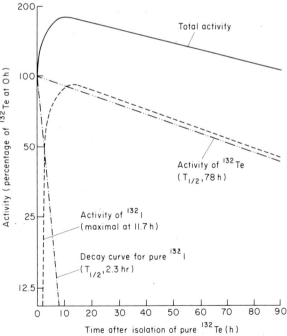

FIG. 28.5. Transient equilibrium in the system $^{132}Te \rightarrow {}^{132}I$.

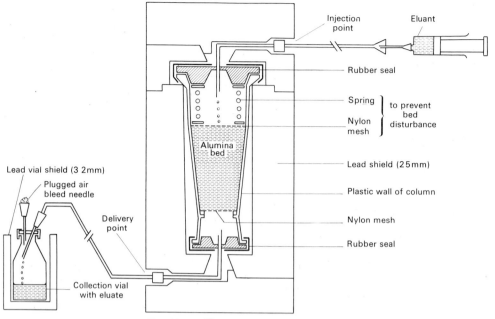

FIG. 28.6. A ^{99m}Te radionuclide generator.

equation (28.4). Alternatively, but less accurately, the logarithm of the activity can be plotted against time, the best line fitted by eye, and the half-life measured or calculated using the equation:

$$t_{1/2} = \frac{0.3010t}{\log_{10} I_o - \log_{10} I_t}, \quad (28.10)$$

where I_o is the initial activity and I_t is the activity after a time t; I_o, I_t and t may be measured from the graph.

Very short or very long half-lives require special techniques for their determination.

A source of error in decay curves is the presence of a second component of different half-life and this results in a curve instead of a straight line (Fig. 28.7). Provided that the half-lives of the two components are sufficiently different the contribution of the shorter lived component becomes negligible and the curve becomes the straight line which characterizes the decay of the longer lived component. This system can be resolved by subtracting the theoretical values for the longer lived component (Fig. 28.7, line CBD) from the observed curve (ABC); this gives the decay curve of the shorter lived component (EF).

Units of Radioactivity

The unit used is the *Curie* (Ci) which is that quantity of any radionuclide which undergoes 3.70×10^{10} disintegrations per second (dps).

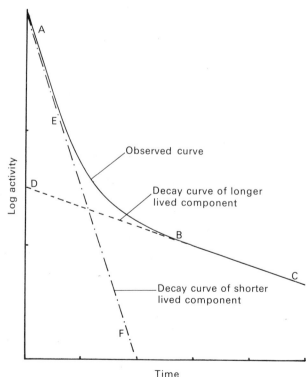

FIG. 28.7. Decay curve of a binary mixture.

The curie is an excessively large unit for most purposes so it is subdivided into the *millicurie* (1 mCi $= 10^{-3}$ Ci $= 3.7 \times 10^7$ dps $= 2.22 \times 10^9$ dpm) and the *microcurie* (1 μCi $= 10^{-6}$ Ci $= 10^{-3}$ mCi $= 3.7 \times 10^4$ dps $= 2.22 \times 10^6$ dpm).

The curie derives from the activity of 1 g of radium in equilibrium with its daughter products, an amount of activity slightly less than the curie as now defined.

The *specific activity* refers both to the proportion of radioactive atoms in an isotope preparation, usually given in terms of mCi/mM, and to the amount of activity in 1 g or 1 ml of a preparation.

The percentage of radionuclide in an isotope preparation can be calculated from the expression:

$$\frac{\text{Specific activity (mCi/mg) of preparation} \times 100}{\text{Specific activity (mCi/mg) of pure radionuclide}} \%$$

The denominator of this expression is calculated as follows.

Specific activity of pure radionuclide

$$= \frac{0.693N}{3.7 \times 10^{10} TA} \text{mCi/mg} = \frac{1.123 \times 10^{13}}{TA} \text{mCi/mg},$$

where T is the half-life in seconds, A is the mass number and N is Avogadro's Number.

MODES OF NUCLEAR DECAY

Alpha-Decay (α-emission)
This occurs with large nuclei, predominantly with nuclides of atomic number greater than 82. It involves the emission of an α-particle (helium nucleus, $^4_2$He), for example,

$$^{226}\text{Ra} \longrightarrow {}^{222}\text{Rn} + {}^4\text{He}$$

Because the α-particle has a mass of about 4 a.m.u. and carries 2 unit positive charges the transformation involves a reduction in both the atomic and mass numbers. The α-particles are emitted with discrete energies, i.e. all the particles emitted from a particular nuclide have the same energy, which is characteristic of that nuclear transformation. The particle energy is related to the decay constant according to the Geiger–Nuttall rule:

$$\log \lambda = A + B \log E,$$

where A and B are constants for the given transformation. Thus nuclides with a short half-life emit particles of greater energy.

Beta-Decay
Negatron emission. Nuclei with excess neutrons gain stability by the conversion of a neutron into a proton plus a β^--particle. The latter are fast negatrons, carrying a unit charge, and possess all the characteristics of normal negatrons, being called β^- particles solely because they are emitted from the nucleus. Since the β^--particle has a very low mass there is no change in the mass number, but the atomic number increases by one unit, for example,

$$^{32}_{15}\text{P} \xrightarrow{\beta^-} {}^{32}_{16}\text{S}$$

$$^{90}_{38}\text{Sr} \xrightarrow{\beta^-} {}^{90}_{39}\text{Y} \xrightarrow{\beta^-} {}^{90}_{40}\text{Zr}$$

The β^--particles emitted in any given nuclear transformation have a continuous energy spectrum (Fig. 28.8) and may have any energy up to a

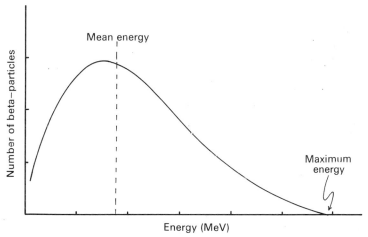

FIG. 28.8. The energy spectrum of β-particles from a pure β-emitter.

maximum (E_{max}) which is characteristic of the nuclide undergoing decay. The values quoted for β^--particle energies are always those of E_{max}. Since the total energy change for a given nuclear transformation must be constant, there must be some means of conserving parity when β^--particles are emitted with energies below E_{max}. This is achieved by the emission of a neutrino (v) which carries the difference between E_{max} and the energy of the β^--particle so that

$$E_\beta + E_v = E_{max}$$

where E_β, E_v are the energies of the β^--particle and the neutrino. Thus the conversion of neutrons into protons may be represented as follows:

$$n \longrightarrow p + \beta^- + v.$$

The neutrinos have extremely small rest mass and no charge and so are not detected by normal counting equipment.

The mean energy of β^--particles falls approximately in the range 0.3 to 0.4 E_{max} (Table 28.3) and

TABLE 28.3

THE MAXIMUM AND MEAN β^--PARTICLE ENERGIES FOR SOME RADIONUCLIDES

Nuclide	β^--energy (MeV) Maximum (E_{max})	Mean ($\bar{E}$)	Ratio ($\bar{E}/E_{max}$)
^{14}C	0.159	0.050	0.31
^{22}Na	0.54	0.225	0.39
^{24}Na	1.39	0.540	0.40
^{32}P	1.71	0.70	0.40
^{36}Cl	0.714	0.30	0.42
^{60}Co	0.31	0.10	0.32
^{82}Br	0.44	0.14	0.32
^{85}Kr	0.67	0.22	0.33
^{89}Sr	1.46	0.56	0.38
^{133}Xe	0.34	0.13	0.38
^{203}Hg	0.21	0.097	0.46
^{210}Bi	1.17	0.33	0.28

(Reproduced by permission of the Radiochemical Centre, Amersham).

is used to calculate the energy absorbed in a system, for example, the radiation dose to a patient in diagnostic or therapeutic procedures using radionuclides. The magnitude of E_{max} determines the maximum range of the β^--particles in matter. There is a relationship between the half-life and the maximum energy given by the expression:

$$t_{1/2} E_{max}^5 = C,$$

where C is a constant. The value of this constant falls into three groups with approximate ratios $1:10:10^2$; nuclear transformations with the smallest

values (and shortest half-lives) are described as *allowed transitions*, i.e. most likely to disintegrate, and those with the higher values are known as *first forbidden* and *second forbidden* transitions. Thus, within each level of forbiddenness, the shorter the half-life the greater the particle energy, a situation qualitatively similar to that which occurs with α-decay.

Positron (β^+) emission. This process is the converse of β^--emission and occurs with neutron deficient nuclei, the deficiency being rectified by the conversion of a proton into a neutron plus a positron. As with β^--emission, positrons are emitted with a continuous energy spectrum and energy conservation is achieved by the emission of an anti-neutrino,*

$$p \longrightarrow n + \beta^+ + v.$$

There is no change in mass number but the atomic number is reduced by one unit, for example,

$$^{22}_{11}Na \xrightarrow{\beta^+} {}^{22}_{10}Ne$$
$$^{58}_{27}Co \xrightarrow{\beta^+} {}^{58}_{26}Fe.$$

Positrons have a very brief existence ($t_{1/2} \sim 10^{-10}$ s) and rapidly annihilate with negatrons to yield two γ-rays each of 0.51 MeV in opposite directions.

$$0.51\ MeV\gamma$$
$$\beta^+ + e^- \rightarrow \quad 180°$$
$$0.51\ MeV\gamma$$

These γ-rays are referred to as the *annihilation radiation* and result from the conversion of the rest masses of the negatron and positron (0.00055 a.m.u. each $\equiv$ 0.51 MeV) into radiant energy.

Electron Capture (EC, K-capture)

This is an alternative form of decay to β^+-emission with neutron deficient nuclei and involves the conversion of a proton into a neutron by capture of an orbital electron (negatron),

$$p + e^- \longrightarrow n.$$

Electron capture may occur concurrently with β^+-emission as an alternative process or as the sole mode of decay when the available energy is less than the 1.02 MeV (0.51 + 0.51 MeV) which is the minimum required for β^+-emission to occur.

The principal source of capture negatrons is from

* Most elementary particles have complementary anti-particles. The difference may be primarily one of charge, as with electrons and positrons, or may result from opposite directions of spin.

the K shell of the atom (hence K-capture) but L shell negatrons may also be captured. In either case capture causes a deficiency in the K or L shells which is made good by the migration of a negatron from one of the outer shells. Since the migrant negatron loses energy in the process, the surplus energy is emitted in the form of X-rays of an energy characteristic of the *product* atom, for example,

$$\ce{^{55}_{26}Fe} + e^- \longrightarrow \ce{^{55}_{25}Mn} + 0.0059 \text{ MeV Mn X-rays,}$$

$$\ce{^{49}_{23}Va} + e^- \longrightarrow \ce{^{49}_{22}Ti} + 0.0045 \text{ MeV Ti X-rays.}$$

The X-rays are characteristic of the product atom since once electron capture has occurred the original nucleus is converted into the product nucleus and negatron migration follows.

As with positron emission the mass number remains unchanged but the atomic number is reduced by unity.

Nuclear Fission

The liquid drop analogy discussed above indicates that large nuclei tend to be unstable and split into two fragments. Although this process can occur spontaneously it is extremely slow and for natural uranium the process has a half-life of about 0.9×10^6 years. However, if large nuclei are irradiated with neutrons of sufficient energy the resultant neutron capture results in a very high degree of instability and fission occurs immediately. This process is the basis of operation of the nuclear reactor (see below), in which a sufficient bulk of fissile material (^{235}U or ^{239}Pu) is brought together so that the neutrons emitted in the occasional spontaneous fission have a high probability of capture by other nuclei. The latter disintegrate promptly to yeild neutrons which are captured in turn, resulting in a self-sustaining chain reaction.

Processes Accompanying Decay

The production of annihilation radiation following β^+-emission and of X-rays after electron capture have been described above and will not be discussed further.

Gamma-emission. Gamma-emission is not usually a form of nuclear transformation but may follow other forms of decay. If the product nucleus is left in an excited state the surplus energy is lost by the emission of one or more γ-rays (electromagnetic radiation of high energy), so that the final energy of the product nucleus is at its ground state (see Fig. 28.8). The γ-rays are emitted with fixed, discrete energies; there is no energy spectrum such as occurs with β^--particles.

Isomeric transition. In some cases radioactive nuclei, in addition to their inherent instability, exist in an excited or *metastable* state which persists for some time. Such nuclides are distinguished by the addition of the letter 'm' to the mass number (^{99m}Tc, ^{110m}Ag, ^{234m}Pa) and decay with different half-lives from the non-metastable nuclides:

Nuclide	Half-life
^{99}Tc	2.1×10^5 years
^{99m}Tc	6 h
^{110}Ag	24 s
^{110m}Ag	253 days
^{234}Pa	6.66 h
^{234m}Pa	1.18 min

Nuclides with the same mass and atomic numbers but different half-lives are described as *nuclear isomers*. This is the only decay process in which γ-rays may be emitted without the emission of particles.

Internal conversion (IC). When the energy of the γ-radiation emitted from a product nucleus is low, a proportion of the γ-rays may not be emitted as such but may react with orbital negatrons and eject them from the atom. Clearly, this process is most probable when the γ-energy (E_γ) is slightly greater than the binding energy of the negatron (E_{BE}). These negatrons are emitted with an energy (E_e) which is given by the expression:

$$E_e = E_\gamma - E_{BE}.$$

Since E_γ and E_{BE} are constants the value of E_e is constant so the negatrons produced by internal conversion are emitted with low, fixed, uniform energies and so are distinguishable from β^--particles, which have an energy spectrum.

Representation of Decay: Decay Schemes

These diagrams are a convenient way of indicating the processes which occur when a large population of nuclei decay. A few representative simple decay schemes are given in Fig. 28.9. The vertical distances represent the energy changes involved, slanting of a line to the right indicates the emission of a negative particle (β^--emission), slanting to the left indicates the emission of a positive particle (β^+- or α-emission) or electron capture, and since

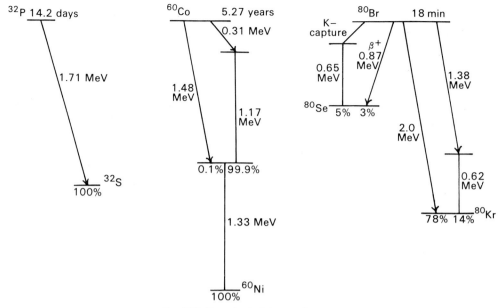

FIG. 28.9. Some typical decay schemes.

γ-emission does not involve the emission of charged particles or a change in atomic number this process is represented by vertical lines. Also the parent and product nuclides are indicated together with the energies involved and, where several modes of decay are possible, the percentage of nuclei disintegrating by each path.

The existence of alternative modes of decay results from the ways in which the energy may be distributed between the nucleons in a nucleus. The probability of the various energy distributions is reflected in the proportions of nuclei decaying by the different routes so that for any given radionuclide the percentages of nuclei decaying by these routes is constant. It should be noted that, whatever the mode of decay, the energy liberated in arriving at a given product nucleus is constant, for example, for ^{60}Co (Fig. 28.9) 0.1 per cent of nuclei decay by the emission of 1.48 MeV β^--particles to yield ^{60}Ni in an excited state and 99.9 per cent of nuclei emit 0.31 MeV β^--particles to yield ^{60}Ni in a doubly excited state (higher energy level). In the latter case the higher energy ^{60}Ni reverts to a lower energy state by the emission of 1.17 MeV γ-radiation and parity of energy is preserved (total change $0.31 + 1.17 = 1.48$ MeV). In either case the ^{60}Ni then reverts to its ground energy state by the emission of 1.33 MeV γ-radiation. This consecutive production of two different energy γ-rays is described as the emission of two γ-rays 'in cascade'.

INTERACTION OF RADIATION WITH MATTER

Specific Ionization

All the types of radiation involved in radioactive decay lose energy in matter by an essentially similar process, namely interaction with the orbital negatrons of atoms. The atom may be ionized by the ejection of an orbital negatron, the residual positive ion and the ejected negatron being described as an *ion pair*, or it may be excited by raising the orbital negatrons to a higher energy state. Ionizations are characteristic of nuclear and X-radiations which are referred to accordingly as *ionizing radiations*: other types of radiation do not possess sufficient energy to produce ionization. There is no general agreement on the relative importance of ionization and excitation but it is probable that the former accounts for at least 50 per cent of the total energy loss.

Specific ionization is defined as the number of ion pairs per millimetre of path length.

The specific ionization increases as particle velocity decreases, since lower velocity particles spend more time in the vicinity of an atom and there is thus a greater probability of interaction. In air about 35 eV is required to produce one ion pair so that about 15 000 ion pairs are created for each 1 MeV of incident energy, assuming that 50 per cent of the energy loss results from ionization.

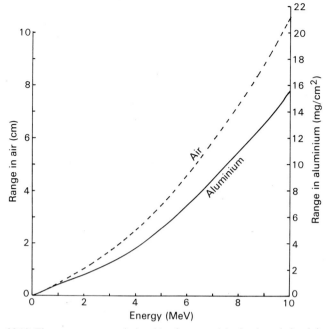

FIG. 28.10. The range-energy relationships for α-particles in air and aluminium.

Particle Range

The range of particles in matter may be expressed in two ways. Most simply this is given as the thickness of material (in cm or mm) which is penetrated. However the energy loss results from interactions with orbital negatrons and the electron density is reflected approximately by the density of the material, so range is usually given in terms of *superficial density*, i.e. the mass of material behind 1 cm^2 of surface.

Superficial density $= \rho x$ g cm$^{-2} = 1000\ \rho x$ mg cm^{-2}, where ρ is the density of the material and x is its thickness in cm.

α-PARTICLES

Most α-particles have energies between 3 and 8 MeV, the corresponding ranges in air being 1.5 and 7.5 cm (Fig. 28.10) and in aluminium 0.01 to 0.4 mm. Thus α-emitters in containers do not represent any hazard to workers since all the energy is absorbed in the walls of the container.

The range of α-particles is related to their energy. The range in air (R) is given by the expression

$$R = 0.32\ E^{1.5}\ \text{cm}$$

where E is the energy in MeV.

However, because of the high mass and charge they produce a high specific ionization of 1 to 6 ions pairs per mm (Fig. 28.11), so the effects produced

in the vicinity of an α-emitter are localized and intense.

β-PARTICLES

These have a small mass and thus a high velocity for a given energy, so they are readily scattered out of a straight line path by other electrons and produce a relatively low specific ionization of about 5 to 10 ion pairs per millimetre of air for β^--particles of 10 to 0.2 MeV respectively.

When β^--particles enter the electrical field of the nucleus a change in velocity results, resulting in the emission of electromagnetic radiation known as

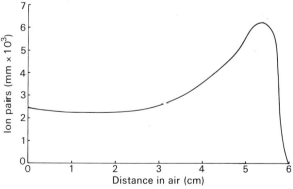

FIG. 28.11. The specific ionization produced in air by 7 MeV α-particles.

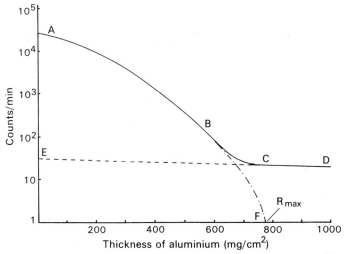

FIG. 28.12. The absorption curve in aluminum for a pure β-emitter (^{32}P).

Bremsstrahlung (braking radiation), which, however, differs from γ-radiation in having a continuous energy spectrum, arising from the wide energy range of the β^--particles affected, and a low energy. About 0.1 per cent of the energy loss of ^{32}P β^--particles in low atomic number material occurs in this way and the amount of Bremsstrahlung production increases with increasing atomic number of the absorbing material. Although the contribution from this source is small it is sufficient to complicate the shape of β^--absorption curves and to create problems in the protection of radiation workers.

The combined effects of the various energy loss processes and of the fact that β^--particles have a continuous energy spectrum lead to an absorption curve of the form shown in Fig. 28.12. This illustrates the absorption curve in aluminium for ^{32}P, which is a pure, mono-energetic β^--emitter. Aluminium is almost transparent to Bremsstrahlung and this results in a tail to the curve almost parallel to the abcissa (line CD). If the Bremsstrahlung contribution (DCE) is subtracted from the observed curve (ABCD), that due to the β^--particles (ABF) is obtained. The maximum, finite range (R_{max}) of the β^--particles can be used to determine their maximum energy using a correlation graph (Fig. 28.13). The ranges and energies quoted are always values of R_{max} and E_{max}, respectively, and these are related by the expressions

$$R_{max} = 0.542\ E_{max} - 0.133\ (E_{max} > 0.8\ \text{MeV})$$

and

$$R_{max} = 0.407\ E_{max}^{1.38}\ (E_{max}\ 0.15\ \text{to}\ 0.8\ \text{MeV}).$$

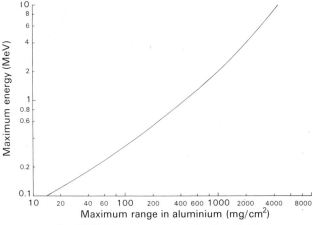

FIG. 28.13. Range-energy curve for β-particles.

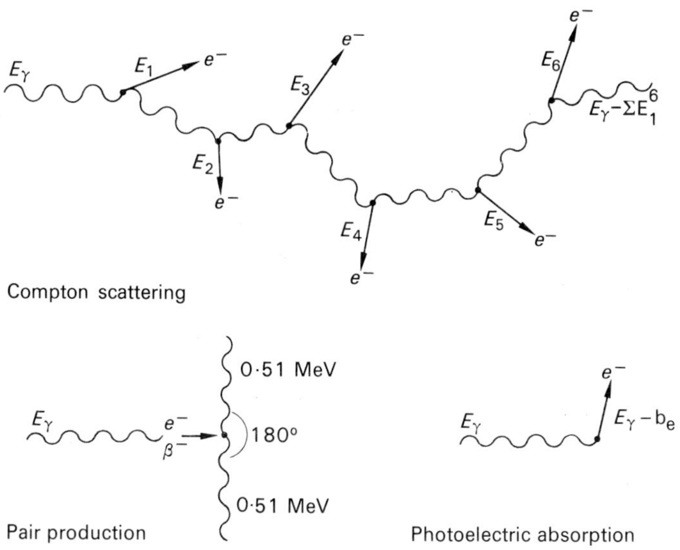

Compton scattering

Pair production   Photoelectric absorption

FIG. 28.14. The processes involved in the loss of energy by γ-radiation. If the initial energy is $E\gamma$ the residual energies are as follows: In Compton scattering, $E\gamma - \sum E_1^6$, i.e. the initial energy less the sum of the energies imparted to the scattered electrons. In pair production, 2×0.51 MeV γ-rays $= 1.02$ MeV: $E\gamma - 1.02$ MeV is the energy lost in creating the positron-electron pair and the kinetic energy lost by the pair before annihilation. In photoelectric absorption the electron has an energy of E minus the binding energy (b_e) of the electron.

γ-RADIATION

Since γ-rays have no charge or mass they interact only weakly with matter, the specific ionization being only about 1 per cent of that for β^--particles. The energy loss processes are more complex than for particulate radiation and are of three types, illustrated in Fig. 28.14.

Photoelectric absorption is important for low energy radiation (up to about 0.5 MeV) and high atomic number absorbers. In this process the entire energy of the incident radiation is absorbed by an atom, which then ejects an orbital negatron, normally from the K or L shells, at about 90° to the direction of the incident radiation.

Compton scattering is the predominant process for radiation of moderate energy (0.5 to 2 MeV) and absorbers of lower atomic number. In this process the radiation loses its energy in a series of elastic collisions with orbital negatrons, the latter being ejected at a variety of angles (greater than 90° to that of the incident radiation) with a corresponding range of energies.

Pair production involves the creation of a negatron–positron pair and is the converse of the annihilation process of positrons referred to above. It follows that the process is impossible below energies of 1.02 MeV and its probability increases

as the radiation energy and the atomic number of the absorber increases.

Despite the complexity of the energy loss processes, the absorption in matter is strictly exponential and

$$I_x = I_0 e^{-\mu x},$$

where I_0 is the intensity of the incident radiation, I_x is the radiation intensity after passing through a thickness x cm and μ is the *linear absorption coefficient*, in units of reciprocal centimetres. From the nature of the relationship it is clear that γ-radiation can be attentuated by a barrier but never completely stopped. This contrasts strongly with the situation obtained with α- and β^--particles, both of which have a finite range.

The half-thickness ($x_{1/2}$) is that thickness of absorber required to attenuate the beam by 50 per cent and

$$x_{1/2} = \frac{0.693}{\mu}.$$

A knowledge of the half-thickness enables the energy of the radiation to be determined (Fig. 28.15) and the thickness of a barrier required to attenuate the beam by any desired amount to be calculated.

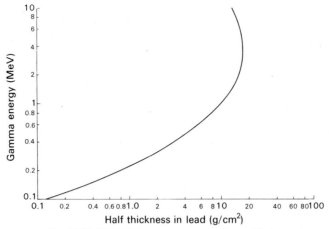

FIG. 28.15. Half-thickness-energy curve for γ-radiation.

Occasionally the *mass absorption coefficient* (μ/ρ) is used when comparing materials of different density, but this is less generally useful.

The relationships between the linear absorption coefficients and energy for different absorbers is shown in Fig. 28.16, from which it is clear that the absorption of γ-radiation depends markedly on both its energy and the atomic number of the absorber.

PRODUCTION OF RADIONUCLIDES

Artificial radionuclides are derived by bombardment of stable target nuclei with neutrons, usually in a nuclear reactor, or with other particles in cyclotrons and by isolation from the spent fuel from nuclear reactors.

Nuclear Reactors

These are devices for producing high fluxes of neutrons. The neutrons in reactors are a mixture of fast neutrons (high energy) and *thermal neutrons*, the latter having an energy similar to the thermal energy of atoms and molecules. Thermal neutrons are obtained by allowing the fast neutrons to pass through a *moderator*, commonly heavy water or graphite, and have a higher probability than fast neutrons of causing nuclear reactions.

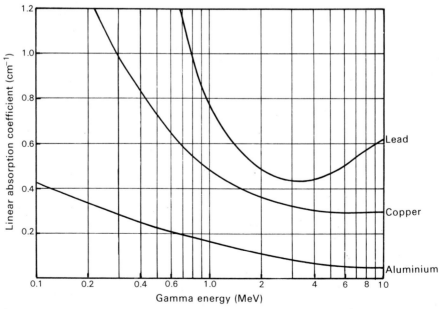

FIG. 28.16. The dependence of the linear absorption coefficients for γ-radiation on energy and atomic number.

The principal reactors used in the United Kingdom for nuclide production are the heavy water reactors DIDO and PLUTO, which are similar in design. DIDO consists of an aluminium tank about 2 m in diameter and 3.3 m deep containing 10 tonnes of heavy water (D_2O) in which are located 25 fuel elements, the total loading being 3.75 kg of enriched uranium fuel. The fuel elements are cylindrical and are designed to provide a very high neutron flux in the central hole and very efficient cooling is achieved by pumping the heavy water through the fuel elements at high velocity. The heavy water system forms a closed loop and the secondary coolant is purified mains water which in turn vents the heat to the atmosphere via a cooling tower. The core tank is surrounded by 60 cm of graphite reflector.

The output of the reactor, normally 12.5 to 15 MW of heat, maximum thermal neutron flux 2.2×10^{14} n/cm^2/s, is controlled by the degree to which cadmium control arms or rods are inserted into the core. Cadmium is a powerful neutron absorber and the further the control rods are inserted the greater the neutron absorption and the lower the power output.

Biological shielding is provided on the sides and bottom by a boral steel tank, 10 cm of water-cooled lead and 1.5 m of barytes concrete. The top shield consists of 2 mm of cadmium, 10 cm of water cooled lead, about 1 m of steel shot concrete and a 35 cm steel top plate.

A variety of experimental facilities is provided so that materials for irradiation can be placed in the centres of fuel elements, in the heavy water or in the graphite. The types of target which may be irradiated are chosen carefully to avoid chemical decomposition and contamination of the reactor.

REACTOR PRODUCTION

Several types of reaction can occur:

The (n, γ) Reaction

This involves the capture of thermal neutrons by the target nuclei to yield a radioactive compound nucleus which is in an excited state due to the binding energy liberated by the capture of a neutron. This surplus energy is emitted as γ-radiation, not to be confused with the γ-emission which may accompany decay of the radionuclide, for example,

$$\underset{11}{\overset{23}{}}Na + n \longrightarrow \underset{\substack{11 \\ \text{Compound} \\ \text{nucleus}}}{\overset{24}{}}Na \longrightarrow \underset{11}{\overset{24}{}}Na + \gamma$$

or more shortly, ^{23}Na (n, γ) ^{24}Na.

The process usually does not yield material of high specific activity since the product is chemically identical to the target and so cannot be separated from it, but high specific activity nuclides may be obtained in some cases, such as ^{56}Mn, ^{170}Tm, ^{192}Ir, ^{198}Au.

Reactions Involving the Loss of Heavy Particles

In these reactions protons or α-particles are emitted from the compound nucleus following neutron absorption. Fast neutrons may be required for these reactions to occur, since considerable energy is needed to expel the heavy particle. Examples of the use of these reactions in radionuclide production are as follows: ^{6}Li$(n, \alpha)^3$H, ^{14}N$(n, p)^{14}$C, ^{32}S$(n, p)^{32}$P, ^{54}Fe$(n, p)^{54}$Mn. In such cases the product is chemically different from the target and can be separated in very high specific activity.

Side Reactions

When compounds are irradiated two or three elements will be present, and each one of these may be a mixture of isotopes. Each isotope may undergo a nuclear transformation so that the product contains a number of radionuclides in addition to that desired. For example, if sodium chloride is irradiated to obtain ^{24}Na the result is as shown in Table 28.4. Some ^{40}K $(1.3 \times 10^9$ years) and

TABLE 28.4

RADIONUCLIDES PRODUCED IN SODIUM CHLORIDE BY IRRADIATION IN A NUCLEAR REACTOR

| Process | Radionuclides (with half-lives) produced from: | | |
	^{23}Na	^{35}Cl	^{37}Cl
n, γ	^{24}Na (15.0 h)	^{36}Cl (3×10^5 years)	^{38}Cl (38 min)
n, p	^{23}Ne (38 s)	^{35}S (87.2 days)	^{37}S (5.1 min)
n, α	^{20}F (11.2 s)	^{32}P (14.3 days)	^{34}P (12.4 s)

^{42}K (12.4 h) are also present due to potassium impurity in the sodium. Fortunately ^{23}Ne, ^{20}F, ^{38}Cl, ^{37}S and ^{34}P decay rapidly and so are not present at the time of use, while ^{35}S and ^{32}P are pure β^--emitters and can be distinguished from the ^{24}Na which is a β-γ-emitter. Because of such complications, ^{24}Na is obtained by the irradiation of sodium carbonate since the product is radiochemically purer.

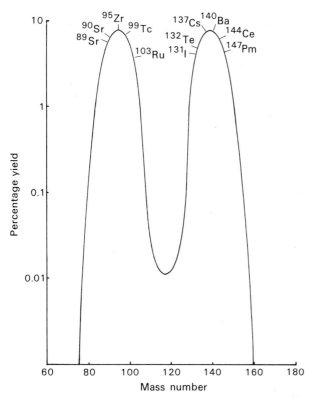

FIG. 28.17. The yield of fission products from uranium-235.

Nuclides from Fission Products

The uranium reactor fuel undergoes fission and, in time, becomes spent and the fuel rods are then removed from the reactor and placed in a deep water tank to 'cool', i.e. to allow the short-lived activity to decay. They are then processed to recover unchanged uranium and to separate the fission products. There is a low probability of central fission of the nucleus and the maximum yields of fission products occur in the region of mass numbers 95 and 138 (Fig. 28.17). Useful amounts of ^{90}Sr, ^{131}I, ^{132}Te, ^{137}Cs and ^{140}Ba are obtained together with many other products.

LABORATORY NEUTRON SOURCES

These provide thermal neutrons at low flux and can be used for the laboratory production of small amounts of short lived radionuclides. The available neutron sources depend principally on the bombardment of a light target element with α-particles, the usual reaction being

$$^{9}_{4}Be + ^{4}_{2}He \longrightarrow ^{12}_{6}C + ^{1}_{0}n$$

since beryllium gives the highest neutron yields.

Suitable α-sources are ^{227}Ac, ^{241}Am, ^{242}Cm, ^{210}Po, ^{226}Ra and ^{228}Th. The neutron emissions vary between 2.5×10^3 and 1.2×10^8 per second, depending on the α-source selected and its activity, and vary in energy between 1 and 12 MeV. Lower energy neutrons (<1 MeV) can be obtained using ^{210}Po with a lithium target.

Monoenergetic 26 KeV neutrons are given by a ^{124}Sb/Be source, which depends on the production of neutrons by high energy γ-rays.

CYCLOTRON IRRADIATIONS

Radionuclides which are deficient in neutrons cannot normally be produced in nuclear reactors but may be obtained by bombarding target nuclei with protons, deuterons or α-particles in a cyclotron.

The principles of construction of a cyclotron are shown in Fig. 28.18. It consists of two flat hollow semi-cylinders, known as 'dees', placed in a very high vacuum chamber and supplied with a source of high frequency voltage. The vacuum chamber is contained between two magnets. When charged particles are injected into the centre of the dees they are induced to follow a spiral path towards the circumference and, in the process, are accelerated to very high energies, about 10 to 20 MeV normally being used for radionuclide production. The beam is deflected from its outermost orbit by the application of an electrostatic voltage and emerges through a window to strike the target material.

The nuclear reactions which can occur are very varied and may be very complex, for example,

(a) proton induced:

^{55}Mn(p, n)^{55}Fe, ^{12}C(p, 3p 3n)^{7}Be,

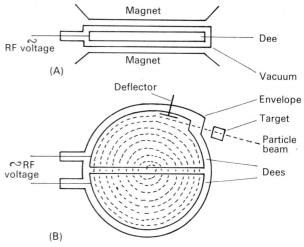

FIG. 28.18. The principle of a cyclotron. A, vertical section; B, horizontal section through the dees.

(b) deuteron induced:
$^{24}Mg(d, \alpha)^{22}Na$, $^{74}Ge(d, 2n)^{74}As$,
(c) α-particle induced:
$^{52}Cr(\alpha, 4n)^{52}Fe$, $^{71}Ga(\alpha, n)^{74}As$.

This is the principal source of nuclides which decay by positron emission or by electron capture.

COUNTING INSTRUMENTS AND THE DETECTION OF RADIATION

Counting instruments depend upon the production of ionization or luminescence by the radiation. Detection may also be achieved by the blackening effect of radiations on photographic film or by the oxidation of chemical systems.

COUNTING INSTRUMENTS DEPENDENT ON IONIZATION

Ion Collection Phenomena

The simplest form of detector is shown in Fig. 28.19. Its functioning depends on the production by the radiation of ion pairs in the filling gas. In the absence of a potential difference between the electrodes the ion pairs recombine but the application of a potential causes the ions to separate, negatrons moving towards the anode and the large cations towards the cathode. Fig. 28.20 shows the relationship between ion collection and the applied potential in such a counter.

With increasing potential there is at first only a *partial colllection* of ions (Fig. 28.20, Region I) but then a point is reached at which all the primary ions produced are collected. A further modest increase in potential has little effect on this situation, so there is a plateau in this region of *saturation collection* (Region II). A further potential rise results in such acceleration of the primary ions that they have sufficient energy to cause secondary ionizations by collision with molecules of the filling gas, a process known as *internal gas multiplication,* so that the number of ions collected may increase

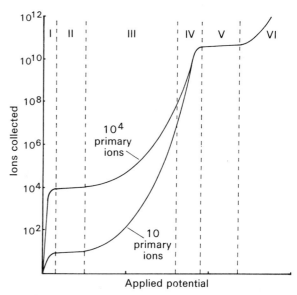

FIG. 28.20. The relationship of charge collected to applied potential in an ionization detector. Regions: I, Partial collection; II, Saturation collection; III, Proportional region; IV, Limited proportionality; V, Geiger region; VI, Continuous discharge.

by a factor of 10^6. The relative increase in the charge collected is proportional to the applied potential so that this section of the curve (Region III) is known as the *proportional region.* A higher potential still results in a *region of limited proportionality* (Region IV) above which the degree of secondary ionization is such that the gas is completely saturated with ions and a second plateau (Region V) occurs in the *Geiger region.* Beyond the end of this plateau the potential is such that the gas ionizes spontaneously and the device goes into *continuous discharge* (Region VI).

Fig. 28.21 illustrates the situations which occur with particles causing a small number of ionizations (β^--particle, say 10 primary ions produced) and a large number of ionizations (α-particle, 10^4 primary ions). In Regions II and III the charge collected is greater with the larger number of primary ions but in the Geiger region both types of particle give identical results since either condition results in total saturation of the gas space with secondary ions.

There are three basic types of detector based on this collection system, ionization chambers (working in Region II), proportional counters (Region III) and Geiger–Müller counters (Region V).

Ionization Chambers

The usual form of these instruments is a hollow cylinder or sphere, which acts as one electrode, with

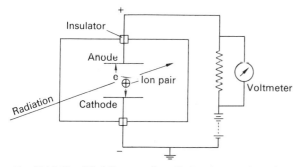

FIG. 28.19. Simplified diagram of a radiation detector dependent on ionization.

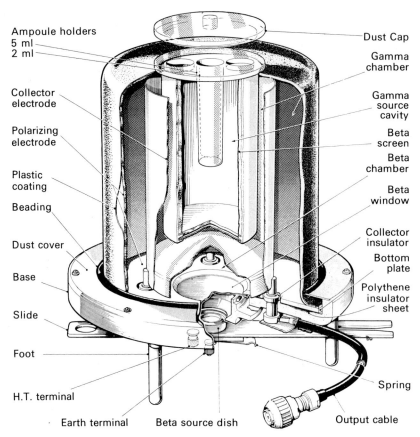

Ampoule holders
5 ml
2 ml

Dust Cap

Gamma chamber

Collector electrode

Gamma source cavity

Polarizing electrode

Beta screen

Beta chamber

Plastic coating

Beta window

Beading

Dust cover

Collector insulator

Base

Bottom plate

Slide

Polythene insulator sheet

Foot

H.T. terminal

Spring

Earth terminal   Beta source dish

Output cable

FIG. 28.21. Cut-away view of the U.K.A.E.A. type 1383A ion chamber (General Radiological type NE 014) (U.K.A.E.A.).

a central, well insulated, oppositely charged electrode. Commonly the outer casing is held at a potential of about 100 V and the central electrode is earthed.

Many ionization chambers permit the radioactive sample to be introduced directly into the sensitive volume of the counter as a solid source or as a gas. The latter arrangement is particularly valuable for very weak β^--emitters (^{3}H, 0.018 MeV; ^{14}C, 0.159 MeV) since this technique avoids absorption of their radiations by the walls of the counter, solid samples or sample mounts.

However, γ-emitters and energetic β^--emitters can be detected as solid or liquid samples, and an ionization chamber designed for this application is illustrated in Fig. 28.21. This instrument is available with calibration certificates issued by the National Physical Laboratory and, being very stable in operation, is a useful standard instrument for the assay of moderately active samples. A very sensitive electrometer has to be used to measure the extremely small ionization currents produced (approximately

6 to 75×10^{-12} A/mCi for γ-emitters, 75 to 450×10^{-12} A/mCi for β^--emitters) and great care must be paid to high quality insulation.

Proportional Counters

These differ in construction from the ionization chambers primarily in having a very much smaller central electrode of fine wire, which is always the anode, so that there is a much higher voltage gradient around it. Also filling gases based on methane or argon are used which have low enough ionization potentials to give good ion collection properties at reasonable operating voltages (1500 to 5000 V).

In a *gas flow counter*, shown in Fig. 28.22, the gas flows through at slightly above atmospheric pressure to exclude oxygen and the sample is within the sensitive volume of the counter, thus giving a high efficiency for low energy β^--particles.

Proportional counters can count at very high rates and since the size of pulse produced depends on the energy of the incident radiation, they can

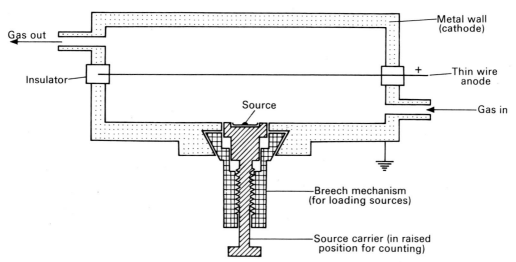

FIG. 28.22. The principle of a gas flow proportional counter.

be used to determine its energy spectrum. However they have found only limited use since the pulses are very small and very stable associated equipment is required, due to both the large variation in output with applied potential and the considerable pulse amplification required.

Geiger–Müller Counters

Characteristics of ion collection. The negatrons produced by the incident radiation in the filling gas are accelerated to the anode wire under a potential such that the gas multiplication factor is of the order of 10^8 and the collection process is complete in 0.05 to 0.3 μs. The collection of this avalanche of negatively charged particles reduces the anode potential to such an extent that the effective field strength drops below the working level and the counter is paralysed temporarily. Over a period of about 100 to 500 μs the larger cations are discharged at the cathode and have sufficient energy to produce ionizations there. If uncontrolled this would result in multiple pulsing, so the filling gas contains a small proportion of a quenching agent which dissociates and absorbs the excitation energy of the cathode. Such *internally quenched counters* may contain organic vapours (ethyl alcohol or ethyl formate) or halogens (chlorine or bromine) and the compositions of typical filling gases are given in Table 28.5.

The reduction in field strength due to ion collection results in the counter being completely inoperative for a period of about 100 μs, the true *dead time*. After a further period of about 100 μs *recovery time* full size pulses will be observed once

TABLE 28.5

CHARACTERISTICS OF ORGANIC AND HALOGEN QUENCHED GEIGER–MÜLLER COUNTERS

	Organic quenched	Halogen quenched
Typical fillings (pressure in cmHg)	Helium 55.0 Argon 9.3 Ethyl formate 0.7	Neon 20.0 Argon 0.02 Chlorine 0.005
Working voltage (range)	1000 to 1600	350 to 700
Minimum plateau length (V)	200	100
Plateau slope (per cent per V)	0.04	0.07
Temperature range (°C)	-20 to $+50$	-55 to $+75$
Useful life (counts)	10^8 to 10^9	$> 10^{10}$
Effect of excessive or reverse voltage	Ruined	May not be permanently damaged
Relative efficiency for β^--particles	100	95

more. This total period of about 200 μs is known as the *paralysis time* (Fig. 28.23), and particles entering the counter during this period may not be counted. Since the paralysis time varies with different counters and with the associated electronic circuitry, a variable, unknown counting loss results. This difficulty may be overcome electronically using a *quenching probe unit* which performs two functions: it gives a small degree of amplification of the pulse, so avoiding counting losses due

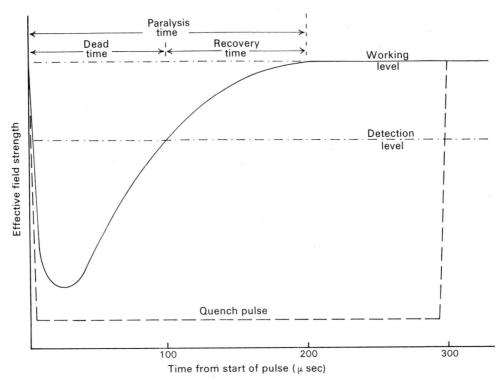

FIG. 28.23. Paralysis in a Geiger–Müller counter.

to pulse attenuation, and it reduces the anode potential of the counter for a predetermined time from the commencement of each pulse, for example, 300 μs (see Fig. 28.24). Corrections may now be made for lost counts due to paralysis since

$$R = R_o/1 - R_o.T,$$

where R_o is the observed counting rate; R is the true counting rate and T is the paralysis time. Provided the counting rates are not excessive, paralysis time corrections may be made by referring to prepared tables.

Parameters of Geiger–Müller counters. The essential components of a Geiger–Müller counting assembly are shown in Fig. 28.24. As the potential (Extra High Tension, EHT) is increased the counter suddenly starts to respond at the *starting voltage* (V_s), each pulse being amplified and recorded as a single count. The counting rate then increases rapidly with EHT until the *threshold voltage* (V_t) is reached, above which the counting rate becomes almost constant throughout a plateau which is about 150 to 200 V long. Further increase in EHT would result in the counter going into continuous discharge ('racing'). This *characteristic curve* is shown in Fig. 28.25. The *working voltage* (V_w) is

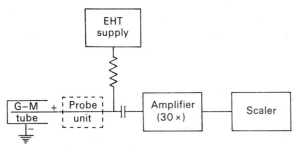

FIG. 28.24. Block diagram of an apparatus for Geiger–Müller counting.

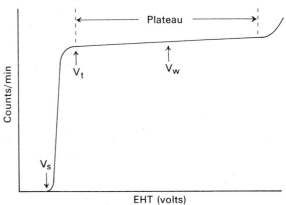

FIG. 28.25. The characteristic curve of a Geiger–Müller counter.

usually 60 to 100 V above V_t, at about the middle
of the plateau where small fluctuations in EHT due
to instability have little effect on the counting rate.

The *plateau slope* should be less than 0.1 per
cent per volt and is smaller for organic quenched
counters than for those quenched with halogens.
The slope tends to increase with age. Counters
should never be allowed to go into continuous
discharge nor be subjected to a reverse voltage.

The characteristics of typical Geiger–Müller
counters are given in Table 28.5.

Types of Geiger–Müller counter. Although many
types are available only two are commonly used
in the laboratory for routine purposes and they are
illustrated in Fig. 28.26. The *end-window counter*
consists usually of a cupped metal body about
2 cm in diameter, used as the cathode, with a fine
wire anode located axially (Fig. 28.26A). The cup
is sealed with a 'window' the thickness of which
determines the minimum energy of β^--particles
which can be counted. The thinnest windows are
of mica (about 2 mg per cm^2) and will just permit
the counting of low energy β^--emitters (^{14}C, 0.159
MeV; ^{35}S, 0.167 MeV) at low efficiency (Fig. 28.28).
Counters with aluminium (7 mg per cm^2) or glass
(20 mg per cm^2) windows can be used only for
higher energy β^--emitters (^{36}Cl, 0.71 MeV; ^{32}P,
1.71 MeV; ^{89}Sr, 1.46 MeV). Counters with ultra-
thin plastic windows are also obtainable.

The geometric efficiency of end-window counters
varies with the source area and its distance from
the counter since the proportion of the emitted
radiation which can enter the counter varies as
these factors are changed. Care must be taken over
these points if reproducible results are to be
obtained.

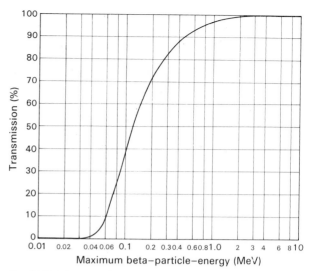

FIG. 28.27. The transmission of β-particles by the 2 mg per cm^2
mica end window of a Geiger–Müller counter.

Liquid counters are of glass construction with a
cylindrical space between the inner wall, which
encloses the electrodes and filling gas and the outer
wall (Fig. 28.26B). This space normally holds 10 ml
of radioactive solution. The inner wall has a thickness of about 25 mg per cm^2 so the counters can
be used only for moderate or high energy radiations.
Since the radionuclide is uniformly distributed
throughout the solution there is a constant geometric efficiency and the liquid counter makes a
useful substandard instrument for assaying sources.

When it is desired to count low energy β^--
particles, *windowless counters* may be used. These
have basically the same construction as the end-
window counter but the window is absent and the
filling gas, which may be argon–propane or a
similar mixture, is made to flow through the
counter at constant speed. To obtain stable operating conditions air must be excluded by maintaining
a slight, fixed, positive pressure of gas in the counter,
so the counter must be positioned very carefully in
relation to a surface to regulate the outflow of filling
gas. If a number of solid samples are to be
counted in this way it is usual to have a special
transfer device to position the counter correctly and
in which samples are gassed out ready for counting
while the previous sample is being counted, so
saving time. Improved stability of operation can be
obtained by having a small open slit in place of the
completely open end and such counters are widely
used for scanning chromatograms since they have
the additional advantage of high resolution due to
the small area being monitored at any one time.

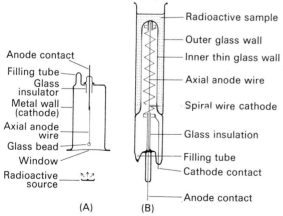

FIG. 28.26. Common forms of Geiger–Müller counter: A, end
window; B, liquid counter.

Geiger–Müller counters have only a low efficiency for the detection of γ-radiation (1 to 2 per cent of that for energetic β^--particles) since γ-rays produce very sparse ionizations in the filling gas and detection depends primarily on their ability to ionize the counter cathode to yield negatrons. Although high efficiency γ-counters are available with cathodes having a high absorption coefficient for γ-radiation (Pb or Cu) other means of detection (scintillation counters, see below) are preferable.

Other Types of Ionization Detector
Semi-conductor detectors have recently become practicable with improved methods of manufacture and the development of associated transistorized and integrated electronic circuitry. The detectors at present available include lithium drifted germanium and silicon diodes which have the advantage, according to type, of very high sensitivity for low energy particles or of exceptional energy resolution. Although in time they may supplant traditional counting devices their principal current use is for high resolution gamma-spectroscopy.

Spark chambers usually consist of a rectangular frame holding a series of close parallel electrode arrays, each array composing two electrodes, a central wire surrounded closely by a tensioned spiral spring. The potential difference is such that ionization of the air gap by radiation causes a spark to jump between the electrodes at the point where the ionization occurred. The sparks may be recorded photographically or electronically. Such counters can be made to cover large areas and are used for the detection of spots of radioactive material on paper and thin layer chromatograms since they can monitor the whole area of the chromatogram simultaneously. This avoids the necessity for the slow stripwise scanning of large areas, as is done at present, and for the complex mechanical devices necessary for such scanning.

SCINTILLATION COUNTERS

It will be recalled that a substantial proportion of the energy lost by radiations in matter results in excitations. Some materials absorb this excitation energy and then emit a proportion of it in the form of blue visible light, the passage of each particle or γ-ray giving a single, minute flash of light. Such materials are known as *phosphors*. Although phosphors exist with which the emitted light can be detected visually, the light intensity is usually so low that the only practicable method of detection is to use a photomultiplier, which is highly photosensi-

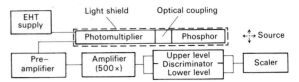

FIG. 28.28. Block diagram of an apparatus for scintillation counting.

tive, converting the light flashes to electrons and amplifying the resultant pulse by a factor of 10^7 to 10^9. There must be good optical coupling between the phosphor and the photomultiplier to avoid light losses by total internal reflection at the interface and coupling may be achieved by cementing the two together or by having a thin film of silicone oil between them. Also it is essential to enclose both phosphor and photomultiplier in a light shield: exposure of the phosphor to visible light often induces chemi-luminescence which causes erroneously high background counting rates, while exposure of the photomultiplier to normally light environments causes excitation of the photosensitive material and, if a high voltage is applied to the tube, to its complete destruction.

The essential units for a set of scintillation counting equipment are shown in Fig. 28.28. The functions of the electronic equipment will be discussed later.

Scintillation Phosphors
The desirable characteristics of a phosphor are that it should have a high efficiency of radiation detection, have as high as possible a light yield for the energy absorbed, have spectral characteristics matching those of the photomultiplier cathode, be as transparent as possible to permit maximum light output to the photomultiplier and the luminescence should decay rapidly so that high counting rates can be obtained.

Generally the light output in a phosphor is proportional to the energy of the incident radiation, so the system can be used for radiation spectroscopy.

Inorganic phosphors. The most popular phosphor of this type consists of a large crystal of sodium iodide containing about 1 per cent of thallium iodide as an activator, normally written NaI(Tl). Because sodium iodide is hygroscopic the crystals are sealed in an aluminium capsule with a transparent glass end which faces the photomultiplier. Its high density (3.7 g per cm^3) and high atomic number (iodine = 53) result in high absorption coefficients for X- and γ-radiation, for which it is the phosphor of choice. NaI(Tl) crystals are characterized also by high light yield and transparency and reasonably short decay times (Table 28.6).

TABLE 28.6

THE PROPERTIES OF SOME SCINTILLATION PHOSPHORS

Phosphor	Peak emission wavelength* (nm)	Relative light yield	Decay time of luminescence ($\times 10^{-9}$ s)
NaI(Tl)	413	230	250
Anthracene	447	100	30
Naphthalene	345	11	80
Stilbene	410	45	6
p-Terphenyl	414	29	10
Liquid	430	75	3
Plastic	430	60	3

* Peak sensitivity of photomultipliers about 420 nm.

Zinc sulphide, normally activated with a trace of silver, can be obtained only in a fine polycrystalline form which thus has very poor optical properties. However it is used as very thin films for the detection of α-particles.

Solid organic phosphors. Many organic compounds possess the properties required for scintillation counting, but because of the relatively low densities and atomic numbers they are unsuitable for detecting X- and γ-radiation, although they have a high efficiency for β^--particles. Among the most efficient organic phosphors is anthracene, which is used as the standard for light output, but it is difficult to grow large crystals of this with good optical properties. Such large crystals are rarely required and it is often used as thin sections cemented to a thin plastic support. The properties of some common organic phosphors are also given in Table 28.6.

Since the efficiency of both organic phosphors and Geiger–Müller tubes for β-particles is the same (100 per cent for all particles which enter the sensitive volume) the extra cost and complexity involved in using solid organic phosphors is justified only in special circumstances, for example, where energy differentiation is required. Another useful application is to have the phosphor in solid solution in a polystyrene or polyvinyltoluene plastic. Such plastic phosphors have excellent optical properties and can be made any desired size and shape.

Liquid phosphors. The detection of very weak β^--radiation presents a special problem, which may be overcome if the sample can be included in the sensitive volume of the counter. Although this can be done with ionization chambers, proportional counters or Geiger–Müller counters, there are considerable technical difficulties. A much simpler technique is to dissolve or suspend the sample in a liquid phosphor, and this is the most favoured method at present.

The commonest liquid phosphors contain p-terphenyl or 2:5-diphenyloxazole (PPO) dissolved in toluene or dioxan. Since the peak wavelength of light emission of such solutions is relatively low a secondary solute is often added to act as a 'spectrum shifter' so that the output matches the photomultiplier, for example, 1:4-di[2-(5-diphenyloxazolyl)]-benzene (POPOP) or 2-(1-naphthyl)-5-phenyloxazole (αNPO).

AUTORADIOGRAPHY

It is well known that radiations blacken photographic emulsions and this is the basis of the use of films as personal dosemeters. Autoradiography involves the use of this phenomenon to record the distribution of radioactivity in a specimen. The quality of the results obtained depends on the type of emulsion used, fine grain size, high grain concentration and thin emulsions all contributing to high resolution, though resolution and sensitivity are inversely related. The quality of the radiation is also important, α-particles and low energy β^--particles giving the best resolution.

Contact Autoradiography

This technique is also known as macro-autoradiography and consists of placing the radioactive specimen in contact with X-ray film for a suitable time. On development the film is blackened in the vicinity of the radiation source and the distribution and extent of blackening indicate the gross distribution of activity in the specimen. Exposures are best determined empirically but, as a guide, the time taken to accumulate 2 to 10×10^6 β^--particles per cm^2 can be calculated, depending on the type of film used.

One useful application of the technique is in the location of the active spots following the paper chromatography or electrophoresis of radioactive solutions and this can be done in tests for the radiochemical purity of preparations of ^{131}I and ^{32}P.

Stripping Film Autoradiography

This technique is sometimes referred to as micro-autoradiography and is used to determine the distribution on a microscopic scale of radioactivity in cells or tissues. In this method a thin (10 to 25 μm) film of wet emulsion is placed in intimate contact with a specimen mounted on a microscope slide, the contact becoming extremely close as the film dries. After prolonged exposure, which may vary from a few weeks to a few months, the film is developed and the specimen is stained by normal techniques, both operations being done without disturbing the location of either on the slide. When dry the blackening of the film is observed microscopically at the same time as the specimen is viewed and the activity can be related to particular cells.

THE CHEMICAL DETECTION OF RADIATION

The fact that radiations cause changes in chemical systems has been known for many years. In aqueous solutions most of the effects result from the radiolysis of water to yield oxidizing agents: hydroxyl and hydroperoxide free radicals (OH, O_2H) and hydrogen peroxide (see the section on the biological effects of radiation below). Thus ferrous sulphate in acid solution is oxidized to the ferric form to an extent which depends on the radiation dose, according to the reaction

$$15.6Fe^{2+} + 3.7O_2 + 15.6H^+ \xrightarrow{100\,eV}$$
$$15.6Fe^{3+} + 7.4H_2O + 0.4H_2$$

The coefficient of 15.6 for Fe^{2+} is known as the G value, the number of ions or molecules which react for each 100 eV absorbed. Determination of the amount of Fe^{3+} produced is normally done spectrophotometrically by measuring the change in optical density at 305 nm. Such systems are of value only for the measurement of very high doses.

One highly sensitive chemical system consists of a mixture of chloroform and a solution of bromocresol purple and makes use of the fact that radiation liberates hydrogen ions from halogenated hydrocarbons, a change reflected in the resultant pH.

ELECTRONIC EQUIPMENT ASSOCIATED WITH COUNTING DEVICES

There is often confusion as to the meaning of the word 'counter', which has been applied to the detector alone and to the detector plus associated electronic equipment. Throughout this text the word counter will be used to signify the detector, and electronic units will be described by their function. It must be emphasized that counters do not themselves count but merely respond to the passage of radiation. The response is observed as an ionization current with ionization chambers and is measured with an electrometer, but with the other principal forms of counter the collection of negatrons results in a fall in the positive anode potential, this negative pulse being amplified and recorded as a single count in a pulse counter (scaler) or as an average counting rate in a pulse integrating device (ratemeter), or in a pulse of light.

The essential units of assemblies for Geiger–Müller and scintillation counting are shown in Figs 28.26 and 28.28.

All counters have a *background* counting rate derived from natural environmental radiation and from radiation in the laboratory. The extent of this background depends on the sensitivity of the counter to the radiation and on counter size, the larger the sensitive volume of the counter the greater its background. Normally counters are supported in a *lead castle* which provides a substantial thickness of lead shielding around the counter and so reduces the background appreciably.

High Voltage Supplies

Apart from ionization chambers, which may be operated with 90 V batteries, all counters require an electronic voltage source, the output being referred to as the Extra High Tension (EHT) or the High Voltage (HV) supply. Most units have a maximum output of about 2500 V, although a 5000 V supply is necessary for some applications, with a positive polarity. The output is stabilized against fluctuations in the mains supply, the stability required varying with the application. The degree of stabilization needed for proportional counters or spectrometric applications, 0.02 per cent or better for 10 per cent mains fluctuation, is not needed for Geiger–Müller counters.

Pre-amplifiers

One important type of pre-amplifier is the quenching probe unit already referred to when describing the characteristic of Geiger–Müller counters. The photomultiplier is also a form of pre-amplifier.

With modern instruments of high input sensitivity a pre-amplifier may not be required provided the length of cable between the counter and the main amplifier is short. However, where the counter is some distance from the main amplifier it is essential to use a pre-amplifier, preferably attached directly to the output contact of the counter, to avoid undue attentuation of the output pulse in the long length of cable. Such pre-amplifiers are usually transistor emitter followers which do not actually amplify the pulse but give a low impedance output of the same phase (negative output for negative pulse input) with which very long cables can be used. Older instruments may use a pre-amplifier which gives phase reversal, a positive output pulse resulting from a negative input.

Amplifiers

For Geiger–Müller counting a simple amplifier with a gain of about $100 \times$ is adequate. Stability is relatively unimportant since all output pulses from the counter are of the same size. Pulses due to background are of the same size as those of interest and background counting rates are low.

With proportional or scintillation counters, however, the output pulses vary in size with the energy of the incident radiation. Also in addition to the 'true' background there is a further contribution due to random pulses which arise in amplifiers and photomultipliers. This is known as *noise* and its amount increases with the applied potential, though the pulses are usually smaller than those of interest. It is essential to be able to discriminate between the background pulses and those from the sample and, where energy discrimination is required, between the differently sized pulses arising from the radiation. Hence *linear amplifiers* which amplify all pulses to the same extent, and so retain the relative sizes of pulses, are essential. Such amplifiers usually have a high gain, up to $10\,000 \times$, to permit the very small pulses from proportional or liquid scintillation systems to be counted.

Discriminators and Pulse Height Analysers

A *discriminator* is an electronic circuit that blocks all pulses below the size selected by the operator and for straightforward counting purposes this is all that is required. With a Geiger–Müller counter the discriminator voltage, described variously as 'Disc', 'Bias', 'Disc Bias' or 'Threshold', is set at a low level which does not interfere with counting, since all pulses are similar in size.

However this arrangement is inadequate for proportional or scintillation counting where it is necessary to select only a part of the range of pulse heights and so distinguish the pulses of interest from those due to background and noise, to distinguish between radionuclides with different

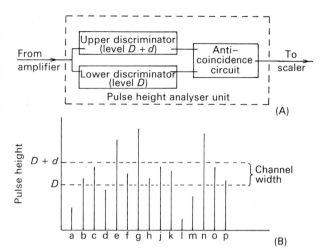

FIG. 28.29. The principle of a single channel pulse height analyser. A, block diagram of the component units; B, pulse selection.

radiation energies or to determine the pulse height (energy) spectrum of the radiations from a single radionuclide. These functions are performed by appropriate settings of a *pulse height analyser* (PHA), the functioning of which is illustrated in Fig. 28.29).

The lower discriminator is set at a level D and the upper discriminator at a level $D + d$, the value of d being fixed. Any pulse smaller than D (Fig. 28.30B, a, d, l, m) will also be smaller than $D + d$ and so is unable to pass either discriminator, so there is no output. Pulses larger than $D + d$ (e, g, n) will give a pulse from both discriminators simultaneously, the pulses being passed to an *anti-coincidence circuit*. The latter is arranged to give no output when pulses arrive simultaneously from both discriminators, i.e. pulses which arrive 'in coincidence', but to pass a pulse which comes from the lower discriminator only, in 'anti-coincidence' with pulses from the upper discriminator. Thus these large pulses are blocked by the anti-coincidence circuit and there is no output from the PHA. However, pulses between D and $D + d$ in size (b, c, f, h, j, k, o, p) pass the lower discriminator only and each gives an output pulse from the PHA. This device is known as a single channel pulse height analyser, the interval d being known variously as the 'channel', 'gate' or 'window' width. Multi-channel analysers are available which examine the counts in all of a large number (400 up to 4096) of channels simultaneously.

Spectrometry by pulse height anlysis. The basic technique used to examine the energy distribution of radiations is to use a system in which the size of the output pulses from the counter is proportional to the radiation energy and to examine the spectrum of pulse heights using a single channel PHA. This may be done by determining the number of counts in each of a series of successive channels or by scanning the entire range mechanically, integrating and recording the output.

When a NaI(Tl) phosphor is exposed to γ-radiation the normal processes of energy loss occur in the crystal, giving a series of Compton electrons of a wide range of energies and photo-electrons of virtually the same energy as that of the incident radiation. Since all the electron energy is absorbed within the crystal the light output, and thus the pulse height, is proportional to the energy of the incident radiation. If the procedure described above is carried out with a series of known radionuclides, the results obtained are illustrated in Fig. 28.30A. The lower energy part of the curve is the *Compton continuum*, followed by a sharp fall in counts immediately before the sharp *photo-peak* due to the photo-electrons. The peak just before the photo-peak results from the fact that near the energy region for photo-electric absorption there is a much higher probability of this process than of scattering. The pulse heights (lower discriminator bias voltages) at which the photo-peaks occur are related linearly to energy so that a standard calibration curve can be drawn for a counting assembly set up in a particular way (Fig. 28.30B). Once the instrument has been calibrated the energy of

unknown γ-emitters can be determined from the discriminator bias voltages at which their photo-peaks occur.

If the γ-energy is high enough for pair production to occur, the pulse height spectrum is somewhat more complex than those illustrated in Fig. 28.31, but the method is still applicable.

Scintillation γ-spectrometry is used as part of the identity tests for all the pharmacopoeial γ-emitting radionuclides and is also used to detect the presence of ^{60}Co impurity as part of the purity tests for cyanocobalamin-^{57}Co and cyanocobalamin-^{58}Co. In the latter case the special technique of coincidence γ-spectrometry is used. This uses two single channel γ-spectrometers operating in coincidence and has the merit of giving a more reliable result than is obtained with a single spectrometer. However, with modern instruments of good resolution there should be no real difficulty in resolving the 0.51 and 0.81 MeV photo-peaks of ^{58}Co (with a small amount of 1.62 MeV radiation) from the 1.17 and 1.33 MeV peaks of ^{60}Co.

Pulse height analysis for the counting of mixed radionuclides. In radioisotope tracer work it is common to have double labelled samples. Typical situations are studies of the adsorption of two different compounds from a complex system, one being labelled with ^{3}H and the other with ^{14}C; investigations of the metabolism of a drug, different groups in the molecule being labelled with ^{3}H and ^{14}C; and determinations of the relative efficiencies of iron utilization when ingested and injected, using ^{55}Fe and ^{59}Fe. In such systems the activities of both radionuclides may be determined simultaneously provided that the energies of the radiations from each are sufficiently different. What is required is that the output from the preamplifier be divided and fed through separate PHAs, the channels of which are arranged to pass pulses of different size.

In the ^{3}H/^{14}C system both components are usually determined by liquid phosphor counting. Although the energies involved are very low, good efficiencies can be obtained, up to 50 per cent for ^{3}H (0.018 MeV) and 90 per cent for ^{14}C (0.159 MeV) and Fig. 28.31 shows how these may be separated into two separate channels of pulse height analysis. This system is so frequently used that there are many commercial instruments available which determine the activities of both components in up to 400 samples automatically.

Data Registration

Pulse counters (Scalers). Usually the pulses which pass the discriminator or PHA are fed into a

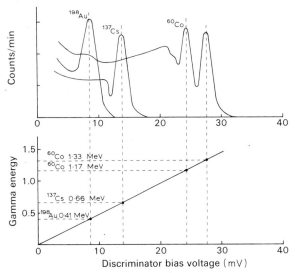

FIG. 28.30. γ-Spectrometry: the relationship of pulse size to the energy of the γ-radiation.

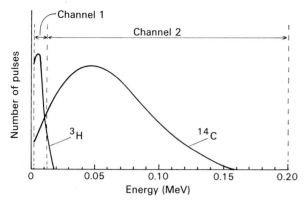

FIG. 28.31. The principle of the simultaneous counting of radionuclides of different β-particle energies (^{3}H and ^{14}C) using two channels of pulse height analysis.

scaler, a device for recording the number of pulses in a given time and so enabling the counting rate to be determined in terms of counts per second (cps) or per minute (cpm).

Simple scalers usually consist of a series of glow number tubes which have ten stable positions, the glow stepping on one unit for each pulse. When the tenth pulse enters the scaler the tube returns to zero and passes a pulse out to the next tube, so that successive tubes count units, tens, hundreds, etc. Such tubes have high *input resolution times* of about 50 or 250 μs, so that they will not record a pulse which arrives within that time from the previous one. Scalers of this type can be used satisfactorily only for routine Geiger–Müller counting where the detector itself has a paralysis time of the same order. They are unsuitable for proportional or scintillation counters which have very short paralysis times and are capable of counting at very high rates without losses due to paralysis. For such applications the current trend is to use transistors or integrated circuits, which have input resolution times of 1 μs or less, combined with indicator tubes which show the condition of the circuits at the end of a count and on which the accumulated counts are displayed.

The scaler also has switches to start the count, to stop counting after a desired interval and to reset the scaler to zero ready for another count. Although these functions may be done manually *autoscalers* which have automatic timing devices are widely used. With an autoscaler it is possible to determine automatically the counts obtained in a preset time or the time required to accumulate a preset number of counts. Integrated scaler/timers display either time or count as desired. Autoscalers are essential if large numbers of samples are to be counted automatically and in such cases the results of each count are printed out or recorded on punched paper or magnetic tape ready for entry to a computer.

Integrating devices (ratemeters). When numerical data are not required the average counting rate may be determined by using an integrating circuit, in which the individual pulses charge up a capacitor shunted by a resistor. The average current developed is then displayed on a meter calibrated in terms of cpm or cps. Ratemeters are used principally to drive chart recorders so that the change of counting rate with time, applied potential or discriminator bias voltage is obtained. The curves shown in Fig. 28.30A may be obtained in this way.

An important application of ratemeters is the *laboratory monitor* which is used to monitor the contamination of hands, clothing, benches, etc. These instruments usually have a loudspeaker which indicates changes in the counting rate by corresponding changes in the sound intensity or frequency, so that if the ratemeter is left switched on in a laboratory there is a continuous audible indication of the level of radioactivity.

PROBLEMS ASSOCIATED WITH COUNTING

Statistical Considerations

The random nature of radioactive decay has already been noted, so it is axiomatic that a series of replicate counts on a single sample under identical conditions will not give identical results, except occasionally by chance. This is a classical case in which statistical techniques must be used to indicate the reliability of the data. A rigorous statistical discussion would be out of place here, so only an outline of the principles involved is given below, assuming some elementary knowledge of statistical techniques.

Radioactive disintegrations and the consequent counts observed are a series of discrete, unit events so a large series of counts derived from a single source will have a *Poisson distribution*. When the *mean* count is low this distribution is markedly skewed, but as the mean increases the distribution becomes progressively more symmetrical until, at a mean of about 20, the shape approximates very closely to that of the *normal distribution*. Since the number of counts observed is invariably considerably greater than 20 it is justifiable to use statistical tests based on the normal distribution. This is certainly so when mean counts are used, since means are normally distributed.

The spread of the distribution curve is defined

by the *standard deviation* (σ), the square root of the *variance* (V), given by the expression

$$\sigma = \sqrt{V} = [\sum (x - \bar{x})^2/n - 1]^{0.5}$$

where x is the value of a count, $\bar{x}$ is the mean count and n is the number of replicate counts done. The mean is the best estimate obtainable of the 'true' counting rate, and deviations from the mean of σ, 2σ and 3σ have probabilities of 0.683, 0.955 and 0.997, respectively, i.e. on 66.3 per cent of occasions a single count x in the set with a mean $\bar{x}$ will lie within the range $\bar{x} \pm \sigma$, etc.

Since the magnitude of σ varies with that of $\bar{x}$, the value of σ is often expressed as a *coefficient of variation* and

$$\text{coefficient of variation} = \frac{100\sigma}{\bar{x}} \text{ per cent}$$

The precision of the mean is defined in terms of the *standard error* (*SE*), which is given by the expression

$$SE_{\bar{x}} = \sigma/\sqrt{n} = [\sum (x - \bar{x})^2/n(n-1)]^{0.5}.$$

If only a single count is done the standard error is the square root of that count (for a Poisson distribution), i.e.

$$SE_x = \sqrt{x}$$

from which it follows that the precision of a count depends on the total number of counts accumulated, the coefficients of variation for counts of 100, 1000 and 10 000 being 10, 3.16 and 1 per cent, respectively. Thus it is essential to count for sufficiently long to achieve acceptably low errors: in biological work the magnitude of other sources of error is such that a coefficient of variation of 2 per cent is acceptable, and this is achieved with a total of about 2500 counts.

Frequently the differences between counts or count ratios are used and it must be noted that variances are additive. If a net count (C) is determined from two counts (X and Y) then if

$$C = X + Y \quad \text{or} \quad C = X - Y$$

it follows that

$$\sigma_c = (\sigma_x^2 + \sigma_y^2)^{0.5}$$

where σ_c, σ_x, σ_y are the respective standard deviations. If

$$C = X/Y$$

then $\quad \sigma_c = (X/Y)(\sigma_x^2/X^2 + \sigma_y^2/Y^2)^{0.5}$

When counting *rates* are being used the time contributing to each rate must be allowed for. If the net counting rate is represented by R and counts X and Y are obtained in times t_x and t_y then

$$R = X/t_x + Y/t_y \quad \text{or} \quad R = X/t_x - Y/t_y$$

and $\quad \sigma_R = (\sigma_x^2/t_x^2 + \sigma_y^2/t_y^2)^{0.5}.$

As usual the significance of the difference between two mean counts is determined by the application of the 't'-test and in experiments where a number of factors are varied the significance of these factors is assessed by *analysis of variance*.

The reliability of a counting assembly is determined most simply from a series of replicate counts using the *chi*-squared (χ^2) test where

$$\chi^2 = \sum [(x - \bar{x})^2/\bar{x}]$$

with ($n-1$) degrees of freedom. Values of χ^2 giving probabilities <0.05 indicate defective equipment and probabilities >0.95 suggest that some factor is operating to suppress the expected variation and give a false impression of reliability.

The application of the statistical techniques outlined above enable the reliability of counts to be estimated, the estimate taking into account not only the errors arising from the random nature of the decay process but also all indeterminate errors, for which corrections cannot be applied. Such errors are the inaccuracy of measurements of volume or weight, the inability to control accurately the area and thickness of sources and their exact location relative to the counter, and variations of counter performance with age, temperature or previous counting rate, of the general level of radioactivity in the laboratory and of the performance of electronic equipment due to mains voltage fluctuations, ageing of components or pickup from other electrical equipment.

Counter Background
The counting rate obtained with an assembly in the absence of introduced radioactivity is the *background counting rate* and is derived from three sources; the natural environmental radiation, radioactive materials in the laboratory and electronic noise. The observed background counting rate must be subtracted from the observed counting rate from a sample to determine the rate appropriate to the active material.

With Geiger–Müller counters the contribution from noise is insignificant and the background counting rate is low, normally about 15 cpm. The background of a liquid Geiger–Müller counter is, however, variable since the walls of the counter are in direct contact with radioactive solutions and variable amounts of activity may be adsorbed and difficult to remove, so that background levels may reach 100 to 150 cpm.

There is an entirely different problem with proportional and scintillation counters. With the latter there is appreciable noise, especially from photomultipliers, although improvements in their design and manufacture have produced tubes with much lower noise characteristics, and the pulse size may be of the same order as that obtained with low energy radiations. Further, the background due to noise increases with the temperature of the photocathode of the photomultiplier and with the applied potential. Fig. 28.32 illustrates both these effects and it is clear that there is a considerable advantage in cooling the photomultiplier, a substantial improvement resulting from cooling to 5° and a further small benefit by cooling to $-10°$. In such situations it is important to decide on the best conditions for counting and there are various criteria of merit used for this purpose. The criterion R_{s+b}^2/R_b, where R_{s+b} is the observed counting rate from the sample including background and R_b is the background counting rate, is independent of source strength but is affected by the energy spectrum of the radiation. This is simpler to calculate than two similar criteria which are often used

and which give similar results, R_s^2/R_b and (efficiency)$^2/R_b$, R_s being the counting rate due to the sample alone. An alternative criterion, which varies with source strength, is $(R_{s+b}^{0.5} - R_b^{0.5})$. Optimal conditions are those at which the criterion of merit has a maximum value, and values of both operating potential and discriminator bias may be chosen with their aid.

From the brief discussion of the statistical aspects of counting given above it is clear that when the counting rate for a sample is large relative to the background ($R_s > 10R_b$) the contribution to the total error of that due to R_b is small. However as the value of R_s approaches that of R_b the error contributed by R_b to the total error is important and the counting time must be increased substantially to obtain acceptable accuracy. For weak sources it is essential to reduce the counter background as far as possible. It is also important to apportion the available counting time to give the minimum error, the proportions being given by the expression

$$t_s/t_b = (R_{s+b}/R_b)^{0.5}$$

where t_s and t_b are the counting times for the sample and background. If $R_s < R_b$ the precision of the determination of R_s is very poor and it is impracticable to make determinations when $R_s < 0.2R_b$, even with long counting times.

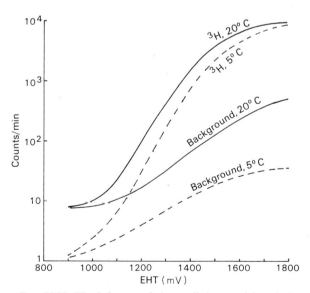

Fig. 28.32. The influence of the applied potential and the operating temperature on the counts from a ^{3}H source and due to background (including noise) in a liquid phosphor scintillation counter.

Low background counting. Several methods for reducing counter backgrounds have already been referred to, namely the reduction of counter size, lead shielding, the use of appropriate discriminator or pulse height anlyser settings and the cooling of photomultipliers. However, these methods are inadequate with sources of very low activity and coincidence or anti-coincidence techniques are used in addition. The principles involved are illustrated in Fig. 28.33.

For Geiger–Müller counting of β^--emitters an end-window counter may be used inside a guard counter, the two being connected in anti-coincidence (Fig. 28.33A). When a β^--particle enters the counter assembly it is absorbed totally in the end-window counter, which gives an output pulse, and since there is no output from the guard counter the anti-coincidence unit passes a pulse to the scaler. However, cosmic and local γ-radiation are very penetrating and such radiation reaches both the guard and end-window counters virtually simultaneously. Both counters thus yield coincident output pulses due to background and these are

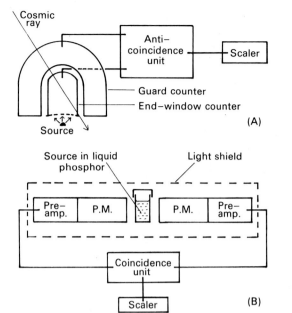

FIG. 28.33. The principles of low background counting.

rejected by the anti-coincidence circuit. The background count of such an assembly is about 1.5 cpm.

In liquid scintillation counting it is possible for the luminescence to be observed by two photomultipliers simultaneously (Fig. 28.33B). A flash of light in the phosphor gives coincident output pulses from the photomultipliers and these are passed by the coincidence circuit as a single count. Noise in the photomultipliers and their associated pre-amplifiers occurs randomly and pulses due to noise are only rarely coincident, so most of these pulses are rejected. Since most of the background in a liquid scintillation counter is due to photomultiplier noise the background is greatly reduced by this technique and may be as low as 10 to 15 cpm.

Counter Efficiency

The intrinsic efficiency of a counter depends on its ability to absorb the radiation energy and respond and it has already been stated that Geiger–Müller, proportional and organic phosphor scintillation counters are most suitable for β^--particles whereas NaI(Tl) scintillation counting is the method of choice for X- and γ-radiation. The overall efficiency depends on a number of additional factors, discussed briefly below.

Physical barriers to the radiation. There are frequently a number of such barriers: the counter window or light shield, the air between the source and the counter and the presence of a source seal.

These are unimportant with γ-radiation but will determine the minimum effective energy of β^--particles which can be detected.

Self-absorption in the source. Low energy β^--particles are absorbed appreciably by the material of the sample itself, e.g. $Ba^{35}SO_4$. As the thickness of a sample of constant specific activity increases, the counting rate at first increases and then becomes constant when the source thickness exceeds the maximum range of the particles in the substance (Fig. 28.34). A source in this latter condition is described as being 'infinitely thick', since all thicknesses above this give identical counts. Such sources are often used with low energy radiations and are satisfactory for comparative purposes. If this is not possible corrections for self-absorption must be applied.

Scattering and back-scattering of radiation. Both β^--particles and γ-radiation are scattered by matter, the effect being smaller with low atomic number materials. The scattering of radiation into the counter from side materials may generally be reduced by placing the source as near the detector as possible. With β^--particles, however, the amount of back-scattering, the scattering into the counter of particles initially travelling away from it, may be appreciable. Back-scattering increases with increasing thickness of backing, being maximal when the thickness is about 0.25 R_{max} (*saturation thickness*), and with increasing atomic number of the backing material.

When the activity of sources is to be compared it is essential that they are mounted on identical thicknesses of the same material and in identical surroundings, so that scattering conditions are constant.

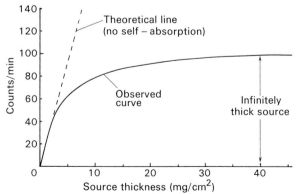

FIG. 28.34. The self-absorption of ^{35}S β-particles by $Ba^{35}SO_4$, sources of constant specific activity.

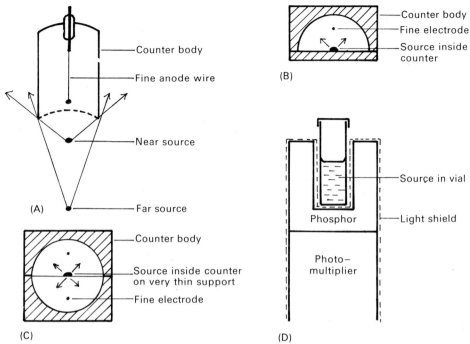

FIG. 28.35. Geometric efficiency in counting. A, With an end-window counter a source near the window gives a higher count than a far source; B, a 2π counting arrangement: 50 per cent geometric efficiency; C, a 4π counter: almost 100 per cent geometric efficiency, but some losses occur by absorption in the source support; D, a well-type scintillation counter: very high geometric efficiency since the source is virtually surrounded by phosphor.

Geometric efficiency.   Normally only a part of the radiation, which is emitted from a source in all directions, enters a counter and the greater the distance between source and counter the smaller is the proportion of the radiation detected (Fig. 28.35A). The intensity of the radiation falls off inversely as the distance squared, if we ignore air absorption, so a much higher proportion of the emitted radiation can be detected if the distance between the counter and the source is reduced to a minimum. The extreme situation is where all the radiation emitted from one side of a source, through a solid angle of 2π radians, enters the counter: this is known as '2π' counting (Fig. 28.35B). Double this efficiency can be obtained if the source is completely surrounded by the counter in a '4π' counting arrangement (Fig. 28.35C), and liquid phosphor counting is a form of this. Very good geometric efficiency is also given by well-type scintillation counters (Fig. 28.35D) which are simple in construction and operation and are used frequently.

Quenching in Liquid Phosphor Counting
The ideal system for liquid phosphor counting is to use a toluene or xylene based phosphor with a low concentration of a sample which is readily soluble in those solvents to give a colourless solution. However, samples are commonly insoluble or coloured and although special techniques are available to overcome these difficulties some quenching of the luminescence is inevitable. Since the degree of quenching increases with sample volume or concentration it is essential to correct for the degree of quenching which occurs with each sample, and several techniques are available.

A tedious, but reliable, method is to count each sample twice, once normally and then to add to it an *internal standard* and count again. The expected increase in count due to the standard is divided by the increase actually observed to give the quench correction factor.

When a single radionuclide is being counted the change in the proportion of the activity in two adjacent or overlapping channels of pulse height analysis may be used: this is the *channels ratio method*, illustrated in Fig. 28.36. The ratio of the counts in the two channels in the absence of quenching is known and as the degree of quenching increases the counting efficiency falls and the channels ratio changes. Corrections for quenching are made from a graph relating the counting efficiency to the channels ratio.

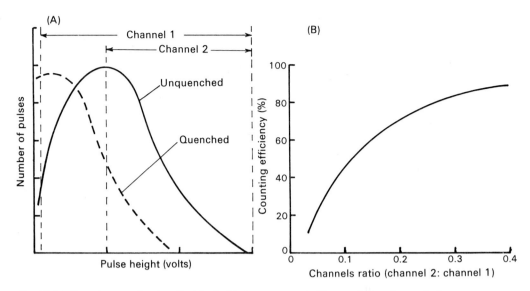

FIG. 28.36. Quench correction is a liquid scintillation counter. A, Unquenched and quenched energy spectra; B. The effect of quenching on the ratio of the counts in two channels of pulse height analysis.

In many commercial automatic instruments *external standardization* is used. After each sample has been counted an external standard source is placed adjacent to it and the counts determined once more. The standard is a γ-emitter giving high energy pulses, so its counting rate is determined in a third channel, widely separated from the others, the count also being reduced by quenching. The correction factor is then obtained from the ratio of the counts in the unquenched and quenched conditions.

SELECTION OF A COUNTING SYSTEM

The most suitable counter is not necessarily that which gives the highest count, since background must also be considered. The criteria of merit, discussed above in connection with counter background, may be used, the most suitable counter having the greatest sensitivity and the highest value for the criterion of merit. An alternative with very weak sources is to use the expression

$$\text{Factor of merit} = M = R_y{}^2 B_1 / R_x{}^2 B_2$$

where R_x, R_y are the sample counting rates for counters 1 and 2 and B_1, B_2 are their respective background counting rates. If $M > 1$ counter 2 is the more suitable.

Other important factors are the physical and chemical form in which the sample can be obtained and the simplicity of sample preparation.

RADIATION HAZARDS AND RADIOLOGICAL SAFETY

This section deals with the problems of radiation dosage and of protection from the harmful effects of radiations and radioactive materials.

DOSE UNITS

The rad. The absorbed dose of any ionizing radiation is the energy imparted to matter per unit mass of irradiated material, the unit being the *rad*.

1 *rad* is that quantity of radiation of any kind which delivers 100 ergs per g of matter.

The term 'dose' as used in the context of health physics refers to the amount of energy absorbed by the tissues. This must not be confused with the dose of a radionuclide (e.g. in millicuries) which may be given to a patient. Although the relationship between the dose in rads and that in millicuries is constant for a given radionuclide, the relationship is different for each.

The röntgen. Although the rad is the unit of absorbed dose it is difficult to measure directly the energy imparted to a given mass of material. Measurements can be made conveniently in terms of the ionization produced in air, the unit used being the röntgen (R).

1 R is that quantity of X- or γ-radiation which produces in 0.001293 g of air ions carrying 1 e.s.u. of charge.

Since 1 e.s.u. is equivalent to 2.1×10^9 ion pairs in air, 1 R is equivalent to an absorption in air of about 88 ergs per g. Since the rate of energy deposition from a given radiation flux depends upon the density of the absorbing material a dose of 1 R corresponds to the absorption by soft tissue of about 97 ergs per g. Thus for most practical purposes exposure doses in air expressed in röntgens can be taken as giving the tissue dose in rads.

The rem.   The biological effects of equal doses, in rads, of different kinds of radiation are not the same since biological damage depends on the specific ionization (local intensity) as well as on the total energy absorption. The *rem* (originally shortened from 'röntgen equivalent for man') is now defined as that dose of radiation which produces in man the effects of 1 rad and is determined by multiplying the dose in rads by a factor (known as the *quality factor*, QF, or the *relative biological effectiveness*, RBE) which expresses the relative efficiencies of different types of radiation in producing biological effects. For all X- and γ-rays, β^--particles and positrons likely to be encountered in pharmacy or medicine the factor is unity, so in these fields of activity

$$\text{dose in rems} = \text{dose in rads.}$$

When radionuclides are deposited in the body their distribution is usually non-uniform and, since the absorbed dose is related to tissue density, this simple relationship no longer holds.

THE BIOLOGICAL EFFECTS OF RADIATION

Mechanism of Injury
The primary event producing injury in a cell is the production of ionization. Excitation plays a relatively small part, since radiations which cause excitation without ionization, such as ultraviolet, are much less effective in causing cell damage. The extent of the initial damage is usually small and a dose of radiation which kills a cell may cause ionization in only one molecule in 10^8. The damage finally observed is much greater than would be expected from the energy absorbed and there are several theories concerning the mechanism by which this situation arises. However, it is generally agreed that under normal conditions of irradiation the damage results from a mixture of direct and indirect effects.

Direct radiation effects are those which result from an ionization or excitation within a biologically functional molecule. The occurrence of an ion cluster within such a molecule releases sufficient energy to make it probable that biological function will be abolished. The principal effects observed with proteins are aggregation and loss of solubility and some degree of fragmentation, while DNA, RNA and polysaccharides exhibit fragmentation and some cross linking. With double-stranded DNA breaks occur principally when both strands are affected in the same region. Although the effects depend to some extent on the fragility of long chain molecules, cross linking is important in the abolition of biological activity since it prevents the uncoiling of closely coiled structures such as DNA and introduces immobile configurations in open chain molecules. It is probable that energy transfer can occur, over a maximum chain length of about 12 carbon atoms, to produce damage in the weakest molecular bonds.

Indirect radiation effects result from the radiolysis of intracellular water, which comprises about 80 per cent of most cells, and of any extracellular water which may be present. The reactions involved are complex and some of the possibilities are summarized in Fig. 28.37. The facts that oxygen generally enhances radiation damage and that many substances which protect against radiation are reducing agents (e.g. cysteamine, cysteine, glutathione) lead to the conclusion that the principal effects are oxidative and oxidations may result from reactions with the hydroxyl and hydroperoxy free radicals, with hydrogen peroxide and, under some conditions, with the hydrogen radicals.

The effect of the rate of cell division.   All cells are vulnerable to radiation damage, though the extent

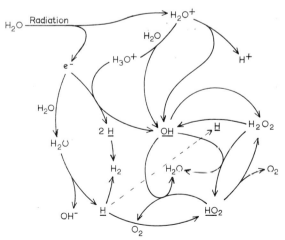

FIG. 28.37. Reactions in the radiolysis of water (free radicals underlined).

varies considerably and depends partly on the rate of cell division. Thus tissues increase in resistance in the following order: lymphocytes, erythrocytes, germinal epithelium, intestinal epithelium, skin, internal organs, brain, muscle, nerve. This indicates that an important part of the damage must be to the nuclear apparatus since any defect here would result in imperfect replication, the effect of which would be multiplied at each cell division, the greater the rate of cell division the greater being the observed damage. Observable effects in radiosensitive tissues (gonads, gut) commence at doses of about 10 rem and are severe at 100 rem. In liver and muscle, which are relatively radioresistant, doses greater than 1000 rem are needed to produce observable effects.

Radiation Effects on the Human Body

Our knowledge of the effects of radiations and absorbed radionuclides on humans is derived from observations on a number of groups of people who have been exposed unwittingly or accidentally. These are radiologists, luminous dial painters, uranium miners, accidentally exposed radiation workers, patients given 'therapeutic' injections of radium and atom bomb survivors. In such cases our knowledge of the doses received may be very limited. Additional information is derived from controlled animal experiments, although extrapolation from results with laboratory animals to predict the situation with humans is unreliable.

The effects of radiation on the entire organism depends on the proportion irradiated, being most severe with whole body exposure and least if only a small mass of relatively insensitive tissue such as the hands is involved. Much depends on the degree to which the harmonious functioning of the various tissues and organs is impaired. Also, for most effects, the dose rate is important and damage will be much less if a given dose is spread out over a long period rather than received in a single, short exposure. Fractionation of a dose permits recovery to occur and in man about 50 and 90 per cent of the dose may be regarded as ineffective after some 20 and 100 days, respectively.

Short term effects. Whole body doses of about 25 rem would produce a transient change in the leucocyte count in most people and nausea in a small proportion. Increasing the dose would result in symptoms of increasing severity, 100 rems causing moderate illness (diarrhoea, vomiting) in about 10 per cent of subjects, and severe illness in about

1 per cent, the syndrome being known as *radiation sickness*. The median lethal dose (LD_{50}) for death in 30 days is about 400 rem and with a dose of 600 rem there would be few survivors. Death from doses of this magnitude is usually the result of gut damage and a loss of resistance to disease, so that infections due to the intestinal microflora proceed unchecked.

Some degree of protection against radiation sickness is afforded by the presence of reducing chemicals (cysteamine, glutathione) and by shielding certain important tissues such as the spleen and the bone marrow. The degree of protection conferred is limited and the LD_{50} is increased two or three times at the most.

Long term effects. The results of exposure, which may appear within a few months or after a latent period of up to 50 years, include permanent skin damage, bone necrosis and an increased incidence of anaemia, leukaemia, cataract and carcinomata. There is also some evidence that there may be a small shortening of life span. At certain stages of its development the human embryo is very sensitive and doses as small as 25 rem may lead to severe abnormalities.

Genetic damage. Mutations may be brought about by quite small doses of radiation and, unlike other types of radiation damage, the effects are independent of dose rate, are cumulative and there is no threshold. Thus any additional radiation dose adds to the mutation load in the population and is undesirable, since it is unlikely that a mutation will introduce improved characters in to a population already well adapted to its environment by the processes of natural selection.

Fortunately most mutations are recessive and many are also lethal, so that the embryo dies at an early stage. However, minor gene modifications may result in the continuous feeding into the population of individuals with disadvantageous characteristics, the number of defective individuals increasing until equilibrium is eventually established. The *doubling dose*, the radiation dose required to double the natural, spontaneous mutation rate, is of the order of 50 rem and if this were maintained for many generations in a large population there would be a serious increase in the proportion of defectives. Doses of this order are insignificant for an individual from the point of view both of observable ill effects and of the probability of producing defective offspring.

BACKGROUND RADIATION

Every individual is continually exposed to radiation which occurs naturally in his environment and arises from cosmic radiation, local γ-radiation from stone and building materials, ^{222}Rn in the air and the natural body burden of ^{14}C, ^{40}K and ^{226}Ra. The average dose rate in Great Britain from this is about 0.1 rem per year and this is of significance only in relation to its possible mutagenic effects. If this is regarded as 100 per cent there are small additions to this from a number of sources. About 1 per cent extra is contributed by nuclear weapon fall-out and a further similar amount from luminous dials and other miscellaneous sources. Both of these contributions are decreasing due to the ban on atmospheric tests of nuclear weapons, to the use of improved luminizing materials and to effective control of devices liable to emit radiations, for example, the virtual disappearance of shoe fitting machines. Another 0.5 to 1 per cent results from occupational exposure and some 20 to 25 per cent from medical procedures. Doses due to these latter sources are increasing with the spread of radioactive work and improved standards of medical care, but the situation is under continual scrutiny to ensure that doses are minimal.

The dose due to background radiation may vary appreciably with the locality and people living at high altitudes receive a substantially greater dose from cosmic radiation than indicated above. Background dose rates may also vary somewhat with the γ-emitting content of local building materials.

THE CONTROL OF RADIATION EXPOSURE

Maximum Permissible Doses

Recommendations as to the maximum radiation doses which are permissible in a variety of circumstances are made by the International Commission on Radiological Protection (I.C.R.P.). The subject is very complex and only a summary of the points of principal interest to radiation workers can be given here.

One maximum permissible dose is that dose which, received in a certain defined period and repeated regularly, is not expected to cause appreciable bodily harm.

Maximum permissible doses have several times been revised downwards and are regularly reviewed as knowledge of the effects of small radiation doses accumulates. The current recommendations are summarized in Table 28.7. Doses resulting from medical procedures are excluded since they are regarded as necessary and beneficial. The relation-

TABLE 28.7

MAXIMUM PERMISSIBLE DOSES FOR RADIATION WORKERS

Organ of interest	Maximum permissible dose (rems)	
	Per year	Per 13-week period
External radiation		
Gonads, blood-forming organs and the lens of the eye	5*	3
Weakly penetrating radiation:		
to the skin (except the hands, forearms, feet and ankles)	30	8
to the hands, forearms, feet and ankles	75	20
Internal radiation		
Limited exposure of internal organs resulting from uptake (other than the thyroid, gonads and blood-forming organs)	15	4
Whole body exposure resulting from generalized uptake	5	3

* This is an average dose rate. The total permissible cumulative dose is given by the expression $5(N-18)$ rems, where N is the age in years, and not more than 60 rem may be accumulated by 30 years of age.

ship governing the total permissible cumulative dose results in an average dose rate of 5 rems per year for persons engaged in radiation work from the age of 18 years. However a dose of 3 rem may be accumulated in 13 weeks, allowing for exceptional procedures involving high dose rates, but if this were to occur subsequent exposure would have to be reduced to ensure that either the average annual dose rate or the total permitted cumulative dose is not exceeded. Rules are laid down for the procedures to be adopted in the event of accidents involving high doses. The I.C.R.P. also recommends for a large range of radionuclides the maximum permissible body burdens and the maximum permissible concentrations in air and water so that the permissible body burdens are not exceeded.

Lower limits of permissible dose are set for the general population, amounting to an addition equal to the natural background dose, and for groups exposed occasionally, such as laboratory maintenance workers.

Estimations of External Dose Rates

The information given below enables dose rates from sources external to the body to be estimated with reasonable accuracy. It is emphasized that such calculations are for planning purposes only and are not intended to provide the final control. The best protection against exposure to external radiation sources is good instrumentation, properly used, and dose rates at working positions should always be measured.

The effect of distance. Radiations are emitted from a source in all directions so with a point source in a non-absorbing medium the inverse square law applies and

$$\text{dose rate} \propto 1/d^2,$$

where d is the distance from the source.

For γ-radiation air is a virtually non-absorbing medium. Provided that the distance from the source is large relative to the source dimensions so that the latter can be neglected, which is normally the case, the inverse square law holds.

With β^--particles there is considerable air absorption and external dose rates are not usually a problem, but application of the inverse square law results in considerable overestimates of dose rates.

γ-dose rates. The specific γ-ray constant (formerly known as the k-factor) is the dose rate produced by the γ-radiation from a radionuclide at a distance of 1 cm from a 1 mCi point source of that nuclide and is given in units of *röngtens per millicurie hour at 1 cm*. Where values of this constant are known this is the most accurate basis for calculating the dose at any distance from a γ-emitting source and the dose constants for some of the radionuclides in common use in medicine are given in Table 28.8. If the dose constant is not known the dose rate may be determined using the decay scheme and Fig. 28.38, the rate contributed by each of the γ-rays emitted by the nuclide being determined separately, with due allowance for the proportions of each γ-ray present, and the whole summed.

For example, ^{48}Va decays giving:

positrons   0.70 MeV (56 per cent)

γ-rays   0.99 MeV (100 per cent)
1.31 MeV (97.5 per cent)
2.25 MeV (2.5 per cent),

but since each positron yields 2×0.51 MeV γ-rays by annihilation, the β^+-emission is equivalent to $2 \times 56 = 112$ per cent of 0.51 MeV γ-rays. The method of calculating the dose rate from this information is given in Table 28.9. Thus the dose rate for ^{48}Va is approximately 15.3 R per h per mCi at 1 cm, which is very near the known value

TABLE 28.8

SPECIFIC γ-RAY CONSTANTS* FOR SOME IMPORTANT RADIONUCLIDES

Nuclide	K	Nuclide	K	Nuclide	K
^{22}Na	12.0	^{59}Fe	6.4	^{131}I	2.2
^{24}Na	18.4	^{60}Co	13.0	^{132}I	11.8
^{42}K	1.4	^{64}Cu	1.2	^{132}Te	2.2
^{47}Ca	5.7	^{24}As	4.4	^{137}Cs	3.3
^{51}Cr	0.16	^{75}Se	2.0	^{182}Ta	6.8
^{54}Mn	4.5	^{82}Br	14.6	^{198}Au	2.35
^{57}Co	0.9	^{85}Sr	3.0‡	^{203}Hg	1.3
^{58}Co	5.5	^{86}Rb	0.5	^{226}Ra†	8.25

* K, R per mCi per hour at 1 cm.
† In equilibrium with daughter products, 0.5 mm platinum screening.
‡ From ^{85m}Rb daughter.
(Reproduced by permission of the Radiochemical Centre, Amersham.)

of 15.6. The slight underestimate in this case results from the fact that 44 per cent of disintegrations are by electron capture, resulting in some additional dose from the resulting 4.5 keV titanium X-rays.

The following approximate formula may also be used:

Dose rate $= 0.5\ C.E$ rad per hour in tissue at 1 m,

where C is the source strength in curies and E is the *total* γ-energy in MeV per disintegration. The total γ-energy must allow for all the energies emitted and the proportion of each, so for ^{60}Co, which emits two γ-rays of 1.17 and 1.33 MeV in

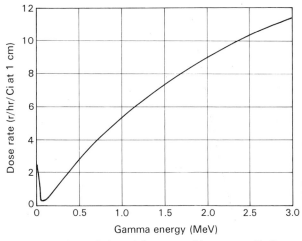

FIG. 28.38. The variation of dose rate with γ-energy (Radiochemical Centre, Amersham).

TABLE 28.9

THE CALCULATION OF THE γ-DOSE RATE AND THE γ-ENERGY PER DISINTEGRATION FOR ^{48}Va

Energy (MeV) (A)	Corresponding dose rate* (B)	Proportion present (C)	Contribution to: Dose rate* (B × C)	Mean energy (MeV) (A × C)
0.51	2.9	1.12	3.22	0.57
0.99	5.3	1.00	5.30	0.99
1.31	6.7	0.975	6.53	1.28
2.25	9.8	0.025	0.24	0.06
Totals	Dose rate* Mean energy (MeV)		15.29 —	— 2.90

* Röntgens per hour per mCi at 1 cm, values under 'B' from Fig. 28.38.

cascade (100 per cent of each), the value of E is 2.5 which would give a dose rate of 12.5 rads per hour in tissue at 1 cm, slightly less than the correct value of 13.0. Again taking ^{48}Va as an example the value of E, calculated as shown in Table 28.9, is about 2.9 MeV and substituting this value in the above formula gives a dose rate of 14.5 rad per hour at 1 cm, a rather lower value than calculated previously but good enough to use in the planning of experiments.

β-dose rates. As already indicated the whole body dose rates due to β^--particles need not be considered since the particles have a limited finite range and can be stopped completely by simple shielding. However some parts of the body, notably the hands and forearms, may be exposed. For a point source of a β^--emitter an approximate estimate of the dose is given by the expression:

Dose rate at 10 cm = 3100 C rads per hour in tissue,

where C is the source strength in curies. The effect of β^--energy is negligible and contributions due to scattering and back-scattering are ignored.

It should be noted that β^--particle doses to the hands may be very large, and the handling of an unshielded 1 mCi source of ^{32}P would give a dose to the hands of about 3 rems per hour, assuming an average distance of 10 cm. This would result in the accumulation of one year's maximum permissible dose in 25 h!

Also the absorption of β^--particles in matter results in the production of Bremsstrahlung and with large amounts of β^--activity the dose arising from this may be appreciable. It is not possible to calculate for this and measurements are always required.

Shielding
It follows from the inverse square law, and the appreciable air absorption of β^--particles, that doses may be reduced appreciably by working at a sufficient distance from a source and this may be adequate with small amounts of radio-activity. With larger amounts of activity shielding is necessary.

Shielding against β-particles. The maximum range of 2 MeV β^--particles in air is about 7.5 m, but ranges in denser materials are much less, the equivalent range in Perspex being about 8.5 mm. Thus 1 cm of Perspex will give effective protection against β^--particles of most energies and such a screen is the simplest method of shielding.

The problem of Bremsstrahlung has been referred to above. Since the amount produced increases with increasing atomic number of absorber, the primary β^--particle absorber should be of as low an atomic number as possible and Perspex fulfils this criterion. About 1 per cent of the β^--energy may be converted into Bremsstrahlung and with large β^--sources additional shielding, as for γ-radiation, may be required.

Shielding against γ-radiation. The extent to which the intensity of a beam of γ-radiation is reduced by a barrier depends primarily on the radiation energy and the atomic number and thickness of the barrier material. The absorption of a *narrow beam* of radiation follows the exponential law already described, but in protection problems narrow beam conditions rarely exist and *broad beam conditions* are usual. In the latter case scattering effects result in a build up of radiation dose which influences principally the first 90 per cent of the absorption.

The *tenth thickness* of an absorber is that thickness required to reduce the intensity of radiation to one-tenth of its initial value and Fig. 28.39 gives the relationships between tenth thicknesses and γ-energy for lead, iron and concrete. The effect of build up is seen in the fact that greater thicknesses are required to reduce doses by the first factor of 10 than are needed for subsequent factors of 10: e.g. for ^{60}Co (mean γ-energy 1.25 MeV) the thickness of lead required to attenuate the dose by a factor of 1000 is approximately $(4.4 + 3.6 + 3.6)$ cm = 11.6 cm.

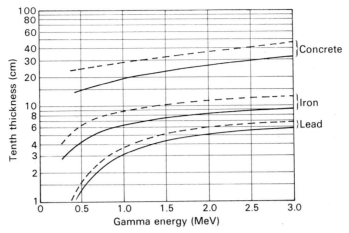

F̲ɪ̲ɢ̲. 28.39. Tenth thickness values for lead, iron and concrete for γ-radiation up to 3 MeV. Broken lines, values for the first tenth thickness; solid lines, values for subsequent tenth thickness. The first tenth thickness is greater due to build-up.

Estimations of Internal Dose Rates

The calculation of the dose rates which arise due to the presence of radionuclides in the tissues is very complex and such estimates are normally required only for patients receiving diagnostic or therapeutic doses of radionuclides or in the case of accidental ingestion by radiation workers.

The factors which influence such calculations are as follows:

(1) The rate of turnover of the element in the body. The effective half-life (T_{eff}) is derived from the actual half-life of the radionuclide ($T_{1/2}$) and the biological half-life (T_b), which defines the turnover rate, and

$$T_{eff} = T_{1/2} \cdot T_b/(T_{1/2} + T_b).$$

(2) The degree of absorption by the body and of selective localization within particular organs and the nature of the organ.

(3) The energy and quality of the radiation, the energy of α- and β^--particles being absorbed wholly within a small volume, whereas only a part of the emitted γ-radiation is absorbed within the body.

The Measurement of Exposure Doses

It is normal to determine exposure doses in a laboratory by two methods which are complementary, personal dosemeters being carried continually by individuals and laboratory monitors being available to determine dose rates at any desired working position from time to time.

Personnel monitoring. The commonest form of monitor for personnel is the *film badge*, which consists of a small piece of wrapped photographic film worn inside a holder, usually as a lapel badge although hand and head badges are useful for particular applications. Except for certain large users who operate their own film badge services, films and holders are distributed in the United Kingdom by the Radiological Protection Service (R.P.S.); one of their holders is illustrated in Fig. 28.40A. The R.P.S. film badge holder is designed to provide six different degrees of shielding of the film; an open window, in which the film is shielded only by its paper wrapping; a thin plastic window (50 mg per cm²); a thick plastic window (300 mg per cm²); and three different types of metal shield. When the film is returned to the R.P.S., normally after two weeks, it is developed under controlled conditions and the pattern of blackening resulting from the different areas of shielding enables the type and energy of the radiation and the dose to be assessed. Although the details of construction of the holder differ, similar principles apply universally for film badge dosimetry.

The principal advantages of the film badge are its cheapness, small size, simplicity in use and ability to integrate radiation doses over a relatively long period. Also it serves as a permanent record of cumulative exposure which is adequate for administrative purposes and is accepted as evidence that an institution has discharged its function of protecting staff from excessive radiation

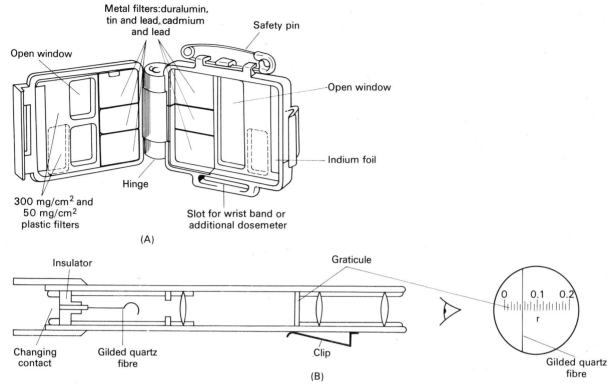

FIG. 28.41. Personnel dosemeters. A, The Radiological Protection Service film badge holder (Radiological Protection Service); B, The principle of the pocket electroscope dosemeter.

exposure. However, it is ineffective for weakly penetrating radiations, owing to the thickness of the film wrapping, it is insensitive to doses below about 0.2 rem, and the dose is not known until some time after the badge has been worn.

When exposure doses are likely to exceed one-half of the maximum permissible dose it is normal to use *pocket ionization chambers* or *pocket electroscope dosemeters*. The former are charged up and read instrumentally and once read require recharging. The electroscope dosemeter (Fig. 28.40B) is designed so that the cumulative dose may be read at any time by looking through the telescope of the dosemeter and observing the position of a gilded quartz fibre on a scale calibrated in röntgens. Various sensitivities are available in the range 0.2 to 500 R. The advantages of the electroscope dosemeter are its robustness, simplicity in use, and ability to indicate the accumulated dose at any time and, providing it has not recorded its full capacity, to continue to record and indicate. Although it is insensitive to β^--particles this is not usually a disadvantage, since shielding is relatively simple in this case, the major protection problems occurring with X- and γ-rays.

Special types of dosemeter are available for use on the fingers or for other special purposes.

It must be emphasized that personal dosemeters can only record the radiation dose in the area of the body where the dosemeter is located. Exposure doses are frequently non-uniform, especially where shielding is used and careful surveys of working positions are essential with sources of moderate or high activity.

Laboratory monitoring. All laboratories which use other than minimal sources for limited purposes should possess a sensitive, accurately calibrated, portable ionization chamber monitor (e.g. Eberline Type R02; Nuclear Enterprises, Type 0030, Fig. 28.41) with which the exposure doses from both β^--particles (energy greater than about 0.2 MeV) and γ-rays at any point in the laboratory may be measured. These monitors may be able to record accumulated doses as well as dose rates.

Pocket electroscopes may also be placed at strategic positions in a laboratory to record accumulated doses.

Biological monitoring. The determination of the total radioactive body burden of radiation workers

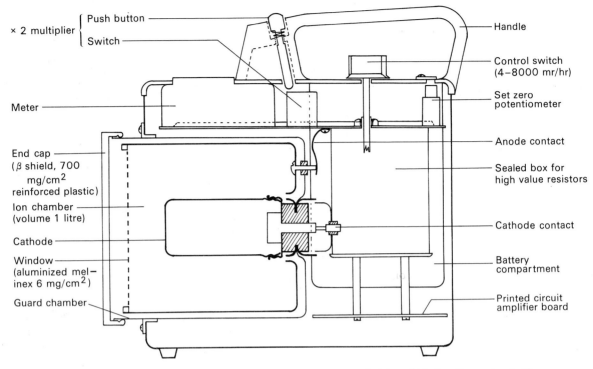

× 2 multiplier { Push button — Switch —

Handle

Control switch (4–8000 mr/hr)

Set zero potentiometer

Meter —

Anode contact

End cap (β shield, 700 mg/cm^2 reinforced plastic)

Sealed box for high value resistors

Ion chamber (volume 1 litre)

Cathode —

Cathode contact

Window (aluminized mel−inex 6 mg/cm^2)

Battery compartment

Guard chamber

Printed circuit amplifier board

FIG. 28.41. An ionization chamber monitor, type 95/0030-1/6 (U.K.A.E.A. and Nuclear Enterprises Ltd.).

is required only in exceptional circumstances. If it is suspected that absorption of significant amounts of a radionuclide has occurred the activity of urine and, less often, faeces may be monitored, though with radionuclides which are firmly bound in particular tissues, as ^{32}P, ^{45}Ca and ^{90}Sr are in bone, the excretion rates are very low once transfer to the tissue concerned has occurred. With radio-iodides the thyroid activity may be monitored using a NaI(Tl) scintillation counter externally. Special facilities are required for whole body monitoring.

Biological monitoring is undertaken principally when radiotracing is used in metabolic studies or medical diagnosis.

THE OPERATION OF RADIOCHEMICAL LABORATORIES

Organization
In any institution all work with radionuclides and radiations should be under the control of a *Radiation Safety Officer*, with adequate training and experience in radiation safety practice, who may be assisted by the persons in charge of individual laboratories or installations. The safety officer is responsible for the following:
(1) The design and approval of laboratories or installations or modifications thereto.
(2) The instruction of personnel in the principles of

radiation safety practice and the procedures to be used for normal working and if accidents occur.
(3) The provision, maintenance and calibration of suitable monitoring devices and the control of dose levels.
(4) The control of ordering, stocks and waste accumulation and disposal.
(5) The provision of adequate medical supervision.
(6) The maintenance of records of the results of monitoring, doses, orders, stocks and waste.
(7) Liaison with police and fire authorities.

Statutory controls. · In Great Britain the operation of radiation laboratories, except those in hospitals, is controlled by the Radioactive Substances Act (1960) and regulations made under its authority. The Act is administered by the Department of the Environment, which grants licences specifying the nature and amounts of radionuclides which may be used in a premises and controlling the accumulation and disposal of waste. Most other countries have similar legislation in force.

Hospitals operating within the National Health Service in Great Britain are exempt from the requirement to register under the Act and the scope of their operations is controlled by a Code of Practice issued under the joint auspices of several

Government Ministries. This exemption does not apply to the corresponding hospitals in Northern Ireland or to other hospitals.

Laboratory Design

The principal criteria are that there should be a safe environment for workers and that radioactivity should be confined within the designated areas. Generally there should be separate provision for decontamination (clothes changing, washing and hand and clothing monitoring), counting, low activity work, high activity work and storage. The counting room and the decontamination area should be inactive areas, without significant levels of radioactivity. If significant amounts of radioactivity are to be used it is common to have physical barriers separating the areas where different levels of activity are handled and these barriers may provide facilities for donning protective overshoes.

It is an advantage to have a more generous provision of fume cupboards than is usual in chemical laboratories. If the fume cupboards are separately and adequately ventilated they provide a valuable means of avoiding contamination of laboratories and personnel and cross-contamination between different experiments or different types of work. Fume cupboard bases should provide shielding against γ-irradiation of the lower part of the body and this may be done by having a 15 cm thick base of heavy (baryta) concrete. The weight of such shielding, of lead walls which may be erected and of the apparatus and local shielding used in counting rooms requires careful attention to possible floor loadings.

The handling of millicurie amounts of pure β^--emitters may require the use of glove boxes, but the dose rate from most γ-emitters is such that millicurie amounts require the use of lead shielding and remote handling tools.

Air conditioning is highly desirable and should provide for a high rate of atmospheric change to minimize airborne contamination in the laboratory. The residual pressure inside the laboratory should be slightly lower than atmospheric pressure to reduce the possibility of the escape of activity to the surroundings. For most purposes it is unnecessary to filter the exhaust from general ventilation or from fume cupboards since the atmospheric dilution is considerable and the resultant concentrations will be below the maximum permissible levels.

The general standards of finish should be high with impervious, easily cleaned surfaces. Floors are best covered with linoleum or vinyl, cemented at edges and joins and well polished, since such coverings can be cleaned readily and are easily removed if they become grossly contaminated. Services should be arranged for simplicity of maintenance, access being preferably from outside the laboratory.

Storage facilities should be so arranged that dose rates are minimal and below the maximum permissible levels. Frequently this means the allocation of a relatively large area, considering the actual bulk of material concerned. Where practicable, source containers should be placed in absorbent packing inside a second receptacle to reduce accidental breakage and to trap any leakage which might occur. Non-rigid plastics are very suitable as the outer container with pure β^--emitters but γ-emitters will usually require lead pots or other types of lead shielding. A standard office safe is very convenient for small containers and gives good security.

Laboratory classification. Three different grades of laboratory are normally distinguished.

Grade C laboratory conditions are provided by a normal good quality chemical laboratory, which is adequate for most biological tracer work and diagnostic medical procedures. The principal hazards in such work arise from the dispensing of individual amounts from stock, for which only a limited amount of shielding is necessary.

For higher levels of activity a *Grade B* laboratory is required, in the design of which special attention is given to the design criteria indicated above and good fume cupboards, substantial shielding and remote handling equipment are essential. Laboratories of this standard are required for handling the amounts of activity involved in the therapeutic uses of unsealed radionuclides, and whenever the volume of work is high, since this involves maintaining large stocks on the grounds of availability, convenience and economy.

Laboratories of *Grade A* are rarely required. They involve massive shielding, complex remote handling equipment and sophisticated ventilation and drainage, so that their design and operation is a matter for experts.

The Toxicity Grading of Radionuclides

Radionuclides are graded in toxicity on the basis of several criteria in relation to the hazards arising from tissue deposition, including the following.

Effective half-life. The effective half-life is the time taken for the body burden to be reduced to one-half. This depends on the physical half-life of the radionuclide and the rate of excretion of the element. Although initial excretion rates following absorption may be high many radionuclides are gradually transferred to organs with very low turnover rates, such as bone. Once locked up in this way it is impracticable to increase excretion rates significantly.

The type and energy of the radiation. In this context α-emitters are the most toxic, since the whole of the energy is absorbed in the immediate vicinity of the source producing intense local damage, β^--emitters are less toxic and γ-emitters the least toxic, as only a part of the γ-radiation is absorbed within the body.

The degree of selective localization within the body. Those nuclides which are concentrated selectively in particular organs or tissues, as are ^{45}Ca, ^{90}Sr and ^{226}Ra in bone and radio-iodides in the thyroid gland, are graded with high toxicity.

Other factors to be considered are the volatility of the compound being handled, its specific activity and its chemical form. The latter point may be important since a radionuclide of low toxicity, e.g. ^3H, ^{14}C, may create considerable hazard if present in a compound such as thymidine which is incorporated into deoxyribonucleic acid, resulting in nuclear damage in newly formed cells.

The toxicity gradings of some important radionuclides are given in Table 28.10. These gradings

TABLE 28.10

THE TOXICITY CLASSIFICATION* OF SOME IMPORTANT RADIONUCLIDES

Class I (high toxicity)
    ^{90}Sr, ^{210}Pb, ^{226}Ra.

Class II (medium toxicity, upper sub-group A)
    ^{22}Na, ^{36}Cl, ^{45}Ca, ^{54}Mn, ^{56}Co, ^{60}Co, ^{68}Ge, ^{89}Sr, ^{90}Sr, ^{110m}Ag, ^{124}I, ^{125}I, ^{131}I, ^{134}Cs, ^{137}Cs, ^{140}Ba, ^{144}Ce, ^{170}Tm, ^{182}Ta, ^{192}Ir, ^{204}Tl, ^{224}Ra, ^{210}Bi.

Class III (medium toxicity, lower sub-group B)
    ^{14}C, ^{18}F, ^{24}Na, ^{32}P, ^{35}S, ^{38}Cl, ^{42}K, ^{43}K, ^{47}Ca, ^{51}Cr, ^{52}Fe, ^{55}Fe, ^{57}Co, ^{58}Co, ^{59}Fe, ^{64}Cu, ^{65}Ni, ^{65}Zn, ^{74}As, ^{75}Se, ^{76}As, ^{82}Br, ^{85}Sr, ^{86}Rb, ^{87m}Y, ^{90}Y, ^{95}Nb, ^{99}Mo, ^{103}Ru, ^{111}Ag, ^{130}I, ^{131}Cs, ^{132}I, ^{132}Te, ^{140}La, ^{141}Ce, ^{147}Pm, ^{177}Lu, ^{197}Hg, ^{197m}Hg, ^{198}Au, ^{203}Hg, ^{206}Bi, ^{222}Rn.

Class IV (low toxicity)
    ^3H, ^{15}O, ^{71}Ge, ^{87m}Sr, ^{99m}Tc, ^{113m}In, ^{133}Xe, natural thorium, natural uranium.

* Based on the International Atomic Energy Agency classification.
(Reproduced by permission of the Radiochemical Centre, Amersham, and the Radiological Protection Service).

TABLE 28.11

THE LEVELS OF ACTIVITY APPROPRIATE TO THE DIFFERENT GRADES OF LABORATORY

Radio-toxicity class	Grade A	Appropriate activity levels* Grade B	Grade C
1	>1 mCi	10 μCi–1 mCi	<10 uCi
2	>100 mCi	1 mCi–100 mCi	<1 mCi
3	>10 Ci	100 mCi–10 Ci	<100 mCi
4	>1000 Ci	10 Ci–1000 Ci	<10 Ci

* Modifying factors for various procedures	
Storage (stock solutions)	× 100
Very simple wet operations	× 10
Normal chemical operations	× 1
Complex wet operations with risk of spills	× 0.1
Simple dry operations	
Dry and dusty operations	× 0.01

are used as a basis for determining the activities which may be handled in the different types of laboratory described above (Table 28.11).

Protection Procedures
Principles. Protection against external radiation hazards depends upon *distance*, and since the inverse square law applies this is the cheapest and simplest form of protection, the *time* of exposure, the total dose being proportional to the time spent in the radiation field, and the use of appropriate *shielding*. Good instrumentation, properly used, is also essential.

The best protection against internal hazards is exceptional cleanliness of working and sensible experimental procedures. The type of rules commonly applied are given in Table 28.12.

TABLE 28.12

TYPICAL RULES FOR A RADIATION LABORATORY

The Radiation Safety Officer for this laboratory is...............
.... Telephone........................

General
1. You are required to familiarize yourself with the laboratory 'Code of Conduct', under which these rules are made.
2. Eating, drinking, smoking and the application of cosmetics, in any part of the laboratories, is prohibited.
3. Only the protective clothing provided may be worn and this must be removed before leaving the laboratories for any reason.
4. Film badges must be worn at all times and other dosemeters as specified for particular personnel.
5. Any exposed unhealed wounds, especially on the hands, must be reported before commencing work. Any wound received in the laboratory must be reported immediately.
6. Before leaving the laboratory the hands must be washed and the hands and clothing monitored. Any residual contamination must be reported immediately.

TABLE 28.12—*continued*

7. No clothing, cases, books or personal belongings other than those essential to the work to be done may be brought into the laboratory.

Safety in Handling
8. Gloves must be worn whenever unsealed sources are handled. Rubber gloves must be decontaminated before removal, disposable plastic gloves are discarded after a single wearing.
9. Pipetting and the performance of any other operation by mouth is strictly forbidden. Damaged or chipped glass apparatus must not be used.
10. All containers of radioactive material must be labelled with the name of the substance, its activity and the date of assay.
11. Radioactive materials must be stored in suitable, secure containers in the specially allocated areas.
12. Operations likely to lead to radioactive dust, vapour or spray must be conducted in a fume cupboard or glove box.

Radioactive Waste
13. Liquid and solid active waste material must be discarded separately into the special containers provided and segregated according to half-life or as instructed. Containers must be labelled adequately.
14. No active waste may be discarded into the sinks or into normal refuse bins without specific authority.

Contamination and Accidents
15. All accidents involving personal injury or radioactive spillage must be reported to the Radiological Protection Officer.
16. The priorities of action following major spillage are as follows.
  First, the protection of personnel.
  Second, the containment of contamination.
  Third, report.
  Fourth, decontamination.
17. Contamination of apparatus, furniture etc. must be marked as to the nuclide and the area involved and the spread of contamination limited by covering with tissues for liquids and with damp tissues for solids.
18. The location of minor spillage must be marked and decontamination carried out promptly.
19. Apparatus contaminated in use must be decontaminated as soon as possible and must not be allowed to dry.

The Counting Room
20. Only sources prepared ready for counting may be taken into the counting room.
21. Where possible all sources must be sealed to prevent the escape of radioactive material.
22. Gloves, overshoes and any protective clothing used in the high activity laboratories must not be taken into the counting room.

The control of contamination. The most satisfactory means of control are a thorough training in appropriate techniques and strict adherence to the laboratory rules. However, some degree of contamination is inevitable and laboratory surfaces and equipment must be checked regularly with a *contamination monitor.* These instruments are of the ratemeter type and give an audible indication of the presence of activity. Although a simple Geiger–Müller assembly is suitable for detecting β^--particles an instrument capable of operating scintillation detectors is desirable since it is more versatile,

different detectors being used according to the type of radiation involved.

A special problem exists in the detection of contamination by low energy β^--emitters. Radiations from ^{14}C, ^{35}S and ^{45}Ca will not penetrate the walls of glassware or other minor barriers and the detection of internal contamination in apparatus must be done by swabbing with a tissue, or rinsing onto a tissue, which is then monitored. Even sensitive monitors have a very low efficiency for these radiations, of the order of 10 to 15 per cent. There is no practicable way of monitoring for ^3H contamination and this may go undetected until it interferes with experimental results.

The procedures used for *decontamination* are very varied and depend on the nature of the contamination and of the contaminated surface. When contamination occurs from aqueous solutions *carriers* may be used. These are dilute solutions of an inactive isotope of the same element in the same chemical form as the radionuclide and remove adsorbed contamination by exchange. Other agents are detergents, complexing agents (oxine, EDTA), organic solvents, dilute or concentrated acids (including nitrosulphuric and chromic acids) and alkalis. Decontamination is commenced with a mild agent and drastic measures are used only when monitoring shows that the mild technique used is ineffective.

Glassware used in radiochemical laboratories should be marked suitably and reserved for use exclusively in those laboratories. In a busy hospital laboratory it may be impracticable to monitor every item of glassware, etc., and decontaminate individually. In such cases it is common to treat all items as contaminated and discard them into cleaning mixture immediately after use.

Handling techniques. The techniques used in the laboratory are onerous, but not especially so, and are comparable in many respects to those used for handling pathogenic microorganisms. Adequate technical skill can be acquired only in the laboratory but a few widely used techniques are outlined below.
(1) Benches, if of wood, should be covered with waterproof paper over which blotting paper may be laid. Self-adhesive sheet plastic can also be used on wood and other types of surface.
(2) Working areas are best defined by using plastic, stainless steel or enamelled trays lined with absorbent paper.
(3) There should be an ample supply of disposable tissues available.

(4) Small volumes of liquid are conveniently measured in automatic zero micropipettes. For larger volumes many designs of safety pipette are available. Alternatively conventional pipettes may be used with an automatic pipette filler or with a syringe attached to the pipette by tubing. Ordinary teats should not be used.

(5) Repetitive dispensing from solutions is best done by self-contained automatic pipettes or burettes.

(6) Balance pans should be protected with cellophane or plastic film.

(7) Solutions should preferably not be boiled but if this is essential it should be done in a fume cupboard and treated as a distillation.

(8) Small volumes of liquid may be evaporated using radiant heat lamps.

(9) Solutions should be sterilized in small batches in bench autoclaves. Very short-lived nuclides may be sterilized as individual doses using a sterile syringe fitted with a membrane filter unit. Syringe attachments giving 6 mm of lead shielding are available.

(10) Sources, beakers, flasks etc. should always be handled with tongs or forceps, especially if γ-emitters are in use, unless it is *known* that the superficial dose rate is negligible.

(11) Contaminated pipettes should never be dipped into a bulk of inactive liquid. A suitable excess volume of the liquid should be placed in a small beaker or, for small volumes, watch glasses of appropriate size. For microvolumes a drop of solution may be placed on a small piece of cellophane.

Waste Control

Most governments exercise statutory control over the accumulation and disposal of radioactive waste. In Great Britain the Department of the Environment issues certificates specifying the general procedures to be adopted.

The accumulation of waste should not result in a hazard to laboratory personnel or the storage of large amounts of activity.

Solid waste, mostly tissues and absorbent paper, is placed in disposable plastic bags in pedal bins. Liquid waste is normally placed in sealable containers, separate ones being used for material with half-lives of less than 14 days, 14 days to 3 months and greater than 3 months. An approximate record should be kept of the radionuclide, its activity and the date, as waste is accumulated.

Waste disposal. Generally small quantities of waste may be discharged into the public sewerage system or the atmosphere, or discarded into the public refuse disposal, provided that there is adequate dilution so that the maximum permissible concentrations in air and water are not exceeded.

Short-lived material (half-life less than 14 days) can be stored for 10 half-lives or until the residual activity is negligible, and this may also be possible with material of up to 3 months half-life. Animal carcasses or tissues contaminated with short-lived material are stored in formalin.

There are considerable problems associated with long-lived materials and it is highly desirable to keep the amounts of waste activity as small as possible and to dispose of it in small quantities as it is generated, rather than accumulate it.

Solid waste which cannot be disposed of by normal refuse disposal may, under suitable control, be buried or incinerated. In the latter case it is preferable to use an existing incinerator, rather than have one reserved for radioactive materials, since this results in dilution with inactive residue.

The incineration of wastes yielding non-volatile, long-lived material should be avoided.

Organic solvent waste is best disposed of by burning, provided the products of combustion are completely volatile and disperse readily in the atmosphere.

The advice and assistance of the controlling authority must be sought if significant amounts of long-lived or highly toxic waste material are accumulated.

Minor disposals of radioactive waste by hospitals under ministerial control are exempted by specific orders made under the Radioactive Substances Act (1960). These exemptions apply also to the premises of medical practitioners and pharmacists but not to other hospitals, to medical schools or to separate medical research units. Disposals of waste other than under the exemption orders are controlled as indicated previously. The excreta of patients undergoing diagnostic or therapeutic procedures involving radionuclides do not normally constitute a problem since the amounts of radioactivity are small or the radionuclides involved are of low toxicity and short half-life so the excreta can be voided to the normal sewerage system, where there is adequate dilution.

RADIOCHEMICAL APPLICATIONS

The subject of radiochemistry covers the use of radionuclides as tracers in chemical and physicochemical systems, analyses using radionuclides or induced radioactivity and radiation chemistry.

Tracer applications may be purely chemical or involve studies of animal and plant metabolism and clinical diagnosis. Radiation chemistry is the study of the effects of radiations on substances or systems and includes therapeutic uses and radiation sterilization.

THE PRINCIPLES OF RADIOTRACER TECHNIQUES

The use of radionuclides as tracers depends on the identity in chemical behaviour of the radioactive and inactive isotopic atoms and the sensitivity with which the radiation can be detected. Until the advent of gas chromatography no other analytical technique approached radio-tracing in sensitivity.

The most important limitations of the method are as follows:

(1) The *isotope effect* results from the difference in mass between the inactive and active isotopes and may be significant with elements of low atomic number, with which small differences in mass are relatively more important. An example is the difference in reaction rates between ^{12}C and ^{14}C.

(2) The *radiation effect*, which results from the effects of radiation on the system, may be appreciable if high energy radiations and high specific activities are used and, in biological systems, if the nuclide is concentrated selectively to give intense local effects, for example, total or partial destruction of the thyroid gland due to the concentration of large amounts of radio-iodide will affect the entire metabolism of an experimental animal.

Generally the stability of a radioactive compound must be regarded as being inferior to that of the inactive compound. Well known examples include: (a) the radiolytic oxidation of solutions of $^{131}I'$ to iodate and periodate; (b) radio-iodide formation from compounds labelled with radio-iodine; (c) the self-destruction of dextran sulphate-^{14}C, presumably due to the radiolytic production of sulphuric acid; and (d) tritiated acetone readily undergoes enolization in alkaline solution with loss of the tritium label, whereas unlabelled acetone is relatively stable under these conditions.

(3) The occurrence of *exchange reactions* between inactive and radioactive isotopic atoms, causing losses of radionuclide from the system. Two simple cases are represented by the following equations:

$$Ba^{14}CO_3 + CO_2 \rightleftharpoons BaCO_3 + {}^{14}CO_2$$
$$C_2H_5{}^{131}I + I' \rightleftharpoons C_2H_5I + {}^{131}I'.$$

Also the hydrogen in some functional groups, such as hydroxyl and amino groups, is rapidly exchangeable in water or hydroxylic solvents and this may lead to the loss of tritium label from the compound.

The applications of radionuclides in analysis are so numerous and varied that a thorough discussion of the subject cannot be attempted here and would be out of place. However a few of the more important uses are described briefly below.

Investigations of Analytical Procedures

The speed and sensitivity of radio-isotope techniques have made them especially valuable in investigations of new analytical or separation procedures and in re-assessments of established methods. Typical examples are studies of ion exchange, chromatographic or gel filtration techniques, especially since continuous recordings of effluent activity can be made, investigations of solvent extraction procedures, determinations of the efficiency of complexing agents and coprecipitation techniques for the concentration or removal of trace elements and examinations of the behaviour of very dilute solutions. Also the effect of different methods of oxidation on the recovery of trace elements from ashed organic materials can be determined.

Radio-isotope Dilution Analysis

Classical analytical methods usually rely on a quantitative isolation of the component of interest in a pure form. Unfortunately the dual aims of purity and quantitative recovery are often incompatible, especially with complex samples or when yields are very small. This problem can often be resolved by the use of radio-isotope dilution analysis, the principle of which is very simple.

It requires a known amount of tracer compound (M_t) of activity C to be added to a mass of sample (M_s) containing an unknown mass (M) of the component of interest. After thorough equilibration a pure sample of the latter is separated and its activity (c) and mass (m) are determined. The mass of the substance of interest in the sample is given by the expression:

$$M = m.C/c - M_t. \tag{28.11}$$

Two important points should be noted. The equilibration step is extremely important and the added radioactive material must be identical in chemical form, combination and distribution with the component of interest so that both behave identically in the separation. Further, any separation technique which yields a pure sample is satisfactory and there is no need for a quantitative yield.

If the mass of tracer added is negligible relative

to that of the component of interest, the expression becomes:

$$M = m.C/c, \qquad (28.12)$$

and in analytical applications the tracer may be regarded as being only a recovery indicator.

The technique has been applied very extensively, examples being the assay of amino acids, hormones, vitamins, antibiotics, insecticides and trace elements.

Recovery indication in analysis. It is often necessary in routine analyses to carry out a preliminary separation of the substance to be assayed and it may be difficult to do this quantitatively due to the occurrence of cumulative losses in complex procedures or to similarities in chemical behaviour between the substance of interest and other components. Losses arising from volatilization or adsorption may also be important with dilute solutions. In all such cases the use of a radioactive tracer as a recovery indicator may reduce substantially the errors involved and the complexity of the procedures used.

The technique is essentially the same as that used in radio-sotope dilution analysis, except that the mass of radioactively labelled material added at the outset is preferably negligible. Since any losses are corrected for, the separation technique need not be quantitative and may be simpler than that which would otherwise be used. The isolated pure component is assayed normally, its radioactivity is measured and the result is calculated using expression (28.11) or (28.12) as appropriate.

Enzyme Assays
A very wide range of radiochemical methods has been developed for the assay of enzymes and the study of the effect of a variety of conditions on enzyme activity. These techniques offer very high specificity, sensitivity and accuracy and are especially valuable in studies of enzyme kinetics, activation and inhibition. The high specificity is useful in assays of crude extracts, even at high dilution, and in the presence of reactions which usually interfere with assays. The high sensitivity permits assays of very low levels of activity, e.g. in the very small amounts of tissue obtained in needle biopsies. Other important applications have been in studies of diseases due to inborn metabolic defects and in investigations of the effects of drugs on enzyme activity.

Activation Analysis
The concentration of many trace elements in drugs, tissues, pathological samples, etc., can often be determined with high sensitivity and accuracy if significant amounts of radioactivity are induced by neutron irradiation.

The growth of activity in a target irradiated in a nuclear reactor is governed by the approximate equation:

$$S = N\varphi\sigma(1 - e^{-0.693t/T}),$$

where S is the induced activity in dps, N is the number of target nuclei present at zero time, φ is the effective neutron flux, σ is the activation cross-section of the target (its probability of capturing neutrons and so undergoing transformation), t is the irradiation time and T is the half-life of the radioactive product. Since σ and T are constants and ϕ and t can be fixed, the induced activity under standard conditions depends solely on N, i.e. the mass of target element present initially.

Usually the sample is placed in a nuclear reactor together with a known mass of a standard sample of the element of interest so that both sample and standard are irradiated identically. Under these conditions:

$$\frac{\text{Activity in sample}}{\text{Activity in standard}} = \frac{\text{Mass of element in sample}}{\text{Mass of standard}},$$

and since the activities of sample and standard can be measured and the mass of the standard is known, that of the sample is calculated readily.

Although it may be possible to assay the sample by γ-spectrometry, without further treatment, a chemical separation of the element of interest is often necessary since radioactivity is usually induced in several components of the sample. Both sample and standard are treated identically, the activities of each are determined, allowing for the chemical yield of the separations, and the radiochemical identity of the isolated material confirmed as a precaution.

An application of interest in forensic medicine is the determination of arsenic in pathological samples, the sensitivity being about 100 times that of normal methods.

Solubility Determinations
The solubility of a slightly soluble substance may be determined readily by preparing a saturated solution of the radioactively labelled substance and comparing the activity of an aliquot of the solution with that of a known weight of the labelled material.

The method can be readily adopted to determine the effects of a variety of conditions on solubility.

A further modification of the technique enables the *specific surface area* of a substance to be determined by making use of the phenomenon of the exchange of ions or molecules between the surface of a solid and a saturated solution of the substance. If the solution is radioactively labelled the extent of this exchange, and so the surface area of the solid, can be determined since at equilibrium:

$$\frac{\text{Number of radioactive atoms on surface}}{\text{Number of radioactive atoms in solution}}$$

$$= \frac{\text{Mass of substance on surface}}{\text{Mass of substance in solution}},$$

The technique can be applied to materials which are normally appreciably soluble, provided that a suitable system offering low solubility can be formulated.

Radioimmunoassay

This technique combines the high specificity of the antigen-antibody reaction with the ease and sensitivity of radionuclide counting to give a uniquely sensitive method for the assay of a variety of compounds, e.g. digoxin, L-thyroxine and insulin, in clinical and other samples. Clinical samples often contain substances which interfere with conventional assay methods but the insulin radioimmunoassay, for example, is capable of detecting c. 0.4×10^{-4} ng (10^{-3} micro units).

The procedure is illustrated in Fig. 28.42. Either a labelled drug is precipitated with immunoglobulin, or with a 'binding agent' consisting of an immunoglobulin-antiglobulin complex. The latter method often gives more rapid and reproducible results. In this latter assay, a range of volumes of sample is mixed with standard preparations of the binding agent and the labelled drug. The labelled standard and the unlabelled drug compete for the binding agent to give a precipitate, the activity of which is measured. The lower the concentration of drug in the sample, the more labelled drug is bound from the standard preparations and the greater is the activity of the precipitated complex and *vice versa*. Thus the amount of drug in the sample is related inversely to the radioactivity precipitated in the complex.

MEDICAL APPLICATIONS

Radionuclides are now widely used in medicine as diagnostic aids, for tumour therapy and in research. The general principles of the various types of application are discussed briefly below and the more common uses of a number of radionuclides and radioactive compounds are summarized in Table 28.13, which is not exhaustive.

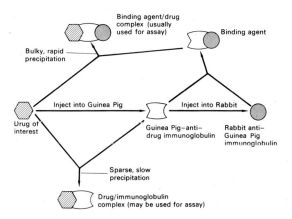

FIG. 28.42. The procedure for radioimmunoassay. Full details are given in the text.

TABLE 28.13

MEDICAL APPLICATIONS OF RADIONUCLIDES

Component or function of interest	Radionuclide or labelled compound used
The determination of body composition and the size of body compartments	
Sodium space and exchangeable sodium	^{24}Na
Exchangeable potassium	^{42}K
Exchangeable chloride, extracellular fluid	^{82}Br*
Body water, oedema	^{3}H
Calcium	^{45}Ca, ^{47}Ca, ^{85}Sr
Body fat	^{85}Kr
Red cell volume	^{51}Cr
Plasma volume	RISA[†]
Heart chamber volumes	^{85}Kr, ^{84}Rb, ^{85}Rb
Pulmonary blood volume	RISA
Metabolism and turnover studies	
Ferrokinetics (loss, absorption, utilization, plasma clearance of iron)	^{59}Fe
Red cell life span, blood transfusion	^{51}Cr, DF^{32}P[†], glycine-1-^{14}C

TABLE 28.13—*continued*

Component or function of interest	Radionuclide or labelled compound used
Sites of red cell destruction	^{51}Cr
Platelet survival	DF ^{32}P, ^{51}Cr, ^{35}S
Leucocyte survival	^{32}P, thymidine-^3H
Calcium metabolism, parathyroid activity, bone turnover, vitamin therapy	^{45}Ca, ^{47}Ca, ^{85}Sr
Sodium turnover	^{22}Na
Chlorine turnover	^{36}Cl
Gastrointestinal haemorrhage	^{51}Cr, ^{32}P
Vitamin B_{12} metabolism	Cyanocobalamin-^{57}Co or -^{58}Co
Fat absorption, sprue, steatorrhoea	Triolein-^{131}I, oleic acid-^{131}I
Folic acid metabolism	Folic acid-^3H
Protein loss	RISA-^{131}I, PVP-$^{131}I^{\dagger}$, $^{51}CrCl_3$, dextran-^{59}Fe
Protein turnover	RISA-^{131}I
Respiration	^{15}O, ^{85}Kr, ^{133}Xe
Thyroid metabolism	^{131}I, ^{132}I
Kidney function	Allyl-inulin-^{131}I or ^{125}I, sodium diatrizoate-^{131}I or -$^{125}I^{\dagger}$, Cyanocobalamin-^{57}Co, EDTA-^{51}Cr
Gall bladder, bile	Iodipamide-^{125}I or -^{131}I
Circulation and blood flow	
Cardiac output	RISA-^{131}I
Coronary blood flow, intracardiac shunts	^{85}Kr, ^{84}Rb, ^{86}Rb
Pulmonary blood flow	^{133}Xe, MAA-$^{131}I^{\dagger}$
Cerebral circulation	^{85}Kr, 4-iodo-antipyrine-^{131}I, ^{133}Xe
Liver blood flow	^{198}Au, sodium idiohippurate-^{131}I
Kidney circulation	^{42}K, sodium iodohippurate-^{131}I, ^{133}Xe, sodium diatrizoate-^{131}I or -^{125}I, sodium iothalamate-^{125}I or -^{131}I
Muscle blood flow	^{24}Na, ^{133}Xe
Skin blood flow, plastic surgery	^{24}Na
Organ and tumour visualization	
Angiography	Sodium iothalamate-^{125}I or -^{131}I
Spleen	Red cells-^{51}Cr, ^{81}Rb, BMHP-$^{197}Hg^{\dagger}$, MPH-$^{197}Hg^{\dagger}$
Liver	Sulphur colloid-^{99m}Tc, ^{198}Au colloid, MAA-^{131}I, ^{113m}In colloid, Rose Bengal-^{131}I, PVP-^{131}I, ^{99}Mo
Gall bladder	Iodipamide-^{125}I or -^{131}I
Pancreas	Selenomethionine-^{75}Se
Stomach	^{131}I
Kidney	Chlormerodrin-^{197}Hg, iron complex-^{99m}Tc
Skeleton	^{18}F, ^{47}Ca, ^{85}Sr, ^{87m}Sr

TABLE 28.13—*continued*

Component or function of interest	Radionuclide or labelled compound used
Brain tumours	^{99m}Tc, chlormerodrin-^{197}Hg, RISA-^{131}I, ^{74}As, ^{113m}In
Thyroid	^{125}I, ^{131}I, ^{99m}Tc
Lungs	MAA-^{131}I, MAA-^{99m}Tc, $Fe(OH)_3$-^{113m}In
Placenta	RISA-^{132}I, albumin-^{99m}Tc
Lymphatic system	Tri-*n*-octylphosphate-^{32}P or triolein-^{131}I in Lipiodol UF
Cartilaginous tumours	^{75}Se
Eye tumours	^{32}P
Therapy	
Solid sources	^{60}Co, ^{90}Sr, ^{90}Y, ^{137}Cs, ^{182}Ta, ^{226}Ra
Colloids	^{90}Y, ^{198}Au
Solutions	^{32}P, ^{131}I

* No convenient chlorine isotope is available.
† RISA, radio-iodinated human serum albumin, labelled with ^{125}I or ^{131}I.
  Di-isopropyl phosphorofluoridate-^{32}P.
  Polyvinyl pyrrolidone, molecular weight 30,000 to 40,000.
  1-Bromomercuri-2-hydroxypropane.
  1-Mercuri-2-hydroxypropane.
  3-Chloromercuri-2-methoxypropyl urea.
  Sodium 3,5-diacetylamino-2,4,6-triazobenzoate.
  MAA, macro-aggregated albumin.

Body Composition and Body Compartments

Studies of the composition of the intact body and the ways in which the amounts of various components are affected by disease and metabolic derangement were previously of great technical difficulty. Clearly, reliable estimates of the concentration and behaviour of body constituents are invaluable in the accurate diagnosis of disease and the management of the condition and its treatment. Such studies have been greatly facilitated by the use of radio-isotope dilution analysis, the principle of which has already been described.

For this purpose the body is considered to be composed of a number of spaces or compartments, such as the 'extracellular space' and the '24 hour sodium space'. This concept has no anatomical or geometric identity and the measurement merely gives the apparent volume of distribution of the substance of interest. The size of a body compartment, or the amount of a component as measured at a given time, is a reflection of the dynamic metabolic equilibrium which existed at the time of sampling. As with other analytical applications the tracer must be equilibrated thoroughly with the system of interest.

One example will serve to illustrate the benefits of radiotracing. In haematology the conventional determinations of haemoglobin and red cell count only give results relative to the total blood volume, and abnormally low or high values may be masked by corresponding changes in blood volume. Thus pseudo-anaemic conditions occur when the red cell volume is normal and the plasma volume is high, a condition which occurs in kidney disease, splenomegaly or congestive cardiac failure, while a low plasma volume may tend to mask the severity of an anaemia arising from a haemorrhagic condition. Although the total blood volume may theoretically be determined by measuring the dilution effect in a sample of whole blood there are a number of limiting factors which make this unreliable and in many conditions it is essential to measure both the red cell volume and the plasma volume. Both measurements may be made simply and simultaneously on the same blood sample, obtained following the injection of red cells labelled with ^{51}Cr and of RISA-^{125}I (radio-iodinated human serum albumin labelled with ^{125}I), the radiations from each being distinguished by the use of a scintillation counter equipped for pulse height analysis.

Metabolism and Turnover

A number of techniques are used in studies of the functioning of various organs. A common method used with discrete organs is to administer a γ-emitting nuclide and to measure the uptake in the organ with a scintillation counter external to the body and located appropriately. Examples of this technique are the uptake of ^{131}I by the thyroid gland, the accumulation of ^{59}Fe and ^{51}Cr in the liver and spleen, the uptake and clearance of sodium iodo-hippurate-^{131}I by the kidney and of Rose Bengal-^{131}I by the liver and measurements of respiratory activity using ^{85}Kr or ^{133}Xe.

Another important method is to measure the urinary or faecal excretion or the activity in the blood, and in some cases all of these parameters may be measured. One application is the determination of thyroid activity by measuring either the amount of labelled hormone (as protein bound iodine) in the blood or the urinary excretion of ^{131}I. The diagnostic value of organ uptake and of plasma iodine measurements is illustrated in Fig. 28.43.

Other applications are studies of the absorption of ^{59}Fe and cynocobalamin (labelled with ^{57}Co or ^{58}Co) in anaemia and the estimation of gastro-intestinal haemorrhage by faecal counting following the injection of ^{51}Cr or ^{32}P.

Circulation and Blood Flow

The principal method used for studies of the circulation is the *clearance method* in which radio-active material is injected and the rate of removal from the site of injection, which is a measure of blood flow rate in the organ, is measured with an external scintillation counter linked to a rate meter and recorder. Examples of the application of this method are the measurement of muscle blood flow using ^{24}NaCl, and of cerebral, coronary and pulmonary blood flow using the inert gases ^{85}Kr

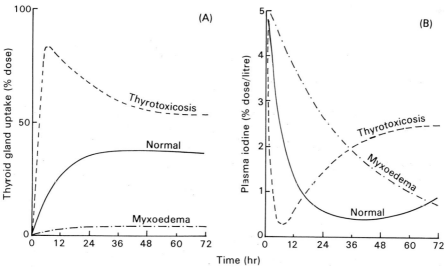

FIG. 28.43. The patterns of iodide utilization in normal subjects and in thyrotoxicosis and myxoedema. A, Uptake in the thyroid gland; B, Changes in the plasma iodine levels with time (modified from data supplied by the Radiochemical Centre, Amersham).

or ^{133}Xe. Measurements of the effect of drugs on the circulation can also be made in this way, observing clearance rates before and after administration of the drug. The inert gases have the advantage that they are almost completely removed from the blood in a single passage through the lungs so that there is virtually no residual activity to complicate the results of repetitive tests.

An unusual technique which has been used to study pulmonary blood flow is to inject macro-aggregated albumin labelled with ^{125}I, ^{131}I, ^{51}Cr or ^{99m}Tc. The albumin is aggregated by shaking and warming at a pH near its isoelectric point. Some 90 per cent of particles in the range 10 to 50 μm are trapped in the lung capillaries and are cleared slowly over a period of several hours. Areas of lung which are poorly perfused, as in pulmonary embolism, trap only a few particles and so show as areas of low activity.

A considerable amount of information can be derived from a single intravenous injection of RISA, recording the activity observed by a scintillation counter carefully aligned over the area of the heart taking a single blood sample after 5 to 10 min, when mixing is complete. This simple procedure yields the cardiac output, the pulmonary circulation time, the pulmonary blood volume, the plasma volume and the blood volume (Fig. 28.44). Further refinements of the technique enable the volumes of individual heart chambers to be determined and the presence of cardiac valvular incompetence or intra-cardiac shunts to be detected.

Organ and Tumour Visualization
Some compounds and elements tend to concentrate in particular organs, for example, iodine in the thyroid gland and strontium in bone, and if the compound is radioactively labelled, or if a radio-isotope of the element is used, the greater activity in the organ of interest relative to that in the surrounding tissue can be observed. Further, if γ-emitters are employed, the radiation may be detected readily by a scintillation counter outside the body.

The principal technique is *radio-isotope scanning* in which a collimated counter is used. Such counters are protected by a heavy lead shield containing one or more carefully defined apertures so that the counter receives the radiation from only a small area at any time. The counter is scanned across the body in a series of adjacent parallel tracks (see Fig. 28.45A) so that the whole of the area of interest is examined. The result may be presented on paper as a dot diagram, in which each dot represents a set number of counts so that the dot density reflects the counting rate, and visualization may be aided by presentation of a colour dot diagram in which the dots are colour coded according to the counting rate. Alternatively, the accumulation of the given number of counts may be used to trigger a flash of light and the dot diagram is then recorded on photographic film. The latter type of scan is shown in Fig. 28.45B in which a brain scan using chlormerodrin-^{197}Hg is superimposed on an X-radiograph of the patient's head, with excellent visualization of a meningioma. The scan can be done in two planes at right angles to give precise location prior to surgery.

An interesting modification of the basic scanning technique is to use a positron emitter (^{18}F, ^{64}Cu, ^{74}As), the annihilation radiation from which yields pairs of 0.51 MeV γ-rays in opposite directions.

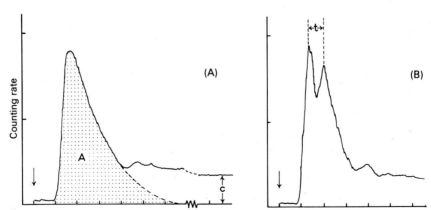

FIG. 28.44. The determination of cardiac output. A, Curve from moderately directional counter. Cardiac output = $F = (cV/A)$, where c is the equilibrium activity, V is the blood volume (determined in the test) and A is the shaded area under the curve; B, Curve from a directional counter, carefully aligned. t, pulmonary circulation time.

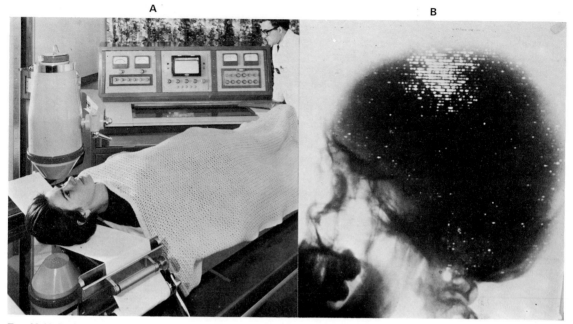

FIG. 28.45. Brain tumour scanning. A, The apparatus, showing two opposing, collimated, NaI(T1) scintillation counters and associated equipment; B, A scintigram of a meningioma obtained with chlormerodrin-^{197}Hg superimposed on an X-radiograph of the skull (Reproduced by permission of St. Bartholomew's Hospital, the National Hospital, Institute of Neurology and the U.K.A.E.A.).

The activity is then scanned with two counters connected in coincidence, one on each side of the body. This arrangement gives very high definition, but has been used to only a limited extent.

Scanning procedures tend to be rather tedious since each scan takes about 20 to 30 min, during which time the patient has to be immobilized. This problem has been overcome by the use of the *gamma camera*, one form of which consists of a large stationary detector comprising a number of crystals and photomultipliers located behind a collimator with several thousand parallel cylindrical holes, each hole viewing a small part of the organ. The gamma camera can produce a picture of the distribution of radioactivity in an organ in a few minutes and makes possible serial determinations of uptake and turnover which may considerably improve diagnostic discrimination.

Organ visualization is used to determine hypertrophy or atrophy, the presence of space-occupying lesions, or displacement, and usually depends on the administration of a radionuclide in a form normally metabolized by the organ, e.g. chlormerodrin-^{197}Hg or hippuran-^{131}I for the kidneys, ^{85}Sr or ^{87m}Sr for the skeleton, red cells labelled with ^{51}Cr for the spleen and colloids of ^{198}Au or ^{113m}In for the liver.

Tumour visualization may depend on a variety of factors. Enhanced uptake due to increased vascularity and metabolic rate occurs with eye tumours (^{32}P) and bone (^{18}F, ^{87m}Sr) whereas increased uptake in brain tumours probably results from breakdown of the normal mechanisms which act as a barrier to the penetration of many substances into brain tissue. However, in many cases the presence of a tumour is inferred from the existence of non-functional masses in organs. Particular advantages of radionuclide tumour scanning are that it will often distinguish between active and inactive lesions (Fig. 28.46) and locate metastases (secondary tumours resulting from the dissemination of cells from a primary malignant tumour), especially with thyroid metastases which often have the ability to concentrate iodide in the same way as normal thyroid tissue.

The technique does not necessarily distinguish between benign and malignant tumours. As with most diagnostic aids the results supplement the information derived from the clinical symptoms and other tests but the value of the technique is beyond doubt.

The chemistry of some radionuclides (^{131}I, ^{99m}Tc, ^{113m}In) enables them to be used as labels for many different substances so that these nuclides have found very wide application.

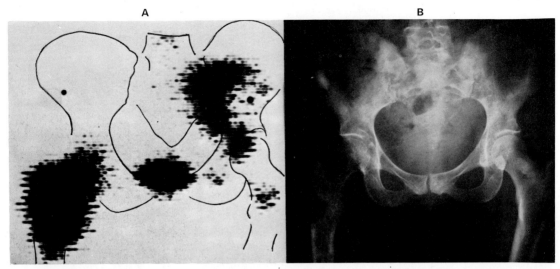

Fig. 28.46. Bone scanning using ^{18}F. A, Scan of pelvis 7 years after the removal of a stomach carcinoma, showing multiple secondary deposits. Excreted ^{18}F shows in the bladder; B, The X-radiograph shows some of the deposits. The dense areas in the right ilium are metabolically inactive since there is no uptake of ^{18}F (Reproduced by permission of Dr V. Ralph McCready and Hospital Medicine Publications Ltd.).

Therapy

Radiation therapy is used principally for the treatment of malignant diseases, damage to the tumour greater than that which occurs to surrounding healthy tissue being obtained by suitable location of solid sources, by suitable adjustment of radiation beams, or by utilizing the ability of certain tissues to concentrate radionuclides. It has already been mentioned that the degree of radiation damage increases with the rate of cell reproduction so tumours, and cells in related conditions which are characterized by uncontrolled growth, tend to be damaged selectively.

Discrete solid sources. Small sources are used for direct implantation into tumours. This has been done for many years with ^{226}Ra and the scope of the technique has been greatly extended by the availability of artificial radionuclides. Removable applicators are used for intracavitary irradiation of the nasopharynx (^{90}Sr), oesophagus (^{60}Co), uterus (^{137}Cs, ^{60}Co), bladder (^{182}Ta, Fig. 28.48) and cervix (^{226}Ra), while foils of ^{90}Sr are applied to small superficial tumours or to the eye (Fig. 28.48). Flexible polythene sheeting impregnated with ^{32}P in the form of red phosphorus or with ^{90}Y as the oxide can be used for the superficial treatment of large areas and for the irradiation of basal cell carcinomas.

An alternative approach is to implant short-lived radionuclides which can be allowed to remain in place since decay results in negligible final radiation doses. This technique is used with ^{198}Au (half-life 2.7 days) in the form of gold grains which are implanted with a special gun (Fig. 28.49) and with ^{90}Y (half-life 64.2 h) rods which are often used for pituitary ablation.

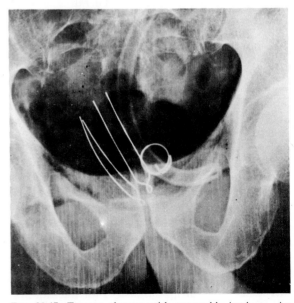

Fig. 28.47. Tumour therapy with removable implants. An X-radiograph of ^{182}Ta hairpins implanted in the bladder. (Reproduced by permission of the Royal Marsden Hospital and the U.K.A.E.A.).

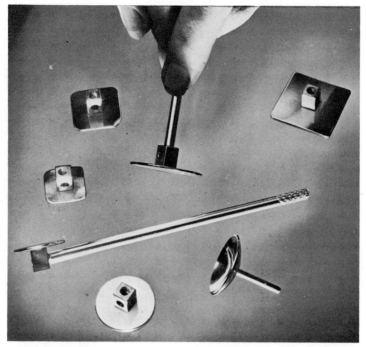

Fig. 28.48. Some ^{90}Sr surface applicators. The spherical sector applicator is for ophthalmic use (U.K.A.E.A.).

Colloids. Colloidal suspensions of appropriate particle size remain located in body cavities or in tissues of low vascularity and this principle is utilized primarily for palliative treatment of the peritoneal and pleural cavities with colloids of ^{198}Au and ^{90}Y, the latter in the form of the silicate or adsorbed onto colloidal ZeoKarb-225. These colloids can also be used in the bladder to treat diffuse growths.

Solutions. Only two radionuclides are widely used in solution form. Inoperable thyroid cancer may be treated with ^{131}I, a form of therapy which is especially valuable if iodine concentrating metastases are present, since these are treated simultaneously.

This nuclide is also used to reduce thyroid activity in thyrotoxicosis, especially when the condition recurs after surgery, and to reduce the basal metabolic rate, and so the demand on the heart, in some cases of intractable cardiac disease. The irradiation of blood-forming tissues by ^{32}P from its absorption sites in bone is the method of choice in the treatment of polycythaemia vera, an excessive production of red cells, and may also be useful in the treatment of myeloid and lymphatic leukaemias, which are characterized by excessive white cell production.

Teletherapy is the irradiation of tissues using powerful radioactive sources located outside the body, the usual sources being γ-emitters, normally ^{60}Co (about 2000 Ci), but ^{137}Cs (about 10 000 Ci) is also used. These are employed similarly to X-ray therapy sets but have the advantages of low operating costs, continuous output, reliability, and cause fewer skin reactions since the maximum dose occurs several millimetres below the skin surface. Also if the source is rotated around the patient in a circle with the tumour as its centre (Fig. 28.50), the dose to the tumour is achieved with a substantially smaller dose than usual to the surrounding tissue. The latter technique is impossible with X-ray generators due to the attachment of the power cables.

Superficial irradiation of the whole body with β^--particles is also used, usually to irradiate the blood as it passes through the skin capillaries, the normal source being an array using about 24 Ci of ^{90}Sr.

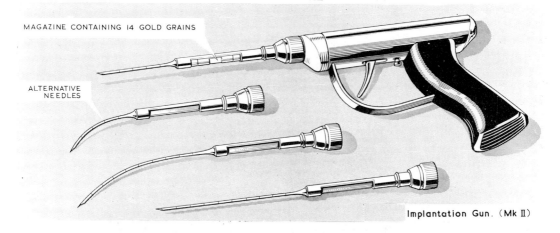

MAGAZINE CONTAINING 14 GOLD GRAINS

ALTERNATIVE NEEDLES

Implantation Gun. (Mk II)

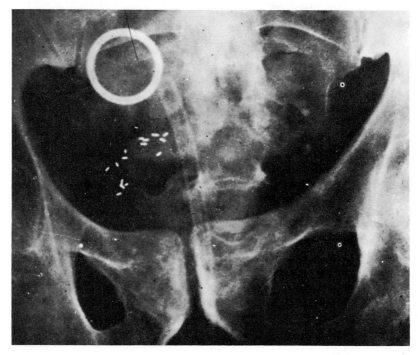

FIG. 28.49. Tumour therapy with permanent implants. A, The gun used for implanting gold (^{198}Au) grains; B, An X-radiograph of gold grains implanted permanently in the bladder (Reproduced by permission of the Royal Marsden Hospital and the U.K.A.E.A.).

RADIATION STERILIZATION

The Sterilization Process
The 'target hit' concept. The basis of the lethal action of radiations on microorganisms is the production of ionizations and, less importantly, excitations when radiation traverses the cell. However, lethally irradiated cells remain intact, respiration continues normally, motile cells retain their motility for some time and, under conditions where reproduction is possible, death may not occur until after one or two divisions of a cell. The extent of these effects in any individual case depends on the extent of damage but it is clear that inactivation is not the result of gross damage but arises from the effects of one or more minor lesions.

The essential particulate nature of ionizing radiations and the fact that they produce discrete ionization loci, the statistical distributions of which can be calculated (Fig. 28.51), have led to the

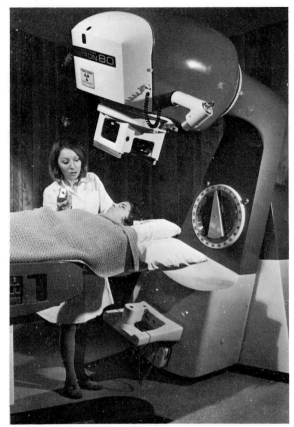

FIG. 28.50. A ⁶⁰Co teletherapy unit. The massive head, containing 4670 Ci shielded with depleted uranium, can be rotated around the patient (Reproduced by permission of the Churchill Hospital and the U.K.A.E.A.).

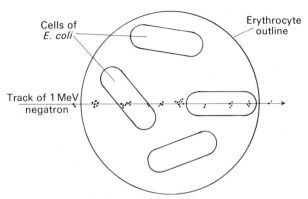

FIG. 28.51. An idealized ionization pattern produced by a 1 MeV negatron superimposed on the outline of cells of *Escherichia coli* and of an erythrocyte (Reproduced by permission of Professor Trump and the Pharmaceutical Press).

radicals and excited atoms, all of which may contribute to molecular damage.

The form of the survivor-dose curve. As with all other sterilizing agents the death of irradiated microorganisms can be described by a probability function, though there is no correlation between the sensitivity of a species to irradiation and any other sterilizing agent. Also, as with other sterilization processes, three types of survival curve may be obtained (Fig. 28.52).

Most survival curves are exponential in form

concept that inactivation is due to 'hits' in specific 'targets'. The hits are specific lesions which individually or cumulatively result in cell death and the targets are the sensitive loci, the integrity of which is essential to viability. The natures of these targets have not been identified but the indications are that they are macromolecular in nature and they have been equated with genes, membranes and other functional entities.

Although this concept appears to place the greatest emphasis on the direct effects of radiation, the indirect effects resulting from the occurrence of primary ionizing events in water are also important because water is the principal component of all cells. Further, cells may be in contact with sufficient water so that appreciable cell wall damage is caused by the free radicals resulting from ionizations in the extracellular fluid. It should be appreciated that within about 10^{-12} s each ionization locus is surrounded by a population of ion pairs, free

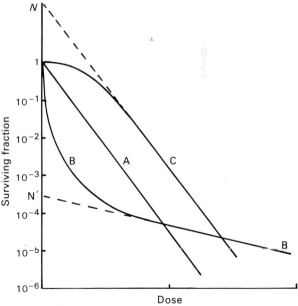

FIG. 28.52. Types of log survivor-dose curves. Type A, exponential (single hit). Type B, curve showing tailing. Type C, multitarget (sigmoidal) curve (Redrawn from data supplied by Dr Margaret Thornley and the International Atomic Energy Agency).

(Fig. 28.52, curve A) and are frequently interpreted as resulting from a 'single hit' inactivation process. Such curves are characterized completely by their slope and a widely used related concept is the D-value, the dose required to reduce the population to one tenth of its initial size. A knowledge of the D-value of such a system enables the dose required for any degree of inactivation to be calculated readily.

The form of the second type of curve (Fig. 28.52, curve C), which is sigmoidal in form when plotted arithmetically, has an initial shoulder and finally becomes exponential. In practical terms this means that there is a threshold dose below which death is not observed. The shape of such survival curves has been ascribed to various causes:

(a) The presence of a number of targets within the cell, all of which have to be inactivated before the cell becomes non-viable (the multi-target model), for example, it has been calculated that 90 hits were required to inactivate a single spore of Cl. botulinum strain 33A.

(b) The necessity for several hits to inactivate a single target, the single target inactivation causing cell death. This multi-hit model would lead to a curve different in form from the multi-target model, though it may not be possible to distinguish between them unless the data are very accurate.

(c) The clumping of cells results in a multi-target type of curve. Since we commonly test viability by the ability to form visible growth and the growth can arise from a single unit or a clump it is necessary to inactivate each unit in the clump to destroy viability.

(d) With some species, such as the naturally resistant M. radiodurans, there is a considerable shoulder, possibly due to the possession of extremely efficient repair mechanisms for radiation damage. Curves of type C can be characterized by two parameters, the D-value derived from the slope of the later, exponential part of the curve and the extrapolation number (N), which is the intercept on the ordinate of the backward extrapolation of the exponential part of the curve. Although the extrapolation number can be interpreted as the number of targets required to be damaged for cell inactivation, this interpretation must be approached cautiously. Instead of the extrapolation number the size of the shoulder may be given. It is possible that exponential curves are a limiting form of the multi-target curve in which the shoulder is negligible since in other situations, such as phenol disinfection, the survival curve shows a shoulder at low concentrations but not at high ones.

The third type of curve (Fig. 28.52, curve B) is not usually amenable to mathematical treatment on the basis of the target theory. In some cases these curves may become exponential in the later stages and can then be characterized by the D-value and the extrapolation number (N'), the latter having a value less than unity. Type B curves may arise by the combination of two or more exponential curves of different slope, e.g. those due to the presence of two strains of widely differing resistance, or two targets of different size. However, such curves are often considered to indicate the occurrence of a population with a markedly skew distribution of resistance, there being an abnormally high proportion of sensitive cells. Inadequate techniques resulting in non-uniformity of dose can also give type B curves.

Factors Affecting the Radiation Sensitivity of Microorganisms

The species. The enormous variation in radiosensitivity between species is the single most important factor in the determination of the sterilizing effect of a given dose. Although the radio-resistance of microorganisms generally increases in the order vegetative bacteria, fungi, bacterial spores, viruses, there are a number of vegetative species of bacteria which are remarkably radio-resistant, notably M. radiodurans. This is clearly illustrated in Fig. 28.53.

Inoculum level. The higher the initial population the greater is the dose required to achieve a given degree of inactivation. This situation arises from the generally exponential nature of the process and is similar to that which occurs when microorganisms are killed by heat or chemicals. This population effect emphasizes the need to keep the initial degree of contamination as low as possible so that the sterilization of articles is achieved with the minimum dose.

Gaseous environment. The presence or absence of oxygen during and after irradiation markedly influences the apparent sensitivity to radiation damage and the overall change in oxygen sensitivity is normally about 3:1 but may be as high as 15:1 in some conditions. There appear to be three different types of radiation damage; one component is totally independent of oxygen, a second (latent) component is observed when anoxic irradiation is followed by exposure to oxygen and the third component (immediate) is involved when irradiations are done in the presence of oxygen.

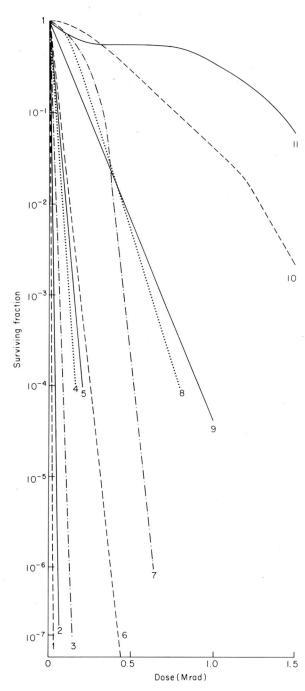

FIG. 28.53. The radiosensitivities of some food spoilage microorganisms. 1, *Pseudomonas* spp.; 2, *Escherichia coli*; 3, *Salmonella typhimurium* in buffer; 4, *Torulopsis famata*; 5, *Bacillus brevis*; 6, *Salmonella typhimurium* in liquid egg; 7, *Streptococcus faecium* strain R53; 8, *Bacillus megaterium* spores; 9, *Clostridium welchii* spores; 10, *Clostridium botulinium* type A spores; 11, *Micrococcus radiodurans*.

Anoxic effects also occur in the presence of reducing agents (H_2S, thiourea) or free radical or oxygen scavengers, such as nitric oxide.

The oxygen effect is usually interpreted on the basis that oxidizing free radicals are formed more readily in its presence, thus increasing the indirect effects, though not all observations fit in with this theory.

Degree of hydration. It is generally accepted that microorganisms are less radiation sensitive under dry conditions than in the presence of water and this is ascribed to the absence of indirect effects arising from the radiolysis of water. Since there may be a 30 per cent change in the inactivation rate over a range of about 20 to 40 per cent relative humidity, there may be an appreciable change of sensitivity within the normal range of ambient humidity.

Temperature. The radiation sensitivity of microorganisms is reduced at, or below, the freezing point of water, due to the immobilization of free radicals and reactive species produced in the water, thus reducing indirect effects.

At temperatures used for sterilization there is a complementary or synergistic effect of temperature and irradiation and sterility may be achieved by a combination of significantly milder treatments of both sterilizing agents. This phenomenon is of potential practical importance in the sterilization of products such as foodstuffs which are both heat and radiation labile.

Stage of cell division. The sensitivity of vegetative bacteria varies during the growth cycle as shown in Fig. 28.54 and the growth phase will clearly affect the dose required if there is the possibility of growth in the material to be sterilized.

Since bacterial spores are considerably more resistant than vegetative cells of the same species there is an abrupt increase in radiosensitivity as spore germination occurs.

Protective and sensitizing agents. A large variety of compounds affect the radiation sensitivity of microorganisms. Protective agents include reducing agents (cysteine, dimethyl sulphoxide, thiourea, cysteamine, β-mercaptoethanol), alcohols and polyhydric compounds (ethanol, glycerol, mannitol) and proteins or complex foodstuffs. The effect of anoxia and free radical scavengers has already been referred to, and most of the protective agents appear to be substances which abolish at least part of the oxygen effect.

The mode of action of radiation sensitizers is obscure. Sensitization has been reported with oxidizing agents (nitrate, nitrite), water soluble stable free radicals (di-*t*-butyl nitroxide), phthalylanilides and phenazinium and *iso*-indolinium compounds. Vitamin K$_5$ has been reported both as a sensitizer and as a protective agent with different bacterial species.

Pretreatment and post-treatment conditions. The physiological condition of an organism at the time of irradiation influences its sensitivity so that the growth temperature, the medium, pH and oxidation reduction potential will all influence the situation. However, there has been little work done on this aspect and most emphasis has been placed on the modifying effects due to variation of the post-irradiation conditions. Post-irradiation treatments which produce reductions in apparent radiosensitivity are: incubation on complex media rather than on simple salt media; the use of more dilute complex media; and retardation of metabolism with metabolic inhibitors or by incubation in distilled water. The effect of incubation temperature varies with the strain of organism, although better survival usually results from the use of temperatures below the optimum for undamaged cells of the same species.

Variation in post-treatments may result in survival curves of different form, indicating that the form of the curve probably reflects the interplay between the revival process after damage and the lethal process. Thus hypotheses concerning the modes of action of lethal agents which are derived from the form of the survival curve should be treated with caution.

It should be noted that the effects of pre- and post-treatment conditions may be related, for example, bacteria grown on a simple salts medium before irradiation have a high concentration of enzymes and may show good recoveries on a complex medium, whereas pre-irradiation growth on a complex medium and the post-irradiation use of salts medium may give the opposite effect due to lack of synthetic ability.

Mutations. In addition to lethal effects, ionizing radiations select radio-resistant mutants from a population and also produce mutations. The degree of radio-resistance appears to be related to the number of cycles of irradiation, isolation and reirradiation so that although the possibility of

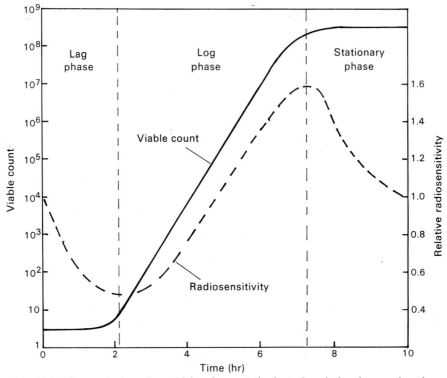

FIG. 28.54. Changes in the radiosensitivity of a vegetative bacterium during the growth cycle.

the emergence of radio-resistant strains must be considered in relation to sterilization practice it is unlikely that this will constitute a major problem.

Determination of the Sterilizing Dose

The selection of the radiation dose required to sterilize various materials depends on several factors: the nature of the species present and their radiation resistance in the particular environment and under the conditions of processing used, the level and the degree of uniformity of the initial contamination and the margin of safety required.

The wide variations in sensitivity between species has already been referred to and the most resistant species likely to occur as a contaminant in the material and the degree of such contamination, are the two most important considerations. Although highly resistant species are relatively uncommon in pharmaceuticals and medical products, which are manufactured under hygienic conditions, the facts that there is a mixed microbial flora of which the exact composition at any time or on any article and the exact degree of contamination are not known precisely, make it essential to assume the worst possible conditions. There is considerable technical difficulty in following the course of the sterilization process at very high inactivation factors since it is impracticable to prepare test microbial suspensions of sufficient concentration to permit the accurate counting of survivors at inactivation factors greater than about 10^9. Also, unless the whole of the dose can be delivered within a very short time the leakage of intracellular material from the high concentrations of damaged cells exerts a protective effect on survivors. However, most inactivation curves seem to be approximately exponential up to high inactivation factors and although the 'tailing' of resistant organisms has been reported, e.g. in irradiations of spores of *Clostridium botulinum* and of yeast and *Salmonella* spp. in dried foodstuffs, the phenomenon may be less important in the irradiation of medical products than of foods.

Although plastic items are frequently sterile at the point of production, subsequent handling results in contamination. Thus disposable plastic hypodermic syringes have an average contamination rate of about 100 microorganisms per article under hygienic conditions, whereas poor handling techniques can result in contamination levels of 10^5 to 10^6 spores per syringe. In contrast with this situation biological materials are inevitably heavily contaminated and thyroid powder has been

reported to contain *Salmonella* spp. and other faecal organisms at a level of 30×10^6 per g.

In the examples referred to above the organisms on plastic syringes would be relatively unprotected by their environment but there would be a considerable protective effect of the thyroid tissues. This latter point is illustrated by some *D*-values reported for *S.typhimurium* in phosphate buffer, canned bacon and canned chicken which were 0.02, 0.16 and 0.33, respectively.

Since the principal type of material sterilized by radiation comprises individual solid items, non-uniformity of contamination is the normal situation and results in a higher dose requirement than if contamination were uniform, since all items have to be treated according to the highest contamination level which occurs.

The margin of safety required depends on the risk of the occurrence of non-sterile articles which is considered to be acceptable for the intended purpose. It has already been noted that the sterilization process is a probability function, so that an inactivation factor of 10^9 coupled with an initial contamination of 10^3 organisms per article would result in residual contamination in an average of one article in 10^6. An increase in the dose, and so in the inactivation factor, gives a lower probability of residual contamination without producing sterility in the absolute sense. This situation is similar to that which occurs with conventional sterilization techniques, though long experience with procedures which are known to produce acceptably safe products and which were developed rather empirically has led to autoclaving being regarded as an absolute sterilization method. The generally accepted autoclaving procedures probably give a residual contamination rate of 10^{-6} and this has been proved acceptable. A widely used concept is that of the '12*D* dose', the dose required to give an inactivation factor of 10^{12}, in order to give a high degree of security even if highly resistant species are present as contaminants, if there is unduly heavy initial contamination or if tailing occurs.

Thus selection of an appropriate sterilizing dose may be difficult and in the absence of precise information about the initial conditions large doses are used, in the range 2.5 to 4.5 Mrad. The 2.5 Mrad dose has been widely accepted but it has been suggested that this may be inadequate. With these high doses, especially at 4.5 Mrad, the effects of irradiation on the material may be important and each type of product requires careful evaluation as to stability, activity, physical properties, storage life and acute and chronic toxicity. However, if it is desired to sterilize a pure culture of known resistance, as in vaccine production, or to eliminate a particular pathogen, e.g. staphylococci from hospital linen or salmonellae from egg products, smaller doses may be acceptable provided that radiation resistant strains are not produced.

Selection of the Sterilizing Process
The criteria for the selection of the type of radiation include the following:
(1) The specific ionization produced should be relatively low. A relatively small number of ionizations within a microorganism is sufficient to cause inactivation so radiations which produce a high specific ionization are less efficient biocides and are more likely to damage the product.
(2) The radiation should be capable of adequate penetration of the material and deliver a reasonably uniform dose therein.
(3) The radiation source should be capable of delivering high doses economically, at the same order of cost as conventional sterilization techniques.
(4) It should be possible to irradiate materials in any physical state.
(5) The dose must be accurately reproducible and capable of accurate measurement and control.
(6) The safety of plant operators should be ensured and radioactivity should not be induced in any irradiated material.

The only types of radiation to meet the above criteria are γ-rays and electron beams. Other radiations have limited and specialised uses.

Plants for γ-irradiation. Virtually all sterilization plants in use at present employ ^{60}Co, the source strength varying from 30 kCi to 2 MCi. Cobalt-60 has the advantages of compactness, high penetration (Fig. 28.55) and high dose rate. Its half-life of 5.26 years necessitates replacement at the rate of about 12.5 per cent per year in order to maintain the desired dose rate.

Although ^{137}Cs could be used and has the advantages of a lower γ-energy, so that shielding problems are less, and a longer half-life (30 years), necessitating a replacement rate of only 10 per cent per 5 years, only one plant using this nuclide has been built (in France), presumably due to the current higher cost of ^{137}Cs.

A typical ^{60}Co irradiation plant (Fig. 28.56) normally has a source consisting of a number of rods built up from ^{60}Co slugs and arranged in the form of a flat plaque around which the packages are circulated. The packages are conveyed past the

source several times so that all packages are irradiated to the same extent and from both sides. Fig. 28.55 illustrates the clear advantage in uniformity of depth dose distribution which is derived from two-sided irradiation. The two irradiations need not be simultaneous since the total energy deposited is the same whether the irradiations of the two sides are concurrent or not and, provided that no changes in the physical or physiological conditions occur between the two irradiations, the effects are identical. Careful attention is paid to the packing density since the uniformity of dose distribution decreases with increasing density and non-uniformity of packing and because the packing density affects the efficiency of operation. Economical operation requires the plant to operate continuously and automatically, the dose being controlled by the source activity and the time of exposure of the package. Protection of the operating personnel is achieved by building the irradiation cell in concrete, a thickness of about 1.75 m being required for a source strength of 100 kCi or about 2.5 m for a 2 MCi source. When maintenance is required, or the source needs replenishing, the source is normally lowered into a water pond, about 6 m depth of water providing adequate protection. The installation is designed for the utmost reliability and to fail safe in the event of any untoward incident.

Electron beam processing. Concentrated beams of high energy electrons (up to about 7 MeV) are produced by van der Graff electrostatic accelerators or by microwave linear accelerators. The penetrative powers of electrons is very much less than that of γ-radiation (Fig. 28.55), so electron irradiation is usually confined to the sterilization of small items such as individual dressings or sutures spread in a thin layer. The objects to be sterilized are passed on a conveyor belt under a focused electron beam which is scanned rapidly (200 cps) to and fro across the conveyor, using electrostatic or electromagnetic deflecting fields, a very high efficiency of utilization of the available energy being obtained. Uniformity of dosage control is achieved by careful regulation of both the electron generator and the conveyor speed. Although the problems of protecting personnel from radiation hazards are much less than with γ-radiation plants there is considerable Bremsstrahlung production, which accounts for most of the biological shielding required.

Comparison of γ-ray and electron beam processes. The relative properties of the two types of irradiation

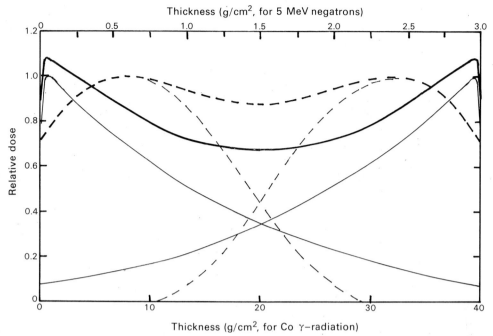

FIG. 28.55. The variation of dose with adsorber thickness for γ-radiation and negatrons. Solid lines, ^{60}Co γ-rays, mean energy 1.25 MeV; broken lines, 5 MeV negatrons; thin lines, single sided irradiations; heavy lines, double sided irradiations.

are given in Table 28.14. Most of the material processed throughout the world is sterilized by ^{60}Co irradiation since increasing utilization of this material has resulted in reduced costs whereas the cost of electron generators has risen in keeping with general inflationary trends. Some γ-irradiations are carried out using the radiation from spent nuclear reactor fuel elements which are held in water ponds to 'cool' to acceptable radiation levels before processing. Such facilities are of low production capacity and are primarily experimental or are used where radiation sterilization is economically non-viable.

Control Procedures

Radiosterilization operations require expert supervision and control and a Code of Practice has been adopted by the International Atomic Energy Agency. The Code specifies high standards of construction and hygiene to ensure the lowest possible initial contamination of articles. It requires sterilized items to be packed to prevent subsequent contamination and sterilized and unprocessed materials to be positively identified and separated. Microbiological control covers the initial levels of contamination, sterility testing and the use of standard strains of bacteria, *Streptococcus faecium*

strain A$_2$-1 (ATCC 19581) and *Bacillus pumilus* strain E601, as a continuous check on the sterilizing efficiency. The methods for checking the dose on initial commissioning and in routine operation are also specified, together with precautions for fail safe operation if any part of the plant does not function correctly, for example, if a ^{60}Co source is incorrectly located, an electron accelerator fails or a conveyor belt stops.

Advantages of Radiosterilization
(1) Highly effective.
(2) Treatment times may be very short.
(3) It is a continuous process suitable for long production runs.
(4) The thermal conductivity of the material is irrelevant.
(5) It is a cold process resulting in a temperature rise of only a few degrees and so is suitable for thermolabile materials.
(6) Materials may be irradiated in the dry or frozen state and under oxic or anoxic conditions.
(7) Products are processed in the final container after packaging with no risk of subsequent contamination until used.
(8) The process may be controlled and monitored accurately.

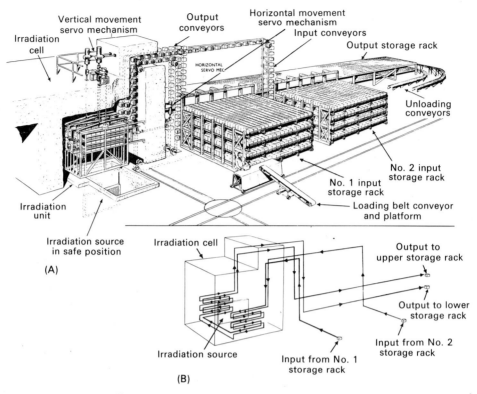

FIG. 28.56. The U.K.A.E.A. ^{60}Co radiation sterilization plant. A, Cut-away diagram; B, The flow pattern past the source; each package undergoes five passes on either side of the source plaque (U.K.A.E.A.).

TABLE 28.14

THE COMPARATIVE PROPERTIES OF γ-RAY AND ELECTRON BEAM PROCESSES FOR RADIOSTERILIZATION

γ-Radiation	Electron beams
1. High penetration	1. Lower penetration, dependent on energy
2. Massive biological shielding and elaborate source storage required	2. Shielding problems are less since the beam has a defined direction and lower range and Bremsstrahlung production is relatively inefficient
3. No directional properties so that the whole of the energy cannot be absorbed within the irradiated material, resulting in maximum efficiencies of about 35 per cent	3. Very high efficiency of utilization of the energy of the scanned beam
4. Large input and output stores required due to relatively long irradiation times and the need to operate continuously for economy	4. Less elaborate storage facilities needed due to high processing capacity
5. Cannot be switched off	5. Can be run at will as required
6. Cannot induce radioactivity	6. May induce radioactivity of energies >10 MeV are used
7. Reliably constant output of energy	7. Energy output requires careful control
8. Low maintenance costs, primarily for ^{60}Co source replacement at a rate of 12.5 per cent per year	8. Liable to breakdown, needing frequent maintenance and has a tube life of about 1000 hr

Applications

The present applications of radiosterilization are confined primarily to those materials for which conventional sterilization methods are unsatisfactory or uncertain (catgut, rubber, certain dressings, oils) or to cheap disposable plastic materials which cannot be heat sterilized. Other medical applications which are being studied intensively are the sterilization of tissue graft materials, such as freeze-dried bone or aorta, the production of vaccines, since antigenicity is generally not affected by sterilizing doses, and the elimination of the virus of serum hepatitis by the irradiation of freeze-dried plasma.

The problems of food sterilization have not been solved, since the products are unacceptable organoleptically, but it is possible that sub-sterilizing doses of radiation may be used to reduce the degree of heat processing or refrigeration required to obtain an acceptable storage life for many foodstuffs. Relatively low radiation doses can be used to eliminate insect infestations of stored foods.

A list of medical products which are known to have been radiosterilized satisfactorily is given below.

Antibiotics of the tetracycline group.
Arterial prostheses.
Atropine eye drops.
Cannulae.
Cardiac valve prostheses.
Chloramphenicol eye ointment.
Dialysis units.
Endotracheal tubes.
Oxygenators for heart-lung machines.
Plastic catheters, gloves, hypodermic syringes (with needles), Petri dishes, tubing.
Rubber catheters and gloves.
Starch glove lubricating cream.
Surgical blades, blood lancets.
Surgical dressings: bandages, gauze, eye pads, swabs, maternity towels.
Sutures: catgut, collagen, silk, polyester, nylon.
Transfusion giving and taking sets.

The question of the economics of the various sterilization processes is probably not as important as has occasionally been implied. There are undoubted differences in cost (the cost of ethylene oxide sterilization, another cold process, has been reported to be about 60 per cent of that for radio-sterilization), but sterilization may account for only 5 per cent of the manufacturer's price and such cost differences are marginal. The real consideration is which sterilization process is the most suitable for the material concerned and gives an appropriate degree of security.

FURTHER READING

ANTHONY, L. J. (1966) *Sources of Information on Atomic Energy.* Oxford: Pergamon Press.

CATCH, J. R. (1961) *Carbon-14 Compounds.* London: Butterworths.

CUNINGHAM, J. G. (1964) *Introduction to the Atomic Nucleus.* London: Elsevier.

EDELMANN, A. (1960) *Radioactivity for Pharmaceutical and Allied Laboratories.* London: Academic Press.

ERRERA, M. & FORSSBERG, A. (eds) (1961) *Mechanisms in Radiobiology,* Vol. 1. London: Academic Press.

EVANS, E. A. (1966) *Tritium and its Compounds.* London: Butterworths.

FAIRES, R. A. & PARKES, B. H. (1960) *Radio-isotope Laboratory Techniques,* 2nd edn. London: Newnes.

INTERNATIONAL ATOMIC ENERGY AGENCY (1964) *International Directory of Isotopes,* 3rd edn. Vienna: International Atomic Energy Agency.

OAK RIDGE INSTITUTE OF NUCLEAR STUDIES (1966) *Radioactive Pharmaceuticals* (A.E.C. Symposium Series 6). Oak Ridge: The United States Atomic Energy Commission.

OVERMAN, R. T. & CLARK, H. M. (1960) *Radioisotope Techniques.* London: McGraw-Hill.

QUIMBY, E. H. & FEITELBERG, S. (1963) *Radioactive Isotopes in Medicine and Biology,* Vol. 1. *Basic Physics and Instrumentation,* 2nd edn. London: Henry Kimpton.

ROTH, L. J. (1965) *Isotopes in Experimental Pharmacology.* Chicago: University Press.

THE RADIOCHEMICAL CENTRE (Amersham, Bucks)
   Radioactive Products 1969/70 (1969)
   The Radiochemical Centre *Reviews*
     No. 1. WILSON, B. J. (1968) *Selected References to Tracer Techniques.*
     No. 3. BAYLY, R. J. & CATCH, J. R. (1968) *The Stability of Labelled Organic Compounds.*
     No. 4. NEWBERY, G. R. (1968) *Standards of Activity.*
     No. 7. BAYLY, R. J. & EVANS, E. A. (1968) *Storage and Stability of Compounds Labelled with Radio-isotopes.*
     No. 8. CATCH, J. R. (1968) *Purity and Analysis of Labelled Compounds.*
   The Radiochemical Manual (1966) 2nd edn.

WANG, C. H. & WILLIS, D. C. (1965) *Radiotracer Methodology in Biological Science.* Englewood Cliffs, New Jersey: Prentice Hall.

WOLF, W. & TUBIS, M. (1967) *J. pharm. Sci.* **56**, 1.

RADIOLOGICAL SAFETY

DEPARTMENT OF EDUCATION AND SCIENCE et al. (1972) *Code of Practice for the Protection of Persons against Ionizing Radiations from Medical and Dental Use.* London: Her Majesty's Stationery Office.

GIBSON, R. (1966) *The Safe Transport of Radioactive Materials.* Oxford: Pergamon Press.

INTERNATIONAL ATOMIC ENERGY AGENCY, VIENNA. *Safe Handling of Radioisotopes (I.A.E.A. Safety Series)*
    No. 1. *Safe Handling of Radioisotopes* (1962).
    No. 2. *Health Physics Addendum* (1960).
    No. 3. *Medical Addendum* (1960).
    No. 6. *Regulations for the Safe Transport of Radioactive Materials* (1961).
    No. 9. *Basic Safety Standards for Radiation Protection* (1967).

INTERNATIONAL COMMISSION ON RADIOLOGICAL PROTECTION (1964) *Radiation Protection. Recommendations of the International Commission on Radiological Protection.* Oxford: Pergamon Press.

MINISTER OF HOUSING AND LOCAL GOVERNMENT et al. (1959) *The Control of Radioactive Wastes* (*Cmnd 884*). London: Her Majesty's Stationery Office.

MINISTRY OF LABOUR (1964) *Code of Practice for the Protection of Persons Exposed to Ionizing Radiations in Research and Teaching.* London: Her Majesty's Stationery Office.

Radioactive Substances Act (1960). 8 & 9 Eliz. 2, 34. London: Her Majesty's Stationery Office.

REES, D. J. (1967) *Health Physics: Principles of Radiation Protection.* London: Butterworths.

WORLD HEALTH ORGANIZATION (1964) *Protection against Ionizing Radiation. A Survey of Existing Legislation.* Geneva: World Health Organization.

COUNTING INSTRUMENTS AND TECHNIQUES

BIRKS, J. B. (1964) *The Theory and Practice of Scintillation Counting.* Oxford: Pergamon Press.

PRICE, W. J. (1964) *Nuclear Radiation Detection*, 2nd end. London: McGraw-Hill.

SHARPE, J. (1964) *Nuclear Radiation Detectors*, 2nd edn. London: Methuen.

SNELL, A. H. (ed.) (1962) *Nuclear Instruments and their Uses.* New York: Wiley.

TURNER, J. C. (1967) *Sample Preparation for Liquid Scintillation Counting* (*R.C.C. Review 6*). Amersham, Bucks: The Radiochemical Centre.

CHEMICAL AND ANALYTICAL APPLICATIONS

BURR, J. G. (1957) *Tracer Applications for the Study of Organic Reactions.* New York: Interscience.

INTERNATIONAL ATOMIC ENERGY AGENCY (1965) *Radiochemical Methods of Analysis.* Vienna: International Atomic Energy Agency.

LAMBIE, D. A. (1964) *Techniques for the Use of Radioisotopes in Analysis: A Laboratory Manual.* London: Spon.

THE RADIOCHEMICAL CENTRE, Amersham, Bucks (R.C.C. Reviews)
    No. 2. GORSUCH, T. T. (1968). *Radioactive Isotope Dilution Analysis.*
    No. 5. GORSUCH, T. T. (1968). *Radioactive Tracers in Chemical Analysis.*
    No. 9. OLDHAM, K. G. (1968). *Radiochemical Methods of Enzyme Assay.*

MEDICAL APPLICATIONS

HOSPITAL MEDICINE PUBLICATIONS (1969) *Diagnostic Uses of Radioisotopes in Medicine.* London: Hospital Medicine Publications.

INTERNATIONAL ATOMIC ENERGY AGENCY (1964) *Medical Radioisotope Scanning*, 2 volumes. Vienna: International Atomic Energy Agency.

INTERNATIONAL ATOMIC ENERGY AGENCY. *Nuclear Medicine. A Guide to Recent Literature.* Vienna: International Atomic Energy Agency, quarterly.†

PATERSON, R. (1963) *The Treatment of Malignant Disease by Radiotherapy.* London: Edward Arnold.

SILVER, S. (1962) *Radioactive Isotopes in Medicine and Biology*, Vol. 2, *Medicine.* London: Henry Kimpton.

SILVER, S. (1965) *New Engl. J. Med.* **272**, 466, 515, 569, 1294.

VEALL, N. & VETTER, H. (1958) *Radioisotope Techniques in Clinical Research and Diagnosis.* London: Butterworths.

THE RADIOCHEMICAL CENTRE, Amersham, Bucks. *Medical Monographs.*
    No. 1. WEST, J. B. (1966) *The Use of Radioactive Tracers in the Study of Lung Function.*
    No. 2. TOTHILL, P. (1966) *Measurement Techniques for the Clinical Application of Radioisotopes.*
    No. 3. HOBBS, J. T. (1967) *Total Blood Volume—Its Measurement and Significance.*
    No. 4. JOEKES, A. M. (1967) *The Radioisotope Renogram.*
    No. 5. GREIG, W. R., BOYLE, I. T. & BOYLE, J. A. (1969) *Diagnosis of Thyroid Disorders using Radioactive Iodine.*
    No. 6. MOLLIN, D. L. & WATERS, A. H. (1968) *The Study of Vitamin B_{12} Absorption using Labelled Cobalamins.*

RADIOSTERILIZATION

INTERNATIONAL ATOMIC ENERGY AGENCY (1963) *Radiation Control of Salmonellae in food and feed products. Tech. Repts. Series* No. 22. Vienna: International Atomic Energy Agency.

INTERNATIONAL ATOMIC ENERGY AGENCY (1966) *Food Irradiation.* Vienna: International Atomic Energy Agency.

INTERNATIONAL ATOMIC ENERGY AGENCY (1967) *Radiosterilization of Medical Products, Pharmaceuticals and Bioproducts. Tech. Repts. Series* No. 72. Vienna: International Atomic Energy Agency.*

INTERNATIONAL ATOMIC ENERGY AGENCY (1967) *Radiosterilization of Medical Products.* Includes the '*Recommended Code of Practice for the Radiosterilization of Medical Products*'. Vienna: International Atomic Energy Agency.

PHARMACEUTICAL PRESS (1961) *Sterilization of Surgical Materials.* London: Pharmaceutical Press.

SILVERMAN, G. J. & SINSKEY, T. J. (1968) The destruction of microorganisms by ionizing radiation. In: *Disinfection, Sterilization and Preservation.* (Ed. by C. A. Lawrence and S. S. Block). London: Henry Kimpton.

SYKES, G. (1965) *Disinfection and Sterilization*, 2nd edn. London: Spon.

Part V

PREPARATIONS OF NATURAL ORIGIN

29

Principles of Microbiology

Microbiology is the study of microscopic organisms, bacteria, algae, fungi, protozoa and viruses. The cells of bacteria and the blue-green algae are *prokaryotic* in structure, the remainder being *eukaryotic*, except for the viruses, which are non-cellular. There is no merit in classifying any of these groups as plants or animals since there are intermediate forms which tend to link the various groups: they are simply microorganisms.

Eukaryotic cells (Fig. 29.1A) are typical of plants, animals and most microorganisms. They have a true nucleus surrounded by a double nuclear membrane with pores, undergo mitotic division with chromosome separation, have a structured cytoplasm with an endoplasmic reticulum and possess mitochondria (and membrane-limited chloroplasts if photosynthetic). Their flagella or cilia are complex, showing a highly structured basal body and within a membrane a ring of nine doublet fibres surrounding a pair of single central fibres.

Prokaryotic cells (Fig. 29.1B) do not have a membrane-limited nucleus, undergo amitotic division (binary fission or budding) with no elaborate mechanism of chromosome separation, have an amorphous, unstructured cytoplasm and the flagella are simple tubes. Photosynthetic species have photosynthetic lamellae without a limiting membrane.

Distribution. Microorganisms are distributed ubiquitously, especially in soil, from which they are transferred to the air, water and plants, and to the skin and body cavities of animals. Most are *saprobes*, being associated with non-living material,

but many live in association with other living forms as *symbionts*. This symbiosis may be *mutualistic*, with both species obtaining some benefit, as with the root nodule bacteria of leguminious plants, or *parasitic*, with only one of the species deriving benefit, as in infectious diseases.

Nomenclature. All microorganisms except viruses are named by the traditional binomial nomenclature consisting of a generic name, always given with a capital letter and abbreviated where there is no possibility of confusion, followed by a specific name which never starts with a capital and is never abbreviated. These names are italicized; e.g. the tubercle bacillus = *Mycobacterium tuberculosis* = *M. tuberculosis*, the pneumococcus = *Diplococcus pneumoniae* = *D. pneumoniae*.

BACTERIA

DEFINITION

Small (0.01–5000 μm^3); prokaryotic; unicellular, filamentous or coenocytic; saprobic, parasitic, non-photosynthetic or photosynthetic without evolution of oxygen; mostly with rigid cell walls containing muramic acid; sterols mostly absent; non-motile or motile by simple flagella, axial filament or gliding motion.

MORPHOLOGY AND ULTRASTRUCTURE

Bacteria may have the following forms, which are illustrated in Fig.29.2

Coccoid, i.e. roughly spherical cells about 1 μm in diameter in chains, pairs, packets of four or eight, or irregular clusters.

433

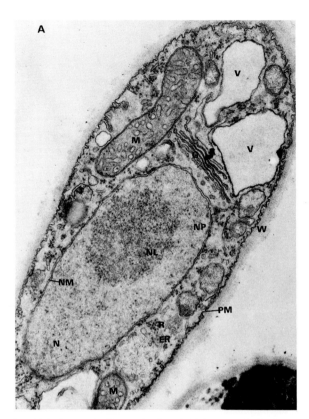
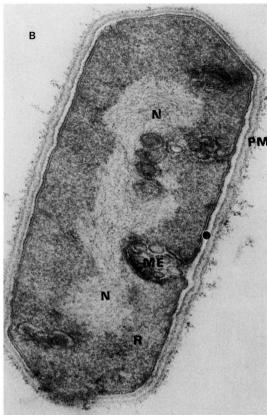

Fig. 29.1. Types of cell organization: A, Eukaryote; B, Prokaryote. V, vacuole; M, mitochondria; G, Golgi Body; W, cell wall; N, nucleus; NM, double nuclear membrane; NP, pore in nuclear membrane; NL, nucleolus; PM, plasma membrane; R, ribosomes; ER, endoplasmic reticulum; ME, mesosome. A by courtesy of Prof. C. E. Bracker, Dr. S. N. Grove and the Indiana Academy of Science; B by courtesy of Dr. P. D. Walker.

Bacillary, i.e. rods, approximately 0.4 to 1.5 μm wide and 1.5 to 8 μm long, occurring singly, in chains or irregular clusters.

Spirillar, i.e. spiral rigid or flexible rods 0.1 to 1 μm wide and 4 to 500 μm long with an axial filament which maintains the spiral structure.

Mycelial, with a mass of fragmented or interlacing slender (1.5 μm) threads and bearing external, asexual spores only, resembling microfungi.

Stalked and Sheathed Forms, mostly aquatic in habitat.

Gliding Forms, flexible rod-shaped forms 0.5 to 1.5 μm wide by 5 to 10 μm long moving by a gliding motion and with complex life cycles.

Staining Reactions

The Gram reaction, introduced by Christian Gram in 1884, divides bacteria into two main classes. Gram-positive cells retain the Gram stain (alkaline gentian violet) after treatment with iodine and solvent, while Gram-negative cells are decolorized

TABLE 29.1.

SOME GRAM-POSITIVE AND GRAM-NEGATIVE BACTERIAL GENERA

Positive	Negative	
Staphylococcus	*Pseudomonas*	*Rhizobium*
Streptococcus	*Escherichia*	*Azotobacter*
Bacillus	*Salmonella*	*Nitrosomonas*
Clostridium	*Shigella*	*Acetobacter*
Mycobacterium	*Enterobacter*	*Neisseria*
Corynebacterium	*Proteus*	*Spirillum*
Lactobacillus	*Vibrio*	*Brucella*
Micrococcus	*Yersinia*	Spirochaetes
Actinomycetes	*Haemophilus*	Rickettsiae
		Mycoplasmas

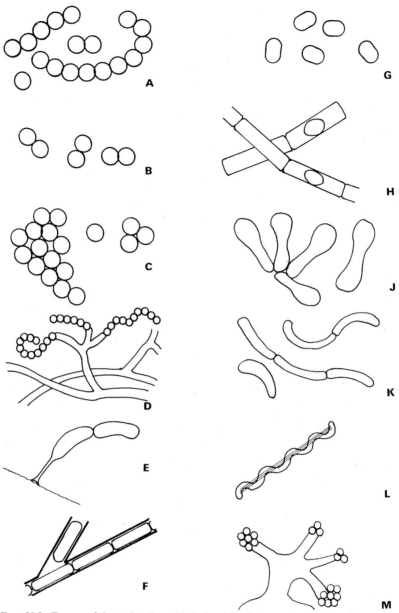

FIG. 29.2. Forms of bacteria. Coccoid (spheroid); A, *Streptococcus pyogenes*; B, *Diplococcus pneumoniae*; C, *Staphylococcus aureus*. Bacillary (rod-shaped); G, *Escherichia coli*; H, *Bacillus anthracis*, with spores; J, *Corynebacterium diphtheriae*. Spirillar; K, *Vibrio cholerae*; L, *Treponema pallidum* with axial filament. Mycelial; D, *Streptomyces griseus* with spores. Stalked; E, *Caulobacter* sp. attached to a substratum by its holdfast. Sheathed; F, *Sphaerotilus natans*, showing rod-shaped cells in a branched sheath largely composed of ferric hydroxide. Gliding forms; M, a myxobacterium, *Chrondromyces* showing the fruiting body with microcysts.

by the solvent. Thus Gram-positive cells are stained purple and Gram-negative cells are red or green according to the counterstain selected. This difference is related to the nature of the cell walls and the outer layers of the cell in the two types (Fig. 29.3) and is used as a primary step in identification.

Some of the genera in the two classes are given in Table 29.1. Only bacteria can be Gram-negative, all other microorganisms are Gram-positive.

In *spore staining* and *acid-fast staining* the endospores and the cells respectively are relatively impermeable to normal stains and are treated

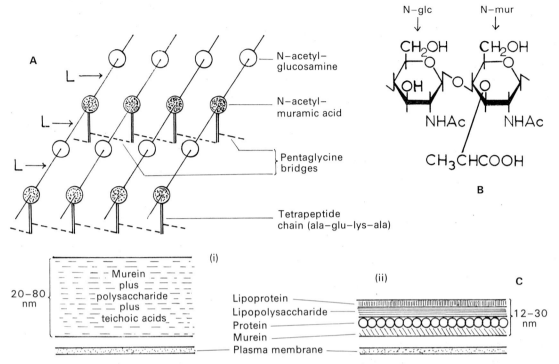

Fig. 29.3. The bacterial cell wall: A, the murein of *Staphylococcus aureus*; B, the N-acetylglucosamine(N-glc)-N-acetyl-muramic acid(N-mur) unit; C, the differences between (i) Gram-positive and (ii) Gram-negative walls; L, point of lysozyme action.

similarly. Hot, concentrated stains are used, followed by sulphite or acid alcohol to decolorize, if possible, and finally staining with a contrasting counterstain. Positive reactions are the retention of the concentrated red or green stain.

The Cell Wall

This confers rigidity on the cell, a property due to the presence of a mucopeptide, *murein*, a polymer based on N-acetylglucosamine and, in Gram-positive species, highly cross-linked by peptide chains (Fig. 29.3A). Several antibiotics (penicillins, cephalosporins, cycloserine, bacitracin, vancomycin) act by interfering with murein synthesis. The cell wall can be removed by the action of lysozymes, enzymes present in lachrymal secretion and eggwhite, the point of attack being shown (L→) in Fig. 29.3A.

Gram-positive walls also contain *teichoic acids*, linear polymers of glycerophosphate or ribitol phosphate with D-alanine or saccharide side chains.

The wall of Gram-negative cells is thinner than that of Gram-positives, but more complex (Fig. 29.3C). The mureins are not major components and do not have peptide bridges between the tetrapeptide chains. The lipopolysaccharides of Gram-negative walls are soluble and act as *pyrogens* if administered intravenously, causing fever and other effects, and are the somatic (0) antigens (see Table 29.14, p. 485).

Some bacteria (mycoplasmas) do not possess a wall, and extreme halophiles, which require concentrated sodium chloride for growth, have a different type of wall structure.

The Plasma Membrane

This has a typical unit membrane structure, does not contain sterols and is the site of the respiratory enzymes, there being no mitochondria. It is semi-permeable, due partly to the presence of systems which actively transport many substances into the cell. These transport systems (permeases) are enzymic in character, may be highly stereospecific and require an endogenous energy source (ATP or phospho-*enol*-pyruvate). They may be *constitutive*, i.e. always present to transport vital materials such as glucose, K^+ or PO_4^{3-}, or *inducible*, i.e. synthesized only when the cell has to do so to obtain a source of carbon or energy, e.g. *E. coli* growing on lactose or glycerol as sole carbon and energy source. Transport systems are distinct from the metabolizing enzymes which mediate utilization of

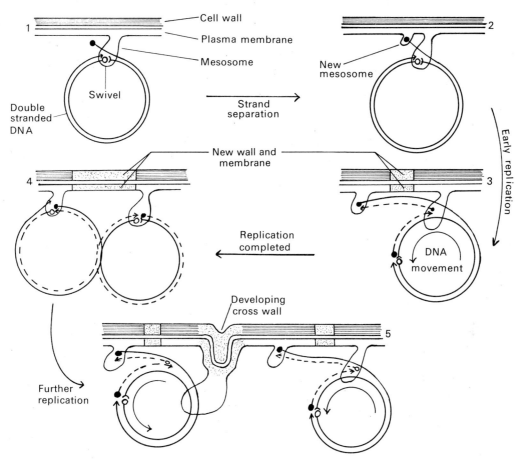

FIG. 29.4. Chromosome replication in bacteria.

the compound after entry into the cell. Compounds not actively transported enter the cell by diffusion processes.

Mesosomes
Mesosomes are membranous invaginations of the plasma membrane (Fig. 29.1) and are probably the sites of synthesis of nuclear material, cell membranes and cell walls.

Nucleus
In many bacteria the nucleus is a single circular chromosome composed of a helix of double-stranded DNA. When the nucleus starts to divide the helix unwinds at the *swivel*, which is attached to a mesosome (Fig. 29.4). The free end of one strand attaches to a newly formed mesosome adjacent to the original mesosome and new complementary strands are synthesized using the existing strands as templates as the chromosome moves relative to the mesosome. At the same time new

membrane and wall synthesis commences between the mesosomes until two complete, separated chromosomes are formed. Finally a new cross wall is synthesized to form two daughter cells. This mechanism ensures the distribution of a complete chromosome replica to each daughter cell.

Cytoplasm
This contains an amorphous mass of ribosomes (the principal sites of protein synthesis), structural proteins and storage granules of polysaccharides (glycogen), polymetaphosphate (volutin) and lipids. Specialized species may have lamellar structures associated with photosynthesis, nitrate reduction, etc. or granules of sulphur. Vacuoles are generally absent.

Endospores
These are formed primarily by members of the genera *Bacillus* and *Clostridium*, in which each vegetative cell forms only one spore and each spore

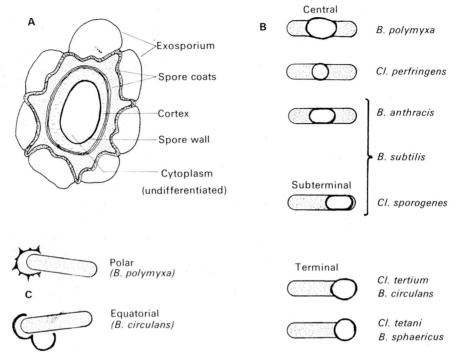

FIG. 29.5. Bacterial endospores: A, a typical spore structure (*Bacillus polymyxa*); B, modes of occurence; C, types of germination.

germinates to form a single vegetative cell. Thus endospores are not a means of reproduction. Mature spores have a very high resistance to heat, chemicals and radiations and it is the presence of spores which determines the treatment required to sterilize materials (see Chapter 30). This high resistance is probably due to the proteins being in a highly protected form resulting from binding to very high concentrations of calcium dipicolinate. Presumably sporulation is an adaptation which permits the cell to survive a variety of unfavourable conditions, e.g. starvation, desiccation and temperature. Germination occurs under favourable conditions, but the germination process is very delicate and is readily inhibited by a variety of conditions, so that the conditions for germination are usually more restricted than those for vegetative growth. The structures of spores and their modes of occurrence and germination may be diagnostic of the species (Fig. 29.5).

Flagella and Motility

Bacterial flagella are relatively long, slender threads 12–20 nm × 3–20 μm) attached to some bacteria, numbers vary from one to about 50 per cell. Electron microscopy shows that they consist of a *basal structure* associated with the plasma membrane and a *hook* region which probably mediates movement of the tubular, wavy *filament* (Fig. 29.6A). Most flagellate bacteria are actively motile, moving at up to 200 μm/s, although some (straight) flagella are non-functional. The spirochaetes possess an axial filament which appears to consist of specially adapted flagella, maintains the spiral form and is responsible for the cell flexions which confer motility. The number and mode of attachment of the flagella are used as characters in bacterial identification (Fig. 29.6B).

Some bacteria, e.g. *Cytophaga* spp. and the myxobacteria do not have flagella but move by a gliding motion the mechanism of which is obscure.

Pili (fimbriae)

These are very fine, short filaments, smaller than flagella, attached to many bacteria, especially Gram-negative rods of enteric origin (Fig. 29.6C). They are of two types: *common pili* are very numerous with 100 to 500 per cell, possibly functioning as organs of attachment to cell surfaces, especially to erythrocytes which are thus precipitated (haemagglutination); *sex pili* occur sparsely on 'male' (F⁺) cells only and enable tham to attach

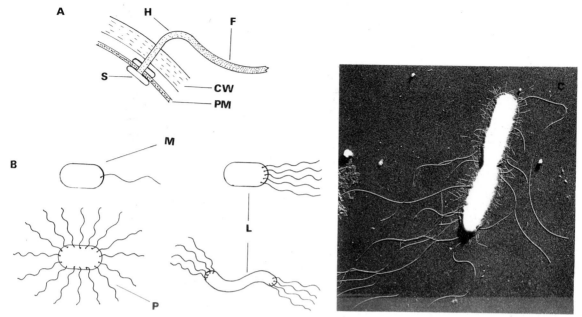

FIG. 29.6. *Bacterial flagella and pili (fimbriae)*. A, the ultrastructure of a typical bacterial flagellum; S, basal structure; H, hook; F, filament; CW, cell watt; PM, plasma membrane. B, modes of attachment; M, monotrichate (*Vibrio cholerae*); L, lophotrichate, cephalotrichate (*Pseudomonas aeruginosa*); P, peritrichate (*Escherichia coli*). C, flagella and pili on cells of *Salmonella typhi*. The electron micrograph shows several long flagella attached peritrichously to two cells of the organism, with numerous short pili projecting from the surfaces of the cells. By courtesy of Prof. J. P. Duguid and the Cambridge University Press.

to 'female' (F⁻) cells. The pilus then contracts to form a cytoplasmic bridge through which genetic material is transferred from the male donor to the female recipient. Subsequent recombination of the donor and recipient genes gives some genetic variation and so confers some of the advantages of the mitotic process of eukaryotes. This mating process is known as *conjugation*.

Capsules

These are well defined, gummy layers formed around some cells (Fig. 29.7) which help to protect the cells against desiccation. Capsules may be polysaccharide (as in *Diplococcus pneumoniae* and *Leuconostoc dextranicum*), polypeptide (*Bacillus anthracis*) or more complex (*B. megaterium*, polysaccharide/polypeptide; *Shigella dysenteriae*, polysaccharide/phospholipid/protein). Capsule formation is a genetic property of the species but depends also on the environment, e.g. the presence of saccharides, CO_2 or serum, and on the age of the culture. In streptococci capsules are formed early in growth and are subsequently destroyed, in *Klebsiella aerogenes* synthesis is prolonged, while in *D. pneumoniae* capsules are formed after active growth has ceased. Capsular structure is highly specific and is used diagnostically.

Encapsulated bacteria give a smooth, glistening

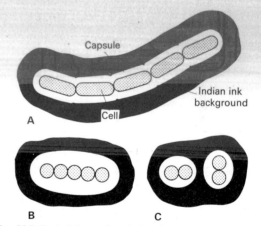

FIG. 29.7. Bacterial capsules. A, *Bacillus anthracis*; B, *Streptococcus pyogenes*; C, *Diplococcus pneumoniae*.

growth on solid media and non-capsulate mutants give a rough, granular growth: this is the *smooth to rough (S→R) variation*. The mutation $S → R$ is associated with a loss of virulence in pathogens and loss of the specificity conferred by the capsule.

Many bacteria, though not capsulate, have a thin, poorly defined *slime layer* surrounding the cell.

Summary of bacterial structure. Fig. 29.8 summarizes diagrammatically the general structure of bacteria.

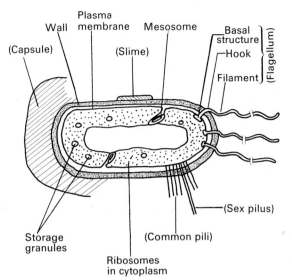

FIG. 29.8. A summary of bacterial structure. Components in brackets are present only in certain species.

FUNGI

DEFINITION

Eukaryotic, filamentous or occasionally unicellular, mostly non-motile, vegetative growth by apical elongation of filaments or by budding, reproduction by asexual and sometimes by sexual spores, plasma membrane contains sterols, require organic carbon for growth, non-photosynthetic.

GENERAL MORPHOLOGY

Usually a mass of branched, interwoven, microscopic tubular filaments, the *hyphae*, the whole structure forming a *mycelium* (Fig. 29.9) from which any specialized fruiting or spore-bearing structures arise. The *yeasts* are generally unicellu-

lar, though some are dimorphic and can also form a mycelium, though this is usually a poorly developed *pseudomycelium*. The hyphae of the lower fungi are non-septate and *coenocytic*, having numerous nuclei embedded in a continuous cytoplasm, but the higher fungi have complete or incomplete septa which divide the hyphae into uninucleate, dinucleate or multinucleate cells.

Although spores, gametes and some primitive species are naked, most fungi have a rigid cell wall consisting of fine fibrils embedded in an amorphous matrix. The wall is primarily polysaccharide in nature (chitin, cellulose, glucan, mannan, galactan, or mixtures of these) but also contains some lipid and protein, the latter sometimes being enzymic.

REPRODUCTION

This is usually by asexual (imperfect) means but sexual spores are sometimes produced. Most species are *eucarpic*, i.e. part of the thallus forms the reproductive structure while the rest continues its normal somatic functions, but some are *holocarpic* and the whole thallus becomes the reproductive structure. Most species show a variety of reproductive methods.

Asexual
The numerous mechanisms, some of which are illustrated in Fig. 29.10, are as follows.

Fragmentation by (a) the random separation of the mycelium due to physical forces (this method is used to make new cultures), (b) the separation of specialized cells which may be oidia (also known as arthrospores, e.g. in *Trichosporum* and *Geotrichum*) or thick-walled resistant chlamydospores (in *Candida albicans*, *Histoplasma capsulatum* and *Fusarium*) or (c) binary fission (in *Schizosaccharomyces*, the fission yeasts).

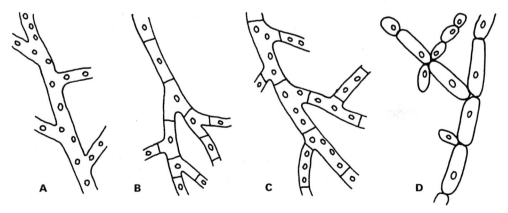

FIG. 29.9. Types of fungal mycelium. A, Coenocytic; B, Septate mononucleate; C, Septate multinucleate; D, Yeast pseudomycelium.

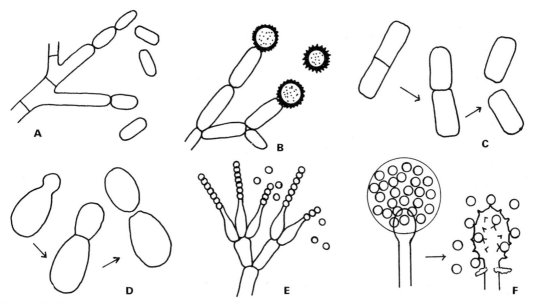

FIG. 29.10. Asexual modes of reproduction in the fungi: A, arthrospores (*oidia*); B, chlamydospores; C, fission; D, budding; E, conidiospores (*Penicillium*); F, sporangiospores (*Mucor*).

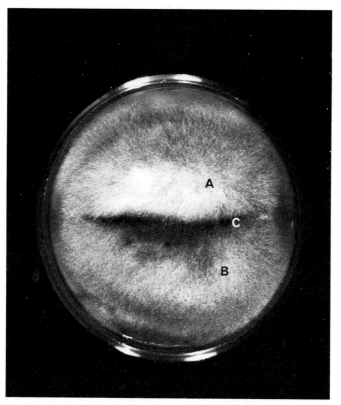

FIG. 29.11. *Heterothallic mating in* Mucor hiemalis *to give sexual zygospores.* The '−' strain was inoculated at one side of the plate (A) and the '+' strain on the other side of the (B). Where the mycelium grew together a line of black zygospores was formed (C).

Budding is the normal method of reproduction in yeasts, e.g. *Saccharomyces cerevisiae*, the common yeast, *Debaromyces* and *Cryptococcus neoformans*. Some dimorphic or polymorphic organisms also show budding in both the unicellular and mycelial forms, e.g. *C.albicans*.

Spore formation may occur in a great variety of ways. Conidia are formed outside the hyphae, either directly or on special branches known as conidiophores, e.g. in *Penicillium* and *Aspergillus*. They are often borne in clusters and are non-resistant and non-motile. Sporangiospores are formed within sacs (sporangia) at hyphal tips or on special hyphal branches (sporangiophores), and

may be motile zoospores, e.g. in *Phytophthora infestans*, which causes potato blight, or non-motile aplanospores, e.g. in *Mucor* and *Rhizopus*.

Sexual

The formation of sexual spores begins with the production of the haploid gametes, male gametes being formed in the *antheridium* and female gametes in the *oogonium*. In some species the male and female gametes are identical. The antheridium and oogonium fuse and the nucleus and part or all of the cytoplasm of the male gamete migrates into the female gamete in the process of *plasmogamy* (cytoplasmic fusion) which yields a binucleate

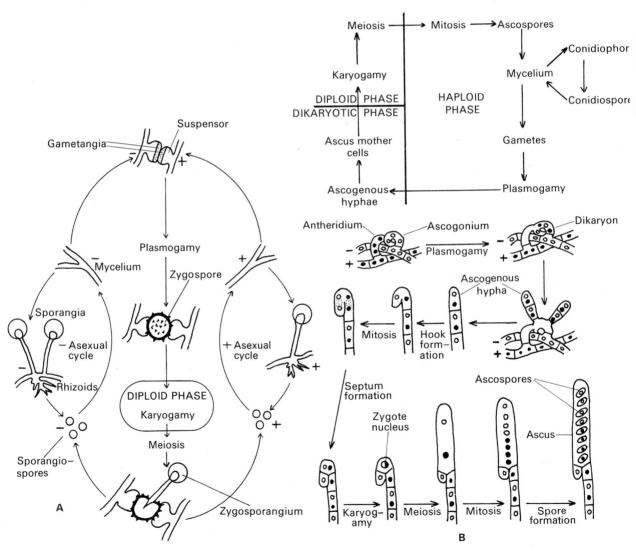

FIG. 29.12. Some typical fungal life cycles. A, *Rhizopus stolonifer*, a heterothallic zygomycete; B, Filamentous ascomycetes, the lower part showing the process of ascospore formation.

dikaryon. This is followed by *karyogamy* (nuclear fusion) to give a diploid *zygote* which then undergoes meiosis and mitosis to form haploid sexual spores.

Some species (*Schizosaccharomyces octosporus, Pythium debaryanum*) are homothallic, i.e. self-fertile, and so can reproduce sexually from a single thallus, whereas others (*Saccharomyces cerevisiae, Rhizopus stolonifer, Mucor hiemalis*) are heterothallic, i.e. each thallus is self-sterile and sexual spores are formed only when two compatible thalli of different mating types (+, −) come into contact (Fig. 29.11).

Fig. 29.12 illustrates some typical fungal life cycles.

PROTOZOA

DEFINITION

Eukaryotic, microscopic to just visible, unicellular, mostly motile, show irritability, no rigid cell wall, all reproduce asexually by fission and some sexually, some with two types of nucleus, most are phagotrophs (particulate feeders) and form resistant cysts.

GENERAL CHARACTERS

There are four major groups, namely the Sarcodina, the Hagistophora, the Ciliophora, and the Sporozoa.

The Sarcodina

These are amoeboid forms moving by pseudopodia, the cytoplasm usually showing an outer, hyaline *ectosarc*, which shows protoplasmic flow during movement, and an inner, granular, more rigid *endosarc*. Some species, e.g. *Naegleria gruberi*, have a flagellate stage in very wet conditions. Because of the normal pseudopodial mechanism of motility they do not have an outer pellicle. Although they have a single nucleus and reproduce asexually, the mode of reproduction may be complex. Most are free living but some are parasitic.

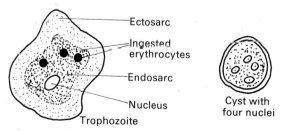

FIG. 29.13. *Entamoeba histolytica.*

Entamoeba histolytica (Fig. 29.13) is the only important pathogen; other species of *Entamoeba*, and species of the genera *Iodamoeba, Endolimax* and *Dientamoeba* are of uncertain pathogenicity. Most species form resistant, multinucleate cysts which are smaller than the vegetative trophozoite.

The Magistophora

These are flagellate forms moving by means of one or more long flagella. They possess a pellicle and a single nucleus and reproduce asexually. Some have a cystic stage. Most are free living but there are a number of important pathogens of man and domestic animals which are of great economic importance in tropical and sub-tropical regions.

Human pathogens may involve the intestine (*Giardia lamblia*), vagina (*Trichomonas vaginalis*), blood (*trypanosomes*) or the tissues (*Leishmania* spp.), the two latter being transmitted by blood-sucking insects. Some of these are illustrated in Fig. 29.14.

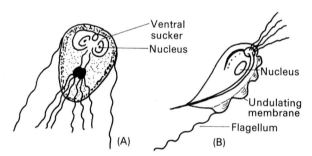

FIG. 29.14. Some pathogenic Magistophora. A, *Giardia lamblia*; B, *Trichomonas vaginalis.*

The Ciliophora

These arganisms have a pellicle and move actively due to the integrated action of rows of short cilia. Most have a *cytostome* (a primitive buccal cavity) and control their osmotic relationships by means of *contractile vacuoles* which collect excess water and pump it out of the cell. Most have a *macronucleus*, which controls feeding, metabolism, excretion and motility, and a *micronucleus* which controls reproduction: several nuclei or compound nuclei may be present.

Most are free living, the best known being *Paramecium*, but one species, *Balantidium coli*, is an intestinal pathogen of man (Fig. 29.15).

The Sporozoa

All the genera in this group are obligate parasites, usually with complex life cycles involving more than one host. There is no specialized locomotive

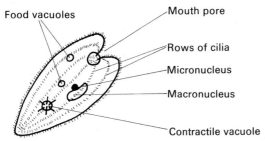

FIG. 29.15. A pathogenic ciliate, *Balantidium coli.*

structure. The most important pathogens of man are species of *Plasmodium* (Fig. 29.16) causing malaria, and of *Toxoplasma*, causing toxoplasmosis. Many other species cause economically important diseases of domestic animals.

NUTRITION AND ENERGY PROVISION

GENERAL REQUIREMENTS

The general chemical composition of microbial cells resembles that of other cells, indicating requirements for inorganic compounds, carbon, oxygen, nitrogen and energy.

Inorganic
Water. This is the major inorganic compound. As water of hydration it is essential for the maintenance of the structure of macromolecular cell components and its complete removal results in cell death. Because of its solvent properties it is the vehicle for entry of substances into the cell, for transport within the cell, for communication between the various enzymes involved in a chain of reactions and for the excretion of waste products. It is also an important reactant in hydrolytic and some oxidative reactions.

Mineral Salts. The principal requirements are for potassium, magnesium and phosphate. Smaller quantities of calcium, iron, manganese, sulphate and chloride are required and also traces of cobalt, copper, molybdenum and zinc. Sodium is not usually required except by *halophiles*. Most of these elements occur naturally in the common growth media, which are prepared from animal or vegetable sources, and their deliberate inclusion is normally necessary only in wholly synthetic media.

All ions show a similar concentration/response relationship, being stimulatory at low concentration and inhibitory at high concentration, with

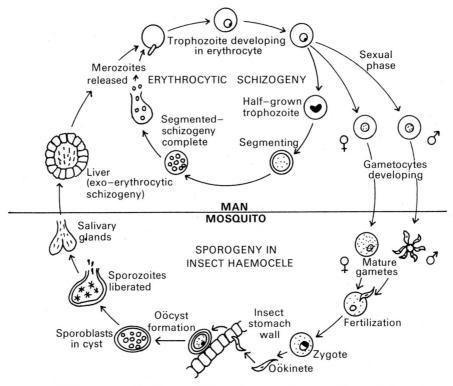

FIG. 29.16. Sporozoa. The life cycle of *Plasmodium vivax*, the agent of benign tertian malaria.

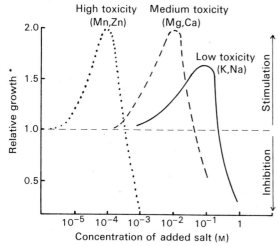

FIG. 29.17. The effect of cations on bacterial growth. Relative to growth without added ions as 1.0.

a well-marked optimum, the differences being in the level at which optimum growth occurs (Fig. 29.17). Minerals may function as constituents of cytoplasm (magnesium ribonucleate), as enzyme components (iron in cytochrome oxidase and catalase) and as enzyme activators (magnesium for isocitratase). Vital roles are played by potassium, in the maintenance of osmotic and pH equilibria, and by phosphate, in carbohydrate metabolism and energy provision.

Oxygen requirements. Oxygen is required for the growth of *aerobic* bacteria but may be toxic to *anaerobic* bacteria which cannot utilize oxygen as final hydrogen acceptor but utilize instead a variety of inorganic compounds. The subject of anaerobiosis is dealt with in more detail on p. 460.

Carbon Sources

Microorganisms may be divided into two main classes on the basis of their carbon requirements. The *autotrophs* will utilize inorganic carbon (CO_2, HCO_3^-) and may be inhibited by organic compounds, whereas the *heterotrophs* require organic carbon. The latter will utilize any of a vast range of compounds; hydrocarbons, acids, alcohols, glycols, monosaccharides, polysaccharides, amines, amino-acids, polypeptides, etc.

Carbon dioxide may be required by some heterotrophs for the synthesis of multicarbon compounds from simpler compounds via the tricarboxylic acid cycle. Usually this is important only in the early stages of growth since subsequent metabolism usually yields ample carbon dioxide.

Nitrogen Sources

Almost any form of nitrogen may be utilized by particular bacteria. Nitrogen fixers utilize atmospheric nitrogen and other species may utilize ammonium compounds, amines, amino acids and polypeptides. Nitrate is utilized primarily by fungi and only to a limited extent by bacteria.

Osmotrophy and Phagotrophy

Most microorganisms are *osmotrophic*, i.e. they obtain their nutrients in soluble form, but many protozoa are *phagotrophic*, i.e. they require particulate food, commonly living organisms, which is taken in by phogocytosis and is digested in food vacuoles in the cell. Phagotrophs may feed on bacteria, on erythrocytes (*Entamoeba histolytica*), on other protozoa (*Stentor, Tetrahymena*), on plants (the shelled amoebae *Arcella* and *Difflugia*) or they may be carnivorous, feeding on comparatively large animals (*Didinium, Dileptus*).

Minor Nutritional Requirements

Many microorganisms can live on relatively simple compounds and are described as *non-exacting*. However many *exacting* species require accessory growth factors, some of which are required in very low concentration and are components of coenzymes or their precursors. These latter are the microbial *vitamins*, which comprise the Vitamin B complex of man. Other growth factors are required in high concentration (haemin, inositol, choline, some fatty acids and amino acids) and are not associated with coenzymes.

Energy Sources

Energy is required for synthesis, growth and reproduction and for motility. Energy provision at the molecular level is provided primarily by ATP, and this aspect will be referred to later. There are two principal energy sources available: the phototrophs utilize light energy and the chemotrophs derive their energy from the oxidation of inorganic or organic compounds.

CLASSIFICATION BY NUTRITIONAL TYPE AND ENERGY SOURCE

The facts described above enable microorganisms to be classified into four main groups (Table 29.2), and subsidiary groups may be formed on various criteria. This scheme is simple but there are inconsistencies, and alternatives have been proposed.

TABLE 29.2

TABLE 29.2

THE CLASSIFICATION OF MICROORGANISMS BY NUTRITIONAL TYPE
AND ENERGY SOURCE

Class	Energy from	Principal carbon source	Examples
Photoauto-trophs	Light	CO_2	Most eukaryotic algae Blue-green algae Green sulphur bacteria Purple sulphur bacteria
Photohetero-trophs	Light	Organic	Some eukaryotic algae Purple non-sulphur bacteria
Chemoauto-trophs	Inorganic oxidation	CO_2	Bacteria only
Chemohetero-trophs	Organic oxidation	Organic	Most bacteria All fungi Most protozoa

THE INFLUENCE OF NUTRIENT CONCENTRATION ON GROWTH YIELD

Nutrient concentration will normally affect both the growth rate and the total bulk of growth similarly: at low concentrations there is a rapid increase and this phase is followed by one in which there is no further increase with increased concentration (Fig. 29.18). However, the effect on growth rate is marked at very low concentrations whereas the effect on yield occurs at much higher concentrations.

FACTORS AFFECTING NUTRIENT REQUIREMENTS AND AVAILABILITY

Requirements
The requirement for a particular nutrient can be influenced by a variety of environmental factors.

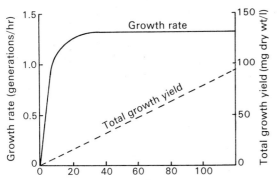

FIG. 29.18. The effect of nutrient concentration on bacterial growth rate and total growth yield.

Metabolic by-pass. Organisms growing on nitrate require molybdenum for the reduction of nitrate to ammonia, but this requirement is abolished if ammonium compounds are provided. Similarly a requirement for tryptophan is abolished if nicotinic acid is provided, since the former is used to synthesize the latter.

Hydrogen ion concentration. At low environmental pH values a higher concentration of K^+ is required to displace H^+ from the cell and maintain the internal pH.

Functional replacement. The absolute requirement for an ion may be reduced if another ion can function in its place, e.g. partial replacement of Na^+ by K^+ with halophiles, Fe or Mn replacing Mg as activators of isocitratase.

Antagonism, balance, synergism. It is well known that ions exert antagonistic actions and that a correct balance is essential for proper cell function and this is the basis for balanced salt solutions e.g. Ringer's solution.

Availability
Ionization and pH. The environmental pH may affect the ionization of nutrients markedly, e.g. p-aminobenzoic acid has pK values of 4.65 and 4.80 and so is largely ionized at physiological pH values (Fig. 29.19). Owing to the predominantly hydrophobic character of the plasma membrane many compounds enter the cell almost exclusively in their unionized (hydrophobic) form. Fig. 29.19 also shows that as the pH increases the total concentration of p-aminobenzoic acid required to give a constant growth yield increases in order to maintain the concentration of unionized molecules.

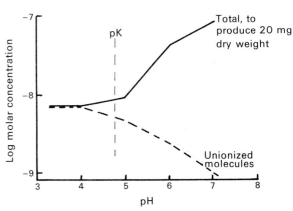

FIG. 29.19. The effect of pH on the ionization of p-aminobenzoic acid and its biovailability for *Neurospora crassa*.

Chemical form. Many compounds which are normally able to pass the plasma membrane will not do so if the molecule is chemically modified, e.g. some bacteria will transport glucose but not glucose-6-phosphate although the latter is a key intermediate in glucose metabolism. Another example is the fact that *Saccharomyces carlsbergensis* is less permeable to pyridoxal phosphate than to unphosphorylated forms of the vitamin and so is less responsive to its presence in the growth medium.

Transport systems and metabolizing enzymes. The utilization of a compound depends on its entry into the cell and its subsequent enzymic modification, and the substance may enter by diffusion or be transported by a specific system (permease). The synthesis of both permease and metabolizing enzymes is under genetic control, but even if the genetic determinants are present the synthesis of both the permease and the metabolizing enzyme may be repressed, e.g. in *E.coli* glucose represses the synthesis of both the lactose permease and the lactase enzyme which splits the lactose into galactose and glucose. Also, mutation may occur to give transport negative and lactase negative mutants and either of these conditions prevents lactose being available to the cell.

Molecular weight. Large molecules are generally unable to enter the cell, for example, pure proteins will not function as nitrogen sources unless extracellular proteases are formed which break down the protein to polypeptides or amino acids which can be utilized. However, some amino acids, e.g. glutamic acid, may enter the cell more readily as peptides.

Chelating agents. Many naturally occurring compounds such as amino acids, function as chelating agents and bind essential cations very strongly. This effect may result in growth restriction, but more usually merely results in considerable uncertainty as to the actual concentration of a cation which is available for growth.

SOME METHODS OF MICROBIOLOGY

A comprehensive account of microbiological techniques cannot be given here. The reader is referred to texts quoted in the bibliography at the end of this chapter.

MICROSCOPY

Light Microscopy

Some methods of differential staining (Gram, acid fast, spore) have al ready been described briefly. Although such techniques permit the shape of cells and their characteristic arrangements to be observed, the relatively drastic fixing and staining methods used inevitably cause some shrinkage and distortion. When it is necessary to avoid these effects unstained cells can be examined using either negative staining or the special microscopical techniques of dark ground illumination, phase contrast or interference microscopy.

Negative staining. A suspension of organisms are mixed with a small amount of the purple dye *nigrosin* which has too large a molecular weight to permit it to penetrate cells. After drying, the cells appear as colourless objects against a uniform purple field (Fig. 29.20A). Nigrosin penetrates

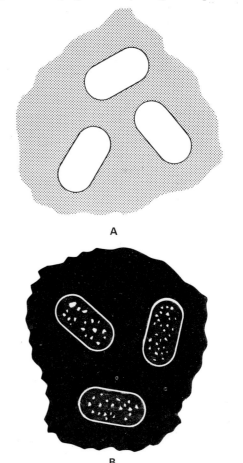

Fig. 29.20. The vizualization of unstained bacteria. A, Negative staining with nigrosin; B, Dark ground illumination.

capsules and so cannot be used to visualize these structures which may be outlined with indian ink or congo red as shown in Fig. 29.7.

Dark ground microscopy. For dark ground microscopy a special illuminator is used in place of the sub-stage condenser. A cone of light is focused in the plane of the object so that in a clear field no light passes into the objective and the field is uniformly black. When cells are present in the field, these reflect and refract the light and appear brightly outlined and with any granular contents visible as bright points of light (Fig. 29.20B).

Phase contrast microscopy. Phase contrast microscopy involves a somewhat similar technique to dark ground illumination, but the undeviated rays enter the objective and pass through an annulus which retards or advances the rays by one quarter of a wavelength relative to the reflected rays. Combination of the undeviated and deviated rays results in colour contrast and the cells may be observed readily. The technique is so simple and convenient that it is often used as a routine method of examination. The only drawback is that objects are surrounded by a halo and the interference by this with observation increases with the object thickness.

Interference microscopy. The apparatus for interference microscopy is more expensive than for phase contrast and so the method is less commonly used, but it has the advantage that haloes are not produced. Also, the interference patterns may be produced to permit measurement of object thickness.

Electron Microscopy
Electron microscopy is the only technique available for examining objects at very high magnifications (greater than about 2000 ×) or for objects beyond the limit of resolution of the light microscope. Extremely high magnifications are possible because the effective wavelength of the electron beam is much shorter than that of visible light. However, the samples must be in very high vacuum and so living cells cannot be examined. Also, the contrast is relatively poor without using special techniques.

Negative staining. The specimen is treated with a high atomic weight salt, such as phosphotungstate or uranyl acetate, which is relatively electron dense. This penetrates between structures and can show in relief the location and arrangement of large molecules. This technique is frequently used to show the details of virus structure (see Fig. 29.40) or to show details in ultra-thin sections (see Fig. 29.1).

Shadowing. To show surface features shadowing is used and the principles are illustrated in Fig. 29.21. A thin film of gold, platinum or other metal is coated onto the specimen under high vaccum at an angle so that a layer builds up on the support grid and on the sides of the object exposed to the metal 'beam'; a shadow being cast where the object protects the grid from the beam.

Scanning electron microscopy. The technique of choice for showing surface features is a scanning type of electron microscope.

CULTIVATION

Transfer of Samples
Small amounts of bacterial culture are transferred using an *inoculating loop* which consists of about 5 cm of platinum or nichrome wire gripped in a holder at one end, the other end being formed into a loop (Fig. 29.22A). Before use the loop and lower end of the holder are sterilized by flaming, i.e. holding almost vertically in a bunsen flame until the loop and wire are red hot. After cooling, the loop is used to pick up small amounts of microbial growth from the surface of a solid medium. Alternatively a sample of a suspension in fluid is taken as a film of liquid held in the loop by

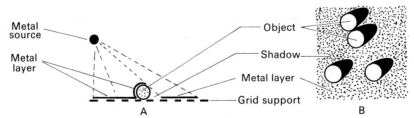

Fig. 29.21. Metal shadowing for election microscopy. A, The technique used; B, The type of result obtained.

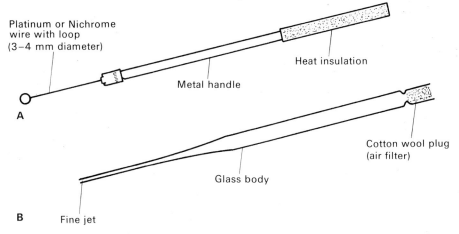

Platinum or Nichrome
wire with loop
(3–4 mm diameter)

Heat insulation

Metal handle

A

Cotton wool plug
(air filter)

Glass body

B   Fine jet

FIG. 29.22. Inoculation devices for small samples. A, The inoculating loop; B, A Pasteur capillary pipette.

surface tension. Larger samples of fluid suspensions are taken using Pasteur (capillary) pipettes (Fig. 29.22B) or graduated pipettes of convenient size.

Aseptic technique is used at all times: this is a technique designed to prevent accidental contamination of sterile materials or pure cultures (containing only a single species or strain) from the environment (air, breath, skin, surfaces, etc.). The details of this technique are out of place here but include procedures such as the use of sterile apparatus and materials at all times, proper closure of containers, the wrapping of apparatus, heating the necks of containers in a bunsen flame, minimal exposure of materials during handling, scrubbing of hands and swabbing benches with antiseptics, the use of protective clothing, carrying out manipulations in special handling cabinets supplied with filtered air, etc. The techniques used for sterilization are discussed in Chapter 31.

Growth Media

Liquid and solid media. In liquid media growth is recognized by the development of a more or less generalized turbidity or of a visible mass of growth (Fig. 29.23A). On solid media the physical nature of the medium causes the progeny of a single cell or of a group of cells to cohere to form a visible mound or mass of growth known as a colony (Fig. 29.23B).

Solid media are usually prepared by adding 1.0 to 1.5 g/litre of agar to a liquid medium. Agar is the agent of choice since few microorganisms attack it and the gel is stable at all incubation temperatures. Although the gel melts only when it is heated at about 100° for some time, it does not solidify until it is cooled to about 40°. Thus it is

normally held molten at about 45°, poured and allowed to set as desired. Normally, viable microorganisms can be mixed with the molten medium at 45° before pouring without causing heat damage to the cells, a technique convenient in counting, antibiotic assay, etc.

For special purposes media may be solidified with gelatin (though the gel melts at 25° and the gelatin is digested by many microorganisms), silica gel, alginate or pectin.

Liquid media are used in test tubes, closed with a non-absorbent cotton wool plug or a slip-on metal or plastic cap, or in screwcapped bottles. Solid media may also be used similarly, either as 'deeps', in which the medium is solidified with the container vertical and which are inoculated by stabbing through the depth of the medium with a straight wire, or as 'slopes', which are prepared by solidifying the medium with the container tilted and which are inoculated on the surface with a loop. A special form of solid culture is the 'agar plate' which consists of a layer of medium poured when molten into a Petri dish, a glass or plastic dish of about 9 cm diameter and 1.3 cm deep and allowed to set. Cultures on both types of media are illustrated in Fig. 29.23.

Routine laboratory media are general media, widely used for the cultivation of non-exacting micro organisms. Bacteriological media normally contain peptone (partially digested protein) and meat or yeast extracts at pH 7.4. Mycological media may be similar but are often supplemented with carbohydrates (glucose, sucrose, malt extract) and may be rather more acid, pH 5.5 to 6.5. Media for algae and protozoa are commonly much more dilute but may require such materials as

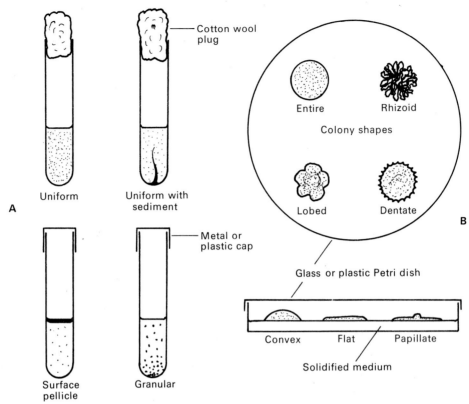

FIG. 29.23. Types of bacterial growth. A, Liquid media showing types of closure used to prevent contamination; B, Colonies growing on the surface of solid medium.

lettuce extract, Casilan and, for phagotrophs, living bacteria or other protozoa. Formulae for a number of routine media are given in Table 29.3.

TABLE 29.3

SOME COMMON MICROBIOLOGICAL MEDIA

Nutrient Broth

Beef extract	0.1*	
Yeast extract	0.2	
Peptone	0.5	
Sodium chloride	0.5	(pH 7.4)

A simple medium for the growth of non-exacting species.

Tryptone Soya Broth

Tryptone	1.7	
Soya peptone	0.3	
Dextrose	0.25	
Sodium chloride	0.5	
K_2HPO_4	0.25	(pH 7.3)

A highly nutrient medium giving luxuriant growth of many fastidious bacteria. It is not suitable for culture maintenance.

Sabouraud Agar

Mycological peptone	1.0	
Dextrose	4.0	
Agar	1.5	(pH 5.2)

A standard medium for the cultivation and identification of fungi.

TABLE 29.3—(*continued*)

Czapek Dox Liquid Medium

Sodium nitrate	0.2	
Potassium chloride	0.5	
Magnesium glycerophosphate	0.05	
Ferrous sulphate	0.001	
Potassium sulphate	0.035	
Sucrose	3.0	(pH 6.8)

A semi-synthetic fluid medium for the cultivation of non-exacting fungi and of those few bacteria capable of utilizing sucrose as sole carbon and energy source and sodium nitrate as nitrogen source.

* All concentrations are given as per cent (w/v).

Enriched media are used for the cultivation of exacting species, enrichments such as blood, serum, liver extract, egg, etc. being used.

Selective and Diagnostic Media. A selective medium is one which is formulated to inhibit the growth of unwanted species. Selective conditions may be provided simply by controlling the nature of the carbon, nitrogen and energy sources, e.g. dark conditions exclude phototrophs, exclusion of combined nitrogen compounds selects for nitrogen fixers and high concentrations of sodium chloride select halophilic species, or by adding inhibitors such as brilliant green to inhibit the growth of Gram-positive organisms or by using the atibiotics nystatin or amphotericin to inhibit the growth of fungi.

It should be noted that almost any conditions of growth exert a selective pressure since no one set of conditions permits the growth of all possible species: any growth is relative to the experimental conditions used.

Diagnostic media give characteristic reactions due to the growth of particular species, e.g. gelatin is digested by *Pseudomonas aeruginosa* but not by *E.coli*, lactose is fermented to give acid and gas by *E.coli* but not by *Salmonella* spp. and lactose media containing an indicator will show this.

However many diagnostic media are also selective. One common example is *MacConkey's Agar* which is formulated as follows:

Component	Concentration (g/litre)	Function
Nutrient broth	—	Nutrients
Bile salts	1.5	Reduces surface tension and tends to select for enteric bacteria
Lactose	10.0	Fermentable carbohydrate
Neutral red	0.03	Indicator to detect the production of acid from lactose fermentation
Agar	15.0	Solidifying agent

This medium is used as a presumptive test for *E.coli* Type 1 (i.e. of enteric origin). Although not itself an important pathogen, *E.coli* may be detected readily by relatively simple tests and its presence is taken to indicate recent faecal pollution, particularly of water and foodstuffs. *E.coli*, being enteric in origin, will grow in the presence of the bile salts and ferment the lactose giving bright pink colonies due to the action of the acid on the neutral red. Many non-enteric organisms are inhibited by the bile salt and enteric, non-lactose fermenters, e.g. *Salmonella* spp., give creamy or yellowish colonies. Since species other than *E.coli* can give similar reactions, the result is only presumptive and must be confirmed by other tests.

If the faecal pollution is of a non-nutrient material such as water, the *E.coli* tend to die, so distant faecal pollution is indicated by the presence of *Clostridium perfringens* which, being a sporing organism, persists for long periods.

Another common diagnostic medium is Brilliant Green agar, which is used for the isolation and recognition of *Salmonella* spp., excluding *Sal.typhi*. In addition to yeast extract, peptone and sodium chloride, as nutrients, and agar, as solidifying agent, it contains lactose and sucrose as fermentable carbohydrates, phenol red indicator and brilliant green as a selective agent. *Salmonella* spp., other than *Sal.typhi*, grow on the medium to give slightly pinkish-white, opaque colonies surrounded by brilliant red medium due to the production of alkali from the peptone. Any lactose or sucrose fermenting organisms which may grow give yellowish green colonies surrounded by an intense yellowish green zone, resulting from acid production. Some strains of *Proteus* also grow on the medium giving red colonies due to ammonia production resulting from urease activity.

From the above brief account of diagnostic media, of which hundreds are available and tens are in common use, it will be seen that none of them are completely specific for a single species. It is always a matter of relatively greater or less exclusion of unwanted organisms. Also, selective media are always inhibitory to some extent even to the species of interest.

BACTERIAL COUNTS

Counts may be made of the number of viable cells or of the total number of viable and dead cells. Differential counts, giving the numbers of organisms of different types, may also be done.

Viable Counts

Plating Methods. These are, in principle, very simple. A measured volume of a suspension of known dilution is inoculated into a solid medium, the solidifying agent keeping individual organisms separate, and the number of colonies is counted after incubation.

This simple proposition is complicated by a number of technical problems. The assumption is that a single cell gives rise to one colony and although this may be true, a colony may result from either a single cell or a clump or chain of cells, so a colony count is a clump count. Further, the degree of clumping varies with the species and its conditions of growth and the way in which the sample has been handled, e.g. shaken vigorously during dilution or not, so there is always a degree of uncertainty in the result. Thus it is common to report results in terms of 'colony forming units (cfu)/cm^3' instead of 'cells/cm^3'. Another factor is that any conditions of medium, pH, incubation temperature are selective, so that the 'true' count is never known, especially if exacting species are present. Bacteria and especially endospores, damaged by heat, chemicals, etc., often show a prolonged lag period before commencing growth, so a count done after 24 or 48 hours incubation may give a falsely low result as compared with a count done after 7, 14 or even 30 days incubation. Damaged bacteria are also very susceptible to variations in medium and composition, pH, temperature, etc., so that conditions suitable for the growth of undamaged organisms may be unsuitable for damaged cells of the same species. Further errors arise in the preparation of dilutions, due to pipetting errors, and the adsorption of cells to the glass surfaces of pipettes and dilution vessels, particularly from dilute suspensions, and of the dishes or bottles in which samples are finally placed together with the medium. Finally, errors occur due to the inherent statistical variability, especially when small number of colonies are being counted, and due to overcrowding if the counts are high.

The best that can be done is to adopt procedures which minimize these effects and enable reliable and reproducible estimates of numbers to be obtained. Such procedures include the following:

(a) adjust the medium, incubation temperature, etc., to give the highest count or to select the particular organisms of interest;
(b) use a rigidly standardized technique at all stages of counting;
(c) minimize adsorption effects by washing out pipettes with the suspensions before sampling and by having the minimum contact time of samples with glassware before the next operation is carried out;
(d) control the expected count, if possible;
(e) replicate counts and apply statistical analysis to the data.

Experienced workers can obtain an accuracy of $\pm$ 5 per cent (P = 0.95) by plating methods.

Whenever possible counting plates and tubes are incubated inverted to prevent the accumulation of condensed water droplets which fall back onto the medium and give a fluid film and resultant confluent growth which invalidates the count.

The *pour plate* technique (Fig. 29.24A) involves placing 0.5 to 1.0 cm^3 of a suspension expected to contain between 50 and 200 viable cfu in a Petri dish, pouring on about 15 cm^3 of molten agar medium at 45°, mixing, allowing to set, incubating inverted and counting the resultant colonies. This method is frequently used but is uneconomical, requiring a considerable amount of apparatus and medium, and has the disadvantage that the sample is exposed to the temperature of the molten medium at 48° and the subsequent slow cooling. This temperature will kill sensitive or damaged cells.

The *roll tube* technique (Fig. 29.24B) is similar to the pour plate except that 0.1 to 0.2 cm^3 of sample is added to 2.5 to 3.5 cm^3 of molten medium in a large test tube or a special bottle. The container is rolled almost horizontally so that the medium forms a film on its walls and is then cooled with water to solidify the film. This is more economical than the pour plate method, the temperature effect is less but the counting procedure is more difficult on the curved surface of the container.

Another similar technique is the *agar drop* method (Fig. 29.24C) in which a number of measured drops of molten medium containing the bacterial inoculum are placed in a plastic Petri dish. On plastic the drops do not spread but solidify coherently and the colonies in the drop can be counted under magification after incubation. This is a very economical method and gives more rapid results since the magnification used and the necessity of avoiding overcrowding effects in the small drop result in short incubation times.

Both economy and avoidance of contact with molten medium are achieved by the *surface viable* and *slide culture* methods. The surface viable method (Fig. 29.40D) uses a sterile agar plate which has been 'overdried' by preliminary incubation with the lid of the Petri dish raised so that liquid drops placed on the surface are absorbed rapidly. Drops of about 0.02 cm^3 of a dilution containing 20 to 50 cfu/drop are placed on the medium, allowed to dry in and the plates, which can have up to 10 drops each, are incubated inverted and the mean number of colonies per drop are counted. Problems with this method are the accurate measurement of the drops, the high sampling error due to the small number of cfu/drop and overcrowding in the small area of the drop. The latter problems can be overcome by using suitable magnification. Slide culture uses the apparatus illustrated in Fig. 29.24E; one loopful (0.015 ml) of a culture containing about 10^{8}cfu/ml is spread on the surface of the medium in the ring, a cover slip is placed on top and the colonies

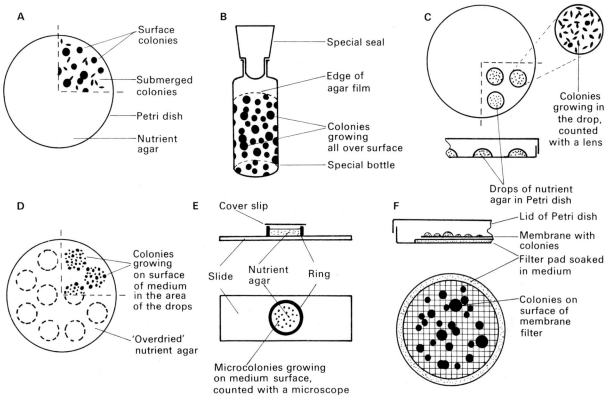

FIG. 29.24. Viable counts on bacteria and yeasts. A, Pour plate; B, Roll tube, using the Astell Laboratory Service Company bottle and seal; C, Agar drop; D, Surface viable; E, Slide culture; F, Membrane filter.

counted under the microscope after suitable incubation. This method has the advantages conferred by direct observation; that the viability can be determined by counting the proportion of cells which reproduce, very short incubation times can be used since the earliest stages of reproduction can be taken as evidence of viability, the degree of clumping can be determined, and differential counts can be done when there are clear morphological differences between cells.

Membrane filter counts are used when the expected count is below about 20 cfu/cm^3. The usual membrane filter is a thin cellulose ester film precipitated under controlled conditions so that the pore size is known and is very uniform. These membranes may be sterilized easily, give very high filtration rates compared with conventional filters and may be obtained in pore sizes (0.22, 0.45 μm) which will retain all bacterial cells on their surface. For counting, a suitable volume of sample, which may be of any size up to several litres provided that the filter does not block, is filtered and the filter placed on the surface of a sterile nutrient agar plate or on a filter paper pad impregnated with a suitable liquid medium. Incubation and counting is done as usual and the filter may be sterilized with formaldehyde vapour, dried and filed for reference purposes. This is rapidly becoming the standard technique in water analysis since viable counts as low as 5/litre may be done. The method is illustrated in Fig. 29.24F.

Dilution Methods are an older method of counting, devised before the introduction of solid media. The method is based on statistical sampling theory, which enables us to calculate the probability of obtaining no viable organisms in a sample of stated size when the count is known. Thus replicate volumes of a sample of low count, inoculated into tubes of liquid medium, will give a pattern of growth and no growth from which the count may be calculated. Tables are available which give the counts corresponding to various sampling regimens and patterns of growth, one of which is reproduced in part as Table 29.4. The count obtained in this way is usually described as a *most probable number* (MPN), since the errors are very large. Despite this lack of accuracy the method is widely used in water bacteriology and is the only method available for those organisms which give a spreading growth on solid media.

TABLE 29.4.

A PARTIAL MOST PROBABLE NUMBER TABLE FOR A DILUTION COUNT

Numbers of positive tubes* from samples of				
10 ml	1 ml	0.1 ml	MPN+	95 per cent confidence limits
0	0	1	2	<0.5–7
1	1	0	4	<0.5–11
2	0	1	7	1–17
2	3	0	12	3–28
3	3	0	17	5–46
4	3	1	33	11–93
5	1	0	33	11–93
5	2	1	70	23–168
5	3	3	175	44–503
5	4	3	278	90–849
5	5	0	240	68–754
5	5	1	348	118–1005
5	5	4	1609	635–5805

* Five tubes were inoculated with each volume of sample, i.e. 5 × 10 ml. 5 × 1 ml. 5 × 0.1 ml.

+ The estimated number of organisms in 100 ml of sample, derived from the number of positive tubes obtained from each sample volume.

Measurement of Metabolic Activity

These methods do not actually count the number of viable cells. Instead, the ability of the cells to metabolize and consume oxygen or reduce dyes is taken as a measure of the count and this may be an adequate measure of viability, especially when it is desired to assess the keeping quality of a product, e.g. milk, which depends more on metabolic activity than on actual numbers. However, non-viable cells may be able to metabolize, e.g. treatment with antiseptics may prevent reproduction yet leave many enzyme systems intact, so results must be interpreted cautiously.

A common method is to measure oxygen consumption by *Warburg manometry* (Fig. 29.25A). This is a semi-micro method in which a small volume of microbial suspension is placed in a flask of about 12 cm^3 capacity attached to a manometer.

Carbon dioxide is absorbed with KOH and suitable substrates or inhibitors are placed in side arms attached to the flask. Different gaseous mixtures can be used if desired. The flask is shaken gently in a water bath and the rate of oxygen consumption measured and related to known population densities. The effect of nutrients or inhibitors can also be studied readily (Fig. 29.25B).

Dye reduction is usually done using resazurin or methylene blue, the time taken for reduction to the colourless leuco-base being determined. The apparatus used is the Thunberg tube (Fig. 29.25C), a buffered sample being placed in the tube and an appropriate substrate or inhibitor in the hollow stopper as required. The tube is evacuated, filled with nitrogen or hydrogen to prevent re-oxidation of the dye, and the stopper closed. After temperature equilibration the contents of tube and stopper are mixed and the time taken to reduce the dye is measured. The greater the microbial population, the shorter the reduction time, so these properties can be related. As with manometry, the effects of nutrients or inhibitors can be assessed.

Other Indirect Measures of Viable Biomass. For special applications numerous methods involving the determination of the amounts of particular cell constituents have been used, e.g. ATP, DNA, alkaline phosphatase, β-galactosidase.

Total Counts

The Coulter Counter. This instrument is a standard method of performing counts on all types of suspensions and is illustrated in Fig. 29.26. For bacteria the orifice diameter is usually 50 μm. The principle is that the resistance is measured between electrodes on either side of the orifice. The suspension is drawn through the orifice at a standard rate and as each particle enters the orifice the resistance is momentarily increased and this change is measured as a single count. It is a very simple matter to count 10^4 cells in a few minutes with high accuracy. Further refinements permit the cell size to be sensed so that single cells can be differentiated from clumps, cocci from bacilli, spores from vegetative cells, etc.

Direct microscopic counting. The only method in this class now used is *Breed's method*, which was developed for milk. A known volume of material is spread evenly over a known area of slide, fixed and stained and the mean number of cells in each field is counted. Knowing the magnification, the original count can be determined. This method is the only one available for turbid samples and has the additional advantages that the morphology, arrangement and staining reactions of the cells can be observed directly.

Other methods of direct microscopy, e.g. counting chambers, are tedious and relatively inaccurate and are now rarely used.

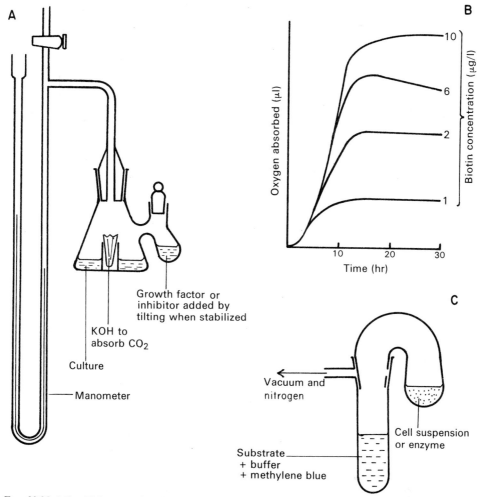

FIG. 29.25. Microbial counts by the measurement of metabolic activity. A, The Warburg manometric apparatus; B, A typical result which might be obtained with a Warburg apparatus, showing the effect of biotin on respiration by an exacting organism; C, The Thunberg tube for dye reduction measurements.

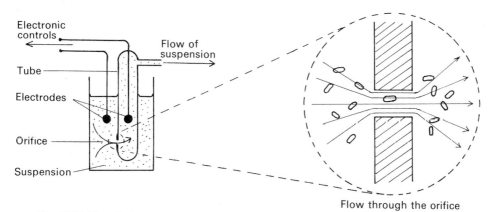

FIG. 29.26. The principle of the Coulter counter method of determining total microbial counts.

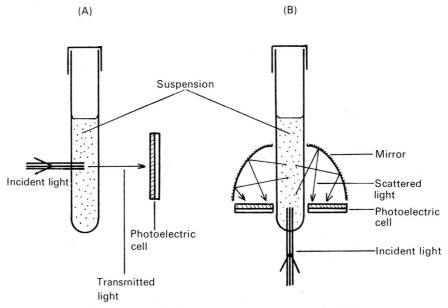

FIG. 29.27. The basic principles involved in the determination of total microbial counts by opacity measurement. A, The absorptiometer method; B, The EEL nephelmeter principle.

Opacity methods. These require careful calibration with a Coulter counter for the species or strains of interest under the precise conditions to be used, since the opacity or light scattering properties of suspensions vary with the growth conditions, the method of preparing suspensions, the suspending fluid, etc.

However, they are widely used for their simplicity and speed. Measurements may be made with a simple colorimeter, but a nephelometer, which measures the light scattered at right angles to an incident light beam is more usual. The principles are illustrated in Fig. 29.27.

Other methods of total counting. Measurements of the total biomass of dense suspensions may be made by centrifugation under standard conditions, by determination of the dry weight of cells, or from the total nitrogen content determined by a micro-Kjeldahl method. These methods are relatively inaccurate but may be adequate for some purposes, e.g. vaccine standardization.

COUNTS OF OTHER MICROORGANISMS

If the organism occurs primarily as individual cells which form colonies on solid media, the methods used for bacterial counts apply.

For non-colonial and filamentous organisms very few of the methods described for bacteria may be used. Fungi form large masses of coherent growth so the wet weight of mycelium is most commonly used, but dry weights, total nitrogen and oxygen consumption are also applied frequently. These methods are also used for filamentous algae but, in addition, colorimetric determinations of chlorophyll content are convenient. With protozoa, particle counting, opacity, wet weight, dry weight and microscopy are the commonest methods.

ISOLATION OF MICRO-ORGANISMS IN PURE CULTURE

The commonest method used for colony forming organisms is streaking. In this, a loopful of a dilute culture is spread over the surface of a sterile agar plate so that there is progressive dilution and, after incubation, well isolated colonies with recognizable morphology are formed. Each colony arises from a single cell, or a small group of cells, and a sample of a typical colony is picked off, diluted and streaked on a second plate. This procedure is repeated until only one type of colony is observed through several isolations, when the culture is assumed to be pure, i.e. consisting of a single, homogeneous species. A successful isolation is illustrated in Fig. 29.28.

Isolation may be assisted using selective conditions, e.g. aerobic, anaerobic, low or high temperature, particular carbon or nitrogen sources, pH, various concentrations of sodium chloride, dyes, surfactants, antiseptics or antibiotics, depending on the properties of the species to be isolated.

Also micromanipulators, which permit the

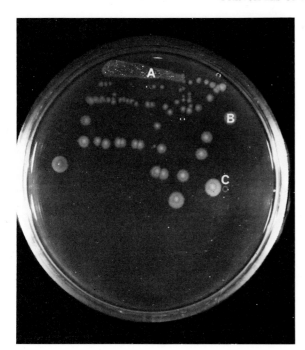

FIG. 29.28. An isolation plate of bacteria prepared by streaking. A, streak of confluent growth; B, a colony of the predominant type; C, two contaminant colonies.

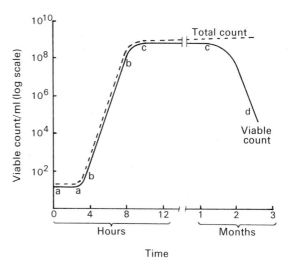

FIG. 29.29. An idealized bacterial growth curve. The growth phases; aa, lag; bb, exponential; cc, stationary; cd, decline. The axes show the approximate magnitudes for the density of growth and the time scale which might be involved, though there is great variation in practice.

inoculation of a single cell into a small drop of medium, can be used.

Normally only pure cultures are used so that studies of the properties of individual species can be made. However, some organisms, notably many protozoa and all viruses, can be grown only in mixed culture with other cells, while obligate parasites are inevitably associated with their host species.

MICROBIAL GROWTH AND REPRODUCTION

POPULATION GROWTH IN LIQUID MEDIA

A typical growth curve obtained when resting bacteria are inoculated into fresh medium is shown in Fig. 29.29. The most important features are the *lag, exponential, stationary* and *decline* phases.

It is important to realize that this curve applies only in a specific context, namely that the organisms are unicellular, the inoculum is of vegetative cells (not spores) derived from the stationary phase and the new growth conditions are identical with those in which the inoculum was grown originally. Also the culture is a batch culture, i.e. a fixed volume of medium, with nothing added or removed during growth.

The following factors affect the form of this curve.

The lag phase. This is a period of adaptation to the new conditions of growth. Any factors, e.g. medium composition, temperature, pH, oxidation–reduction potential, which tend to favour growth will reduce the length of lag, and conversely. Lag is also reduced by using rapidly growing cells from the exponential phase (cells from the stationary, decline and lag phases giving longer lag phases, in that order) and with large inocula, the length of lag being roughly proportional to the logarithm of the inoculum size. Cells which have been damaged by antiseptics, heat, etc. tend to give long lag phases. Long delayed growth may also result from the use of spore inocula and fully dormant spores may take weeks or months to germinate, though germination may be triggered by 'heat shock', i.e. heating at 80° for 10 minutes and in other ways. The lag phase is not a period of dormancy but of active metabolism and cell enlargement. Individual cells increase to a certain critical size and then start to divide, possibly when the concentrations of essential metabolites reach critical levels. However, the term growth normally refers to reproduction and population growth and not to the increase in size of individual cells.

The exponential phase. This is a period of constant growth rate which is most rapid under optimal environmental conditions. The optimal growth rate is a genetic property of the strain, e.g. with *E.coli* the population may double in 20 minutes whereas with *M.tuberculosis* doubling takes several hours, even under the most favourable conditions.

The growth rate may be defined in terms of the *doubling time*, the time taken for the population to double in size, or in terms of the *mean generation time* (MGT), the average time taken for a single cell to produce two daughter cells. Under favourable conditions these two parameters are identical, but if some daughter cells are non-viable the MGT is less than the observed doubling time.

If at zero time the population is N_o, then after one doubling time the population is $2N_o$, after two doubling times is $4N_o = 2^2 N_o$ and after n doubling times is $2^n N_o$, i.e. the population at time $t = N_t = 2^{t/td} N_o$, where td is the doubling time, therefore:

$$\log N_t/N_o = (t/t_d) \log 2$$

i.e. $t_d = 0.301\, t/(\log N_t - \log N_o) = $ MGT (under favourable conditions). The growth rate constant (k) in doublings/hour is the slope of the growth curve in the exponential phase and is given by the expression:

$$K = {}^1/t_d = (\log N_t - \log N_o)/0.301\, t$$

The stationary phase. After a variable period of exponential reproduction, growth slows and ceases, usually owing to exhaustion of available oxygen (in aerobic cultures) and by auto-intoxication, i.e. the production of metabolites by the cell which inhibit its own growth, the best known examples of which are the production of alcohol by yeast and of lactic acid by lactobacilli. Exhaustion of food material occurs only rarely and under conditions of very low nutrient concentration. A further possibility is that, under a particular set of conditions, each organism has a characteristic maximum population which is controlled by the packing density of the cells.

The length of the stationary phase is very variable and depends markedly on the species (indefinitely long with sporing organisms) and on the environment, notably temperature. Optimum growth temperatures tend to give short stationary phases, cultures preserved by refrigeration usually gives extended times.

The decline phase. This is produced by a variety of factors, e.g. auto-intoxication and unbalanced metabolism due to enzyme activity under conditions preventing growth, resulting in the production of lytic enzymes. The rate and extent of decline varies considerably with the species and environmental conditions, many cultures becoming sterile within a few days or weeks.

THE CHANGE OF TOTAL COUNT DURING POPULATION GROWTH

With most species growing under good conditions, the total count is very similar to the viable count, at least during exponential growth (Fig. 29.29), but during the stationary phase the total count tends to increase and normally remains constant from the end of the stationary phase and during the decline phase, unless the cells lyse and break up. The increase in total count during the stationary phase while the viable count remains constant shows that all the cells are not inactive, but that some are reproducing, though reproduction is balanced by death of an equivalent number.

CONTINUOUS CULTURE

In a batch culture, described above, growth occurs in a closed system, but this does not result in uniform conditions. As reproduction occurs, nutrients are utilized, metabolic products accumulate and the oxidation–reduction potential falls. This results in continually changing conditions in the culture and it is known that the composition of the cell wall and the concentrations of a number of cytoplasmic components vary as growth proceeds.

However, the growth rate of a culture, and so its physiological condition, may be maintained absolutely constant by the process of continuous culture, usually in a *chemostat* (Fig. 29.30). In this the desired conditions of temperature, gas mixture, pH, nutrients, etc., are maintained constant. Fresh medium is added at a predetermined rate with efficient mixing and the excess culture overflows at the same rate as fresh medium is added. Under these conditions the growth rate may be fixed within wide limits by the rate of addition of fresh medium.

This system is of the utmost importance since it is the only one which allows detailed studies of the effects of individual factors on the physiology and biochemistry of microorganisms and is the standard technique for such studies.

FACTORS INFLUENCING GROWTH AND VIABILITY

Temperature
With most microorganisms three cardinal temperatures can be identified. The optimum temperature and the maximum temperature at which

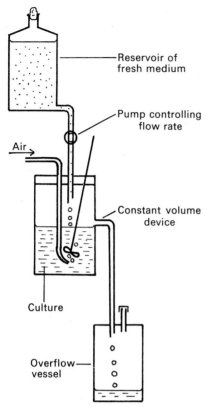

FIG. 29.30. The principle of the chemostat.

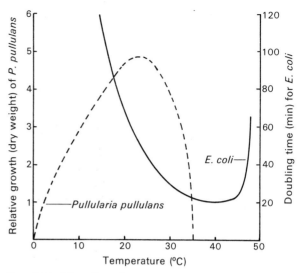

FIG. 29.31. The effect of temperature on the growth of a bacterium (*Escherichia coli*) and a mould (*Pullaria pullulans*).

in form for all types of microorganisms, though the optima may be very different.

TABLE 29.5.

THE APPROXIMATE TEMPERATURES AND pH VALUES FOR OPTIMUM GROWTH OF A RANGE OF BACTERIA, TOGETHER WITH THEIR GROWTH RANGES

Family or Species	Temperature values (°C)			pH values		
	Opti-mum	Mini-mum	Maxi-mum	Opti-mum	Mini-mum	Maxi-mum
M.tuberculosis	37	30	40	7.3	4.5	8.4
C.diphtheriae	37	15	15	1.4	6.0	8.0
Ps.aeruginosa	37	5	42	6.8	4.4	8.8
Ps.fluorescens	25	0	37	—	—	—
V.cholerae	37	16	42	7.2	5.6	7.6
N. meningitidis	37	30	—	7.5	6.1	7.8
N.gonorrhoeae	37	30	38.5	7.3	5.8	8.3
Strep.faecalis	37	10	45	—	4.8	11.0
Staph.aureus	37	12	45	7.5	—	—
Proteus spp.	—	—	—	6.5	4.3	9.5
E.coli	37	15	45	6.5	4.3	9.5
Sal.typhi	—	—	—	7.6	4.0	9.6
Yersinia pestis	27	−2	45	7.2	5.0	9.6
Thiob.thio-oxidans	—	—	—	3.5	0.6	9.8

growth will occur and, less precisely a minimum growth temperature (Table 29.5). The optimum temperature is normally taken as that at which growth is most rapid, though other criteria may be used, and three groups are distinguishable on the basis of this optimum.

Group	Optimum temperature
Mesophiles	25 to 40°C
Thermophiles	Above 45°C
Psychrophiles	Below 25°C

However, the temperature ranges for growth vary widely. Above the normal range there is a rapid fall in growth rate and lethal temperatures are reached rapidly (Fig. 29.31), whereas below the normal range the growth rate gradually falls towards zero, though *low temperatures are not lethal*. Thus refrigeration is used to preserve foods, and often microbial cultures, from spoilage and high temperatures are used for sterilization (see Chapter 31). Fig. 29.31 also shows that the temperature/growth rate curve is essentially similar

Desiccation

Drying in air is often lethal, though the effect depends markedly on the species, e.g. *Neisseria gonorrhoeae* survives in air about 3 hours, *Streptococcus pyogenes* for several days, *Myobacterium tuberculosis* for several months and bacterial spores for many years. The lethal effect also depends on the temperature, the rate of drying and on the presence of protective materials such as proteins, sugars and reducing agents.

Lyophilization is the standard method of preserving most bacterial and fungal cultures.

Acidity and Alkalinity (pH)

As with temperature, minimum, optimum and maximum pH values for growth may be identified. Broadly speaking bacteria have pH optima around neutrality (range pH 5—8.5) while fungi have optima about pH 5.5 (range pH 2—9), though individual species vary widely in pH tolerance (Table 29.5). Protozoa and algae tend to be more restricted in pH range in the region of neutrality.

The influence of pH on the availability of *p*-aminobenzoic acid has already been mentioned, but pH similarly affects the activity of inhibitors so that the total effect of pH depends upon the nutrients and inhibitors present and their pK values. Low environmental pH values are dealt with in bacteria by exchanging K^+ for H^+, i.e. K^+ is taken up and H^+ is excreted, so maintaining the internal pH within physiological limits, provided that the pH is not too low and enough K^+ is available.

Oxidation–Reduction (O/R) Potential

Oxidation can be defined as a loss of electrons, reduction as a gain of electrons, e.g. $Fe^{2+} \rightarrow Fe^{3+}$. The O/R potential ($E$) is defined by the Nernst equation

$$E = E_o + (RT \ln[ox]/[red])/nF$$

where R is the gas constant, T is the absolute temperature, [ox] is the concentration of oxidized component, [red] is the concentration of reduced component, F is the Faraday and n is the number of electrons transferred in the reaction. E_o is the *standard (normal) electrode* potential, i.e. the O/R potential of the 50 per cent oxidized system, and is an indication of the oxidizing power of a system. At 18°, constant pH and single electron transfer

$$E = E_o + (0.058 \log[ox]/[red]).$$

The O/R potential may be determined potentiometrically, but in the usual microbiological media the electrodes tend to become poisoned and indicators are used. Usually these are methylene blue, blue when oxidized and colourless when reduced, or resazurin, a blue dye which undergoes irreversible reduction to pink, which is then reversibly reduced to the colourless leuco-base. Resazurin is often preferred as being less toxic than methylene blue. The relationship of the percentage reduction to O/R potential is shown in Fig. 29.32A.

Bacteria and O/R Potential. Three classes of bacteria are distinguishable in relation to O/R potential (Fig. 29.32B).

Aerobes, e.g. *Bacillus* spp., will initiate growth at values of $E > +0.2$ volt, and tend to reduce the value to -0.02 to -0.04 volt.

Anaerobes, e.g. *Clostridium* spp., will initiate growth only at values of $E < +0.1$ volt and growth reduces the value to about -0.4 volt.

Microaerophiles, e.g. *Lactobacillus* spp., grow only slowly at values of $E > +0.1$ volt.

Facultative organisms, e.g. *E.coli* and *Staph. aureus*, will grow under either aerobic or anaerobic conditions, though aerobic growth is more vigorous since respiration yields more energy than fermentation.

Methods for Producing Anaerobiosis

There are two basic methods, the removal of oxygen from the medium and environment and the addition of reducing substances to the medium. In the McIntosh and Fildes (Fig. 29.32C) and 'Gas-Pak' anaerobic jars, the oxygen in the atmosphere is removed by catalytic combination with hydrogen. Reducing substances which are widely used are thioglycollic acid ($HS.CH_2COOH$) and cysteine ($HS.CH_2.CHNH_2.COOH$); glutathione (3-glutamyl-cysteinyl-glycine), sulphites and glucose are also used. These media normally contain an O/R indicator. Another valuable medium uses a layer of granules of defatted meat, which contains a variety of reducing systems. To prevent access of oxygen to the reduced medium it is common to add a low concentration of agar, about 0.1 per cent, which increases viscosity and so reduces carriage of oxygen into the medium by convection, and to seal the surface of the medium with vaspar (equal parts of soft and liquid paraffins).

The formulae of media of this type are given in Table 29.6. (See p. 462.)

Reasons for Anaerobiosis

Absence of cytochromes. Most anaerobes do not possess the complete cytochrome system and so cannot utilize oxygen as the final hydrogen acceptor. This results in the accumulation of reduced NAD ($NADH_2$) and, since there is a limited supply of NAD, metabolism ceases unless the cell can oxidise $NADH_2$ using an alternative hydrogen acceptor to oxygen.

Sulphydryl enzymes. Many enzymes depend on sulphydryl groups ($-SH$) for activity, especially enzymes in anaerobic organisms. Under oxidizing conditions the sulphydryl groups form disulphides and the enzymes are inactivated.

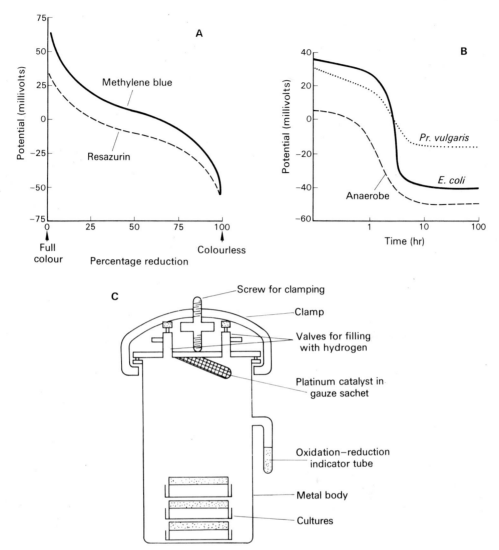

FIG. 29.32. Oxidation-reduction potential and bacterial growth. A, the relationship of oxidation–reduction potential to the reduction of indicator dyes; B, The change in oxidation–reduction potential with time in bacterial cultures; C, One type of McIntosh and Fildes anaerobic jar.

Absence of catalase. Peroxidase enzymes yield hydrogen peroxide, which is toxic. Aerobes possess catalase, which breaks down the peroxide to oxygen and water, but this enzyme is generally absent from anaerobes, which are thus inhibited by hydrogen peroxide toxicity.

Oxygen toxicity. Anaerobic metabolism is specifically inhibited by oxygen, and this is the basis of the 'Pasteur effect' i.e. fermentation reactions cease abruptly when a culture is aerated.

Although these reasons are widely quoted, it should be noted that there are exceptions and

anomalies to the first three of these, so it must be concluded that the precise reasons for anaerobic growth are still obscure and understanding of anaerobes is limited. However, if it could be shown that anaerobic operator genes (see p. 468) are specifically repressed by oxygen, or a substance produced under oxidizing conditions, many outstanding problems would be clarified.

Osmotic Pressure
Hypotonic environments do not affect microorganisms unless the concentrations of salts or nutrients is so low that growth cannot occur.

TABLE 29.6

SOME COMMON ANAEROBIC MEDIA*

Cooked Meat Medium (Robertson's Medium)

Defatted granules of	
beef heart	3.0
Peptone	1.0
Beef extract	1.0
Sodium chloride	0.5
0.2 per cent of dextrose is often added.	

The medium should be freshly prepared or freshly steamed. It is one of the most valuable of all anaerobic media.

Fluid Thioglycollate Medium USP

Yeast extract	0.5	} Nutrients
Casein peptone	1.5	
Sodium chloride	0.25	
L-Cystine	0.05	Source of sulphur
Dextrose	0.55	Nutrient and mild reducing agent
Agar	0.075	Increases viscosity and prevents aeration by convection
Sodium thioglycollate	0.05	Reducing agent
Resazurin	10^{-4}	Oxidation–reduction indicator

Recommended by the USP for sterility tests, especially if heavy metals are present.

Reinforced Clostridial Medium

Yeast extract	0.3	} Nutrients
Beef extract	1.0	
Peptone	1.0	
Sodium chloride	0.5	
Soluble starch	0.1	Detoxifies inhibitors of spore germination
Dextrose	0.5	Mild reducing agent, growth promoter
Cysteine hydrochloride	0.05	Reducing agent
Agar	0.05	Increases viscosity and prevents aeration by convection
Sodium acetate	0.03	Nutrient favouring anaerobic growth

A semi-solid medium giving excellent growth of fastidious anaerobes. A solid medium is available.

* Concentrations are given as per cent (w/v)

Hypertonicity also has little effect until the osmotic pressure of the environment becomes very high. Microorganisms can maintain a suitable internal osmotic pressure even if the external osmotic pressure varies widely, either by transport of ions, notably K^+, into and out of the cell, or by special mechanisms, e.g. the contractile vacuole in many protozoa.

High concentrations of sodium chloride (30 per cent), sugars (70 per cent), and glycerol (50 per cent) inhibit cells and may cause plasmolysis, and these substances are used extensively as preservatives, but there is no lethal effect and contaminants grow when the solutions are diluted. Many bacteria and fungi, especially yeasts, are osmotolerant and will cause spoilage of products preserved in this way, a notable example being Syrup, unless additional preservatives are present.

Spoilage of salted meat and fish products results from the activities of *halophilic organisms*, i.e. those which *require* high concentrations of sodium chloride for growth, e.g. *Halobacterium* spp. need 20–30 per cent w/v NaCl. These are distinguished from *halotolerant* organisms, such as *Staph.aureus*, which will grow in the presence of 10 per cent w/v NaCl, but do not require it for growth.

Electromagnetic Radiations

The harmful effects of these increase as the wavelength decreases, the order of increasing biological activity being as follows: infrared (4×10^5 to 750 nm), visible light (750 to 400 nm), ultraviolet (300 to 100 nm) and X- and γ-radiations (10 to 0.0005 nm).

The effects produced are mutations and lethal damage, due both to the direct effect of the radiations on DNA and to indirect effects on DNA from the production by the radiation of H_2O_2 and oxidizing radicals from water.

Gamma-radiations are widely used for the sterilization of thermolabile products and ultraviolet radiation of wavelength 260 nm is used to a limited extent for the sterilization of atmospheres and water (see Chapter 28).

Surface Tension

Low surface tension inhibits the growth of many bacteria, bile salts and Teepol being used as selective agents for the cultivation of the enteric bacteria, which normally live in the presence of bile salts. Other effects are the production of more generalized growth in liquid media with organisms which tend to produce a granular or adherent cell mass, e.g. *B.subtilis*, and the formation of elongated cells of bacterial rods.

Surfacants may be inherently biostatic or biocidal and may potentiate the activity of other antimicrobial agents.

Ultrasonic Energy

This is carried by sound-waves of frequency > 20 000 Hz. Very high frequencies (320–680 kHz) may sterilize cultures, but they are used only as a research tool.

Pressure

Very low pressures kill cells due to desiccation but high pressures have little effect unless they cause inhibition by the solution of excessive oxygen or carbon dioxide in the cytoplasm. Very high pressures inhibit most cells.

ENERGY YIELDING METABOLISM

FERMENTATION AND RESPIRATION

Except in photosynthesis all energy yielding reactions are oxidations at the expense of a suitable reductant, e.g.

$$AH_2 + B \longrightarrow BH_2 + A.$$
$$\underset{\text{donor}}{\text{Hydrogen}} \quad \underset{\text{acceptor}}{\text{Hydrogen}}$$

Fermentation is oxidative metabolism in which both the hydrogen donor and hydrogen acceptor are organic.

Respiration is oxidative metabolism with an inorganic hydrogen acceptor, the hydrogen donor being either organic or inorganic.

The function of both processes is to link the oxidation to the production of ATP which can be used either directly for energy requiring reactions or indirectly for the synthesis of alternative energy yielding phosphates, e.g. phospho-*enol*-pyruvate, or of energy rich stores, e.g. creatinine phosphate.

GLUCOSE FERMENTATION

The three main pathways of glucose utilization are outlined in Fig. 29.33 and are the Embden-Meyerhof-Parnas (EMP), Entner-Doudoroff (ED) and hexose monophosphate (HMP) pathways. The net ATP yield is two molecules per molecule of glucose in the EMP pathway, which is the commonest, and is one ATP in the HMP and ED pathways The former of these occurs in many organisms but the latter only in bacteria.

All the pathways yield pyruvate oxidatively at the expense of NAD as hydrogen acceptor, the $NADH_2$ being oxidized to yield ATP in the process of oxidative phosphorylation. The pyruvate is then broken down in various ways by different species to yield products of diagnostic or industrial interest (Fig. 29.34)

Pyruvate is also a key compound in many biosynthetic reactions.

ENERGY FROM RESPIRATION

The principal types of microbial respiration are shown in Table 29.7. Aerobic respiration with organic hydrogen donors goes in two main steps; the production of pyruvate and its stepwise oxidation to carbon dioxide via the tricarboxylic acid

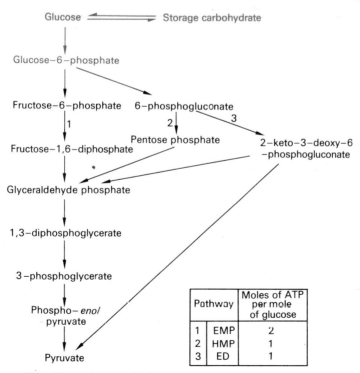

FIG. 29.33. Glucose fermentation in cells. The Embden-Meyerhof, hexose monophosphate and Entner-Doudoroff fermentation pathways.

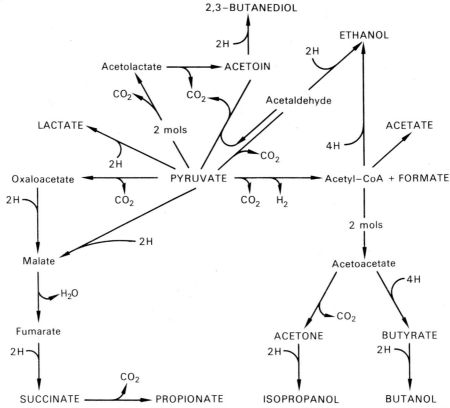

Fig. 29.34. Some compounds resulting from the metabolism of pyruvate. End products are shown in capitals.

TABLE 29.7.

THE PRINCIPAL TYPES OF MICROBIAL RESPIRATION

Type	H_2 accep-tor	H_2 donor		Example	
Aerobic	O_2	Organic		\All plants and animals / Most bacteria	
		Inorganic	H_2 NH_4^+ NO_2^- Fe_2^+ S cpds.	Hydrogenomonas Nitrosomonas Nitrobacter Ferrobacillus Thiobacillus (some) Beggiatoa	
Anaerobic	SO_4^{2-} NO_3^- CO_2	H_2 Organic H_2 H_2		Desulfovibrio Fungi, many bacteria Mic.denitrificans Methane bacteria	

All genera and species quoted are bacterial.

(TCA, Krebs, citric acid) cycle (Fig. 29.35A) yielding $NADH_2$, and finally the oxidation of the $NADH_2$ by the stepwise transfer of hydrogen to oxygen, a process known as electron transport or oxidative phosphorylation (Fig. 29.35B), the principal source of ATP.

Electron transport in eukaryotes occurs in the mitochrondria, all organisms having similar mechanisms, but in prokaryotes the more varied components are associated with the plasma membrane or the mesosomes.

OTHER PROCESSES YIELDING ATP

Many other reactions are used to produce ATP, the principal ones being amino acid fermentations, other conversions, e.g. citrulline–ornithine, and photosynthesis.

DNA FUNCTIONS AND SOME CELLULAR CONTROL MECHANISMS

ASPECTS OF DNA FUNCTION

Protein Synthesis
The basic unit of the chromosome is the gene, a unique series of nucleotides. Each gene specifies a particular polypeptide; the sequence of amino acids in the polypeptide, i.e. the primary structure of

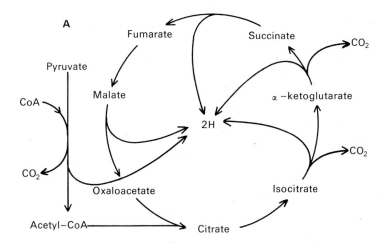

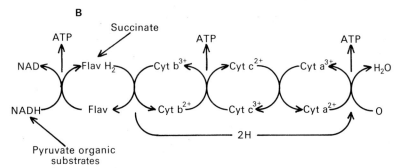

FIG. 29.35. Respiration and energy production. A, The elements of the tricarboxylic acid (TCA, Krebs, citric acid) cycle; B, The production of ATP by the action of the election transport chain. Flav, flavin nucleotide.

the final protein, being determined by the nucleotide base sequence in the gene and each amino acid being coded for by a nucleotide triplet, known as a *codon*, e.g. the triplet AAT* is the codon for leucine, the codon for alanine being GCC and for proline GGT. There are also codons for chain termination (UAA, UGA or UAG) and for chain initiation (UAG or GUG after a termination codon).

Polypeptide synthesis involves firstly the *transcription* of the DNA into *messenger RNA* (mRNA) and then the *translation* of the mRNA information into the polypeptide chain. Transcription is directed by RNA polymerase, the base sequence complementing that of one strand of the DNA. Translation of the mRNA occurs at the *ribosome* (Fig. 29.36A), several ribosomes becoming attached to one mRNA molecule to give a *polyribosome* on which several identical polypeptides are synthesized simultaneously. Each amino acid is

*A, adenylic acid; G, guanylic acid; T, thymidylic acid; C, cytidylic acid; U, uridylic acid.

carried to the polyribosome by a specific *transfer RNA* (tRNA, Fig. 29.36B).

The sequence of events is illustrated in (Fig. 29.37). The mRNA consists of an initiation codon (IC), the codons specifying the number and sequence of amino acids and the termination codon (TC).

A ribosome is formed on the beginning of the mRNA molecule and a tRNA carrying N-formyl methionine (NfMet), is attached to the first ribosome at the IC recognition site: N-formyl substitution directs chain growth in the right direction. A second tRNA, carrying the first amino acid (A1) of the polypeptide chain attaches at codon 1 and a transferase attaches NfMet to A1. The ribosome moves along one codon and a third tRNA, carrying the second amino acid (A2), attaches at codon 2, the growing peptide chain is transferred as before and the tRNA for NfMet detaches from the ribosome and is recycled. As the procedure is repeated to build up the polypeptide chain, more ribosomes attach to the mRNA to

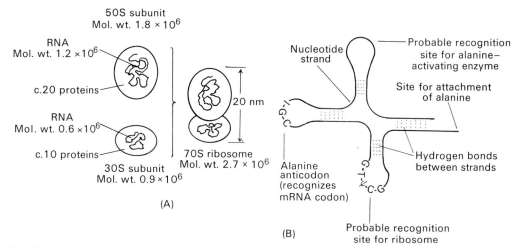

FIG. 29.36. Some compounds involved in protein synthesis in prokaryotic cells. A, The 70s ribosome; B, The probable configuration of alanine tRNA (from Holley, R. W. et al. (1965) *Science*, **147**, 1462).

form a polyribosome, a further molecule of the polypeptide being synthesized on each ribosome. Finally, the polypeptide is terminated at the TC site on the mRNA, the polypeptide and the ribosome are released and the ribosome sub-units recycled. The NfMet bond is hydrolysed to leave the polypeptide which then coils and cross-links to form the secondary structure of the protein, further coiling and binding yielding the active protein with its tertiary structure.

The Control of Protein Synthesis

For protein to be synthesized two conditions must be fulfilled: the appropriate gene must be present and it must be *expressed*, i.e. no factor is operating to prevent the gene being translated into protein. One such factor is mutation, and a mutated gene either produces a different protein or is non-functional. Gene expression is also carefully controlled in response both to environmental factors and the state of cell metabolism.

The classic example of the control of gene expression is the β-galactoside transport and utilization systems of *E.coli*, in which the enzymes for glucose transport and utilization are always present (i.e. *constitutive*) but those for lactose (β-galactosides) are present only if required (i.e. *inducible*), though the genes controlling lactose permease and lactose hydrolysis are always present in non-mutant strains.

If *E.coli* is grown with a limited amount of glucose and any amount of lactose as sole carbon sources, it utilizes the glucose preferentially. Once all the glucose has been metabolized, there is a lag

during which the lactose permease and the β-galactosidase are synthesized and growth is then resumed utilizing the lactose. Thus glucose *represses* the lactose permease and β-galactosidase genes, the mechanism for this being illustrated in Fig. 29.38. The basis for this is presumably economy of energy resources. In the presence of glucose, the enzymes for which are constitutive, there is a readily available carbohydrate and there is no point in using energy to synthesize the enzymes which transport and hydrolyse lactose, so the latter are synthesized only when they are essential for growth to continue.

The Operon Theory states that the basic unit of DNA function is the operon, which consists of an *operator gene* plus the adjacent *structural genes*. There is also a nearby *promoter gene*, the site of attachment of the RNA polymerase which catalyses the synthesis of the mRNAs on the structural gene patterns, and a *regulator gene*.

In the presence of glucose the regulator gene controls the synthesis of a soluble repressor protein which either attaches to the operator gene and blocks RNA polymerase attachment or prevents RNA polmerase activity, so no mRNAs are synthesized on the structural genes.

Also glucose, or an intermediate of glucose metabolism, may act directly on the operator gene to prevent mRNA synthesis. In this state the genes at the *lac* locus are *repressed*. In the absence of glucose the RNA polymerase can attach to the promoter site, the lactose causes the production of inactive repressor protein, so mRNA is synthesized on the structural genes and can be translated into

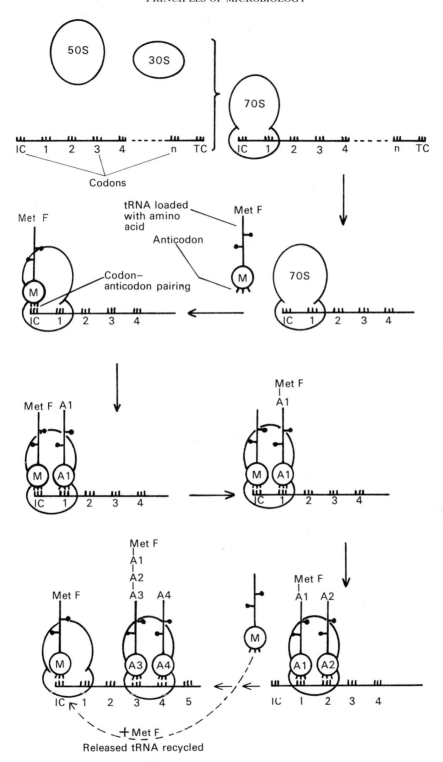

Fig. 29.37. The sequence of events in protein synthesis. IC: initiation codon, n: the number of amino acids in the protein, TC: termination codon, MetF: N-formylmethionine, A1, A2 etc., successive amino acids in the peptide chain.

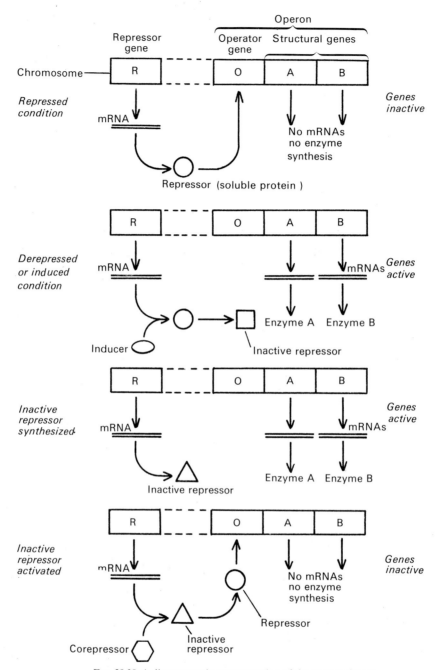

FIG. 29.38. A diagrammatic representation of the operon theory.

the appropriate enzymes in the cytoplasm. This is the *derepressed* or *induced* condition.

In some cases, e.g. alkaline phosphatase synthesis, the repressed state is normal and the regulator gene codes for an *activator* protein which causes derepression and enzyme synthesis.

ALLOSTERIC CONTROL OF ENZYME ACTIVITY

It is well known that the supply of an end product of a synthetic chain, or the build up of a high concentration of the end products due to metabolism, will suppress the synthesis of that end product. This is *end product repression* or *feed back*

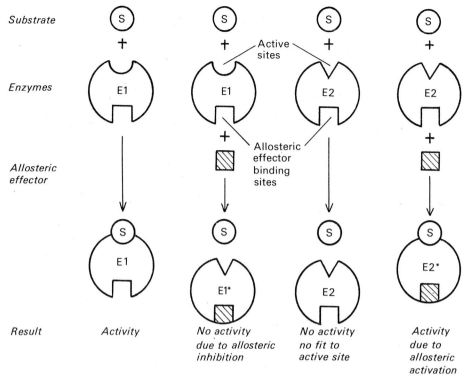

Substrate

Enzymes

Allosteric
effector

Result   Activity   No activity   No activity   Activity
                               due to allosteric   no fit to   due to
                               inhibition   active site   allosteric
                                                                       activation

FIG. 29.39. Metabolic control by allosteric effectors. *Enzyme modified by combination with an allosteric effector.

inhibition, e.g. supplying histidine prevents its own synthesis, and supplying tryptophan represses the tryptophan synthetase and induces tryptophanase.

Although it was once thought that these effects were due to mass action, it is now known that they are primarily produced by specific *allosteric effectors*, i.e. compounds which inhibit or activate enzymes, not by attaching to the active site but by attaching to another site on the enzyme molecule and so modifying the configuration of the active site. This is illustrated in Fig. 29.39. Hence the term allosteric, 'another shape', one not fitting the active site yet affecting activity.

The effects may be very complex and sensitive. In the EMP glucose pathway phospho-enol-pyruvate (PEP) may accumulate and this compound then acts as an allosteric inhibitor of the pathway and also as an allosteric activator for the conversion of glucose into glycogen, i.e. the cell switches from glucose metabolism to glycogen storage. When the concentration of PEP falls, both of these effects are removed and the cell switches from glycogen synthesis to glucose utilization.

VIRUSES

CHARACTERISTICS

Viruses are the simplest entities capable of self-replication and are distinguished from all other microorganisms by being non-cellular. They possess the following unique characters.

1. Contain only *one* kind of nucleic acid, RNA or DNA but never both.

2. Other components are a limited range of proteins and sometimes small amounts of lipid, carbohydrate and polyamines.

3. There is no cell wall, no plasma membrane, no cytoplasm.

4. They have no independent metabolism.

5. The mode of replication is unique, there being no growth of all parts followed by budding or division but the nucleic acid and protein components are synthesized separately in the host cell and then assembled into numerous replicate complete viruses.

Additional features, which are not unique to viruses, are as follows.

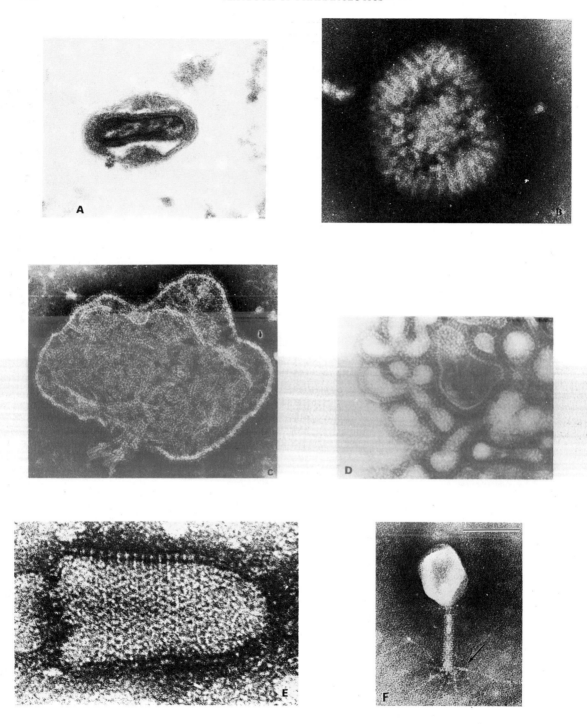

FIG. 29.40. *Some typical viruses.* A and B, two forms of vaccinia virus, A showing the central *nucleoid* surrounded by a membrane, two ovoid *lateral bodies* and the outer membrane. By courtesy of Prof. E. L. Medzon and Academic Press. C, measles virus, showing the outer capsid and extensive helical nucleocapsid (escaping through the ruptured capsid). By courtesy of Dr. A. F. Howatson and Academic Press. D, influenza virus, showing the flexible nature and the surface projections. By courtesy of Prof. A. P. Waterson. E, rabies virus, showing the bullet shape and surface projections. By courtesy of Prof. K. Hummeler and the American Society for Microbiology. F, T$_4$ coliphage, the details of which are shown in Fig. 41. By courtesy of Dr. L. D. Simon, Dr. T. F. Anderson and Academic Press.

6. They are small, in the range 25 to 300 nm, and may pass bacteria-proof filters, though filterability is an outdated criterion.

7. Obligate intracellular parasites causing death of the host, extensive cell damage or excessive cell proliferation (hyperplasia). They are highly host and tissue specific.

8. Insensitive to all the usual antibiotics. Antibiotic sensitivity may indicate that an organism is not a true virus.

9. Many are very liable to mutation.

STRUCTURE AND COMPOSITION

The intact virus particle, the *virion*, consists of an internal *nucleocapsid*, based on RNA or DNA, protected by a protein shell (*capsid*) composed of a number of *capsomers*. The capsomers are globular protein sub-units and may be arranged regularly so that the structure is icosahedral (herpes simplex, polio), helical (influenza, rabies), or more complex (smallpox). The bacteriophages (usually shortened to *phage*) are viruses which infect bacteria and these may have a very complex symmetry. Also, some viruses (mumps, influenza) have a lipoprotein outer membrane, the *peplos*. Small amounts of enzymes, carbohydrates and polyamines may also be present. The structures of some typical viruses are illustrated in Fig. 29.40 and an idea of size and composition is conveyed in Table 29.8.

REPLICATION

The Replication of Phage

The details of phage replication are very well known, so the replication of the T4 coliphage, (structure Fig 29.41) a DNA virus which attacks *E.coli*, will be described as illustrating the general pattern (Fig. 29.42) although the details differ for each virus.

The phage comes into contact with a bacterium at random and *attachment* occurs via the tail fibres. The fibres contract and bring the tail plate into contact with the host cell wall, which is dissolved locally by a lysozyme. The tail sheath then contracts and *penetration* occurs by injection of the phage DNA through the tail tube into the host, and host metabolism ceases very soon. The phage DNA is then transcribed into 'early' viral mRNA which utilizes the cellular ribosomes and energy for translation into a variety of enzymes, e.g. deoxyribonuclease to break down host DNA, and DNA replicase and polymerase which produce new *viral* DNA. When new viral DNA starts to appear, 'late' viral mRNA and 'late' enzymes are synthesized. These result in the synthesis of new viral capsids, in the production of a condensing protein which condenses the separately synthesized DNA and capsid into new phages in the *maturation* phase, and in the production of phage lysozyme which causes *lysis* (bursting) and the liberation of numerous mature phages from the bacterium.

Lysis usually results in complete host destruction and when this occurs in a confluent sheet of bacterial growth on the surface of a medium, there are areas of clearing of this growth around the infected cells which are called *plaques*. The number of phage particles released per bacterium on lysis is known as the *burst size* and may vary from a few to several hundred.

TABLE 29.8.

THE SIZES AND COMPOSITIONS OF SOME TYPICAL VIRUSES

	Agent	Per cent			M. Wt × 10⁶		Sizes§	Shape
		RNA	DNA	Pr	NA	Virion	(nm)	
Animal	Vaccina*	—	5	89	150	2000	220 × 280	Cuboid
	Influenza†	1	—	70	1	280	80	Spherical
	Poliovirus	25	—	75	2.2	3.6	27	Icosahedral
	Adenovirus	—	13	87	23	177	75	Icosahedral
Plant	TMV	6	—	94	2.1	40	300	Helical rod
	Tomato	17	—	83	1.7	11	—	Helical rod
Insect	Tipula iridescent	—	—	—	—	—	130	Icosahedral
Bacterial	T₄ phage	—	50	50	120	300	95 × 65 110 × 25	Head and tail
	φx 174	—	26	74	1.7	6.2	30	Icosahedral

* Vaccinia; lipid, 6 per cent.
† Influenza; carbohydrate, 23 per cent; lipid, 5 per cent.
§ For comparison; haemoglobin molecule, 15 × 3 nm; *Staph. aureus* cell, 1000 nm.

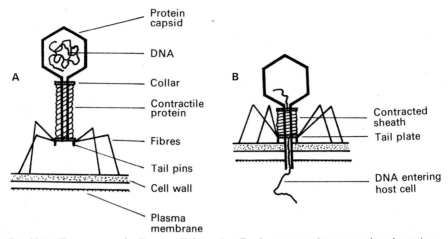

FIG. 29.41. The structure of a T-even coliphage. A, a T_4 phage at attachment to a host bacterium; B, penetration showing contracted protein tail sheath.

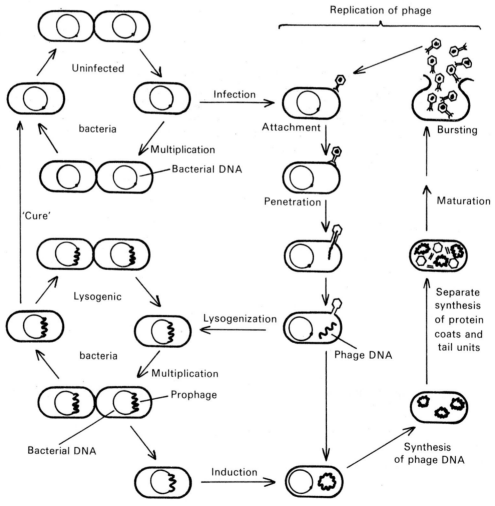

FIG. 29.42. The stages involved in phage replication and lysogenization.

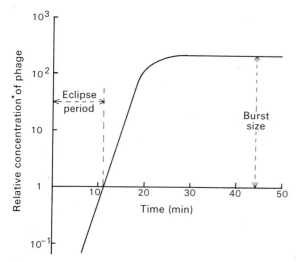

FIG. 29.43. The one step growth curve for a T_4 coliphage concentration relative to the initial count as 1.0. The subsequent steps have been inhibited. The stepwise nature of the curve is lost rapidly since phage is not released synchronously, as shown by the slope on the rising part of the curve.

The mode of replication described results in a stepwise increase in the phage count (Fig. 29.43). In the period immediately following infection, no phage can be detected if the cells are disrupted. This is the *eclipse phase*, during which the host cell metabolism is being switched to phage directed synthesis and no mature phage particles or infective DNA are present in the cell.

Lysogeny. The replication cycle just described is that of a virulent phage. Some types of *temperate phage*, e.g. *E.coli* phages λ, P1, P2, infect the host but the capsid genes are repressed, so no new phage is produced. Instead, the phage genome either attaches to the cell membrane or becomes incorporated into the host cell genome, often at a specific site, and replicates synchronously with the host cell genome as a *prophage*. Each daughter host cell carries a prophage replica. The host is thus described as being *lysogenized* by the phage, and the culture as *lysogenic*. The prophage may be *induced* to virulence by exposure of the lysogenic culture to low doses of ultraviolet radiation or to chemicals (alkylating agents, mitomycin, certain carcinogens), or may occur spontaneously. In either case the normal cycle of vegetative phage replication is completed. Prophage may also be lost (*cured*) either spontaneously or by treatment with chemicals such as acridines.

The relationship between lysogeny and vegetative reproduction is illustrated in Fig. 29.42.

Lysogenization results in changes in the host cells since there is additional genetic information present, examples being toxin production by *Corynebacterium diphtheriae*, non-lysogenic cultures being non-toxigenic and avirulent, and modification of the surface structure in *Salmonella typhimurium*.

Transduction. In some cases of infection with a temperate phage, the phage may carry a fragment of the host genome of variable size to a new host cell, a process known as *transduction*. The transduced DNA can then undergo *recombination* with the new host DNA to yield a mutant host, e.g. genes specifying antibiotic resistance may be transduced in this way.

The Replication of Other Viruses

The general process is believed to be similar to that described above. The mode of entry into the cell may be rather different and, with a very specific attachment process, entry may be mediated by specific enzymes e.g. neuraminidase with influenza virus, or entry may be by a pinocytosis type of mechanism in which the peplos, being derived from the original host cell membrane, may play a key role by fusing with the membrane of the new host cell. The details of viral NA synthesis and replication clearly differ depending on whether the NA is single or double stranded and is RNA or DNA, but these details are beyond the scope of this chapter. The viral components may be synthesized either in the cytoplasm (influenza, vaccinia, polio) or in the nucleus (herpes simplex, influenza, adenoviruses), sometimes producing characteristic *inclusion bodies* which are of diagnostic value. The effects of infection may be gross tissue damage analogous to phage lysis, as in smallpox, major inflammatory reactions, as with measles, or hyperplasia, i.e. excessive and sometimes uncontrolled cell multiplication, resulting in warts, benign tumours, or cancer and leukaemia.

Many viruses can exist in a latent form analogous to prophage in lysogenic bacteria. This is well known with herpes simplex, yellow fever and serum jaundice. One theory of the way in which a wide range of diverse chemicals can cause cancer is that the carcinogens are simply cytotoxic and damage cells infected with latent virus, so inducing the virus to the vegetative, virulent state.

CULTIVATION

There are three methods available: tissue culture, embryonated eggs and whole host inoculation.

Tissue Culture

The basic technique. A tissue culture consists of a suitable living host tissue (animal, plant, insect) plus a suitable nutrient fluid for the *tissue* cells, the formulation of which may be very difficult. The tissue is incubated and agitated, the virus is inoculated into the tissue at a suitable time and, after further incubation, the virus may be harvested from the fluid.

Types of tissue culture. The *roller culture* consists of cultivation in a series of test tubes placed in a drum and rotated so that the tubes are almost horizontal. This method is useful for small scale work, research or analytical procedures. In the *rocker culture* the culture vessels are large glass bottles laid on their sides in a rack, the whole rack being rocked gently to obtain good mixing and gas exchange, a procedure widely used in large scale cultivation, e.g. for vaccines. Where very large scale production is required a *submerged culture* is used, the tissue cells being suspended in a large bulk of medium which is carefully stirred and aerated. There are many difficult technical problems with submerged cultivation, but the technique is the only suitable way of achieving very large scale virus cultivation.

Fragment cultures simply consist of minced tissue suspended in the nutrient fluid. The fragments do not normally grow during incubation but live for the two to three days necessary for virus growth. Frequently, *cell cultures* are prepared by digesting tissue with trypsin and the isolated cells, or small clumps of cells, used as *suspended cell cultures* or as *monolayer cultures*. In the latter case the cells are allowed to grow as a single sheet of cells on the glass surface of a tube, bottle or dish. If only a small number of virions is inoculated into a monolayer culture each virus produces plaques of lysed cells, similar to phage plaques (Fig. 29.45), or characteristic local cytopathogenic effects which are of diagnostic value. *Organ cultures* are small fragments of a selected organ, e.g. embryonic respiratory epithelum, in a thin layer of nutrient medium in a Petri dish. Such cultures will often grow fastidious viruses which will not grow in other types of culture.

Embryonated Egg Culture

This is a special type of whole host cultivation used for animal viruses. The method uses a fertile hen's egg after 7 to 12 days' incubation (Fig. 29.44), the virus being inoculated onto or into a suitable embryonic tissue or fluid, e.g. chorio-allantois, vaccinia; allantoic fluid, influenza; embryo, rabies, yellow fever; yolk sac, rickettsiae (see below). After further incubation the virus is harvested from the appropriate tissue and purified by differential centrifugation.

Whole Host Inoculation

This method is usually used only when the technical problems of tissue or embryonated egg culture cannot be solved or when the virus becomes attenuated or mutates in such cultures. The technique is widely used for many vaccines, notably smallpox (sheep or calves) and rabies (sheep or rabbits).

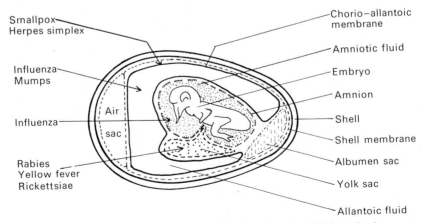

FIG. 29.44. The tissues of the embryonated hen's egg at about 10 days development, together with the routes of inoculation of various viruses, indicated by arrows.

Advantages and disadvantages of Virus Culture Methods

Method	Advantages	Disadvantages
Tissue culture	Adaptable to a large range of viruses Can be used for large scale production, e.g. vaccines No antibodies formed	Technically difficult. Virus may become attenuated during cultivation Unsuspected virus may be present, e.g. SV40 tumour virus from monkey kidney tissue
Embryonated eggs	No unsuspected viruses or bacteria No antibodies formed Simple and inexpensive	Not all viruses will grow Adaptation to growth in the embryo may cause attenuation Some viruses cause extensive damage and are difficult to separate High labour costs if used for large scale cultivation
Whole host inoculation	No attenuation May be only method available	Contamination almost inevitable Antibodies produced (by animals) Can have major handling problems (especially with large animals) Elaborate and expensive facilities may be required

ENUMERATION OF INFECTIVE VIRUS

There are three basic methods: plaque counts, pock counts and dilution counts.

Plaque counts. This involves counting the number of plaques produced from a suitably dilute viral suspension inoculated into a sensitive bacterial culture, which is then transferred to an agar plate, or into a suitable monolayer tissue culture (Fig. 29.45).

Pock counts. This method is used primarily for animal viruses if they will grow on the chlorio-allantoic membrane of the chick embryo. A dilute suspension of virus is inoculated onto the membrane. After incubation the membrane is covered with a series of pocks, each being a focal point of infection (Fig. 29.46). Plant viruses which produce localized necrotic lesions of plant leaves may be counted similarly.

Dilution counts. The principle of this method is exactly as for counting bacteria by dilution (see p. 453) but in this case the serial dilutions are inoculated into a series of host plants or animals or into a series of tissue cultures or bacterial cultures. In all cases the presence or absence of infection is sought, rather than examining for growth as with bacteria.

REACTION TO ENVIRONMENTAL CONDITIONS

Viruses are inactivated by most of the conditions which kill other microorganisms, e.g. heat at 56–60° for 30 minutes (poliovirus and serum hepatitis virus are more resistant), oxidizing agents,

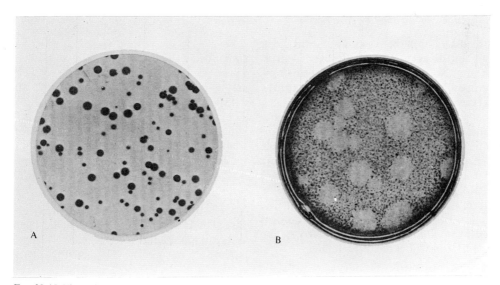

FIG. 29.45. Virus plaques. A, phage plaques, showing four different types distinguished by size and turbidity; B, poliovirus plaques in rhesus monkey kidney monolayer culture (adapted from part of Fig. 22-9 of *Principles of Microbiology* by B. D. Davis, R. Dulbecco, H. N. Eisen, H. S. Ginsberg and W. B. Wood Jr. by courtesy of Hoeber Division, Harper & Row).

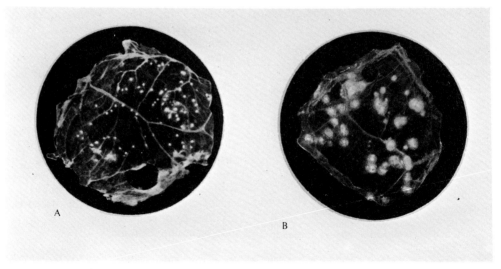

FIG. 29.46. Viral counts by pock counting on the chick embryo chorioallantoic membrane. Each dense white circular area (pock) is a focus of viral growth and different viruses give pocks of different appearance. A, vaccinia; B, herpes simplex (by courtesy of *The Glaxo Volume*).

halogens, formaldehyde, glutaraldehyde, ethylene oxide, β-propiolactone, ultraviolet and ionizing radiations.

Viruses with a peplos, which is lipoid, are consequently sensitive to solvents such as ether and to surfacants.

They are resistant to the actions of agents which attack cellular integrity or interfere with metabolism, e.g. many atiseptics, especially phenols, glycerol and antibiotics.

CHEMOTHERAPY OF VIRUS INFECTIONS

The close association between virus and host means that most agents which prevent virus replication are also highly toxic to the host. Only methisazone (N-methylisatin-β-thiosemicarbazone) has found significant systemic application in the prophylaxis of pox virus infections, notably smallpox and complications of smallpox vaccination, if given early enough after known contact with infection. It is useless once overt infection has occurred. IUDR (5-iododeoxyuridine) inhibits DNA synthesis and though too toxic for systemic use has a possible application in the topical treatment of spreading skin and corneal lesions due to smallpox, vaccinia and herpes. The status of interferon will be dealt with later.

CLASSIFICATION OF VIRUSES

There is no universally agreed system, but most authorities use the following criteria: type of nucleic acid and number of strands, capsid architecture, size, presence of peplos, nuclear or cytoplasmic synthesis, host specificity. The principal type of virus on this basis are listed in Table 29.9.

OTHER OBLIGATE PATHOGENS

Rickettsiae
These are small spherical or ovoid organisms ($0.2 \times 0.6 \mu$m), Gram-negative and mostly arthropod borne. Members of this group cause epidemic typhus, scrub typhus, murine typhus, spotted fever, trench fever and Q fever.

Chlamydiae (Bedsoniae)
These are generally similar to the rickettsiae but are spherical, a small (0.3μm) form alternating with a large (0.5 to 1.0μm) form in the life cycle. They are highly unstable outside their hosts, in which they cause psittacosis and ornithosis, trachoma, inclusion conjunctivitis, lymphogranuloma venereum and cat scratch disease.

Mycobacterium leprae
This is the causative agent of leprosy and is acid fast, like *M.tuberculosis*. It has never been isolated on artificial media

Bdellovibrio bacteriovorus
This is a small highly motile organism, parasitic on Gram-negative bacteria, notably the Enterobacteriaceae.

TABLE 29.9.

SOME IMPORTANT GROUPS OF ANIMAL VIRUSES

Group	Type of NA	Icosa-hedral	Helical	Other archi-tecture	Site of synthesis	Relative size (nm)	Tumour Produc-tion	Peplos	Other characters	Examples
Adenoviruses	2 DNA	+	−	−		75	Many	−	Latent lymphoid infections	Numerous numbered types
Papovaviruses	2 DNA	+	−	−		50	Some	−		Polyoma, Papilloma, SV40
Herpes viruses	2 DNA	+	−	−		c. 100	−	+	Often give latent infection	Herpes simplex (cold sores), Varicella-zoster (chickenpox and shingles)
Poxviruses	2 DNA	−	?	?		c. 300	Myxoma Fibroma	+	Epidermal tropism	Smallpox, Vaccinia
Picornaviruses	1 RNA	+	−	−		25	−	−	Enteric and respiratory infection	Polio, coxsackie, Rhinoviruses Foot & mouth
Reoviruses	2 RNA	+	−	−		75	−	−	Asymptomatic respiratory and enteric infections	
Arboviruses	1 RNA	?	−	−			−	+	Arthropod-borne	Yellow Fever, Equine encephalitis
Myxoviruses	1 RNA	−	+	−	N	80−200	−	+	Cause haemagglutination. Many filamentous	Influenza
Paramyxo-viruses	1 RNA	−	+	−	C	100−180	−	+	Haemolytic	Mumps, Distemper Parainfluenza
Rhabdoviruses	RNA	−	+	−		60 × 200	−	+	Bullet-shaped	Rabies

SOME RELATIONSHIPS BETWEEN MICROORGANISMS AND THE HUMAN BODY: MICROBIAL DISEASES AND IMMUNOLOGY

THE COMMON BODY FLORA

There is a large ectosymbiotic population of bacteria, fungi, protozoa, helminths and even mites, living on the surfaces and in the body cavities, but not in the tissues. The skin between the waist and the knees is usually heavily contaminated with intestinal organisms, which represent a special hazard during surgery in that area. Most of the symbionts are *parasites*, since the host apparently derives no benefit from their presence, although the parasite has a controlled temperature environment with an ample supply of water and food. However, some are *mutualistic* symbionts, both species deriving benefit e.g. the lactobacilli in the vagina produce lactic acid which effectively prevents most other organisms from becoming established and intestinal bacteria produce some of the normal human daily intake of vitamin B complex. Thus there is normally a balance between the various parasites and also between these and their host. Breakdown in this balance leads to *infection*.

INFECTION AND PATHOGENICITY

Pathogens are organisms capable of causing infection, i.e. the growth of micro-organisms causing damage to the host. Damage, however, slight, is essential and the mere presence of organisms does not constitute infection. Normally harmless symbionts may be *facultative* pathogens and produce infections after injury or act as secondary invaders in the wake of a primary infection.

Carriers carry and transmit pathogens but do not themselves show any symptoms. The carrier state is common during recovery from infection or due to sub-clinical (silent) infection, but is usually only temporary, but persistent carriers of *Salmonella typhi, Staph.aureus* and other organisms are common.

Virulence is the degree of pathogenicity (non-pathogenic = avirulent) and can be defined only in statistical terms, i.e. virulence is the likelihood of producing a severe infection rapidly. Although some organisms, such as *Bacillus anthracis* and *Clostridium tetani* are always pathogenic, most show a very variable ability to produce infection between strains, e.g. *Corynebacterium diphtheriae* has three distinct strains producing mild, moderate and severe infections. Apart from strain variation, virulence also depends on the route of infection, e.g. *B.anthracis* is characteristically a wound pathogen but also produces a violent pneumonia if inhaled and intestinal symptoms if ingested, whereas *Salmonella typhi* produces infection *only* if ingested. Other important factors are the invasiveness and toxigenicity of the pathogen and the reaction of the host to infection.

Invasiveness
Invasiveness is the ability of a pathogen to invade and penetrate the host tissues and has a number of components.

Aggressins are microbial substances which counter host defences in various ways, e.g. by preventing leucocyte chemotaxis (*M.tuberculosis*), by resisting phagocytosis (the capsules of *B.anthracis* and *D.pneumoniae*) and by destroying phagocytes (*Staph. aureus*, streptococci).

Diffusion factors are enzymes which assist penetration into tissue, e.g. the collagenases of various clostridia, the hyaluronidases and kinases of streptococci and the coagulase of staphylococci. However, the exact role of some of these in the disease process is not clear.

Organ tropism is the selective attack of a pathogen on a particular organ or tissue within that organ. Thus *Neisseria meningitidis* invades the meninges of the brain to cause meningitis and *Bordetella pertussis* attacks ciliated bronchial mucosa, causing whooping cough.

All viruses show marked tissue tropism.

Toxigenicity
Many bacteria produce toxic substances and these fall into two classes, the *exotoxins* which are proteins, many being enzymes, and the *endotoxins* which are lipopolysaccharide–protein complexes.

Exotoxins. The general properties of exotoxins are as follows: they are usually liberated during active growth in media, and mostly show specific tissue affinities. They are highly toxic and antigenic, thermolabile and photolabile. On standing they spontaneously form toxoids, non-toxic compounds with a similar antigenic specificity. Table 29.10 lists a number of diseases in which exotoxins are implicated.

TABLE 29.10

SOME DISEASES IN WHICH BACTERIAL EXOTOXINS ARE IMPLICATED

Disease	Species	Mode of action
Diphtheria	*Corynebacterium diphtheriae*	Inhibits protein synthesis giving muscular (cardiac) paralysis*
Tetanus	*Clostridium tetani*	Neurotoxin damages anterior horn cells and blocks inhibitory synapses*
Botulism	*Cl.botulinum*	Neurotoxin blocks acetyl choline release and inhibitory synapses*
Gas gangrene	*Cl.perfringens*	Lecithinases† (give membrane damage)
	Cl.novyi	Necrotoxic proteases§
	Cl.septicum	Collagenases†
Anthrax	*B.anthracis*	Two components†
Plague	*Yersinia pestis*	Two components†
Cholera	*Vibrio cholerae*	Promotes formation of cylic AMP from ATP† causing massive excretion of Na^+, Cl^- and H_2O
Dysentery	*Shigella dysenteriae*	Affects CNS small blood vessels, causing paralysis and haemorrhage. Neurotoxic§
Skin, systemic, enteritis	*Staph.aureus*	Leucocidal, haemolytic, necrotic, enterotoxic§
Skin, systemic	*Strep.pyogenes*	Leucocidal, haemolytic, erythrogenic§
Wound, systemic	*Ps.aeruginosa*	Necrotic proteases§

* Toxic effects account for all of the pathology of the disease.
† Toxic effects account for some of the pathology of the disease.
§ The toxins have an uncertain role in the pathology.

Endotoxins. These are components of the cell wall of all Gram-negative pathogens. They are relatively thermostable, are less potent than exotoxins, are relatively non-specific and do not form toxoids. The actual toxic component is the phospholipid and its parenteral administration causes inflammation, shock and diarrhoea.

Also it is an indirect pyrogen, acting on the polymorphs to cause the release of an endogenous pyrogen which affects the thermoregulatory centre of the brain to cause fever. The pharmacopoeias require Water for Injections to be free from pyrogens (i.e. endotoxins) which, being non-volatile, can be removed by a distillation process.

Endotoxins also cause a fall in resistance to infection after about 5 hours followed by an increase in resistance after about 20 hours. Continual reinforcement of this resistance by intestinal Gram-negative bacteria may contribute to human resistance to infections by these organisms.

Other Mechanisms of Pathogenicity

Apart from toxicity the detailed mechanisms of pathogenicity are little understood. They include mechanical lesions due to necrosis, including damage to vital organs, interference with nutrition or metabolism of the host, e.g. impairment of detoxification in the liver, and hypersensitivity reactions (see p. 487).

HOST DEFENCES AGAINST INFECTION

The defences are of two types, constitutive and inducible.

Constitutive Defences

These are the inborn, normal defence mechanisms of the host species and are present under a wide variety of environmental conditions, though each species shows a different range of susceptibility and resistance.

The initial barriers are the skin and mucous membranes which physically exclude microorganisms and also secrete antimicrobial compounds. Once microorganisms enter the tissues the secondary barriers are provided by the *circulatory system* and the *phagocytes*. The blood and lymph contain antibacterial substances and also phagocytic cells (neutrophils, monocytes, fixed macrophages) which ingest foreign particles. Fixed macrophages are also present in the liver, spleen and bone marrow. Wandering macrophages (histiocytes) occur in connective tissue.

Inflammation is an extremely important basic mechanism of resistance. It is characterized by local capillary dilation and increased capillary permeability. This results in increased blood flow through the site and local reddening, swelling and temperature rise. There is also pain. Initially polymorphs, and later monocytes, are able to pass through the capillary walls and move to an infective focus by chemotaxis. The syndrome is produced by a variety of irritants, not merely microorganisms, which cause the release of histamine, 5-hydroxytryptamine, etc., from cells and platelets.

The results are phagocytosis of invading particles, an increased flow of antimicrobial serum factors, release of cellular antimicrobial factors from dead tissue, reduced oxygen tension and an increased concentration of lactic acid. These collectively act to kill invading cells, the mass of dead and moribund microorganisms, phagocytes and tissue cells forming *pus*.

Individual resistance is markedly affected by *age*, e.g. newborn infants are especially susceptible to gastorenteritis whereas old people are especially liable to respiratory disease. The *health* of an individual may also be crucial, the following factors increasing susceptibility, often by suppressing leucocyte activity: damaged skin and mucous membranes, a diet deficient in vitamins A and C and protein, excessive alcohol consumption, fatigue, breathing impure air, radiotherapeutic or immunosuppressive treatments.

Inducible Defences: Acquired Immunity

Definition. The acquisition by the body of means of eliminating foreign substances, known as *antigens.* The response may be *humoral,* (i.e. due to the presence of circulatory *antibody* (immunoglobulin, Ig), or *cellular,* i.e. due to the action of sensitized lymphocytes.

Antigens are substances which, when introduced unaltered into the tissues, stimulate the production of specific neutralizing proteins (antibodies or immunoglobulins) or cells.

To act as an antigen (Ag) a substance must be foreign to the animal, colloidal (minimum molecular weight c 5000) and present within the tissues. The natural antigens are usually proteins or conjugates of protein with polysaccharides, lipids or both.

A single Ag may have a number of different *determinant* groups, each about five to ten amino acid residues in size, each of which will stimulate the production of a specific Ig. Some compounds, such as nucleic acids and some bacterial lipids and polysaccharides, will not stimulate the production of Ig but will combine with homologous Ig which has already been produced. These substances are partial antigens or *haptens.*

TABLE 29.11.

THE PROPERTIES OF THE IMMUNOGLOBULINS

(approximate values)	IgG	IgM	IgA	IgD	IgE
Molecular weight	15×10^4	90×10^4	$15–60 \times 10^4$	15×10^4	20×10^4
Sedimentation constants	7S	19S (18–23)	7, 9, 11, 13, 17S	7S	8S
Sugar content (per cent)	3	12	11	?	11
Concentration in serum mg/100 ml	1200	100	250	3	4×10^{-4}
Allergic reagin	−	−	−	−	+
Mostly formed in: primary response	−	+	−	−	−
secondary response	+	−	−	−	−
Binds complement	+	+	−	?	−
Passes placenta	+	−	−	− ?	−
Production in fetus	(+)	+	−	?	?

Immunoglobulins. There are 5 classes of Ig which are all glycoproteins namely IgG* (gamma-globulin), IgM (macroglobulin), IgA, IgD and IgE. These can be distinguished on the basis of their physicochemical and other properties (Table 29.11), but the different Igs within each class can only be distinguished immunologically, by their reaction with the specific stimulating Ag, and by the fact that they themselves act as highly specific Ags in another species of animal and stimulate the production of homologous Igs.

It is generally assumed that any Ag will elicit a homologous Ig, so that an individual can produce upwards of 10^6 specific Igs. The most likely current theory to account for this diversity is that of *clonal selection*, which states that the Ig producing cells can undergo extensive random mutation to give a large number of germ cells, each with the potentiality of producing a different Ig. Contact with Ag stimulates the germ cells capable of producing the homologous Ig to reproduce and synthesize large amounts of that Ig.

The IgG molecule consists of two 'light' chains (mol. wt. *c.* 25,000) linked to two 'heavy' chains (mol. wt. *c.* 50,000) by a number of disulphide bridges, the heavy chains also being linked by disulphide bridges.

The N-terminal ends of both chains, consisting of about 110 amino acid residues in each is the *variable* portion ·which confers the different speci-

* An alternative terminology replaces Ig with γ, giving γG, γM, etc.

ficities on the Igs and are the Ag binding sites. The remainder of the molecules, one half of the light chains (107 amino acids) and three quarters of the heavy chains (3×107 amino acids), at the C-terminal ends are of *constant* composition and are the same in all IgGs. The molecule can be split by papain into three fragments, two identical, non-crystallizable Ag binding fragments, call Fab, and a crystallizable fragment, Fc, which does not bind Ag but binds complement. These features are illustrated in Fig. 29.47.

Immunoglobulin Production
The time course of production. The situation is shown in Fig. 29.48. Before contact with a particular Ag no homologous Ig is detectable in the serum. At a first contact with Ag there is a lag period of 5 days to a few weeks when Ig cannot be detected, and the serum titre of Ig then rises to a low level and falls. This is the *primary response*. If there is a second contact with Ag at this stage there is no lag but a prompt and rapid rise in Ig titre, to above the immunity level in the case of a pathogen, thus conferring immunity (protection) against the disease. Any subsequent contact with the same Ag will produce a similar, prompt *secondary response* which is the basis of immunity to disease. If very sensitive methods of detection are used it can be seen that Ig production starts at the very first contact with Ag and that there is no real difference between the primary and secondary responses.

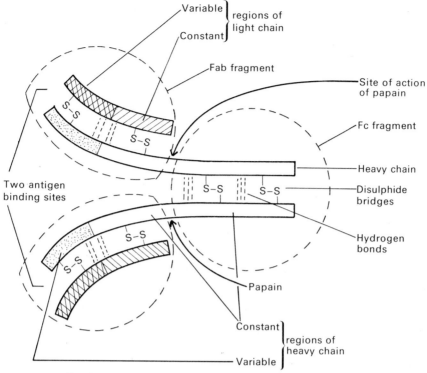

FIG. 29.47. A diagrammatic representation of the structure of IgG.

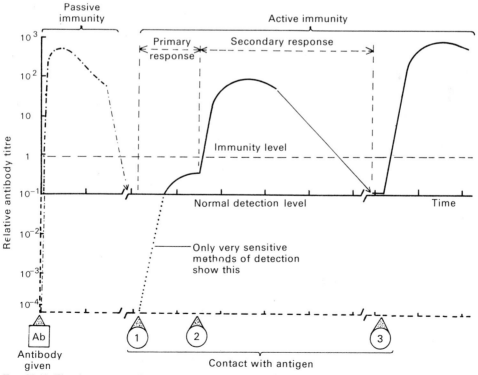

FIG. 29.48. The time course of immunoglobin production and the difference between active and passive immunity.

The site of immunoglobulin synthesis. The Igs are produced by the *plasma cells* of the blood and lymphoid tissues since the number of plasma cells increases after immunization, the Ig titre is proportional to the number of the cells, Ig can be shown to be present in the cells and isolated plasma cells synthesize homologous Ig. Also, in patients suffering from hypogammaglobulinaemia, an inability to produce significant amounts of Ab, there is a deficiency of plasma cells and their numbers do not increase after immunization.

What appears to happen (Fig. 29.49) is that the Ag is taken up by the macrophages and other phagocytic cells which then attract small lymphocytes to cluster round them. Cytoplasmic bridges are formed between the macrophages and the lymphocytes and RNA, or RNA plus bound Ag ('activated Ag') is transferred to the lymphocytes which are thus stimulated to form immunoblasts. These divide rapidly and differentiate, some to form short lived *plasma cells* which actively produce Ig, but most forming first *large lymphocytes* which mature into a clone of sensitized *small lymphocytes* ('memory cells') which can respond rapidly to a further contact with the same Ag by producing large amounts of Ig. In this secondary response the macrophages are probably not essential. Each plasma cell produces only one type of Ig.

Immune Tolerance

Uptake of Ag will prevent an immune response if given in low doses to a fetal or neonatal animal, to an adult treated with X- or γ-radiation, immunosuppressant drugs and corticosteroids, or if given in raised doses to a normal adult. Thus tolerance results from a very high concentration of Ag relative to the number of plasma cells synthesizing homologous Ab. The mechanism probably explains why individuals do not normally synthesize Ig against their own tissues.

The Use of Immunological Products in Medicine

Active and passive immunity. The primary and secondary Ig responses described above lead to *active immunity* in an individual, i.e. the individual's own tissues respond to produce protective levels of Ig.

The stimulus may be *natural*, due to contact with an infective agent or other Ag, or *artificial*, when antigenic preparations (vaccines) are given to produce artificial active immunity. The types of preparation used are given in Table 29.12. Provided that the vaccine used has a suitable antigenic content which is not impaired by the method of preparation, the effect of immunization and of the natural infective agent are similar giving a long

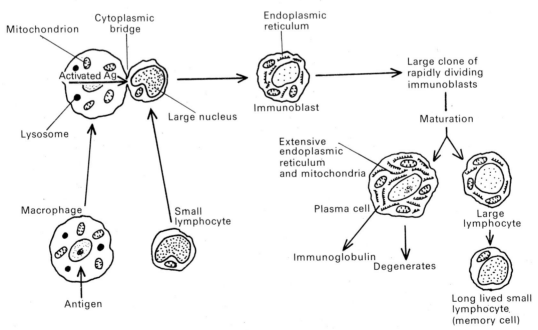

FIG. 29.49. A hypothetical scheme for the differentiation of small lymphocytes into immunoglobin producing plasma cells and into memory cells.

Type of antigenic material	Examples	Comments
Attenuated living organisms	*Naturally occurring* Brucella strain 19, Yellow Fever virus strain 17D Vaccinia virus *Artificially produced* BCG (for tuberculosis), poliomyelitis, rabies	Usually a highly satisfactory type of agent. The natural mode of infection is mimicked giving a high grade, long lasting immunity, provided the antigenic structure of the material is satisfactory
Killed micro-organisms	*Bacterial* Typhoid, whooping cholera *Viral* Influenza, measles, foot and mouth disease, canine distemper	Killing normally damages the antigenic structure, so only limited protection is produced
Toxoids (detoxified bacterial exotoxins)	Diptheria Tetanus	Give very high grade, long lasting immunity
Endotoxins	Cholera	The most satisfactory material so far for this disease
Unmodified agents	Rubella (German measles)	Unmodified agents rarely used. It is possible in this case because of the low virulence and the benefits arising from infection.

lasting, highly effective immunity to the agent. If, as often happens, the vaccine is not wholly effective, booster doses can be given at intervals of 6 months, 1 year or 5 years, as appropriate, to maintain a high level of immunological reactivity in the patient.

The responsiveness of the patient may be increased by the addition of one of a variety of *adjuvants* to the vaccine, such as aluminium hydroxide or phosphates with toxoid preparations and influenza vaccine emulsified with mineral oil, though the latter has not been approved for human use. The ability of Pertussis Vaccine to act as an adjuvant and enhance the response to Diphtheria Vaccine is well known, so these preparations are always administered together. Active immunization is used solely as a prophylactic measure, except in the case of rabies, where

the disease has a very long incubation period, and active immunization is the method of choice for conferring immunity.

However, if a patient especially at risk has been exposed to infection, or if a patient has an overwhelming infection which does not respond to chemotherapy, *passive immunization* may be used. This involves giving preformed Ab prepared from the serum of other patients or of suitably immunized animals. Although immunity so acquired is rapidly established, it is short lived, with a half-life of about 7 days in humans, and immunologically competent plasma cells are not produced, so on a subsequent contact with the infective agent only a primary response results. This situation is illustrated in Fig. 29.48. Passive immunity may also be acquired naturally in humans by transfer of Igs from the mother's blood across the placenta and possibly also via the breast milk. This natural passive immunity protects the infant for the first few months of life, the half-life of the parental Igs being about 30 days. The child then starts to produce its own Igs, normal adult levels being attained by about 4 years of age

ANTIGEN–ANTIBODY REACTIONS

The principal types of reaction are listed in Table 29.13

Most Igs are divalent though IgM is pentavalent. In contrast most Ags are multivalent since each possesses a number of the same or different antigenic determinants, to all of which specific Igs may be produced. The reaction between the Ag and the homologous antiserum results in the formation of a complex lattice structure with some or all of the Igs present locking together molecules of Ag. If the antigen is cellular, e.g. bacteria, foreign erythrocytes, there are a number of Ags present, but the same basic mechanism still applies. Lattice development continues until very large complexes which precipitate are formed. The bonds between Ag and Ig may be ionic, hydrogen bonds and, especially, hydrophobic bonds: the more non-polar the Ag the stonger the binding.

In addition to their importance as a mechanism of protection the Ag/Ig reactions are invaluable for the identification of microorganisms, for the exact diagnosis of disease, for tracing the source of an epidemic infection and, through the techniques of radioimmunoassay, for assaying traces of enzymes, drugs, etc. in tissue and fluid samples.

TABLE 29.13.

THE PRINCIPAL TYPES OF ANTIGEN–ANTIBODY REACTION

Type of Antibody	Reaction	Typical Antigen	Sensitivity*
Reactions with soluble antigens			
Precipitin	Precipitation of insoluble complex	Pneumococcal capsule	20–60
Antitoxin	Neutralization of toxicity	Dipheria and tetanus toxins	10^{-4}
	Precipitation of insoluble complex (flocculation)		20
Reactions with particulate antigens			
Agglutinin	Clumping of cells (agglutination)	Salmonella O and H	0.01 – 0.1
Lysin	Death and lysis of bacteria	Gram-negative bacteria	1
	Haemolysis	Erythrocytes	
Opsonin	Increased phagocytosis	—	—

* Minimum amount of antibody detectable, μg/cm^3.

Precipitation and Flocculation

Both these processes result in the precipitation of Ag/Ig complex as a visible precipitate, precipitation being maximal and most rapid when the components are present in equivalent concentration. An electrolyte must be present for complete precipitation to occur.

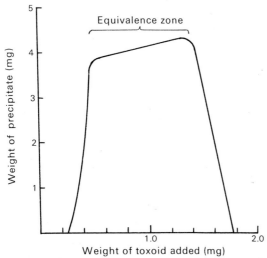

FIG. 29.50. The flocculation of antitoxin (data of Pappenheimer, A. M., jun., Robinson, E. S. (1937) J. Immunol., **32**, 291).

Flocculation is a special term applied to the precipitation of exotoxins and arose historically before the true nature of the reaction was understood. Additionally, the first effect of the reaction between exotoxin and the homologous antitoxin is neutralization of toxicity. Fig. 29.50 illustrates the importance of equivalence in flocculation.

The Quellung Reaction is the capsular swelling which occurs when an encapsulated bacterium is treated with homologous antiserum, the capsule appearing much larger and more clearly defined due to the precipitation and altered refractility.

Gel Diffusion Techniques (*The Ouchterlony Plate*). The original technique is illustrated in Fig. 29.51. Various Ag and Ab preparations are placed in wells cut in a plate of plain agar gel. The Ags and Abs diffuse towards each other and precipitation bands occur between the wells if homology exists. If identical Ags or Igs are present in two of the wells a continuous symmetrical precipitation band results.

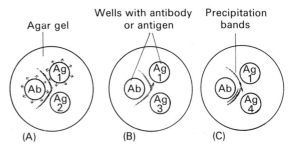

FIG. 29.51. Gel diffusion techniques for demonstrating precipitation reactions. The Ouchterlony plate. A, Continuous symmetrical precipitation band, Ag1 and Ag2 are the same; B, Partial symmetry, Ag1 and Ag3 are related; C, Complete assymmetry, Ag1 and Ag4 are different.

Immunoelectrophoresis is an elegant variation of the original technique and is illustrated in Fig. 29.52. In this, use is made of electrophoresis to separate the components in a complex mixture of Ags or Igs in serum. Following electrophoretic separation the diffusion technique is used to give the appropriate precipitation bonds.

Agglutination

Agglutination is the precipitation of clumps of cells (bacteria, protozoa, erythrocytes, etc.) plus homologous Ig and, apart from the fact that cellular Ags are involved, is basically similar to precipitation.

The antigenic structure of the genus *Salmonella* has been elucidated in great detail because of their importance as agents of enteric fevers (typhoid,

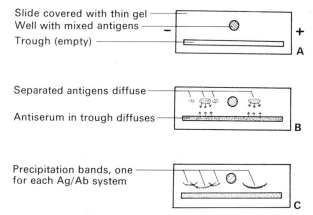

Slide covered with thin gel
Well with mixed antigens
Trough (empty)

Separated antigens diffuse
Antiserum in trough diffuses

Precipitation bands, one
for each Ag/Ab system

FIG. 29.52. Immunoelectrophoresis. A, Before electrophoresis; B, After electrophoresis antigens are separated and antiserum is placed in the trough; C, Finally precipitation occurs between homologous antigens and antibodies.

paratyphoid) and of food poisoning. These bacteria have three types of Ag, *flagellar* (H) and two types of *somatic* Ag, i.e. Ags associated with the body of the cell. These are the O-Ags, which correspond to the endotoxins, and the Vi-Ag, so called because of a presumed association with virulence, which is more superficial than the O-Ags, thus masking them. Strains which possess Vi-Ag are attacked with extreme specificity by phages, which are thus very useful for typing *Salmonella* spp. The resultant situation in the agglutination of *Salmonella* spp. is outlined in Table 29.14.

TABLE 29.14.

SOME AGGLUTINATING ANTIGENS OCCURRING IN SALMONELLA

A. *The general properties of the Salmonella antigens*

	Somatic		Flagellar
	O	Vi	H
Chemical nature	Lipopolysaccharide	Polysaccharide	Protein
Thermolability	−	+ + +	+ (80–100°)
Stability to:			
Formaldehyde	−		+
Alcohol	+	+	−
Dilute acids	+	−	+
Phenols	+	−	+
Special properties		Prevent O-agglutination	
		Phage attack is highly specific on Vi + strains	

TABLE 29—14 (continued)

B. *The antigenic structures of specific strains*

Sub-group	Species	Somatic		Flagellar	
		Characteristic	Other	Phase 1	Phase 2
A	*S.paratyphi* A	II	(I), XII ...	a	—
B	*S.paratyphi* B	IV	(I), (V), XII ...	b	1, 2, ...
	S.abortus-equi	IV	XII ...	—	e, n, x
C	*S.paratyphi* C	VI	VI₂, VII, (Vi)	c	1, 5 ...
D	*S.typhi*	IX	XII, (Vi) ...	d	—
	S.gallinarum	IX	XII ...	non-flagellate	
E	*S.anatis*	III	X, XXVI	e, h ...	1, 6 ...

Note that several strains may share common somatic or, less often, flagellar antigens. Such strains cross-react with multivalent agglutinating sera and special techniques are necessary to distinguish between them.

Lysis and Complement Fixation

Complement (C′) is a component of normal serum and consists of a complex of 11 proteins, some enzymic (C′1 is an esterase) and some being thermolabile, C′1 and C′2 being destroyed by heat at 56° for 5 minutes, C′4 and C′5 being inactivated after 30 minutes at 56°. The various components act in a complex sequence to cause a variety of immunological reactions.

In *lysis*, C′ acts on the complex between erythrocytes or Gram-negative bacteria and the homologous Ab (*lysin*) to cause lysis of the cells.

Erythrocytes + lysin + C′ ⟶ haemolysis.

Gram-negative bacteria + lysin + C′

$$\xrightarrow[\text{Ca}^{2+}]{\text{Mg}^{2+}} \text{lysis of bacteria.}$$

However, although C′ is bound (*fixed*) by Gram-positive bacteria/lysin complexes, these cells are not lysed, i.e.

Gram-positive bacteria + lysin + C′

⟶ no lysis (but C′ is fixed).

In all cases C′ binds to the C-terminal end of the Ig molecule and this fixed C′ is not available for any other reaction. Complement fixation is used as an indication of Ag/Ig reactions, especially with viruses, one application being the *Wasserman test for syphilitic Ab* which is applied to blood products to ensure that the donor is not suffering from syphilis. In this test, since it is difficult to cultivate and handle the causal agent, *Treponema pallidum*, an artificial antigen known as *cardiolipin* is used,

TABLE 29.15

WASSERMAN TEST

Type of serum	Reaction	Components	Result
Syphilitic	1	Cardiolipin + Syphilitic serum (heated at 56°) + Known amount of C	C′ fixed
		Add to the first system	
	2	Sheep erythrocytes + Anti-sheep serum (heated at 56°)	No haemolysis
Non-syphilitic	1	Cardiolipin + Serum (heated at 56°) + Known amount of C′	No reaction
		Add to the first system	
	2	Sheep erythrocytes + Anti-sheep serum (heated at 56°)	Haemolysis

Other Reactions Induced by Complement are summarized below

Cells + Ab + C′1, 4, 2, 3 → Opsonization, i.e. cells are more readily phagocytosed.

Cells + Ab + C′1, 4, 2, 3, 5 → Polypeptide (anaphylatoxin) causing histamine release from mast cells.

Cells + Ab + C′1, 4, 2, 3, 5, 6, 7 → Polymorph chemotaxis → phagocytosis of complexes and reactions important in allergy (see p. 487).

prepared by extraction of heart muscle and with lecithin and cholesterol added. The test is carried out in two parts. In the first the patient's serum, heated to 56° to destroy C′, is mixed with cardiolipin and known amount of C′. No reaction is visible but if C′ has been fixed this may be ascertained by using an indicator reaction consisting of sheep erythrocytes and anti-sheep serum prepared in rabbits and heated to destroy C′. If C′ was fixed in the first reaction, no haemolysis of the sheep erythrocytes occurs; if C′ was not fixed, haemolysis occurs, i.e. *no haemolysis* is the *positive* reaction, *haemolysis* is the *negative* reaction. This is shown diagrammatically in Table 29.15.

Immunoflourescence

This is an extremely valuable technique in which Ag is conjugated with flourescein or rhodamine B, so that Ag/Ig complexes can be observed as brightly flourescent under the ultraviolet microscope. The technique is highly versatile and can be used to identify microorganisms, to detect contaminant yeasts in brewing, to observe the location of viruses in cells and to detect particular pathogens in the presence of large numbers of similar organisms, such as are enteropathogenic *E.coli* 0127 in faeces.

IMMUNITY IN VIRUS DISEASES

It is well known that with many viruses a single attack causes a life-long, high grade immunity, as in measles or smallpox, while with other viruses, such as influenza or the common cold, repeated infection is the rule. Good immunity results from antigenically stable viruses which come in contact with Ab in the blood. Poor immunity occurs with

highly unstable viruses which throw up variants so different antigenically that a population immune to the former strains is sensitive to the variant and when transmission is along the epithelial mucous membranes so that there is little contact with high Ab titres.

A special immunity mechanism which is important in *recovery* from viral infection is *interferon*. Interferons are low molecular weight proteins (human, Mol. Wt. 26 000) produced by the cells of the host in response to certain viral infections and are host specific and not virus specific. Interferon acts on other host cells to induce the synthesis of a protein which inhibits the condensation of viral mRNA with host cell ribosomes and so blocks the synthesis of new viral components. Fig. 29.53

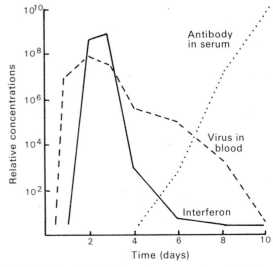

FIG. 29.53. The role of interferon in recovery from viral disease.

shows that interferon acts to reduce the viral titre before sufficient Ab has been produced to affect the course of an infection, though the Ab is responsible for final recovery. There is hope that artificially produced interferon can be used as a therapeutic agent for some of the many virus infections for which no effective control has yet been found.

UNDESIRABLE IMMUNOLOGICAL REACTIONS

The immunity mechanism does not always have the beneficial protective action described above, but may cause a range of pathological effects. Sometimes this may be an abnormal reaction to antigens, a condition known as *hypersensitivity*, or antibodies may be produced against the body's own tissues, resulting in *autoimmune disease* of varying severity. Also, the normal rejection of antigens may frustrate attempts at therapy, as in *blood transfusion* and *organ and tissue transplantation*.

Hypersensitivity

Hypersensitivity includes the phenomenon of *allergy*. There are two basic forms of reaction, *immediate type* reactions are mediated by circulatory Ab, while delayed type reactions are mediated by sensitized lymphocytes or macrophages. The terms, which are of historical origin, are confusing since not all immediate type reactionns occur promptly and though many do appear within minutes others evolve more slowly over several days.

Immediate type reactions. These are typical Ab responses and require a primary induction with Ag. A second contact with the Ag usually results in the appearance of symptoms within minutes. The reaction is mediated by IgE (reaginic Ab) only, which becomes bound to mast cells and platelets by the C-terminal ends of the heavy chains, leaving the binding sites free to react. The Ag/Ig reaction then occurs on the cell surfaces, damaging the cell and causing the release of histamine, 5-hydroxy-tryptamine, bradykynin and other substances which produce a marked physiological response. This reactivity can be passively transferred by the injection of the Ab.

The clinical symptoms may be very varied, and depend on the site of the reaction and the absolute and relative concentration of the pharmacological mediators.

Generalized *anaphylaxis* is a major, transient (30–60 minute) reaction ivolving collapse charac-terized by shock, capillary leakage, bronchial constriction and *angioneurotic oedema*, and it may prove fatal. It is a not an uncommon sequel to the administration of viral vaccines or antisera, due to traces of egg protein or horse serum in them, of drugs such as penicillin and of intravenous X-ray contrast media. It can also occur following insect bites or stings.

The intradermal injection or penetration of Ag may result in *cutaneous anaphylaxis* and local or more widespread wheal and flare reactions in the skin, while *organ anaphylaxis* is characterized by smooth muscle spasm in a particular organ.

Serum sickness is a syndrome characterized by fever, headache, malaise, local inflammation and occasionally by vomiting and diarrhoea and results from the administration of vaccines or sera. On a first contact there may be no reaction or a reaction may appear after 7 to 14 days, when Abs have been synthesized. On a second contact with the same Ag there is an accelerated reaction, symptoms appearing in 3 to 4 days.

Idiosyncrasy (atopy) is sensitivity to Ags which are normally encountered in daily life and this may be manifested as hay fever, asthma, eczema and urticaria. *Hay fever* is characterized by sneezing, a running nose and eye irritation and is usually caused by inhalation of pollen, dust, etc., while in *asthma* there is acute bronchial spasm of varying severity, sometimes causing asphyxiation. The skin is the organ affected in *urticaria* the symptoms being irritation, rash and wheals, either localized or generalized, and in *eczema*.

Delayed type reactions. These are usually induced by prolonged contact with Ag, tuberculosis and contact dermatitis being classic examples. A second contact with the Ag causes a slow response with a peak reaction after 24 to 72 hours. The reaction, which is inflammatory in nature, is mediated by sensitized lymphocytes and circulating Ab is not involved, and the condition can be passively transferred by circulating lymphocytes.

Typical examples are reactions to a variety of microbial infections, e.g. tuberculosis, brucellosis, leprosy, lymphogranuloma venereum, dermatomycosis, measles, and reactions to many drugs. Drugs can also induce *contact dermatitis* when applied to the skin, as can also many dyes, a variety of plant exudates and many high atomic weight ions, e.g. Hg, I, Ni, Co, Pt. Many of the inducing agents are not antigenic but become attached to skin proteins or lipids, induce a response and subsequently act as haptens.

Treatment of hypersensitivity. A variety of treatments are in use, with very variable benefit to the patient. Apart from a few agents giving symptomatic relief, such as adrenaline, salbutamol and terbutaline, it is difficult to get drugs into the sensitive organ in sufficient concentration without causing unwanted side effects. *Antihistamines* are widely used for the treatment of hay fever (allergic rhinitis) and urticaria and the latter condition may also be relieved by *corticosteroid* lotions. Corticosteroid aerosols or insufflations alleviate the symptoms of allergic rhinitis and bronchial ashthma, and avoid the dangers of systemic corticosteroid therapy. However, the drug of choice in bronchial asthma in *disodium cromoglycate* which has produced a revolution in the treatment of the disease. It probably acts by blocking the release of pharmacological mediators. The other main drug used is *adrenaline*, the only effective treatment for generalized anaphylaxis and angioneurotic oedema. *Desensitizing injections* are used in the prophylaxis of allergic rhinitis and a variety of food allergies, the techniques being to inject initially very small doses of the Ag concerned at intervals, alum precipitated pyridine extracts being most effective, and gradually work up to large doses. The main effect is the induction of large amounts of circulatory IgG which reacts with any allergen to neutralize it before it can produce allergic symptoms: the circulating Ab is known as *blocking Ab*.

AUTOIMMUNE DISEASE

An autoimmune disease is one which results from an immune reaction to ones own tissue components. These diseases are now believed to be relatively common, though whether all such attributions are correct remains to be seen. There are three basic mechanisms for the occurrence of the condition. A well known mechanism is tissue damage releasing 'secluded Ag' which does not usually come in contact with the blood and so is regarded as foreign by the body. This occurs with the lens and fluids of the eye, damage to one eye sometimes leading to loss of both eyes due to *allergic ophthalmitis*, with spermatozoa, leading to sterility, and to various thyroid gland components, resulting in *Hashimoto's disease, primary myxo-edema* and *thyrotoxicosis.*

Autoimmune disease can also occur as a sequel to a variety of infectious diseases. Hepatotropic virus may leave a condition of chronic *allergic hepatitis*, while neurotropic viruses may cause death due to a *demyelinating encephalitis*, in which the myelin sheath of nerve fibres is destroyed. The commonest bacterial origin of autoimmune disease is streptococcal infection, which frequently results in *rheumatic fever*, in which there is a reaction to cardiac tissue, especially the heart valves, and in *acute glomerulonephritis*, in which there is auto-immune destruction of the glomerular basement membrane. Probably several mechanisms are responsible for such phenomena, the infective agent may damage tissues to release sequestered Ag, microbial components may attach to certain body cells to create 'foreign' Ag or there may be a cross reaction between certain tissues and some microbial Ag. A third mechanism is a genuine breakdown of self-tolerance, though the reason for this is unknown. Autoimmune diseases believed to come in this latter class are *acquired haemolytic anaemia, idiopathic thrombocytopenic purpura* (excessive platelet destruction), *leucopenia*, some forms of *pernicious anaemia, rheumatoid arthritis, disseminated lupus erythematosus* (destruction of leucocyte nuclei), *primary thyroiditis, idiopathic Addison's disease, ulcerative colitis* and *male sterility*. However, the first three of these diseases can be induced by drugs and it is possible that some form of external agency is involved in the others.

BLOOD GROUP ANTIGENS

These are isoantigens which are present in some individuals of a species but not in others. There are ten major systems of blood group Ags, involving about 60 different antigen types which are important in forensic medicine, but only two are of major interest in blood transfusion. The first of these is the ABO system in which the red cells may have one of two mucopolysaccharide iso-antigens, or none, and the serum contains IgM isoantibodies to the isoantigen which is absent from the red cells. Thus there are four basic groups, as follows:

Red cell type   : A : B : AB : O

Antibodies in the serum: Anti-B : Anti-A : None : Anti-AB.

The Rh system is complex but basically about 85 per cent of the poulation of Western Europe are Rh + and 15 per cent Rh −. Antibodies to Rh Ags do not occur naturally but are induced during pregnancy or by blood transfusion. If a pregnant mother is Rh − and the father is Rh +, the child will be Rh + and the mother will develop Abs against the fetal erythrocytes. In a first pregnancy this is often unimportant but in subsequent pregnancies the fetus develops 'haemolytic disease of the newborn' (erythroblastosis fetalis) and usually aborts unless intrauterine total blood relacement is possible. If the fetus is carried to full term, neonatal blood replacement is usually essential for survival. A similar situation can also arise with the ABO system.

In blood transfusion the patient's blood is cross matched with the donor blood to get a correct match for both ABO and Rh systems. If blood of the same group is not available then group O, Rh− may be used as an emergency procedure. Blood transfusion is successful since most erythrocyte Ags are only feebly antigenic, whole blood or erythrocytes are not often transferred and careful attention is paid to matching and to any previous history of transfusion.

Transplantation Immunity
Grafts of tissues or organs are used extensively for the repair and replacement of damaged or diseased tissues. *Autografts*, taken from one area of the body and grafted onto another area of the same individual, as in skin replacement, take perfectly unless the technique is inadequate. *Isografts*, between identical twins, also take very well. However, the usual type of graft is an *allografts*, in which an organ or tissue is taken from another individual of the same species as the recipient. In such cases there is a delayed hypersensitivity reaction and the graft is rejected. The greater the differences genetically between donor and recipient, the more rapid the rejection. True tolerance of an allograft results from the occurrence of certain 'privileged' sites, primarily the cornea, but the normal practice is to use careful tissue typing to ensure as good a match as possible between the two types of tissue, together with immunosuppressive treatment.

Immunosuppression
There are numerous methods of preventing the immune response. Lympholytic agents, such as cyclophosphamide and busulphan, destroy lymphocytes and are used in the very early stages, whereas in the inductive phase (immunoblast formation) antimetabolites are used. Most of the latter are purine or pyrimidine analogues and are too toxic for general use, although one purine analogue, *azathioprine*, is widely used, as is the folic acid antagonist, *amethopterin*. The antibiotics actinomycin D, which prevents RNA synthesis on a DNA template, and chloramphenicol, which blocks protein synthesis, have also been used. Other techniques are to give large doses of 11-oxycorticosteroids, to give a substantial radiation dose to damage the

small lymphocytes, or to use antilymphocytic serum.

There are major difficulties with all these techniques since many of the agents used are relatively toxic and there are important side effects, such as the effect of corticosteroids on electrolyte metabolism. Also, as a direct result of the suppression of the immune response the patient has a markedly increased susceptibility to infection and requires highly skilled nursing and elaborate facilities for the exclusion of potential pathogens. Normally a combination of treatments is used to take advantage of the additive effects while reducing considerably the dosage for any one form of treatment.

EPIDEMIOLOGY

Some Definitions
Prevalence. The total number of cases in an area.
Incidence. The number of new cases occurring.
Vector. An animal or other carrier of disease. A typical example is the transmission of plague from rats to humans by fleas, rats providing the reservoir of disease and fleas being the vectors.
Endemic. A disease is said to be endemic when it is constantly present in a particular area, giving a steady incidence of low grade infection.
Epidemic. An epidemic disease is characterized by the occurrence within an area or community of an unusually high incidence of infection. An epidemic may occur when a virulent parasite is imported into the community, when carriers are present with easy routes of transmission of the disease, when sanitation breaks down, e.g. after floods or an earthquake, if a parasite mutates to virulence and when the proportion of susceptibles in the population is high. That the last factor may be crucial has been shown for many diseases, e.g. with diphtheria the effect of immunization improves markedly when the proportion of susceptibles falls below 50 per cent.

An endemic disease may epidemic in another area, e.g. smallpox, cholera and typhoid are endemic in India and Pakistan but the outbreak of a few cases is regarded as an epidemic in the U.K.
Pandemic. This is the world-wide spread of epidemic disease. The prime example is influenza, for which the prevalence in the 1957/58 epidemic is believed to be about 80×10^6 and only some Pacific islands were unaffected.

Factors Influencing the Spread of Disease
Until 1850 there was little that could be done to prevent the spread of disease in a community, but

the introduction of sewage systems, better nutrition, education and sanitation produced a marked improvement in the position; then vaccines and sera, and, finally, the introduction of antibiotics and chemosynthetic antimicrobial agents brought a substantial improvement. There are three groups of factors involved.

Natural factors, such as the virulence of the organism, the susceptibility of the population and the presence of suitable vectors and reservoirs of infection.

Social factors, including the quality of nutrition, sanitation and education, especially health and hygiene education, the existence of fast, simple means of travel and the extent to which quarantine and regulations concerning the immunization of travellers are enforced.

These are possibly the most important factors in reducing the prevalence of disease in a population.

Technical factors, primarily medical procedures which can be used to prevent the spread of disease, including immunization and the use of antibiotics, chemotherapeutic agents and biocides.

However, the extent to which antimicrobials modify the situation is doubtful, since suppression of the normal flora may permit resistant strains or secondary infections to occur.

Some Potentially Epidemic Diseases
Poliomyelitis. This is caused by a small picorna virus, 27 nm in diameter and with icosahedral symmetry. The D-Ag, which corresponds to whole infective virus particles, is unstable chemically and occurs in three serological types, known as 1, 2 and 3; type 1 virus causes most clinical infections.

The disease occurs in four clinical forms. *Subclinical* (silent) infection causes no overt symptoms, though its occurrence is known from antibody surveys. *Abortive poliomyelitis* is a mild febrile illness and is unlikely to be diagnosed as poliomyelitis. *Non-paralytic* disease is a febrile illness but characterized by stiffness and pain in the back and neck. The disease lasts from 2 to 10 days and there is usually complete recovery. In all the above types of infection the virus remains confined to lymphatic tissue (Peyer's patches, lymph nodes) and the blood, with little neural involvement, but in severe infections invasion of the CNS causes *paralytic poliomyelitis*. This form starts with the typical symptoms of non-paralytic disease which subside after 3 to 5 days to be followed after a further 2 to 3 days by paralytic symptons, i.e. a flaccid paralysis, incoordination, painful spasm of unparalyzed muscle and, sometimes, respiratory and cardiac failure.

Symptoms occur in only 1 per cent of all cases and only a fraction of those show paralytic symptoms. Paralysis may be provoked by any sort of trauma which occurs during the incubation and early stages of the disease, so care must be taken over energetic exercise, tonsillectomy and injections. Most notably 'provocation poliomyelitis' may be induced by prophylactics containing alum (e.g. diphtheria and tetanus vaccines).

The disease was known as infantile paralysis in the 19th century and is still an endemic disease of children in the less developed countries with a low level of nutrition and sanitation. In one North African city 50 per cent of children were immune (i.e. had been infected) by 14 months of age and 100 per cent were immune at 5 years, an effect which is beneficial in that community. The pattern was similar in Western Europe and North America in the 19th Century and serological surveys indicate that 86 per cent of children in the U.K. were immune by the age of 5 and paralytic disease was common. However, in the 1948 epidemic the main incidence was at 12 to 14 years and in the 1957 epidemic more than 35 per cent of cases were over 15 years of age. This arises from the high standards of hygiene and nutrition and highly protective child rearing so that there is a basically non immune adult population. The result is an epidemic form of the disease rather than the endemic form.

The scale of the U.K. epidemic in 1957 is typical, with an incidence of about $10\,000/10^6$ of the population with deaths at about $750/10^6$. The occurrence and severity of epidemics has declined markedly since the introduction of the killed vaccine in 1956 and the living attenuated virus vaccine in 1962, so that poliomyelitis is no longer an important disease in highly developed countries.

Influenza. The influenza virus is predominantly a roughly spherical, easily deformed virus about 70 nm in diameter with an outer membrane about 8 nm thick and an inner helical nucleocapsid containing single-stranded RNA. The surface bears numerous 10 nm projections of glycoprotein which are the sites of the neuraminidase, the enzyme which aids attachment of virus and which produces haemagglutination.

The disease spreads by droplet infection and after 1 to 2 days causes a severe respiratory infection which is normally self-limiting in about 3 to 7 days, some 10 per cent of cases having limited lobar consolidation. If death occurs it is due usually to secondary bacterial bronchopneumonia.

There are three antigenic types, known as A, B

and C, which are determined by the core, and about 20 antigenic determinants associated with the surface macromolecules, so that there can be, for example, a basically Type A virus with several different sub-types. Most epidemics are associated with Type A, of which epidemics occur at about 3 year intervals, Type B virus causing sporadic, localized outbreaks, while Type C is epidemiologically unimportant.

In the U.K. only occasional mild epidemics occurred up to 1890, probably mostly due to Type A_2. The first severe recorded epidemic occurred in 1890 (Type A) and caused some 500 deaths/10^6. Subsequently the prevalence increased markedly, with about 4 epidemic peaks per decade. In 1918 and 1919 there was a major pandemic (Type A, 3129 deaths/10^6) largely affecting women and children, the cause for this being ascribed to poor nutrition during the war. Subsequently the mortality in epidemics declined to about 250/10^6 and remained roughly at the same level until 1947, when Type A_1 appeared to be succeeded by the Asian Type (A_2). Although Type A_2 persists there was a marked change in antigenic structure in 1964.

Vaccination with the killed saline vaccine is of doubtful value in view of the variability of the virus, the occurrence of hypersensitivity reactions and the short lived nature of the immunity. An attenuated living virus vaccine is used in the U.S.S.R. and seems promising but is not used in the U.K., and purified viral protein and vaccines prepared with mineral oil adjuvants also seem to be promising but are not generally available. Antamidine HCl prevents the penetration of A_2 into cells and provides a possibility for chemotherapy if given early enough.

Cholera. The causative agent, *Vibrio cholerae*, is a curved or straight Gram-negative, facultative anaerobic bacterium with a single polar flagellum. Under natural conditions it is exclusively a human pathogen. The disease has an incubation period of 2 to 5 days; the toxin produced then affects the intestinal epithelium and promotes the formation of cyclic adenosine monophosphate with a resultant fall in the level of available, energy providing, ATP. This causes a massive loss of sodium and water into the bowel and up to 12 litres/day may be lost with consequent dehydration, anuria, haemoconcentration, acidosis, toxaemia and shock. The severity of symptoms varies widely and in severe cases death may result in 12 hours from the onset of symptoms, although if it is possible to give adequate fluid replacement it is usually possible to prevent death. The natural fatality rate is 25 to 50 per cent.

The disease is frequently water borne, as was first shown by the London physician Snow in 1854, but may also be spread by contaminated food, by flies and by direct contact. Chronic carriers do not occur but patients who recover are infective for 3 to 4 weeks. Since the organism is non-invasive and remains confined to the gastrointestinal tract, infection followed by recovery gives only a limited immunity whereas the vaccine, prepared from whole cells or a lipopolysaccharide fraction, gives significant protection. There are four principal strains, *El Tor* originated in the Arabian peninsular, *Inaba* occurs mostly in Japan, *Ogawa* is characteristic of the Indian sub-continent and *Hikojima* is primarily Chinese. The strain at present causing concern is a modified El Tor which arose in the Celebes Islands in 1961. Since then it has spread steadily: 1962, Borneo; 1963, Malaya and Indo-China, South-eastern China, Korea; 1964, Assam; 1965/1966, India and the whole of south-west Asia; 1970, the Middle East, south-western Russia, Arabia and central and eastern North Africa; 1971, the whole of North Africa and Spain. In 1973 there was a minor epidemic in Italy, with about 10 reported deaths and although it is doubtful that there could be anything other than sporadic cases in western and northern Europe, including the U.K., because of the high standards of hygiene, the speed of modern travel means that an infected person may travel home and be in contact with his local community long before overt symptoms arise. Clearly, the utmost vigilance is necessary.

ANTIMICROBIAL AGENTS: MODES OF ACTION AND RESISTANCE

Numerous modes of action have been proposed for various compounds, but they have been elucidated completely for only a limited number, notably some antibiotics, for example, the nature of the cellular lesion in the case of phenol is still not known certainly after some 100 years of use.

Substances Affecting Metabolism

General poisons. These are mostly highly reactive compounds which cause widespread damage to the cell, e.g. azide and cyanide bind with the iron of cytochromes and prevent oxidative phosphorylation, while dinitrophenol is an uncoupling agent and prevents oxidative phosphorylation without stopping fermentation. Other compounds in this class are halogens, especially hypochlorites, formaldehyde, hydrogen peroxide and alkylating agents.

Substances disrupting membranes. Since biological membranes contain lipids, the membrane structure can be damaged by hydrophobic compounds, lipid solvents and surfactants. Typical agents in this group are acetone, ether, toluene, the quaternary ammonium biocides, e.g. cetrimide and domiphen bromide, and probably phenols and related compounds.

Chemical mutagens. These modify the DNA structure chemically. Since most mutations are lethal the modifications usually result in death, after allowing a period for cell division to occur. Mutagens in this class are the alkylating agents, such as nitrogen mustard, and nitrous acid.

Metabolite analogues. These are compounds which are structurally similar to natural metabolites and either displace the natural compound from the active site of an enzyme or mask the active site, or are incorporated in place of the natural metabolite to give a non-functional final product. Examples of the first type are the sulphonamides, which antagonize p-amino-benzoic acid, and of the second type are 5-bromouracil and 5-fluorouracil which antagonize thymine and uracil respectively.

Agents affecting cell wall synthesis. The first agent of this kind was penicillin and all the penicillins act in this way, as do some of the chemically related cephalosporins. Other antibiotics in this class are bacitracin, cycloserine and vancomycin. Gentian violet affects wall synthesis but it is not known whether this is its primary site of action, since it has more general effects also. These drugs are effective chemotherapeutic agents because mucopeptide is found only in bacteria so that the drug has no action in humans. The principal effect of the drug in the animal host is to act as an allergen.

Agents affecting cell membranes. Membrane damage is usually inferred when leakage of cell contents occurs, a condition produced in bacteria by polymyxin and novobiocin. The precise mechanism of attack is not known, though in some cases there is good evidence that permeability to K^+ is increased. Fungal cell membranes contain sterols (virtually absent from bacteria) so only the former are damaged by nystatin and amphotericin, which are inactive against bacteria.

Agents affecting nucleic acid funtion. Some compounds with this type of activity have been mentioned already as chemical mutagens. A more subtle effect is caused by the acriflavine dyes, which appear to function as *intercalating agents*. The structure of these enables them to fit into a groove in the DNA helix and bond to adjacent purine and pyrimidine bases. The DNA is thus distorted producing mutations which are lethal to the cell. Mitomycin C cross links the two strands of the DNA helix and so prevents uncoiling and therefore replication of the DNA. Another type of action is shown by actinomycin, which binds to DNA and prevents mRNA synthesis.

Agents affecting protein synthesis. Any substance affecting DNA function will eventually affect protein synthesis. However, many antibiotics affect protein synthesis directly, often exerting the action at ribosomal level. Since bacterial ribosomes are smaller than host ribosomes (70S and 80S respectively) this means that effective chemotherapeutic agents are possible. Streptomycin, neomycin and kanamycin are related chemically and act by combining with the 30S sub-unit of the ribosomes to cause misreading of mRNA, resulting in inactive proteins. A different mode of action is shown by chloramphenicol and the tetracyclines, which inhibit different steps in the peptide chain elongation. Puromycin is actually a structural analogue of aminoacyl-tRNA and so blocks the binding of tRNA to the ribosome and prevents protein chain elongation.

DRUG RESISTANCE IN BACTERIA

Biochemical Mechanisms
Decreased penetration of the drug. This was the first type of drug resistance observed, when it was observed that the resistance of trypanosomes to arsenicals increased during treatment. The uptake ratio (resistant/susceptible) may be as high as 500. With amino acid analogues resistance is due to blockage of the transport system, so that the cell becomes exacting for the natural metabolite. Differences in permeability between Gram-positive and Gram-negative cells may be a reflection of wall differences, as in the case of actinomycin which is stopped by the Gram-negative cell wall but not by the Gram-positive wall. This mechanism is also concerned in the resistance of some organisms to chloramphenicol, fucidin, streptomycin and tetracyclines.

Enzymic destruction of the drug. The most familiar example of this type of resistance is the induction of a β-lactamase which destroys many penicillins. In fact the cells are inherently sensitive, so small populations are sensitive to penicillin but large populations, which rapidly produce large amounts of β-lactamase are resistant. Similar mechanisms are involved in the resistance of some organisms to chloramphenicol, dihydrostreptomycin, kanamycin and mitomycin C.

Increased production of natural metabolite or enzyme. The resistance of staphylococci, streptococci, gonococci and *E.coli* to sulphonamides is due to increased *p*-aminobenzoic acid (PAB) synthesis. Since the sulphonamides competitively inhibit PAB, increasing the amount of PAB displaces the sulphonamide from the enzyme. In *Staph.aureus* there may also be more efficient conversion of PAB into folic acid. It is important to note that more than one mechanism may operate simultaneously in the same organism.

Increased enzyme production is found in cells showing resistance to psicofuranine, (enzyme, xanthine 5'-phosphate aminase), D-cycloserine (alanine racemase) and 2-thiazolealanine (histidine enzymes).

Production of enzyme or organelle with decreased affinity for the drug. A resistant enzyme with decreased sulphonamide affinity, dihydropteroate reductase, is concerned in sulphonamide resistance. Altered ribosomal configuration is often the basis of resistance, and reduced binding to the 50S subunit occurs in erythromycin and tetracycline resistance, while reduced binding to the 30S sub-unit results in resistance to kanamycin A, neomycin C and streptomycin. In the case of streptomycin another modification of the 30S sub-unit can cause streptomycin dependence in organisms which are normally sensitive or resistant.

Reduction or loss of enzyme activity. Purine or pyrimidine analogues must be converted, first into nucleotides and then nucleic acids before they can exert their activity. Resistance to the analogues 6-mercaptopurine and 8-azaguanine results from loss of the corresponding phosphorylases, though the cells then become exacting for the corresponding nucleotides.

Other mechanisms. The following occur infrequently: the synthesis of an enzyme with decreased affinity for an antimetabolite relative to the natural metabolite, as in the *p*-fluorophenylalanine/alanine system; development of alternative metabolic pathways to by-pass the normal pathway (tetracyclines); and decreased requirement for a metabolite (antagonists of folic acid precursors).

This last mechanism is the reason why sulphonamides and trimethoprim can be used therapeutically since a sensitive pathogen synthesizes its own folic acid from precursors and is inhibited by these compounds, whereas man requires preformed folic acid and so is not affected by agents preventing its synthesis.

The Genetic Basis of Drug Resistance

The basis of drug resistance, no matter what the biochemical mechanism involved, is the presence of appropriate genes. There are three ways in which the appropriate genes may be acquired.

Mutation involves the modification of an existing gene. There is no evidence that this occurs during treatment to an extent to make it important in the emergence of drug resistance.

Transformation involves the leakage of soluble DNA from a naturally resistant organism and absorption of the DNA by a sensitive organism which then incorporates the resistance genes from the donor cell into its own DNA. This is a well-established phenomenon in the laboratory and probably provides one way of spreading resistance in a bacterial population.

Transduction is the carrying of resistance factors from a donor to a number of recipients by phage. Many bacteria are lysogenic and carry prophage either incorporated in their chromosome or attached to the cell membrane. Induction of the prophage often results in the released phages carrying a variable amount of host bacterial DNA to new hosts which they infect. This is known to be an important mechanism for spreading resistance.

Conjugation is probably the most important mechanism of all. Many enteric bacteria have sex pili, there being 'male' and 'female' cells. Similarly, some bacteria have a *resistance transfer factor* (RTF) which promotes transfer of *resistance* (R) *factors* from a donor to a recipient cell, following attachment by a pilus. This pilus shrinks to form a cytoplasmic bridge between the two cells, through which the R-factors pass to the recipient cell, which then incorporates these R-factors into its own DNA and becomes resistant. Reproduction of the newly resistant recipient results in daughter cells each of which carries the R genes. In some species, e.g. *Proteus mirabilis*, the resistance factors can be replicated to produce as many as 30 sets of resistance genes within the cell. Further, R-factor transfer can occur between different bacterial genera, e.g. transfer from *Klebsiella* to *Pseudomonas* is known to have occurred in the course of the prolonged antibiotic treatment of burn patients.

The R-factors are one form of *plasmid*, an extra-chromosomal inheritance factor which may be attached to the cell membrane or become incorporated in the chromosome. Plasmids often carry resistance to a number of drugs simultaneously, so that recipients become multiply resistant in a single step.

THE CLINICAL PROBLEM

Although conjugation is known to occur during antibiotic therapy to cause the emergence of resistant populations, the principal source of resistant cells is the small proportion of naturally resistant organisms, perhaps $1/10^8$ of the initial population. Antibiotic therapy exerts a selective pressure, the sensitive population is inhibited and the resistant cells can grow to become dominant. Fortunately, the resistant cells are usually less well adapted to their environment so that if treatment is stopped and the selective pressure is removed, the population frequently reverts slowly to its original state. However, resistance often persists so that the majority of *Staph.aureus* now encountered in hospitals are penicillin resistant.

As each new drug is introduced, resistant bacteria are found after a short while, and there is no reason to expect any different pattern in the future. The inference is clear: antibiotics should be used only for conditions where the clinical picture or laboratory tests indicate clearly that the drug will be beneficial. The routine use of broad spectrum antibiotics either prophylactically or for trivial conditions is highly undesirable and there should be a rational use of antibiotics. Rotation in use, may help to reduce the emergence of resistant strains to a minimum.

THE IDENTIFICATION OF MICROORGANISMS

Several different approaches to the identification of microorganisms have been used and they depend on criteria which have been found to be reasonably simple and reliable in practice.

It must be stressed that the aims of identification and taxonomy are very different. Identification aims at determining the place of an organism in an existing taxonomic framework so that an appropriate name can be given to it which all other workers will recognize and which informs as to its principal characters and previously published work. In clinical work it may be necessary to do this very rapidly with as few tests as possible so that the causal agent of a disease can be recognized and appropriate treatment instituted immediately. Taxonomy aims to place all organisms into their correct position with regard to all other organisms, in a genus, family or tribe. For this, speed is of no consequence and the completeness of information and the logic of the taxonomic system are paramount. Thus, taxonomy is a specialist study, whereas identification is something which all bacteriologists have to do at some time.

Eukaryotic Microorganisms

These are identified primarily on morphological criteria, biochemical characters being used usually only to identify sub-species or species, though with fungi the composition of the cell wall is an important character.

Viruses

The main characteristics, which have already been indicated (Table 29.9), are as follows:
1. The type of nucleic acid and whether single-stranded or double-stranded.
2. The capsid morphology, whether helical, icosahedral or more complex, if naked or enveloped (lipid membrane) and the number of capsomers.
3. Size.
4. Susceptibility to inactivation by various agents.
5. Whether replicated in the nucleus or cytoplasm (inapplicable to phage).
6. Secondary criteria include the host range, specificity to particular organs or tissues, the mode of transmission and the immunological characters.

Bacteria

Prokaryotic microorganisms show such a restricted morphological range that only gross features such as coccus or bacillus are used.

There are numerous keys to bacterial identification, the best available at present for bacteria of medical interest is that of Cowan and Steel (1974). Their (first stage) approach is to determine the Gram reaction and then to observe the results of a limited series of morphological tests and biochemical reactions which enable a worker to assign the bacterium to a single genus or to two possible genera (Fig. 29.54). For the second stage the worker is referred to an appropriate table in which the individual species are identified primarily by a series of biochemical tests, involving such things as sugar fermentations, the production of indole and H_2S, the presence of urease, gelatinase, amylase, urease, etc.

Unfortunately, Cowan and Steel set out with the limited objective of including bacteria of medical importance or bacteria likely to be encountered by medical bacteriologists. Within this context it functions excellently, though it necessarily excludes many bacteria of industrial importance. No satis-

factory key exists for the latter, though Skerman (1959) has a key based on *Bergey's Manual*, 7th ed (1957). For many groups, *Bergey's Manual* is unsatisfactory, though it is hoped that some, at least of the problems will be elucidated in the eighth edition, publication of which is expected shortly. Further, it is becoming increasingly difficult to define a genus or species since DNA can be transferred between species and genera, for example

FIG. 29.54. Typical tables for identification of the common medical bacteria using the system of Cowan and Steel (1974).

First-stage table for Gram-negative bacteria

	1	2	3	4	5	6	7	8	9	10	11	12	13	14	15	16	17	18
Shape	R	S	S	S	S/R	R	R	R	R	R	R	R	R	R	R	R	R	R
Motility	−	−	−	−	−	−	+	+	−	+	−	−	+	D	−	−	+	−
Growth in air	−	−	+	+	+	+	+	+	+	+	+	+	+	+	+	−*	−†	+
Growth anaerobically	+	+	−	−	−	−	−	−	−	+	+	+	+	+	+	+	−	+
Catalase	d	D	+	+	+	+	+	+	+	+	+	−	+	+	D	−	D	−
Oxidase	−	×	+	+	−	+	+	+	+	+	+	+	+	−	−	+	+	−
Glucose (acid)	D	−	+	−	+	−	+	−	+	+	+	+	+	+	D	−	−	+
Carbohydrates [F/O/−]	F/−	−	O	−	O	−	O	−	O	O	F	F	F	F	NT	−	−	F

	1	2	3	4	5	6	7	8	9	10	11	12	13	14	15	16	17	18	
Bacteroides	+																		7.2
Veillonella		+																	
Neisseria			+																
Branhamella				+															7.3
Acinetobacter					+														
Moraxella						+													
Brucella						+													7.4
Bordetella						+													
Chromobacterium lividum							+												7.5
Alcaligenes								+											
Flavobacterium									+										7.6
Pseudomonas										+									
Actinobacillus											+								
Pasteurella											+								7.7
Necromonas											+								
Cardiobacterium												+							
Chromobacterium violaceum													+						
Beneckea													+						
Vibrio													+						7.8
Plesiomonas													+						
Aeromonas													+						7.9
Enterobacteria														+					
Haemophilus															+				
Eikenella																+			
Campylobacter																	+		
Streptobacillus‡																		+	7.10
Mycoplasms																		+	

* No growth in air; growth in air $+ CO_2$. × Not known.

† No growth in air or anaerobically; growth in 5–6% O_2. NT Not testable by usual methods. Fermentative (Sneath & Johnson, 1973).

‡ Also *Shigella dysenteriae* 1 (Shiga's bacillus). Typical form.

FIG. 29.54—(continued)

Second-stage table for differentiation of the enterobacteria (majority reactions)

	1	2	3	4	5	6	7	8	9	10	11	12	13	14
Motility	D	+	D	−	+	+	+	+	+	+	+	+	−	−
Growth in KCN medium	−	−	−	−	D	−	−	+	+	+	+	+	D	+
Citrate as C source	−	−	−	−	+	+	+	−	+	+	+	+	+	d
Gas from glucose	D	+			+	D	−	+	D	+	d	+	D	D
MR test	+	+	+	+	+	+	−	+	+	−	d	−	D	+
VP test	−	−	−	−	−	−	d	−	d	+	+	+	D	−
Indole	+	+	−	d	D	−	−	+	D	−	−	−	D	−
Gelatin	−	−	−	−	−	D	+	−	D	−	+	(d)	D	−
Urease	−	−	D	−	D	−	−	+	D	−	d	d	+	d
Phenylalanine	−	−	−	−	−	−	+	+	+	−	−	−	−	−
H₂S from TSI	−	+	−	−	D	+	.	−	D	−	−	−	−	−
Lysine decarboxylase	+	+	−	−	−	+	−	−	−	+	d	D	+	d
Ornithine decarboxylase	d	+	D	D	d	D	−	+	D	+	D	+	−	−

1 *Escherichia coli*; A–D group
2 *Edwardsiella tarda*; Asakusa biotype; Bartholomew group
3 *Yersinia* spp.
4 *Shigella* spp.
5 *Citrobacter* spp.; *Levinea* spp.
6 *Salmonella* spp. and serotypes

7 *Erwinia herbicola*
8 *Morganella morganii*; *Proteus morganii*
9 *Proteus* spp. (including Providence group)
10 *Hafnia alvei*
11 *Serratia* spp.

12 *Enterobacter* spp.
13 *Klebsiella aerogenes*; *K. atlantae*; *K. edwardsii*; *K. oxytoca*; *K. pneumoniae*
14 *Klebsiella ozaenae*; *K. rhinoscleromatis*

Details of sub-groups 1–5, 6–9 and 10–14 in Third-stage tables.

resistance factors between *Klebsiella* and *Pseudomonas*.

To solve some of these problems many taxonomists have resorted to simple forms of genetic analysis, e.g. the percentage of guanine and cytosine in the DNA (the G-C ratio), the ability of single-stranded DNA from two organisms to hybridize or of hydridization between the DNA and mRNA. Such experiments are difficult and are little used at present for indentification, though they are of great value for the taxonomist.

FURTHER READING

Elementary Texts

ALEXOPOULOS, C. J. & BOLD, H. C. (1967) *Algae and Fungi*. London: Macmillan.

SISTROM, W. R. (1971) *Microbial Life*. 2nd ed. London: Holt, Rinehart & Winston.

VICKERMAN, K. & COX, F. E. G. (1967) *The Protozoa*. London: Murray.

Standard Microbiology Texts

JAWETZ, E., MELNICK, J. L. & ADELBERG, E. A. (1972) *Review of Medical Microbiology*. 10th ed. Los Altos: Lange.

STANIER, R. Y., DOUDOROFF, M. & ADELBERG, E. A. (1970) *General Microbiology*. 3rd ed. London: Macmillan.

Reference and Advanced Texts

ALEXOPOULOS, C. J. (1962) *Introductory Mycology*. 2nd ed. New York: Wiley.

BROCK, T. D. (1970) *Biology of Microorganisms*. London: Prentice Hall International.

DAVIS, B. D., DULBECCO, R., EISEN, H. N., GINSBERG, H. S. & WOOD, W. B. Jr. (1967) *Microbiology*. New York: Harper & Row.

INGOLD, C. T. (1973) *The Biology of Fungi*. 2nd rev. ed. London: Hutchinson.

PELCZAR, M. J. Jr. & REID, R. D. (1972) *Microbiology*. 3rd ed. Maidenhead: McGraw Hill.

SMITH, G. (1969) *An Introduction to Industrial Mycology*. 6th ed. London: Edward Arnold.

STEWART, F. S. (1968) *Bacteriology and Immunology for Students of Medicine*. 9th ed. London: Ballière, Tindall & Cassell.

Protozoa and Parasitology

WATSON, J. M. (1965) *An Introduction to Parasitology* Pharmaceutical Monographs, Vol. 2. Stenlake, J. B. ed. London: Heinemann Medical.

BLACKLOCK, D. B. & SOUTHWELL, T. (1966) *Guide to Human Parasitology*. London: Lewis.

Viruses

COHEN, A. (1969) *Textbook of Medical Virology.* Oxford: Blackwell Scientific.

FENNER, F. J. & WHITE, D. O. (1970) *Medical Virology.* London: Academic Press.

Epidemiology

BURNET, M. & WHITE, D. O. (1972) *The Natural History of Infectious Disease.* 4th ed. London: Cambridge University Press.

Antibiotic Action and Resistance

GALE, E. F., CUNDLIFFE, E., REYNOLDS, P. E., RICHMOND, M. H. & WARING, M. J. (1972) *The Molecular Basis of Antibiotic Action.* London: Wiley.

Practical Microbiology

MEYNELL, G. G. & MEYNELL, E. (1965) *Theory and Practice in Experimental Bacteriology.* London: Cambridge University Press.

NORRIS, E. J. & RIBBONS, D. W. Eds (1969) *Methods in Microbiology.* London: Academic Press. (Numerous volumes.)

Classification

BERGEY'S MANUAL (1957) *Bergey's Manual of Determinative Bacteriology.* 7th ed. (under revision). Breed, R. S., Murray, E. G. D. & Smith, N. R. (eds). Baltimore: Williams and Wilkins.

COWAN, S. T. & STEEL, K. J. (1974) *The Identification of Medical Bacteria.* 2nd ed. London: Cambridge University Press.

MICROBIAL CLASSIFICATION (1962) *Soc. gen. Microbiol. 12th Symposium.* London: Cambridge University Press.

SKERMAN, V. B. D. (1967) *A Guide to the Identification of the Genera of Bacteria*: 2nd ed. Baltimore: Williams & Wilkins.

30

Disinfection

DEFINITIONS AND TERMINOLOGY

Much confusion exists in the terminology applied to disinfectant action. The following definitions (marked*) are based on the British Disinfectant Manufacturers' Association list of agreed definitions (1970):

Bactericide—a chemical agent capable of killing bacteria, but not necessarily bacterial spores.

Bacteriostat—a chemical agent capable of preventing the growth of bacteria but not of killing them. Reproduction and multiplication are prevented.

Fungicide—a chemical agent capable of killing fungi, including their spores.

Fungistat—a chemical agent which prevents fungal proliferation.

Germicide—usually applied to an agent which kills all microorganisms.

Virucide—an agent which kills viruses.

Sporicide—an agent which kills spores.

Algicide—an agent which kills algae.

Antibiotic—a term suggested by Waksman (1942) for antibacterial substances produced by moulds and bacteria, e.g. penicillin, streptomycin, oxytetracycline, etc.

Disinfection—the destruction of microorganisms, but not usually bacterial spores: not necessarily killing all microorganisms but reducing them to a level not harmful to health. This term is applied commercially to treatment of inanimate objects and materials, although in some literature disinfection is analagous to bactericidal action on skin and living tissues.

The term disinfectant usually implies a substance with bactericidal action. Sanitization is a term which appears in much American literature and implies disinfection combined with a cleansing process.

Antisepsis—the destruction of microorganisms, but not bacterial spores on living tissues: not necessarily killing all microorganisms but reducing them to a level not normally harmful to health. The action of an antiseptic should be lethal to microorganisms, not, as implied in some literature, static.

Many substances can act both as lethal agents and static agents, depending on their concentration, the time of contact, and the temperature of the reaction. If graphs are plotted of log viable counts against time (see Fig. 30.1) the three main situations growth (A), bacteriostasis (B), and bactericidal action (C) are shown.

Disinfection implies elimination of infection, but not necessarily a complete killing effect.

DISINFECTANTS

Disinfectants have been used empirically from the time of the ancient Egyptians. They used antibacterial oils, spices and balsams in the embalming of bodies. Alcock, in 1827, in the *Lancet* referred to the use of chlorine compounds as 'powerful, disinfecting agents'. During the first half of the nineteenth century compounds employed as disinfectants included chlorine gas, silver nitrate (the antibacterial properties of silver and copper had been used by the Persians and Romans), phenol,

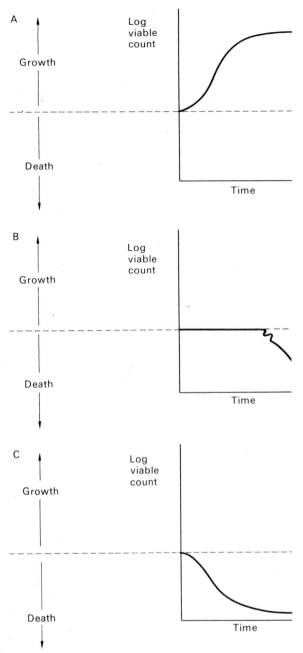

Fig. 30.1. Growth, bacteriostatic and bactericidal effects on bacteria. A, Bacteria inoculated into nutrient medium. Normal initial stages of growth curve shown; B, Bacteriostatic environment viable, population remains constant, but falls after prolonged time; C, Bactericidal environment. Sigmoid death curve often shown.

zinc compounds, and iodine. Semmelweiss, in Vienna in 1861, used a solution of chlorinated lime for hand disinfection, and this produced a marked fall in the incidence of puerperal infection in his hospital. Pasteur showed that putrefaction was due to microorganisms, and following the work of Lister in 1865 onwards, disinfection was put on a rational basis, and antiseptic surgery started. Koch (1881) tested the action of different disinfectants on pure cultures.

Many disinfectants are often described as 'general disinfectants'. The term is a misnomer as it is impossible to prepare a disinfectant that will serve best for such different purposes as disinfecting sinks, drains, linen, intact and broken skin, mucous surfaces, body cavities, etc. An ideal disinfectant would have the following properties:

High potency under the conditions of use.

Ready solubility in, or miscibility with, water at effective antimicrobial concentration.

Non-caustic with a low degree of toxicity and without harmful or sensitizing effects on delicate tissues.

No deleterious effect on linen and metals.

Complete compatibility with other antimicrobial agents being used and with other components of the disinfectant formulation.

Stable on storage. Often long-term stability over a wide range of temperature may be be required.

Reasonably cheap.

No offensive odour, taste (oral disinfectants), or colour.

No ideal disinfectant exists.

The disinfectants used at present can be conveniently divided into 10 main groups:

(1) Phenols   (6) Halogens
(2) Alcohols   (7) Metals
(3) Aldehydes   (8) Guanidines and
(4) Dyes   Amidines
(5) Surface-active   (9) Furan derivatives
    compounds   (10) Quinoline and
                                  isoquinoline
                                  derivatives.

A number of compounds are used as aerial disinfectants, e.g. glycols, α-hydroxycarboxylic acids, and ethylene oxide (see gaseous sterilization).

MODE OF ACTION OF DISINFECTANTS

The mode of action varies according to the type of disinfectant used and the microorganisms involved. Excellent reviews of modes of action are given by Hugo (1967, 1970) and these are summarized in Table 30.1.

Phenolic disinfectants, in low concentrations, disrupt the cytoplasmic membrane causing leakage of bacterial cellular constituents (Gale & Taylor 1947) and also affect membrane permeability (Hugo

TABLE 30.1

SUMMARY OF MODES OF ACTION OF DISINFECTANTS (BASED ON REVIEWS BY HUGO (1967, 1970)

Action	Some disinfectants involved
PRIMARY DRUG/CELL INTERACTIONS	
Adsorbtion—not generally lethal but leads to secondary reactions, which are often bacteriostatic or bactericidal	Phenols, Iodine, Chlorhexidine, Basic dyes, some surface-active compounds.
Electrophoretic mobility changes—bacteria in water normally have a negative charge, and thus migrate to the cathode when a potential is applied. This migration may be slowed or accelerated, stopped or even reversed by disinfectants.	There is an increase in the rate of migration with increase in concentration with phenols and halogenated phenols acting on *Aerobacter aerogenes*. Chlorhexidine causes decrease in migration rate (*E.coli, Staph.aureus*).
SECONDARY DRUG/CELL INTERACTIONS	
Cell permeability modification and leakage of cell constituents (partial lysis).	Hexylresorcinol, Cetyltrimethylammonium bromide, and Phenol. Chorhexidine (at low concentrations).
Lysis	Phenol, Aldehydes, Mercuric Chloride, Hypochlorites.
Irreversible general coagulation of cytoplasmic constituents, e.g. protein precipitation. Usually produced by high concentrations of disinfectant.	Phenols, Cetyltrimethylammonium bromide, and Chlorhexidine.
General metabolic effects, e.g. inhibition of succinate dehydrogenase, and interference with enzyme systems.	Alcohols, Phenols, and Surfactants.
DRUG/CELL INTERACTIONS WHERE MECHANISM IS KNOWN WITH SOME PRECISION	
Interaction with thio(sulphydryl) groups. Two main mechanisms: (a) Combination; (b) Oxidation	Mercury, silver and copper compounds, Halogens, Potassium permanganate.
Action as metal binding agents, thus depriving bacteria of metals essential for their metabolism.	8-hydroxyquinoline.
Interaction with amino groups.	Formaldehyde. Some halogens, in addition to their oxidizing action.
Interference with oxidation reduction systems.	Nitrofuran.
Reaction with acidic groups in the cell, inhibition of glutamine, or inhibition of bacterial cell wall synthesis. (The latter being the action of crystal violet).	Triphenylmethane dyes.
Interference with nucleic acid function.	Acridine dyes.

1956). At high concentrations they act as protoplasmic poisons (Hugo 1957).

Alcohols have the ability to denature proteins. This denaturation is much more marked in the presence of water, and hence concentrations of 60 to 90 per cent v/v are usually used for disinfection (Archer 1945). Actions of alcohols are discussed by Sykes (1965) and Salton (1961).

Aldehydes usually act by combining with the amino groups of proteins, while halogen compounds halogenate or oxidize vital cell components.

Specific combination with thiol ($-SH$) groups accounts for the activity of mercury, silver, and copper, although in high concentrations they are protein precipitants. The toxic part, in the case of mercury, is the mercuric ion Hg^{2+}. This ion reacts as follows with thiol groups in enzymes and structural proteins:

$$\text{Enzyme}\begin{matrix}SH \\ \\ SH\end{matrix} + HgCl_2 \longrightarrow$$

$$\text{Enzyme}\begin{matrix}S \\ \\ S\end{matrix}Hg + 2HCl$$

(Fildes 1940).

Basic dyes (triphenylmethane dyes) inactivate bacteria by reacting with acidic groups in the cell, although inhibition of glutamine synthesis is the

TABLE 30.2

LETHAL ACTIVITY OF DISINFECTANTS (A GENERAL OUTLINE)

	Gram-positive organisms	Gram-negative organisms	Acid-fast bacilli	Bacterial spores	Fungi	Viruses**
Phenols	S	S	MR*	R	MS	V
Alcohols	MS	S	S	R	V	V
Aldehydes (formaldehyde and glutaraldehyde)	S	S	S	S	S	S
Halogens	S	S	MR (Chlorine compounds) S (Iodine compounds)	MR (Chlorine compounds) S (Iodine compounds)	MS	S
Metals	S	MS	R	MR	S (Cupric salts)	R
Dyes	S	MS	R	R	R+	R
Cationic surfactants	S	MS	R	R	MS	R+
Guanidines and Amidines	S	S	R	R	S (Amidines) MS (Guanidines)	R
Furan derivatives	S (Nitrofurans)	S (Nitrofurans)	V	V	S	R
Quinoline and isoquinoline derivatives	S	R	S	R	S	MR

Code: S = Sensitive; MS = Moderately sensitive; MR = Moderately resistant; R = Resistant; V = Variable results.
** see Morris & Darlow (1971). Many agents are virucidal in vitro, but difficult to assess in vivo.
* except to Lysol.
+ Resistant to acridines. Crystal violet is fungistatic, and virucidal. Brilliant green has virucidal activity.

bactericidal action in the case of *Staph.aureus* (Fry 1957). Gentian violet is thought to inhibit cell wall synthesis. Acridines impair the function of cellular DNA, thus interfering with reproduction of bacteria. Albert (1951) gives a general review of the acridines.

The main action of the surface-active agents, particularly the positively charged quaternary ammonium compounds, is that they are strongly adsorbed onto the negatively charged bacterial surface. This is followed by damage to the cell membrane and cytoplasmic leakage.

Hugo and Longworth (1964, 1965, 1966) conclude that chlorhexidine, the main guanidine disinfectant, disrupts and finally destroys cytoplasmic membrane function. The mode of action of amidines used in therapy is uncertain, although a similar chemical compound, pentamidine (an antiprotozoon drug) is thought to inhibit amino acid transport linked with phospholipid synthesis.

Suggested reasons for the antibacterial activity of the nitrofurans include inhibition of hydrogen and electron transfer enzyme systems, reduction of nitrofurans (thus reducing the capacity of the reductive enzymes in metabolism), and controversial evidence of inhibition of cell wall synthesis. No definite mode of action has yet been established.

8-hydroxyquinoline (oxine) chelates with iron or copper to form a toxic complex, which is thought to oxidize essential thiol groups (Rubbo & Gardner 1965).

PROPERTIES OF DISINFECTANTS

These will be dealt with for each of the 10 main groups of disinfectants mentioned earlier. Lethal activity is shown in Table 30.2.

Phenols
Phenols used as disinfectants include phenol itself (carbolic acid), cresol and chlorocresol (*p*-chlor-*m*-cresol), xylenols (the *m*-isomer being most active),

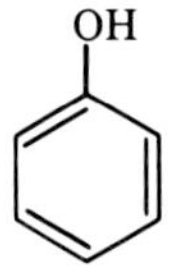

Phenol

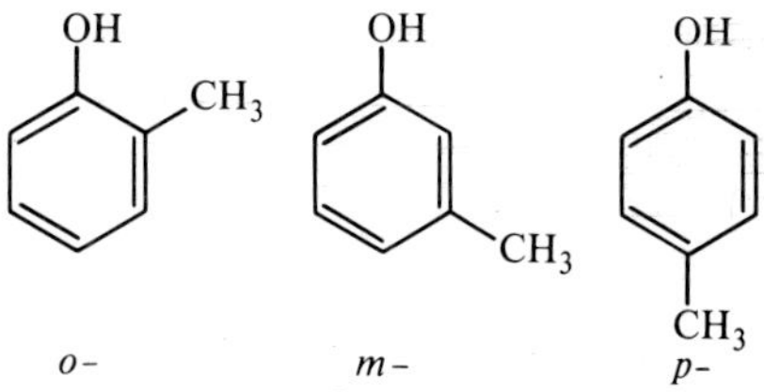

Cresol

Cresol BP is a mixture of these

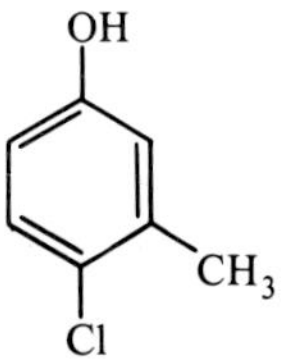

Chlorocresol
(parachlorometacresol or
6-chloro-3-hydroxytoluene)

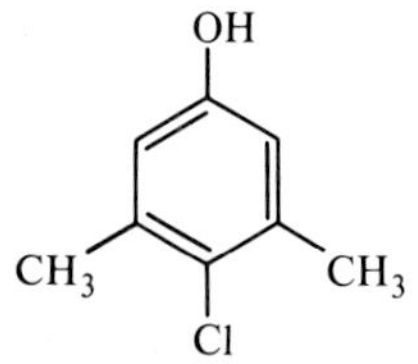

Chloroxylenol
(parachlorometaxylenol or
2-chloro-5-hydroxy-1,3-dimethylbenzene)

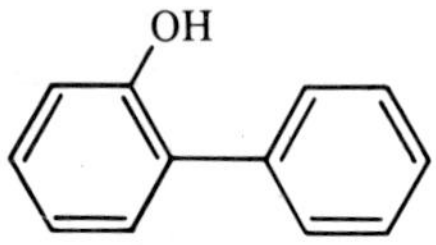

o-phenylphenol
(an arylphenol)

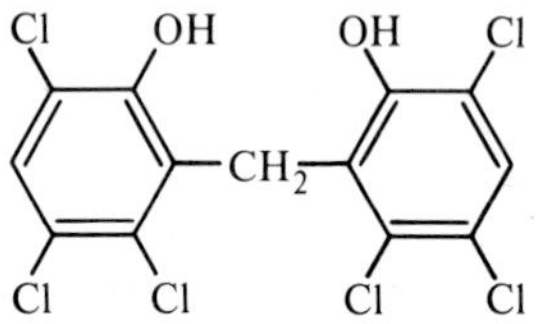

Hexachlorophane
(a bisphenol, also named
di-(3,5,6-trichloro-2-hydroxyphenyl)
methane or 2,2′-methylene-bis-
3,4,6-trichlorophenol)

FIG. 30.2. Chemical structures of the more important phenolic disinfectants.

chlorophenols, and chloroxylenols. Many are produced from coal tar distillates, e.g. cresols and xylenols, while more costly chlorinated phenols are produced synthetically. Other important phenols include arylphenols, e.g. *o*-phenylphenol, and bisphenols, e.g. hexachlorophane. The chemical structures of the more important phenols are given in Fig. 30.2.

With the exception of hexachlorophane the activity of phenols diminishes markedly with dilution. Activity generally increases with an increase in temperature, and they are more active at an acid pH (the phenate ion being much less active than the free phenol). Organic matter diminishes the bactericidal action of phenols, but the extent of the reduction depends on the amount and nature of the organic matter and the type of phenol concerned. Usually the higher the phenol coefficient (see section on disinfectant evaluation) the greater is the reduction of bactericidal activity due to organic matter (see Table 30.20). The organic matter simply adsorbs the phenol, and thus reduces its concentration.

The simple phenols are readily soluble in water, but the chlorinated phenols, e.g. chlorocresol and chloroxylenol, have poor water solubility. The chlorinated phenols have the advantage, however, that they are more potent, less toxic and less caustic than simple phenols. Most phenols are readily soluble in alcohol, the alcohol often enhancing their activity, but such solutions are extremely toxic to tissues and when diluted with water the phenolic material is thrown out of solution. Phenols have high oil-water coefficients, so the presence of oily material in the environment to be disinfected will markedly reduce the disinfectant action of the phenol. Oily solutions of phenol are devoid of bactericidal action.

Activity may be increased by the presence of soap in the formulation, e.g. Lysol (Cresol and Soap Solution BP) and Roxenol (Chloroxylenol Solution BPC).

Simple phenols are corrosive, cause tissue damage, and if adsorbed systematically (this may occur by adsorption from tissues) are very poisonous.

Phenol (carbolic acid). Its germicidal properties were discovered by Lister in 1867. Since many of its derivatives are less toxic and less caustic, the main uses of phenol itself are as a standard against which other germicides are compared; as an added bactericide to multi-dose injections (0.5 per cent w/v); in gargles (see BPC), and mouthwashes; in ear drops (6.4 per cent w/w, but the caustic action is lessened by the use of glycerin as solvent—this preparation should never be diluted with water), and as an oily injection (this is used as a sclerosing agent for internal haemorrhoids). For full details of the uses of this disinfectant and others mentioned in this chapter see Martindale (1972).

Cresol. This is a mixture of *o*-, *m*-, and *p*-cresols, in which the meta-isomer predominates, and other phenols obtained from coal tar. It has similar caustic and toxic properties to phenol, but has the disadvantage of being less soluble in water (1:50), though it is more strongly bactericidal than phenol.

Cresol and Soap Solution BP (Lysol). This is a useful disinfectant, in which cresol is solubilized with soap. Its corrosive action on living tissue has restricted its use, although similar formulations using ethylphenols and xylenols in place of cresol can be used on the skin and yet have comparable properties to lysol (Finch 1963). Bacterial spores (especially spores of clostridia) are resistant to lysol, but most pathogenic bacteria are susceptible, including acid-fast bacteria (mycobacteria). It forms a clear solution on dilution with water. Between 2 to 5 per cent is recommended for disinfection of contaminated surfaces. The higher concentration is recommended for killing mycobacteria, Report to the Public Health Laboratory Service, 1958.

Chlorocresol. It is used in the sterilization process 'heating with a bactericide', and as an added bactericide to multi-dose injections (0.2 per cent w/v for the sterilization process, and 0.1 per cent w/v as an added bactericide). It is only soluble 1:260 in water.

Chloroxylenol. This is even less soluble than chlorocresol. Solubility is 1:3000 in water, but it can be solubilized with soap (Roxenol BPC). It is used in many proprietary disinfectants, e.g. 'Dettol'.

It is active against streptococci, less active against staphylococci, and almost devoid of action against some Gram-negative organisms, e.g. *Pseudomonas aeruginosa*, and against bacterial spores.

Chloroxylenol Solution BPC (Roxenol). The chloroxylenol is solubilized by soap, but the formulation also includes terpineol (an oily carrier which helps solubilize the chloroxylenol in the form of a complex emulsion on dilution, and gives the formulation a pine-like odour) and alcohol. Doubts have been expressed about the effectiveness of the diluted form of this disinfectant. (Whittet, Hugo & Wilkinson 1965).

Black Fluids and White Fluids. These are cheaper than Chloroxylenol and similar solutions. Both fluids are defined in British Standard B.S. 2462: 1961. Black fluids are homogeneous solutions of coal tar acids, or similar crude petroleum acids. They are usually solubilized by soaps (made from interaction of resin acids with sodium hydroxide, or of sodium hydroxide with sulphonated oils). An example of a modified black fluid is 'Jeyes' Fluid'. White fluids are finely dispersed emulsions, not solutions, of coal tar or similar crude petroleum acids, and are more stable on dilution than black fluids. An example of a modified white fluid is 'Izal Germicide'. Black and white fluids are usually used for the disinfection of drains, agricultural and horticultural equipment, etc.

Bisphenols. Examples of these are *o*-phenylphenol and hexachlorophane. The former has antibacterial and antifungal properties, with similar potency to chloroxylenol, although its activity against *Pseudomonas aeruginosa* is superior to that of chloroxylenol. Hexachlorophane, until recently, widely used in soaps, dusting powders and skin preparations, as a deodorant and disinfectant, is practically insoluble in water. Use of hexachlorophane was curbed in 1972, due to its toxic side-effects, particularly in preparations for infants. It has a relatively weak effect against Gram-negative bacteria. The activities of bisphenols against *Staph. aureus* are listed by Gump and Walter (1960).

Alcohols

These have a fairly rapid bactericidal action against vegetative bacteria when diluted to concentrations of 60 to 70 per cent v/v with water (the water potentiates the denaturation of bacterial proteins by the alcohol). Both ethanol (60 to 70 per cent v/v) and isopropanol (50 to 60 per cent v/v) are used as skin disinfectants, while methanol vapour has been used as a fungicide. Ethanol is not self-sterilizing, and if required for surgery and similar purposes must be sterilized by filtration before use. Alcohols are used as preservatives in some vaccines, e.g. 25 per cent ethanol used in T.A.B. Vaccine BP, and in tinctures. 2-Phenoxyethanol is useful, as it is particularly active against *Pseudomonas aeruginosa* (*pyocyanea*), even in the presence of serum. It has a water solubility of 1 in 43, and is usually used as a 2.2 per cent w/v solution. Phenylethyl alcohol (0.25 to 0.5 per cent w/v) is active against Gram-negative organisms, except *Ps.aeruginosa*, and is used, usually with another bactericide, to preserve ophthalmic preparations. Chemical structures of the more important alcoholic disinfectants are given in Fig. 30.3. Chlorbutol (2,2,2-Trichloro-1,1-dimethylethanol hemihydrate) has limited applications in the preservation of eye-drops and parenteral injections (0.5 per cent w/v). It is rather unstable on heating, is thrown out of solution at low temperatures, and decomposes in alkaline solutions.

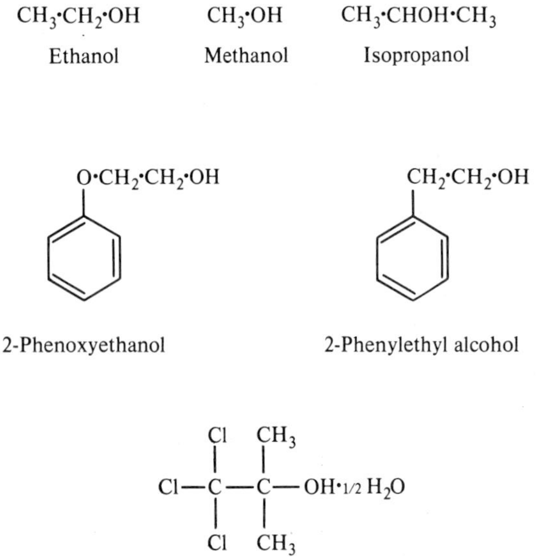

$$CH_3 \cdot CH_2 \cdot OH \qquad CH_3 \cdot OH \qquad CH_3 \cdot CHOH \cdot CH_3$$

Ethanol   Methanol   Isopropanol

2-Phenoxyethanol   2-Phenylethyl alcohol

Chlorbutol (2,2,2-Trichloro-1,1-dimethylethanol hemi-hydrate)

FIG. 30.3. Chemical structures of more important alcoholic disinfectants.

Aldehydes

Formaldehyde (H.CHO) is the main aldehyde used for disinfection. It is effective as a gas or as an aqueous solution (Formaldehyde Solution BP, or Formalin) containing 34 to 38 per cent w/w of CH_2O. Formaldehyde tends to polymerize to form paraformaldehyde. This solid polymer may be vapourized to yield formaldehyde. Formaldehyde is sporicidal. It is irritant to tissues and eyes, and causes hardening and wrinkling of the skin. Alcohol is usually included in solutions to prevent poymerization, and borax may also be included to prevent rusting of metal instruments. Virus infectivity can be destroyed by formaldehyde without destruction of antigenic properties, and it is therefore used to prepare certain viral vaccines, e.g. Poliomyelitis Vaccine (Inactivated) BP and Influenza Vaccine BP.

Glutaraldehyde ($CHO.CH_2.CH_2.CH_2.CHO$) is a dialdehyde with rapid sporicidal and tuberculocidal action (Rubbo, Gardner & Webb 1967). It is used as a 2 per cent aqueous solution, buffered with sodium bicarbonate to pH 7.5 to 8.5.

Dyes

In general, basic dyes are more effective bactericides than acidic dyes. Two main classes are used as disinfectants: *acridine* dyes and *triphenylmethane* dyes.

Acridine dyes. Most of these dyes are orange-yellow, with the exception of the non-staining aminacrine. They are useful skin disinfectants, as they are not inactivated by serum and are not adsorbed on dressings. Apart from aminacrine hydrochloride, the main acridine dyes in use are acriflavine and proflavine. Problems encountered with acridine dyes include their relatively slow action and the development of bacterial resistance to them. Their chemical structures are shown in Fig. 30.4.

Triphenylmethane dyes. Due to their intense staining action these compounds are only of limited use as antiseptics. They are not inactivated by serum but are readily adsorbed by dressings. They inhibit staphylococci and streptococci, but high concentrations are required to inhibit Gram-negative organisms. The three main dyes used in medicine are brilliant green, crystal violet (also known as gentian violet or methyl violet) and malachite green. Crystal violet agar (containing 1 in 100 000 crystal violet) inhibits staphylococci but not streptococci and is used as a selective medium. Aqueous solutions of single dyes or combinations of dyes are used to treat staphylococcal and mycotic skin infections. Chemical structures are shown in Fig. 30.4.

Acridine dyes

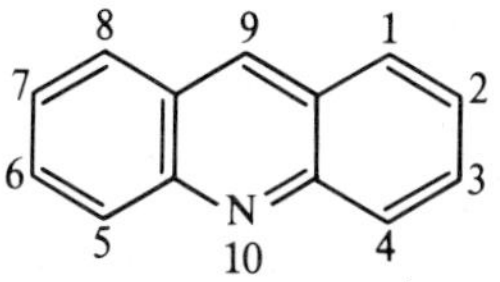

This shows the ring
numbering in the current BP and BPC

Acridine

Acriflavine (mixture of two dyes below)

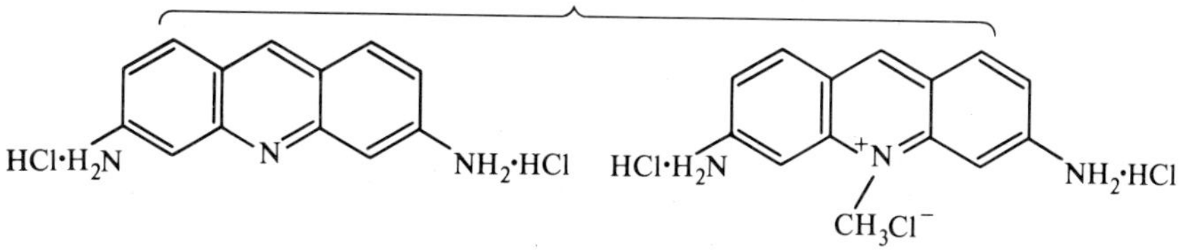

3,6-Diaminoacridine dihydrochloride

3,6-Diamino-10-methylacridinium chloride

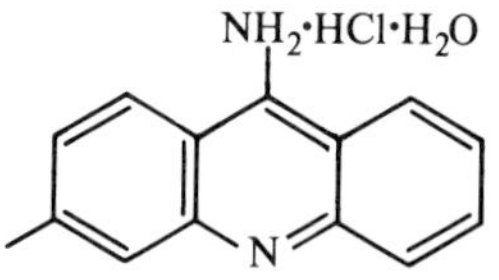

Aminacrine hydrochloride
(9-Aminoacridine hydrochloride)

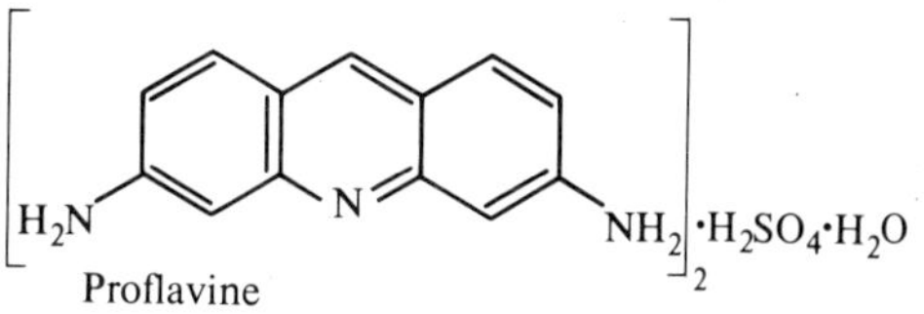

Proflavine
(3,6-Diaminoacridine hemisulphate)

Triphenylmethane dyes

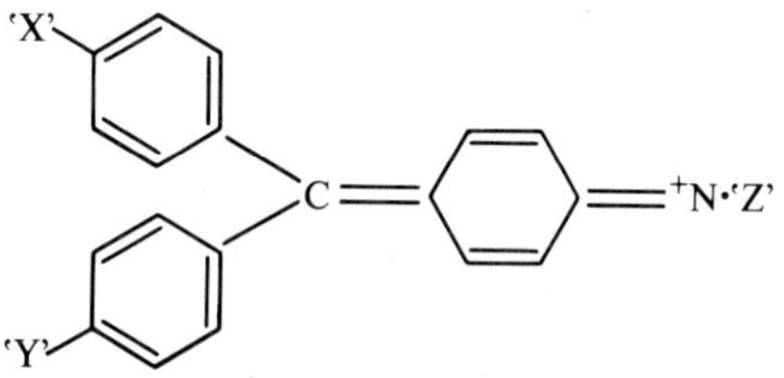

Basic structure

Crystal violet
'X' = $(CH_3)_2N$, 'Y' = $(CH_3)_2N$,
'Z' = $(CH_3)_2 \cdot Cl^-$

Brilliant green
'X' = $(C_2H_5)_2 N$, no group at 'Y',
'Z' = $(C_2H_5)_2 \cdot HSO_4^-$

Malachite green
$(CH_3)_2N$, no group at 'Y',
'Z' = $(CH_3)_2 \cdot Cl^-$

FIG. 30.4. Chemical structures of more important antibacterial dyes.

Surface-active Compounds

There are four basic types of compound; these are:
anionic, e.g. soaps (sodium stearate)—slightly antibacterial; *cationic*, e.g. Cetrimide—bactericidal;
non-ionic, e.g. Sorbitan mono-oleate—devoid of
antibacterial activity; and *amphoteric or ampholytic*,
e.g. 'Tego' compounds—bactericidal and fungicidal. Only cationic and amphoteric or ampholytic types are important disinfectants.

Cationic compounds. The compounds used are
quaternary ammonium compounds (QACs or
QUATs), and have the general formula:

$$\left[\begin{array}{c} R_1 \\ | \\ R_4 - N - R_2 \\ | \\ R_3 \end{array} \right]^+ \quad Hal^-$$

They are incompatible with soaps, and are represented in the BP by Cetrimide, Cetylpyridinium
chloride and Domiphen Bromide. Benzalkonium
chloride is listed in the *International Pharmacopoeia*. Many are inactivated by non-ionic
surface-active agents such as Tween 80 and Lubrol
W. In water they ionize into the halide ion (anion)

and the long-chain ion (cation). The latter is hydrophobic and endows the compound with its surface activity. They are strongly adsorbed onto negatively charged surfaces, e.g. bacterial cells, where they cause damage to the cytoplasmic membrane and hence leakage of cytoplasmic material. They are widely used for skin and wound disinfection where their cleansing action in the presence of oil and grease are particularly useful. Their action is markedly reduced by organic matter. Unlike the phenols, the quaternaries are more active in alkaline solution but are incompatible with alkali hydroxides. At pH 3 many quaternaries are practically devoid of activity.

The chemical structures of some cationic disinfectants are given in Fig. 30.5.

Amphoteric or ampholytic compounds. These compounds contain both cationic and anionic groups in the same molecule. Their ionic properties therefore depend on the pH as shown below:

Acid solution	$R.\overset{+}{N}H_2CH_2CH_2COOH$	Cationic
Iso-electric point	$R.\overset{+}{N}H_2CH_2CH_2COO^-$	Non-ionic
Alkaline solution	$R.NH.CH_2CH_2COO^-$	Anionic

They have the detergent properties of anionic surfactants combined with the disinfectant properties of cationic surfactants. In general these materials are said to be compatible with quaternary ammonium compounds and phenolic disinfectants. Examples are the 'Tego' compounds. The structures of the main surfactants used as disinfectants are given in Fig. 30.5.

Halogens

Both chlorine and iodine derivatives, as well as chlorine and iodine themselves, are widely used as disinfectants. Chlorine is used universally in the treatment of water supplies, in the disinfection of swimming pool water, as a disinfectant and deodorant in sewage, and in the disinfection of dairy equipment. In medicine, hypochlorites are used in the treatment of wound infections.

Chlorine and hypochlorites react rapidly and powerfully with organic matter and are efficient bactericides, even in quite low concentrations. A chlorine content of 0.2 to 1.0 part per million gives a wide margin of safety to drinking water. Because it reacts so readily with organic matter, much of its bactericidal activity is lost in the presence of the latter. A solution of chlorine in water contains hypochlorous acid, and it is thought that the undissociated form of this acid is responsible for the activity of chlorine against bacteria. Chlorine is sporicidal and fungicidal, although some spores are moderately resistant.

The activity of hypochlorites is markedly affected by pH. They are most active at low pH values and activity declines with increasing pH, although stability increases. Increase in pH produces an increase in ionization of the hypochlorous acid.

The main chlorine disinfectants include chlorine gas, chlorinated lime and preparations from this, hypochlorites, and inorganic and organic chloramines. The main iodine disinfectants include various solutions and iodophors (where iodine is complexed with surface-active agents).

Chlorinated lime. This is a cheap, powerful disinfectant and deodorant. It is used to disinfect faeces, urine, and utensils. Eusol and Dakin's Solution

$$(CH_3)_3N^+(C_nH_{2n+1})Br^-$$

Cetrimide or alkyltrimethylammonium bromide. It is a mixture with n = 12, 14 or 16.

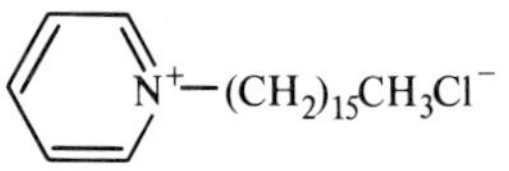

$$\text{N}^+\!\!-\!(CH_2)_{15}CH_3Cl^-$$

Cetylpyridinium chloride

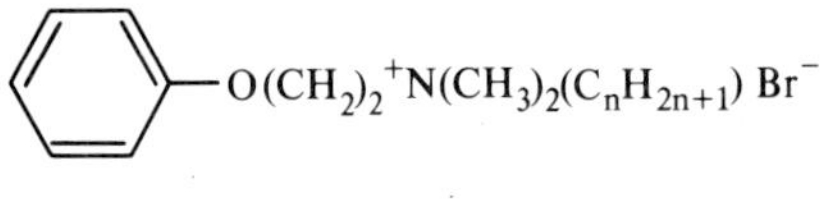

$$-O(CH_2)_2{}^+N(CH_3)_2(C_nH_{2n+1})\ Br^-$$

Domiphen or phenoxyethyldimethylalkylammonium bromide. n = 12 to 14.

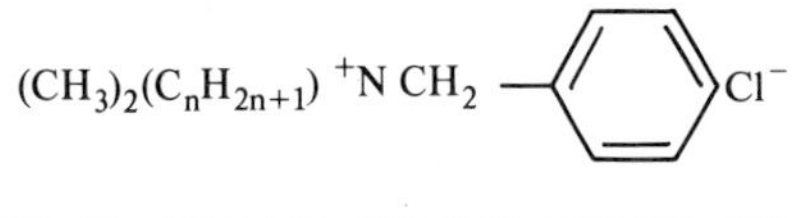

$$(CH_3)_2(C_nH_{2n+1})^+N\ CH_2-\!\!\!\!\!\!\!\text{Cl}^-$$

Benzalkonium chloride. n = 8 to 18.

$$C_{12}H_{25}.NH.C_2H_4.NH.C_2H_4.NH.CH_2.COOH$$

'Tego 1305'—amphoteric or ampholytic

Fig. 30.5. Chemical structures of the main surfactant disinfectants.

are both prepared from chlorinated lime and contain hypochlorites. Both solutions deteriorate on storage but Dakin's Solution is somewhat more stable than Eusol.

Organic chloramines. Those used in medicine include Chloramine, Dichloramine, and Halazone. Their structures are shown in Fig. 30.6. Solutions of these compounds are more stable than those prepared from chlorinated lime. Halazone is used for sterilization of drinking water (4 mg/litre, left for 1 h). The taste of residual chlorine can be removed by adding sodium thiosulphate, usually in tablet form (5.5 mg).

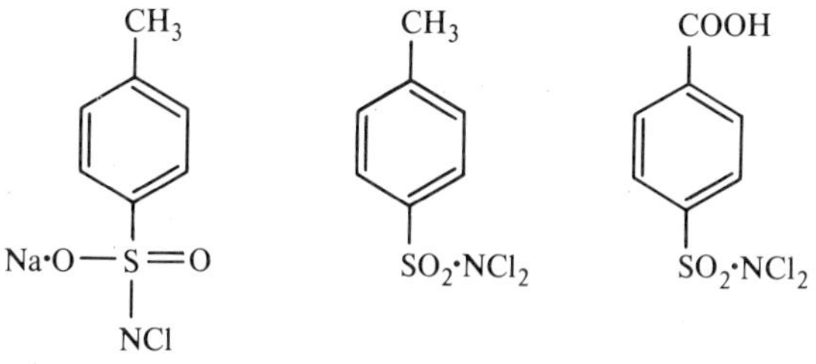

FIG. 30.6. Chemical structures of main organic chloramines.

Iodine disinfectants. Iodine itself is a good disinfectant in aqueous or alcoholic solution. It is remarkably non-selective in its action. It is sporicidal, fungicidal, and active against many viruses. It is used as a skin disinfectant and for cold sterilization of surgical sutures. Formulations include Weak Iodine Solution BP (2.5 per cent Iodine) and Aqueous Iodine Solution BP (Lugol's Solution—5.0 per cent Iodine). Iodophors, in which the iodine is complexed with surface-active agents, e.g. polyvinylpyrrolidone-iodine are said to be more stable in dilute solutions, and are non-staining and non-irritant. Iodine itself has to be used with care on sensitive skins.

Iodoform has weak antibacterial properties, but is chiefly used as a deodorant.

Metals
Metal disinfectants include *mercury* compounds; *silver* compounds; and *copper* compounds.

Mercury compounds. There are two types: simple inorganic compounds, e.g. mercuric chloride, and more complex organic compounds such as the phenylmercuric compounds. Many mercurial compounds are only slowly bactericidal and fungicidal, and this limits their use as disinfectants. Mercuric

chloride solution (0.1 per cent), although a rapid bactericide, is highly toxic, corrosive to both tissues and metal instruments, and is thus rarely used. Mercuric oxycyanide, which is far less toxic than mercuric chloride, is used at a concentration of 0.1 to 0.2 per cent in the treatment of conjunctivitis. Ammoniated mercury (NH_2HgCl) is used in ointments, often in conjunction with coal tar phenols and salicylic acid, to treat skin infections. Yellow mercuric oxide has been used in eye ointments. Mercurochrome, a vivid red dye, is a comparatively feeble germicide, and has lost popularity. Thiomersal (Merthiolate) has similar bactericidal potency to phenylmercuric compounds, but it is unstable in acid solutions and is therefore only used in solutions of pH 7 upwards. It is used as a preservative (0.01 to 0.02 per cent) for bacterial and viral vaccines, as a fungicide and as a skin disinfectant.

Phenylmercuric nitrate and phenylmercuric acetate are both effective antibacterial and antifungal agents. The acetate has the advantage that it is slightly more soluble than the nitrate. Both the nitrate and the acetate can be used, at a concentration of 0.002 per cent, in the sterilization process 'heating with a bactericide'. They can be used as preservatives for parenteral injections at a concentration of 0.001 per cent. The activity of mercurials is modified by organic matter.

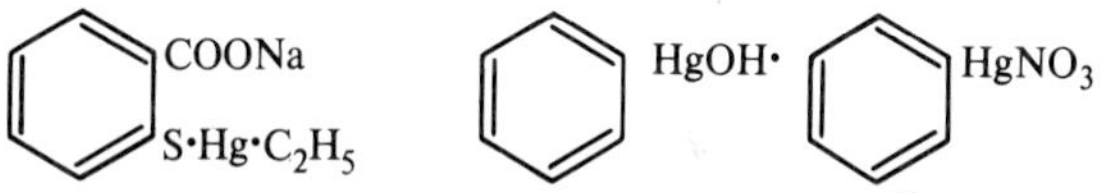

Thiomersal   Phenylmercuric nitrate (basic)

The disinfectant action of phenylmercuric compounds is due to complex phenylmercuric ions; they do not ionize into phenol ions and mercuric ions.

Silver compounds. Silver nitrate solutions of 0.2 to 0.6 per cent have been used to treat eye infections. Silver protein derivatives (Silver Protein, and Mild Silver Protein BPC) have antibacterial properties, due to the presence of low concentrations of ionized silver, and are also used in eye-drops.

Copper compounds. These are mainly used as fungicides and algicides.

Guanidines and Amidines
The main guanide disinfectant is chlorhexidine, and is available as a digluconate, diacetate, or dihydrochloride of 1:6-di(N-*p*-chlorophenyldiguanido)-hexane.

Chlorhexidine. It is bactericidal against a wide range of Gram-positive and Gram-negative vegetative bacteria, but is ineffective against acid-fast bacteria, bacterial spores, and viruses. It is nevertheless a very good skin disinfectant. Variation in

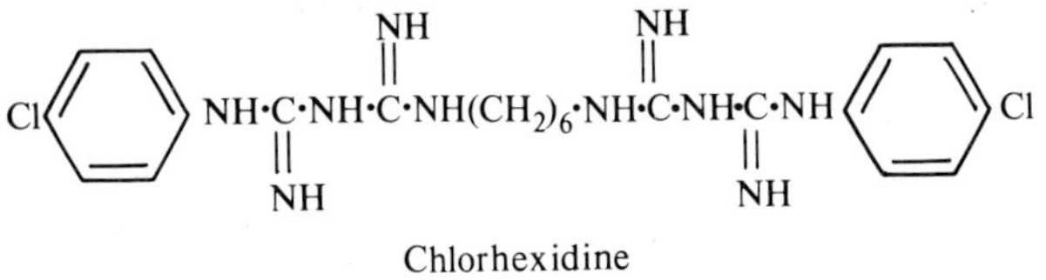

Chlorhexidine

resistance occurs in the *Pseudomonas* and *Proteus* spp. Chlorhexidine is most active in neutral or slightly alkaline pH, but its activity is reduced by blood and organic matter. The gluconate and hydrochloride are mainly used. The acetate is used for preservation of eye-drops. The hydrochloride has the longest antibacterial action.

The main amidines are Dibromopropamidine isethionate BP and Propamidine isethionate BPC 1949. Resistance to the amidines develops and this limits their use. The action of these two amidines

Dibromopropamidine isethionate

is not affected by tissue fluids, serum or pus, and they are used in eye-drops and antiseptic creams.

Furan Derivatives

Nitrofurazone is the main derivative of interest, as it has antibacterial action against a number of vegetative bacteria. Formulations are usually applied topically and include creams, ointments, solutions, and ear-drops.

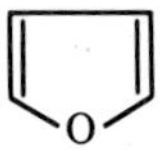

Furan 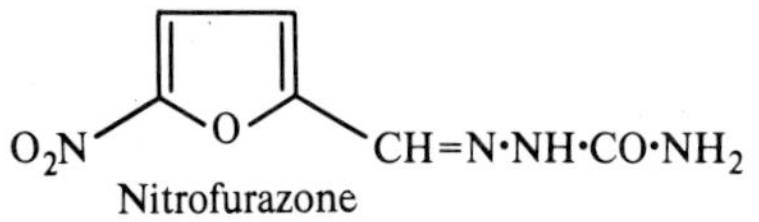   Nitrofurazone

Quinoline and Isoquinoline Derivatives

8-Hydroxyquinoline is both bactericidal and fungicidal, but its activity is entirely dependent on the presence of traces of divalent metals, e.g. copper and iron. The lethal agent is a metal oxine complex (oxine is another name for 8-hydroxyquinoline), although the ratio of concentrations of oxine to metals affects the toxicity of the complex.

Dequalinium chloride ('Dequadin') and dequalinium acetate are both antibacterial and antifungal. Their action is little affected by serum. The main use of the chloride is in lozenges for treatment of mouth and throat infections.

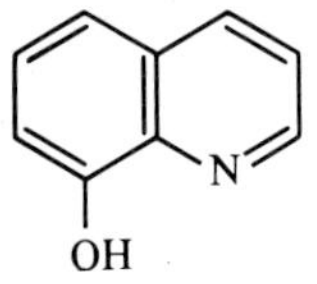

8-Hydroxyquinoline

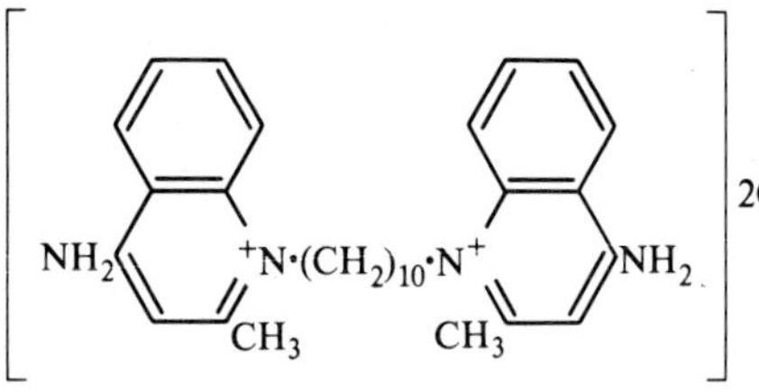

'Dequadin'
(Decamethylene-bis-(4-aminoquinaldinium) chloride)

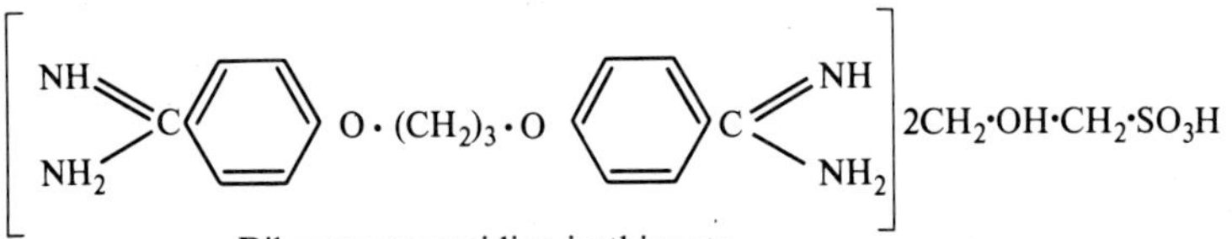

In addition to these ten groups of disinfectant compounds, there are a number of specific antifungal agents, e.g. undecenoic acid and salts, tolnaftate, chlorphenesin, etc.

FACTORS AFFECTING DISINFECTANT ACTION

Some of the main factors affecting disinfectant action are:
Time of contact.
Concentration of disinfectant.
Temperature.
The type of organism present, its numbers and condition.
The presence of organic matter, and other inactivators.
Hydrogen ion concentration.
Surface tension.
The formulation of the disinfectant.
The chemical structure of the disinfectant.
The nature of the surface to be disinfected.
Potentiation, synergism, and antagonism of disinfectants.

Time of Contact

A plot of the viable count of a bacterial population against time, when the population is subjected to a lethal environment, will give a death or mortality curve. Madsen and Nyman (1907), and Chick (1908), working independently, showed the course of disinfection to approximate that of a unimolecular reaction. It was shown that the principles of first-order kinetics could be applied to the disinfection process, and that the rate or velocity constant, k, was a measure of the efficiency of the disinfectant.

$$k = \frac{1}{t} \log \frac{B}{b}$$

where t = time for the viable count to fall from B to b.

B = initial number of organisms.

b = final number of organisms.

Since this early work the disinfection process has been widely studied (Withell 1938, 1942; Jordan & Jacobs 1944; Berry & Michaels 1947; Jacobs 1960; Prokop & Humphrey 1970). The main conclusion of these workers is that the survivor/time curve is not constant, its shape being influenced by a number of factors, especially the concentration of the disinfectant being used. This is shown in Fig. 30.7.

Three main types of death curve are shown in disinfection processes, and these are given on Fig. 30.8.

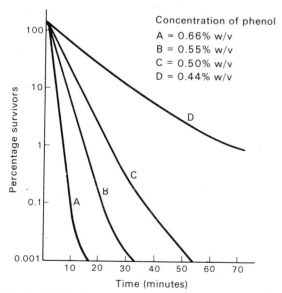

FIG. 30.7. Effect of concentration of phenol on survivor/time curves of *Escherichia coli*.

Concentration of phenol

A = 0.66% w/v
B = 0.55% w/v
C = 0.50% w/v
D = 0.44% w/v

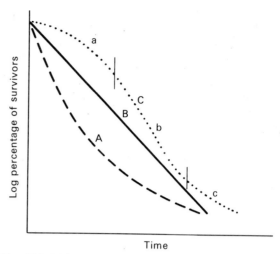

FIG. 30.8. Main types of death curve shown in disinfection processes. A, Disinfection process obeying first order kinetic law (sometimes obtained); B, Sigmoid curve is most usually obtained. The process can be divided into 3 stages: (a) a slow initial kill, mainly of sensitive or susceptible members of the population, (b) a faster 'near-linear' rate of kill showing a similar pattern to a first order reaction. In this stage organisms of average resistance are mainly killed, (c) a slower death rate of resistant members; C, This curve is often obtained with high concentrations of disinfectant.

Concentration of Disinfectant

The relationship between concentration and the time taken to kill the organisms, at a given temperature, is exponential, i.e. doubling the concentration considerably more than halves the rate if the concentration exponent is greater than 1. This can be expressed in the equation:

$$C^n.t = \text{a constant}$$

where C = concentration

n = concentration exponent or dilution coefficient for the disinfectant

t = death time

The equation may be written:

$$n \log C + \log t = \text{a constant}$$

If therefore a graph is plotted of $\log t$ against $\log C$ a straight line is usually obtained, and the slope of the line is the concentration exponent (Fig. 30.9). The value of n may therefore be obtained graphically or by substitution in the equation:

$$n = \frac{\log t_2 - \log t_1}{\log C_1 - \log C_2}$$

where t_1 is the death time with disinfectant concentration C_1.

t_2 is the death time with disinfectant concentration C_2.

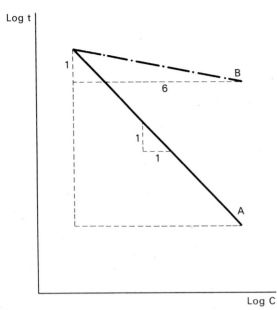

FIG. 30.9. Graphical determination of concentration exponent n, of disinfectants. A, slope of graph 1/1, n = 1; B, slope of graph 1/6, n = 6.

The approximate values of n for common bactericides are given in Table 30.3.

TABLE 30.3

VALUES OF n FOR COMMON BACTERICIDES

Bactericide	n	Bactericide	n
$HgCl_2$	1	Thymol	4
$AgNO_3$	0.75	Resorcinol	5
HCl	1	Phenol	6
HCHO	1	o-cresol	7.5
NaOH	1.5	p-cresol	8.5
H_2O_2	2	ethanol	11.5
Lysol	2.5	butanol	12

The value of n is affected by the factors which influence disinfection, e.g. temperature, type of organism, environmental factors, and the formulation.

A knowledge of the approximate concentration exponent is useful in determining the effect of dilution on the disinfectant, as shown in Table 30.4.

TABLE 30.4

COMPARISON OF INCREASED AND DECREASED CONCENTRATION ON KILLING RATES OF PHENOL AND FORMALDEHYDE AGAINST *E.coli*

Phenol (n = 6) 0.7% kills in 100 min	Formaldehyde (n = 1) 0.7% kills in 100 min
(A) Effect of doubling concentration 1.4% kills in $\dfrac{100}{2^n} = \dfrac{100}{2^6}$ = 1.6 min	1.4% kills in $\dfrac{100}{2^1}$ = 50 min
(B) Effect of halving concentration 0.35% kills in 100×2^n $= 100 \times 2^6$ $= 6400$ min	0.35% kills in 100×2^1 $= 200$ min

This explains why phenolic disinfectants are rapidly inactivated by dilution, but disinfectants such as formaldehyde or mercurials are much less affected by changes in concentration.

Temperature

An increase in the temperature of a bactericide increases the velocity of the bacterial reaction just as it does the velocity of a chemical reaction. As the temperature increases arithmetically the activity of a given concentration of bactericide against a standard inoculum of bacteria increases geometrically, the relation between temperature and extinction time being shown in Fig. 30.10.

The relation between temperature and the velocity of a bactericidal reaction may be expressed by the equation:

$$\theta^{(T_2 - T_1)} = \frac{k^2}{k_1}$$

where k_1 = reaction velocity at temperature T_1
k_2 = reaction velocity at temperature T_2
θ = temperature coefficient

The reaction velocity, k, is proportional to

$$\frac{1}{\text{extinction time}}$$

Thus, providing the inoculum level is the same, the above equation becomes:

$$\theta^{(T_2 - T_1)} = \frac{k_2}{k_1} = \frac{t_1}{t_2}$$

where t_1 = extinction time at T_1°
t_2 = extinction time at T_2°
(extinction time is the time at which no living cells can be detected in the sample taken)

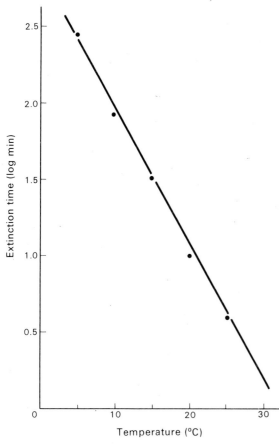

FIG. 30.10. Relation between temperature and extinction time of *Salmonella paratyphi* in 1.0 per cent phenol solution.

The following example illustrates the use of the equation to determine the value of the temperature coefficient per degree rise in temperature. In an experiment with ethylene glycol monohexyl ether, the test organisms (*E.coli*) were killed in 62 min at 20°C and in 10 min at 30°C.

$$\theta^{(30-20)} = \frac{62}{10} = 6.2$$

$$10 \log \theta = \log 6.2$$

$$\log \theta = \frac{0.7924}{10}$$

$$\theta = 1.20$$

The temperature coefficient may also be calculated from the percentage of survivors knowing:

$$k_1 = \frac{1}{t_1} \cdot \log \frac{B_1}{b_1} \quad \text{and} \quad k_2 = \frac{1}{t_2} \cdot \log \frac{B_2}{b_2}$$

Some values for θ for different bactericides are shown in Table 30.5 below. Also recorded are θ^{10} or ϕ_{10} values—the increase in activity for 10° rise in temperature. All figures refer to temperature in the range 20 to 30°C.

TABLE 30.5

VALUES OF θ FOR COMMON BACTERICIDES

Bactericide	θ	ϕ_{10}
Phenol	1.15	4.0
o-cresol	1.18	5.1
p-cresol	1.19	5.8
resorcinol	1.22	7.1
ethylene glycol	1.34	18.0
n-butanol	1.41	31.0
ethanol	1.46	43
ethylene glycol monoethyl ether	1.76	291

In practice the ϕ_{10} value is most useful, and bactericides may be grouped according to this value. The effect of increasing the temperature of phenol from 20° to 30° is to increase its activity four-fold. The effect of increasing its temperature from 20° to 100° is theoretically to increase its activity $1.15^{80} \equiv 70\,000$-fold, providing the value of θ is constant over the range of 80°, which is unlikely. Nevertheless, increasing the temperature of a phenol from room temperature to 100° will increase its activity very appreciably and, in addition, the high temperature itself will have an adverse effect on microorganisms. The combined effect of temperature and increase in reaction velocity at the higher temperature is utilized in the BP sterilization process of Heating with a Bactericide.

The Test Organism

The type of organism, the number, and the condition of the organisms all affect the disinfection process. The lethal activity of disinfectants against the main groups of microorganisms is given in Table 30.2. It can be seen that most vegetative bacteria, with the exceptions of acid-fast bacilli, are rapidly killed by most chemical disinfectants. Apart from acid-fast bacilli many *Pseudomonas* spp. are highly resistant to antimicrobial substances. Bacterial spores are difficult to destroy but some aldehydes are sporicidal. Aldehydes and halogens, together with β-propiolactone are most active virucides. Antifungal activity varies considerably and many disinfectants have a limited spectrum of activity.

The success of disinfection is often dependent, in part, on the degree of initial contamination. A large number of microorganisms initially often leads to longer disinfection times, or greater concentrations of disinfectant are required to achieve a satisfactory killing effect.

Resistance of microorganisms varies with their age and the conditions under which they are grown. A detailed review of the influence of inoculum history on the response of microorganisms to inhibitory and destructive agents is given by Farewell and Brown (1971).

In any description of disinfectant action the inoculum size, age, and past history should be stated.

The Presence of Organic Matter and Other Inactivators

Organic matter often exerts a marked influence on antimicrobial activity. The protective action may be due to mechanical protection of the cells against the action of the antimicrobial agent or to the combination of this with the organic matter. Chemically active compounds, e.g. the hypochlorites and formaldehyde, react readily with extracellular protein with a consequent fall in their bactericidal potency. The presence of oils and fats markedly reduces the disinfecting ability of phenolics. Mercurial disinfectants react with thiol groups in the environment. Adsorption and inactivation reduce the amount of disinfectant available to react with the cells, and the interfering substance may form a protective coat around the cell preventing penetration to the site of action.

Hydrogen Ion Concentration

The pH during the disinfection process affects:
  (a) the rate of growth of the microorganisms,
  (b) the degree of ionization of the antimicrobial substance and hence its potency,
  (c) the adsorption of the antimicrobial substance at the cell surface.

The optimum pH for bacterial growth is in the range 6 to 8. Outside this range, growth may be inhibited to some extent.

Some compounds, e.g. phenol, benzoic acid, salicylic acid, are most active in the unionized form. These compounds have pK_a values of 9.9, 4.2, and 3.0 respectively, and are least ionized and least active at an acid pH. Phenol, with a pK_a value of 9.9, is about 55 per cent ionized at pH 10, and since it is the unionized molecule which is active, has little activity at pH 10. Other examples are given in Table 30.6.

TABLE 30.6

EFFECT OF pH ON IONIZATION OF DISINFECTANTS

Phenol	Benzoic Acid
pK_a 9.9	pK_a 4.2
% ionized at various pH values	
pH 10–55	pH 7—over 99
pH 8–1.24	pH 3—6
pH 7–0.126	pH 2.2—1

Thus phenolic and acidic antimicrobial agents usually have greatest activity in acidic conditions. In the acridine compounds, however, it is the cation which is the active agent, and hence these are most active in the ionized form. Most acridines used as skin and wound antiseptics are well ionized at pH 7.0. Basic dyes, e.g. crystal violet, brilliant green, and cationic surfactants, e.g. cetrimide, increase in antibacterial activity with increase in pH. A review of the effects of pH on antibacterial activity is given by Albert (1973).

Surface Tension and Effect of Formulation

Many surface-active compounds and in particular the cationic quaternary ammonium compounds such as cetrimide are highly bactericidal themselves, but they can also affect the bactericidal efficiency of other substances. Alexander and Tomlinson (1949) have shown that the addition of small amounts of an anionic surface-active agent to phenol solution reduces the surface tension of the latter and reduces the extinction time of E.coli (Fig. 30.11), because of faster penetration of the bacteria by the phenol molecules.

Soaps can be used and the more soap that is added, the lower the surface tension and the extinction time, until the soap concentration is equivalent to the critical concentration for micelle formation. In excess of this concentration the surface tension remains almost constant, but the extinction time increases, due to phenol leaving the aqueous phase and entering the interior of micelles. For a review of effects of surface tension on antibacterial activity Berry (1952) should be consulted.

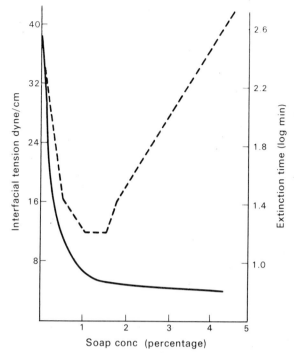

FIG. 30.11. Relation between extinction time of *Escherichia coli* and the interfacial tension of 0.5 per cent phenol/soap mixtures. (After Alexander & Tomlinson 1949).

Often disinfectants may be formulated in either aqueous solution or in 70 per cent alcohol, e.g. chlorhexidine and some quaternary ammonium compounds. The alcoholic formulation often increases penetrating power and leads to enhanced antimicrobial activity.

It has already been mentioned that the activity of phenol varies with the organism concerned, is reduced by oil and organic matter, and is highest when the phenol is in the non-ionized form, i.e. in acidic pH conditions. In addition the presence of a solubilizing or emulsifying agent and the type and concentration markedly affect the activity of the phenol (Berry & Stenlake 1942).

In simple saponaceous solution, the soap acts as a solvent for the phenols. If the phenol is partially soluble in water, a marked increase in its overall solubility in the soap solution occurs at the critical micelle concentration of the soap; if the phenol is almost water-insoluble then virtually no phenol goes into solution below the critical concentration. The differential solubility of chloroxylenol in potassium laurate is shown in Fig. 30.12. A sharp increase in the differential solubility of chloroxylenol occurs at 0.02 M potassium laurate, the critical concentration; above about 0.04 M potassium laurate, when the micelles are fully formed, there is no further increase in the differential solubility with increase in soap concentration. The shaded area in Fig. 30.12 is an area of solubility and the unshaded area an area of insolubility. An arbitrarily chosen point (X) within the area of solubility describes the composition of a solution since the position of the point indicates the soap concentration and the number of molecules of chloroxylenol present per molecule of soap. If the solution represented by X is diluted with water, the composition of the solutions produced by increasing dilution is represented by points along a line drawn from X parallel to the abscissa. The broken line in Fig. 30.12 shows the bactericidal activity against *E.coli* of solutions produced by dilution of X. A maximum activity (minimum extinction time)

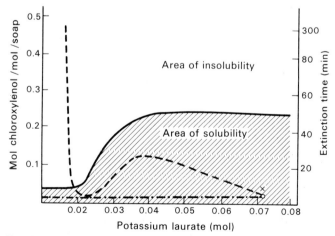

FIG. 30.12. Influence of soap concentration on the extinction time of *Escherichia coli* in soap/chloroxylenol mixtures. Solid line indicates solubility and the dotted line extinction time (Bean 1961).

is obtained in solutions in which the soap concentration is approximately 0.02 M (the CMC) and a minimum of activity in solutions in which the soap concentration is about 0.04 M. At 0.02 M potassium laurate the micelles are just forming and are small. Between 0.02 M and 0.04 M the micelles increase in size and reach maximal size at 0.04 M. For solutions having a constant chloroxylenol/ potassium laurate ratio the percentage saturation of the micelles by the chloroxylenol decreases as the soap micelles increase in size. That is, the decrease in activity which occurs in spite of an increase in the concentration of both the chloroxylenol and the soap is due to a decrease in the saturation of the micelles. Since the chloroxylenol is partitioned between the micelles and the water, the decrease in the concentration in the micelles is accompanied by a decrease in the water. Thus the bactericidal activity of simple saponaceous solutions of halogenated phenols is independent of the overall concentration in the system. It is dependent upon the concentration in the micelles which, in turn, controls the concentration in the water (Bean & Berry 1953). For further interpretations of similar systems reference should be made to papers by Berry, Cook and Wills (1956), Berry and Briggs (1956), Cook (1960) and Mitchell (1964).

Further evidence for the above explanation is provided by Alexander and Tomlinson (1949) who added a surfactant (dihexyl sodium sulphosuccinate) to 0.5 per cent phenol solution. Solutions containing about 1 per cent of the soap are more bactericidal than those containing either a higher or lower concentration (Fig. 30.11). The increase in bactericidal activity as the surfactant concentration is increased from zero to 1.0 per cent is due to the reduction of the surface tension of the system which reaches a minimum at about 1.0 per cent soap concentration, the critical concentration for micelle formation. On increasing the soap beyond this critical concentration, micelles are formed and there is competition between the micelles and the water for the phenol. The concentration of the phenol in the water gradually drops from the original 0.5 per cent as the micelles are formed, and there is progressive loss of bactericidal activity. Thus, the bactericidal activity of phenol in the surfactant solution is maximal at the CMC.

For convenience and economy it is essential to formulate a disinfectant solution to be as concentrated as possible and suitable for dilution with water immediately before use. The user cannot be relied upon to dilute the disinfectant to the critical concentration of the soap. Insufficient dilution

would cause loss of activity and over-dilution would probably result in phenol being thrown out of solution. The difficulty is solved by the inclusion of an oily carrier which is a solvent for the insoluble phenol, e.g. in Chloroxylenol Solution BPC. When Chloroxylenol Solution is diluted with water a complex system is formed. An o/w emulsion of terpineol is produced by part of the soap; the remainder of the soap is dispersed as micelles or is in solution in the water. The chloroxylenol is distributed between the terpineol droplets (most is in this oily carrier), the soap micelles and the water in accordance with the partition coefficients. The concentration in the carrier influences the concentration in the water, and thus selection of a carrier which gives maximum concentration of the chloroxylenol in water must be carefully made. Many organisms have been shown to be resistant to the diluted forms of formulated chloroxylenol preparations.

The Chemical Structure of the Disinfectant

A review of the effect of chemical structure on the activity of phenols is given by Suter (1941). A summary of this review is given in Table 30.7.

TABLE 30.7

EFFECT OF CHEMICAL STRUCTURE ON ACTIVITY OF PHENOLS

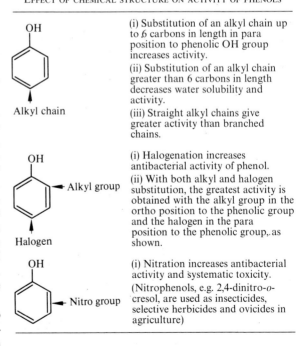

OH — Alkyl chain	(i) Substitution of an alkyl chain up to 6 carbons in length in para position to phenolic OH group increases activity. (ii) Substitution of an alkyl chain greater than 6 carbons in length decreases water solubility and activity. (iii) Straight alkyl chains give greater activity than branched chains.
OH — Alkyl group — Halogen	(i) Halogenation increases antibacterial activity of phenol. (ii) With both alkyl and halogen substitution, the greatest activity is obtained with the alkyl group in the ortho position to the phenolic group and the halogen in the para position to the phenolic group, as shown.
OH — Nitro group	(i) Nitration increases antibacterial activity and systematic toxicity. (Nitrophenols, e.g. 2,4-dinitro-o-cresol, are used as insecticides, selective herbicides and ovicides in agriculture)

The Nature of the Surface to be Disinfected

Uneven, porous or cracked surfaces resist chemical disinfection, due to the inaccessibility of the microorganisms. Often, deeply situated bacterial flora on the skin remain unaffected by disinfectants applied to the skin surface. Thus bactericides work effectively on hard, clean, impenetrable surfaces. Tests should be made to ensure that the disinfectant does not react adversely with the surface, does not leave detrimental residual effects which cannot be easily eliminated, and, in the case of living tissues, is not toxic to underlying cells.

Potentiation, Synergism, and Antagonism of Disinfectants

Potentiation of a disinfectant (usually by inactive substances) leads to enhanced antimicrobial activity. Synergistic effects are often shown by two antimicrobial agents working together and either giving an increased activity (i.e. more than their additive effect) or an increased spectrum of activity (i.e. lethal to a greater range of organisms). Examples of potentiation and synergism have been reported in many types of disinfectant. A few examples are given in Table 30.8.

Different p-hydroxybenzoate esters show synergistic activity, and mixtures are often used to obtain adequate preservation. Phenolic disinfectants are inactivated by dilution and other factors.

Antagonism leads to decreased antimicrobial activity, and use is made of antagonists in the elimination of antimicrobial properties of materials which are being tested for sterility. If the substance or preparation to be tested has antimicrobial properties, such properties must be counteracted either by inactivation with an antagonist, dilution, or by filtration and washing, using a membrane filter with an average pore diameter not exceeding 0.470 nm.

DISINFECTANT EVALUATION

A comprehensive review of the laboratory assessment of antibacterial activity has been published by Spooner and Sykes (1972). Different tests are used to assess bacteriostatic and bactericidal activity. A summary of the tests used is given in Table 30.9.

TABLE 30.8

POTENTIATING AGENTS AND ANTAGONISTS FOR DISINFECTANTS

Disinfectant	Potentiating agent	Antagonist
Benzalkonium chloride Chlorexidine diacetate	Low concentrations of non-ionic surfactants*	
p-Hydroxybenzoates	Polysorbate 80**	
Chlorine compounds	Bromine (or iodine) compounds***	
Halogens		Sodium thiosulphate
Quaternary ammonium compounds		Anionic agents, e.g. Lubrol W + lecithin; Soaps; Milk
Mercurials and arsenicals		Thioglycollic acid; sulphydryl compounds
Chlorhexidine		Lubrol W + lecithin
Formaldehyde		Morpholine + dimedone

  * Brown & Richards (1964)
  ** Brown (1968)
*** Shere, Kelly & Richardson (1962)

TABLE 30.9

TESTS FOR DISINFECTANT ACTIVITY

Substance tested	Bacteriostatic tests	Bactericidal tests
Liquid disinfectants	Serial dilution in fluid media	End-point or extinction time methods
	Serial dilution in solid media	Counting methods
	Cup-plate, fish-spine bead, and filter-paper methods	Turbidometric assessment
	The gradient-plate method	'In use' and other tests
	The ditch-plate technique.	In addition, 'in vivo' tests are applied
	All methods can be used quantitatively; the final method is usually used qualitatively	
Semi-solid antibacterial formulations, e.g. creams, ointments, pastes and gels	Cup-plate methods	Modified end-point or extinction time methods
	The ditch-plate technique	In addition, 'in vivo' tests are applied (e.g. skin tests)
Solid disinfectants, disinfectant powders	Inhibition on seeded agar	Modified end-point or extinction time methods
Aerial disinfectants		Use of slit-sampler in test chamber

TESTS APPLIED TO LIQUID DISINFECTANTS

Assessment of Bacteriostatic Activity
Serial dilution in fluid media. In this method, graded concentrations of the test substance in a nutrient medium are inoculated with the test organism and incubated. The minimum concentration preventing detectable growth (Minimum Inhibitory Concentration or MIC) is taken as a measure of bacteriostatic activity. Since the MIC varies considerably with inoculum size, medium used, and incubation conditions, these factors should be noted with each MIC obtained. Assessment of bacteriostatic activity can be observed quantitatively, and microscopically by a microcultural technique (Quastel 1966; Posthate 1969). Alternatively, the effect of a single concentration of antimicrobial on the rate of growth, as compared to the normal growth shown by a control experiment, can be used to assess bacteriostatic activity (Spooner & Sykes 1972).

Serial dilution in solid media. A suitable volume of double strength nutrient agar is diluted with an equal volume of bacteriostatic solution and poured into a sterile petri dish. When solidified the surface is dried by incubating at 37°C for 1 h with the lid slightly raised. Drops of 24-h broth cultures of the test organisms are placed on the dried surface and incubated for 2 to 3 days. Up to 27 cultures can be tested on each plate if a multi-point inolulator (Hale & Inkley 1965) is used. A separate petri dish is used for each concentration of bacteriostatic. Choice of the correct inoculum density is important. The main uses are for turbid bacteriostatic solutions, or solutions which give turbidity with fluid nutrient media. Solid media also offer the advantage of economy, since a number of different organisms can be accommodated on a single petri dish. A fair degree of correlation between serial dilution on solid and fluid media was shown by Cook (1954).

Cup-plate, fish-spine bead, and filter paper methods. These methods are very similar to those used in the assay of antibiotics. In these methods the agar is melted, cooled suitably, inoculated with the test

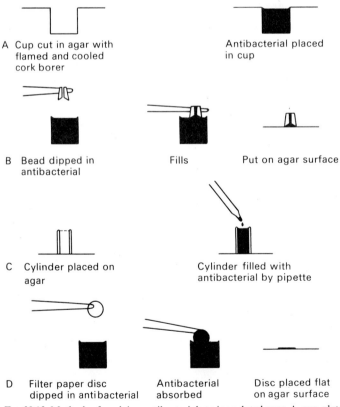

A Cup cut in agar with
   flamed and cooled
   cork borer

Antibacterial placed
in cup

B Bead dipped in
   antibacterial

Fills   Put on agar surface

C Cylinder placed on
   agar

Cylinder filled with
antibacterial by pipette

D Filter paper disc   Antibacterial   Disc placed flat
   dipped in antibacterial   absorbed   on agar surface

FIG. 30.13. Methods of applying antibacterials to inoculated agar. A, cup-plate method; B, fish-spine head method; C, cylinder method; D, filter paper method.

organism and poured into a sterile petri dish. In the cup-plate method, when the inoculated agar has solidified, holes about 8 mm in diameter are cut in the medium with a sterile cork borer. In the fish-spine bead, filter paper, and the cylinder method the antimicrobial agent is applied to the surface of the solidified, inoculated agar, and in the cup-plate method it is placed directly in the holes (Fig. 30.13). In all cases zones of inhibition may be observed, the diameter of the zones giving a rough indication of the relative activities of different antimicrobial substances against the test organism, or the effects of different concentrations of anti-microbial substance. A diagram showing the effect is given in Fig. 30.14. The method can give false indications because the development of an inhibition zone is dependent on the ability of the anti-microbial substance to diffuse through the agar.

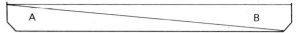

FIG. 30.15. Assessment of bacteriostatic activity by gradient-plate method. Wedge A; 10 ml of nutrient agar with anti-microbial, Wedge B; 10 ml of nutrient agar with no antimicrobial. After overnight incubation diffusion occurs to give a concentration gradient across the plate with a maximum on the left and minimum on the right. Wedges A and B may be reversed, the plate immediately streaked and then incubated.

where MIC is the minimum inhibitory concentration

C = concentration, in mg/ml, in total volume (i.e. volume of wedges A and B),
x = length of growth, in cm,
y = total length of possible growth, in cm (i.e. length streaked).

The ditch-plate technique. An agar plate is poured, allowed to solidify, and a trough or ditch cut out of the agar. A solution of the antimicrobial substance or a mixture of this with agar is carefully run into the ditch so as to about three-quarters fill it. A loopful of each test organism is then streaked outwards from the ditch on the agar surface. Organisms resistant to the antimicrobial grow right up to the ditch whereas susceptible organisms show a zone of inhibition adjacent to the ditch (see Fig. 30.16). The width of the inhibition zone gives an indication of the relative activity of the anti-microbial substance against the various test organisms.

Similar methods of testing are used for assessment of both antibacterial and antifungal activity. In the latter case suitable media for use in the test

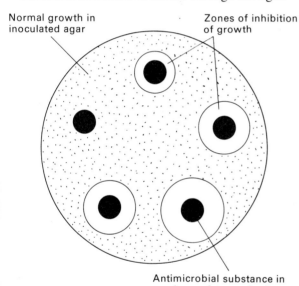

Normal growth in inoculated agar

Zones of inhibition of growth

Antimicrobial substance in cup (cup–plate method) or applied to agar surface (fish–spine bead, cylinder, or impregnated filter paper disc).

FIG. 30.14. Assessment of bacteriostatic activity by cup-plate, fish-spine head and filter paper methods.

The gradient-plate method. Two layers of agar are poured as shown in Fig. 30.15 (Szybalski & Bryson 1952). The plates are then incubated overnight to allow diffusion of the antimicrobial substance. The agar is streaked in the same line as the slope of the agar (i.e. along the concentration gradient) and reincubated. An approximate MIC can be obtained from the following equation:

$$\text{MIC} = C \times \frac{x}{y} \,\text{mg/ml}$$

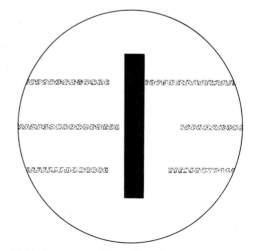

FIG. 30.16. Assessment of bacteriostatic activity by the ditch-plate technique. The six different test organisms show varying degrees of susceptibility to the antimicrobial in the ditch.

include Sabouraud medium and Czapek Dox medium. The effect of combining two (or more) antimicrobial agents may be examined by a filter paper strip method (King, Knox & Woodroffe 1953), or by a gradient-plate method combined with filter paper strips (Streitfield & Suslaw 1954). The main effects obtained by combining antimicrobial agents are:

Antagonism—leading to reduced activity.

Potentiation—leading to increased activity.

Synergism—literally a 'working together'—often leads to increased activity or a broader spectrum of activity.

Indifference—neither antimicrobial substance has any effect on the other.

Assessment of Bactericidal Activity

End-point or extinction time methods. There are two types of extinction time method; (a) in which the extinction time is fixed and the concentration of disinfectant needed to kill in the specified time is estimated, and (b) in which the concentration of bactericide is fixed and the extinction time is estimated. The former group (a) are referred to as phenol coefficient type tests and include: the Rideal-Walker Test (B.S. 541: 1934), the Chick-Martin Test (B.S. 808: 1938), the United States Food and Drug (FDA) Method (U.S. Dept. of Agric., Circular 198), the Crown Agents' Test (B.S. 2462: 1954), and the US Association of Official Agricultural Chemists (AOAC) Phenol Coefficient Test.

Phenol coefficient tests. The Rideal-Walker Test uses:

Standard Rideal-Walker Broth,

Salmonella typhi No. 786—standard subcultures are specified,

Standard apparatus, e.g. inoculating loop, glassware, etc., must conform to the specification given in the Standard.

Dilutions of the test disinfectant and phenol are inoculated with 0.2 ml of the 24-h culture of the organisms, the reaction mixture being kept at $17.5° \pm 0.5°$. Subcultures of each reaction mixture are taken and transferred to broth after $2\frac{1}{2}$, 5, $7\frac{1}{2}$ and 10 min (Fig. 30.17). The broth tubes are incubated at 37°C for 48 to 72 h and are then examined for the presence or absence of growth. The Rideal-Walker coefficient of the test disinfectant is then calculated as follows:

R.W. coefficient

$$= \frac{\text{dilution of disinfectant killing in } 7\frac{1}{2} \text{ but not in 5 min,}}{\text{dilution of phenol killing in } 7\frac{1}{2} \text{ but not in 5 min.}}$$

A typical result of the experiment described above might be:

		Minutes culture exposed to disinfectant			
Dilution		$2\frac{1}{2}$	5	$7\frac{1}{2}$	10
	1 in 1000	+	−	−	−
Test	1 in 1100	+	+	−	−
Disinfectant	1 in 1200	+	+	+	−
	1 in 1300	+	+	+	+
Phenol	1 in 105	+	+	−	−

(+ = growth; − = no growth)

$$\text{R.W. coeff.} = \frac{1100}{105} = 10.47.$$

The idealized result shown above may not be obtained on every occasion, because the loopfuls of reaction mixture transferred to the broth tubes represent random samples from the reaction mixture in which the mortality of the organisms is approaching 100 per cent. A few organisms of abnormal resistance in the reaction mixture, or the absence of organisms possessing the normal resistance of the last survivors, would influence the result. Thus, although not specified in the Standard, the test ought to be replicated. Since the replicates

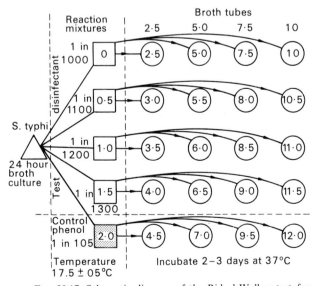

FIG. 30.17. Schematic diagram of the Rideal-Walker test for disinfectants.

are liable to indicate slightly different coefficients the latter would be more accurately expressed as a range rather than by a single value. Some typical Rideal-Walker coefficients quoted by manufacturers are given in Table 30.10.

TABLE 30.10

RIDEAL-WALKER COEFFICIENTS

Phenol 1% in water (by definition)	1
Lysol	3–4
Roxenol	5–5.5
White fluid	10–11
Black fluid	14–15

The other main phenol coefficient tests are given in Table 30.11.

As can be seen from the table the Chick-Martin test contains suspended yeast in the reaction mixture which tends to make the test more severe as the activity of some bactericides is markedly depressed by organic matter, together with a longer contact time of 30 min. In the Crown Agents' test the reaction mixture is prepared with artificial sea-water. Thus the test is unsuitable for disinfectants formulated with soap such as the so-called

Black Fluids and disinfectants of the Chloroxylenol type.

Merits of Phenol Coefficient Tests:
(1) The tests are thoroughly described and rigorously controlled by the appropriate standards. The results they yield are reasonably reproducible, not only from time to time in any one laboratory but also between laboratories.
(2) The tests are quickly and cheaply carried out and involve no great outlay in time, materials or labour.
(3) The tests provide a 'yard-stick' by which disinfectants can be sorted into those possessing activity and those which are worthless.
Deficiencies of Phenol Coefficient Tests:
(1) Use of single strain of organisms—all of the tests specify *Salmonella typhi* as the test organism. The AOAC test and the Rideal-Walker *Staphylococcus aureus* test (British Standard Institution, 1961) permit *Staph.aureus* to be used as an alternative test organism. The use of *S.typhi* is undoubtedly due to the fact that phenol coefficient tests originated in 1903 when the typhoid organism was a much greater menace than it is in modern times. The knowledge that a disinfectant has a specified phenol coefficient against the typhoid organisms is today of little more than academic interest. In any case, the typhoid organism is not

TABLE 30.11

ESSENTIAL DIFFERENCES BETWEEN PHENOL COEFFICIENT TESTS

	Rideal-Walker	FDA	Chick-Martin	AOAC	Crown agents
Medium pH	7.3–7.5	6.8	7.3–7.5	6.8 before autoclaving	7.3–7.5
Volume medium	5.0 ml	10.0 ml	10.0 ml	10.0 ml	5.0 ml
Volume reaction mixture	5.0 ml	10.0 ml	5.0 ml	5.0 ml	5.0 ml
Diluent for test disinfectant	Water	Water	Yeast suspension	Water	Artificial sea-water
Reaction temperature	$17.5 \pm 0.5°$	$20°$	$30°$	$20°:37°$	19.0 ± 1.0
Organism	*S.typhi*	*S.typhi*	*S.typhi*	*S.typhi Staph.aureus*	*S.typhi*
Sampling times	$2\frac{1}{2}$, 5, $7\frac{1}{2}$, 10 min	5, 10,15 min	30 min	5, 10, 15 min	10 min
Calculation of coefficient	Dilution test killing in $7\frac{1}{2}$ but not 5 min divided by same for phenol	Dilution test killing in 10 but not 5 min divided by same for phenol	Mean of highest phenol concentration inhibiting and lowest permitting growth divided by same for test	Greatest dilution of test killing in 10 min divided by same for phenol	Greatest dilution of test killing in 10 min divided by same for phenol

usually particularly resistant to disinfectants. The use of a more resistant organism would provide a much more stringent test for any disinfectant. A disinfectant which possesses high activity against the typhoid organism does not necessarily possess a similar activity against different species. Some bactericides are very selective, and the tests would be much more valuable if they were performed with several species of organisms. Another source of error is variation in susceptibility of the test organism to the test disinfectant.

(2) Tests compare activity of bactericides at only one concentration with a fixed death time—the dilution of both standard phenol and test disinfectant killing in a specified time is determined. Thus each test only ascertains the performance of one concentration of the test disinfectant. This would not matter if all disinfectants possessed the same concentration exponent. Fig. 30.18 shows the log concentration–log extinction time regression lines for two disinfectants X and Y (the slopes represent the concentration exponents of the two disinfectants). If the two bactericides are compared by determining the dilutions which kill at time a, Y

is seen to be the better bactericide. If the time is fixed at b, identical concentrations of both bactericides are needed and the phenol coefficient would be 1. If the time is fixed at c, X appears to be the better bactericide. Hence phenol coefficients can be changed by altering the arbitarily chosen reaction time.

(3) Tests compare activity of bactericides at only one temperature—the phenol coefficient tests are usually performed at one fixed temperature, whereas in practice disinfectants are likely to be used at widely different temperatures. The activity of a bactericide at the temperature specified for the test may be quite different from its activity at the temperature at which it is used. Every bactericide has its characteristic temperature coefficient and the knowledge that a particular bactericide has a certain phenol coefficient at 20° gives no information about its performance at any other temperature.

(4) Most phenol coefficient tests give no indication of the activity of the bactericide in the presence of organic matter—with the exception of the Chick-Martin test, the commonly used phenol coefficient tests are performed in the absence of organic matter, whereas in practice most disinfectants and bactericides are used in the presence of organic matter. Different disinfectants are affected to different extents by the same type of organic matter. The activity of phenol is not seriously affected by the presence of as much as 10 per cent blood serum, whereas the activity of some emulsified disinfectants is seriously affected. Formaldehyde and oxidizing agents such as hydrogen peroxide, chlorine, and permanganates react vigorously with organic matter whereas the acridines retain their activity in the presence of organic matter. Thus any phenol coefficient test which does not include organic matter is inadequate.

(5) Phenol coefficient tests give no indication of tissue toxicity—although Lysol and Roxenol-type disinfectants have similar phenol coefficients the former would never be considered for use on the body due to its tissue toxicity. The latter are relatively non-toxic to tissue. The phenol coefficient test thus gives no indication of the suitability of a bactericide for a specific purpose.

(6) Phenol coefficient tests give no indication of the effects of dilution on the activity of the disinfectant.

(7) Phenol coefficient tests can only logically be used to evaluate phenolic disinfectants—to use this type of test, with phenol as a standard, to evaluate non-phenolic disinfectants contravenes the basic principle of a biological assay of testing

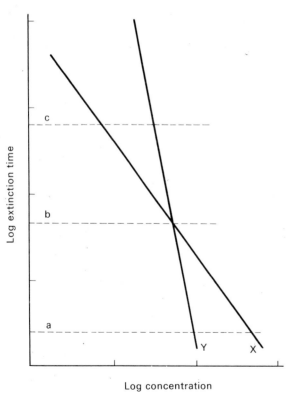

FIG. 30.18. Influence of selection of extinction time on apparent activity of two bactericides X and Y.

'like' against 'like'. Despite this fact phenol coefficient tests are used to test the performance of many formulated disinfectants.

(8) Sampling errors are large in phenol coefficient tests—a very small volume is sampled from a large volume containing a small number of survivors, which may be in clumped aggregates. The error in the sampling is dealt with in detail by Dodd (1969).

(9) Recovery conditions in phenol coefficient tests may not be suitable for 'damaged' organisms.

Despite their limitations, phenol coefficient tests are widely used in preliminary disinfectant evaluation. The Chick-Martin test was used up to 1970 as a test for disinfectants for agricultural use. A new Order for disinfectants for agricultural use was made in 1970 (Statutory Instrument 1970, No. 1372) in which disinfectants are approved according to their intended use.

Determination of mean death time or mean single survivor time. In these tests the extinction time is measured for several different concentrations of bactericide. Berry and Bean (1954) developed a method of this type. The reaction mixtures were each distributed, immediately after preparation, into a series of sterile tubes in which the reaction proceeded at a controlled temperature until it was quenched by the addition of broth. Apart from its simplicity the advantage of the method was that the samples were taken before the reaction mixture had become heterogeneous due to the clumping of the dying organisms. Berry and Bean performed their experiments in replicate, a typical result being shown in the Table 30.12.

A between-experiment variation is immediately obvious and stresses the need for replication. A

TABLE 30.12

BACTERICIDAL ACTIVITY OF 1% PHENOL AGAINST *E.coli.*

Experiment	Exposure time (min)								Estimated Extinction Time (min)
	40	50	60	70	80	90	100	110	
1	+	+	+	+	+	–			90
2	+	+	–	–	–	–	–	–	60
3	+	+	+	–	–	–	–	–	70
4	+	+	+	+	–	–	–	–	80
5	+	+	+	–	–	–	–	–	70
							Total		370

$$\text{Mean death time} = \frac{370}{5} = 74 \text{ min}$$

closer examination shows the results to be less haphazard than at first glance. At each successive sampling time there is a reduction in the number of samples containing live organisms. For example, after 40 minutes' exposure to the phenol, live organisms were recovered in all five experiments; after 60 minutes' exposure live organisms were recovered in only four of the experiments and after 80 min in only one experiment. The between-experiment variations are called 'sampling errors' and are largely due to the survivors being too few to ensure at least one live organism being in each sample. The observation led to the development of a statistical treatment (Mather 1949) for extinction-time data and the calculation of the 'mean single survivor time' which is the time needed to reduce the number of viable organisms to an average of one per sample volume. The mean single survivor time is somewhat shorter than the mean death time because the mortality level involved is slightly lower. An example of the calculation of the mean single survivor time (MSST) is given by Cook and Wills (1954).

Counting methods. A consideration of the Rideal-Walker and similar end-point methods shows the difficulty of determining the exact end-point. In the RW test the end-point lies somewhere between 5 and $7\frac{1}{2}$ min; taking extreme cases, the dilution of phenol might kill in, say, 5.1 min and the disinfectant under test in 7.4 min; both subcultures will show no growth after $7\frac{1}{2}$ min. The results at the standard time of $7\frac{1}{2}$ min are therefore purely arbitrary. The disadvantages are avoided if the rate of death is followed by viable counts. Rates of death can only be determined by counting in *dilute* solutions of germicides, i.e. in solutions from which it is possible to withdraw samples at accurate intervals of time. *Viable counts are not reliable with organisms that clump or form long chains.* Quaternary ammonium compounds, e.g. cetrimide, promote clumping and BS 3286: 1960 deals specifically with evaluation of the disinfectant activity of this type of compound. In many cases the problem of clumping can be overcome by the use of a non-ionic surfactant. Berry and Michaels (1947) give examples of statistical methods applied to the results. Comparison of reaction rates may be made (Davis, 1940) as shown in Fig. 30.19.

Other methods of estimating bactericidal activity from viable count data are available, including comparison of LT_{50}s—the time taken to kill 50 per cent of the test organisms. Withell (1942) suggested

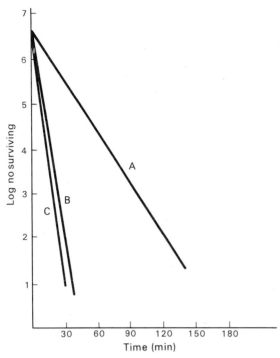

FIG. 30.19. The germicidal effect of 0.5 per cent phenol; A, 0.05 per cent chlorocresol; B, 0.05 per cent chlorobuto; C, on *Staphylococcus aureus* in watery suspension at 19° to 20.5° (Davis 1940).

that a bactericide should be evaluated by determining:

LT_{50} for phenol and the bactericide at suitable concentrations.

LT_{50} for phenol and the bactericide at other concentrations (in order to determine the concentration coefficients).

the temperature coefficient, θ, by similar methods. Since the majority of the organisms will possess average resistance, the LT_{50} is determined by a large number of organisms whereas the extinction time is determined by the comparatively few organisms possessing maximal resistance to the bactericide. Thus the LT_{50} is more dependable and more representative than the extinction time.

Turdidimetric methods. Berry and Cook (1950) developed this method for evaluating the bactericidal action of solutions of phenols in potassium ricinoleates. They discuss the accuracy of the method; for further details the original papers should be consulted.

'In-use' and other tests. A more versatile evaluation of disinfectants is often required, particularly

in hospitals, where the type of organisms, disinfection period, presence of various organic soiling materials, and other factors can vary considerably. The basis for a more adaptable test appears in British Standard 3286: 1960 and allows variation in the test culture(s), disinfection period, presence of organic matter, and other factors. In 1965, Kelsey, Beeby and Whitehouse produced a capacity use-dilution test. The main aim of this test was to measure the capacity of the disinfectant to deal with successive bacterial contamination. Instead of determining the ability of the disinfectant to cope with one large inoculum, inocula are made in six increments.

From the British Standard 3286: 1960 and the Kelsey, Beeby and Whitehouse test was developed the Kelsey and Sykes test (1969), which incorporates the advantages of both tests. This test is worthy of mention in more detail.

Kelsey and Sykes test (1969)—the test organisms are *Staph.aureus* NCTC 4163 and *Ps.aeruginosa* NCTC 6749. *Proteus vulgaris* NCTC 4635 and others, such as *E.coli* can be added.

Disinfectant dilutions are made in water of 300 p/m hardness. Any number of dilutions can be made, but it is important to include:
(a) the dilution recommended by the manufacturer,
(b) a dilution 20–25 per cent weaker than (a), and
(c) a dilution 20–25 per cent stronger than (a).

'Clean' and 'dirty' conditions are simulated in the test. In both cases the final concentration of bacterial cells should be about 10^9/ml. 'Clean' conditions are simulated by using broth as the suspending fluid, and 'dirty' conditions by the use of a yeast suspension or inactivated horse serum as suspending fluid. The basic procedure is outlined in Table 30.13.

The samples taken at 8, 18 and 28 min are then incubated at 30 to 32°, and the number of tubes showing growth or the number of colonies/drop from surface plate culture is recorded.

A disinfectant is satisfactory for use at the initial concentration if: (a) no growth occurs in 2 or more of the 5 tubes of the 18 min samples, i.e. subcultures taken after second incremental addition of bacteria; or (b) there are not more than 5 colonies from the 5 drops on the agar plate.

Tubes of disinfectant reaction mixture should be kept for 5 days, without further inoculation, and further samples taken to confirm that undetected surviving cells have not developed. The main source of error in this test is due to organism variation, but this test will show the stability of disinfectant dilutions and their long term effectiveness. An

TABLE 30.13

PROCEDURE FOR KELSEY AND SYKES TEST

Time from start (min)	Procedure
0	Inoculate 3 ml of the disinfectant dilution with 1 ml of bacterial suspension in broth, yeast or serum, and shake gently. (This gives a bactericide/bacteria reaction mixture).
8	Remove sample from above reaction mixture with a 50 dropper pipette. Transfer 1 drop to each of 5 tubes of liquid recovery media, or 5 drops to the surface of a nutrient agar plate.
10	To bactericide/bacteria reaction mixture, prepared at start (time 0), add a second 1 ml of bacterial suspension.
18	As for 8 minutes (reaction mixture now contains 2 ml of bacterial suspension).
20	Add third incremental addition of 1 ml of bacterial suspension to original bactericide/bacteria reaction mixture. (A total of 3 ml has now been added.)
28	As for 8 minutes.

improved Kelsey-Sykes test for disinfectants has been described by Kelsey and Maurer (1974). They defined more precisely the conditions of the test without altering the general principles or end results.

An 'in-use' test was described by Kelsey and Maurer (1966). In this test samples are taken from situations in which the disinfectant is used, e.g. liquid from mops, storage and rinse liquids for urine bottles, etc. One ml of the liquid is diluted with 9 ml of one-quarter strength Ringer's solution (plus inactivator if necessary) and 10 drops are placed on the surface of an agar plate with a 50 dropper pipette. If not more than 5 out of the 10 drops show growth after 48 h at 30 to 32°, the disinfectant is considered adequate.

In addition to the four main types of test for assessing bactericidal activity, 'in vivo' tests must be applied if the antibacterial is intended to be used on living tissue. If it is to be used on the skin, the disinfectant action can be evaluated by placing the test organism on the back of the hand, subjecting it to the disinfectant, then swabbing the infected area of the hand to ascertain if disinfection has occurred. Details of in vivo tests are given by Spooner and Sykes (1972). Assessment of systemic toxicity should be applied to wound disinfectants. The nature of the surface to be disinfected may also affect the choice of a method of evaluation.

TESTS APPLIED TO SEMI-SOLID ANTIBACTERIAL FORMULATIONS

These include creams, ointments, pastes and gels. The base used for the formulation often markedly affects the antimicrobial activity of the disinfectant substance (Kolstad & Lee 1955).

Assessment of Bacteriostatic Activity

In the original method proposed by Reddish (1927) sample portions of the formulation were placed on the surface of agar seeded with *Staph.aureus* and the zones of inhibition, if any, measured. The technique was later modified by the incorporation of 10 per cent horse serum in the agar. The cup-plate or ditch-plate techniques can equally well be applied to these types of formulation.

Assessment of Bactericidal Activity

Modified phenol coefficient type tests can be used. The test organism must be well mixed with the semi-solid formulations, samples taken at appropriate intervals, and placed in a broth which is capable of dispersing the base and nullifying the antimicrobial activity of the disinfectant compound. Sampling errors using a loop are large, and a method of transferring the mixture to a hypodermic syringe and ejecting small volumes into suitable media was proposed by Foter and Nisonger (1950).

Skin tests should also be made.

TESTS APPLIED TO SOLID DISINFECTANTS

In these formulations the disinfectant compound is often mixed with an inert substance such as talc or kieselguhr to form a disinfectant powder.

By dusting the powders onto inoculated plates, using the inert diluent as a control, the extent of inhibitory action can be ascertained. British Standard (B.S. 1013: 1946) gives details of the determination of the Rideal-Walker coefficient for disinfectant powders. A weighed sample is shaken with distilled water at 18° for 30 min and the suspension used for the Rideal-Walker test.

TESTS ON AERIAL DISINFECTANTS

Although the lethal process is very similar to that in the liquid environment, the mechanism of disin-disinfection is quite different. A concise summary of the evaluation of air disinfectants is given by Bourdillon et al. (1948), Whittet, Hugo and Wilkinson (1965) and Sykes (1965).

For the basic evaluation a closed room of approximately cubic dimensions and 1000 cu ft capacity should be used. Fans should be incorporated to ensure uniform mixing of bacteria and bactericide. *Staph.albus* is often used as the test organism as it is a non-clumping strain. Dispersion of the organisms into the air can be done with a Collison inhaler, and samples of the air taken at suitable intervals with a slit sampler. Obviously, the room must be initially free from extraneous microorganisms (this is done by careful cleaning and use of ultraviolet light disinfection of the air), and the temperature and humidity of the air carefully controlled, although, in practice, such ideal conditions do not occur naturally. A bactericide achieving an 85 per cent (or more) kill in 4 to 6 min (RH 55 to 65 per cent, temperature 20°C) is considered satisfactory. Cyclopentanol-1-carboxylic acid has been suggested as a reference standard for air disinfection.

REFERENCES

ALBERT, A. (1951) *The Acridines.* London: Edward Arnold.

ALBERT, A. (1973) *Selective Toxicity.* London: Chapman & Hall.

ALEXANDER, A. E. & TOMLINSON, A. J. H. (1949) *Surface Activity.* London: Butterworths.

ALCOCK, T. (1827) *Lancet* i, 643.

ARCHER, G. T. L. (1945) *Brit. med. J.* 2, 148.

BEAN, H. S. & BERRY, H. (1953) *J. Pharm. Pharmacol.* 5, 632.

BEAN, H. S. (1961) *Bentley's Text-book of Pharmaceutics,* Ed. H. Davis, London: Bailliere, Tindall and Cox.

BERRY, H. (1952) *J. appl. Bact.* 15, 138.

BERRY, H. & BEAN, H. S. (1954) *J. Pharm. Pharmacol.* 6, 649.

BERRY, H. & BRIGGS, A. (1956) *J. Pharm. Pharmacol.* 8, 1143.

BERRY, H. & COOK, A. M. (1950) *J. Pharm. Pharmacol.* 2, 217, 311, 565.

BERRY, H., COOK, A. M. & WILLS, B. A. (1956) *J. Pharm. Pharmacol.* 8, 425.

BERRY, H. & MICHAELS, I. (1947) *Quart. J. Pharm.* 20, 331.

BERRY, H. & STENLAKE, J. B. (1942) *Pharm. J.* 148, 112.

BOURDILLON, R. B., LIDWELL, O. M. & LOVELOCK, J. E. (1948) *Studies in Air Hygiene.* London: HMSO.

BRITISH DISINFECTANT MANUFACTURERS' ASSOCIATION, D5/D7, 1080/70, London, 1970.

BRITISH STANDARDS INSTITUTION (1934) *Technique for determining the Rideal-Walker coefficient of disinfectants.* B.S. 541: 1934 (with amendments).

BRITISH STANDARDS INSTITUTION (1938) *Specification for the modified Chick-Martin test for disinfectants.* B.S. 808: 1938 (with amendments).

BRITISH STANDARDS INSTITUTION (1946) *Disinfectant and sanitary powders.* B.S. 1013: 1946.

BRITISH STANDARDS INSTITUTION (1960) *Method for the laboratory evaluation of quaternary ammonium compounds by suspension test.* B.S. 3286: 1960.

BRITISH STANDARDS INSTITUTION (1961) *Specification for black and white disinfectant fluids.* B.S. 2462: 1961.

BRITISH STANDARDS INSTITUTION (1961) *The Crown Agents' Test.* Appendix A, B.S. 2462: 1961.

BROWN, M. R. W. (1968) *J. pharm. Sci.* 57, 389.

BROWN, M. R. W. & RICHARDS, R. M. E. (1964) *J. Pharm. Pharmacol.* 16, *Suppl.,* 51T.

CHICK, H. (1908) *J. Hyg. Camb.* 8, 92.

CHICK, H. & MARTIN, C. J. (1908) *J. Hyg. Camb.* 8, 654.

COOK, A. M. (1954) *J. Pharm. Pharmacol.* 6, 629.

COOK, A. M. (1960) *J. Pharm. Pharmacol.* 12, 197.

COOK, A. M. & WILLS, B. A. (1954) *J. Pharm. Pharmacol.* 6, 638.

DAVIS, H. (1940) *Quart. J. Pharm.* 13, 32.

DODD, A. H. (1969) *The Theory of Disinfectant Testing.* London: Swifts.

FAREWELL, J. A. & BROWN, M. R. W. (1971) *Inhibition and Destruction of the Microbial Cell,* Ed. Hugo, W. B. London: Academic Press.

FILDES, P. (1940) *Brit. J. exptl. Path.* 21, 67.

FINCH, W. E. (1963) *Pharm. J.* 170, 59.

FOTER, M. J. & NISONGER, L. L. (1950) *Ann. N.Y. Acad. Sci.* 53, 112.

FRY, B. A. (1957) *J. gen. Microbiol.* 16, 341.

GALE, E. F. & TAYLOR, E. S. (1947) *J. gen. Microbiol.* **1**, 77.

GUMP, W. S. & WALTER, G. R. (1960) *J. Soc. Cosmet. Chem.* **11**, 307.

HALE, L. J. & INKLEY, G. W. (1965) *Lab. Pract.* **14**, 452.

HUGO, W. B. (1956) *J. gen. Microbiol.* **15**, 315.

HUGO, W. B. (1957) *J. Pharm. Pharmacol.* **9**, 145.

HUGO, W. B. (1967) *J. appl. Bact.* **30** (1), 17.

HUGO, W. B. (1970) *Disinfection*, Ed. Bernarde, M. A. New York: Marcel Dekker Inc.

HUGO, W. B. & LONGWORTH, A. R. (1964) *J. Pharm. Pharmacol.* **16**, 655, 751.

HUGO, W. B. & LONGWORTH, A. R. (1965) *J. Pharm. Pharmacol.* **17**, 28.

HUGO, W. B. & LONGWORTH, A. R. (1966) *J. Pharm. Pharmacol.* **18**, 569.

JACOBS, S. E. (1960) *J. Pharm. Pharmacol.* **12**, 9T.

JORDAN, H. & JACOBS, S. E. (1944) *J. Hyg. Camb.* **43**, 275.

KELSEY, J. C., BEEBY, M. M. & WHITEHOUSE, C. W. (1965) *Mon. Bull. Minist. Hlth.* **24**, 152.

KELSEY, J. C. & MAURER, I. M. (1966) *Mon. Bull. Minist. Hlth.* **26**, 110.

KELSEY, J. C. & MAURER, I. M. (1974) *Pharm. J.* **213**, 528.

KELSEY, J. C. & SYKES, G. (1969) *Pharm. J.* **202**, 607.

KING, M. B., KNOX, R. & WOODROFFE, R. C. (1953) *Lancet* **i**, 573.

KOCH, R. (1881) *Mitt. Reichgesunh. Amt.* **1**, 234.

KOLSTAD, K. & LEE, C. O. (1955) *J. Am. pharm. Ass.* **44**, 5.

MADSEN, T. & NYMAN, N. (1907) *Z. Hyg. Infect. Kr.* **57**, 388.

MARTINDALE (1972) *The Extra Pharmacopoeia*, 26th ed. London: The Pharmaceutical Press.

MATHER, K. (1949) *Biometrics* **5**, 127.

MITCHELL, A. G. (1964) *J. Pharm. Pharmacol.* **16**, 533.

MIURA, K. & RECKENDORF, H. K. (1967) *Progress in Medicinal Chemistry*, Vol. 5, 320, Eds. Ellis, G. P. & West, G. B. London: Butterworths.

MORRIS, E. J. & DARLOW, H. M. (1971) *Inhibition and Destruction of the Microbial Cell*, Ed. Hugo, W. B. London: Academic Press.

POSTGATE, J. R. (1969) *Methods in Microbiology*, Vol. 1, Eds. Norris, J. R. & Ribbons, D. W. London: Academic Press.

PROKOP, A. & HUMPHREY, A. E. (1970) *Disinfection*, Ed. Bernarde, M. A. New York: Marcel Dekker Inc.

QUASTEL, J. H. (1966) *J. gen. Microbiol.* **45**, xiv.

REDDISH, G. F. (1927) *J. Am. pharm. Ass.* **16**, 652.

REPORT TO THE PUBLIC HEALTH LABORATORY SERVICE (1958) *Mon. Bull. Minist. Hlth.* **17**, 10.

RUBBO, S. D. & GARDNER, J. F. (1965) *A Review of Sterilization and Disinfection.* London: Lloyd-Luke (Medical Books) Ltd.

RUBBO, S. D., GARDNER, J. F. & WEBB, R. L. (1967) *J. appl. Bact.* **30**, 78.

SALTON, M. R. J. (1961) *Bact. Rev.* **25**, 77.

SEMMELWEISS, J. P. (1861) *Die aetiologie der Bergriff und die prophylaxis des kindbettfiebers*, Vienna: Pest.

SHERE, L., KELLY, M. J. & RICHARDSON, J. H. (1962) *Appl. Microbiol.* **10**, 538.

SPOONER, D. F. & SYKES, G. (1972) *Methods in Microbiology*, Vol. 7B, Eds. Norris, J. R. & Ribbons, D. W. London: Academic Press.

Statutory Instrument 1372 (1970). London: HMSO.

STREITFIELD, M. M. & SUSLAW, M. S. (1954) *J. lab. clin. Med.* **43**, 946.

SUTER, C. M. (1941) *Chem. Rev.* **28**, 269.

SYKES, G. (1965) *Disinfection and Sterilisation.* London: E. & F. N. Spon.

SZYBALSKI, W. & BRYSON, V. (1952) *J. Bact.* **64**, 489.

WAKSMAN, S. A., HORNING, E. S., WELSCH, M. & WOODRUFF, H. B. (1942) *Soil Sci.* **54**, 281.

WHITTET, T. D., HUGO, W. B. & WILKINSON, G. R. (1965) *Sterilisation and Disinfection*, Ed. Stenlake, J. B. London: W. Heinemann Medical Books Ltd.

WITHELL, E. R. (1938) *Quart. J. Pharm.* **9**, 736.

WITHELL, E. R. (1942) *J. Hyg. Camb.* **42**, 339.

31

Sterilization

Definitions

Sterility. Sterility may be defined as the absence of living organisms from any given milieu. Strictly speaking, it is an absolute concept and cannot be qualified in any way. Expressions such as 'virtual sterility' and 'partial sterility' are contradictions in terms and the sanction for their use arises purely from the practical difficulties, examined later in this chapter, of determining with certainty the point at which sterility has been attained.

Sterilization. Sterilization is the total process by which sterility is achieved. Whether it is effected by physical or by chemical agencies, it is an orderly process proceeding to extinction, and the dynamics of this process are the same as those which have been examined in Chapter 30, Disinfection. The latter term, however, is used whether the lethal process is complete, resulting in sterility, or whether it proceeds to some intermediate stage, and it is often restricted to the destruction of pathogenic and non-sporing organisms (Reddish 1957, Rubbo & Gardner 1965). Sterilization, on the other hand, is a process by which all microorganisms may be assumed to have been killed.

THERMAL RESISTANCE OF MICROORGANISMS

Thermal Death Time

The *thermal death time* is defined as the time required to kill a particular species or strain of microorganism at a given temperature, under specified conditions. The usefulness of the statistic is, however, greatly reduced by the fact that it is influenced not only by controllable environmental factors, e.g. temperature, pH, presence of bactericides, etc., but also by uncontrollable factors such as the number of contaminating organisms and their resistance to heat, which may vary even within recognized strains, due to the age of the cells and the conditions of growth prior to heat treatment.

Table 31.1 gives some approximate values of thermal death times. It will be seen that there is a considerable variation between different types of organism, the spores of many bacterial species being much more resistant than non-sporing bacteria, or the thinner-walled, larger and more structured moulds. Although the spores of the latter are more resistant than their hyphal forms, only one mould spore, that of *Byssochlamys fulva*, shows any marked resistance to heat and, although it is quite easily killed by the treatment normally employed for sterilizing pharmaceutical products, it can cause trouble in the food industry, e.g. in the canning of soft fruits, some of which will withstand heat treatments only slightly more severe than that required to kill the spores of the mould.

It might be supposed therefore that an adequate margin of safety can be secured by taking care that the temperature used and the time for which it is applied will exceed those indicated by the known thermal death times of the most resistant species expected to be present. A common practice is to increase the time of exposure indicated by the thermal death time by 50 per cent, though Darmady, Hughes & Jones (1958) suggest that, for dry heat, the thermal death time used for the calculation should be that obtained at a temperature 10° lower than that used for sterilization.

TABLE 31.1

APPROXIMATE THERMAL DEATH TIMES OF MICROORGANISMS

Group	Organism	Boiling water °C 100	Autoclaving °C 115	120	130	Dry heat °C 120	150	160	180
Highly sensitive	Non-sporing bacteria. Viruses. Moulds and yeasts (including spores)	2	—	1	< +	—	—	3	<1
Slightly resistant	*Byssochlamys fulva* (spores) *Cl. perfringens* (spores)	5	—	2	< +	—	—	4	<1
Moderately resistant	*Cl. welchii* (spores) *B. anthracis* (spores)	5–45 2–15	4 —	1 —	— < +	50 180	<5 6–120	— 9–90	3
Resistant	*Cl. tetani* (spores)	5–90	—	5	1	—	30	12	1
Very resistant	*B. stearothermophilus* (spores) *Cl. botulinum* (spores) Soil bacteria (spores)	300 >300 >500	— 10–40 15	12 4–20 6–30	2 2 4	— 120 —	30 30 180	— 20 30–90	5 5–10 15

However, the inaccuracy of thermal death times, (see below) makes their use suspect.

Death Rate of Microorganisms

It is not possible to determine exactly, by direct method, the point in time when sterility is first achieved, because shortly before this is reached the number of surviving organisms is so small that accurate determination of it becomes impossible, due to the very high sampling errors involved. Reliance is therefore usually placed on extrapolation of the plot of log survivors against time, because in many cases this is found to be linear over a large part of its range. However, this relationship, as in the case of disinfection by chemicals (see Fig. 30.8) is not always linear and may prove under some circumstances to be sigmoid in character, finally approaching the zero survivor level in an assymptotic manner (Hansen & Riemann 1963). This has been ascribed to the presence of a few very resistant organisms, although Rahn (1945) denied this and regarded it as entirely due to sampling error. Under such conditions, extrapolation of the linear part of the curve may give a thermal death time that is too low, and Vas and Proszt (1957) suggest that in these circumstances the destruction characteristics can only be described numerically by the mean destruction time and its standard deviation. It is generally assumed, however, that provided conditions are so arranged that the death rate is sufficiently rapid, a linear log/survivor/time relationship can be assumed to hold effectively down to the zero survivor level and that

the thermal death time can be determined without undue error. For this reason, Rubbo and Gardner (1965) recommend that the sterilization process employed should be as rapid as possible, having regard to the ability of the materials being treated to withstand the temperature selected.

Decimal Reduction Time (D)

If one assumes that a linear log/survivor/time relationship will hold, a graphic method can be used for determining the thermal death time. Alternatively, making the same assumption, one can use data from the earlier, assuredly linear, part of the curve to calculate functions which can be taken as indicators of the efficiency of the process, without using the end-point itself. One such function is the *decimal reduction time* or D Value (Schmidt 1950). This is the time in minutes required to reduce the number of viable organisms by 90 per cent, i.e. the time corresponding to one log cycle on the survivor/time curve. Numerically it is also the reciprocal of the velocity constant k of the reaction, calculated from the equation:

$$k = \frac{1}{t} \log_{10} \frac{N_o}{N_t}$$

Inactivation Factor

The *inactivation factor* is the degree to which the viable population of organisms is reduced by the treatment applied, and is obtained by dividing the initial viable count by the final viable count. Alternatively, where the complete survivor/time data is not available, but the D value for the organism is known, it can be calculated from the equation:

$$\text{Inactivation Factor} = 10^{t/D}$$

where t = treatment time in minutes
    D = D value for the same temperature and conditions

z Value

This is defined as the increase in temperature required to reduce the D value by 90 per cent (Ball 1923 quoted by Schmidt 1957); it is used as an indicator of the relative heat resistances of the organisms under tests, organisms with high z values being the most resistant. Most non-sporing organisms have z values of about 4 to 6°, while for spores it may be as high as 16 to 20° (Hansen & Riemann 1963).

Choice of Test Organism

From Table 31.1, it might be supposed that in all cases, spores of a soil bacterium would be most suitable for testing the efficiency of sterilization procedures. Other factors besides heat resistance must be considered, however. The organism must be easily cultivated and have a distinctive colonial morphology which will enable it to be recognized and counted. This rules out most clostridial spores which are difficult to culture, and many of the genus Bacillus, because they produce indistinguishable, spreading colonies.

It may also be useful to relate the requirements for the test organism to conditions in which it is normally found and to the sterilization process employed. Thus, for dry heat sterilization of instruments and syringes, Darmady, Hughes & Jones (1958) argue that a suitable pathogen should be used, and advocate the use of Clostridium tetani, while Quesnel et al. (1967) reject this argument and advise the use of strains of Bacillus subtilis, considering heat resistance and cultural characteristics to be more important than pathogenicity. One of the organisms they used, Bacillus subtilis var. niger (B.globigii) produces distinctive brown colonies and was first recommended for testing sterilization with ethylene oxide, by Phillips (1949). Because they represent natural contamination, soil samples themselves have often been used for testing autoclaving procedures, but with unidentified organisms in mixed culture, erratic results may be expected to occur. For this reason Kelsey (1959) suggested the use of Bacillus stearothermophilus spores. For radiation sterilization, Powell (1961) recommended the use of a strain of B.pumilis, but Quesnel et al.

(1967) found it to have only moderate heat resistance. The Pharmaceutical Handbook (1970) gives a useful summary of current practice and advocates the use of B.stearothermophilus for testing both moist heat and dry heat processes, B.pumilis for ionizing radiations, and B.subtilis var. niger for ethylene oxide.

ACCEPTABLE STANDARDS FOR STERILIZATION PROCEDURES

Terminology

The difficulties of ascertaining with certainty the point at which sterilization is first achieved have led to a change in attitude concerning the use of the term 'sterility'. Although it is an absolute concept, it is nevertheless one of immense practical importance and in order to retain the word 'sterility' in describing the practical situation it has been found necessary to sacrifice terminological rectitude to functional necessity. Consequently, the term 'virtual sterility' is sometimes used to indicate the achievable end-point of sterilization of large volumes of air (Elsworth 1972). The Pharmaceutical Handbook (1970) redefines the term 'sterile' as 'free from demonstrable forms of life', and suggests that sterilization can be regarded as being associated with a definite degree of risk, acceptable levels of which must be decided arbitrarily if methods are to be standardized in codes of good practice.

Methods of Assessment

One way of defining this risk would be to decide that a given inactivation factor should suffice. Thus, Powell (1961) suggested that for radiation sterilization a dose of 2.5 megarads, corresponding to an inactivation factor of 10^7 to 10^{12} would be suitable, and Sykes (1969) gives a factor of 10^{15} to 10^{20} as being acceptable for steam sterilization, while admitting that a lower level of 10^8 to 10^9 would be necessary for sterilization with ethylene oxide. Rubbo and Gardner (1965), however, point out that the residual contamination depends not only on the inactivation factor, but also on the original population of contaminants. Thus, if the inactivation factor is 10^7 and the original contamination is 10 organisms per article, there is a risk of one unsterile article remaining in every million processed; but if the original contamination is 10^5 organisms per article there would be a risk that one in every hundred articles would be unsterile. Clearly the latter situation is unacceptable, but it remains a matter of opinion whether the risk of one unsterile article per million is acceptable or not. Fortunately, for most purposes pharmaceutical materials do not carry a very high number of contaminants before sterilization, though surgical dressings can prove the exception to this and they also pose a number of special problems which will be referred to later.

The z value has also been used to determine the temperature required to produce effective sterility within a predetermined, convenient time, when data is only available for performance at a different temperature.

All such calculations, carried out using a single type of organism, must be treated with caution when considering the requirements for overall standards for sterilization procedures, and most of the official methods at present in use (see below) were developed from a consideration of end-point data rather than from the use of derived functions such as D and z values. It must also be realized that other factors such as the nature of the material being sterilized, its volume and method of packing, all affect the efficiency of the process, so that the criteria that have become accepted for the sterilization of pharmaceutical preparations have been derived from practical experience in the working situation rather than from isolated laboratory experiments. In view of the many factors operating, it is not surprising that the evidence obtained has been conflicting and that different standards have been officially adopted in different countries. It is known, for example, that spores of some soil bacteria will survive the sterilization procedures laid down in the *British Pharmacopoeia*, but despite this Sykes (1965) claims that pharmaceutical products are unlikely to contain such resistant organisms and hence the British official requirements have proved satisfactory in practice. Thus the evidence available from the use of both survivor levels and of end-point assessments is sufficiently variable to require a final arbitrary judgement regarding the standards which should be set.

Nevertheless, the abandonment of the goal of complete sterility in favour of a very low level of residual contamination associated with an acceptable level of risk, makes quantitative estimation of sterilization efficiency both possible and valid and the accumulation of data for a wide range of organisms and sterilizing conditions could lead to a more precise formulation of acceptable standards.

STERILIZATION PROCESSES

The processes used to effect sterility of pharmaceutical preparations may be classified as:

Processes involving the use of Physical Means. These may involve the utilization of heat in the presence or in the absence of moisture, or the application of ultraviolet, or ionizing radiations (see Chapter 28).

Chemical Processes. For most purposes the application of chemicals in solution to e.g. surfaces of utensils or to skin, does not produce sterility, and this disinfectant activity has already been considered in Chapter 30. A chemical bactericide can however be used in solution together with the application of heat for the sterilization of certain thermolabile injectables and this method is permitted in the *British Pharmacopoeia* 1973, in some cases. Bactericidal gases may also be used for the sterilization of apparatus and materials which might be damaged by heat.

Mechanical Processes. In these, the organisms are not killed in situ, but are removed by filtration.

STERILIZATION WITH MOIST HEAT

Immersion in Boiling Water

Table 31.1 shows that, while boiling water will kill non-sporing organisms quickly, most spores are considerably more resistant, and some remain viable for 5 h or more, though these are generally non-pathogenic. As boiling is only used as an emergency sterilizing procedure for surgical instruments, it could be argued that pathogenic spores alone are of significance, but these too are fairly resistant, some strains resisting boiling for about 95 min. As has been said already, such a figure derived from end-point determinations of the death time, can show wide variation, and indeed Kelsey (1958), assuming a z value of 10°, calculated that to obtain the equivalent of killing in 5 min at 121°C, which he regarded as offering a reasonable margin of safety, boiling for 5 h would be required. It is not surprising therefore that in hospitals the method has largely been abandoned and replaced with the use of sterile, individually wrapped, instruments, from a central sterile supplies depot, or from commercial sources producing disposable, sterile units. Some vaccines are sterilized by heating in water at a temperature of 55 to 60°C. The vaccine is, or should be, a suspension of known organisms and should be free from spores, and the low temperature is used to kill the organisms present without impairing their antigenic properties.

Treatment with Steam at Elevated Pressure

Although steam at atmospheric pressure can be used for the sterilization of, for example, heat sensitive culture media, the process is unreliable and can often be avoided. For many media prepared from dried granules, for rubber gloves, glass apparatus or containers with rubber fittings or liners, for aqueous injections and for surgical dressings, treatment with steam at a pressure greater than that of the atmosphere is generally used. This process is known as autoclaving.

AUTOCLAVING

Principles of Steam Sterilization
If water is boiled in an open vessel, i.e. at atmospheric pressure, and if the vessel is then closed and heating of it continued, the temperature of the water and its vapour will rise above the normal boiling point and the pressure will also rise. Assuming that all air has been swept out of the vessel before it is closed, the temperature/pressure relationship will be as shown in the phase diagram Fig. 31.1. In this, the pressure is recorded in kgf/cm^2 above atmospheric pressure, and the phase boundary is the boiling point curve where steam and water are in equilibrium and the steam is said to be saturated. Columns 1 and 2 of Table 31.2 give figures which correspond to points on the curve.

Saturated Steam
When steam is saturated, it has its maximum capacity for condensing out. In doing so it gives

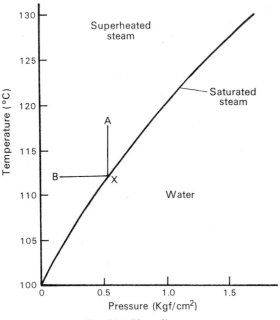

FIG. 31.1. Phase diagram.

TABLE 31.2

EFFECT ON TEMPERATURE/PRESSURE RELATIONSHIP OF DILUTING STEAM WITH AIR

Steam Pressure (above atmospheric)		Temperatures of mixtures of saturated steam with percentage (by volume) of air shown.				
		0%	20%	40%	60%	80%
$0\ lbf/in^2$	$0\ kgf/cm^2$	100	94	86	76	61
$10\ lbf/in^2$	$0.70\ kgf/cm^2$	115	108	100	89	72
$15\ lbf/in^2$	$1.05\ kgf/cm^2$	121	114	104	92	74
$20\ lbf/in^2$	$1.40\ kgf/cm^2$	126	118	110	98	81
$30\ lbf/in^2$	$2.10\ kgf/cm^2$	134	126	118	106	87

up its latent heat to the materials on which it condenses. The heat-up of objects being sterilized at temperatures of 115° to 135° is therefore rapid, because the heat energy liberated is about four to four and a half times that retained in the same amount of condensed water. The condensed water also assists in the sterilization process by hydrating the microorganisms present and allowing them to be easily killed (see p. 539). Moreover, when the steam condenses, a very considerable contraction occurs and more steam is drawn into the area to re-establish the pressure, so continuing the build-up of local heating until condensation is complete.

Superheated Steam
If the conditions of temperature and pressure are such that their effect is shown by a point above the phase boundary in Fig. 31.1, then the steam will be less than saturated, and is said to be *superheated*. Saturated steam may become superheated if it is isolated from contact with excess liquid water and either heated further or caused to expand by reducing the pressure, or by a combination of both provided that the above conditions are met. This will, of course, always be so if the temperature rise takes place at constant pressure, or the pressure falls while the temperature is held constant, as shown by the lines XA and XB in Fig. 31.1. Conversely, if steam is cooled or the pressure allowed to rise, condensation will occur if conditions traverse the phase boundary to a point lying beneath it.

Steam can also become superheated if mixed with air at constant pressure, for the partial pressure of the water vapour will thereby be lowered and the ability of the water molecules to condense will be reduced. Table 31.2 shows the effect of such dilution on the temperature of saturated steam at different overall pressures. If an unknown proportion of air is present in an autoclave, neither temperature readings nor pressure reading taken alone will reveal it. But if both readings are taken together, it can then be seen that the conditions do not correspond with those for pure water vapour, and suitable action can be taken. Industrial autoclaves are therefore fitted with both temperature and pressure recorders, and careful attention must be paid to these to ensure that sterilizing conditions are attained. The importance of this was shown in an incident which occurred in 1971 (Clothier, Committee of Enquiry, 1972) where the readings of the temperature recorder were ignored because it was assumed to be faulty, though its low readings really signified the presence of air which had not been voided from the autoclave.

Superheating can also be produced if local hot spots occur e.g. close to the chamber walls of a jacketed autoclave if the jacket is maintained at a temperature above that of the chamber, or by the interaction of the water vapour with the material being sterilized when the heat of adsorption is positive. Such an interaction occurs when cotton fibres adsorb and absorb moisture from steam, for the water is in effect bound as a liquid and the heat of adsorption will be equal to the sum of the latent heat and the residual heat of the liquid water. The fibres will therefore be rapidly heated, but superheating may occur. However, this only becomes appreciable if the cotton material has previously been dried to a moisture content of less than 1 per cent (Knox, Penikett & Duncan 1960). As cotton fabrics and dressings normally contain about 5 per cent of moisture, the heat of adsorption usually produces a negligible level of superheating.

Tolerable Degrees of Superheating

So far we have considered the equilibrium existing between water vapour and pure water. If, however, a substance is dissolved in the water, its vapour pressure will be lowered and the solution can exist in equilibrium with steam that would be superheated with respect to water. Savage (1937) proposed that the bacterial substances could be regarded in this way and that it could equilibrate with steam showing some degree of superheating, so that condensation could still take place. He tested the efficiency of steam having varying degrees of superheat in killing spores and found that the degree of superheat that could exist and still provide satisfactory sterilizing conditions rose as the temperature itself rose. At the usual autoclaving temperatures, i.e. 115° to 120°, sterilization could be achieved

within the normal time schedule, even though two or three degrees of superheat existed. Savage advocated this procedure in order to ensure that dressings would be dry after sterilization, but the Medical Research Council's Working Party (1959) suggested that superheating could occur within the dressings due to heat of adsorption and that therefore no further superheating should be tolerated. They recommended that steam should be admitted to the chamber without any superheating and that the practice then current, of holding the jacket at a temperature about 10° higher than the chamber should be abandoned.

Wet and Dry Steam

When steam is produced from a boiler, it contains a large number of entrained droplets of water. If such 'wet' steam is used for sterilization, it will reduce condensation of water vapour so that less latent heat will be made available to produce a rapid heat-up. Moreover, if the objects to be sterilized are absorptive, e.g. surgical dressings, paper wrappings, they will become sodden. Before admission to the autoclave, therefore, the excess moisture is removed by suitable baffles in a *separator*. The resultant steam, freed from its water droplets, is referred to as 'dry' steam.

DESIGN AND OPERATION OF AUTOCLAVES

Portable Autoclaves

A portable, or bench, autoclave is essentially very similar to the familiar domestic 'pressure-cooker'. It consists of an upright aluminium or stainless steel, cylindrical vessel, of about 15 litres capacity, fitted with a lid which can be firmly secured. In one type the lid is held down with eight screw clamps and carries a pressure gauge, an air vent and an adjustable safety valve. The externally fitted lid ensures that the whole of the capacity of the vessel can be used, but the arrangement has disadvantages. If one of the clamps should fracture, the strain imposed on others may cause these to fail successively and an explosion will then follow. It is therefore essential that all the clamps should be firmly secured and that they should be carefully maintained. The lid itself is heavy and does not carry a thermometer as this would be likely to be damaged when the lid is put down, as it cannot be easily inverted. Conditions within the autoclave are therefore indicated solely by the pressure gauge. Although saturation will always be maintained by the excess water at the bottom of the autoclave, it is essential that all air should be expelled before the vent is closed, otherwise the reading of the pressure gauge will indicate a temperature higher than that attained.

A more satisfactory arrangement is that shown in the autoclave illustrated in Fig. 31.2. The lid is fitted under the lip of the opening at the top of the stainless steel vessel. This offers maximum safety, because increase of pressure will only secure the lid more firmly. Both lid and opening are oval in shape so that the lid can be inserted diagonally with its narrow axis presented to the wider part of the opening. It is then rotated into its correct position under and aligned with the opening and secured by a cross-bar passed through the handle. The bar carries a clamping screw at one end which can be screwed down on to the lip, thus raising the bar and the lid suspended from it. The lid is surrounded by a rubber rim and this is brought tightly against the underside of the lip of the vessel; it carries only a spring-loaded safety valve and a pressure gauge and is quite light and easy to handle.

The thermometer, with its bulb shielded, is inserted through the lip and not through the lid, so that it is not damaged when the latter is withdrawn or inserted. The lip also carries a thermostat which can be pre-set to maintain any required temperature in the autoclave, and this can be adequately monitored because both temperature and pressure

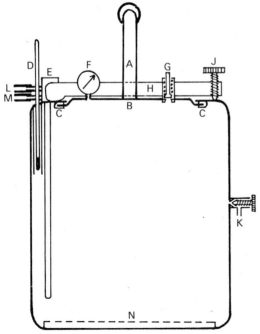

FIG. 31.2. Bench autoclave. A, handle of lid; B, lid; C, gasket; D, armoured thermometer; E, thermostat; F, pressure gauge; G, spring safety valve; H, crossbar; J, screw for tightening lid; K, blow-off valve; L, gas inlet; M, gas outlet to burner (not shown); N, perforated stand.

readings can be made. This type of autoclave is generally designed to be heated on a gas ring, but electrically heated models are also available. If relatively large objects are to be sterilized, e.g. infusion bottles, these are placed on a perforated plate which rests on the bottom of the autoclave. This arrangement gives the maximum head room, which is necessary as the insertion of the lid reduces this. Smaller articles can be placed on a wire basket the legs of which keep them above the water.

A blow-off valve is fitted at the side of the autoclave in order to void air. Owing to the turbulence created by the boiling water, air and steam are well mixed and the rather low position of the valve is therefore no detriment. Unlike the model first described, the valve is not attached to a siphon tube inside the vessel. This was used to blow off the excess water and then the steam at the end of autoclaving in order to create 'dry' conditions. This is really of importance only when dressings are sterilized and portable autoclaves are not suitable for this. A siphon tube is therefore not required.

Operation. The operation of this type of autoclave is very simple. About two litres of water is placed in the vessel, the objects to be sterilized are loaded into it, and the lid is fitted in place. The air vent is left open and the heat turned on. If solutions in unsealed containers, e.g. bacteriological cultures in plugged tubes, are being sterilized, they should not be put in the autoclave until the water has started boiling, otherwise concentration of the solution may occur during the heat-up period. When steam has issued freely from the vent for about 5 min, the latter is shut. The temperature and pressure then rise till the former reaches that controlled by the thermostat. When this is seen to be so, heating is continued for the required time and the autoclave is then allowed to cool. As soon as the pressure in the autoclave drops to that of the atmosphere, the vent is opened in order that the gauge should not be damaged by the vacuum that would otherwise result. This might also cause some evaporation of liquids in unsealed containers. Injections in ampoules may be removed almost immediately, but intravenous infusions in large bottles, because heat transfer from them is poor, cool down more slowly than the autoclave itself. They therefore retain a pressure higher than that of the atmosphere for some time and, if removed too early may explode.

If the autoclave is temperature controlled by a thermostat, it is not absolutely necessary to vent the air from it, for the correct temperature will be reached and maintained and saturation will always occur due to the reserve of water present. Venting, however, decreases the risk of pockets of air remaining between or within the objects to be sterilized, and ensures a satisfactory penetration of steam into them.

Horizontal Large Scale Autoclaves

The portable autoclaves described above can only be used for small loads of vaccine bottles or for one or two transfusion bottles. For large loads, horizontal autoclaves are used of the general design shown in Fig. 31.3.

Main steam is passed through a reducing valve A to bring the pressure down to that required for operation, and then through a separator B to remove water droplets. The steam line is then bifurcated, one branch passing to the jacket surrounding the chamber, the other leading to the top of the chamber itself where steam is admitted through the baffle F. The chamber is fitted with a pressure gauge P and a spring-loaded safety-valve C, a relief valve D and also an air inlet E, guarded by a sterile, bacteria-proof filter. It is drained at G and the drain pocket carries an armoured thermometer H and a probe for a recording thermometer I. The drain line then passes through a strainer J, a non-return valve K and a steam-trap L. The jacket drain also carries a steam-trap M. Both steam-

traps drain into a common waste through U-bends, but an air-break is maintained between these and the main drainage system so that no water can be sucked back when the chamber is cooled or exhausted, and the exit of condensed water can be observed. The chamber may also be fitted with an exhaust line O passing to an ejector operated by water or steam, or by a water-sealed rotary pump. These give only a moderate vacuum, but where a higher vacuum is required, a water ring pump may be used to suck air through a special ejector (Whittet, Hugo & Wilkinson 1965), or an oil-sealed pump with means to remove condensed water may be employed.

Operation. The mode of operation may depend on the type of material to be sterilized. In the case of porous materials, particularly surgical dressings, it is necessary to draw a vacuum to remove air, not only from the chamber itself, but also from the interstices of the materials being sterilized. For non-porous materials this is not necessary and use of high vacuum cycles is inappropriate for bottled liquids (Sykes 1969); downward displacement with steam is therefore generally used. In this case, it is not necessary that the autoclave should be provided with a steam-jacket, provided that it is properly lagged, but it is of course often a matter of convenience to use a jacketed autoclave for all purposes.

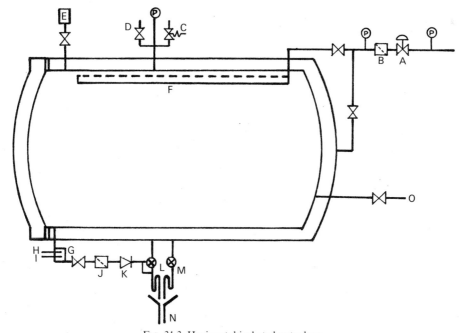

FIG. 31.3. Horizontal jacketed autoclave.

Loading. The load must be carefully stacked in the autoclave so that channels are left between the articles to allow the maximum penetration of steam. None of the articles should touch the chamber wall, and if packed in containers, these must allow free drainage of air downwards through the pack and out at its base. The load is often carried on a wheeled rack with perforated shelves, and this may be partially withdrawn from the chamber on to a detachable gantry for ease of operation. When loading is completed, the door is shut and secured either with shackled clamps arranged peripherally or, for cylindrical chambers, by radial bolts actuated by a wheel placed centrally on the door.

Removal of air. The next stage consists of admitting steam to the chamber and removing air from it. As has been said, this can be done in two ways.

Downward displacement. Steam is admitted to the chamber through F, the baffles of which are designed to ensure that steam is directed to the top of the chamber in a turbulent state, so that an air pocket is not formed there. The steam, being slightly lighter than air at the same temperature, gradually displaces the air and air-stream mixtures below it and forces them out through G. When this process is complete the temperature recorded at G should have risen to that of saturated steam at the pressure indicated by the chamber pressure gauge. In practice a low vacuum can be drawn before admission of steam even for bottled fluids and can assist in removing part of the air before steam is admitted to remove the remainder (Clothier Report 1972).

High pre-vacuum process. In this process the air is removed by reducing the vacuum pressure to about 20 mmHg. The vacuum may be applied continually while the steam is gradually admitted (Alder 1970), but usually the application of vacuum and admission of steam are made to alternate; two periods of evacuation being often employed, each followed by admission of steam. A vacuum of 20 mmHg (absolute) is drawn (Knox & Penikett 1958), followed by a short burst of steam to raise the pressure to just above atmospheric. The vacuum assists penetration of the fibres by the steam which raises their temperature somewhat, but the subsequent inrush of steam also entrains air and carries it back into the fibres, so that as the steam condenses, small pockets of air are formed. A second vacuum is then necessary to remove these and, this is assisted by the 'boiling-out' of the condensate.

Wilkinson and Peacock (1961) showed that in closely packed materials, e.g. hospital towels, better results were obtained if the jacket temperature was held at 135° and during the first steam burst the pressure was raised to 200 mmHg. Enough high temperature steam was drawn into the fibres to raise their temperature to 45° and to provide good boiling-out facility when the second vacuum of 20 mmHg was applied. At the end of this, the temperature of the fibres dropped only to 40° and steam was readmitted to give 2.11 kgf/cm² (30 lbf/in²) gauge for only 3 min. This high prevacuum, high temperature process greatly reduces the time taken for a complete sterilization cycle as each stage is of short duration, but it is not suitable for fabrics which have become either very dry or moisture-laden before sterilization.

Henry and Scott (1963) showed that 'boiling-out' occurred more readily with full loads than with an autoclave in which a large air-space was left and suggested that to obviate difficulties with light loads a high vacuum of better than 15 mmHg should be drawn with a steam-jacketed, oil-sealed pump.

Heat-up time. When large bottles of liquid are sterilized, this may be considerable, as heat penetration through the individual items items of the load is slow. The actual time required will vary with the volume of each bottle and the steam temperature employed, and the rate of heat penetration should therefore be determined by placing thermocouples in specimen loads. The recording of the chamber drain thermometer is often used, but it gives only a crude estimate of the conditions in the autoclave. For a 500 ml transfusion bottle the heat-up time, using steam at 115° is about 15 min (*Pharmaceutical Handbook* 1970).

When the high-vacuum process is used for porous loads, the rapid penetration of the steam quickly raises the temperature of the articles being sterilized and it is not necessary to allow for any further heat-up time.

Sterilization period. When all air has been removed from the chamber and from the load in the case of porous objects, and when the whole of the load has been raised to the sterilizing temperature, this is held for the required time. Appendix 29 of the *British Pharmaceutical Codex* 1973 lists the following temperature-time combinations which are based largely on those proposed by the Medical Research Council Working Party (1959). Choice of the combination used will depend on the ability of the material being sterilized to withstand the conditions imposed.

Temperature (°C)	Corresponding nominal pressure in excess of atmospheric (kgf/cm²)	(lb/in²)	Recommended minimum holding time (min)
115–116°	0.70	10	30
121–123°	1.05	15	15
126–129°	1.40	20	10
134–138°	2.25	32	3

Drainage of air and condensate. During downward displacement of air, this is vented through the drain at the bottom of the chamber. To prevent excessive loss of steam at the same time a steam-trap is inserted in the exit line. This may be a bellows operated trap of the type shown in Fig. 31.4. The flexible capsule contains a liquid mixture which boils at a temperature slightly lower than that of water. When air passes through the valve the capsule is not extended, but after the air is voided and the steam enters the trap it raises the temperature, causing the capsule to expand and close the exit. The trap should open within 3° and close within 2° of the saturated steam temperature and is therefore referred to as a 'near-to-steam' trap. The fact that the capsule is flexible subjects the liquid inside it to the same pressure as that of the atmosphere surrounding it: the liquid will then boil at a higher temperature if the pressure is raised so that near-to-steam conditions are maintained. Such traps will vent air, air and steam mixtures and

small volumes of condensed water and can be successfully used during the downward displacement of air, but during the sterilization period, heavy loads of non-porous articles, e.g. bottles of liquid, can produce copious condensation and the bellows-operated trap is unable to cope with it. A float-operated trap of the type shown in Fig. 31.5 may be used for this purpose, but Barson, Peacock Robins and Wilkinson (1958) showed that under their test conditions neither bellows-operated nor float-operated traps were fully satisfactory. The former are insensitive to small amounts of air and the latter can only be used to control the expulsion of water. Barson et al. suggested that the bellows-operated valve should be provided with a small permanent by-pass and that the whole unit should be incorporated inside the body of a float-chamber so that both valves and the by-pass were all operative.

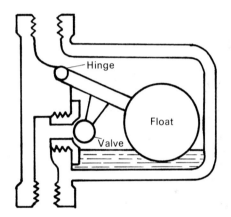

FIG. 31.5. Float operated steam trap (after Whittet, Hugo & Wilkinson 1965).

Cooling down period. When the sterilization period is completed, the inflow of steam to the chamber is stopped and the autoclave is allowed to cool. Where large volume bottles of liquid have been sterilized, these may take some time to cool and the pressure round them must not be allowed to fall too quickly or they may burst. The steam is therefore vented slowly through the drain or a by-pass. The contents of the autoclave are then left until the temperature of the bottled fluids falls below 100° so that the autoclave can be opened and the load removed without danger to the operator. When dressings are sterilized, no such considerations arise and after sterilization is complete the steam is removed by the pump and a vacuum is drawn to remove residual moisture from the load. The jacket temperature is maintained

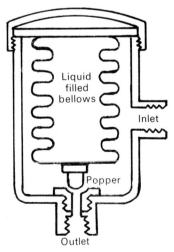

FIG. 31.4. Bellows operated steam trap.

meanwhile to prevent local condensation. Penikett, Rowe and Robson (1958) suggested that a vacuum of 50 to 200 mmHg held for less than 3 min would produce suitably dry dressings. At the end of this period the vacuum is broken by admitting sterile air through the bacteria-proof filter and the load can then be removed.

The cooling period for bottled fluids can be greatly reduced by spraying them with jets of warm water (Bowie 1959). Wilkinson, Peacock and Robins (1960) found that, if excessive breakage of bottles was to be avoided, the spray must form a mist fine enough to prevent localized cooling and thermal shock, and a small volume of air must be admitted concurrently to prevent too rapid a reduction of pressure around the bottles. The object of spray-cooling is not only to shorten the time of cooling as an economic measure, but also to reduce the hazard of exploding bottles by ensuring that they are cool enough before the door of the autoclave is opened. However, both Beverley, Hambleton and Allwood (1974) and Myers (1974) showed that contamination could occur of the outer surface of the bottle closure and of the interface between the neck of the bottle and the aluminium screw-cap used to confine the closure. If then the contents of the bottle are poured out for topical use, or if the closure is pierced by the cannula of a giving set, infection of the sterilized fluid can occur. Beverley et al. found that direct contamination of the contents occasionally occurred during sterilization and spray-cooling, but in these cases the bottle closures were sufficiently defective to permit the entry of water in volume large enough to be obvious. Although the Rosenheim Committee (1972) in its interim report suggested that contamination could be prevented by adequate bottle closures, Myers considers that the present specifications for infusion bottles (BS 2463, 1962) and the DHSS standard for bottles for non-injectable sterile water, are inadequate and it is necessary to provide improved designs for bottles to be used in spray-cooled autoclaves.

Automatic Process Control
In view of the heavy responsibility that rests upon process workers carrying out sterilization procedures to ensure that every stage is adequately monitored and performed, automation of the control procedure offers an attractive refinement and provision is made for it in British Standard 3970/2 (1966). Each stage of the process is under automatic control and the temperature/time combination is controlled by an integrator operating

from a probe placed within the load and can be varied to give suitable conditions for the sterilization of different loads, e.g. dressings, surgical gloves, instruments and bottled fluids. To allow for variations in atmospheric pressure at different times or places, the switch controlling the vacuum pump is barometrically compensated. The door mechanism must be so arranged that steam cannot enter the chamber before the door is locked, and the door cannot be opened until the chamber pressure is reduced to 0.2 kgf/cm^2 and the chamber is vented to the atmosphere. Alarm systems are also arranged to give warning if failures occur at any stage.

Performance Tests
Although the monitoring of the sterilization procedure by careful observation of the temperature and pressure within the chamber gives some indication that the process has been properly carried out, it is necessary to perform additional tests to ensure the sterility of the products because it cannot necessarily be assumed that the observed conditions are those which have obtained in the depths of the load, for this can depend on the nature, moisture content and packing of the articles being sterilized. It is necessary therefore to carry out routine tests to ensure that full sterilizing conditions have been attained and maintained throughout the load.

One way of doing this is by testing random samples of the load for sterility and this is discussed later in this chapter. Another is to make estimates of conditions in the load itself. This can be done in several ways.

Instrumental methods. Temperature conditions within the load can be sensed by thermocouples or thermistors inserted into it at various places. In the case of liquids, the probe is placed in representative bottles and in the case of dressings it is inserted well into specimen packs. The autoclave must be fitted with ports to take the leads for the probes and these are connected to recorders which give a continuous tracing. The method does not, however, give any direct information on the humidity conditions and the possible existence of superheating within porous loads such as surgical dressings.

Bacteriological methods. The use of resistant bacterial spores is regarded by some workers as providing the only satisfactory evidence of the effectiveness of a sterilization process and the choice of suitable test organisms has already been discussed. The spores are usually dried onto strips or discs of filter paper or aluminium foil (Kelsey

1961, Beeby & Whitehouse 1965, Cook & Brown 1965), each test piece carrying about 10^6 spores. Kelsey (1961) found that with such an inoculum of *B. stearothermophilus* a test piece would require sterilizing for about 10 min at 121°. For use, the test pieces are placed in special envelopes and embedded in the centre of dressings or other materials to be sterilized. After the sterilization process has been completed, they are removed and aseptically withdrawn from the envelopes and cultured in a medium which will give maximal growth conditions. One disadvantage of the method is that incubation of the recovered spores must be continued for several days. Kelsey (1951) found that very few positives occurred after three days and chose five to give a margin of safety, but even this means that the result may not be known until after the sterilized material is required, and bacteriological tests of this kind are therefore more useful as indicators of satisfactory routine conditions than as safeguards in the processing of a particular batch.

Chemical indicators. The earliest of these, called 'witness tubes', consisted of single crystalline substances of known melting point contained in glass tubes, e.g. sulphur (115°), acetanilide (116°), succinic anhydride (120°), benzoic acid (121°). A dye could be included to show more clearly that the crystals had melted. Such a device, of course, only indicates that a certain temperature has been reached, but attempts have been made to indicate the exposure time by putting the crystals in one end of an 'hour-glass' tube, the volume of the crystals and the diameter of the constriction of the tube being adjusted so that the time for transfer of the melt is the same as that required for sterilization at the required temperature. If, however, the designated temperature is exceeded during sterilization, the liquid in the tube will flow through the constriction more quickly and the new time-temperature relationship will not necessarily correlate with that required for sterilization. A modification of this process was devised by Simpkins and Wilkinson (1964), in which they used a filter paper strip laminated with an adhesive to aluminium foil acting as a heat distributor. One end of the strip is impregnated with a 2-4 dinitrophenylhydrazone of suitable melting point and on melting, the liquid travels along the paper strip at a controlled rate. The device is sealed in a perforated polypropylene envelope through which it is observed.

A slightly different method is used in Browne's tubes (A. Browne, Leicester, Ltd.), in which a controlled chemical reaction is involved in the change of colour of a red liquid through amber to green. For autoclaving, two types are available: Type I changes to full green in about 16 min at 120° and in 10 min at 125°, Type II also changes in about 10 min at 120°. These conditions accord reasonably well with those officially demanded by the *British Pharmaceutical Codex*, but at lower temperatures they give an inadequate margin of safety. Because the result is dependent on a chemical reaction, it can still be produced by longer exposure to sub-lethal temperatures, so that if extra time is allowed for the sterilization of a particular load, the results can be misleading. Unlike the methods which involve the melting of a pure substance, the chemical system employed introduces an inherent instability and careful storage in a cool place is required before Browne's tubes are used (Brown & Ridout 1960).

Chemical methods are also available in which the colour of adhesive tape (3M's Ltd) or sheets of paper marked with sensitized strips (E. S. & A. Robinson Ltd.) changes when moist heat is applied, but these are only useful when a high autoclaving temperature (134°) is employed with a holding time of not more than 3.5 min (Alder 1970).

Kelsey (1958) constructed a diagram to show the characteristics of available indicators. An adapted form of this is shown in Fig. 31.6. Kelsey first plotted the thermal death times for resistant pathogens which had a z value of about 10°. He advocated the use of an indicator which would show the same slope for time/temperature dependency as that given by the death time curve of the pathogens. The line representing the characteristics of this ideal indicator should lie above that given by the death times of the pathogens but below that indicating the approved schedules for sterilization, for Kelsey argued that if the indicator showed complete change under conditions corresponding too closely to those used for sterilization, too many false negatives would be recorded. Simpkins and Wilkinson chose indicators, the characteristics of which corresponded very closely with the official sterilization conditions. Kelsey's ideal indicator certainly reacts at too low a temperature to ensure absolute sterility, for, if a mean curve is fitted for known resistant non-pathogenic spores it lies well above that for the indicator and indeed above the lower part of the curve provided by the official sterilization schedules, but reference has already been made to the view of Sykes (1969) that the occurrence of such resistant organisms in pharmaceutical materials is too rare to warrant concern. Kelsey's diagram also shows that the slope for

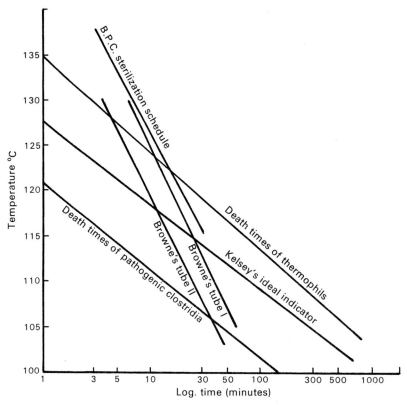

FIG. 31.6. Performance of indicators of sterilization efficiency.

Browne's tubes is much greater than that of the pathogens or of the official sterilization schedules, so that only at the higher temperatures could they ensure sterility.

Other Autoclaving Methods

Low pressure method. In this method steam is admitted to a previously evacuated autoclave to give a negative pressure of about 360 mmHg, resulting in a temperature of 80°. These conditions are maintained for 10 min in order to kill all vegetative bacteria. The effectiveness of the process can be increased by adding formaldehyde vapour to the steam and spores can then be killed if conditions are held for 2 h (Alder 1970). Residual formaldehyde is removed at the end of the sterilization period by applying a further vacuum. The method has been used for sterilization of woollen blankets and of heat-sensitive surgical instruments such as endoscopes, and materials such as plastic tubing.

Counterpressure method. Sykes (1969) has pointed out that when sealed containers of liquid are sterilized, air is not eliminated from them and it is not always necessary to remove all the air from an autoclave. Doing so has two advantages; it provides the maximum condensation conditions from the saturated steam present, and it enables temperature and pressure conditions to be easily correlated. These advantages can be offset by using unsaturated steam at a higher pressure, provided that the conditions in the autoclave chamber are registered by adequate temperature recordings and not from pressure readings. However, as Savage (1959) pointed out, local condensation in an autoclave can cause steam and air to separate into two layers, so that air pockets can occur in which sterilizing conditions are not attained. If therefore a high-pressure air-steam mixture is used, it must be continually mixed by the inclusion of a fan in the chamber. One advantage claimed for the method is that the higher pressure surrounding sealed bottles of liquid reduces breakage during sterilization. In this technique a pressure of 2.11 kgf/cm^2 (30 lbf/in^2) is used, the air-steam mixture being adjusted to give a temperature of 115° by alternately pulsated jets of steam and air, under automatic control.

OTHER METHODS OF STERILIZATION WITH MOIST HEAT

Tyndallization. This method consists of heating the material at 80° for 1 h, or at 100° for less, on three successive days. It was based on the supposition that after vegetative cells have been killed in the first heating, spores will germinate before the next, when they also will be killed. However, some spores may remain dormant for long periods and heat-damaged spores may be slow to germinate, so the method cannot guarantee sterility, and although it was included in the *British Pharmacopoeia* 1932, it was eliminated in the Addendum of 1941, Davis (1940) having shown it to be unsuitable for injections.

Heating with a bactericide. Davis (1940) in his investigation of tyndallization of injections had shown that the method could succeed if the medicament itself was bactericidal. Since the efficiency of bactericides in solution was known to increase with temperature, an obvious development was to include a substance of known bactericidal activity in the injection. Coulthard (1939) found chlorocresol and phenylmercuric nitrate effective when heated at 100° for 30 min and Berry et al. (1938) confirmed this, pointing out also that the bactericide must be free from toxicity, compatible with the medicament and stable under the conditions of sterilization and storage. The method was adopted by the *British Pharmacopoeia* to replace tyndallization for the sterilization of injections and is still official. It consists of heating the injection solutions in their final containers in boiling water or in a steamer at 98 to 100° for 30 min, the permitted bactericides being 0.2 per cent chlorocresol and 0.002 per cent phenylmercuric nitrate. The method must not be used for intrathecal, intracysternal or peridural injection, where the bactericides would exhibit toxicity, nor in intravenous injections greater than 15 ml in volume where toxicity would arise from the total amount of injected bactericide, nor of course is it applicable to the sterilization of culture media. The method is also used for the preparation of eye-drops; the permitted bactericides being those specified in Chapter 27 as preservatives (see p. 360). The same principle is involved in the sterilization of canned fruit, where the natural acidity permits sterilization at lower temperatures than would be required in neutral solution. It was also invoked in the now outmoded method of sterilizing surgical instruments in solutions of sodium carbonate or borax.

Pasteurization. Although this is not strictly a method of sterilization, since all organisms present are not necessarily killed, it may be briefly mentioned here. It was devised by Pasteur to improve the keeping qualities of wine and is now applied to the processing of milk in order to kill pathogenic organisms without significantly affecting the taste, nutritional value, or emulsification of milk. Two methods are used:
The Holding Method; in this the milk is heated in tanks at 62.8°C for 30 min, the milk being mixed by gentle agitation. A jet of steam is used to disperse foam on the surface.
High Temperature—Short Time, or Flash Process; the milk is passed at a controlled rate through heat exchangers which rapidly raise its temperature to 71.6°C and hold it so for 15 s, after which it is as rapidly cooled in a second heat exchanger. By decreasing the severity of the conditions the process can be used for the sterilization of large volumes of culture media, which can then be fed directly to fermentors (Whitmarsh 1954).

DRY HEAT STERILIZATION

Resistance to Dry Heat

Reference to Table 31.1 shows that sterilization by dry heat requires higher temperatures and longer exposure times than those required when moist heat is used. Rahn (1945) assumed that this was due to a difference in the fundamental processes involved and ascribed the lethal effect of dry heat to oxidation, whereas he postulated that the sterilizing action of moist heat was due to protein denaturation. Hansen and Riemann (1963), however, consider that the difference is due to the presence or absence of water of hydration attached to the protein molecules, and interstitial water held between them. When heat is applied in the presence of sufficient water, disulphide bonds and hydrogen bonds between the protein strands can be broken and the strands have sufficient mobility to form new linkages resulting in the denaturing of the protein, which, if it is part of an enzyme, will render it inactive. In the absence of sufficient water, rearrangement of the protein is more difficult and more energy is required to denature it. Hansen and Riemann applied their argument only to non-sporing organisms, which are only slightly more resistant to dry heat than to moist heat. Spores, however, unlike vegetative cells, contain demonstrable amounts of dipicolinic acid (DPA), an it has been suggested that their greater heat resistance is due to the manner in which the proteins are bound to calcium dipicolinate (Brown & Melling 1973), the complex formed having considerable stability and protecting the protein against thermal displacement.

Official Requirements

The minimum treatment prescribed by the *British Pharmacopoeia* is to hold the material to be sterilized at 150°C for 1 h: this applies to fixed oils and oily solutions, and is also recommended by the *British Pharmaceutical Codex* for ethyl oleate, liquid paraffin and glycerol. Many workers regard this regimen as barely sufficient to ensure sterility and it is used only because higher temperatures may decompose the substance being sterilized. For glassware, the *British Pharmacopoeia* demands that 160° should be used for 1 h, while the *British Pharmaceutical Codex* suggests the alternative, in addition, of 180° for 11 min. The United States Pharmacopoeial requirements are more severe, involving the use of 180° for 2 h.

The Hot Air Oven

The hot air oven is the equipment most commonly used for dry heat sterilization. It may be heated by gas or electricity, but electrically heated, thermostatically controlled, ovens are generally employed because of their greater convenience and the fact that the heaters can be placed in the side walls as well as under the floor, giving the best distribution of heat.

Articles or materials placed in the oven can receive heat by direct transfer from the hot air circulating in the oven, by radiation from the oven walls, and by conduction.

Direct transfer of heat from circulating air. Owing to its low specific heat, air is a poor heating agent, and considerable amounts of it must pass over the articles in order to raise their temperature to that of the oven. In the absence of a fan, circulation of the air over the heating surfaces and then over the articles to be sterilized, is due entirely to convection which not only promotes the movement of too little air but may also distribute it unevenly. The oven is therefore usually fitted with a fan or turboblower, placed in the back wall. Air from the oven is drawn through the fan and recirculated over the heaters before it is passed back into the oven cavity. There is thus a continuous forced circulation of the hot air in sufficient volume to impart an effective amount of heat to the articles in the oven.

Radiation. A considerable amount of heat is radiated from the heated walls of the oven and this will heat those surfaces which are accessible to it. Newman (1955), using paper strips covered in heat sensitive paint, concluded that radiation is much more efficient than the air as a heating agent but, while articles near the wall will be easily heated, they will screen others and in a heavily loaded oven the contribution of radiation to the total heating may be lost.

Conduction. Conduction will occur to a limited extent along the shelves on which the articles are placed, but contact will usually be too limited to provide for efficient heating. The articles being sterilized will themselves be penetrated by heat at a rate dependent upon their own composition and structure. In the case of liquids this will be assisted by convection within the material, but in the case of solids which are poor conductors of heat, e.g. powders, or loosely packed materials containing entrapped air, the heat-up time may be prolonged.

Performance characteristics of the oven. These are specified in British Standard No. 3421: 1961 which requires that the oven should work within the temperature range 140° to 180°, that its heat-up time for a rise of 140° should not exceed 135 min, and that temperature variations during the heat-up and subsequent holding periods should not exceed given limits. A test load of glass jars is used to determine temperature distribution in the oven, the four corner jars and the central one on each shelf carrying thermocouples immersed in liquid.

Loading. From the foregoing, it is evident that proper loading is of the greatest importance. Channels for circulation of the heated air must be left and if articles must be placed on top of each other they should be staggered. If sufficient room is available, articles should be so placed that each can receive the maximum radiation from the walls and no articles should be left in contact with these, or overheating and possibly charring may occur. To ensure adequate internal transfer of the heat, the bulk of each article or unit should not be too great. Rubbo and Gardner (1965) recommend that packages should not exceed $4 \times 4 \times 12$ inches and that the depth of powders, oils and waxes should not be greater than half an inch.

Operation. The oven should be brought up to operating temperature before the load is placed in it, in order to reduce the heat-up time to a minimum. Since it cannot be assumed, at least for larger articles, that they will heat up as quickly as the oven itself, the thermometer measuring oven temperature will not satisfactorily indicate when the load has reached the required temperature throughout its bulk. It will then be necessary to carry out a pilot test, using thermocouples placed inside the articles being sterilized by which the rise in temperature at the centre of the articles can be recorded. The lag or heat penetration time for each load can then be assessed and it must be added to the normal heat-up time of the oven to give an extended heat-up time after which the temperature within the load should remain the same as that of the oven. This condition is maintained for the required Holding Time and the current is then switched off and the oven and its contents allowed to cool. During the cooling period, of course, non-sterile air may enter the oven, so articles must be wrapped in paper, or placed in metal boxes, or as in the case of culture tubes plugged with cotton wool or closed with aluminium caps.

Performance tests. As with autoclaving, routine performance tests should be carried out when the hot air oven is used for sterilization. Similar tests to those already described can be carried out using instrumental, bacteriological and chemical indicators. The use of instruments is exactly the same as in autoclaving and the choice of suitable bacteria has already been discussed on p. 528, but the carriers for the spores must, of course, be able to withstand the higher temperature of the oven and are usually made of metal, glass or ceramic. Browne's tubes Type III are available for use with hot air sterilization.

Forced-draught ovens. Quesnel et al. (1967) reported on the use of an oven in which hot air was forced in a linear stream from the top, through the load and out at the bottom, where it passed over the control and recording temperature probes. The principal object of this was to overcome the viscous drag of the air adherent to the surface of the articles in the load by using an air flow of 700 ft^3/min at a temperature of 200°. Both the relatively high speed of flow of the air and its high temperature would assist in sweeping away the static air film and improving heat transfer. At the end of the sterilization period the heaters were turned off and the incoming air was passed over water-cooled coils to hasten the cooling of the load, all stages being automated. Metal strips could be heated in an overall time of about 20 min, sputum cups took about twice as long, and glass jars, presumably because of their lower conductivity, somewhat longer.

Infra-red Conveyor Ovens

Darmady, Hughes and Tuke (1957) described the use of a conveyor oven heated by infra-red projectors, for sterilizing syringes. These were passed at a controlled rate, on a conveyor belt, through a shallow tunnel over which the heaters were placed, the articles to be sterilized being arranged in a single layer in open trays. Each syringe was contained in a glass or metal tube or box. These receive the heat radiated from the projectors and convey it to the syringes by conduction. Consequently the rate at which heat is transferred will vary with the material used for the container, and its surface. It is quickest with glass and slower for metal containers. The surface finish of the latter is important: a bright shiny surface reflects much of the radiation it receives and gives a heat-up time about twice that of a dull black one. Darmady et al. recommended a holding time of about 11 min, but different passage times are required for different loads and each load should consist of similar articles so that the conditions can be pre-set to suit them. The method has the advantage of being a continuous process and because of the short heat-up time has a considerable throughput. It can be used for small instruments such as forceps and scissors: penetration of steam between the blades of the latter can sometimes prove difficult to achieve (Quesnel 1967) and infra-red heating offers a useful alternative without the hazards of ionizing radiations and the specialized equipment for using them.

The conveyor oven is, however, unsuitable for bulky instruments of varying dimension. For sterilizing these, Darmady et al. (1961) devised an infra-red oven in which a high vacuum could be drawn and maintained during the sterilization period. Removal of the air means that no heat is lost in warming it up, the instability produced by convection currents is absent and oxidation of metal is avoided. Sterile nitrogen is admitted during the cooling down period to minimize this. A very high temperature of 280° is used and an exposure time of only 7 min is therefore possible.

Thermal Heating Blocks

Although in hospitals instruments are generally supplied from a central sterile supplies depot, it may be necessary sometimes to carry out emergency sterilization of syringes or small instruments. This used to be done by boiling in a 'fish-kettle' sterilizer, but as has been explained, this is unreliable. Darmady, Hughes, Jones and Tuke described a method in which an aluminium block with holes bored horizontally into it was fixed to an electric hot-plate. The holes were made the right size for the insertion of syringes and a tray was fitted to the top of the block for small instruments. The whole block was surrounded by a cover during heating. Darmady et al. used a temperature of 190° for 22 min to achieve sterilization.

Radio-Frequency Induction Heating

In this process a radio-frequency current, generated by a suitable oscillator, is passed through a hollow copper coil surrounding the work piece to be sterilized. Trotman (1969) advocated its use for the in situ sterilization of the handling equipment, e.g. metal pipettes and wire loops, of automatic diagnostic systems. The object to be sterilized must, however, be a conductor and this must limit the use of the method, although Trotman suggested that it could be adapted for general use by passing the articles through a horizontal coil on a conveyor belt. Non-conductors could be attached to a conducting susceptor which would heat the non-conductor by contact.

STERILIZATION BY FILTRATION

Sterilization by passage through a bacteria-proof filter is used for thermolabile solutions and gases including air. Thermolabile solutions would suffer damage if subjected to heat sterilization. The process is also used occasionally as an alternative to heating methods for the sterilization of thermostable solutions. The process consists of three main stages for solutions:
(1) Passage of the solution to be sterilized through a previously sterilized filter-unit.
(2) Aseptic transference of the filtrate to sterile containers which are then sealed aseptically.
(3) Tests for sterility are carried out on the filtered product.
The third stage is part of the process since there are a number of hazards in filtration sterilization. For the same reason a bacteriostatic is usually included in the solution.

The disadvantages of the process often outweigh the advantages as shown in the following:

Advantages. (a) No heating used, thus ideal for thermolabile solutions.
(b) Removes all bacteria and fungi, and often clarifies the solution.
(c) Useful process for sterilization of large volume solutions.
(d) Useful for eye-drops, as dropper bottles do not withstand heating processes well.

Disadvantages. (a) Aseptic technique required. This requires highly trained staff and sterile equipment and facilities.
(b) Sterility tests are required. Except in emergency, issue is not permitted until tests have been passed. Deterioration can occur in the 7 days required.
(c) Viruses, filtrable forms of bacteria, and bacterial products, such as toxins and pyrogens, are not removed or destroyed.
(d) Filter may break down either suddenly or gradually in use. Gradual faults may be undetectable immediately.
(e) Filtration unit may leak and permit entry of non-sterile air. Thus filter units should have as few joints as possible. Use of positive pressure (i.e. forcing the solution through the filter with compressed air) has an advantage over negative pressure (i.e. sucking the solution through the filter by vacuum) as leaks of air into the solution which has been filtered do not occur.
(f) Adsorbtion can occur with some filters, e.g. candles and fibrous pads.
(g) Some filters yield fibres or alkali, e.g. fibrous filters, but neutralized alkali-free filters are available.
(h) Clogging can occur with prolonged filtration, although this can be minimized by use of suitable prefilters. Bacteria may grow through some types of filters, with lengthy filtration runs.
(i) Filtration cannot be used for sterilizing suspensions.
(j) Oxidation may occur on larger filters, and the medicament must be stable in the solvent.

Two main types of unit are available. These are the positive pressure type, where the solution is forced through the filter by compressed air, and the negative pressure (or vacuum) type where the solution is sucked through the filter. The former has more advantages than the latter, but both are used.

Advantages of positive and negative pressure systems

Positive pressure	Negative pressure (vacuum)
Unsterile air does not enter via leaking joints.	Loose joints are tightened.
Evaporation and foaming of the filtrate is reduced.	A closed system is not required.
On large scale, an aseptic transfer from vacuum vessel to point of use is not required.	
Pressure differential is only limited by equipment, not to a maximum of 1 atmosphere as in negative pressure system.	

Bacteria-Proof Filters for Solutions

Various types of filter are available for sterilization. They can be divided into four basic classes:

Ceramic filters—usually made of porous porcelain or kieselguhr.

Fibrous pads—containing asbestos and wood cellulose.

Sintered (Fritted) glass filters—made from powdered borosilicate glass.

Microporous plastic or membrane filters—prepared from cellulose esters, particularly the acetate and nitrate.

Apart from the above basic classes several filters are available which incorporate the advantages of two or more classes. An example of this is the submicron filter composed of micronized glass and asbestos fibres bound in epoxy saturant. This filter (Cox M-780) has many of the advantages of membrane filters, while being less prone to clogging. Depth and screen filters are compared in Table 31.3.

Ceramic filters. One of the earliest ceramic filters was the Pasteur-Chamberland, introduced in 1884. They are made of either porous porcelain or kiesel-guhr. They are usually encountered as cylindrical candles with comparatively thick walls. These are depth filters with cellular walls and are available in various sizes and a number of grades of porosity, some types are shown in Fig. 31.7. Examples of the porcelain candle are manufactured by Doulton & Co. Ltd., and the kieselguhr type are produced by British Berkefeld Filters Ltd. The Mandler filter is the American equivalent of the Berkefeld filter. Kieselguhr filters have a greater pore density than do porcelain ones and are therefore more permeable to aqueous liquids. Kieselguhr filters are rather softer than the porcelain variety and have a thicker wall. Berkefeld filters are sold for water sterilization, and an allegedly 'self-sterilizing' Berkefeld filter ('Sterasyl' filter) has been developed. This filter is similar to the standard kieselguhr filter but has been impregnated with ionic silver. Doubts have been expressed about its self-sterilizing ability (Sykes 1965). Both porcelain and kieselguhr filters may be fitted with nozzle mounts. These mounts may be glazed porcelain or cemented metal and the jointing is one of the weaknesses of these filters. During cleaning and sterilization cracks and

TABLE 31.3

COMPARISON OF DEPTH AND SCREEN FILTERS

	Depth Filters	Screen Filters
Examples	Fibrous pad ('Seitz', 'Carlson-Ford') Ceramic candles ('Doulton', 'Berkefeld') Sintered glass (and metal)	Cellulose membrane ('Oxoid', 'Millipore', 'Sartorius' etc.)
Filtration	Particle may be forced through filter Particles stop at point where resistance is equal to driving force. Increase in pressure will drive particle deeper and sometimes through filter. This is particularly true when large pressure fluctuations occur.	Particles Filtrate Particles larger than the pore size are mechanically 'sieved' from solution, and are retained on the surface of the filter. Increase in pressure, and pressure fluctuation does not cause particles to pass through the filter.
Advantages	Fibrous pad filters are less prone to clogging than screen filters. The chemical resistance is high.	The 0.22 μm filter will retain all bacteria on its surface. No bacterial 'grow-through' occurs. No pH change. Very low adsorbtion. High flow rate with solutions containing few particles.

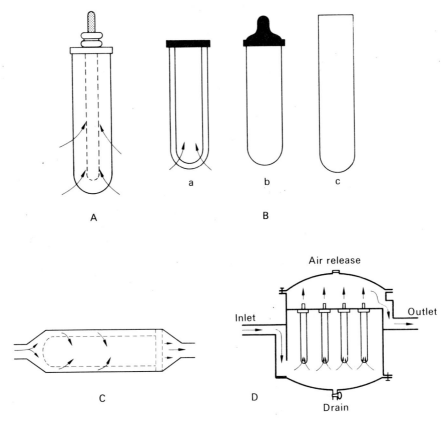

FIG. 31.7. Ceramic filters. A, Kieselguhr filter (metal nozzle); B, unglazed porcelain filters (a and b have glazed mountings); C, pipeline candle filter; D, large supply filter using a number of filter candles.

leaks may develop at these joints. Unglazed and unmounted porous porcelain candles are available but are less easily fitted into filtration units.

It is an advantage to filter on to the outside of the filter as this is easier to clean than the inside. The porcelain filters can be cleaned by scrubbing the exterior with a nail brush, or more thoroughly by the use of strong sodium hypochlorite solution. The softer texture of the kieselguhr filters means that a softer brush must be used for scrubbing, or the hypochlorite treatment used. They can then be dry heat sterilized, although care must be taken to gradually increase the temperature and allow the filters to cool slowly, to prevent cracking. Strong acids should not be used to clean Berkefeld filters, and chromic acid should never be used to clean ceramic or sintered glass filters because chromic ions are strongly adsorbed by the filter, cannot be removed by washing, and may oxidize or react with the medicament on subsequent use of the filter.

Advantages. (a) Relatively inexpensive, and (b) ranges of porosities available.

Disadvantages. (a) Not very robust, particularly kieselguhr candles; (b) adsorbtion is high, particularly with kieselguhr candles; (c) easily clogged and blocked; (d) regular complicated cleaning needed; (e) relatively high pressure needed for filtration; (f) leaks often occur at nozzle joints; and (g) difficult to fit into filter units.

If these filters are used for oily products they are slow, not very efficient, become more susceptible to breakage and are very difficult to clean (Avis & Gershenfeld 1955).

Fibrous pad filters. The pads used are approximately 3 mm thick, usually round for most filter units, but square sheets are used in filter-presses. They are composed mainly of asbestos fibre, compressed with mixtures of other fibrous material such as wood cellulose to give adequate porosity, together with binders and fillers. Various types are shown in Fig. 31.8. The original German filters were sold under the trade name of Seitz (grade EK being used for filtration sterilization), and are available in this country from Carlson-Ford Ltd. in over 40 grades and in several hundred cut sizes (Carlson-Ford filter sheet grade EKS is most often used for sterilization of pharmaceuticals). They are pliable and fragile when wet, and must be supported on a perforated metal, plastic or glass disc. Care is needed in sterilization by autoclaving to avoid distortion.

Advantages. (a) A new pad is used for each filtration, so that filtrate is not contaminated with previous filtration residues or cleaning agents; (b) pads are inexpensive; and (c) filtration is rapid with less tendency to clogging. They are better than ceramic and sintered glass filters for viscous solutions.

Disadvantages. (a) Filtration and adequate removal of bacteria depends on the pad fibres taking up water and swelling to reduce interstitial space in filter. Thus fibrous pads are not suitable for sterilizing non-aqueous products, e.g. alcoholic and oily preparations; (b) pads may release alkali, causing precipitation of alkali-sensitive medicaments (Browne 1942). Alkali-free pre-sterilized filters are available; (c) pads may shed fibres. These can be removed from the filtrate by means of a sterile grade 3 or 4 sintered glass filter; (d) adsorbtion is high, particularly at the start of filtration; and (e) fluctuating pressure may damage the wet pads.

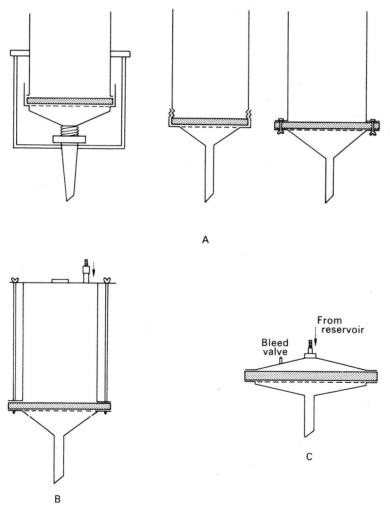

FIG. 31.8. Fibrous pad filters. A, negative pressure fibrous pad filter; B, positive pressure fibrous pad filter; C, large-scale fibrous pad filter.

Sintered (Fritted) glass filters. Sintered glass filters were first made by Jena Glassworks, Germany. Borosilicate glass is finely powdered in a ball mill and particles of the required size are separated by air elutriation. The selected powder is packed into disc moulds and heated until suitable adhesion takes place between the granules. The sintered discs are finally fused into funnels of suitable size and shape (Fig. 16.4) or into line filters (Fig. 31.9). Sintered glass filters are available in several different porosities, but for filtration sterilization a number or grade 5, or 5 on 3, must be used. Specifications for quality, pore size and permeability are given in a British Standards Specification BS 1752: 1963. Filtration through a thick grade 5 (maximum pore size 2 μm) filter is slow, but thinner grade 5 filters are very fragile and thus the 5 on 3 filter was developed with a thin grade 5 filter supported on a thicker layer of grade 3 filter (pore size 15 to 40 μm). The manufacture and uses of sintered glass filters are described by Smith (1944) and their care by Cooper (1951) and Sykes (1958). Microorganisms do tend to grow through sintered glass filters if left in contact for more than 18 h (Morton 1943). They are easily cleaned by passing a reverse stream of water through the filter after use. Organic matter may be removed by passing strong sulphuric acid with 1 per cent of sodium nitrate through the filter. Chromic acid should not be used (see ceramic filters). All filters must be thoroughly washed after chemical treatment.

Advantages. (a) Easily cleaned; (b) they yield no fibres, alkali, etc. to filtrate; (c) adsorbtion is very low; (d) filtrate retention by the filter is less than ceramic filters; and (e) they can be fused into filtration units thus reducing risk of leaks.

Disadvantages. (a) They are relatively expensive; (b) they have a small area of filtration; and (c) they are fragile.

Membrane filters. A review of membrane filter techniques is given by Mulvany (1969). They are composed of various types of cellulose and cellulose esters and are marketed by Gelman Instrument Company, the Millipore Filter Corporation, Oxo Ltd., Sartorius-Membrane Filter, and a number of other companies. A vast range of grades and pore sizes are available, together with membranes developed for specialized uses. They are very thin (Oxoid filters are 120 μm thick) and need careful handling. The pore sizes most often used for sterilization are 0.45 μm $\pm$ 0.02 μm (Millipore grade HA) or, particularly where very small bacterial contaminants (e.g. certain pseudomonads) are likely to occur, preferably 0.22 μm $\pm$ 0.02 μm (Millipore grade GS). They are sterilized by autoclaving, in the holder, or packed between thick filter pads to prevent curling. They are also available ready sterilized (by ethylene oxide or ionizing radiation). As with fibrous pad filters membrane filters are supported on a rigid base of perforated metal, plastic, or coarse sintered glass. If the solution to be filtered has a high content of unwanted suspended particulate matter the membrane filter, which acts like a sieve trapping particles on its surface, will rapidly become clogged. To avoid clogging preliminary filtration through a suitable depth filter (e.g. glass fibre filter) will extend the usage of the membrane filter. The membranes have a high and uniform porosity permitting a rapid rate of filtration. The HA grade will filter approximately 65 ml/min/sq cm (GS 22 ml/min/sq cm) with a differential pressure of 70 cm mercury across the membrane. The membranes can be stored indefinitely in the dry state, but are brittle when dry, although fairly tough when wet. They are screen filters.

Advantages. (a) Bacteria are mechanically sieved from solution. Thus no bacteria pass through the filter with prolonged filtration and there is no

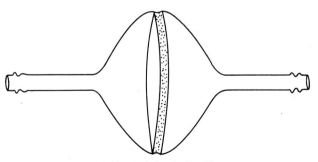

FIG. 31.9. Sintered glass in-line filter.

bacterial growth through it as occurs with depth filters; (b) membranes are disposable. No cross contamination occurs between filtered products; (c) adsorbtion is negligible, although some occurs with phenols; (d) rapid filtration rate; and (e) they yield no fibres, alkali etc. to contaminate the filtrate.

Disadvantages. (a) Tendency to clog—not a problem with most pharmaceutical solutions; and (b) they have less chemical resistance to certain organic solvents such as chloroform, ketones, and esters, although, as mentioned earlier specialized filters (e.g. Millipore Solvinert) have been developed to overcome this problem.

Details of the setting up of a small-scale 'Swinnex' syringe membrane filter for preparation of eye drops is given in Chapter 27. Fig. 31.10 shows some other types of units used.

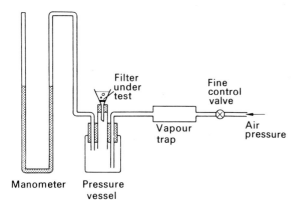

FIG. 31.10. Suitable apparatus for determination of maximum pore size of bacteriological filters.

Other filters. Many other types of filters have been developed for sterilization purposes, but only a few can be mentioned here. Sintered metal filters are the metallic counterpart of sintered glass filters. They are usually made from sintered bronze or stainless steel. They have great mechanical strength but are liable to attack by the solutions passing through them (Newman 1954). Nitrocellulose (collodion) filters have now been replaced for most purposes by cellulose acetate and mixed cellulose ester membrane filters. Many descriptions of filtration units were given in the *Pharmaceutical Journal* in the 1930s and early 1940s, and an enclosed unit for sintered glass or fibrous pad filters is described by Barfield (1955). Use of centrifugal force to filter small volumes of material is employed in the Hemmings filters (Wyllie 1955).

Mechanisms Involved in Filtration Sterilization
Mechanical sieving. The membrane filters have pores, the diameter of which are less than the dimensions of the bacteria and it is obvious that they remove bacteria from solutions by a simple sieving mechanism. However, although this may be part of the filtration mechanism in other filters, other mechanisms must also play a part since the majority of pores in ceramic, sintered glass, and fibrous filters are larger than the bacteria, e.g. ceramic filters have a maximum pore size up to 2.5 μm and yet can be relied upon to hold back *Serratia marcescens*, the dimensions of which are usually less than 1.0 μm.

Electrostatic attraction or adsorbtion on filter. Support for this hypothesis is found in the observation that filters which have been 'insulated' with oil may not retain the organisms from a subsequently filtered aqueous suspension of bacteria (Sykes & Royce 1950). Evidence for adsorbtion is given by Wyllie (Sykes 1965), with photomicrographs showing adsorbtion of yeasts on asbestos fibres. Since ceramic, sintered glass, and asbestos pad filters are negatively charged and the charge on the bacterial surface is also negative, repulsion rather than attraction may prevent the bacteria entering the pores. However, the nett negative charge on the bacterium may be less important than the attraction between the filter and local positively charged basic groups on its surface. Both attractive and repulsive forces may play a part in filter efficiency.

Retention in irregular cellular structure. Liquid filtering through a depth filter does not pass a 'straight-through' pore but, due to the cellular structure, has to negotiate up to 2000 bends per cm of thickness. Each short path may contain pockets in which organisms can be lodged. Thus, in its course through a filter an organism would have a very considerable number of chances of being trapped but on theoretical grounds can be expected to ultimately pass through the filter. This accounts for the fact that depth filters occasionally allow bacterial contamination to pass, especially when used for prolonged filtration. The thicker the filter the greater the delay. The effect of wall thickness and pore size on the efficiency of filtration is recorded by Royce and Sykes (1950).

Standardization and Testing of Filters
It is necessary to show that the filter will retain organisms, and that its flow rate is satisfactory.

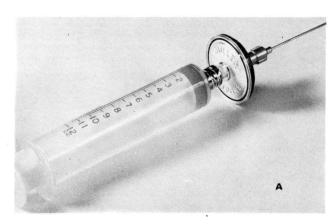

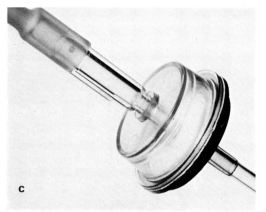

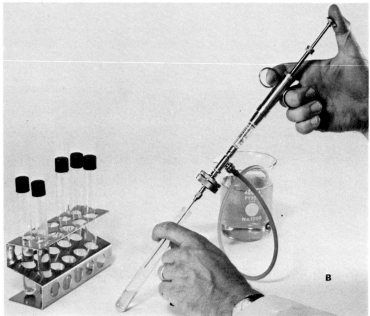

FIG. 31.11. Bubble-pressure. A, Millex filter unit; B, microsyringe filtering and dispensing system (Swinnex, Millex and Swinny) units can be used as filtering system; C, Ivex filter unit (Millipore Filter Corporation Ltd.).

The retention ability of the filter can be tested indirectly by means of bubble pressure techniques and directly by bacteriological techniques.

Bubble pressure techniques. Direct measurement of the pore sizes in a bacterial filter is not practicable and an indirect method of measuring the 'bubble pressure' is employed. This consists of immersing the candles in water (or other liquid) or filling the funnel with the liquid in the case of a sintered glass filter, and very gradually applying an increasing air pressure until the first bubble is seen at the filter/liquid interface. A suitable apparatus is shown in Fig. 31.10. The pressure reading can be converted to the approximate pore size by means of the Becbold formula; useful equivalents are given below:

| Bubble pressure in water | | Approx pore size |
mmHg	lbf/sq in	μm
413.7	8	5.3
620.5	12	3.5
775.7	15	2.8
930.9	18	2.3

The results are reproducible and it is possible to distinguish between filters with a pore size difference of 0.25 μm. Mulvaney (1969) describes a suitable apparatus for testing line filters. The trend is for manufacturers of ceramic filters to standardize on a bubble pressure of 17 lbf/in^2. This pressure is equivalent to a maximum pore size of 2.5 μm which will hold back *Serratia marcescens* in aqueous suspension for at least 6 to 7 h.

The bubble pressure method is adopted by a British Standard (BS 1752: 1963) for the measurement of pore size. The pressure when the first bubble is seen indicates the maximum pore size of the filter. The latter is calculated from the equation

$$D = \frac{30\gamma}{P}$$

where D = diameter of pore, in microns,
γ = surface tension of the test liquid (dynes/cm),
P = bubble pressure (mmHg).

Bacteriological techniques. In spite of the apparent reliability of the bubble pressure test, the *British Pharmaceutical Codex* requires bacteria-proof filters to comply with a bacteriological test. A diluted broth culture of *Serratia marcescens* (*Chromobacterium prodigiosum*) is filtered through a previously sterilized filter and unit, employing a pressure difference across the filter of not less than 400 mmHg. At least 50 ml of the filtrate is incubated for 5 days at 25°C, the optimum temperature for growth (and pigment production) of the organism. The use of a good chromogenic (pigment-producing) strain is advised since the appearance of a pink colour in the incubated broth instantly confirms the presence of *Serratia* and the failure of the filter. The appearance of growth without pigment suggests contamination after passage through the filter, or some leak in the unit. The organism chosen is particularly useful since it is small (0.3 to 1.3 μm long and 0.3 to 0.4 μm wide), aerobic, non-pathogenic, and grows vigorously to produce a red to pink pigment at 25°.

FILTRATION OF AIR

Sterilization of large volumes of air has become important due to the development of deep culture fermentation processes in the manufacture of antibiotics and other products of microbial metabolism. Many modern drugs require aseptic handling and various laminar-flow devices producing clean air environments are available. The principles and applications of laminar-flow devices are described

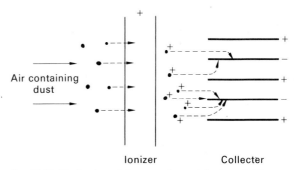

Fig. 31.12. Mechanism of electrostatic precipitation of airborne particles.

by McDade (1969). Treatment of process air for deep culture is discussed by Elsworth (1969), and factors affecting bacterial survival in air and gases by Sykes (1963).

Methods available for air sterilization are: (a) mechanical filtration; (b) electrostatic precipitation; (c) heating methods; (d) ultraviolet light; and (e) use of chemicals.

Before dealing with mechanical filtration, which is the most widely used method for air sterilization, the limitations of the other methods will be outlined. Electrostatic precipitation is a costly method, but is extremely efficient. The mechanism of removal is shown in Fig. 31.12. Heating methods are costly and of marginal importance in air sterilization. Heat sterilizers are described by Elsworth, Morris and East (1961). Ultraviolet light has poor penetrating power, and thus does not kill bacteria embedded in particles. It also suffers from other disadvantages, such as its harmful effects on the eyes and skin, high initial and replacement costs, and relatively low efficiency at low humidities. The use of aerial chemical bactericides is limited by their slow action, problems of 'carry over' of chemical to the fermentation plant, and their erratic action. Examples of aerial bactericides are glycols (propylene and triethylene), phenols (resorcinol and hexylresorcinol) and sodium hypochlorite.

As with filtration sterilization of solutions both depth and screen filters are available for air sterilization. A comparison of the two types of filters for high-volume air sterilization is given by Russell (1971). Russell indicates the unreliable nature of polytropic compression of air (a heating method), and states that filter selection depends on the nature of the contamination to be removed. Often depth and screen filters are used in a complementary situation, as in the 'Millitube' cartridge filter (Fig. 31.13).

The main types of depth filters for air sterilization

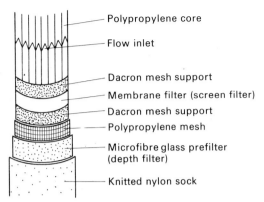

Polypropylene core

Flow inlet

Dacron mesh support

Membrane filter (screen filter)

Dacron mesh support

Polypropylene mesh

Microfibre glass prefilter
(depth filter)

Knitted nylon sock

FIG. 31.13. Section of 'Millitube' filter.

are: *granules*, e.g. activated charcoal; *fibrous pads*, e.g. cotton wool, slag wool, and glass wool; and *filter papers*, cellulose-asbestos, or glass fibre. Filters for air sterilization should be steam-sterilizable, reproducible in quality, and preferably absolute (showing 100 per cent efficiency). Depth filters cannot be classed as absolute, but steam-sterilizable resin-bonded glass fibre is useful as an alternative to membrane filters.

GASEOUS STERILIZATION

Chemical vapours have a limited use in cold sterilization of some thermolabile solid medicaments, and thermolabile hospital equipment, such as plastic equipment, electrical and rubber articles and blankets. Formaldehyde was originally used, but ethylene oxide is the main gas now used for sterilization. According to the Medicines Commission Report on the prevention of microbial contamination of medicinal products (1973) the process of ethylene oxide sterilization does not lend itself to physical methods of measurement, and consequently stringent microbiological controls and test procedures must be applied. The Commission Committee accepted the value of ethylene oxide but stated that application to medical products should have due regard to the risks of chemical incompatability and the production of toxic residues and to its inefficacy against organisms occluded in crystals or otherwise protected from the gas (Abbott, Cockton & Jones 1956).

Although ethylene oxide is the most widely used gaseous sterilant in the pharmaceutical and medical fields other chemicals used are: (a) formaldehyde; (b) beta-propiolactone; and (c) propylene oxide. In addition to these, various glycols, methyl bromide and alcohol have been used for room sterilization.

ETHYLENE OXIDE

Use of ethylene oxide is a recognized method of sterilization in both the 1973 *British Pharmacopoeia* and the *British Pharmaceutical Codex*. In the *British Pharmacopoeia* it is among the procedures for sterilization of certain powdered substances.

Properties and action. It is a volatile cyclic ether with the structure:

$$CH_2 \underset{O}{-\!\!-\!\!} CH_2$$

Its boiling point is 10.8°C and it can be easily liquefied. It forms explosive mixtures with air, but this disadvantage can be overcome by using mixtures of 10 per cent ethylene oxide with 90 per cent carbon dioxide or halogenated hydrocarbons, or by removing 95 per cent of the air from the apparatus before use of the ethylene oxide. The latter method of exposure at sub-atmospheric pressure is preferred by Mayr (1961) in his discussion of equipment for ethylene oxide sterilization. It is irritant and vesicant, and thus rubber gloves and similar articles should be aired in a sterile air stream for 24 h before use. Its antimicrobial action, like that of other gaseous antimicrobial agents, is due to its ability to alkylate $-SH$, $-OH$, $-COOH$, and NH_2 groups in enzymes, proteins, and nucleic acids (Bruch 1961) for example:

$$PROTEIN\text{--}NH_2 + C_2H_4O \rightarrow PROTEIN\text{--}NH\text{--}(C_2H_4OH)$$

$$PROTEIN\text{--}SH + C_2H_4O \rightarrow PROTEIN\text{--}S\text{--}(C_2H_4OH)$$

Factors Affecting Sterilizing Efficiency
Concentration of the gas. Sterilization rates depend on the partial pressure of the gas within the load. The partial pressure of the gas may be lowered by absorbtion by the load e.g. by blankets, rubber and plastics, and packaging materials (Royce 1959). Royce gives examples of absorbtion by various materials after contact with a gas concentration of 200 mg/litre for 24 h at 25°. A few examples are given below:

Material	Amount absorbed (mg/g)
Polythene	2
Polyvinylchloride	19.2
Cardboard	10.4
Non-absorbant cotton wool	4.1
Neoprene rubber closures	15.2

Concentrations used for sterilization range from 200 to 1000 mg/l, and these concentrations certainly appear adequate if compared with the work of Phillips (1961). Phillips determined the activity of ethylene oxide against spores of *Bacillus subtilis* var. *globigii* (dried on cloth) at 25°. Some of the results are given below:

Ethylene oxide concentration (mg/l)	Exposure time required to obtain no recoverable organisms (hours)
44	24
88	10
442	4
884	2

Thus it can be seen that if the concentration is doubled the exposure time is approximately halved.

Temperature of the load. A rise in temperature increases the activity. The temperature coefficient (see Chapter 30) is 2.7 for each 10° change in temperature, but since ethylene oxide is mainly used for thermolabile materials the usual range of use is 20 to 60°.

Effect of moisture. According to Phillips some moisture is necessary 'but a little was better than a lot'. The state of hydration of the micro-organisms on the surfaces to be sterilized seems to be of more importance than the relative humidity of the gas. A relative humidity of approximately 30 to 33 per cent seems to be favoured (Kaye & Phillips 1949). Dry organisms are much more resistant than moist ones. The type of surface also affects the sterilization. Organisms dried on hard impermeable surfaces, such as glass, plastic and metal, are less easy to kill than those dried on absorbant surfaces, such as paper and cloth (Opfell, Hohmann & Latham 1959; Royce & Bowler 1961).

Time of exposure. This will depend on the type of material being sterilized and the concentration of the gas. Various combinations have been used successfully including:

850–900 mg/l for 3 h at 45°
450 mg/l for 5 h at 45° (Perkins & Lloyd 1961)
200 mg/l overnight for 16–18 h (Royce 1959).

The exposure time is dependent also on the power of penetration of the gas. Paper and fabrics are freely permeable, but some of the polyesters are

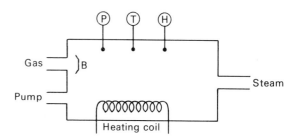

FIG. 31.14. Generalized diagram of an ethylene oxide sterilizer (based on diagram from Kelsey, 1967).

not. Polythene and most rubbers are freely permeable. The *British Pharmaceutical Codex* states that hydration and heating of the load can be more reliably achieved by conditioning in a suitable atmosphere prior to sterilization.

The condition and accessibility of the organisms. Dried organisms are slow to rehydrate and thus difficult to sterilize (Gilbert et al. 1964). Organisms may be protected within hard crystals (Abbott, Cockton & Jones 1956; Royce & Bowler 1961; Beeby & Whitehouse 1965).

Apparatus and Techniques for Ethylene Oxide Sterilization

Specially designed sterilizers are commercially available. As shown in Fig. 31.14 they consist of:
(a) A gas-tight sterilizing chamber capable of withstanding the necessary changes in pressure.
(b) The chamber is fitted with an efficient vacuum pump.
(c) Valve regulated gas admittance, linked with controls. Gas is introduced from canisters or cylinders after evacuation of the chamber by the pump. Baffles (B) prevent damage of the load by liquid ethylene oxide.
(d) Control devices such as a pressure gauge, P, thermostatic control, T, and humidity control, H are included.
(e) Humidity can be provided from a damp sponge or steam.
(f) A heating coil or heating jacket.
However sophisticated the apparatus, variation in loads means that very careful microbiological monitoring of the process is essential. Particular attention should be paid to keeping microbial contamination of materials to be sterilized to a minimum. Some typical cycles used commercially in ethylene oxide sterilizers are quoted by Kelsey (1967) (see Table 31.4).

TABLE 31.4

TYPICAL CYCLES IN ETHYLENE OXIDE STERILIZERS

Concentration of ethylene oxide %	(mg/l)	Pressure (atm)	Temperature (°C)	Time (h)
90	1500	<1	25	18
10	400	2	50	4
10	1800	6	60	1

Perkins and Lloyd (1961) and Mayr (1961) describe equipment for ethylene oxide sterilization.

Advantages. (a) Few materials damaged; (b) low temperature can be used, e.g. room temperature; (c) penetration into porous materials and some plastics good; (d) little residual effect; (e) effective at low humidities; (f) bactericidal, not bacteriostatic; (g) effective against all organisms.

Disadvantages. (a) Some plastic and nylon wraps must be left open and sealed aseptically (this is a disadvantage compared with radiation sterilization); (b) slow; (c) control of RH and hydration of organisms is critical; (d) cost is higher than heat processes; (e) it requires special sophisticated equipment; and (f) toxic and inflammable.

Rubbo and Gardner (1965) give a list of articles for which ethylene oxide sterilization is suitable. They consider the gas unsuitable for disposable transfusion sets (dried organisms on plastic surfaces occasionally survive gassing), vitamins (which may be destroyed), and hypodermic needles (as gas cannot penetrate between the plunger and the barrel).

Control of the Process
The process must be monitored bacteriologically—it is not sufficient to rely on physical monitoring. The bactericidal efficiency is monitored by:
(a) Insertion of a minimum of 10 bacteriological test pieces in different parts of the load, particularly those most inaccesible to the gas. These test pieces consist of aluminium foil on which has been dried a suspension of at least 10^6 spores of *Bacillus subtilis* Camp Detrick strain NCTC 10073 (*B.subtilis* var. *globigii*). This organism is chosen as it is fairly resistant to ethylene oxide.
(b) Routine random sterility tests on the load.
Royce and Bowler (1959) have described an indicator control device for ethylene oxide sterilization.

OTHER GASEOUS STERILANTS

These are less important than ethylene oxide in the pharmaceutical and medical fields.
Propylene oxide (see Rubbo and Gardner (1965) for sterilizer design); it is less effective than ethylene oxide, but less explosive.
Formaldehyde; this is now mainly used for fumigation of rooms and hospital blankets. It has poor penetrating power, polymerizes to paraformaldehyde, and is irritant and pungent. It is readily inactivated by proteins and organic matter. It must be used at high humidities in excess of 75 per cent, and high concentrations are difficult to maintain. Further information is given in the Public Health Lab. Report 1958.
Beta-propiolactone; this has a boiling point of 163°, and thus a heated plate vaporizer must be used. Again, as with formaldehyde, RH of at least 75 per cent is required, and its penetrating power is low. It is highly virucidal, but is irritant, vesicant, and carcinogenic to animals, and thus needs expert handling.
Glycols; these are used as aerial bactericides at a concentration of 0.2 to 0.5 mg/l.
Methyl bromide and methyl alcohol; the former is used as an insecticide, and the latter for fungal decontamination of incubators and cold rooms.

THE PREPARATION OF STERILE MEDICAMENTS

TYPES OF STERILE MEDICAMENT

Pharmaceutical preparations and materials are sterilized and supplied in a sterile condition when they are to be injected, or applied to wounds or mucous surfaces, because body fluids and tissues provide a good substrate for the growth of many microorganisms.

Preparations for injection may consist of solutions sterilized in their final containers or, if the aqueous solution has very limited stability, of powders sterilized in containers to which Water for Injections can be added to dissolve the solids. Sterile liquids or gels may also be required for use in surgical operations, for irrigation of the urethra, bladder or vagina, or for lubrication of catheters. Sterile solids may be implanted under the skin. Other preparations described elsewhere are: preparations for the eye (Chapter 27), powders to be applied to wounds or cavities (Chapter 26), surgical dressings (Chapter 31), absorbable haemostatics (Chapter 35) and ligatures and sutures (Chapter 36).

Parenteral Injections

A parenteral injection is one which is injected under one or more layers of the skin or mucous membranes into a specific region of the body. The following types are available:

Intradermal or intracutaneous injections. These are injected into the skin between the epidermis and the underlying dermis, usually into the flexor aspect of the forearm. The volume is therefore small, usually being 0.1 to 0.2 ml. Such injections are used as diagnostic agents to test susceptibility to certain diseases, e.g. diphtheria (Schick test), tuberculosis (Old Tuberculin, Tuberculin Purified Protein Derivative).

Subcutaneous or hypodermic injections. These injections are made beneath the skin into the subcutaneous tissue. The upper arm is most usually used and the volume does not normally exceed 1 ml. Larger volumes can be accommodated if hyaluronidase is added to the injection: it hydrolyses the hyaluronic acid which holds the cells together so that the injection can drain away quickly without causing undue swelling; no permanent damage to the tissue is caused because the enzyme action is reversible. The method is called hypodermoclysis and is sometimes used in place of intravenous infusion if this is contraindicated, and it is possible to administer as much as 3 to 4 l per day. Conversely, a vasoconstrictor such as adrenalin may be added to ensure a local effect with, e.g. local anaesthetics.

Intramuscular injections. These are injected directly into a muscle, using a longer needle than that required for subcutaneous injection. The muscles selected are usually those of the thigh, buttock or shoulders. The *British Pharmaceutical Codex* 1973 directs that the volume should not normally exceed 4 ml. Being made into firm tissue, such injections can cause pain if the process is carried out too quickly. Both aqueous and oily solutions and also suspensions can be administered by the intramuscular route, and by controlling the formulation the rate of absorption can be controlled. Thus suspensions of the medicament can be made of different particle size, the largest particles providing the slowest absorption. An even slower rate of absorption may sometimes be obtained by dissolving the medicament in oil from which it is partitioned into the body fluids, or by making a suspension of a compound of the medicament of low solubility.

Intravenous injections. These are injected directly into the lumen of a vein, the median basilic vein on the inner forearm being most commonly selected. They are nearly always aqueous solutions, but a few consist of oil-in-water emulsions (e.g. Phytomenadione Injection, BP), where the oily medicament is dispersed in a sufficiently fine emulsion to prevent damage. The volume injected may be quite small and in that case the solution can be sufficiently concentrated to be hypertonic without causing ill effect, because when it is injected slowly it is easily carried away and diluted by the blood stream. If a single-dose volume is greater than 15 ml no bactericide must be added. Much larger volumes, of 500 ml or more, are given by intravenous infusion to replace blood fluids lost as a result of shock, injury, or surgical operation, or body fluids lost by severe diarrhoea, e.g. in cholera. The infusion is fed by gravity from a bottle placed above the patient's bed, at the rate of about 50 drops per min, which is monitored by means of an in-line drip-tube. Such large volume injections must not only be free from added bactericide but also from pyrogens (see below), and they are usually made isotonic with blood serum.

Intraarterial injections. These are less commonly used than intravenous injections and are used when an immediate action is required in a peripheral area. They also must not contain any added bactericide.

Intracardiac injections. These are aqueous solutions to be injected directly into the cardiac muscle or ventricle for emergency treatment and must also be free from added bactericide.

Intrathecal or subarachnoid injections. These are injected into the subarachnoid space which surrounds the spinal cord. The cord narrows just above the third lumbar vertebra, being continued as the filum terminale, and the space around this is sufficiently wide for a needle to be inserted without undue danger of injuring the spinal cord. The injection is usually made between the third and fourth, or between the fourth and fifth lumbar vertebrae, and is used for spinal anaesthetics. The density of these is sometimes adjusted in order to concentrate them above or below the site of injection. Intrathecal injections normally do not exceed 20 ml, must be dispensed from single-dose containers, and must contain no added bactericide. Lumbar puncture is also used for the reverse process of withdrawing samples of cerebrospinal fluid for diagnostic examination.

Intracisternal injections. At the base of the brain the subarachnoid space widens into the cisterna magna and injections can be made into this. Entry is however difficult and not without danger of damaging the brain, and although occasionally used for the administration of antibiotics, is more usually used for the withdrawal of cerebrospinal fluid. Intracisternal injections are subject to the same official requirements as intrathecal injections.

Peridural injections. A narrow space exists between the dura mater which encloses the cerebrospinal fluid, and the vertebrae. Peridural injections can be made into this space in the thoracic, lumbar and sacral regions. The space is, however, narrow and much skill is required to locate the needle acurately. Peridural injections are subject to the same official requirements as intrathecal injections.

Pyrogens

Any substance which on injection causes a rise of temperature can be called a pyrogen, but the name was originally coined by Seibert (1923) for those which are derived from the cell walls of bacteria, and is usually applied specifically to such. They generally consist of lipopolysaccharides, of which the lipid portion appears to be the active pyrogen. On its own, however, it is insoluble in water, but it is solubilized by its attachment to the polysaccharide and is then active. It has been proposed that the lipid is attached to 2-keto-3-deoxyoctonic acid which is the terminal unit of a common non-specific phospholipid-polysaccharide core, to the other end of which is linked another specific polysaccharide chain characteristic of the organism producing it (Ridgway 1973). The whole lipopolysaccharide appears to be excreted from the cell as a complex with protein (Work 1971).

When bacterial pyrogen is injected there is usually a short latent period after which a small temperature rise is shown. This subsides a little and is then succeeded by a rapid and more extended rise showing a peak after about 4 to 8 h. This led to the hypothesis that the bacterial pyrogens or endotoxins do not themselves provoke fever, but that they liberate an *endogenous pyrogen* from polymorphonuclear leucocytes and possibly from other cells. The composition of this endogenous pyrogen is not precisely known though it has been suggested that it is of protein or lipoprotein composition. It is active in minute amounts and

there is considerable evidence that it acts upon the thermoregulatory centres of the hypothalamus, possibly by raising the level of 5-hydroxytryptamine. The sodium/calcium ion balance in the hypothalamus may also be involved (Feldberg 1961).

Removal of pyrogens. Bacterial pyrogens are fairly easily hydrolysed by dilute acid and alkali, but are resistant to the action of heat and often cannot be inactivated by autoclaving, though some have been found to be thermolabile (Palmer & Whittet 1961). They easily pass through the normal bacterial filters, though some special filters have been made which will remove them. These filters probably act by adsorption and ion exchange rather than by simple filtration (Ridgway 1973) and the use of ion-exchange columns has been advocated for the production of apyrogenic water (Cook & Saunders 1962). The method is permitted by some pharmacopoeias, but while ion-exchange resins efficiently remove pyrogens, they easily become contaminated by live bacteria and the method is not permitted by the *European Pharmacopoeia*, 1973. The official method is therefore distillation, since the pyrogens are non-volatile. It is necessary to include an adequate baffle system in the still-head to prevent entrainment of droplets or particles which may carry over pyrogens into the distillate.

Test for pyrogens. The official test for pyrogens with which Water for Injections and some prepared injections must comply, is now contained in the *European Pharmacopoeia*, 1973. It is a limit test, consisting essentially of injecting the test liquid into the ear vein of rabbits and measuring the rectal temperature rise with thermocouples or thermistors. Three rabbits are used initially, and if the summed temperature rise of all three lies below a specified value the sample passes, while if it exceeds a higher specified value it fails. If the summed response lies between the specified values the test is repeated with three more animals and the summed response of all six similarly tested against two further specified values which give a lessened tolerance. If the temperature rise again falls between the specified limiting values, a third test may be carried out in the same way, the tolerance being again smaller for the larger sample involved. A fourth and final test may also be given, but in this the specified values become coincident and the sample either passes or fails. No animal must be reused for a test within three weeks of the last and care is required to see that the animals are healthy and not subjected to any excitation which would itself raise their body temperature. All glassware, syringes and needles must be pyrogen free and are sterilized by dry heat at 250° for 30 min or 200° for 60 min.

A limit test of this kind lacks the precision of a biological assay because no controls are applied. To do this would require the use of a stable and reproducible standard preparation. Such preparations have been produced, the aim being to obtain a bacterial lipopolysaccharide free from protein by extracting dried enterobacteria with phenol followed by alcoholic precipitation. One such preparation was approved by the National Centre for Antibiotics and Insulin Analysis of the American Food and Drugs Administration as a standard in 1970, but stocks of a similar British preparation have become exhausted. Such preparations are active in amounts as low as 5 μg/kg and so must be highly purified and therefore expensive to produce. It can reasonably be argued that for the purpose of protecting the patient the limit test suffices, but a standard preparation would be necessary for the satisfactory investigation of pyrogenic mechanisms and for the biological assay of antipyretic drugs.

Water for Injections (*Aqua iniectabilia, EP*)

Water for Injections was included in the *British Pharmacopoeia* 1973, but did not appear in the *European Pharmacopoeia* until the Supplement of 1973. Distillation is the only method of preparation permitted, and pyrogens must be removed by an effective device to prevent entrainment of droplets, because although the presence of minimal amounts of pyrogen may not always matter in small-volume injections, their virtual absence is very necessary in the case of infusion fluids given in large volume; patients receiving these are often dangerously ill and the danger may be significantly increased if a fever is induced. After distillation, the water is distributed into ampoules or bottles and sterilized by heat. The *British Pharmacopoeia* also permits filtration but, since the object of sterilization is to deal with the odd organism or two which may have accidently contaminated the receiver, there would seem to be no point in using a sterilization method involving a further final aseptic transfer which carries a risk of contamination.

ASEPTIC TECHNIQUE

An aseptic technique is one which is designed to prevent contamination of materials, instruments, utensils, or containers, during handling. Its importance has already been stressed in this chapter with regard to filtration sterilization and in Chapter 29 with regard to the manipulation of cultures, and it is equally important when sterile liquids or solids are distibuted from bulk into final containers.

Sources of Contamination

The air. This carries a mixed population of microorganisms, the density of which varies greatly with circumstances. The majority of the bacteria present are hardy saprophytes such as micrococci and sarcinae from natural waters, some enterococci, and spores of soil organisms of the species *Bacillus* and *Clostridium*, but some pathogenic clostridia may also occur. In a dry period, the ground may become dusty and the dust can be swept up into the air by winds, carrying with it the attached bacteria. Droplets expelled from the mouths of human beings and animals will also carry bacteria with them: the heavier drops may settle to the ground but the smaller ones, carried on the air currents, will dry out till the residual 'droplet nuclei' are dispersed as solid specks. Mould spores are also abundant as most of these are produced on aerial structures specifically designed to promote dispersal by wind currents. They are therefore often naked and not attached to dust particles. Yeasts, although not ejected by the dehiscence of a fruiting body from a parent structure, can be blown off the leaves of plants which often form their natural habitat.

The breath. During coughing and sneezing droplets can be ejected from the mouth and can be propelled a considerable distance. Apart therefore from their contribution to the atmospheric flora, direct contamination of articles being handled is possible. Staphylococci and haemolytic streptococci may thus be distributed.

The skin. Although the sebaceous secretions exhibit some antibacterial activity, the skin usually has a resident population of non-pathogens located in its folds and in the hair follicles and even sebaceous glands. In addition, a transient population may contaminate the skin, particularly of the hands, as a result of touching non-sterile objects. Pathogens as well as non-pathogens may be picked up when attending the toilet or blowing the nose.

The hair. Dust can easily settle on the hair and become enmeshed in it. If it is dry, shaking the head or simply disturbing the hair may detach considerable numbers of dust particles.

Clothing.   This also, unless freshly laundered, may carry a heavy load of dust particles which can easily be disturbed.

Working surfaces.   Dust will, of course, settle and collect on horizontal surfaces and to a lesser extent on vertical ones, and if present this dust may contaminate materials being handled.

Methods of Minimizing the Contamination Level
Having recognized the possible sources of contamination, it requires no more than the application of common sense to devise methods which will minimize the risk arising from them.

Airborne contamination.   This can be guarded against by working in a room fitted with a fan drawing in air through a suitable filter and maintaining a slight positive pressure within the room so that dust cannot be blown into it from outside. To prevent a sudden inrush of air when entering or leaving the room, an entrance porch fitted with doors at each end is usually provided. Ledges on which dust can accumulate should be avoided when designing the room.

To avoid contamination from the breath, gauze masks can be worn, but these must fit closely to the face or they may simply deflect the breath downwards onto the working area, and they cannot be fine enough to provide complete filtration of droplets which will build up on the gauze, dry out and finally be discharged through the mask. This must therefore be frequently changed if working for long periods.

As an alternative to the use of masks, or as a supplement to it, the working area can be covered by a screen. Articles placed under it must be free from dust, as must the interior of the screen itself, which can be swabbed with a disinfectant solution. Simple screens like that illustrated in Fig. 31.15 can

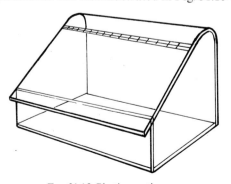

FIG. 31.15. Plastic aseptic screen.

be used effectively if care is taken to see that the operator's head does not sink to a position in which he blows continually into the space intended to accommodate his arms. To prevent this, screens have been devised in which the arms are inserted through ports which if necessary can be sealed with long rubber gloves. Special screens (laminar-flow cabinets) are also available: filtered air is fed into the screen through a carefully designed baffle system to prevent turbulence which might disturb particles of dust or of powders being distributed. The interior can be sterilized either by ultraviolet light or with ethylene oxide.

Contamination from the skin.   It is impossible to sterilize the skin without using heroic measures which may be injurious to it. Careful washing will remove most of the transient flora and some of the resident organisms, but those embedded deeply in crevices or ducts will not be removed even by extensive scrubbing, though this can be effectively used to clean away dirt lodged under the nails. Before commencing an aseptic operation the nails should therefore be scrubbed and the hands and forearms washed thoroughly with detergent solution. A bactericide can be added to this, though its effectiveness is somewhat doubtful. Obviously the hands must not be allowed to touch any part of the apparatus or utensils which will come into contact with the sterile material being handled. Direct contamination in this way can therefore be avoided by careful attention to technique, and it could be argued that the chief advantage of scrubbing up is to make the hands moist and so prevent the dislodgement of dirt and dried skin particles. It would therefore seem more important to add a humectant to the washing water than a bactericide; alternatively a suitable cream could be applied.

Hair and clothing.   Since the principal problem here is to prevent the detachment of dust, the obvious course of action is to cover both with freshly laundered material. Overalls or gowns should be worn over normal clothing and the sleeves should be rolled up above the elbow so that they do not pick up any foreign dirt from unclean surfaces. A cotton cap should be worn on the head, but if the hair is frequently washed to remove dirt, skin particles or dandruff, and particularly if an oily dressing is applied to it there is no great risk of contamination if the aseptic manipulations are carried out under a screen. Long hair should be tied back for obvious reasons.

Working surfaces. Before commencing operations, the surfaces of the working bench should be swabbed down with a bactericidal solution. Cetrimide solutions are useful for this as they have both bactericidal and detergent activity. This treatment does not, of course, sterilize the surfaces and, as in the case of skin, cleanliness and the laying of dust are the most important considerations, but it is not necessary for this purpose to provide a permanent pool of disinfectant. The surfaces of walls and ledges above the actual working surface must also be kept clean and the floor should be frequently swabbed to prevent dust rising from it.

Apparatus and equipment. Glass vessels, containers and equipment, when freshly removed from the sterilizer, will have those parts covered which may come into contact with sterile materials. They should be stored in dust-free cupboards and the exposed parts should be wiped down before use.

Containers for Parenteral Injections

Parenteral injections may be dispensed in single- or multiple-dose containers. Single doses up to about 10 ml are usually dispensed in ampoules and single-dose injections of large volumes, such as perfusion fluids, are dispensed in blood or MRC bottles. Multiple-dose injections are dispensed in vaccine bottles.

Ampoules

Ampoules are thin glass single-dose containers, the capacity ranging from 0.5 to 50 ml. After filling, they are sealed by fusion of the glass before being sterilized. The contents can then be expected to remain sterile until they are used. Specifications for ampoules are given in BS 795: 1961, and requirements for the quality of glass used are discussed in Chapter 39. Ampoules provide the most satisfactory form of container for most injections and are mandatory when the air above the solution is replaced by nitrogen or other inert gas. Spinal injections may only be packaged in ampoules because the inclusion of bacteriostatics is not permitted, and such injections may not be dispensed in multiple-dose containers.

Glass ampoules do, however, suffer from one major defect: they must be opened by snapping off the neck after marking it with a file, and although they have proved in practice to be very reliable, there exists always the possibility of glass spicules dropping into the solution and being taken up by the syringe. Special glass ampoules are made with prescored or preweakened necks which can be snapped off cleanly without having to be filed, and plastic ampoules are also made in which the contents are removed by inserting the syringe directly through the shoulder (*Pharm. J.*, 1973, **210**, 110).

A number of devices have been produced to cut down the time taken by assembling a syringe and using it to withdraw the contents of an ampoule. One such device is the injection cartridge (Fig. 31.16) consisting of a length of glass tubing closed at both ends with tight-fitting rubber plugs. The cartridge is inserted into a metal holder forming in effect the barrel of the syringe. The holder is equipped with a plunger which fits into one of the rubber plugs which then acts as the piston, while at the other end the needle mount is prolonged inwards as a short, strong needle which pierces the other plug of the cartridge, forming a seal. Plastic syringes are also available with the injectable solution already in situ, while in other designs the use of a syringe is avoided altogether. In the automatic injector shown in Fig. 31.17 the solution

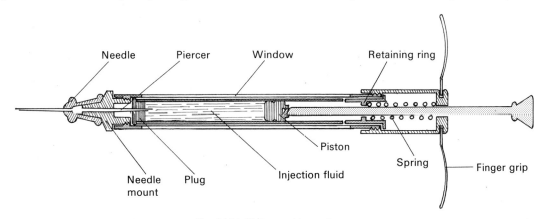

FIG. 31.16. Viule cartridge syringe.

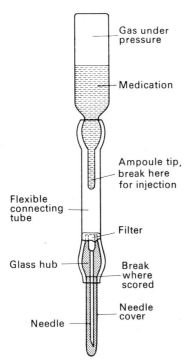

Gas under
pressure

Medication

Ampoule tip,
break here
for injection

Flexible
connecting
tube

Filter

Glass hub

Break
where
scored

Needle
cover

Needle

FIG. 31.17. The 'Ampin' automatic injector.

is contained in a glass ampoule the residual space of which is occupied by an inert gas under pressure. The ampoule tip is broken by bending the plastic tube after the needle has been inserted into the recipient: any glass fragments are retained by the filter.

Filling ampoules. As supplied by the manufacturer, ampoules for liquids are usually sealed to exclude dust, having previously been washed and dried. For use, the ampoule is filed above the neck and the sealed end broken off, care being taken to prevent glass spicules from falling inside. The length of neck remaining should be sufficient to provide adequate leverage when the completed ampoule is opened. Preliminary sterilization is not essential if the contents are to be subjected to a final heating process after sealing, but if the contents are thermolabile, the empty ampoules must be sterilized before filling them. In order that the ampoules may be dry, it is best to sterilize them in a hot air oven, but if they are to be used for aqueous liquids they can be sterilized by autoclaving provided that they are well drained. For small batches, filling is usually carried out under a screen using a syringe, while for slightly larger batches a burette fitted with a hypodermic needle covered by a hood can be used.

The necks may then conveniently be sealed with a twin-jet burner. On a large scale, of course, automatic filling, sealing and labelling machines are employed.

Single-Dose Containers for Large Volumes
Perfusion fluids are often required in volumes of 500 to 1000 ml. Specifications for suitable bottles are given in BS 2463: 1962 (amended) which describes tests for the mechanical strength, thermal resistance and hydrolytic resistance of the glass to water, saline and citrate solution. They are made of good quality glass, stout enough to resist breakage and capable of repeated use. All bottles before filling should be scrupulously clean and entirely free from solid particles internally. Chemical cleanliness alone is necessary if the contents are to be autoclaved, but if the solution is not to be heated, the bottles must be sterile.

Most of the common perfusion fluids are sterilized in the autoclave in the final sealed containers. Containers made of plastics are now widely used. They are flexible and collapse as the fluid is delivered, so that it is not necessary to have a sterile air inlet filter. A plastic giving set is attached to the plastic bag before sterilization, avoiding the necessity of aseptic assembly. The plastics used are permeable to water vapour molecules and to avoid loss of fluid the bag containing the injection is surrounded by another. Nevertheless, the pack has a limited shelf life and Myers (1974) found that 'ballooning' sometimes occurred between the inner and outer bags. Injections supplied in plastic containers of not less than 500 ml capacity must comply with the limit test for toxicity of the *British Pharmacopoeia* 1973.

Multiple-Dose Containers
Multiple-dose containers are used for subcutaneous, intramuscular and, occasionally intravenous injections (e.g. sclerosing agents). The vials used may contain from 2 to 25 ml and are usually closed with a flanged rubber bung which is secured by an aluminium capping. This is turned in under the lip of the neck of the vial and its central portion is cut away to expose the top of the rubber bung, so that a needle can be passed through it. The exposed area is protected from dust by a cap which either simply slips over the closure or is screwed onto a thread on the bottle neck. As with ampoules, the glass must conform to necessary standards and similarly the rubber seal must comply with BS 3263: 1960 (see Chapter 39).

Although multiple-dose containers are convenient in use, they have several disadvantages, the chief of these being the risk of contamination from the insertion of a non-sterile needle or from leakage, and the possibility of measuring the wrong dose. The contents should normally be used quickly because, as doses are removed, the increased air-space may accelerate oxidation of the contents and it may be necessary to add an antioxidant to the injection. Vials are however useful for the packaging of sterile, thermolabile powders (e.g. antibiotics) which are dissolved in Water for Injections prior to use, because the material can be dried from solution in the final container.

Multiple-dose injections must contain a bactericide in sufficient concentration to prevent multiplication of any organisms accidentally introduced during the withdrawal of successive doses. The *British Pharmacopoeia* 1973 recommends the use of cresol 0.3 per cent w/v, chlorocresol 0.1 per cent w/v, or phenylmercuric nitrate 0.001 per cent w/v. Injections which are sterilized by the official process of Heating with a Bactericide need no further addition.

Choice of Sterilizing Method

Autoclaving. This is the method of choice for the sterilization of most aqueous injections, provided that they will withstand the time-temperature combination used. In the case of substances which readily oxidize, sodium metabisulphate may be included in the formulation, e.g. adrenalin, procainamide. Alternatively, the air in the sealed container may be replaced with nitrogen, e.g. for promazine and its derivatives, soluble sulphonamides. Sodium Bicarbonate Injection is gassed with carbon dioxide before sealing the ampoules or bottles, in order to prevent conversion to the normal carbonate. Sodium lactate injections are made by neutralization of lactic acid and the autoclave is used as a convenient method of heating them to ensure completion of the reaction prior to adjustment of pH and sterilization by a second autoclaving procedure. Autoclaving is the only method applicable to the sterilization of bulky cotton dressings or fabrics and the special problems associated with them have already been discussed. Oily injections cannot, of course, be autoclaved. In the absence of moisture the process would amount to no more than using dry heat at a temperature too low to be effective.

Glassware can be autoclaved provided that the steam can reach both internal and external surfaces, but as the articles are usually required to be dry,

they are generally sterilized in a hot air oven. Some plastic materials can be autoclaved, but not all, and natural rubbers will also withstand normal autoclaving temperatures. Delicate rubber articles like surgeons' gloves are liable to perish, however, unless care is taken to remove all residual moisture by applying an effective vacuum after sterilization.

Sterilization by dry heat. This is used for all oily vehicles, e.g. soft and hard paraffins, ethyl oleate and waxes and for a number of oily injections, e.g. those containing steroids in solution. If the medicament dissolved or suspended in such a vehicle will not withstand the temperature used, it must be sterilized separately by treatment with ethylene oxide or ionizing radiations or by dissolving it in a volatile solvent which, after passage through a bacterial filter, can be removed. The sterile solid is then mixed aseptically with the sterilized vehicle. Oily suspensions can be sterilized by dry heat, but in some cases the suspended solid may dissolve at the higher temperature and recrystallize in larger aggregates on cooling and care must be taken to minimize this. Glycerol can also be sterilized by dry heat and is used in Phenol and Glycerol Injection BP.

Dry heat is also useful for the sterilization of a number of non-injectable articles. Paraffin gauze dressings can be sterilized in their final containers by heating in an oven, and implants of steroids which have melting points higher than 150° can be made by sterilizing the material in an oven and then either pouring it aseptically into sterile moulds or allowing it to crystallize and then tabletting the crystals by heavy compression.

Silicone rubber can be sterilized by autoclaving, but where completely dry conditions are required, it can be sterilized by dry heat. Similarly, syringes and some surgical instruments can be sterilized by autoclaving, but it is usually more convenient to use dry heat, especially where the process can be made continuous as with the infra-red tunnel sterilizer. Sterilizable Maize Starch can also be sterilized in the hot air oven and the method is the only suitable one for dusting powders containing talc. On the small scale the talc is set out in shallow layers in the oven in order to get adequate heat penetration. Large amounts of talc are however used by the pharmaceutical and toiletry industries and sterilization of it is greatly assisted by its refractory nature. Because it can be heated to a high temperature without deteroration, large volumes can be heated in a furnace so that even if there is a considerable temperature gradient through the material the innermost regions still reach the necessary temperature. Some absorbable haemostatics which are prepared by freeze drying, and therefore have a very low moisture content, are sterilized by heating at about 130° for 3 h e.g. Human Fibrin Foam.

Dry heat *must not* be employed for the sterilization of aqueous fluids. The explosive power generated by even a few ml of water heated to 150° in a sealed ampoule is enormous and potentially lethal.

Gaseous sterilization. This can be used for thermolabile materials which will not withstand the conditions imposed by autoclaving or heating in an oven. Ethylene oxide is generally used and the limitations on its use have already been discussed. It can be effectively employed for sterilizing some surgical instruments and equipment made wholly or partly of plastics where these cannot be sterilized by autoclaving or ionizing radiations. The method has been used for absorbable dusting powder, for rubber gloves and for oxidized cellulose. Formaldehyde is still occasionally used for sterilizing rooms, but its principal application is in the formaldehyde-steam process for sterilizing woollen blankets.

Sterilization by heating with a bactericide. This process is permitted by the *British Pharmacopoeia* as an alternative to filtration for a few relatively heat-sensitive alkaloids, e.g. morphine, emetine, and also for mersalyl and sodium aurothiomalate. It is also officially approved for sterilizing suxamethonium chloride, but not for the bromide, the injection of which must be made by dissolving the sterile solid in the vehicle. Dimenhydrinate Injection contains benzyl benzoate as an ingredient and no further bactericide is required. Similarly, some acid solutions e.g. Procaine and Adrenaline Injection BP and some alkaline solutions e.g. Phenobarbitone Injection BP provide adequate conditions for sterilization at 98° to 100° without additional bactericide.

Sterilization by ionizing radiations. This process has been discussed in Chapter 28. Either high-speed electrons from an accelerator or γ-rays from a radioisotope may be used to give the necessary penetration and the method is particularly useful for some ready-packed disposable surgical equipment such as catheters, intravenous giving sets and plastic syringes. It is necessary to choose the right type of plastic or glass for the purpose. Some materials which would otherwise be difficult to sterilize can be treated effectively by irradiation, e.g. catgut, graft tissues and adhesive dressings.

Sterilization by filtration. Where none of the foregoing methods is applicable, filtration remains the only available method of sterilization. This may involve the filtration of the final solution followed by aseptic distribution into containers, or if the medicament is unstable in aqueous solution it may be dissolved in a non-aqueous solvent and passed through a bacterial filter, the solvent being then removed by distillation, if required under reduced pressure, or by freeze drying, e.g. antibiotics, hormones and enzymes. Paraldehyde Injection BPC may not be subjected to heat sterilization and must be sterilized by filtration: it must be supplied in single-dose ampoules, contact with rubber or plastics being contraindicated.

Aseptic operation. As has already been pointed out, some thermolabile solids are prepared in a sterile condition and injections are made from them by redissolving them in a sterile vehicle. In a few cases aseptic dilution of a stronger solution is prescribed e.g. Noradrenaline Injection BP. Insulin Injection BP is sterilized by filtration, but a test portion is then withdrawn aseptically and assayed, and the remainder is then adjusted to volume with sterile diluent and distributed aseptically into the final containers. Cortisone Injection BP and Hydrocortisone Acetate Injection BP are sterile suspensions prepared by aseptic technique. Vaccines, sera and blood products are also prepared aseptically from an original source assumed to be sterile, and the final product must therefore be adequately tested for sterility.

REFERENCES

ABBOTT, C. F., COCKTON, J. & JONES, W. (1956) *J. Pharm. Pharmacol.* **8**, 709.

ALDER, V. G. (1970) In *Microbiological Methods*, 3rd edn. Ed. Collins, C. H. & Lyne, R. M. London: Butterworths.

AVIS, K. E. & GERSHENFELD, L. (1955), *J. Am. pharm. Ass. (Sci. Edn)* **44**, 682.

BALL, C. O. (1923) *Natl. Research Council Bull., Pt. I*, No. 37 cited by Schmidt, A. B. (1957).

BARFIELD, J. C. (1955) *Pharm. J.* **174**, 9.

BARSON, T. E., PEACOCK, F., ROBINS, E. L. & WILKINSON, G. R. (1958) *J. Pharm. Pharmacol.* **10**, 47T.

BEEBY, M. M. & WHITEHOUSE, C. E. (1965) *J. appl. Bact.* **28**, 349.

BERRY, H., JENSEN, E. & SILLER, F. K. (1938) *Quart. J. Pharm.* **11**, 729.

BEVERLEY, S., HAMBLETON, R. & ALLWOOD, M. C. (1974) *Pharm. J.* 306.

BLISS, A. B. (1934) *Science* **79**, 38.

BOWIE, J. H. (1959) In *The Operation of Sterilizing Autoclaves.* London: Pharmaceutical Press.

BROWN, M. R. W. & MELLING, J. (1973) *J. Pharm. Pharmacol.* **25**, 478.

BROWN, M. R. W. & RIDOUT, C. W. (1960) *Pharm. J.* **184**, 5.

BROWNE, H. H. (1942) *J. Bact.* **42**, 315.

BRUCH, C. W. (1961) *Ann. Rev. Microbiol.* **15**, 245.

BRITISH STANDARDS INSTITUTION, LONDON
   BS 1752: 1963 *Laboratory sintered or fritted filters*
   BS 3421: 1961 *Performance of electrically heated sterilizing ovens*
   BS 3970 Pt. 1: 1966 *Sterilisers for porous loads*
   BS 2463: 1962 *Transfusion Equipment for Medical Use*
   BS 3263: 1960 *Rubber Closures for Injectable Products*
   BS 3970 Pt. 2: 1966 *Sterilisers for bottled fluids*
   BS 795: 1961 *Specification for Ampoules*

CHAMBERLAND, C. (1884) *Compt. rend. Acad. Sci.* **99**, 247.

CLOTHIER COMMITTEE OF ENQUIRY (1972) Command Paper. Cmnd. 5035. London: HMSO.

COOK, A. M. & BROWN, M. R. W. (1965) *J. Pharm. Pharmacol.* **17**, Suppl. 7S.

COOK, A. M. & GILBERT, R. G. (1968) *J. Pharm. Pharmacol.* **20**, 803.

COOK, A. M. & SAUNDERS, L. (1962) *J. Pharm. Pharmacol.* **14**, 83T.

COOK, A. M. & WILLS, B. A. (1954) *J. Pharm. Pharmacol.* **6**, 638.

COOPER, P. (1951) *Pharm. J.* **167**, 439.

COULTHARD, C. E. (1939) *Pharm. J.* **142**, 79.

DARMADY, E. M., HUGHES, K. E. A. & TUKE, W. (1957) *J. clin. Path.* **10**, 291.

DAVIS, H. (1935) *Quart. J. Pharm.* **8**, 361.

DAVIS, H. (1940) *Quart. J. Pharm.* **13**, 14.

ELSWORTH, R. (1969) In *Methods in Microbiology*, Vol. 1, Ed. Norris, J. R. & Robins, D. W. London: Academic Press.

ELSWORTH, R. (1972) In *Safety in Microbiology*, Ed. Shapton, D. A. & Board, R. G. London: Academic Press.

ELSWORTH, R., MORRIS, E. J. & EAST, D. N. (1961) *Trans. Inst. Chem. Engrs* **39**, A47.

FELDBERG, W. (1971) In *Pyrogens and Fever* Ed. Wolstenholme, A. B. & Birch, A. B. London: Churchill-Livingstone.

GILBERT, G. L., GAMBILL, V. M., SPINER, D. R., HOFFMAN, R. K. & PHILLIPS, C. R. (1964) *Appl. Microbiol.* **12**, 496.

HANSEN, N.-H. & RIEMANN, H. (1963) *J. appl. Bact.* **26**, 314.

HENRY, P. S. H. & SCOTT, E. (1963) *J. appl. Bact.* **26**, 234.

KAYE, S. & PHILLIPS, C. R. (1949) *Am. J. Hyg.* **50**, 296.

KEALL, A. (1973) *J. appl. Bact.* **36**, 35.

KELSEY, J. C. (1958) *Lancet* **i**, 306.

KELSEY, J. C. (1959) In *The Operation of Sterilising Autoclaves.* London: Pharmaceutical Press.

KELSEY, J. C. (1961) *J. clin. Path.* **14**, 313.

KELSEY, J. C. (1967) *J. appl. Bact.* **30**, 92.

KNOX, R. & PENIKETT, E. J. K. (1958) *Brit. med. J.* **i**, 680.

KNOX, R., PENIKETT, E. J. K. & DUNCAN, M. E. (1960) *J. appl. Bact.* **23**, 21.

MAYR, G. (1961) In *Symposium on the Sterilisation of Surgical Materials.* London: Pharmaceutical Press.

MCDADE, J. J. (1969) In *Methods in Microbiology*, Vol. 1, Ed. Norris, J. R. & Robins, A. B. London: Academic Press.

MEDICINES COMMISSION REPORT (1973) *Report on the Prevention of Microbial Contamination of Pharmaceutical Products.* London: HMSO.

MORTON, H. E. (1943) *J. Bact.* **46**, 312.

MEDICAL RESEARCH COUNCIL (1959) Report by the Medical Research Council Working Party on pressure-steam sterilisers. *Lancet* **i**, 425.

MULVANY, J. G. (1969) In *Methods in Microbiology*, Vol. 1, Ed. Norris, J. R. & Robins, A. B. London: Academic Press.

MYERS, J. A. (1974) *Pharm. J.* **212**, 308.

NEWMAN, F. H. (1954) *May & Baker Pharmaceutical Bulletin* **3**, 140.

NEWMAN, F. H. (1955) *May & Baker Pharmaceutical Bulletin* **4**, 134.

OPFELL, J. B., HOHMANN, J. P. & LATHAM, A. B. (1959) *J. Am. pharm Ass. (Sci. Edn)* **48**, 617.

PALMER, C. H. R. & WHITTET, T. D. (1961) *J. Pharm. Pharmacol.* **13**, 62T.

PENKIETT, E. J. K., ROWE, T. W. & ROBSON, E. (1958) *J. appl. Bact.* **21** (2), 282.

PERKINS, J. J. & LLOYD, R. S. (1961) In *Symposium on the Sterilization of Surgical Materials*, 76. London: Pharmaceutical Press.

PHARMACEUTICAL HANDBOOK (1970).

PHILLIPS, C. R. (1949) *Am. J. Hyg.* **49**, 280.

PHILLIPS, C. R. (1956) *Am. J. Hyg.* **50**, 280.

PHILLIPS, C. R. (1961) *Symposium on the Sterilisation of Surgical Materials*, 59. London: Pharmaceutical Press.

POWELL, D. B. (1961) *Symposium on the Sterilisation of Surgical Materials*, 59. London: Pharmaceutical Press.

PUBLIC HEALTH LABORATORY REPORT (1958) *J. Hyg. Camb.* **56**, 485.

QUESNEL, L. B. (1967) *J. appl. Bact.* **30**, 529.

QUESNEL, L. B., HAYWARD, J. M. & BARNET, J. W. (1967) *J. appl. Bact.* **30**, 518.

RAHN, O. (1945) *Bact. Rev.* **9**, 1.

REDDISH, G. F. (1957) Ed. *Antiseptics, Disinfectants, Fungicides and Chemical and Physical Sterilization*, 2nd edn. London: Kimpton.

RIDGWAY, K. (1973) *Proc. Biochem.* **8**, (7), 9.

ROSENHEIM COMMITTEE (1972).

ROYCE, A. (1959) *Publ. Pharm.* **16**, 235.

ROYCE, A. & BOWLER, C. L. (1950) *J. Pharm. Pharmacol.* **11**, 294T.

ROYCE, A. & BOWLER, C. L. (1961) *J. Pharm. Pharmacol.* **13**, 87T.

ROYCE, A. & SYKES, G. (1950) *Proc. Soc. appl. Bact.* **13**, 146.

RUBBO, S. D. & GARDNER, J. F. (1965) *A Review of Sterilization and Disinfection.* London: Lloyd-Luke.

RUSSELL, J. H. (1971) *Proc. Biochem.* **6**, (9), 25.

SAVAGE, R. M. (1937) *Q. J. Pharm.* **10**, 451.

SAVAGE, R. M. (1959) In *Symposium on the Operating of Sterilising Autoclaves.* London: Pharmaceutical Press.

SCHMIDT, C. F. (1957) In *Antiseptics, Disinfectants, Fungicides and Chemical and Physical Sterilization*, 2nd Edn. London: Kimpton.

SEIBERT, F. (1923) *Am. J. Physiol.* **67**, 90.

SIMPKINS, D. E. & WILKINSON, G. R. (1964) *J. Pharm. Pharmacol.* **16**, Suppl. 108T.

SMITH, I. C. P. (1944) *Pharm. J.* **152**, 110.

SYKES, C. H. (1958) *Publ. Pharm.* **15**, 163.

SYKES, G. (1963) *J. appl. Bact.* **26**, 287.

SYKES, G. (1965) *Disinfection and Sterilisation* 2nd edn. London: Spon.

SYKES, G. (1969) In *Methods in Microbiology*, Ed. Norris, A. B. & Robins, A. B. London: Academic Press.

SYKES, G. & ROYCE, A. (1950) *J. Pharm. Pharmacol.* **2**, 639.

TROTMAN, R. E. (1960) *J. appl. Bact.* **32**, 297.

WHITMARSH, J. M. (1954) *J. appl. Bact.* **17**, (i), 27.

WHITTET, T. D., HUGO, W. B. & WILKINSON, G. R. (1965) *Sterilisation & Disinfection*, Ed. Stenlake, A. B. London: Heinnemann.

WILKINSON, G. R. & PEACOCK, F. G. (1961) *J. Pharm. Pharmacol.* **13**, 67T.

WILKINSON, G. R., PEACOCK, F. G. & ROBINS, K. L. (1960) *J. Pharm. Pharmacol.* **12**, 197T.

WORK, A. B. (1971) In *Pyrogens and Fever*, Ed. Wolstenholme, A. B. & Birch, A. B., 23. London: Churchill-Livingstone.

WYLLIE, D. M. (1955) *Pharm. J.* **175**, 492.

32

Microbial Contamination Control and Sterility Testing

Microbial contamination may be important in three ways. In injections, eye drops and certain dressings and lavage solutions sterility is essential since any contaminants may cause infections and the products of contaminants (pyrogens) have caused harmful and even lethal reactions. Also, infection may result from contaminated oral and topical preparations, the most serious incident being the occurrence of typhoid fever as a sequel to the ingestion of contaminated thyroid tablets. Finally, excessive microbial contamination may cause more or less extensive deterioration of the product, but can be dealt with by a combination of hygienic preparation and preservation (see below and Chapter 37).

QUALITY CONTROL

The hygienic production of pharmaceuticals and the sterilization processes for the production of sterile materials are aspects of the quality control operation. The same conditions apply to both hospital and industrial production and there is no reason to apply different standards in these two situations, though the methods and equipment used to achieve satisfactory products will clearly differ.

It must be understood that quality control does not consist simply of a few analytical procedures carried out by a laboratory at the end of a production run, but is a series of procedures which start at the inception of plans for a new product and continue well beyond the despatch of each batch. The quality of a product can be no better than that of the weakest link in the production chain. General guidance to U.K. manufacturers is given in the *Guide to Good Pharmaceutical Manufacturing Practice* produced by the Department of Health and Social Security and its appendices.

Principles

The establishment of a proper managerial structure is probably the most important aspect. Everyone connected with quality control and production must know clearly what their duties are, what is the chain of command and how they fit into that chain. A quality controller must be a senior manager, independent of production and with access to the highest levels of management. He must be consulted on the location, design and maintenance of the buildings, on the selection of the equipment to be used and in setting the standards of hygiene and cleanliness appropriate to buildings, equipment and personnel. Personnel training and retraining are also important. Further, he will specify exactly what records and documentation are required to check adequately the various aspects of each process.

Once production has commenced, under the direction of a production manager independent of the quality controller, the quality control laboratory will conduct chemical and other analyses as well as routine checks on the levels of microbial contamination of the starting materials, the buildings and their atmospheres, personnel and equipment and on the product at various stages of production. These checks include chemical, physico-chemical and biological methods and also the surveillance of those aspects of production which contribute to contamination. Biological methods include determinations of the nature and extent of microbiological contamination of any non-sterile materials used, and sterility testing, the details of the latter being dealt with below. Also, aseptic filling procedures can be verified by filling a nutrient medium in place of the product, incubating the filled containers and checking for the presence of microbial growth.

If quality control procedures are be reliable it is essential that sampling is done exclusively by quality control staff and not by production workers and that sampling is properly randomized, for example, by the use of tables of random numbers.

It must always be assumed that human errors will occur, so the checks introduced at suitable stages in production are designed to monitor this possibility.

Finally, all documentation relevant to each batch, from starting materials to finished product, is collated, checked and filed for future reference and samples of each batch are retained and checked at intervals until all the batch has certainly been used.

THE MICROBIAL CONTAMINATION OF NON-STERILE PRODUCTS

Interest is focused on two points: the extent of the contamination and its nature. The establishment of standards is not easy but should be fixed by what is attainable by good manufacturing practice and with regard to the nature of the preparation, so that the standards which are set can be achieved at the point of use.

The Extent of Contamination
Standards. The USP XVIII is one of the few pharmacopoeias which sets standards for the numbers of aerobic bacteria in a variety of products, e.g. gelatin, aluminium hydroxide gel. No standards limiting the total bacterial population appear in the BP 1973. An FIP Working Party (Report, 1972) indicated levels of the order of 10^6 to 10^9/g in substances of animal or vegetable origin and of 100/g in synthetic or purified substances, while some materials, e.g. vitamins, lactose, talc, kaolin, posed special problems (Table 32.1). The Report also gives recommended standards and methods applicable to various classes of non-sterile medicaments.

The methods laid down in the USP XVIII are standard bacteriological counting methods. For clear miscible products the total number of viable aerobic bacteria is determined by the pour plate method, but with suspensions or emulsions in which turbidity makes colony counting difficult or

TABLE 32.1

LIMITS SUGGESTED BY THE FIP WORKING PARTY (REPORT, 1972) ON PERMISSIBLE LEVELS OF MICROBIAL CONTAMINATION OF NON-STERILE MEDICAMENTS

(The procedures are a compromise between the limits for numbers of revivable organisms[†] and fixing limits for the exclusion of specified pathogens.)

Product	Numerical tolerance limit of bacteria	Totally excluded species or genera
Injectable	Nil	All
Ophthalmic preparations, large volume lavage solutions for sterile cavities, burns, ulcers	None in 1 g or 1 ml	—
Topical preparations (for damaged skin, nose, throat, ear)	10^2/g or 10^2/ml	Entero-bacteriaceae* Ps.aeruginosa Staphylococcus aureus
Other preparations	10^3/g or 10^3/ml (10^2/g or 10^2/ml of yeasts and fungi)	Entero-bacteriaceae* Ps.aeruginosa Staph.aureus

* Some materials based on natural sources must be allowed to contain Enterobacteriaceae, e.g. to the extent of 20/g, but in such cases strict limits must be applied on the numbers of *E.coli*, salmonellae and *Shigella*.
[†] No general norms can be laid down for starting materials, but (a) synthetic compounds or pure substances of non-biological origin usually contain <100/g,
(b) crude products of biological origin may contain 10^6–10^9/g,
(c) exceptionally lactose, calcium lactate, steroids and mixed earths may be contaminated with a mostly saprophytic microflora but including *Bacillus*, *Micrococcus*, *Staphylococcus*, *Streptococcus* group D, *Cl. tetani* (in talc), and fungi.

impossible the count may be done by the dilution method (most probable number, MPN or multiple tube method), although the accuracy of this is very poor.

If the preparation contains antimicrobial agents, either naturally or as added preservatives, the inhibitory effect must be removed by dilution, chemically or by filtration prior to testing. The latter is done using a sterile membrane filter which is washed free of inhibitor and the filter can then be incubated directly on a nutrient medium.

Methods (USP XVIII). A 10 g or 10 ml sample is derived from not less than 10×1 g or 10×1 ml samples, taken from different containers and blended, and dissolved or suspended in 90 ml of phosphate buffer. Gelatin is treated similarly, except that further dilution is usually necessary. Hydrophobic materials are emulsified with polysorbate

80. Two 1 ml samples of the final suspension, diluted further if necessary, are then counted by the normal pour plate technique, using soybean-casein digest (tryptone soya) agar. Colonies are counted after 48 to 72 h.

If the diluted sample is a suspension, or an emulsion too turbid to permit colony counts, a multiple tube (MPN) method may be used, the count being determined by reference to a MPN table similar to that given in Table 29.4. If it is difficult to decide whether growth is present or not, the contents of the tubes are subcultured into fresh medium.

All samples must be tested to ensure that they do not contain inhibitory substances; if they do the procedure is modified to remove or neutralize the inhibitory action.

The Nature of the Contamination

Only four species are looked for routinely. *E.coli* is used universally as an index of faecal pollution of food and water and can fill this role since it is probably exclusively human in origin, occurs in large numbers in faeces and survives well outside the body. Thus there are numerous, rapid, well-proved methods for detecting this species which is widely used as an index of hygienic production.

There are numerous *Salmonella* species comprising the agents of typhoid and paratyphoid fevers (enteric fever), and many of the common causal agents of food poisoning. Direct attempts to isolate these are not usual in water bacteriology since they may be of animal origin, are present in relatively small numbers in the intestines of infected patients and the methods are of doubtful sensitivity. Presumably, interest has focused on these species since they frequently infect animals and invade the blood stream after slaughter, so products derived from animals are likely to be infected. Indeed, several cases of typhoid fever in Sweden were traced back to infected thyroid tablets.

Staphylococcus aureus is carried by many individuals in the nose and throat and sometimes on the skin, as a harmless parasite. Under appropriate conditions it can cause wound infections which may be difficult to treat and is a common cause of food poisoning if some foods infected with it are left so that the organism can grow and produce exotoxin. It is thus another index of hygienic production.

Although *Pseudomonas aeruginosa* is of relatively low virulence it is a common wound pathogen since it establishes itself readily in damaged tissue or in debilitated patients. It has been reported as the causal agent of deaths in burns units, and of loss of sight, and may also cause systemic infections. Further, the organism is resistant to most antibiotics, apart from carbenicillin and colistin, and readily acquires resistance by the transfer of resistance factors. Other pseudomonads are very common in water and although these will not ordinarily grow above 30° (*Ps.fluorescens, Ps.putida*) they are very versatile biochemically and can break down many compounds including antiseptics.

Other organisms such as anaerobic bacteria and fungi, may be important in particular cases, so reputable manufacturers test products appropriately. The official standards are to be regarded, in this as in all other cases, as *minimum requirements* which manufacturers augment as necessary.

Methods

E.coli. The BP 1973 recommends that samples should be inoculated into nutrient broth and incubated. Tubes showing growth are then subcultured into MacConkey broth and again incubated at 37°. Any tubes showing acid and gas production are subcultured into both MacConkey broth and tryptone water, which are then incubated at $44° \pm 0.5$. Production of acid and gas in the former medium and indole from the latter is presumptive of *E.coli*.

The USP XVIII requires a 10 g or 10 ml sample to be added to a lactose broth and incubated. If growth is present a loopful is streaked on a plate of MacConkey agar. Brick red colonies of Gram-negative rods are streaked on Eosin Methylene Blue agar for confirmation. Blue-black colonies with a metallic sheen are presumed to be *E.coli* and confirmed by further tests as above.

The methods given above do not conform to current practice in water bacteriology, in which samples are incubated in Minerals Modified Glutamate (MMG) medium and positive (acid and gas) tubes are subcultured into Lactose Ricinoleate (LR) broth and Tryptone water and incubated at $44°C \pm 0.2$. Growth and lactose fermentation to give acid and gas in the former medium and indole production in the latter is considered presumptive of *E.coli*. These latter methods have been introduced because selective media generally, and MacConkey medium in particular, are frequently inhibitory to the very organisms which they are intended to select. In water analysis MMG and LR media have been shown to give a higher number of positive with a minimum of false positive reactions (Report, 1969), but whether this applies also to pharmaceuticals is not known.

Salmonella spp. The method given by the BP 1973 is to enrich the culture by incubating the sample with nutrient broth, and to add heavy inocula from the enrichment culture into Selenite F and Tetrathionate media. After further incubation samples from each tube showing growth are streaked onto Brilliant Green, Desoxycholate Citrate and Bismuth sulphite agars. Any suspect colonies are confirmed by inoculation into Triple Sugar Iron and Urea media. The USP XVIII uses the remainder of the lactose broth culture prepared for the *E.coli* test and adds portions to Selenite–Cysteine and Tetrathionate media. After 12 to 24 h at 30–35° portions of each enrichment culture are streaked on Brilliant Green, Xylose–Lysine–Desoxycholate, and Bismuth Sulphite agars. Suspect colonies are confirmed on Triple Sugar Iron agar, final confirmation being done by further biochemical tests.

The requirement to use both selenite and tetrathionate media is a reflection of the inhibitory nature of these media to *Salmonella* spp. and therefore the results should be viewed with caution since counts may be low.

The colony characters used to characterize these and other organisms are given in Table 32.2.

TABLE 32.2

COLONIAL AND MORPHOLOGICAL CHARACTERS OF CONTAMINANTS OF INTEREST IN NON-STERILE PHARMACEUTICALS

Organism	Gram reaction and morphology	Medium	Colonial characters
Staphylococcus aureus	Positive Cocci in clusters	Vogel–Johnson agar	Black, surrounded by a yellow zone
Pseudomonas aeruginosa	Negative Slender rods	Cetrimide agar	Generally greenish, fluorescent
Escherichia coli	Negative Short rods	MacConkey agar	Brick red to bright pink, usually halo of precipitated bile acids
Salmonella spp.	Negative Short rods	Brilliant Green agar	Small, transparent, colourless or pink to white, opaque, frequently surrounded by pink to red zone.
		Xylose–Lysine–Desoxycholate agar	Red, sometimes with black centres.
		Bismuth Sulphite agar	Black or green

Staphylococcus aureus. The BP 1973 does not give any tests for the presence of this organism. The USP XVIII directs that samples should be incubated in Soybean–Casein Digest (Tryptone Soya) broth followed by subculture from tubes showing growth onto Vogel–Johnson agar. Black colonies of Gram-positive cocci surrounded by a yellow zone are presumptive of *Staph.aureus* and this is confirmed by a positive coagulase test, thus i.e. cultures are able to coagulate rabbit serum.

Ps.aeruginosa. The BP 1973 recommends inoculation into 0.03 per cent cetrimide broth, incubating at 30° for 72 h and then streaking from this onto 0.1 per cent cetrimide agar. All colonies showing green pigmentation are tested by the oxidase test and Gram staining. The oxidase test consists of spreading a colony on paper saturated with N.N′-*p*-aminodimethylaniline hydrochloride, when oxidase positive organisms, e.g. *Ps.aeruginosa*, give a purplish colour.

The USP XVIII uses the same primary culture as for *Staph.aureus* and then streaks onto an agar medium containing 0.03 per cent cetrimide. All 'generally greenish' fluorescent colonies are presumed to be *Ps.aeruginosa* and are tested by the oxidase test. Oxidase positive organisms are presumed to be *Ps.aeruginosa*, which may be confirmed by further biochemical tests.

The USP is generally safer than the BP since it defines the composition of its cetrimide agar fairly closely. The selective effect of the cetrimide depends markedly on the nature of the ingredients of the medium, and pigmentation is similarly sensitive. Several pigments may be produced, pyocyanin which is blue-green, fluorescein which is pale yellowish-green and fluorescent and the red pigment, pyorubin. Melanin may also be produced. Thus the pigmentation may be anything from pink to purple or black. The production of visible pigment is unreliable and it is generally accepted that growth plus fluorescence is the best guide. Also, about 10 per cent of strains are non-pigmented. Finally, incubation at 30° will permit the growth of saprobic pseudomonads, which produce the fluorescent pigment only, and other Gram-negative rods (*Flavobacterium*) which cannot be differentiated from pseudomonads by the tests described above. Thus it is essential to test each batch of media with known strains to ensure that the proper growth patterns are produced. This is also desirable for all the procedures described for all four organisms and is the procedure given by the BP, which lists the strains to be used for controlling the tests for *E.coli*, *Salmonella* spp. and *Ps.aeruginosa*, though whether the range of test strains is adequate is open to doubt.

The most satisfactory medium for *Ps.aeruginosa* so far devised is that of Lilly and Lowbury (1972), based on a controlled formula containing 0.02 per cent cetrimide and nalidixic acid. These workers used growth and fluorescence as their criteria.

Ophthalmic Ointments

These are required to pass tests for total bacterial count and for freedom from *Staph.aureus* and *Ps.aeruginosa*. The technique used is to dissolve 1 g of bulked sample in 100 ml of sterile isopropyl myristate and to filter the solution through three 0.22 μm membrane filters. Each membrane is then washed with 5 × 100 ml portions of peptone/beef extract broth containing (*p-tert*-octylphenoxy)polyethoxyethanol as a solubilizing agent for isopropyl myristate and residual ointment base. The membranes are then incubated on Soybean–Casein Digest (Tryptone Soya) agar and the colonies developing on the surfaces of the membranes are counted. Finally the colonies are streaked onto Vogel–Johnson and Cetrimide agar media to test for the presence of the specific contaminants.

STERILITY TESTING

In the main, sterility tests are applied to products intended to be sterile to check that the products are free from detectable contamination, both bacterial and fungal. Additionally, the test is applied to products known to contain viable microorganisms, such as Smallpox Vaccine, oral Polio Vaccine and BCG Vaccine, to ensure freedom from extraneous microorganisms.

The central proposition of the sterility test is extremely simple: samples are inoculated into suitable media and the media are incubated and examined for growth. However, on examining this proposition in greater detail, numerous problems occur.

Sample Size

The European Pharmacopoeia Vol. II and the USP XVIII specify the sample sizes to be used and these are given in Table 32.3.

It is doubtful whether there is any logic in such specifications except where the volume tested is one human (or animal) dose since what we need is security that the dose as administered in its entirety is unlikely to cause infection or other untoward effects. Thus the simple proposition should be to

TABLE 32.3

PHARMACOPOEIAL RECOMMENDATIONS ON SAMPLE VOLUMES TO BE TAKEN IN STERILITY TESTING

Authority	Container content	Minimum volume of sample	Minimum volume of medium
USP XVIII	10 ml or less	1 ml or total content if less than 1 ml	15 ml
	From 10 ml to 50 ml	5 ml	40 ml
	More than 50 ml	10 ml	80 ml
EP Vol. II	Less than 1 ml or 50 mg	Whole contents in each of bacterial and fungal tests	
	1 ml (50 mg) or more but less than 4 ml (200 mg)	Half the contents in each of the tests	Not less than 10 times the volume of sample
	4 ml (200 mg) or more but less than 20 ml	2 ml (100 mg) in each of the tests	
	20 ml or more	10 per cent of the contents in each of the tests	

test one human dose. However, this is impracticable where products have a very small dose, e.g. 0.1 ml, so that when tuberculin, eye drops, Schick test toxin and certain insulin preparations, etc., are tested, a volume larger than one dose must be tested and this gives additional security.

If a single aerobic/anaerobic medium is used in testing for bacteria, it is clear that the sample volumes must be doubled to give the same security of testing as if two media had been used.

Statistical Considerations

The argument over sample size in reinforced when the statistics of sampling are examined.

The distribution which fits the sterility test system is the hypergeometric distribution, and Knudsen (1949) has shown that the chance of detecting even a heavily contaminated batch is small, that the probability of detection depends primarily on sample size and that batch size is almost irrelevant in the range 50 to 10^4 items (Fig. 32.1).

A good approximation to the hypergeometric distribution is given by the *binomial distribution*, which is much easier to handle mathematically.

The probabilities of $0, 1, 2, ..., n$ defectives in a sample of n items, drawn at random from a batch

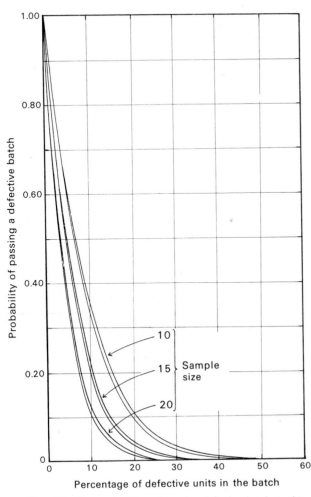

FIG. 32.1. The probability of passing defective batches with different levels of contamination, for different batch and sample sizes (hypergeometric distribution).

TABLE 32.4

THE PROBABILITY OF PASSING A BATCH WITH 10 PER CENT CONTAMINATED ITEMS, USING A SAMPLE OF FOUR ITEMS (BINOMIAL DISTRIBUTION)

Number contaminated	0	1	2	3	4	Total
Term of expression*	q^4	$4q^3p$	$6q^2p^2$	$4qp^3$	p^4	$(q+p)^4$
Probability of observation	0.6561	0.2916	0.0486	0.0036	0.0001	1.000
Probability of acceptance	0.656					—
rejection	—		0.344			—

* q, proportion sterile, 0.9; p, proportion contaminated, 0.1; n, sample size, 4.

It must be emphasized that both the statistical treatments discussed above assume that the whole of the contents of each container will be tested. However, sampling from containers is permitted (Table 32.3) and if samples are taken from containers in a sterility test, e.g. 1 ml samples from a 500 ml infusion fluid, the probability of detection falls to even poorer levels than those indicated above.

Finally the optimum number of items to be taken to detect particular levels of contamination, or to give acceptable levels of safety to the patient, must be considered. These two aims are not identical. To satisfy the requirement to detect contaminated batches with reasonable security it can be shown that the probability of detection increases rapidly with the number sampled at first, but then decreases, there being no worthwhile benefit in taking more than 40 items. To give a minimum risk of passing an unsatisfactory batch, Bentzon (WHO Report, 1960) showed that the sample size should equal the square root of the number of items in the batch.

However, it is unrealistic to take large proportions from small batches or to take a very large number of items from a large batch, in view of the low probability of detecting contamination. Compromises are therefore made and the numbers of items required to be taken by some pharmacopoeias are given in Table 32.5. Even at these reduced levels the cost of testing may be a major part of the total cost of production and any suggestion of increased sample sizes is strongly resisted by manufacturers.

Media

The media used must be capable of supporting the growth of small numbers of exacting micro-organisms.

with a proportion of defective (contaminated) items p and a proportion of satisfactory (sterile) items q, are given by the successive terms of the expansion of $(q+p)^n$. Thus the probability of n contaminated is p^n, of n sterile is q^n and of some contaminated is $(1-q^n-p^n)$. E.g., if $n = 4$, $q = 0.9$, $p = 0.1$, the result given in Table 32.4 is obtained, which shows that with 10 per cent of contaminated items in a batch and a sample of four, about 66 per cent of samples will contain no contaminated items, i.e. the batch will be accepted. From this it is again clear that when sampling by attributes (pass/fail), a small sample gives a very crude estimate of the proportion contaminated, even if this reaches the exceptionally high level of 10 per cent.

Further, since the probabilities depend only on p and n, the conclusion of Knudsen that batch size is irrelevant is substantiated.

TABLE 32.5

SAMPLE SIZES TO BE TAKEN IN STERILITY TESTING

European Pharmacopoeia Vol. II

Number of containers in the batch	Number of items to be taken
Not more than 100	10 per cent or 4, whichever is the greater
More than 100 but not more than 500	10
More than 500	2 per cent or 20 whichever is the less

United States Pharmacopoeia

Sterilization method	Number of items to be taken
Autoclaved at 121° for 15 min (minimum conditions)	10
Sterilized in final container but not autoclaved at 121° for 15 min	20
If a biological indicator is used	10
Nor sterilized in final container	30
If the bulk has already passed a test for sterility	20

What this means is often not defined precisely, for example in the USP XVIII, but the EP Vol. II suggests tests with *Staphylococcus aureus* (an aerobic bacterium), *Clostridium* (*Plectridium*) *sphenoides* (an anaerobic bacterium) and *Candida albicans* (a yeast). The WHO Report (1960) also includes *Streptococcus pyogenes* (Group A). However, it is well known that damaged bacteria are especially fastidious in their growth requirements, (Harris 1963b) though this does not seem to apply to fungal spores (Chauhan & Walters 1962). No pharmacopoeia has attempted to tackle this problem and adequate tests for media capable of growing small members of damaged organisms will be difficult to devise.

The USP XVIII recommends the following media and should be consulted for details. It also requires each batch of medium to be tested for growth-promoting properties using two nutritionally exacting strains.

Fluid Thioglycollate Medium is an anaerobic medium with resazurin as oxidation–reduction indicator, and is intended for use with clear, fluid products. Inoculations into anaerobic media must always be made into the (reduced) depths of the medium with a Pasteur pipette.

Alternative Thioglycollate Medium is similar in formula to Fluid Thioglycollate Medium but does not have the resazurin or the agar and is used for testing turbid or viscous products. It must be recently boiled and cooled to remove oxygen before use.

Soybean-Casein Digest Medium is a medium giving rich growth of many organisms and is recommended for detecting small numbers of aerobic bacteria and fungi. The formula is identical with that for 'Oxoid' Tryptone Soya broth.

The EP Vol. II makes no recommendations on the formulae of media, but requires them to be adequately sensitive and nutritive. The WHO Report (1960) gives the formulae for additional media, including cooked meat medium, probably the most satisfactory of all the anaerobic media.

No pharmacopoeia lays down any requirements for tests for viruses, rickettsiae or chlamydiae because of the technical difficulties involved and because they have a low heat resistance and so are unlikely to be present in the majority of sterilized products, but tests are applied to specific viral and rickettsial vaccines according to the hazards involved.

Samples possessing Inherent or Added Antimicrobial Activity
Where samples falling into this category are to be tested they have to be treated so that the antimicrobial activity is abolished completely. This may be done by neutralization, inactivation or removal and the principal recommended techniques are given in Table 32.6. However, none of the methods given is sacrosanct and, since it is known that non-ionic detergents inactive phenols and most biocides and biostats there is no reason why Letheen (Lecithin plus Tween 80) or Lubrol media should not be used for most preparations, provided that it could be proved that this was at least as effective as the recommended methods.

Membrane filtration. This is now the method of choice for sterility testing since it permits virtually the complete removal of any antimicrobial agent, the testing of large volumes of sample and the testing of oily preparations and certain soluble powders.

The membrane filter is a thin disc of mixed cellulose esters of a closely controlled pore size, 0.45 μm being commonly used, though 0.22 μm membranes may be used for special purposes.

Hydrophilic materials may be filtered directly or dissolved or diluted in peptone water, the solution

Antimicrobial agent	Neutralization method*
Quaternary ammonium compounds and other surfactants	Medium with non-ionic surfactant (Lubrol or Tween 80/lecithin)
Sulphonamides	Medium with p-aminobenzoic acid
Phenolic compounds	Dilute to less than 0.01 per cent or as for quaternary ammonium compounds
Halogens	Neutralize with thiosulphate
Ethyl alcohol Isopropyl alcohol Glycerol	Dilute to less than 1 per cent
Acids and alkalis	Neutralize
Heavy metals (Hg, As, Cu, Ag, Zn)	Medium with sulphydryl compound (thioglycollate, cysteine)
Dyes	Membrane filtration
Formaldehyde	Neutralize with bisulphite, membrane filtration
Penicillin	Incubate with penicillinase
Other antibiotics	Membrane filtration

* Membrane filtration is the method of choice for all tests on products containing antimicrobial agents. Where indicated as the sole method it is the only possible one.

then being filtered through a sterile membrane, adding if necessary, substances such as penicillinase or other antimicrobial inhibitor. In the latter cases the membrane is washed with portions of 0.1 per cent w/v peptone water to remove any traces of inhibitor. Since substances are often absorbed in the margin of the membrane where it is trapped in the filter unit, the use of membranes with a hydrophobic edge may be desirable. The procedures suggested by the USP XVIII are summarized in Table 32.7.

It is then often recommended that the membrane be divided and that half should be added to aerobic/anaerobic bacterial medium and the other half to aerobic mycotic medium. However, this is open to the same objection as was voiced previously about the use of samples taken from large volume containers and it is preferable to filter the whole of the contents of one container, add the membrane to aerobic bacterial medium, and then filter the contents of two more containers, the mem-

branes being incubated in mycotic and anaerobic media. This procedure gives adequate one-dose test security, though at the expense of additional samples, membranes, media, etc.

The testing of hydrophobic products (powders, oils, lecithin, soft paraffin products) presents special difficulties both in physical handling and in attempting to ensure the complete recovery of revivable organisms from the product. Some approaches are also suggested in Table 32.7.

Further problems occur with insoluble powders due to blockage of the membrane and this may be overcome by layering the membrane with sterile Hyflo filter aid, a special diatomaceous earth, and adding further Hyflo to the suspension before filtration.

It will be clear that sterility testing in general and the membrane filter technique in particular requires an exceptional degree of skill and knowledge and is not to be undertaken lightly. The question of controls has still to be mentioned and successful control procedures are an integral part of the whole sterility test procedure, whether conducted by membrane filtration or otherwise.

TABLE 32.7

A SUMMARY OF THE MEMBRANE FILTER PROCEDURES OF THE USP XVIII

Nature of sample	Procedure
Non-viscous homogeneous	Filter directly
Viscous liquid	Dilute with Fluid A* and filter
Has inherent bacteriostatic properties	Filter and wash with one to three 100 ml portions of Fluid A
Contains lecithin	Filter and wash one to three 100 ml portions of Fluid B†
Ointments and oils (not containing soft paraffin)	Dissolve 1 g in 100 ml of sterile isopropyl myristate. Filter and wash with 2 × 200 ml Fluid B and 100 ml Fluid A. Transfer membrane to medium containing TOPPE
Products containing soft paraffin	Dissolve is isopropyl myristate and filter. Wash with 3 × 100 ml of special rinse medium§. Transfer membrane to medium containing TOPPE
Insoluble solids and suspensions	Dilute if necessary, filter and wash as appropriate

* Diluting Fluid A; 0.1 per cent peptone water
† Diluting Fluid B; 0.1 per cent peptone, 0.1 per cent (p-tert-octylphenoxy)polyethoxy ethanol (TOPPE)
§ Special Rinse Medium; 0.05 per cent peptone, 0.03 per cent beef extract, 0.1 per cent (p-tert-octylphenoxy)polyethoxy ethanol.

Controls

Two types of control are used. Positive (growth) controls are intended to ensure that the sterility test system, i.e. medium plus sample plus inhibitor (plus membrane filter if appropriate) will support the growth of fastidious microorganisms and is therefore likely to detect all potentially viable contaminants. Negative controls ensure the sterility of all materials, media and apparatus used in the test.

When tests are set up on several items from a single batch these must be done separately, but it is necessary to set up only one set of controls. The EP Vol. II requires the positive controls to be done in duplicate.

Control organisms may vary widely according to the particular application, but the organisms suggested by the EP Vol. II have been referred to already under 'Media', and tests for *Mycobacterium tuberculosis* may be controlled with strain H37RV. The use of *Staphylococcus aureus* as an aerobic control organism may be criticised since it is a facultative anaerobe and a strictly aerobic exacting *Micrococcus* would be preferable. For positive controls small numbers of organisms, about 100, should be used.

It is clear from what has been said that although sterility tests by membrane filtration require three membranes for each test, one for aerobic bacteria, one for anaerobic bacteria and one for fungi, six membranes are required for each set of controls if the requirements of the *European Pharmacopoeia* are to be complied with, two each for aerobic bacteria, anaerobic bacteria and fungi. If proof of sterility is required, further membranes are necessary.

The Time and Temperature of Incubation

The incubation temperature and time are important, since the temperature must be suitable for growth and the time must be long enough for visible growth to be achieved even with slowly germinating spores or damaged bacteria, which are known to have very long lag phases. The WHO Report (1960) recommended for bacteria either incubation at 15 to 22° *and* 35 to 37° or, if only one temperature is used, 30 to 32°. The EP Vol. II follows the second procedure while the USP XVIII requires temperatures of 30 to 35°. In the test for mycotic sterility the WHO Report and the USP XVIII both give an incubation temperature of 20 to 25°C.

Regrettably there is no real rationale behind these decisions, except convenience, since it is

known that damaged bacteria usually revive best at temperatures different from the optimum temperature for the growth of undamaged cells of the same species (Harris, 1963a).

So far as the time of incubation is concerned the EP Vol. II follows the recommendation of the WHO Report (1960) and requires an incubation period of 7 days for bacteria, though the USP XVIII specifies periods varying from 7 to 14 days. A period of 14 days is usual for fungi. The times used are undoubtedly a compromise between the need to give ample opportunity for growth, and the desire to avoid undue cost to the manufacturer. In fact, most manufacturers would tend to use rather longer incubation periods, if experience shows that this is desirable, to protect the quality of their products.

The EP Vol. II lays down 37° for 42 days for tests for *Mycobacterium tuberculosis*.

Recording and Interpretation of the Test

The following information must be recorded clearly. The nature, size, composition and origin of each item in the sample, the method of testing and the nature and volume of media and of any neutralizing agents employed (if necessary) and the results of all tests and controls. The presence of growth may be detected at periodic inspection by turbidity, centrifugation and microscopy of the sediment and by subculture.

The sample passes the test if all 'tests' and the negative controls show no growth and all positive controls show growth. Note that samples are *not* reported as sterile due to the statistical and technical uncertainties of the procedure.

The sample fails the test if one or both 'tests' show growth, the negative control shows no growth and the positive controls show growth.

The test is invalid, and should be repeated after investigation of the causes, if a negative control shows growth or if one or more of the positive controls shows no growth.

The EP Vol. II, but not the USP XVIII, permits a sample which fails the first test to be retested. If growth of the same microorganism occurs in the second test the sample fails, but if a different microorganism grows in the second test, the test may be repeated for a third time. If no growth occurs on the third occasion the sample passes the test. Such a procedure, previously permitted in the BP 1968 and earlier editions, is very unsound and any manufacturer using such a practice would be taking considerable risks both with the health of users of the product and with their own reputation, especially since even the theoretical basis for the procedure is very dubious. The same comments naturally apply to products produced in the hospital service.

Special Modifications of Technique
Tests for Mycobacterium tuberculosis in BCG vaccine. This is a special hazard since the virulent organism grows under the same conditions as the attenuated BCG and carriers of the virulent organisms are not uncommon. Accidental contamination with virulent *M.tuberculosis* would give a dangerously toxic product. The test involves low speed centrifugation of 25 ml of product, suspending in saline or preservative inhibitor, centrifuging again, resuspending in saline and inoculating into 10 tubes each of liquid and solid medium of proven growth capacity. Incubation is at 37° for 42 days.

Sutures. Containers are sterilized externally and tested for leakage simultaneously by immersion in an antiseptic dye solution before opening the tubes and transferring the sutures directly to suitable media. The test is made more rigorous by applying and releasing a vacuum while the containers are in the solution. Any leaky containers are regarded as contaminated and set aside for bacteriological examination. Non-leakers are then tested for sterility. However, most sutures are nowadays sterilized by irradiation in a foil pack. Those which will not withstand radiation sterilization, e.g. polypropylene, are sterilized with ethylene oxide and transferred to foil packs aseptically. There is now no preservative included in any packing fluids, except some sutures which are tubed in alcohol, but this is diluted out on transfer of the suture to medium. Prolonged incubation periods are not required, though 14 days is commonly used.

Devices. The whole device should preferably be incubated in an aerobic/anaerobic medium. Failing this, crucial parts could be incubated or the article could be rinsed through with sterile medium and the rinsings tested.

Dressings. The whole dressing up to 500 g, or up to 2×50 g portions from the innermost part of the sample, are transferred to media.

The technical difficulties of sampling from large dressing packs are such that it is often recommended (e.g. BPC 1973) that technical controls should be carried out, sampling from, say, 20 'oversterilized' packs to assess the probability of chance contamination. It is doubtful whether this is necessary under modern conditions using laminar flow cabinets, with which the level of technical contamination is very low.

Paraffin gauze. The testing of this product is a controversial subject. The USP XVIII method involves shaking a sample with fluid thioglycollate medium plus agar and gelatin at 52° to melt the soft paraffin, cooling, breaking the paraffin seal and incubating and 20 to 25° for 7 days before further subculture. However, heating presumably damaged organisms at 52° is likely to render potentially viable cells non-viable.

An alternative procedure would be to dissolve the soft paraffin away from the gauze using *isopropyl myristate* and to test the resulting solution by membrane filtration and the residual gauze by direct inoculation into media.

Biological indicators. When articles are awkward to sample or too large to test satisfactorily, e.g. large dressings, bronchoscopes, a useful procedure is to include test pieces contaminated with resistant microorganisms, such as soil or the spores of *B.globigii*, *B.subtilis* var. *niger*, *B.pumilus*, *B.stearothermophilus* or *Cl. botulinum* Type E, according to the application. The test piece is then checked for sterility, assuming that if the test piece is sterile then the actual article is also sterile. Although there are dangers inherent in such a proposition, the technique can work well under skilled supervision.

When products are sterilized in their final containers by a method other than autoclaving at 121°C for 15 min and biological indicators are used to monitor the sterilization process, the USP XVIII permits the number of units taken for the sample to be reduced from 20 to 10.

REFERENCES

British Pharmacopoeia (1973). London: HMSO.

British Pharmaceutical Codex (1973). London: Pharmaceutical Press.

Chauhan, N. M. & Walters, V. (1962) *J. Pharm. Pharmacol.* **14**, 605–610.

Clothier Committee (1972). Report of a Committee Appointed to Enquire Into the Circumstances, Including the Production, which Led to the Use of Contaminated Infusion Fluids in the Devonport Section of Plymouth General Hospital. Command Paper, *Cmnd.* 5035. London: HMSO.

EUROPEAN PHARMACOPOEIA VOL. II (1971).

GROVES, M. J. (1973) *Parenteral Products.* London: Heinemann Medical.

GUIDE TO GOOD PHARMACEUTICAL MANUFACTURING PRACTICE (1971). Department of Health and Social Security. London: HMSO.

HARRIS, N. D. (1963a) *J. Pharm. Pharmacol.* **15**, 196T.

HARRIS, N. D. (1963b) *J. appl. Bact.* **26**, 387.

KNUDSEN, L. F. (1949) *J. Am. pharm. Ass.* **38**, 332.

LILLY, H. A. & LOWBURY, E. J. L. (1972) *J. med. Microbiol.* **5**, 151.

PHARMACOPOEIA OF THE UNITED STATES OF AMERICA, XVIIITH REVISION (1970). Including the First U.S.P. XVIII Supplement (1971).

REPORT (1960) *Requirements for Biological Substances. 6. General Requirements for the Sterility of Biological Substances. Wld. Hlth. Org. techn. Rep. Ser.* 200. Geneva: WHO.

REPORT (1969) *The Bacteriological Examination of Water Supplies. Reports on Public Health and Medical Subjects,* No. 71. London: HMSO.

REPORT (1972) *J. Mond. Pharm.* **15**, 88.

ROSENHEIM, THE LORD (1972) Interim Report on Heat Sterilized Fluids for Parenteral Administration. Medicines Commission. London: HMSO.

33

Vaccines and Sera

HISTORICAL REVIEW

Vaccines and sera are the pharmacologically useful derivatives of the science of immunology. Both may be used for the prevention of infectious disease and, in addition, sera may be used in the treatment of several established conditions. The pharmacological activity is, in almost all instances, due to the modified γ-globulins present in the serum after vaccination or serum treatment.

The first vaccine was developed in 1798 by the Gloucestershire naturalist and physician, Edward Jenner (Jenner 1798), who tested the folk belief that an attack of the relatively innocuous and localized disease, cowpox, provided immunity from the disfiguring and often fatal smallpox. Jenner took a sample of the lymph from a cowpox pustule on the hand of a milkmaid and scratched it into the arm of a boy. The boy developed a cowpox pustule as expected, but when later challenged with lymph from a smallpox pustule he was found to be completely immune. Jenner's technique became the accepted method of smallpox prophylaxis and it was from the Latin for cowpox, *vaccinia*, that the word 'vaccine' was derived. Almost a hundred years later Louis Pasteur was to extend the meaning of the word to indicate not only the vaccine lymph used for the prevention of smallpox, but all microbial preparations intended for the prevention of infectious disease.

Despite the success of smallpox vaccination, progress towards the development of vaccines to prevent other infectious diseases was insignificant until the last 25 years of the nineteenth century. Then, as men came gradually to accept the microbial theory of infectious disease, the conditions matured for new developments and the significant advances recorded in the diagram (Fig. 33.1). Louis Pasteur, bearing in mind the work of Jenner, developed strains of chicken cholera, anthrax, and even rabies microbes, so attenuated in virulence as to be quite innocuous when injected into animals but capable of inducing immunity to the respective infectious diseases (Pasteur, Chamberland & Roux 1881). Three years later, in America, Daniel Salmon and Theobald Smith (1884) showed that the same effect could be obtained by the injection of killed microbes and between 1895 and 1898 in Britain, Almroth Wright used a suspension of killed typhoid bacilli as a typhoid vaccine. Since that time vaccines made from killed microbes have been used for the prophylaxis of many diseases for, unlike the attenuated vaccines of Pasteur, they are free from the danger of reversion to virulence and the disasters which such a change would inevitably entail. It is interesting to note, however, that the latest virus vaccines (poliomyelitis, measles, rubella and mumps) are all made from living attenuated viruses manipulated with such care that the possibility of reversion to virulence is very small.

While Pasteur and his followers were devising vaccines to prevent diseases caused by the multiplication of microbes which characteristically invade the tissues of their hosts, other workers were engaged on prophylactics to prevent the clinical manifestations of the powerful toxins secreted by certain bacteria, the most important of

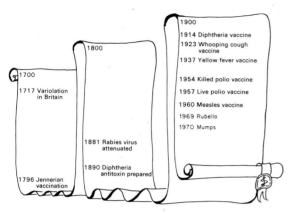

1700
1717 Variolation in Britain
1796 Jennerian vaccination

1800
1881 Rabies virus attenuated
1890 Diphtheria antitoxin prepared

1900
1914 Diphtheria vaccine
1923 Whooping cough vaccine
1937 Yellow fever vaccine
1954 Killed polio vaccine
1957 Live polio vaccine
1960 Measles vaccine
1969 Rubella
1970 Mumps

FIG. 33.1. Significant events in the history of vaccination and serotherapy.

which were the diphtheria bacillus, isolated by Loeffler (1884), and the tetanus bacillus, isolated by Kitasato (1889). The isolation of these two organisms was quickly followed by the separation of the respective toxins and thus to the great discoveries of von Behring and Kitasato (1890). These workers injected animals with sub-lethal doses of the toxins and later found in the animals' sera neutralizing substances specific for each of the toxins. These substances, the antitoxins, were of immense importance; prepared in large volumes in horses, they were the first specific drugs for the treatment of either diphtheria or tetanus. Diphtheria antitoxin, in addition to its use in the treatment of diphtheria, was also used to detoxify diphtheria toxin. The non-toxic toxin–antitoxin floccules formed in this reaction were used with relative safety as a vaccine for humans. Vaccines of this toxin–antitoxin type, however, were regarded by many as potentially dangerous, because of the possibility of dissociation with the release of toxin, and after a time they were superseded by vaccines containing antitoxin combined with toxin that had been converted by the action of formaldehyde to non-toxic 'toxoid'. Later the antitoxin was omitted and the immunizing power of the toxoid was improved by the addition of an alum salt (Glenny et al. 1926). Still further improvements included the use of highly purified toxoid and the use of aluminium phosphate (Holt 1950) or aluminium hydroxide (Schmidt & Hansen 1933) instead of alum.

The need for technical developments held up the progress towards the production of vaccines capable of preventing virus diseases and it was not until 1937 that a third virus vaccine suitable for general use was developed (Theiler & Smith 1937). It was

yellow fever vaccine prepared from virus grown in fertile hens' eggs and was followed in 1944 by an effective influenza vaccine made from influenza virus grown in the same way (Salk, Menke & Francis 1945). The need for living cells in which to propagate the viruses required for these vaccines, however, proved a continuing obstacle to rapid progress and it was not until 1949 that this problem was overcome by John Enders and his colleagues (Enders, Weller & Robbins 1949) who grew poliomyelitis virus in tissue cultures of human embryo. By so doing they pioneered the way in which tissue cultures could provide the vast quantities of virus needed to make all the various types of virus vaccine that are available today.

THE IMMUNE STATE

Immunity is resistance to attack by microorganisms. Apart from the natural resistance which most animal species have to certain of the diseases which attack other species, immunity depends on the presence in the serum of the immune individual of modified γ-globulins known as antibodies. Such antibodies, and the immunity they provide, may be acquired either naturally as the result of a biological event or artificially as the result of medication.

Natural immunity is the usual consequence of infection, either overt or inapparent. The presence of the invading microbes within the tissues of the host stimulate the production of antibody, which not only eliminates the infection but provides subsequent immunity to a further infection by the same species of microbe. Since the immunity which follows infection is a response of the host to the invading microbes it is known as active immunity. Antibodies produced as a consequence of infection are transferred during pregnancy across the placenta from mother to fetus so that a newborn infant is immune to those infections to which the mother is immune. However, since there is no production of antibody by the infant this form of natural immunity is known as passive immunity.

Artificial immunity, like natural immunity, may be either active or passive. Active artificial immunity is the immunity which develops as a consequence of vaccination; following successful vaccination, the presence of the vaccine in the tissue of the host stimulates the production of antibody in much the same way as a natural infection. On the other hand the injection of antibody-containing serum obtained either from man or animals induces a state of artificial passive immunity and it is on this technique that serum prophylaxis and therapy are based.

NATURAL RESISTANCE

Some animals are naturally resistant to certain bacteria and viruses although these same microbes may be highly lethal to other animal species. Humans are unaffected by the myxomatosis virus so lethal to rabbits and, conversely, a herpes virus (B virus), endemic and benign in some species of monkey, is lethal to man. It is interesting to note also that Old World monkeys are susceptible to poliomyelitis viruses but New World monkeys are naturally resistant. Herpes zoster and chickenpox viruses infect man alone, and fowl leucosis viruses are unique to the domestic fowl; on the other hand there are few, if any, mammals resistant to rabies virus.

Just as several viruses are restricted to specific hosts there are many examples of virus specificity in cell cultures. Poliomyelitis virus infects simian and human tissue whether in primary or continuous culture, but is without effect on rabbit tissue. An even more subtle differentiation is shown by a simian virus (SV40) which does not cause marked changes in rhesus monkey kidney tissue but is easily recognized in African green monkey kidney cell cultures in which it causes complete destruction. The isolation of rhinoviruses had to await the production of human cell cultures since many will not grow in cells derived from other sources.

IMMUNITY AFTER INFECTION

The immunity remaining after infection by viruses can vary from transient to permanent. Second attacks of measles, smallpox or yellow fever, for example, are very rare whereas multiple attacks of influenza and the common cold are well known. This may be due, in part, to the many different serotypes causing the cold syndrome and a series of colds may be caused by immunologically unrelated agents. Thus, against antigenically stable viruses, antibodies are generally effective but when the antigenic structure alters (influenza in man, foot-and-mouth in animals) the immunity, based on antibody, may fail. The same is true for some bacterial infections. With cholera for example there are two serological strains, Ogawa and Inaba and each has the El Tor biotype differentiated by biochemical reactions. Indeed the bacterial infections that have been most successfully mastered by immunological methods are those caused by an exotoxin of the organism for which the toxoid may be used as the specific prophylactic.

In the early days of virology it was a common belief that infection with a virus altered the cell susceptibility, thus having a marked effect on reinfection, but the work of the last 20 years has given much more weight to the importance of protection by specific antibodies. In many careful studies with herpes, measles and poliomyelitis, immunity to the disease coincides with the appearance of antibodies and passive immunity which can reduce the severity of or completely abort disease can be effected by injecting convalescent serum. This is the basis of globulin therapy practised in the U.K. and on a much larger scale in the U.S.A.

It is not yet clear why immunity to some virus infections is permanent or, indeed, why high antibody titres are maintained for years. In studies with bacterial infections a high antibody response is obtained to a reinforcing stimulus by the antigen. It has been postulated, therefore, that the antibody titres after measles and yellow fever, for example, could be maintained only by a continuous antigenic stimulation, but its source is not always evident. After the majority of virus infections or injection of a virus vaccine, however, the initial high antibody titre falls but there is a rapid response to a booster dose.

ACTION OF HUMORAL IMMUNITY

Antibodies, whether antitoxic or antibacterial, play a major role in immunity to bacterial infections; in the first case the toxin is neutralized, in the second the bacterium is rendered more susceptible to phagocytosis. Similarly humoral immunity plays an important part in protection against viral diseases. It is now common practice to measure responses of man to virus diseases and vaccine by neutralization tests in which a constant test dose of virus is mixed with serum dilutions and, after a suitable incubation time, inoculated into susceptible animals or cell cultures. Infection or cytopathic effect occurs when the serum has been diluted beyond the point of neutralization. Agglutination or precipitation of virus by antiserum and complement fixation are other serological techniques by which immunity may sometimes be measured. Combination of virus and antibody undoubtedly occurs, making the virus non-infectious but immediately after mixing the virus and antiserum the majority of the virus particles can be recovered as infectious entities. This has been shown both by diluting the mixtures to decrease the neutralizing power of the serum (Bedson 1928; Todd 1928; Andrewes 1928) and by centrifuging the virus particles out of such mixtures (Sabin 1935). With many viruses a period of hours and sometimes days at temperatures of 25° or higher is required before complete neutralization occurs (Bedson & Crawford 1928; Andrewes 1930).

Interaction of virus and antibody has been studied in cell cultures and it has been shown that the addition of antiserum to cell cultures before the addition of virus, or the mixing of the virus with antiserum before addition to cell cultures, will prevent infection of the cells. No amount of antiserum added after the virus has been in contact with the cells, however, will protect the culture (Andrewes 1930). The antibody, in combining with the virus particle, in some way prevents entry into the cell. This combination is most effectively demonstrated in the haemagglutination test with influenza virus, which has the property of attaching itself to mucoprotein receptors of red blood cells; aggregates are formed and the red cells are agglutinated. The addition of specific antiserum to the virus prevents this haemagglutination since it coats the virus and blocks the initial combination of virus and red cells.

In general it is clear that, whatever the protective mechanism against disease may be, antibodies play a most significant part and attempts at prophylaxis are concerned with obtaining the greatest antibody response and maintaining circulating antibody throughout life.

Passive immunity induced by the transference of preformed antibody, although useful in an emergency, is not a procedure that can be used for the elimination of disease from a community. Frequent injections would be needed and furthermore the passive immune host may be infected and become a carrier of the disease without showing any clinical symptoms. Active immunity is the only means of eradication of a disease, and the time at which the antigenic stimulus should be given and the nature of the antigen used are important considerations.

RESPONSE OF THE SUBJECT

There is much to be said on psychological grounds for immunizing infants during the first months of life. At this time the mother is anxious to have her baby protected against diseases and the baby experiences very little discomfort. On scientific grounds it is also worth considering because a basal immunity and a reinforcing dose of vaccine can both be given before the child is exposed to an infectious environment. Two factors, however, militate against successful vaccination at this time.

Maternal Antibody Inhibition

A baby is born with antibody concentrations equal to those of his mother and these maternal antibodies are lost at the rate of 50 per cent every three weeks. Working with poliomyelitis vaccine, Perkins, Yetts & Gaisford (1958) showed that infants with high maternal antibody titres at the time of primary vaccination had no increase in antibody titre after two doses of vaccine, whereas some infants with low or no antibody titre before vaccination responded (Fig. 33.2). In the absence of and observable rise in antibody titre it was not possible to say whether the maternal antibody had completely inhibited or merely masked a response.

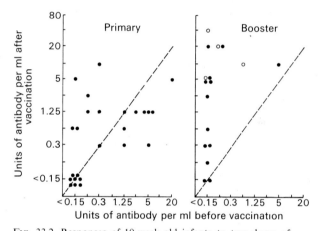

Fig. 33.2. Responses of 10-week-old infants to two doses of inactivated poliomyelitis (type 1 component) and their responses to a booster dose given 10 to 12 months later. The open circles represent infants giving a primary response.

The infants were recalled (Perkins, Yetts and Gaisford 1959a) ten to twelve months later (Fig. 33.2) when the maternal antibody had been lost and their responses to a reinforcing dose observed. Clearly a high maternal antibody titre at the time of primary immunization completely inhibited the response, an intermediate level of maternal antibody permitted some response and a low level of maternal antibody had no inhibitory effect.

These findings are not unique to poliomyelitis antigens, for Butler, Barr and Glenny showed in 1954 that maternal antibody inhibited the response to diphtheria toxoid and Gaisford, Feldman and Perkins (1961) have shown this to be so for responses to whooping cough vaccine. This phenomenon has not, however, been observed with tetanus toxoid.

Age of the Infant

By selecting infants of different ages, all of whom were without maternal antibody, Perkins et al.

(1959b) observed that the proportion of older children responding was higher than that of young infants and, furthermore, the older children gave higher antibody titres (Fig. 33.3). The reason for this is a delay in production of γ-globulin which does not begin to appear until the fourth to twelfth week of life and does not reach normal levels for at least six months (Gitlin, Gross & Janeway 1959). Since there is a close association between antibody and γ-globulin, it is not surprising therefore that the young infant does not respond as well as the one year-old child.

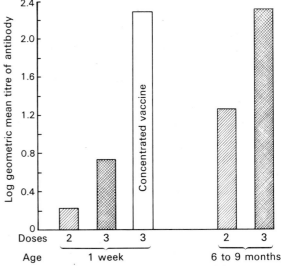

FIG. 33.4. The effects of the number of doses and concentrate of antigen on the response of infants to poliomyelitis vaccine. The figures at the top of each column denote percentage of children responding.

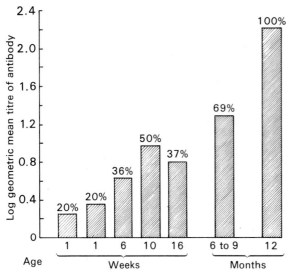

FIG. 33.3. The effect of age of infants on their responses to poliomyelitis vaccine. The figures at the top of each column denote percentage of children responding.

NATURE OF THE ANTIGEN

Concentration

For all antigens in all animals there is a dose–response relationship; the more antigen given the higher the response until a maximum is reached. Thus the inhibition by maternal antibody and the poor response of the young infant may be counteracted by the use of a greater quantity of antigen, either by giving an additional dose of vaccine or by increasing the concentration of antigen in the vaccine (Perkins et al. 1959c) (Fig. 33.4).

Studies using inactivated poliomyelitis vaccine which contains the antigens of Types 1, 2 and 3 viruses, have indicated a qualitative difference between the antigens. In young infants both the proportion responding and the mean titres have been highest for Type 2, not so high for Type 3 and lowest for Type 1. Beale (1961) measured the concentration of antigen in the vaccines and, in order to obtain similar antibody responses to the three viruses, a much greater concentration of Type 1 antigen was required than of Type 3, which, in turn, required a larger dose than Type 2.

Adjuvants

As long ago as 1926 Glenny and his colleagues found that when alum was added to diphtheria toxoid a very much better antitoxin response was induced. Since that time adjuvants such as aluminium hydroxide and aluminium phosphate have been used on a large scale to give enhanced responses to both toxoids and bacterial vaccines.

The mode of action of an adjuvant is not clearly understood but efficient adjuvants appear to be irritants as well as allowing only a slow release of the antigen into the body, thus giving a prolonged and continuous antigenic stimulus. More recently, antigens have been effectively adjuvanted by incorporation into a water in oil emulsion, and the antibody response to inactivated influenza virus is both greater and longer lasting when incorporated in such an emulsion.

The inability of a young infant to respond to an antigenic stimulus can also be successfully overcome by use of an adjuvant. Osborn, Dancis and Julia (1952) showed that infants under two weeks of age responded as well as older children to a single dose of adsorbed tetanus toxoid.

Live or Dead Antigens

When sufficient antigen can be produced and contained in a single, painless, reaction-free potent injection, this is certainly the method of choice of vaccination. For some antigens, however, this has not been possible and the alternative has been to produce a vaccine from the living microorganism which has been manipulated in such a way that the infection it causes will not progress to the untoward or sometimes fatal sequelae of the natural disease. Thus smallpox vaccine is made from an attenuated strain grown in the skin of animals and yellow fever vaccine is a living attenuated strain grown in fertile eggs. Furthermore immunity to tuberculosis is given by a particular living bovine strain of the tubercle bacillus.

Immunization against poliomyelitis was the first occasion on which there was a choice of living vaccine given by mouth or dead vaccine given by injection. The obvious reason for the development of the living vaccine was a deliberate attempt to simulate a natural infection using a safe strain of virus but there has been considerable discussion concerning the advantages of the live poliomyelitis vaccine. For a number of years vaccination with killed vaccine was practised in several countries, and although the incidence of paralytic poliomyelitis fell dramatically, there have been small sporadic local outbreaks of the disease. These cases almost always occurred in non-vaccinated subjects or in those having an inadequate number of doses of vaccine.

Because of the more acceptable method of administration, many countries used live vaccine given orally on a mass scale as soon as it became available, and this always resulted in elimination of the disease from the community. From 1962 live vaccine has been used in this country as a routine immunization procedure, and although the disease has not been entirely eliminated, the number of cases since 1965 has been the lowest of the century and has remained at a low level.

IMMUNE SERA

Immune sera have the great advantage that they provide the individual into whom they are injected with an immediately effective supply of antibacterial or antiviral antibodies, or antitoxins. Consequently, immune sera can be useful prophylactically in unvaccinated persons exposed to infection, and therapeutically in persons with established infectious disease. In general, antitoxic sera have proved far more effective than either antibacterial or anti-viral sera and thus it has been in the prophylaxis and treatment of diphtheria and of tetanus that serotherapy has been most used. The incidence of both these diseases, however, has been much reduced during the last quarter of a century by active immunization and thus the demand for diphtheria and tetanus antisera is now relatively small.

The production of diphtheria, tetanus and gas gangrene antitoxins is almost always carried out in horses. Healthy horses are immunized with a series of injections of the appropriate toxoid and, when a trial bleed shows that a satisfactory amount of antitoxin is present, the animals are bled from the external jugular vein. The blood is separated into cells and plasma and the plasma partly digested with pepsin. The antitoxin is then precipitated from the digest with ammonium sulphate, dialysed against water, concentrated by ultrafiltration, brought to the desired concentration and filled into containers.

Serotherapy as a method of prophylaxis suffers from two serious disadvantages. The first is that immune horse serum injected into a human is immediately recognized as foreign protein, and is eliminated from the body so rapidly that even a large dose is unlikely to provide protection for longer than a few weeks. Moreover, as the proteins of horse serum are antigenic in the human they stimulate the production of antibodies against themselves and thus a second injection of horse serum given at a later date is eliminated even more rapidly. The second disadvantage is the occasional reaction which certain individuals suffer following the injection of foreign protein. Reactions to horse serum are particularly likely to occur in individuals who have received an earlier injection of this therapeutic agent and they may vary in severity from a trivial rash to immediate death from anaphylactic shock.

In the serotherapy of established disease the necessity to neutralize circulating toxin usually outweighs the risks attendant on the administration of immune horse serum. Immune sera, therefore, still have a part to play in the treatment of both diphtheria and tetanus, but it is usual for these therapeutic agents to be administered only after tests have shown that the individual to whom it is intended to administer the serum is tolerant of horse serum proteins. For victims of tetanus sensitive to horse serum proteins, antitoxic serum prepared in sheep is available and in recent years human tetanus immunoglobulin has also become available.

In countries where venomous snakes abound it is customary for antisera to be prepared against the venoms of the indigenous species. Such sera are generally used to infiltrate the area of the bite and, by intravenous injection, to neutralize circulating venom. The bites of the only species of venomous snake in the U.K., *Viper berus*, are not sufficiently dangerous to justify the injection of antisera containing large amounts of horse serum protein.

POTENCY ASSAY OF IMMUNE SERA

The potency of an antitoxin is determined by comparing its neutralizing power with that of an accepted standard antitoxin to which an arbitrary potency in units has been assigned. The comparative test is performed in two stages and in the case of diphtheria antitoxin may be carried out as follows.

In the first stage of the test a series of dilutions of diphtheria toxin is made and to each dilution is added 1.0 unit of the standard diphtheria antitoxin. The toxin and the antitoxin in the mixtures are allowed to react for an arbitrary time and then each mixture is injected subcutaneously into a guinea pig. The guinea pigs are examined four days after injection and those injected with the mixtures containing the largest amounts of toxin are found to have died and those which had the mixture with the smaller amounts of toxin have survived. It is thus possible to determine the smallest dose of toxin which, when mixed with 1.0 unit of antitoxin, is sufficient to cause the death of a guinea pig; this dose is known as the L+ (Limes Tod or death limit) dose. In the second part of the test a series of dilutions of the antitoxin which is to be compared with the standard antitoxin is made and each dilution is mixed with 1.0 L+ dose of the toxin as determined in the first part. After standing as before the mixtures are again injected into guinea pigs and after four days it is again possible to observe which mixture contained just sufficient free toxin to kill the guinea pig into which it was injected. Since this mixture contains the L+ dose as determined in the first part of the test it must also contain 1.0 unit of antitoxin. The concentration of antitoxin in the material being tested may then be calculated from the dilution factors involved. In everyday practice the L+ dose is seldom employed on account of the extravagant amounts of antiserum and toxin used and it is usually replaced with the L+/10 dose which provides equally satisfactory results. Furthermore the accuracy of the test is improved if several guinea pigs are injected with each mixture. Since diphtheria toxin is erythrogenic, however, it is possible to perform the same type of test using erythema of guinea pig skin as the end point rather than death. The dose of the toxin in this type of test is known as the Lr (Limes Reaktion) dose and it is usually used at the Lr/1000 level. The intradermal tests give results which are in accord with the lethal test but has the advantage of considerable economy for as many as 20 mixtures may be injected into the depilated flanks and back of a single animal.

Complementary to the in vivo methods for the titration of diphtheria antitoxin is the in vitro flocculation technique. In this method serial dilutions of antitoxin, usually in the range 20 to 40 units per ml are mixed with a constant amount of toxin. The mixtures are partly immersed in a water bath at 44°C so that convection currents ensure continuous mixing and after a variable time the union of antitoxin and toxin produces readily visible flocculation. The time taken for flocculation to appear is dependent on the relative concentrations of the two reagents and in the tube that flocculates most rapidly the reagents are said to be in optimal proportions. Such a mixture is said to contain a number of Lf of toxin equivalent to the number of units of antitoxin in that mixture. If serial dilutions of an antitoxin of unknown potency are then mixed with the same amount of toxin under the same conditions, and the mixture that flocculates first is again observed, this mixture will contain antitoxin and toxin in amounts equivalent to the amounts of these reactants in the tube that flocculated first in the first part of the test, and thus the potency of the antitoxin can be calculated.

Tetanus antitoxin can be titrated for neutralizing and flocculating potency by methods similar to those used for diphtheria antitoxin except that, since tetanus toxin is not erythrogenic, the intradermal test cannot be used. However, since tetanus toxin readily kills mice, considerable economies can be made by using mice instead of guinea pigs. Gas gangrene antitoxins are titrated by the lethal method using mice and an intravenous technique for the injection of the mixtures.

VACCINES

LABORATORY CONTROL

When a licence to sell a vaccine is granted to a laboratory under the Medicines Act 1968, the manufacturer is obliged to allow representatives of the Licensing Authority to inspect his premises. The care and attention invested in the design of the production facilities is almost always reflected in the final product and it is essential to know where and by whom each vaccine is made. The production of each immunological product must be carried out in a separate area and, if two different vaccines are being made on the same premises, there must be physical separation of the two processes.

Even with these precautions there are some products that should *never* be made in the same building since accidental contamination may have serious consequences. For example, tetanus vaccine should always be made in a separate area and a living infectious vaccine given by the oral route (e.g. oral poliomyelitis vaccine) should not be made in the same building as a vaccine given parenterally.

Buildings are expensive and the problem of using a single building for the production of several substances is often overcome by sequential production. After a sufficient quantity of any particular vaccine has been made, the building is sterilized with such chemicals as formalin or ethylene oxide, washed down or redecorated, and the production of a second vaccine begun.

The safety tests applicable to any biological substance are determined by the potential hazards that may arise in the course of production and in considering vaccines it is suitable to discuss these under (1) the seed strain, (2) the substrate, and (3) tests for adventitious agents and safety tests.

Although the production of bacterial and virus vaccines have several principles in common, these are better considered separately.

Bacterial Vaccines and Toxoids

Less than twenty years ago the name 'vaccine' would have been more closely associated with a toxoid or pertussis vaccine and less likely to bring to mind a virus vaccine, yet in spite of the enormous modern developments in virus vaccines little change has taken place in bacterial vaccines in this time. The two toxoids (diphtheria and tetanus), pertussis (a killed bacterial vaccine) and Bacillus–Calmette–Guérin (BCG, a living bacterial vaccine) are the only successes, whereas vaccines against staphylococci, typhoid and cholera are less satisfactory. In general, the control of bacterial vaccines is not so complicated as that of the virus vaccines.

The Bacterial Seed Strain

Since toxoid production preceded the manufacture of bacterial vaccines, great stress was placed on a search for the bacterial strain giving the greatest yield of toxin and, thereafter the strain was maintained without alteration of its biological properties.

Provided that no contaminants grow in the culture and introduce unwanted by-products, the problems of control are reduced to a minimum. In the case of toxins which are filtered from the culture and toxoided, the yield of toxin is most important but the inherent safety of the original bacterial strain has little significance. Even with the bacterial suspension vaccines, in which the bacteria are killed, there is much greater emphasis on the immunogenicity of the strains than on their toxicity, and the only danger to man lies in the quantity of protein injected in the human dose. All the bacterial vaccines give some local reactions but these are regarded as being more uncomfortable than dangerous.

With living bacterial vaccines such as BCG, however, the situation is much more like that of virus vaccines, and safety tests are applied to ensure that the vaccine strain does not differ from the original material shown to be safe by clinical trials in man (Medical Research Council 1958). Any deviation must be regarded as dangerous and the rate of growth, bacterial size and reaction of guinea pigs to intradermal injection are significant tests.

The Substrate for Bacterial Growth

The production of bacterial toxins presents few difficulties from the point of view of safety of the substrate. Peptones are used as growth media and if serum is not used in the growth of the organisms there is little of the substrate present in the final purified product. Even with bacterial vaccines the organisms are invariably washed free from culture medium before heat or chemical inactivation. The large quantity of protein present in the form of the bacterial suspension far outweighs any traces of proteins from the substrate in the final product. The only concern in a killed bacterial suspension vaccine is the presence of an endotoxin, the concentration of which may be affected by the substrate, and intradermal tests in animals can control this.

Safety Tests of Bacterial Vaccines

The toxoids have simple controls since animal tests to ensure complete toxoiding, adequate potency and freedom from abnormal toxicity and in vitro tests to ensure bacterial sterility suffice.

Killed bacterial vaccines have tests similar to the toxoids with the additional safeguard against excessive protein in a single human dose. Thus a lower limit is placed on potency and an upper limit on bacterial concentration. With the living BCG vaccine, however, strict control of the approved strain is exercized and care is taken to prevent its contamination by prohibiting work on other strains in the production area. Control of the bacterial count is essential, as are tests to ensure that the course of infection on animal inoculation follows its usual pattern.

Virus Vaccines

Testing virus vaccines, both inactivated and live attenuated, is much more time consuming and extensive than testing bacterial vaccines. The production of virus vaccines involves the use of complex biological systems and demands the constant attention of experts. Overall responsibility must be taken by qualified scientists, and all persons signing any section of a production protocol must be registered with the Licensing Authority.

The Virus Strain used for Vaccine Production

When a killed virus vaccine is made, the only demands placed on the seed strain are that it shall be killed in a regular manner and shall be immunogenic. The reason why killed poliomyelitis vaccine was several years under development was because all early attempts to kill the virus also destroyed antigenicity. However, once the critical concentration of formalin was found which killed the virus and retained antigenicity, no additional requirement for the use of a particular strain was necessary. Extensive tests were made with a number of strains for each virus type and the most immunogenic were selected. With an infection such as influenza, however, the problem is quite different because new antigenic variants are constantly appearing. Since it is important to prepare vaccine from the virus strains involved in the most recent epidemics, the composition of influenza vaccines is constantly under review.

For vaccines prepared from living attenuated viruses the data required for the approval of a seed strain are much more complex. Invariably the originally isolated wild virus is attenuated in cell cultures (e.g. monkey kidney tissue incubated at 35°C was used for poliomyelitis viruses whereas chick embryo fibroblast cultures were used to attenuate measles virus). A change in pathogenicity of the virus as shown by some laboratory animal tests (e.g. attenuated poliomyelitis viruses no longer paralysed monkeys and attenuated measles virus no longer produced a rash in monkeys) gives an indication that the virus may now be subjected to a small pilot clinical trial to test reactivity in man. This is followed by larger trials to prove safety and immunogenicity and general acceptability when used on a wide scale. Having carried out

such courageous and carefully controlled trials, leading to the approval of the particular strain for vaccine production, it is important that the control tests ensure that the approved seed virus has not changed during production of the vaccine. It is essential to ensure that the attenuated strain has not reverted to the wild strain, which may be dangerous, and it is equally important to ensure that the strain has not become further attenuated and possibly less immunogenic.

Having selected the seed strain and tested the seed pool for the presence of extraneous agents or an undesirable biological property the 'seed virus system' is rigidly applied. In such a system the seed pool is kept frozen or dried in suitable aliquots and each production batch of vaccine originates from the approved seed. For the live attenuated vaccines the production batch must not be more than a limited number of passages from the seed strain, the absolute number of which is determined by the genetic stability of the virus. For example, measles vaccine may be as many as ten passages from the seed virus whereas Type 3 poliomyelitis virus must not exceed two passages.

Tests on Cell Substrate

It is far better to prevent extraneous viruses from contaminating the vaccine than to attempt to detect a few contaminant viruses in the presence of a large population of vaccine virus or indeed to attempt to eliminate the contaminating viruses. Thus a certain proportion (about 25 per cent) of the tissue prepared for vaccine production is set aside as uninoculated controls and the tissue and fluids are examined for extraneous viruses (Fig. 33.5).

The control tissue and the tissue used for vaccine production are incubated under identical conditions and the fluids are taken for examination at the time the production tissue is used for virus inoculation and harvest. In addition, the control tissue is incubated for 10 to 14 days after the virus is harvested from the production tissue and a further search is made for extraneous viruses.

Tests on Virus Harvest

The virus harvest from the cell cultures shown to be free from contaminating viruses is also subjected to stringent tests for extraneous agents. These tests differ from those of the control cell cultures since there is now a large population of vaccine virus which must be neutralized with monospecific serum before a search is made for extraneous viruses. Tests in a number of different cell cultures and in

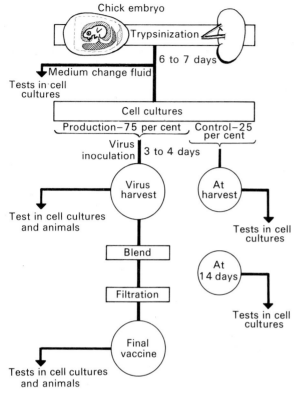

FIG. 33.5. Diagrammatic representation of the testing of live virus vaccines.

a specific time of inactivation, tests are done to ensure complete inactivation and further searches made for extraneous agents.

All 'in process' tests applied during vaccine production can be made only by the manufacturer but all tests on the final bulk material are done by both the manufacturer and the control laboratory. These tests for extraneous agents are the most expensive and time consuming part of safety testing. No test can be taken as an absolute guarantee of freedom from extraneous agents and the confidence limits are dependent upon the plating efficiency of the cell system. It is quite likely that they are no better than those of a bacterial sterility test.

The pattern of safety testing of virus vaccines is now almost stereotyped and the stages are shown in the summary in Fig. 33.6.

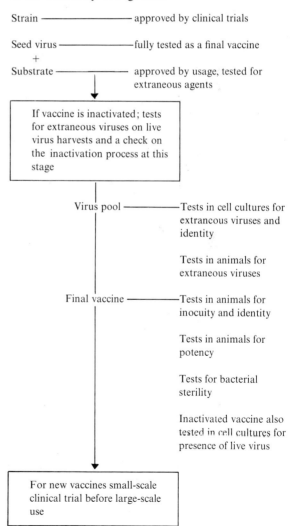

FIG. 33.6. Stages in the testing of a virus vaccine.

small animals are done in an attempt to cover all possible contaminating viruses.

Extraneous agents are detected by cytopathic effects, by interference effects in cell cultures, or by clinical signs in animals and there are a number of techniques available to detect the presence of unknown contaminants. Not all viruses cause cytopathic degeneration of cell cultures and some (e.g. the fowl leucosis viruses and rubella virus) may be detected only by their ability to make the infected cell cultures resistant to challenge by a second virus normally causing cytopathic degeneration in uninfected cultures—hence the name of interference. Some viruses may also be detected by staining the cell sheets with nucleic acid fluorescent stains, and others may be revealed by the examination of cell cultures under the electron microscope.

Contaminating viruses are most likely to be isolated at the time of virus harvest because it is at this stage that some vaccines are killed by the addition of formalin or β-propiolactone. With killed vaccines it is essential to follow the course of virus inactivation and any deviation from the normal must be regarded as a danger signal. After

Potency Tests

The clinical effectiveness of vaccines is assessed by various potency tests, most of which are based on the responses of groups of animals to fractional doses of the vaccine. The responses measured are in all cases antibody responses although the method of measurement varies from test to test. In some tests the measure is the result of challenge of the vaccinated animals with live microbes of the type against which the vaccine is intended to protect, in others it is the measurement of antibody titres, and in yet others it is screening of the sera of the vaccinated animals for an arbitrary level of antibody. All these methods depend on the relationship which exists between the logarithm of the dose of the antigen administered and the magnitude of the antibody response. This relationship, known as a dose–response curve, is generally sigmoid in character (Fig. 33.7). The middle range of the response, however, is sufficiently linear to be used to compare the potencies of any two vaccines of the same type which have slopes of the same steepness.

An example of a potency test which involves the challenge of vaccinated animals is the Kendrick test used in the potency assay of pertussis vaccine (Kendrick et al. 1947). In this test three doses of vaccine separated by five-fold dilution steps are used to immunize three groups each of sixteen mice. At the time when the vaccine on test is injected, three further groups of mice are immunized with comparable dilutions of a standard vaccine. Fourteen days later all the mice are challenged intracerebrally with live pertussis microbes, and

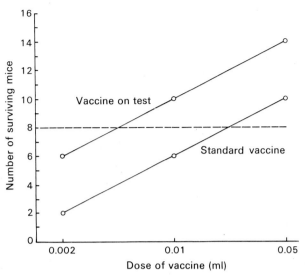

FIG. 33.8. The Kendrick test: estimation of the immunogenic potency of a pertussis vaccine by comparing part of its dose response curve with that of a standard vaccine.

after a further fourteen days the survivors in each group are counted and a graph constructed as shown in Fig. 33.8. The graph is then used to calculate the doses of each of the vaccines which would protect half the mice from death due to the challenge, so comparing the vaccine on test with the standard vaccine—in this case a five-fold difference.

If for technical reasons the response is measured by antibody titration rather than by the results of lethal challenge, the determination of two complete dose–response curves as in the Kendrick test tends to be extravagant with animals and very time consuming. A more economical but less statistically valid method is to use only a part of the dose–response curve. The potency assays of diphtheria and tetanus toxoids as described in the British Pharmacopoeia are examples of this type of test. Both tests involve immunization of a group of guinea pigs at a single point on the dose–response curve. The criterion of adequate potency in tests of this type is a fixed and arbitrary level of antibody response which, in the case of diphtheria toxoid (plain), is determined from the results of intradermal challenge with a standard dose of diphtheria toxin and, in the cases of diphtheria toxoid (adsorbed) and tetanus toxoids, involves measurement of the antibody titres of the sera of the inoculated animals.

A test which is similar in principle but rather different in execution is frequently used for the assay of the potency of killed poliomyelitis vaccine. In this test groups of chickens are immunized with

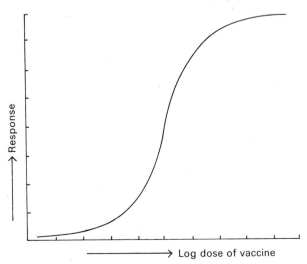

FIG. 33.7. The antibody responses of animals to increasing doses of vaccine.

serial dilutions of vaccine and after six days the animals are killed and bled out. The chicken sera are then screened for antibody at a single arbitrary level and the dilution of vaccine calculated which evokes in 50 per cent of the chickens an antibody response equivalent to the level at which the screening is operated. By this method the potency of all three antigenic components of a poliomyelitis vaccine may be compared with the potency of the corresponding standard vaccines.

The potencies of live vaccines such as BCG, smallpox, poliomyelitis vaccine and measles vaccine cannot be assayed by dose–response curve methods as the microbes of each of these vaccines either infect or fail to infect the individuals to whom they are given and thus they evoke an 'all or none' response. However, since larger doses of live vaccines generally produce a larger percentage of infections, the efficacy of vaccines of this type may be estimated approximately by counts of viable particles. These are performed by colony counting methods on bacteriological media in the case of BCG vaccine, and by infectivity titrations or plaque counting methods in eggs or on cell monolayers in the case of the virus vaccines.

VACCINES USED IN PROPHYLAXIS

BACTERIAL VACCINES

Bacterial vaccines are made either from the whole organisms or from the exotoxin which has been shown to be responsible for the clinical symptoms of the disease. They are:

Disease	Type of vaccine
Anthrax	Killed organisms
Cholera	Killed organisms
Diphtheria	Toxoid
Leprosy	Living organisms (BCG)
Plague	Living attenuated or killed organisms
Tetanus	Toxoid
Tuberculosis	Living organisms BCG
Typhoid	Killed organisms
Whooping cough	Killed organisms

In the case of the toxoids it is clearly established that these antigens stimulate the production of antibody which provides protection from the disease. With whole bacterial vaccines, however, it is not known which part of the bacterium is the important antigen. Clinical trials of vaccines in areas where the disease is endemic are the only means of obtaining such information, but as these are difficult to arrange progress tends to be slow. The salient features of each vaccine are as follows.

Anthrax
Anthrax is a highly infectious disease of animals, especially ruminants, caused by *Bacillus anthracis* and it may be transmitted to man either directly or indirectly through the handling of animal products, in particular wool or hide. The disease in this country is confined to the carpet, tanning and agricultural industries and may take the form of cutaneous or pulmonary anthrax. In general the disease is treated with antibiotics, but vaccines consisting of killed organisms have been prepared for those in high risk groups.

Cholera
Cholera is caused by *Vibrio cholerae* and is spread by the ingestion of water or foods contaminated by the faeces of infected subjects.

Cholera vaccine is prepared by growing in separate cultures the Ogawa and Inaba strains and their El Tor biotypes. The microbes are killed with formaldehyde or phenol and a mixed suspension is prepared with a total bacterial count of 8000×10^6 per ml.

Diphtheria
Diphtheria is an infectious bacterial disease caused by *Corynebacterium diphtheriae*. Active immunization with diphtheria toxoid is effective protection against the disease.

The toxoid is made by growing a high toxin producing strain (usually Park Williams 8 strain) in a suitable liquid medium. After incubation of the cultures at 34°C to 37°C for 7 to 10 days the organisms are filtered off. The filtrate containing the toxin may be purified at this stage and then toxoided by formaldehyde or toxoided before any purification takes place. The purification involves precipitation by ammonium sulphate in an attempt to obtain a highly immunizing antigen giving no untoward reactions.

When it is necessary to determine whether a person is naturally immune to diphtheria or whether an immunization course has been effective, it is usual to perform a Schick test on the subject. This test involves the intradermal inoculation of that amount of toxin that would be neutralized by $\frac{1}{1000}$ i.u. of diphtheria antitoxin. A person having sufficient circulating antitoxin to neutralize the toxin shows no reaction (Schick negative) whereas a person having no immunity to diphtheria shows an area of inflammation greater than 1.0 cm at the site of the injection (Schick positive).

Leprosy

Leprosy is a chronic mildly contagious infectious disease caused by *Mycobacterium leprae*. Drugs (such as sulphones, thiosemicarbazones or ethyl mercaptan derivatives) are used in the treatment of leprosy and BCG has given encouraging results.

Plague

Plague is a rapidly progressing acute febrile disease caused by *Pasteurella pestis*. Streptomycin and sulphonamides have been used in treatment, but a prophylactic vaccine made from a living attenuated strain of organisms has been shown to increase resistance to the disease. A vaccine made from killed organisms also protects against the disease but immunity is short-lived and a booster dose is required each year.

Tetanus

Tetanus is an acute infectious disease caused by *Clostridium tetani* and characterized by tonic spasms of voluntary muscles caused by the tetanus toxin. Immunization with the toxoid protects against the disease. The preparation of toxoid is similar to that for diphtheria to which reference should be made.

For many years the treatment of an individual injured in circumstances likely to be associated with infection with *Cl.tetani* has included the injection of antitoxin, but recently some physicians have relied on débridement and the bactericidal effects of penicillin. This régime has occasionally proved dangerous, since some tetanus spores may survive and give rise to the disease after subsequent trauma. The modern treatment is passive immunization with tetanus antitoxin (preferably human tetanus immunoglobulin) together with the first dose of toxoid in a course of active immunization. It is important to ensure that the course of active immunization is completed.

Tuberculosis

Tuberculosis is an acute or chronic communicable disease caused by *Mycobacterium tuberculosis*.

The vaccine is a suspension of living attenuated BCG organisms shown to multiply at the site of intradermal inoculation and to produce protection against tuberculosis without causing any of the dangerous sequelae of the natural disease. The salient feature of the production in the U.K. is the use of a particular liquid medium giving growth in small groups or single organisms rather than the large pellicles so characteristic of the growth of tubercle bacilli in the majority of liquid media. The freeze drying is carefully controlled so that the final vaccine has a predictable viable count (in the U.K. the vaccine has a count between 4 and 9×10^6 organisms per ml).

The immune status to tuberculosis is shown by an intradermal inoculation of old tuberculin or PPD (purified protein derivative) prepared by extracting tuberculin from tubercle bacilli with hot trichloracetic acid. Injection of five to ten tuberculin units produces redness, induration and oedema of the subcutaneous tissue 48 to 72 hours later in the immune patient (tuberculin positive). A negative reaction (tuberculin negative) indicates absence of immunity and a need for BCG vaccination.

Typhoid

Typhoid fever (enteric fever) is an acute generalized infection caused by *Salmonella typhi*. Vaccines are prepared from killed bacilli and usually contain *S.typhi*, *S.paratyphi A* and *S.paratyphi B*. Clinical trials have given conflicting results concerning the best method of killing the organisms and at the same time preserving the protective antigen. Some trials have shown that phenolized vaccine is better than that made from alcohol killed organisms and more recent trials have shown that acetone killed and dried vaccine may be the most effective. None of the vaccines is ideal and protection does not last long.

Whooping Cough

Whooping cough is an acute, highly communicable infectious disease caused by *Bordetella pertussis*. In some countries infection with *B.parapertussis* is reported as giving rise to the same clinical symptoms as those of whooping cough.

The vaccine is made by growing separately freshly isolated strains of *B.pertussis* either on solid medium or in suitable liquid medium. The organisms are harvested, washed, killed and blended into a suspension with a maximum bacterial count of 20×10^9 organisms per human dose. The vaccine is given mixed with diphtheria and tetanus toxoids as D.T.P. (diphtheria, tetanus and pertussis vaccine). If parapertussis is known to be endemic in a community, the vaccine may contain these organisms also.

VIRUS VACCINES

Influenza

Influenza is a highly infectious acute disease caused by influenza viruses.

Both killed and live attenuated vaccines have been used to immunize against influenza, but the assessment of their value has been complicated by the appearance of antigenic variants to the different virus strains. The first influenza A strain was isolated in 1933 and antigenic variation within this strain was recognized when viruses recovered from different epidemics were not antigenically identical. In 1946 an antigenic variant of influenza A appeared in Australia. This spread throughout the world and all epidemics for the next few years were caused by the A1 (A prime) strain until in 1956 another new A variant named A2 or Asian virus appeared. This A2 strain was responsible for the pandemic of 1957. The antigenic differences between the influenza A viruses are small compared with the marked difference in the antigenic properties of a virus which caused influenza in New York in 1940 and, for differentiation, was called Type B. Antigenic variants of Type B have also been found since 1940 although the differences between them are not so marked as those between the Type A strains. In 1949 a virus from a sporadic case of influenza was isolated and found to be antigenically distinct from Types A and B and was termed influenza Type C; this strain, however, has been found only in minor respiratory cases and has not been involved in any epidemic.

The production of an effective prophylactic requires the inclusion of strains of both Types A and B isolated during the most recent epidemic and unless a new variant appears there is much evidence to show that the vaccine will be effective. Influenza virus for vaccine manufacture is prepared in embryonated hens' eggs. The vaccine is prepared by harvesting the allantoic fluid at a suitable time after the virus inoculation of the allantoic cavity (Fig. 33.9). The harvested material is purified, killed with formalin and usually concentrated by centrifugation. The Type A and Type B components are standardized by haemagglutination titrations before dilution and blending into a vaccine. In some vaccines a mineral carrier or oil adjuvant is incorporated and although such vaccines have stimulated higher antibody responses they have not received general acceptance.

A second method of immunization is that

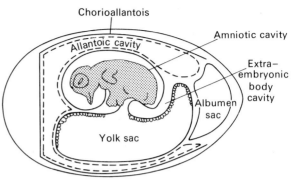

Fig. 33.9. Membranes and activities of a 12- to 15-day-old chick embryo.

developed in the U.S.S.R. where living attenuated virus is sprayed into the nose. The vaccine is an egg or tissue culture preparation of a strain passaged in eggs or cell cultures and selected because of its ability to multiply in the nose and appear in nasal secretions. Unlike the killed vaccine this live prophylactic is said to be effective even when used during an influenza epidemic. Clinical reactions are minimal in adults but may be severe in young children.

Recent findings show that the isolated haemagglutinin of the virus is immunogenic and does not give rise to the febrile and toxic reactions seen after vaccination with the whole virus.

Parainfluenza

This virus is the cause of some respiratory diseases in children. Experimental killed alum-adsorbed vaccines have been found to give good antibody responses in man but their protective efficacy has not been evaluated.

Respiratory Syncytial Virus

Respiratory syncytial virus (RSV) is a cause of both upper and lower respiratory tract illnesses in young children. Alum-adsorbed killed vaccines give an antibody response in man but their protective value is not yet known.

Adenovirus

Both killed and live vaccines have been used in the U.S.A. on a large scale, particularly in military units, and have given good protection. Recently, however, it has been shown that some serotypes of this group (including 3, 7, 12, 18 and 31) are oncogenic (tumour-producing). Although an enteric coated capsule of adeno 4 living virus vaccine is still being used with success, the other vaccines may have to await purification of the virus components.

Rhinovirus

Rhinoviruses are the main cause of common colds in adults and of both upper and lower respiratory tract disorders in children. Already over a hundred distinct serotypes have been isolated and, with the numbers increasing rapidly, the possibility of controlling the infections with a vaccine is remote.

Smallpox

Smallpox is an acute highly infectious disease caused by variola virus. Passive immunization with adequate doses of γ-globulin prepared from the plasma of recently vaccinated donors may be expected to protect unvaccinated household contacts of smallpox or persons last vaccinated many years previously. Generalized vaccinia and vaccinial infections of the eye may also be controlled by γ-globulin; the dose varies from 500 mg to 2.0 g depending upon the age of the patient.

Smallpox vaccine is generally prepared from the vesicular eruption scraped from the skin of animals, e.g. calves, water-buffaloes or sheep. To each gram of pulp 1 ml of trifluorotrichloroethane (Arcton 113) is added and a 10 per cent (w/v) suspension of the vaccinial material is made by mechanical homogenization in dilute buffer solution (pH = 7.4) containing 0.5 per cent (w/v) phenol. During subsequent slow centrifugation up to 70 per cent of the non-virus material is sedimented in the Arcton fraction (specific gravity = 1.5). The supernatant fluid is incubated at 25°C for 24 hours to reduce the bacterial count and when the bacterial contamination of the extract is within the permitted limits, glycerol and peptone are added to give concentrations of 40 and 1 per cent respectively. The bulk vaccine is assayed for potency and stored at -15°C. Before issue it is assayed again and the potency adjusted to 5×10^8 pock-forming units per ml by dilution with a solution of glycerol and peptone to which has been added brilliant green dye to a concentration of 5 g per litre. Vaccinia virus may also be grown in chick embryo chorioallantoic membranes or monolayer cultures of chick embryo or rabbit kidney cells. The resulting vaccine is bacteriologically sterile and equal in prophylactic value to the conventional product.

Chickenpox (Varicella)

Chickenpox is an acute infectious disease caused by a virus having a close relationship to herpes zoster. The virus can be recovered from the vesicles and grown in human embryonic cell cultures. At this moment the virus yield is not adequate for the purposes of vaccine production.

Convalescent serum has been used in the prevention of varicella but the results have been conflicting. Good results have been claimed with use of γ-globulin but controlled trials have not substantiated these claims.

Herpes Simplex (Febrillis)

Herpes simplex is a recurrent virus infection. There is some indication especially from America that in cases of disseminated herpes γ-globulin is effective but in England it is thought that no specific preventive measures are practical.

Yellow Fever

Yellow fever is an acute infectious virus disease occuring in tropical and sub-tropical zones. The vaccine is prepared by grinding up chick embryos infected with the living attenuated 17D strain and drying from the frozen state. The vaccine is reconstituted in sterile normal saline and a single dose, usually 0.5 ml, is injected subcutaneously. All reconstituted vaccine not used within 30 min should be discarded because of the instability of the virus. Administration of the 17D vaccine by scarification although possible is not as effective as by subcutaneous injection. Two scratch vaccinations separated by an interval of 14 days using a mouse brain 17D vaccine have been shown to give 98 per cent protection and may soon be acceptable for general use.

Western Equine Encephalomyelitis (WEE) and Eastern Equine Encephalomyelitis (EEE)

These viruses are found in the west and east of America, Venezuela and the Caribbean region.

Vaccines against western equine encephalitis and eastern equine encephalitis have been prepared by formalin treatment of the virus grown in chick embryo tissue. Although these vaccines, containing one or both strains, are mainly used to prevent the disease in horses, two injections being given annually, they have also been used for laboratory workers in contact with the viruses. The incidence of outbreaks is so low, however, that general use of these vaccines is not indicated. The causal agent of the sporadic encephalitis of Great Britain is unknown.

Japanese B. Encephalitis (JBE)

This disease is the new form of encephalitis occurring in Japan, so-called to distinguish it from von Economo's disease, or epidemic encephalitis lethargica which is called Japanese A encephalitis. A vaccine consisting of a 10 per cent suspension of infected mouse brain in normal saline with the virus killed by 0.2 per cent formalin at 4°C was given to hundreds of thousands of American troops in the Far East between 1942 and 1945. In 1942 the Russians used a similar vaccine which was effective against Russian autumn (Japanese B) encephalitis. A chick embryo vaccine was used over a 3-year period in children in an endemic area in Japan and a reduced incidence of illness resulted in the vaccinated group.

The use of this vaccine has been abandoned by the United States Armed Forces and a more purified mouse brain preparation (protamine-treated) is being used for the vaccination of children in Japan and some other countries. Recently the virus has been attenuated by workers in Japan and the USA; the attenuated strain is grown in hamster kidney cells in a serum-free medium and the killed vaccine prepared from it is believed by some to be safer and more antigenic.

Russian Spring Summer Encephalitis (RSSE) or Tick-borne Encephalitis (TBE)

This tick-borne disease was first described in 1953 occurring in forest areas of the far eastern U.S.S.R. and later is Siberia and western U.S.S.R. A formalin-treated vaccine prepared from a suspension of infected mouse brains has been used successfully in both man and animals. In man, incidence of the disease amongst the vaccinated was reduced to 10 per cent and there were no fatal cases in this group.

Recently an aluminium adsorbed killed vaccine grown in chick fibroblast cell cultures has been used on a large scale.

Dengue

Low passage mouse-adapted strains of dengue virus Types 1 and 11 have produced a modified disease in man giving solid homologous immunity and an immunity lasting a few months against heterologous strains. A more attenuated Type 1 strain has also provided protection. No data are available on the transmissibility of the vaccine strain from man to man by *Aëdes aegypti*.

Epidemic haemorrhagic fever of unknown aetiology has occurred in North Korea and Manchuria and the acute disease was treated with convalescent serum. Recent epidemics in Bangkok, Singapore and Calcutta were associated with dengue viruses; and in South India Chikungunya virus was isolated from all but a few cases (Myers et al. 1965). Attenuated vaccines of the type mentioned above may possibly be useful prophylactics of this disease in the future.

Rift Valley Fever

A killed vaccine grown on monkey kidney or hamster kidney cell cultures and killed with formaldehyde, has been shown to be safe and immunogenic, apparently giving protection to scientists working with this infectious agent.

Louping-Ill

Formalin treatment of infected mouse brains has produced a vaccine which invokes a high titre of neutralizing antibodies in immunized laboratory workers. Propagation of the virus in tissue culture and inactivation by ultraviolet light and β-propiolactone suggest that it may be possible to produce a suitable vaccine.

Poliomyelitis

Poliomyelitis is an acute virus infection in which only a small proportion of those infected show clinical symptoms. Passive immunization against this disease is certainly not the method of choice. When a paralytic case occurs in a family it is more than probable that the family contacts were exposed to the disease simultaneously or are already well into the incubation period and γ-globulin may not be effective. There are data, however, to suggest that γ-globulin may help to neutralize the viraemia when administered in the early stages of the disease before the virus has infected the nerve cells. There are special cases where γ-globulin may be used; children who have recently undergone tonsillectomy are at special risk, as are nurses and medical students entering an infectious area. A dose of 500 mg of γ-globulin for infants under 1 year, 1 g for children 1 to 6 years and 1.5 g for children 7 years and older should be used.

Poliomyelitis is now a preventable disease and the advantages and disadvantages of the killed and live attenuated prophylactics have already been discussed earlier in this chapter. These vaccines have been subjected to more stringent controls than any other prophylactic and both vaccines are undoubtedly safe.

The killed vaccine is produced by infecting monkey kidney cell cultures separately with each type of poliomyelitis virus (Brunenders Type 1, MEF-1 Type 2, Saukett Type 3). The virus suspensions are harvested 3 days later, killed with formalin and blended to make a trivalent vaccine. A full course of immunization consists of two doses given by the intramuscular route at an interval of 4 to 6 weeks followed by a third similar dose given 9 to 12 months later. A fourth dose is recommended 5 to 6 years later but nothing is known of the necessity for further booster doses to maintain lifelong immunity. The killed vaccine can be incorporated with diphtheria, tetanus and pertussis prophylactics into a quadruple vaccine.

The live vaccine is also made by infecting monkey kidney or human embryo lung fibroblast cell cultures but with attenuated virus strains shown to be safe by large-scale clinical trials. The virus suspensions are harvested 3 days later and stringent control procedures ensure, as far as possible, that no changes have taken place from the original strains during the course of production. In many countries the vaccine is given orally as monovalent virus in the order Type 1 followed by Type 3 and finally Type 2 with an interval of 6 weeks between each dose. In this country, in Canada and in Russia three doses of trivalent vaccine are given at 6 to 8-week intervals and a reinforcing dose is given at school entry. In Russia a dose of vaccine is given each year to children between 2 months and 3 years and little is known about the period of immunity following primary immunization.

Rabies

Rabies is an acute infection of mammals caused by *rabies virus*. Clinical rabies (hydrophobia) is fatal in man. The infection usually has a long incubation period after the introduction of the virus by the bite of a rabid animal. If a high level of immunity can be stimulated while the virus is slowly travelling centrally via peripheral nerves its establishment in the brain may be prevented. Modern practice combines passive and active immunization to attain a high concentration of antibody as rapidly as possible. The majority of rabies vaccines used today consist of suspensions of virus infected sheep, rabbit or mouse brain tissue (usually 5 per cent w/v) and the virus may be inactivated by exposure to phenol (Semple type), β-propiolactone or ultraviolet irradiation. In the wet state rabies vaccine has a limited life even when stored between 2°C and 5°C. Lyophilized vaccine is more stable, but only a very small proportion of the total output of rabies vaccine is dried. The presence of nerve tissue in the vaccine makes it potentially dangerous since it may induce demyelination in the patient analogous to the 'allergic' experimental encephalomyelitis which can be produced in experimental animals by the injection of either homologous or heterologous brain tissue. The reported incidence of this complication of anti-rabic treatment varies from country to country, but is probably between 1:4000 and 1:10000 of the patients treated. In any case, even a 'light' course of treatment produces extremely painful local reactions to the later injections.

Anti-rabic treatment, therefore, must not be embarked on without careful consideration, but if it is decided that treatment is necessary, every effort must be made to ensure that it is successful. Bites and other wounds should be given local treatment by thorough washing with soap or detergent and water. Bites by wild vectors (wolves, foxes, skunks, bats, mongooses, etc.) or severe exposure (multiple or face, head, neck or finger bites) call for the immediate application of anti-rabies serum, some of which should be infiltrated around and beneath the wound if this is possible. The recommended dose of serum is not less than 40 I.U. per kg body weight. At least fourteen daily doses of vaccine should be given (up to twenty-one after severe exposure); and where serum is given, supplemental doses of vaccine should be given 10 and 20 days after the completion of the treatment. If possible the supplemental vaccine should be non-encephalitogenic.

Vaccine prepared from non-neural tissue should be free from encephalitogenic material. To this end rabies virus strains have been adapted to growth in chick and duck embryos. Live avianized vaccines of attenuated virulence are not widely used because of the difficulties in producing batches of uniformly adequate potency. However, virus grown in duck embryos and inactivated by β-propiolactone appears to be reasonably effective. A different approach to the preparation safe rabies vaccine is to grow the virus in the brains of very young animals. Infected brains harvested before the start of myelination are a rich source of fixed rabies virus, but the brains appear devoid of encephalitogen when tested in guinea pigs. Vaccines prepared in Chile, the U.S.S.R. and Holland from brains of suckling mice, rats and rabbits have had very satisfactory potencies by the usual tests. Human subjects immunized with them have developed higher concentrations of neutralizing antibody than controls immunized with conventional nervous tissue vaccines. However, the large numbers of immature animals needed and the difficulties associated with their care make it improbable that this type of vaccine will displace the more usual Semple type, except for limited use in special circumstances.

Rabies antiserum is usually produced in horses. The animals are primed by a course of injections of inactivated fixed virus in nervous tissue and subsequently hyperimmunized by repeated courses of fully infectious fixed virus. Plasma from hyperimmune horses may be concentrated and refined by the same methods used for antitoxic sera, including peptic digestion. In practice, reactions to even refined globulins have about the same incidence as reactions to other refined antisera of animal origin, and the usual precautions should be taken to avoid them.

Active immunization against rabies will remain an unsatisfactory procedure until highly potent, safe, inactivated vaccines are available. Current research on the suitability of human diploid cells and other types of cell culture as substrates for the growth of high concentrations of rabies virus is now showing great promise and safe vaccines will be available in the foreseeable future.

Hepatitis

Hepatitis occurs sporadically or in epidemics and is caused by a virus spread by ingesting food and water contaminated with faeces.

Epidemics of infectious hepatitis (viral hepatitis A) have been successfully controlled by an injection of γ-globulin prepared from normal adult serum although this has been relatively ineffective against serum transfusion hepatitis (viral hepatitis B). Prophylactic γ-globulin is recommended to all contacts of infectious hepatitis, especially pregnant and post-menopausal women, as early as possible after exposure and confers protection even if given as late as 6 days before the onset of symptoms. The dosage is 250 to 750 mg for subjects under 10 years of age and 500 to 1500 mg for older subjects. Modern production methods ensure that the γ-globulin is virus free; in the absence of γ-globulin, plasma or serum should on no account be substituted. There have been a number of reports of the isolation of hepatitis virus in tissue culture but none has been confirmed and no vaccine is available.

Measles (Rubeola)

Measles is a highly infectious acute disease caused by measles virus. The disease can be attenuated or completely prevented by γ-globulin prepared from pooled adult serum.

Early attempts to produce a killed vaccine by formalin treatment of virus grown in either monkey kidney or dog kidney cell cultures met with little success. The antibody responses to such a vaccine were very poor although a single dose of killed vaccine, even in the absence of antibody response, was able to protect against the rash and febrile reaction caused by the injection of a live attenuated vaccine. Concentration of the killed vaccine and especially the addition of a mineral carrier has greatly improved the antibody responses but the duration of immunity is short.

Several attenuated strains of reduced pathogenecity have been developed. These vaccines, though provoking a lower incidence of reaction, give antibody responses in as high a proportion of vaccines as some less attenuated strains. The immunity to the disease given by the live attenuated vaccines used in the U.K. has lasted without signs of waning for a least 9 years (the duration of the trial up to 1974).

German Measles (Rubella)

German measles is an exanthematous contagious disease caused by the German measles virus.

There is a well-recognized connection between maternal rubella during the first 3 months of pregnancy and miscarriages, stillbirths and congenital defects such as mental retardation, deaf mutism, cardiac abnormalities and cataract. Although γ-globulin is not very effective in treatment it has been used successfully to prevent infection in contacts. The best results were obtained with 1.5 g given within a week of exposure. Delay should be avoided and where there is more than one exposure at intervals of longer than 2 or 3 weeks a further dose should be given after each contact. Administration of γ-globulin is unnecessary after the first 3 months of pregnancy as rubella rarely infects the fetus in the later months.

In 1966 Meyer, Parkman & Panos in America announced the successful attenuation of the rubella virus after 77 passages in African green monkey kidney cell cultures (HPV 77 strain). The attenuated virus was given to children in a nursery with some uninoculated children serving as controls. Antibody appeared in all inoculated children but in none of the controls. Although the virus could be isolated from some of the inoculated children all specimens from the control children were negative.

Vaccines are now available prepared from any of three strains:
(i) the HPV 77 further attenuated in either duck embryo fibroblast cells HPV 77 DE 5 or dog kidney cells HPV 77 DK 12,
(ii) the Cendehill strain isolated in monkey kidney tissue and attenuated in rabbit kidney cells, and
(iii) RA27/3 strain isolated and attenuated in human diploid embryonic lung fibroblast cell cultures.

All vaccines give good antibody response with little reaction in children and it is hoped that protection against the disease will last many years. In adults, however, the HPV 77 DK 12 vaccine has given an unacceptably high incidence of reactions and this vaccine has been withdrawn from the market. In the U.K. vaccine is being given to girls between the ages of 11 and 13 years.

Mumps (*Infective Parotitis*)

Mumps is an acute infectious generalized virus disease caused by mumps virus.

γ-Globulin prepared from adult donors is valueless. γ-Globulin prepared from mumps convalescent serum given in 20 ml doses within 24 hours after the onset of illness has reduced the incidence of orchitis to 7.7 per cent as compared with 27.4 per cent in controls.

A live attenuated vaccine has been grown in chick cell tissue and the results are encouraging. Only a really effective and lasting immunity to mumps would justify the use of a mumps vaccine in children since a transient or partial immunity would leave them susceptible to the disease after puberty when complications such as orchitis would be harmful. There is every prospect that this will be realized with the use of the live attenuated vaccine.

Trachoma

Trachoma is a chronic contagious viral conjunctivitis and is the greatest single cause of progressive loss of sight in the world. The agents, causing trachoma and inclusion conjunctivitis (TRIC) are closely related, belong to the genus *Bedsonia* and the vaccines so far tested in man have been prepared in the yolk sacs of chick embryos. In most trials killed vaccines have been used, but there are indications that live vaccines may be more effective. The latest conclusions are that TRIC agents are poor antigens and a fully effective vaccine is not available.

BALANCE OF RISKS

No vaccination or form of serum therapy is free from all risk. Thus the acceptability of protection against a disease is an assessment of the balance of the risk against the benefits expected from it.

Each disease must be considered separately for its severity and communicability and each vaccine and antiserum must be judged for its efficacy and the severity of undesirable reactions. These factors differ from place to place, time to time and in different social and economic groups. Reactions to a vaccine giving good immunity against a serious disease would certainly be tolerated whereas protection against a mild disease requires a vaccine free from reaction.

Although safety must be a cardinal factor in the development of vaccines, tests must be based on fact and not on theoretical considerations which may hinder progress. It is equally important, however, that the need for a vaccine is also assessed on facts, and not on speculation.

REFERENCES

ANDREWES, C. H. (1928) *J. Path. Bact.* **31**, 671.

ANDREWES, C. H. (1930) *J. Path. Bact.* **33**, 265.

BEALE, A. J. (1961) *Lancet*, 1166.

BEDSON, S. P. (1928) *Br. J. exp. Path.* **9**, 235.

BEDSON, S. P. & CRAWFORD, G. J. (1928) *Br. J. exp. Path.* **8**, 138.

VON BEHRING, E. & KITASATO, S. (1890) *Dtsch. med. Wschr.* **16**, 1113.

BUTLER, N. R., BARR, M. & GLENNY, A. T. (1954) *Br. med. J.* **i**, 476.

ENDERS, J. F., WELLER, T. H. & ROBBINS, F. C. (1949) *Science, N.Y.* **109**, 85.

GAISFORD, W., FELDMAN, G. V. & PERKINS, F. T. (1961) *J. Pediat. St Louis* **58**, 493.

GITLIN, D., GROSS, P. A. M. & JANEWAY, C. A. (1959) *New Engl. J. Med.* **260**, 21.

GLENNY, A. T., POPE, G. C., WADDINGTON, H. & WALLACE, V. (1926) *J. Path. Bact.* **29**, 31.

HOLT, L. B. (1950) *Developments in Diphtheria Prophylaxis.* London: Heinemann.

JENNER, E. (1798) *An Inquiry into the Causes and Effects of the Variolae Vaccinae.* London: Low.

KENDRICK, P. L., ELDERING, G., DIXON, M. F. & MISNER, J. (1947) *Am. J. publ. Hlth.* **37**, 803.

KITASATO, S. (1889) *Z. Hyg. Infec.-Kr.* **7**, 225.

LOEFFLER, F. (1884) *Mitt. Reichsgesundt. Amt.* **2**, 421.

MEDICAL RESEARCH COUNCIL (1958) *Brit. med. J.* **i**, 79.

MEYER, H. M., PARKMAN, P. D. & PANOS, T. C. (1966) *New Engl. J. Med.* **275**, 575.

MYERS, R. M., CAREY, D. E., REUBEN, R., JESUDASS, E., RANTZ, C. D. S. & JADHAV, M. (1965) *Ind. J. med. Res.* **53**, 694.

OSBORN, J. J., DANCIS, J. & JULIA, J. F. (1952) *Pediat. Springfield* **9**, 736.

PASTEUR, L., CHAMBERLAND, C. & ROUX, E. (1881) *C. R. hebd. séanc. Acad. Sci Paris* **92**, 1378.

PERKINS, F. T., YETTS, R. & GAISFORD, W. (1958) *Br. med. J.* **11**, 68.

PERKINS, F. T., YETTS, R. & GAISFORD, W. (1959a) *Br. med. J.* **i**, 680.

PERKINS, F. T., YETTS, R. & GAISFORD, W. (1959b) *Br. med. J.* **ii**, 530.

PERKINS, F. T., YETTS, R. & GAISFORD, W. (1959c) *Br. med. J.* **i**, 1083.

SABIN, A. B. (1935) *Br. J. exp. Path.* **16**, 70, 84, 158, 169.

SALK, J. E., MENKE, W. J. Jr & FRANCIS, T. Jr (1945) *Am. J. Hyg.* **42**, 57.

SALMON, D. E. & SMITH, T. (1884) *Proc. Soc. biol. Wash.* **3**, 29.

SCHMIDT, S. & HANSEN, A. (1933) *Acta. path. microbiol. scand.*, Suppl. **16**, 407.

THEILER, M. & SMITH, H. H. (1937) *J. exp. Med.* **65**, 787.

TODD, C. (1928) *Br. J. exp. Path.* **9**, 244.

34

Antibiotics

Microorganisms produce a great diversity of metabolites with structures as simple as that of ethanol or as complex as that of a polypeptide antibiotic. The biological activity of these metabolites has been long known; Pasteur in 1877 observed that the growth of *Bacillus anthracis* was inhibited by contamination with other bacteria and in 1896 Gosio found that *Penicillium brevi-compactum* produced a substance, mycophenolic acid, which although bacteriostatic towards the anthrax bacillus was too toxic for clinical use.

In 1929 Fleming observed that *Penicillium notatum* produced a substance which inhibited the growth of *Staphylococcus aureus* and other Gram-positive organisms. He suggested that the culture filtrate, which was non-toxic, could be used for the treatment of infections and named the active constituent penicillin. With the facilities then available, Fleming was not able to isolate and purify penicillin and it was not until after the outbreak of war in 1939 that the potential of this substance was fully appreciated and it received the intensive investigation necessary to isolate, purify and elucidate its structure. This work was carried out at many centres in the UK and the USA and the results were published in *The Chemistry of Penicillin* (Clarke, Johnson & Robinson 1949).

In 1944 Waksman isolated streptomycin from a culture of *Streptomyces griseus*; the value of this antibiotic lay in its broad spectrum of activity against Gram-positive and negative organisms and *Mycobacterium tuberculosis*. This discovery accelerated the search for other antibiotics, and soil samples from all over the world were screened

TABLE 34.1

COMMON ANTIBIOTICS

Antibiotic	Source	Spectrum of activity
Penicillin (1929)	*Penicillium notatum*	Gram-positive
Griseofulvin (1939)	*Penicillium griseofulvum*	Anti-fungal
Streptomycin (1944)	*Streptomyces griseus*	Broad, *Mycobacterium tuberculosis*
Chloramphenicol (1947)	*Streptomyces venezuelae*	Broad, some *Rickettsia*
Polymyxin (1947)	*Bacillus polymyxa*	Gram-negative
Cephalosporin (1948)	*Cephalosporium brotzu*	Broad
Chlortetracycline (1948)	*Streptomyces aureofaciens*	Broad
Neomycin (1949)	*Streptomyces fradiae*	Broad
Oxytetracycline (1950)	*Streptomyces rimosus*	Broad
Erythromycin (1952)	*Streptomyces erythreus*	Gram-positive, some *Rickettsia*, some viruses
Novobiocin (1956)	*Streptomyces spheroides*, *Streptomyces niveus*	Gram-positive, some negative
Fusidic acid (1962)	*Fusidium coccineum*	Broad, penicillin resistant staphylococci
Gentamicin (1963)	*Micromonospora purpurea*	Broad, particularly Gram-negative

594

for the production of biologically active metabolites. Many thousands of moulds and bacteria have been examined and activity has been found in several thousand strains. From many of these the active substance has been isolated and its structure elucidated by chemical degradation and physical studies. Some of the more common antibiotics found in this way are given in Table 34.1.

ANTIBIOTIC RESEARCH AND PRODUCTION

The production of antibiotics proceeds along well-defined lines and the general principles apply for all; details differ, but much of this information is either unpublished or contained within the patent literature and cannot be included here.

THE SEARCH FOR A NEW ANTIBIOTIC

Most antibiotics are obtained either directly by fermentation, or by chemical modification of a fermentation product. The first stage in the search for a new antibiotic is the screening either of pure cultures obtained from a collection, or of soil samples which contain bacteria and moulds in abundance. In the latter case, soil suspensions are plated out into petri dishes containing different media, and after incubation selected colonies are transferred to a nutrient agar slope to establish the culture. To test these or the pure cultures for antibiotic activity they are then grown in agar media and when growth has been established plugs are cut out and incubated on large agar plates seeded with a test organism (frequently *Staphylococcus aureus*). Where the culture has produced an antibiotic and inhibited the bacterial growth, a clear zone is obtained. Alternatively, the organism may be grown in a liquid medium and the filtered brew placed in cups cut into a seeded agar plate, again giving zones of inhibition similar to those shown in Fig. 34.5.

Having established that an organism produces an antibiotic, it is tested against a range of bacteria in order to obtain an indication of its possible clinical value and the extent to which the activity is novel.

The next stage in the study is the growth of the organism on a laboratory scale, using 5- or 10-litre vessels (Fig. 34.1) to define some of the conditions required for its production by deep culture. These studies include the effects of medium composition, pH, fermentation time, aeration and stirring rates and inoculum size. Methods for the isolation of the metabolite are also studied, the usual method being extraction with a variety of water-immiscible solvents over a range of pH. Purification may be

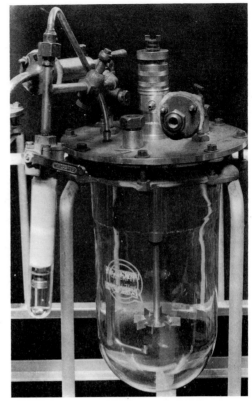

FIG. 34.1. Laboratory fermenter.

achieved by crystallization of a suitable salt, ion-exchange chromatography or adsorption followed by extraction, but in the case of a mixture, or an intractable product, it is sometimes only possible to obtain a freeze-dried extract at this stage.

Before proceeding to large scale production it is necessary to carry out pilot plant studies in 100- to 2000-litre vessels (Fig. 34.2) to optimize the conditions and to give sufficient material for the extensive pharmacological and toxicological investigations which have to be carried out before any clinical studies can be started. At the same time the structure of the antibiotic is established and possible variants prepared chemically.

A continual search is made for strains of the mould or bacterium which will produce greater yields of the antibiotic; for this purpose mutants are produced by X-ray or ultraviolet irradiation or treatment with radiomimetic substances such as nitrogen mustard.

ANTIBIOTIC PRODUCTION

Originally penicillin was produced by surface culture, the mould being grown in small static containers, the mycelium forming a mat on the surface

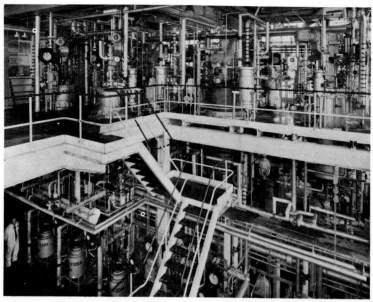

FIG. 34.2. Fermentation pilot-plant.

of the medium. In spite of the extremely cumbersome nature of the process it was used for all the early production of penicillin in the UK. The production of penicillin was revolutionized by the discovery at Peoria, that a strain of *Penicillium chrysogenum* (obtained from an over-ripe Cantaloupe melon) would produce high yields of penicillin under conditions of deep or submerged culture. The growth of a mould is aerobic and, in surface culture, growth and production of antibiotic is limited by the rate at which oxygen can diffuse into the medium. In submerged culture the mould is grown in an agitated tank and supplied with a continuous flow of air to give non-limiting conditions.

The medium used in fermentation will vary for the particular antibiotic being produced but all media contain a source of carbon, which may be lactose or glucose, nitrogen as ammonium salts and trace elements such as phosphorus, sulphur, magnesium, iron, zinc and copper. In addition, corn-steep liquor is added for penicillin production and soya bean meal and dried distillers residues for streptomycin; these provide various factors which increase the yield of product. Before use, the medium as well as the fermentor and associated equipment is steam sterilized, since bacterial contamination could destroy the antibiotic.

The selected culture is transferred from storage as the master culture first to an agar slope, then to culture to give a seed suspension, and finally it is grown in seed vessels in the plant for 24 to 48 h before transfer to the main fermentors (Fig. 34.3). Fermentation is continued for 3 to 5 days during which period the vessel is cooled to keep the temperature between 23° and 27°, stirred and aerated with sterilized air. The introduction of large volumes of air causes frothing which is controlled by the addition of antifoams such as lard oil, octadecanol or silicones.

When fermentation is complete the mycelium is removed on a rotary filter and the antibiotic extracted with an organic solvent, after adjustment of the pH. Alternatively, as with streptomycin, the brew is passed through a carboxylic acid resin from which it is subsequently removed with dilute acid. The extracted antibiotic is converted into the particular derivative which is to be used, products for injection being rendered sterile by passage of their solution through sterilizing filters followed by final crystallization or precipitation under sterile conditions.

ANTIBIOTIC ASSAY

When a new antibiotic has been isolated it is essential to have an assay method available in order to follow the processes of purification, its distribution within the blood and tissues when given to animals and finally humans, and also the potency of the various formulations used. In the absence of a chemical method, a biological assay against a standard sample of agreed potency is performed, using a suitable test organism. A biological assay

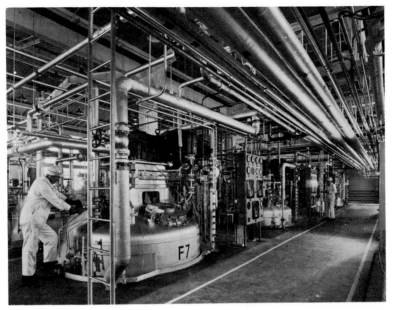

FIG. 34.3. Production fermenters.

is also used for the determination of low concentrations of an antibiotic, such as are obtained in blood and urine, where a chemical assay might be insufficiently sensitive.

The cup-plate method, which is preferred, requires the test organism to be very sensitive to the antibiotic, giving clear zones of inhibition with well marked changes in zone diameter with small changes in concentration. The antibiotic must also diffuse readily through the agar medium; if this is not so, assay is carried out using serial dilution or turbidimetric methods to measure its effect upon the test organism.

Petri dishes or rectangular glass trays are filled to a uniform depth, with nutrient agar medium which has been inoculated with a suitable organism. The *British Pharmacopoeia* 1973 lists organisms to be used, e.g. *Bacillus pumilus* for erythromycin, *Bacillus subtilis* for novobiocin, etc. When the agar has solidified, sterile cylinders of glass, stainless steel, porcelain or aluminium 5 mm in diameter are placed on the surface. Alternatively, holes 5 to 8 mm in diameter are cut into the medium using a sterile borer. Solutions of various concentrations of the standard and also solutions of the preparation under test, presumed to be of similar concentration, are placed in the holes. When petri dishes are used (Fig. 34.4) the standard and test solutions are alternated in the dishes, and when rectangular trays are used (Fig. 34.5) the solutions are arranged in

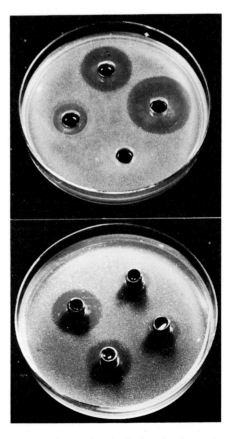

FIG. 34.4. Cup-plate (top) and cylinder-plate (bottom) assay.

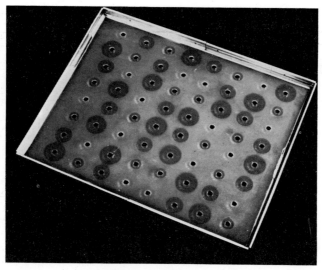

FIG. 34.5. Cup-plate assay in a tray.

the form of a randomized Latin square. The plates are then maintained at room temperature for 2 h to allow the antibiotic to diffuse into the medium.

If the agar is uniform, diffusion of the antibiotic will occur uniformly around the cup and a concentration gradient will be established around it and at a certain distance from the cup, depending upon the concentration of the antibiotic within it, the concentration in the agar will be just sufficient to inhibit the growth of the organism. When the plates have been incubated at a suitable temperature (usually 37° to 39°) for 16 h, each cup will be surrounded by a clear zone of inhibition, the diameter of which is proportional to the logarithm of the concentration of antibiotic in the cup. By plotting zone diameter against concentration for both standard and test, the potency of the test relative to the standard may be obtained by measuring the horizontal displacement between the two lines which should be parallel. Any lack of parallelism indicates either that the test was faulty or that another antibiotic was present with a different dose response curve.

PENICILLINS

From 1940 on, the penicillins were the subject of considerable investigation at a number of industrial and university laboratories in the UK and in 1943 this collaboration was extended to the USA. During the early days of this research, considerable differences in analytical and degradative results were obtained from different laboratories. These were resolved when it was demonstrated that the mould produced six different penicillins. In the UK the medium used was synthetic and penicillin F was the main product while in the USA corn-steep liquor was added to increase the yield of penicillin and here penicillin G was the major product. Early studies on the structure of penicillin were hampered by the low yields and purity of the unstable product. Later when crystalline material became available, the structure was elucidated by degradation and partial synthesis and confirmed by X-ray crystallographic analysis.

The molecule was shown to contain a carboxyl group, a β-lactam ring (four membered cyclic amide) fused to a thiazolidine ring (five membered ring containing nitrogen and sulphur) and an acyl-amino group, and the various penicillins differed only in the structure of the acyl-group, R, of the side-chain. The general structure is:

Of the natural penicillins only G, benzylpenicillin, ($R = C_6H_5.CH_2{}^-$) is used therapeutically and this compound has been the most extensively studied both in its chemistry and in improving methods of production. The stimulation of yield by corn-steep liquor was shown to be due to the presence of β-phenylethylamine and this provided the side-chain phenylacetyl group. Subsequently, it was found that the addition of phenylacetic acid greatly enhanced the yield of benzylpenicillin and this is now added as a regular practice.

PENICILLIN BREAKDOWN

The presence of the intact β-lactam ring in the penicillin molecule is essential for antibiotic activity. The structure is, however, reactive and it is at this

A penicillenic acid

ring that attack can occur to give a variety of products the structure of which depends on the particular conditions.

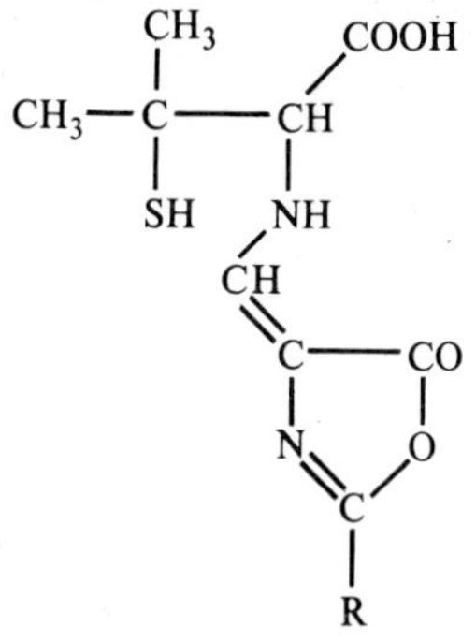

Penicilloic acids are readily formed by hydrolysis under alkaline conditions or in the presence of the bacterial enzyme penicillinase (more correctly β-lactamase) and it is the secretion of this enzyme which can be responsible for the resistance to penicillin by bacteria, for example, some strains of *Staph. aureus.*

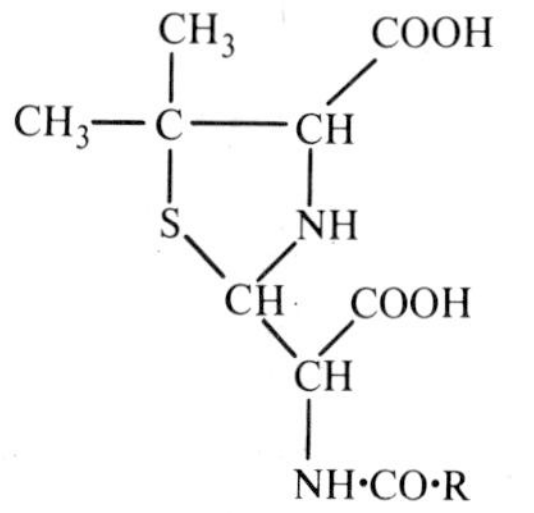

A penicilloic acid

Applications of Benzylpenicillin

Benzylpenicillin acts specifically on bacteria by interfering with the mechanism of cell-wall synthesis; it is of very low mammalian toxicity and consequently has been used for the treatment of a wide range of infections. Almost all the Gram-

positive and some of the Gram-negative pathogens are sensitive, e.g. *Staph. aureus, Strep. pyogenes, Strep. pneumoniae, C. welchii, B. anthracis, N. gonorrhoeae.*

In moderately acid solution the carbonyl-group of the side-chain reacts with the β-lactam ring to give a penicillenic acid while at a lower pH, and particularly in the presence of heavy metals, a penillic acid is formed by such a reaction followed by a complex series of rearrangements. Because of the ready decomposition of most penicillins under acid conditions they are usually administered as their neutral salts.

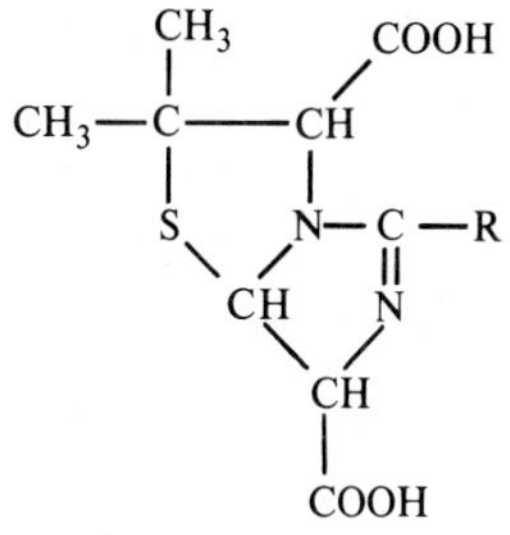

A penilloic acid

N.meningitidis. As it is rapidly destroyed by acid and poorly absorbed from the stomach it is almost invariably administered by injection, although occasionally it is given orally.

Forms of Benzylpenicillin

Benzylpenicillin is official in the *British Pharmacopoeia* as its sodium and potassium salts which give high blood levels for only a few hours unless administered repeatedly. In order to obtain prolonged, but lower, blood levels, the water-insoluble salts with procaine (diethylaminoethyl *p*-aminobenzoate) and benzathine (*N*:*N'*-dibenzyl-ethylenediamine) are used. Procaine penicillin will give detectable blood levels after 24 h and benzathine penicillin after several weeks.

Assay of Benzylpenicillin

The basis of the chemical assay for benzylpenicillin is that penicillins do not react with iodine in neutral aqueous solution, but their penicilloic acids consume a quantity of iodine, which although non-stoichiometric is reproducible under constant conditions. Thus the difference between the amount of iodine consumed by a sample in neutral solution and one which has been hydrolysed to the penicilloic acid is proportional to the amount of penicillin present. A sample of known potency is assayed concurrently in order to obtain the actual potency of the sample under test.

PHENOXYMETHYLPENICILLIN

When it was discovered that phenylacetic acid added to a penicillin fermentation was incorporated in the molecule as benzylpenicillin, large numbers of substituted acetic acids were screened to discover if they were incorporated and if so whether the resulting penicillin had desirable properties. As a result of this investigation, it was found that phenoxyacetic acid was accepted by the mould and the resulting phenoxymethylpenicillin (penicillin V) was acid stable.

Although there was no great change in the antibacterial spectrum or its sensitivity to penicillinase, this represented a considerable advance in convenience since it could be administered orally in tablets, capsules or syrups.

Phenoxymethylpenicillin

Applications of Phenoxymethylpenicillin
The spectrum of activity of phenoxymethylpenicillin is similar to that of benzylpenicillin but it is slightly more active against resistant staphylococci since it is more slowly destroyed by penicillinase, slightly less active against streptococci and much less active against Gram-negative bacteria. It is particularly useful in the oral treatment of Gram-positive infections.

Forms of Phenoxymethylpenicillin
Phenoxymethylpenicillin is official as the free acid, its calcium and potassium salts and in the form of tablets and capsules.

Assay of Phenoxymethylpenicillin
The total penicillin content of phenoxymethylpenicillin is determined iodometrically against a standard sample. As phenoxymethylpenicillin may contain traces of other penicillins, the phenoxymethylpenicillin content is also determined photometrically.

SEMI-SYNTHETIC PENICILLINS

The range of structures accepted by the *Penicillium* mould as precursors is limited to acetic acid derivatives and, of the penicillins which can be prepared by this process, only pencillin V is of therapeutic value. Batchelor et al. (1959) showed that in the absence of any added precursor *Penicillium chrysogenum* produced 6-aminopenicillanic acid, which could be isolated using ion-exchange resins and subsequently it was found that this compound could also be prepared by the enzymic de-acylation of penicillin G or V.

6-Aminopenicillanic acid

Although 6-aminopenicillanic acid itself has only very slight antibiotic activity, it can be acylated chemically to give a penicillin of any desired structure which could not be prepared by the precursor technique. A very large number of penicillins have been prepared and it has been shown that with a suitable side-chain it is possible to obtain compounds which are stable to acid, such as phenethicillin; resistant to penicillinase, such as methicillin and cloxacillin, or with a broad spectrum of activity including Gram-negative organisms, such as ampicillin and carbenicillin, the last having particular value as it is also active against *Pseudomonas aeruginosa*. Further penicillin derivatives are given in Table 34.2.

Applications of the Semi-Synthetic Penicillins
Phenethicillin. This analogue of phenoxymethylpenicillin shows a similar antibacterial spectrum but is better absorbed and so gives higher blood levels. It is always administered orally.

Methicillin. Highly resistant to staphylococcal penicillinase and is consequently clinically effective against penicillinase-producing and penicillin-sensitive strains of *Staphylococcus aureus*. It is readily destroyed by acid and has to be administered parenterally.

TABLE 34.2

PENICILLIN DERIVATIVES

R	Penicillin
$CH_3 \cdot \overset{*}{CH} —$ $\mid$ OC_6H_5 DL-configuration	Phenethicillin DL-α-phenoxyethylpenicillin
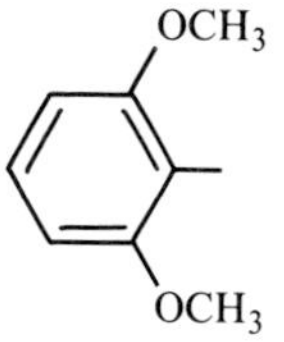 OCH$_3$ / OCH$_3$ (2,6-dimethoxyphenyl)	Methicillin 2:6-dimethoxyphenylpenicillin
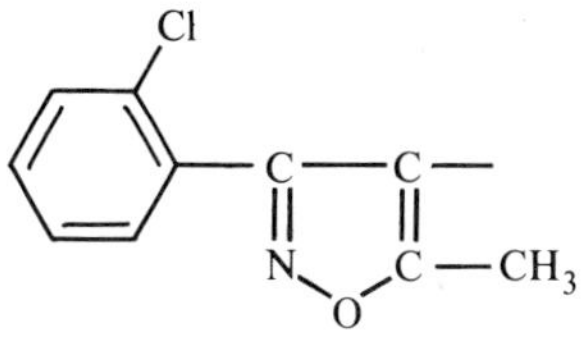 Cl-phenyl-isoxazole-CH$_3$	Cloxacillin 3-(2-chlorophenyl)-5-methyl-4-isoxazolylpenicillin
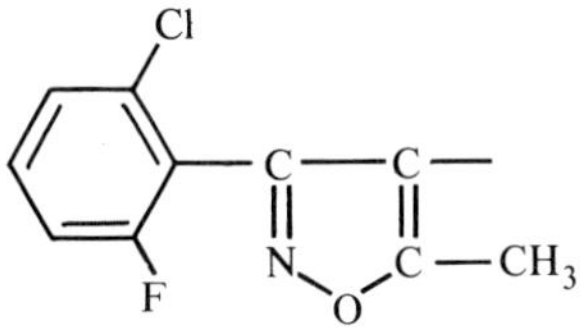 Cl, F-phenyl-isoxazole-CH$_3$	Flucloxacillin 3-(2-chloro-6-fluoro-phenyl)-5-methyl-4-isoxazolylpenicillin
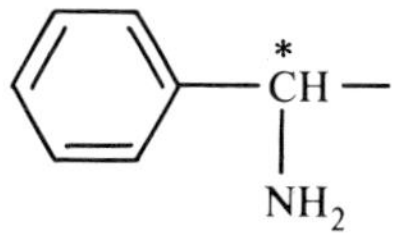 phenyl-$\overset{*}{CH}$— $\mid$ NH$_2$ D(-) configuration	Ampicillin D(-)-α-aminobenzylpenicillin
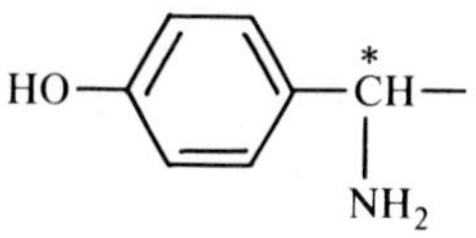 HO—phenyl—$\overset{*}{CH}$— $\mid$ NH$_2$ D(-) configuration	Amoxycillin D(-)-α-amino-p-hydroxybenzyl-penicillin
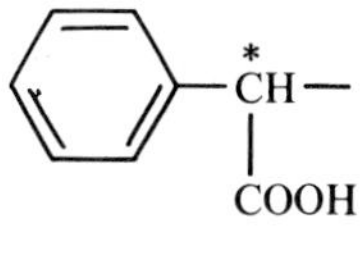 phenyl-$\overset{*}{CH}$— $\mid$ COOH DL-configuration	Carbenicillin DL-α-carboxybenzylpenicillin

* Assymetric Carbon

Cloxacillin. Resistant to penicillinase and acid, used orally and parenterally for the treatment of Gram-positive infections particularly those due to penicillinase-producing staphylococci.

Flucloxacillin. Similar in properties to cloxacillin but considerably better absorbed when given orally.

Ampicillin. Slightly less active than benzyl-penicillin against Gram-positive but much more active against Gram-negative bacteria, e.g. *Haemophilus influenzae, Salmonella* and *Shigella* species, most strains of *E.coli* and non-penicillinase producing strains of *Proteus mirabilis.* Ampicillin is highly resistant to acid and is administered orally as its zwitterion of low water solubility or by injection as its soluble sodium salt.

Amoxycillin. Similar in activity to ampicillin but much better absorbed from the gastrointestinal tract, giving considerably higher blood levels. Administered orally as its zwitterion.

Carbenicillin. Broad spectrum with predominantly Gram-negative activity extending to *Escherichia coli*, *Pseudomonas aeruginosa* and strains of *Proteus vulgaris*, *Proteus rettgeri* and *Proteus morganii*. Carbenicillin is not absorbed orally and is administered parenterally as its highly soluble disodium salt.

Forms of the Semi-Synthetic Penicillins
Phenethicillin. This is official as the potassium salt and in the form of tablets and capsules.

Methicillin. This is official as the sodium salt which is used for injection.

Cloxacillin. This is official as the sodium salt which is used for capsules and injection.

Flucloxacillin. Is used as its sodium salt for oral and parenteral administration.

Ampicillin. The free acid exists in two forms, as a trihydrate and the anhydrous compound, both of which are official and may be formulated into capsules. The sodium salt is used for injection.

Amoxycillin. The free acid is used as the trihydrate which may be formulated into capsules and a dry syrup mix to which water is added before use.

Carbenicillin. This is official as the disodium salt which is used for injection.

Assay of the Semi-Synthetic Penicillins
Phenethicillin, methicillin, cloxacillin and flucloxacillin. Are assayed by heating with an excess of a known amount of alkali. The penicilloic acid produced by the hydrolysis of the β-lactam ring consumes an equivalent amount of alkali which is determined by titrimetric estimation of the amount remaining. As the formation of the penicilloic acid is stoichiometric this assay is absolute and does not require the use of a standard.

Ampicillin. Determined by acid hydrolysis in the presence of a copper catalyst to give α-amino-benzylpenillic acid which is estimated photometrically against a standard sample of ampicillin of known potency.

Carbenicillin. Assayed by iodometric assay for total penicillins with correction for the trace of benzylpenicillin, produced by decarboxylation, by agar-gel electrophoresis.

CEPHALOSPORINS

In 1945, Brotzu isolated from a sewage outfall in Sardinia a strain of *Cephalosporium* which produced metabolites with some activity against typhoid. Studies by Abraham and Newton (Abraham 1967) showed that the mould produced a complex mixture of antibiotics one of which, cephalosporin C, was active against Gram-negative and penicillinase producing organisms. Chemical degradation followed by X-ray crystallographic analysis showed that the structure was related to the penicillins in that it also contained a β-lactam ring bearing an acylated amino-group but it was fused to a dihydrothiazine ring instead of the thiazolidine ring present in penicillins.

Cephalosporin C

The side-chain of cephalosporin C cannot be removed enzymically, but this can be accomplished chemically, for example with nitrosyl chloride to give 7-aminocephalosporanic acid which like 6-aminopenicillanic acid can be acylated to give a whole range of semi-synthetic cephalosporins. In addition to acylation, the group at carbon 3 can be modified to improve the properties of the compounds. A large number of cephalosporins have been prepared, of which those in common use are given on following pages.

Applications of Cephalosporins
Cephaloridine. This shows activity against all strains of staphylococci and streptococci, except *Streptococcus faecalis*. Of the Gram-negative bacteria *Neisseria* species are highly sensitive, *Haemophilus influenzae*, *Escherichia coli*, *Proteus mirabilis*, *Salmonella* and *Shigella* species less so. Cephaloridine is not absorbed orally and is administered parenterally.

Cephalothin. Similar spectrum of activity to cephaloridine but frequently slightly less active against certain organisms.

R·CO·NH·CH— CH$\overset{S}{\diagdown}$CH$_2$
CO— N$\diagup$C$\diagdown$C —R^1
COOH

R	R^1	
(thiophene)CH$_2$—	—CH$_2$—N$^+$(pyridine)	cephaloridine
(thiophene)CH$_2$—	—CH$_2$·O·CO·CH$_3$	cephalothin
C$_6$H$_5$—$\overset{*}{C}$H— NH$_2$ D(-) configuration	—CH$_2$·O·CO·CH$_3$	cephaloglycine
C$_6$H$_5$—$\overset{*}{C}$H— NH$_2$ D(-) configuration	—CH$_3$	cephalexin

Cephaloglycine. Active against many Gram-negative bacteria but enterococci, indole-positive *Proteus* and *Enterobacter* are usually resistant, *Pseudomonas* invariably so. Absorbed from the gastrointestinal tract sufficiently well to be used for urinary tract infections. Metabolized to the desacetyl compound which also has antibacterial activity.

Cephalexin. Similar in spectrum of activity to the parenteral cephalosporins but less active against resistant staphylococci. Well orally absorbed in man, most of the compound being excreted unchanged in the urine.

Forms of the Cephalosporins
Cephaloridine. Official as the betaine (α or δ form) for injection.

Cephalothin. Official as the sodium salt for injection.

Cephaloglycine. Available as zwitterion dihydrate.

Cephalexin. Official as the monohydrate in the form of capsules and tablets.

Assay of Cephalosporins
The β-lactam portion of the molecule is assayed · iodometrically by a procedure similar to that used for benzylpenicillin. The pyridine content of cepha-loridine is determined by reaction with bromine and potassium cyanide to give a red colour which is estimated photometrically.

CHLORAMPHENICOL

Chloramphenicol was isolated in 1947 from a culture of *Streptomyces venezuelae* and chemical degradation showed that the structure was D($-$)-*threo*-2-dichloroacetamido-1-*p*-nitrophenyl-1:3-propanediol. The most surprising feature of this relatively simple compound was the presence of an aromatic nitro-group which was previously unknown in nature.

O$_2$N—(benzene)—$\overset{\overset{H}{|}}{\underset{\underset{OH}{|}}{C}}$—$\overset{\overset{NH·CO·CHCl_2}{|}}{\underset{\underset{H}{|}}{C}}$—CH$_2$·OH

Chloramphenicol

Although chloramphenicol was originally obtained by fermentation, a number of syntheses have been devised and it is now exclusively prepared synthetically. Numerous analogues of chloramphenicol have been synthesized but these have shown reduced activity or increased toxicity.

Applications of Chloramphenicol
Chloramphenicol is bacteriostatic to a broad spectrum of organisms being particularly valuable for the treatment of typhoid and rickettsial infections. It is now less used than formerly since very high doses can produce granulocytopenia and aplastic anaemia. Chloramphenicol is well absorbed orally but it has an intensely bitter taste. To overcome this, the primary hydroxyl group is esterified with palmitic acid to give a bland ester which is very suitable for use in syrups. The water-soluble mono-sodium salt of the hemi-ester of succinic acid is used parenterally.

Forms of Chloramphenicol
Chloramphenicol and chloramphenicol Capsules are official in the *British Pharmacopoeia*. It is assayed photometrically.

POLYPEPTIDE ANTIBIOTICS

The polypeptide antibiotics all consist of amino acids linked by peptide bonds into cyclic structures of some considerable complexity containing unusual amino acids and saturated aliphatic acids.

BACITRACIN

Bacitracin was isolated in 1945 from cultures of *Bacillus licheniformis* obtained from the leg wound of a young girl. It has been shown to be a mixture of five related polypeptides, the material which is produced commercially by deep fermentation being predominantly bacitracin A.

Applications of Bacitracin
Bacitracin is active against Gram-positive organisms particularly certain strains of clostridia. Its nephrotoxicity limits its parenteral use but as it is not absorbed its main use is topical, it has been used for sterilization of the gut. It is official as the zinc salt.

POLYMYXIN

Polymyxin was isolated in 1947 from *Bacillus polymyxa* in a soil sample. Like the other members of this class of antibiotic, polymyxin was found to be a mixture of five antibiotics each of which is separable into two closely related substances. Of the polymyxins only B and E (colistin) are used therapeutically, the other members of the group being too toxic.

Polymyxin B.   This is basic and forms a water-soluble sulphate which is used in the treatment of Gram-negative infections such as *E.coli* and *Ps.*

pyocyanea. It is administered orally, topically and by injection. The sulphate is official.

Colistin.   Its use is similar to polymyxin B, being administered orally as tablets of its sulphate or by injection as the sodium salt of its tetramethane-sulphonate (colistin sulphomethate) prepared by reacting the free amino compound with formaldehyde and sodium bisulphite. Colistin sulphate and sulphomethate sodium are official.

THE CARBOHYDRATE ANTIBIOTICS

This group, of which the most important members are streptomycin and neomycin, is produced by streptomycetes. They are basic compounds giving crystalline, water-soluble salts and consist of sugars and amino sugars linked glycosidically.

STREPTOMYCIN

Streptomycin was isolated by Waksman in 1944 from a culture of *Streptomyces griseus* obtained from a chicken's throat. Two years earlier, streptothricin had been isolated from *Streptomyces lavendulae* and although it possessed a broad spectrum of activity, it was too toxic for use. Streptomycin was far less toxic and in addition to its Gram-negative activity it was found to be the first useful antibiotic active against *Mycobacterium tuberculosis.*

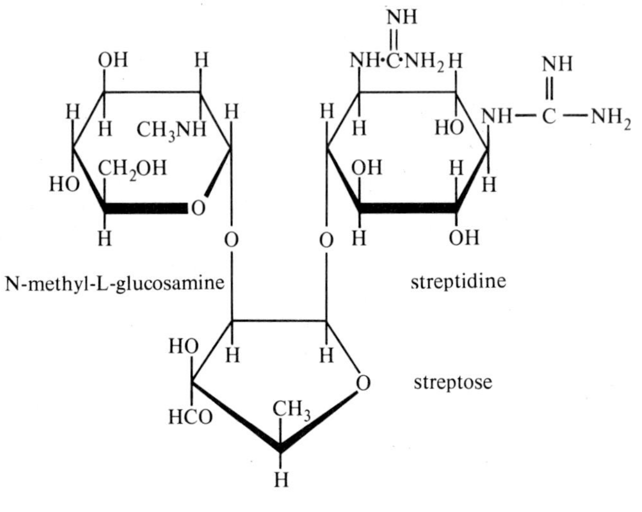

N-methyl-L-glucosamine

streptidine

streptose

Streptomycin

Streptomycin is a triacidic base consisting of three units; streptidine, a diguanidino derivative of inositol; streptose, an aldose, and *N*-methyl-*L*-glucosamine.

Early production of streptomycin was by surface culture, meat extract, peptone and sodium chloride being added to the medium. Subsequently, it was found that deep culture techniques were applicable, the meat extract could be replaced by a much cheaper extract of soya bean meal and distillers' soulbles and this process is now used on a large scale. After fermentation and clarification of the broth, the antibiotic is absorbed on to a carboxylic acid ion-exchange resin and then eluted from the washed resin with dilute acid. The concentrated streptomycin salt solution so obtained is then purified by crystallization of the complex formed between two molecules of streptomycin trihydro-chloride and one of calcium chloride. From this purified salt the sulphate is prepared, either crystal-line for oral use, or sterile for injection.

Catalytic hydrogenation of the aldehyde group in streptomycin gives the corresponding alcohol, dihydrostreptomycin which was thought to be less toxic than the parent compound; this is now believed not to be so and the compound is no longer described in the *British Pharmacopoeia*.

Applications of Streptomycin
Streptomycin is chiefly used in the treatment of tuberculosis, particularly in combination with other drugs such as isonicotinic hydrazide or *p*-amino-salicylic acid, which delay the development of resis-tance by the bacterium. It is also used for the treatment of plague and tularaemia. Although well absorbed by injection, it is not absorbed orally and has been used for the treatment of gastro-intestinal infections and sterilization of the gut prior to abdominal surgery. The most serious side effect of streptomycin is on the eighth nerve causing vertigo and also deafness.

Assay of Streptomycin
Streptomycin may be assayed biologically using *B.subtilis*, or chemically by heating with sodium hydroxide, when the streptose fragment of the molecule rearranges to give maltol which is esti-mated colorimetrically by the purple colour pro-duced with ferric ammonium sulphate.

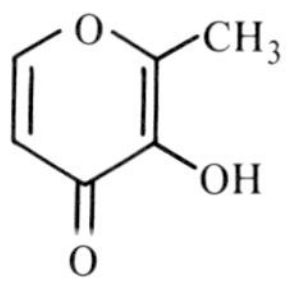

Maltol

NEOMYCIN

Neomycin is a mixture of three closely related antibiotics (neomycins A, B and C) first isolated

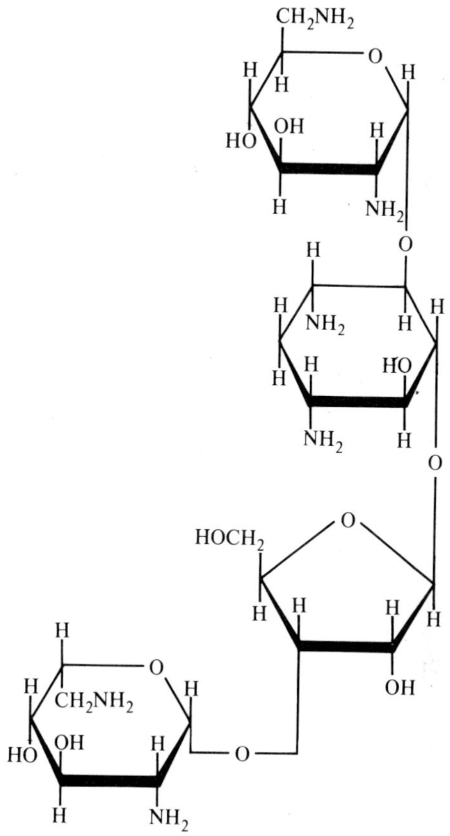

Neomycin B

from *Streptomyces fradiae* in 1949. It consists of three basic sugars and D-ribose linked glycosidically.

Applications of Neomycin
Neomycin has a broad spectrum of activity and as it is not absorbed orally its sulphate is used for sterilization of the gut and for the treatment of intestinal infections. It is of considerable value for the topical treatment of infections due to staphylococci and Gram-negative bacteria, and is frequently used in combination with polypeptide antibiotics to prevent the development of resistant strains.

KANAMYCIN

Kanamycin was isolated in 1957 by Umezawa from a culture of *Streptomyces kanamyceticus* obtained from soil collected in Nagarov in Japan. It is a mixture of predominantly kanamycin A together with kanamycins B and C.

Kanamycin A has the structure shown below, B

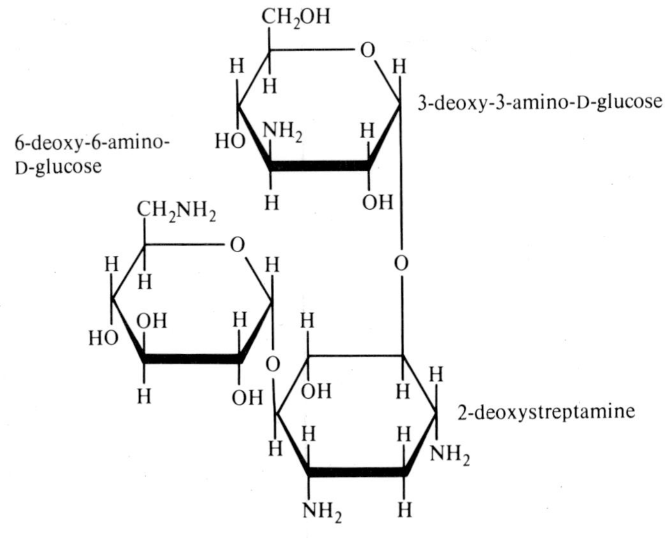

Kanamycin A

and C differ in the structure of the amino sugar linked to the 2-deoxystreptamine ring. The structures of all three compounds have been confirmed by total synthesis.

Applications of Kanamycin

Kanamycin has a spectrum of activity similar to the other carbohydrate antibiotics against Gram-positive and negative organisms. It is not usefully absorbed from the alimentary tract and hence is used for the treatment of infantile gastroenteritis and for sterilizing the gut. Although it does exhibit some ototoxicity it can be administered by repeated intramuscular injection particularly for the treatment of tuberculosis.

Kanamycin is administered as its readily water-soluble monosulphate (official).

GENTAMICIN

Weinstein in 1963 isolated gentamicin, a mixture of water-soluble basic antibiotics from *Micromonospora purpurea* and *M.echinospora*. The mixture of components is complex but the structures of gentamicins A and C have been elucidated; A having been prepared in a pure crystalline form has been shown to consist of paromamine (a component of the neomycin analogue paromomycin) linked to a novel 3-methylamino-3-deoxy-pentapyranose (gentosamine). Gentamicin forms salts with mineral and strong organic acids, the sulphate (official) being used clinically.

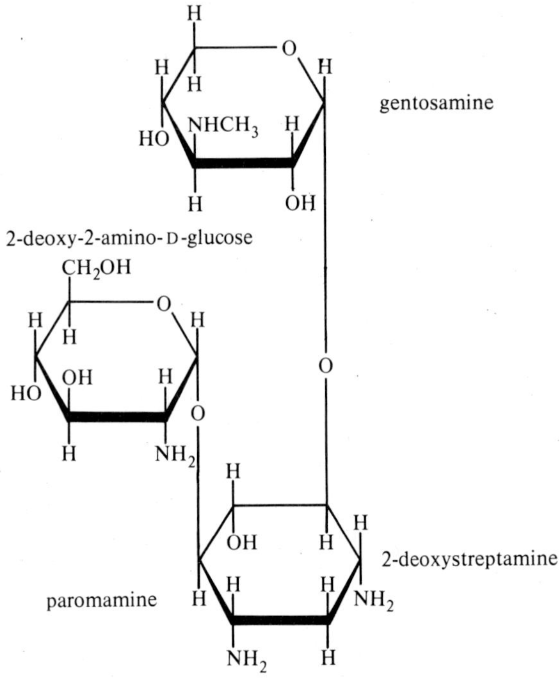

Gentamicin A

Applications of Gentamicin

An antibiotic with Gram-negative activity particularly against *Aerobacter*, *Escherichia*, *Klebsiella*, *Salmonella* and some *Proteus* species. Its most significant activity is against *Pseudomonas aeruginosa* and it is largely used for the treatment of infections caused by this organism.

Like all the other carbohydrate antibiotics it is not absorbed orally and must be administered by intramuscular injection as its sulphate (official).

THE TETRACYCLINES

The tetracyclines are a group of broad spectrum antibiotics possessing a hydronaphthacene skeleton bearing a wide variety of functional groups. They are amphoteric, forming crystalline salts with strong acids and bases and chelates with many metal ions and it has been suggested that this last property is responsible for their antibacterial action. They are prepared by deep culture fermentation of streptomycetes and have been isolated by a number of methods; as their calcium or mixed barium and magnesium salts, as their iron chelates or as salts with cationic surfactants.

Because of the clinical value of the tetracyclines and the number of functional groups capable of modification, many have been synthesized in attempts to obtain maximum antibiotic activity and blood levels, modified absorption excretion patterns and improved chemical stability (Blackwood & English 1970). At least eight tetracyclines are produced commercially of which half are obtained by chemical modifications of fermentation products. The most important at the present are chlortetracycline, oxytetracycline, tetracycline, demethylchlortetracycline, doxycycline and methacycline.

CHLORTETRACYCLINE

The first member of this group to be isolated was chlortetracycline in 1948 from *Streptomyces aureofaciens*. Its structure was established shortly after Woodward elucidated that of oxytetracycline in 1953. Chlortetracycline hydrochloride is a yellow crystalline solid which is assayed biologically against *B.pumilus* and is usually administered orally in capsules.

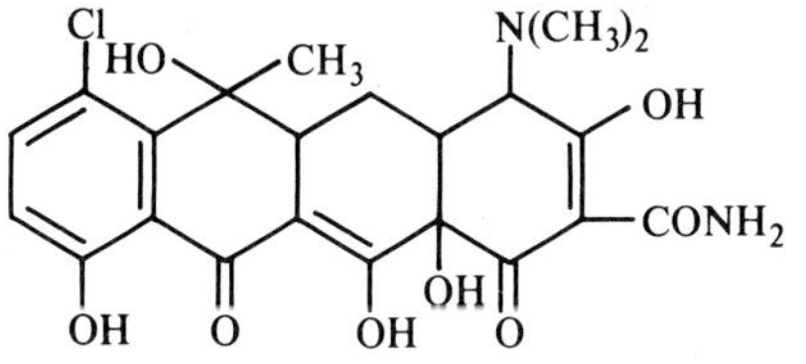

Chlortetracycline

OXYTETRACYCLINE

Oxytetracycline was isolated in 1950 from the soil organism *Streptomyces rimosus*. As may be seen it differs from chlortetracycline in the absence of a chlorine and the presence of an additional hydroxyl group. The total synthesis of DL-oxytetracycline has been performed by Muxfeldt and the product shown to possess 50 per cent of the biological activity of the natural, optically active, material (Muxfeldt et al. 1968).

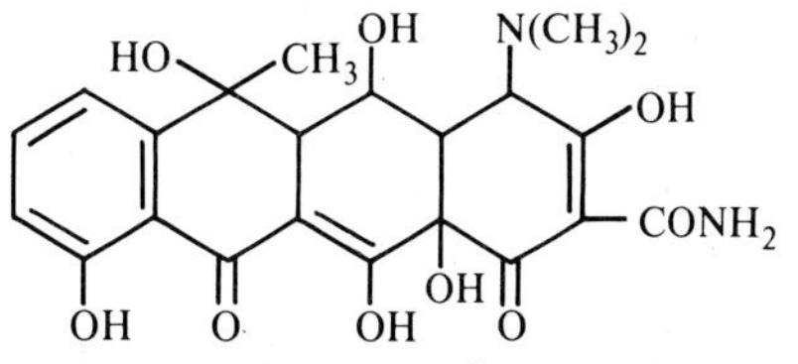

Oxytetracycline

Oxytetracyline is used as its hydrochloride in injections and capsules and as the less soluble dihydrate of the free base in tablets.

TETRACYCLINE

Tetracycline was originally prepared by hydrogenolysis of chlortetracycline or later from oxytetracycline. More recently mutant strains of *Streptomyces* have been isolated which produce tetracycline directly. The antibacterial spectrum of tetracycline is similar to the 'chloro' and 'oxy' derivatives but it is better absorbed orally. Tetracycline hydrochloride is administered orally or by injection.

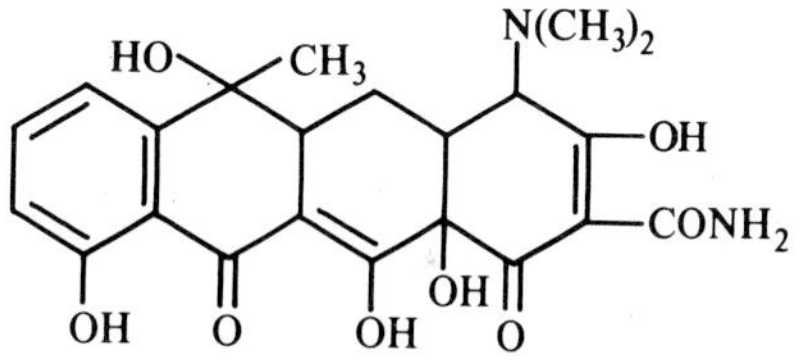

Tetracycline

DEMETHYLCHLORTETRACYCLINE

This antibiotic was isolated in 1957 from a mutant strain of *Streptomyces aureofaciens* and its structure was soon established by degradation and comparison of its ultraviolet spectrum with that of chlortetracycline.

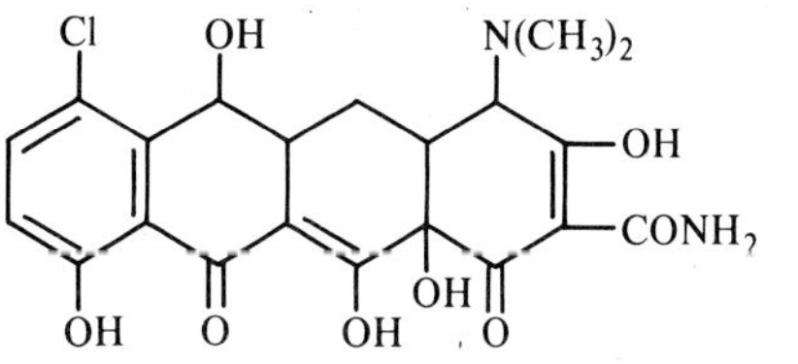

Demethylchlortetracycline

DOXYCYCLINE

Chemical modification of oxytetracycline or methacycline yields doxycycline (α-6-deoxytetracycline) which is more active against most bacteria than tetracycline and in addition is well absorbed orally with a prolonged serum half-life.

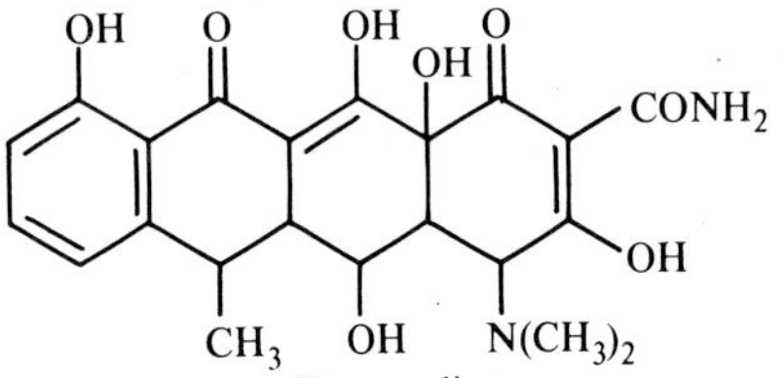

Doxycycline

METHACYCLINE

Methacycline is prepared synthetically from oxytetracycline, its activity and absorption characteristics are similar to those of demethylchlortetracycline with slightly higher blood levels during the first eight hours after administration.

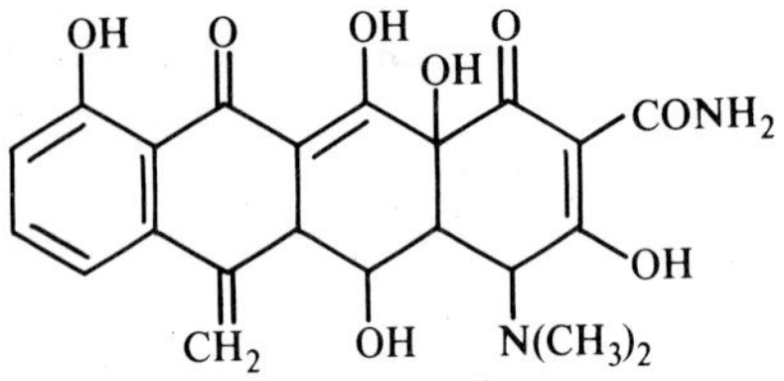

Methacycline

Methacycline is official as its hydrochloride and is administered in capsules.

Applications of the Tetracyclines
The tetracyclines as a group are of considerable value by virtue of their activity against a wide range of Gram-positive and Gram-negative bacteria, rickettsiae, actinomycetes, spirochaetes and the psittacosis virus. The various members differ slightly in their pharmacological properties but all have a low toxicity and are well absorbed orally. They are used particularly for the treatment of brucellosis, chronic bronchitis and other respiratory infections.

Forms of the Tetracyclines
Chlortetracycline. Hydrochloride, capsules.

Oxytetracycline. Hydrochloride for injection and in capsules. The dihydrate of the free base in tablets.

Tetracycline. Hydrochloride capsules, tablets and for injection.

Demethylchlortetracycline. Hydrochloride, capsules.

Doxycycline. Hemihydrate, hemiethanolate of the hydrochloride, capsules.

Methacycline. Hydrochloride, capsules.

ERYTHROMYCIN

This antibiotic, discovered in 1952, is prepared by the fermentation of the soil organism *Streptomyces erythreus*. It is a basic compound consisting of three linked units, a basic sugar, desosamine; a neutral sugar, cladinose; and a large ring lactone, erythronolide.

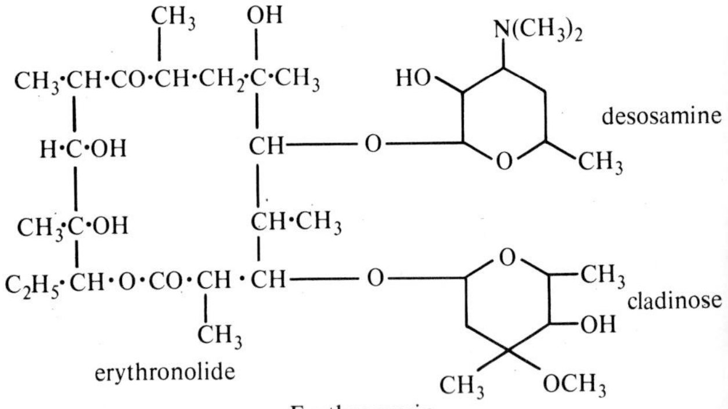

Erythromycin

Erythromycin is a crystalline compound with a bitter taste, only slightly soluble in water, and activity rapidly destroyed at a low pH. In order to overcome the flavour problem and improve absorption by delaying attack by gastric acid, the hydroxyl group in the desosamine ring can be esterified to give the stearate, propionate or estolate (the lauryl sulphate salt of the latter). Water-soluble salts for injection are obtained with glucoheptonic or lactobionic acids.

Applications of Erythromycin
Erythromycin is an antibiotic of low toxicity with an antibacterial spectrum similar to benzylpenicillin. It is active against many Gram-positive and some Gram-negative bacteria such as *Neisseria*, *Haemophilus* and *Brucella* strains; also some activity against *Rickettsia*. It was particularly valuable before the advent of penicillinase resistant penicillin, since it is unaffected by this enzyme. Erythromycin is usually administered orally: for parenteral use a soluble salt is used.

Forms of Erythromycin
Erythromycin tablets, erythromycin stearate tablets, erythromycin estolate capsules.

NOVOBIOCIN

Novobiocin has at various times been isolated from several different strains of streptomycetes and is now prepared from *Streptomyces niveus*. Novobiocin has been shown to consist of a coumarin linked to a substituted benzoic acid and a neutral nitrogen containing sugar.

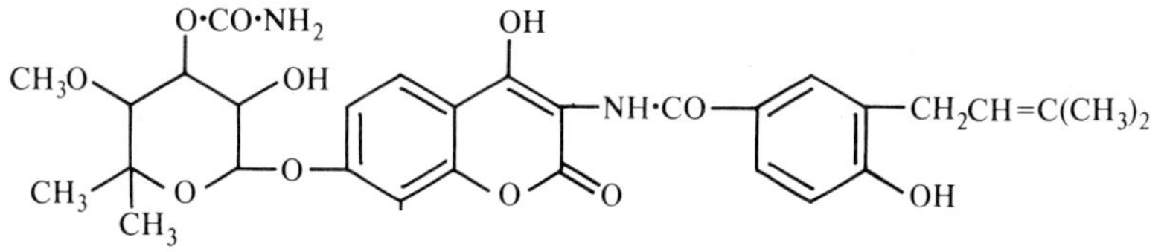

Novobiocin

The hydroxyl group in the coumarin portion of the molecule is acidic and gives salts with strong bases such as sodium or calcium which are used in tablet formulations. Novobiocin is well absorbed orally and is well tolerated and has been used in the treatment of infections due to Gram-positive bacteria resistant to other antibiotics.

FUSIDIC ACID

Fusidic acid was isolated in 1962 from a strain of *Fusidium coccineum* found in monkey droppings in Japan. The structure of fusidic acid is unusual in that antibiotic activity is rarely associated with steroids or triterpenes although recently the antibiotics cephalosporin P_1 and helvolic acid have been shown to possess similar structures.

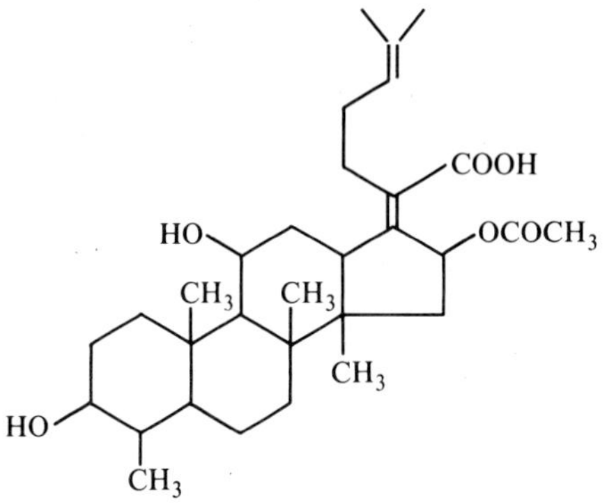

Fusidic acid

Fusidic acid is sparingly soluble in water but the crystalline sodium salt is readily soluble and is administered in capsules.

Applications of Fusidic Acid
Fusidic acid is active against Gram-negative cocci and Gram-positive bacteria particularly *Staphylococcus aureus*. It is of low toxicity, well absorbed orally and has been principally used for treatment of severe staphylococcal infections.

GRISEOFULVIN

Griseofulvin was isolated in 1939 from the mycelium of *Penicillium griseofulvum* and has been used clinically since 1958. It is now prepared commercially by deep fermentation of *Penicillium patulum*.

Griseofulvin is a spiran and its structure has been established by degradation, X-ray diffraction studies and synthesis. Many analogues have also been synthesized but none has so far proved superior to griseofulvin against dermatophytes.

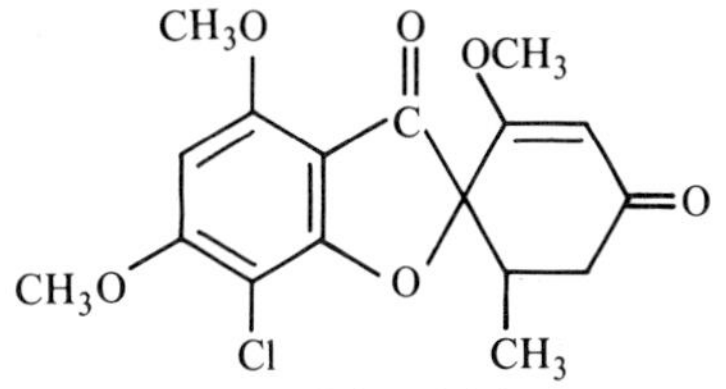

Griseofulvin

Griseofulvin is only very slightly soluble in water and in order to ensure absorption when given orally, it is essential for the material to be very finely divided, the *British Pharmacopoeia* requires a particle size of less than 5 μm.

Applications of Griseofulvin
Griseofulvin has no antibacterial action but it is very active against the dermatophytes that affect animal and human hair, nail and skin such as *Microsporum audouini*, *Trichophyton rubrum* and *Trichophyton mentagrophytes*. It is administered orally in tablets.

Assay of Griseofulvin
Griseofulvin is assayed photometrically at a wavelength of 291 nm.

LINCOMYCIN

Lincomycin was isolated in 1962 from cultures of *Streptomyces lincolnensis* var. *lincolnensis*. Chemical degradation to *trans*-1-methyl-4-*n*-propyl-L-proline, D-allothreonine and D-galactose has indicated the structure shown below, which has been confirmed by synthesis.

Lincomycin is a basic antibiotic forming a readily water-soluble hydrochloride which is used orally and parenterally. The hydrochloride monohydrate is official in capsules and injection.

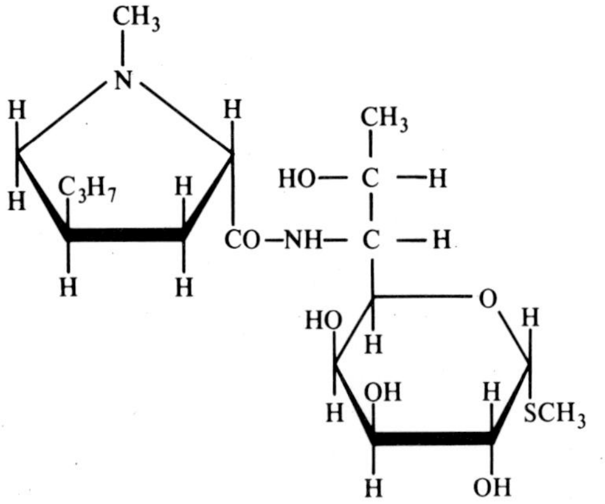

Lincomycin

Applications of Lincomycin

Lincomycin resembles erythromycin in its activity against Gram-positive organisms, particularly the haemolytic streptococci, pneumococci and staphylococci including those producing penicillinase. It is readily absorbed orally with a low toxicity and is generally used where benzylpenicillin is contraindicated.

CLINDAMYCIN

Modification of lincomycin by the insertion of chlorine into the allothreonine moiety has yielded clindamycin (7-chloro-7-deoxylincomycin) which is considerably more active than the parent compound against staphylococci and pneumococci and of at least comparable activity against other sensitive species. The compound is well absorbed orally and is administered as the hydrochloride hydrate in capsules, as the palmitate ester hydrochloride in syrup formulations and as the phosphate for parenteral use.

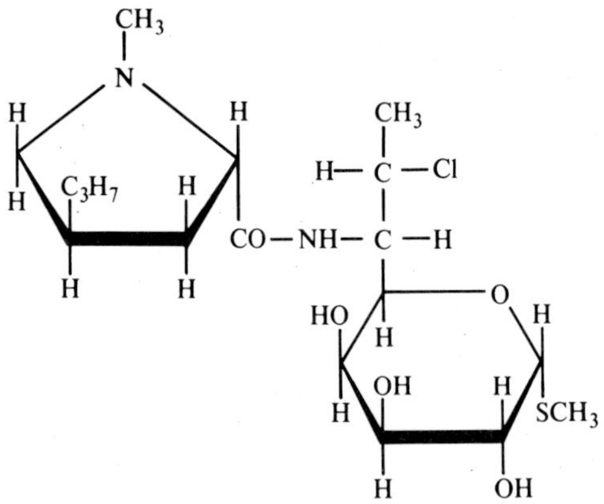

Clindamycin

VANCOMYCIN

Vancomycin was isolated in 1955 from *Streptomyces orientalis*. It is an amphoteric substance but little is known of its structure. Hydrolysis yields a number of amino acids, glucose and a compound containing chlorinated phenyl residues.

Applications of Vancomycin

Vancomycin is bactericidal to many Gram-positive cocci, including *Staphylococcus aureus*, by inhibition of bacterial cell wall biosynthesis. It is not absorbed orally and on intramuscular injection it tends to produce pain and necrosis, hence it is usually administered intravenously. It is mainly used for the treatment of septicaemia caused by staphylococci or streptococci resistant to other antibiotics.

Vancomycin is administered as its hydrochloride (official).

RIFAMPICIN

In 1959 rifamycin B was isolated from a culture of *Streptomyces mediterranei*, it was active against Gram-positive bacteria, *Mycobacterium tuberculosis* and some Gram-negative organisms. The compound was poorly absorbed from the alimentary tract and caused local irritation when injected. In addition, its solution was unstable, increasing in potency on storage. It was established that this change was due to oxidation and hydrolysis to give a quinonoid compound, rifamycin S, which could be reduced with ascorbic acid to the phenolic rifamycin SV. This compound was more active and less toxic than the parent. Over 400 semi-synthetic rifamycins have been prepared by chemical modification in order to obtain optimal activity and oral absorption. A Mannich reaction between rifamycin S, formaldehyde and dimethylamine followed by ascorbic acid reduction yields the 3-dimethylaminomethyl derivative of rifamycin SV [$R^1 \equiv H$, $R^2 \equiv -CH_2N(CH_3)_2$] from which the aldehyde [$R^1 \equiv H$, $R^2 \equiv -CHO$] is obtained by oxidation. The orally absorbed hydrazone, rifampicin, is obtained by reaction of the aldehyde with 1-amino-4-methyl-piperazine.

Rifampicin acts as an antibiotic by blocking the initiation of ribonucleic acid synthesis, and because of this the compound is also active against various pox and adenoviruses.

Applications of Rifampicin

Rifampicin is well absorbed orally and is used for the treatment of tuberculosis, respiratory, urinary tract and Gram-positive infections.

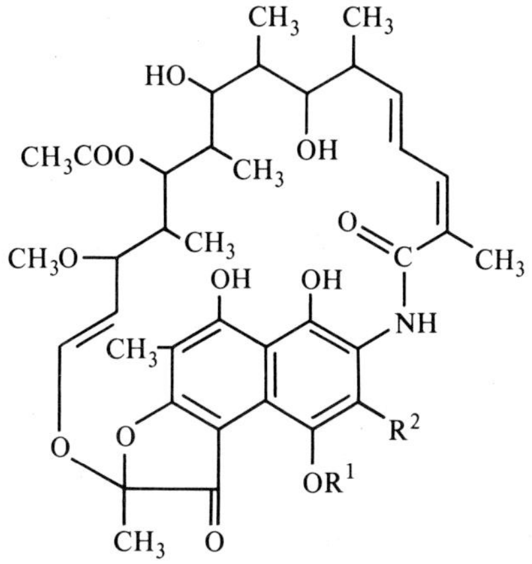

Rifamycin B	$R^1 \equiv CH_2COOH$
	$R^2 \equiv H$
Rifamycin SV	$R^1 \equiv R^2 \equiv H$
Rifampicin	$R^1 \equiv H$
	$R^2 \equiv -CH=N-N\bigcirc N-CH_3$ 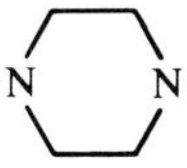

The rifamycins

REFERENCES

ABRAHAM, E. P. (1967) *Q. Rev.* **21**, 231.

BARRETT, G. C. (1963) *J. pharm. Sci.* **52**, 309.

BATCHELOR, F. R. et al. (1959) *Nature, Lond.* **183**, 257.

BLACKWOOD, R. B. & ENGLISH, A. R. (1970) *Adv. appl. Microbiol.* **13**, 237.

CELMER, W. D. (1966) *Antimicrobial Agents and Chemotherapy*—1965, 144.

CHILDRESS, S. J. (1967) *Topics med. Chem.* **1**, 109.

CLIVE, D. L. J. (1968) *Q. Rev.* **22**, 435.

DOYLE, F. P. & NAYLER, J. H. C. (1964) *Adv. Drug Res.* **1**, 1.

FLEMING, A. (1929) *Br. J. exp. Path.* **10**, 226.

GROVE, J. F. (1963) *Q. Rev.* **17**, 1.

HOCKENHULL, D. J. (1960) *Progr. indust. Microbiol.* **2**, 131.

MUXFELDT, H. et al. (1968) *J. Am. Chem. Soc.*

UMEZAWA, S. et al. (1969) *Bull. Chem. Soc. Japan*, **42**, 529.

WILKINSON, S. (1967) *Antimicrobial Agents and Chemotherapy*, 651.

FURTHER READING

CAIN, C. K. (Ed.) (1965 and onwards) *Annual Reports in Medicinal Chemistry*. Academic Press, New York.

CLARKE, H. T., JOHNSON, J. R. & ROBINSON, R. (1949) *The Chemistry of Penicillin*. Princeton: Princeton University Press.

EVANS, R. M. (1965) *The Chemistry of the Antibiotics Used in Medicine*. Oxford: Pergamon Press.

FLYNN, E. H. (1972) *Cephalosporins and Penicillins, Chemistry and Biology*. New York: Academic Press.

GARROD, L. P. & O'GRADY, F. (1971) *Antibiotics and Chemotherapy*. Edinburgh: Livingstone.

KORZYBSKI, T., KOWSZYK-GINDIFER, Z. & KURYLOWICZ, W. (1967) *Antibiotics, Origin, Nature, Properties*, Vols I and II. Oxford: Pergamon Press.

KUCERS, A. (1972) *The Use of Antibiotics* (*A Comprehensive Review with Clinical Emphasis*). Philadelphia: J. B. Lippincott.

SOCIETY OF CHEMICAL INDUSTRY (1965, 1967) *Reports on the Progress of Applied Chemistry*. London: Society of Chemical Industry.

STEEL, R. (1958) *Biochemical Engineering*. London: Heywood & Co.

UMEZAWA, H. (1967) *Index of Antibiotics from Actinomycetes*. Tokyo: University of Tokyo Press.

35

Blood Products and Plasma Substitutes

While blood may in many respects be regarded as a 'therapeutic substance', and is listed in its alphabetical position in the *British Pharmacopoeia*, it has, relative to other entries, certain unique properties. These derive from the fact that the red blood corpuscles are living cells. They are not capable of growth and reproduction but they contain a complex intracellular structure and a multiplicity of enzymes and enzyme systems. If, after transfusion, the corpuscles are to perform their basic physiological role of oxygen transport, it is necessary that their structural and functional integrity should be maintained. Because of this, and other related factors the collection and preservation of blood presents considerable problems, and its administration involves risks to the patient which cannot be completely eliminated. These risks fall into four categories.

Deterioration during Storage

Red cells may be damaged or haemolysed by exposure to heat, by freezing, by excessive agitation, by hypertonic or hypotonic solutions, by incorrect environmental pH, or by storage beyond the specified dating period. Incorrect collection procedures may cause clotting of the blood. In normal circumstances some small clots may be present, and blood must always be administered through a suitably designed 'giving' or 'recipient' set (as defined in British Standard 2463: 1962, Transfusion Equipment for Medical Use). This type of set includes a filter with a large surface area, which will remove clots, but will not easily be blocked during the transfusion.

Bacterial Contamination

Blood cannot be sterilized by heat or by chemical agents without causing irreparable damage to the red cells and plasma proteins; nor can it be sterilized by filtration. The prevention of bacterial contamination of whole blood prepared for transfusion therefore depends upon the use of properly sterilized equipment, a meticulous technique of collection, and storage at 4° to 6° at all times, including transportation. Even when thus collected a small proportion of donations contain a few viable organisms derived from the donor's skin. With few exceptions these die out, or are prevented from proliferating to a dangerous level by storage at 4° to 6°. Rarely, blood may be contaminated by cryophilic Gram-negative organisms which grow at 4°, usually without causing macroscopic changes. Depending on the number of organisms present, transfusion of such blood may cause a mild, severe or rapidly fatal reaction.

Transmission of Disease from the Donor

Certain diseases, for example syphilis, malaria and hepatitis, can be transmitted by blood transfusion. A serological test for syphilis is always made, but a negative test is not a complete safeguard. Apart from this test, whether or not a donor is free of disease transmissible by transfusion is decided from his medical history. The greatest risk is that of transmitting hepatitis B (serum hepatitis), a serious illness with a significant mortality rate. It has been found that a high proportion of hepatitis carriers can be identified by the presence in their blood of hepatitis B surface antigen (previously termed Australia antigen), which can be detected by immunological tests (Prince 1968; Blumberg et al. 1969; Ling & Overby 1972; Reesink et al. 1973; Cayser et al. 1974). All blood donations are now screened by such tests. The number of symptomless donors in the U.K. who carry the antigen is estimated to be about 0.1 per cent.

Sensitization to Blood Group Antigens

The transfusion of blood has been described as a kind of homograft, that is, the transfer of living tissue from one individual to another. As with other homografts the body may react to the introduction of the foreign tissue. Antibodies develop in the plasma, which reject red cells of the type introduced, by reacting with antigens on the cell surfaces. In the case of the ABO blood group antigens, isoantibodies are present in the blood even when there has been no previous transfusion of blood, and will react with cells of the wrong group if these are transfused.

The rejection reaction caused by the action of antibodies on red cells results in intravascular agglutination, lysis or disruption of the cells transfused, and may have a serious or fatal effect on the patient. Therefore, before blood is used, it is tested and labelled according to its blood group; the patient is grouped and blood of the appropriate group selected; as a further check, a compatibility test is performed, i.e. the cells to be transfused are tested against the patient's serum to confirm that it contains no antibodies that will agglutinate or lyse the cells. In order to avoid blood of the wrong group being transfused in error, it is necessary to maintain an elaborate system of labelling, record-keeping and cross-checks.

On account of the risks attaching to the use of blood, and of the consequent legal implications, the supervision of a hospital blood bank and of associated laboratory work should always be the direct responsibility of a pathologist fully trained in haematology. Responsibility for the storage and issue of blood (and of plasma and plasma fractions should not be given to or accepted by pharmacies.

Bleeding. To obtain blood, an area of the donor's arm over the antecubital vein is thoroughly cleansed and swabbed with an antiseptic solution. A local anaesthetic is then injected, and the sterile needle of a blood donor set is inserted in the vein. The needle connects, via the tubing of the set, to a bottle or plastic bag containing 2.0 to 2.5 g

disodium hydrogen citrate, 3 g dextrose and water to 120 ml (acid-citrate–dextrose or 'ACD' anticoagulant). Volumes of 420 ml of blood are usually collected, with appropriate mixing with the solution in the container, and two samples are taken, one for syphilis and blood group tests before the blood is issued, and one for the 'compatibility' test which is made before the blood is given to a particular patient. The citrate, by binding calcium ions, prevents the clotting of the blood which would otherwise occur within a few minutes of collection. Dextrose preserves red cells, increasing their 'life' in storage from 4 to 7 days in citrate alone, to 21 days in ACD. Other anticoagulants are also, for example, citrate phosphate dextrose (CPD).

On standing, the cells sediment to form a dark red layer occupying about half the fluid volume, with a yellowish layer of plasma above. The latter may be clear or cloudy depending on the amount of lipid ingested by the donor in his meals before giving blood. Blood which is contaminated, or haemolysed through improper storage, may be visibly abnormal and a careful inspection should always be made before blood is given to a patient.

British Pharmacopoeia requirements for Whole Human Blood include the following:

1. That the blood is cooled to 4° to 6° immediately after withdrawal from the donor and is maintained at that temperature throughout its dating period of 21 days, except for short periods, not exceeding 30 min, which are necessary during transportation or testing.
2. That the haemoglobin concentration of blood–anticoagulant mixture is not less than 9.7 g/dl.
3. That the ABO blood group is determined by examination of both the corpuscles and the serum, and the Rh group by an examination of the corpuscles.
4. That the blood should meet the *British Pharmacopoeia* requirements for sterility testing. It is not practicable to test the sterility of the blood before it is transfused and the usual practice is to test a proportion of containers of blood older than 21 days as a check on the technique of collection and storage.
5. That the label should state the ABO and Rh groups, the volumes of blood and anticoagulant solution present, the date on which the blood was collected, the expiry date and required storage conditions, that the contents must not be used if there is any visible sign of deterioration, and a number or code by which the history of the preparation can be traced back to the original donor.

Uses. Whole Human Blood is transfused to replace red blood cells, clotting factors or other normal constituents partly or completely missing from the patient's blood, or to restore blood volume after acute haemorrhage.

For further information concerning the preparation, grouping, storage and use of Whole Human Blood see Bowley and Dunsford (1967), Mollison (1972).

CONCENTRATED HUMAN RED BLOOD CORPUSCLES BP

To obtain this preparation most of the upper plasma layer is removed from harvested blood in containers which have been left standing, or have been centrifuged. The quantity of fluid removed is not less than 40 per cent of the total volume. In the case of centrifuged blood, a certain amount of plasma is left so that the cell preparation is not too viscous for administration. The blood from which the concentrate is prepared meets the Pharmacopoeia requirements for Whole Human Blood and is not more than 14 days old. The haemoglobin concentration of the final preparation is not less than 15.5 per cent w/v.

Concentrated red cells from blood collected in glass bottles should be used within 12 h of preparation because of the risk of bacterial contamination during the separation of the plasma. The concentrate should be stored at 4° to 6° pending transfusion. Blood from each of the donors contributing to the concentrate must have been grouped and compatibility-tested against the blood of the intended recipient. Labelling requirements are generally similar to those for Whole Human Blood, but include in addition a statement of the date and time of removal of the plasma. Red cell concentrates are used principally in the treatment of anaemia.

CONCENTRATES OF PLATELETS AND WHITE BLOOD CORPUSCLES

By centrifugation under controlled conditions the red blood cells can be sedimented from fresh blood, leaving the platelets suspended in the supernatant plasma. The separated upper layer is used in treatment, or is recentrifuged at high speed and the resulting deposit suspended in a small volume of plasma, to give a highly concentrated platelet preparation. Such concentrates are used primarily to prevent haemorrhage in patients suffering from thrombocytopenia and to treat patients with leukaemia who are undergoing immunosuppressive therapy. White blood cell concentrates, similarly prepared, are not as yet in general use.

PLASTIC TRANSFUSION EQUIPMENT: PLASMAPHERESIS

In recent years disposable plastic blood bags or packs have become available and have some advantages over glass bottles. In the form of 'double' or 'triple' packs they are convenient for preparing separated blood components. The double pack consists of two bags, one fitted with a blood collecting tube and both with 'ports' for the insertion of a giving set. The two bags are joined by tubing. One bag contains standard ACD anticoagulant, in which the blood is collected. The complete double unit is then centrifuged. The connecting tube between the two bags is opened and a proportion of the upper plasma layer is expressed from the bag containing the blood into the empty one. The tubing is then sealed and cut, giving a unit of red cell concentrate and a unit of platelet-rich plasma. This plasma can be used as it is or processed further to give platelet concentrate and plasma. The latter can be utilized as such or fractionated.

A further application of plastics equipment is in the technique known as 'plasmapheresis', in which red cell concentrates prepared by the above procedure are returned to the donor, who thus has in effect donated plasma without any significant loss of his red cells. It has been found that healthy donors can give relatively large quantities of plasma, provided that red cells are not harvested at the same time; as much as one litre of plasma per week has been removed from a single donor over a period of years without untoward effect (Simson et al. 1966). This procedure can be applied to donors whose plasma has a high content of a protein of a particular therapeutic value, for example coagulation Factor VIII, anti-D antibody or tetanus antitoxin.

PLASMA, SERUM AND PLASMA FRACTIONS

During storage the red corpuscles progressively lose their capacity to survive in the circulation of the transfused recipient. When blood 21 days old is transfused approximately 70 per cent of the cells remain in the patient's circulation 24 hours later. Blood older than 21 days is thus not normally considered suitable for transfusion. However the plasma proteins are more stable and the normal procedure is to aspirate the plasma from the sedimented red cells of time-expired blood and to use it for therapeutic products. Freshly collected blood is centrifuged to provide fresh plasma for preparing certain labile components, which cannot be recovered in active form from time-expired blood.

It should be noted that plasma and certain fractions made from it, even when prepared, as is now the practice, from blood screened for hepatitis B surface antigen, may carry the virus of hepatitis B (Berg et al. 1972). They should thus be used only when the benefit likely to accrue to the patient outweighs the risk of transmitting heptatitis. These fractions should not be transfused merely as a vehicle for administering a drug or other substance. Dried plasma and serum are being replaced as volume expanders by albumin preparations which do not carry this risk (see below).

Proteins are complex macromolecules and are easily damaged or 'denatured' by exposure to heat, so that storage requirements must be strictly observed. Because of their instability in solution some protein-containing products are issued as a freeze-dried powder, sealed in presence of dry nitrogen. Such preparations are hygroscopic and may become unstable or insoluble if moisture gains access, for example through a loose or faulty seal.

The *British Pharmacopoeia* contains sections relating to plasma, serum and plasma fractions, and should be consulted for detailed specifications. Requirements are laid down with respect to sterility, identity, freedom from pyrogens, total protein content, electrolyte content, the presence of preservatives and stabilizers, and, in the case of freeze-dried preparations, solubility and residual moisture content. In addition special requirements for individual plasma proteins define required protein composition, as determined by electrophoretic analysis or other procedures. General labelling requirements apply to these products. The label must include: (i) the correct name of the product; (ii) an identifying batch number; (iii) information concerning potency or concentration; (iv) name and address of manufacturer or authorized distributor; (v) date of manufacture; (vi) expiry date; (vii) required storage conditions; and (viii) nature and concentration of any added bacteriostatic agent. Any additional labelling requirements are given below.

Products used in blood volume replacement therapy, including plasma, human albumin preparations and solutions of various substances used as plasma substitutes have been reviewed by Gruber (1969).

DRIED HUMAN PLASMA BP

The plasma of some donors contains haemagglutinating antibodies of the ABO system which on transfusion into patients of certain blood groups may cause intravascular agglutination and haemolysis. This risk can be avoided by neutralization of the haemagglutinins with the soluble blood group substances present in the plasma of other donors of appropriate blood groups. Plasma is pooled from donations of blood selected so that the normal distribution of ABO groups is represented; thus a ten-donor pool contains plasma from about equal numbers of A and O donations, together with at least one B or AB donation.

It was shown many years ago that when plasma pools were restricted to ten donors the risk of transmitting hepatitis B was low; such 'small-pool plasma' is issued for use in this country, the risk of transmitting hepatitis being about one in 500 patients transfused. Attempts to inactivate the virus with ultraviolet irradiation or with β-propiolactone have been unsuccessful. A combination of ultraviolet irradiation and β-propiolactone inactivates the agent, but plasma so treated shows electrophoretic and other abnormalities.

Plasma is difficult to filter and it is not practicable to sterilize large numbers of small pools by filtration. As whole blood cannot be assumed to be sterile it is therefore necessary to test each ten-donor pool for sterility. Pools which have passed these tests are then redistributed in transfusion bottles in quantities suitable for freeze-drying (Greaves 1946). The dried plasma is a light to deep cream-coloured powder, free from streaks of red or pink indicative of red cells or haemoglobin. It is reconstituted to the original volume with Water for Injection at room temperature and dissolves completely in less than 10 min to give a cloudy solution. The protein content is not less than 45 g/l. Addition of 17 g/l calcium chloride to 1 ml should cause coagulation, demonstrating the presence of fibrinogen.

Storage. Under dry conditions; below 50°; protected from light.

Labelling. In addition to general requirements the label states: (i) the names and percentages of anticoagulant and other added substances; (ii) the quantity of Water for Injections required to reconstitute to the original volume; (iii) the protein content of the reconstituted liquid; and (iv) that the contents must not be used more than 3 h after reconstitution.

Uses. For the restoration of plasma volume in patients suffering from burns, scalds or crush injury.

In emergencies, to restore blood volume when whole blood is not available or while awaiting the results of compatibility tests. In an emergency, when fibrinogen concentrate (see below) is not available, dried plasma, reconstituted to one third or one quarter of the original volume, may be used in the treatment of acute fibrinogen deficiency. The dried residue from 400 ml plasma contains about 1 g fibrinogen. Dried plasma prepared from time-expired blood does not contain useful amounts of labile clotting factors such as Factor V and VIII.

FRESH FROZEN PLASMA

Plasma prepared by centrifugation from Whole Human Blood within a few hours of its collection from the donor is stored in the frozen state, preferably below $-30°$. If it is not pooled it must be labelled, and used, according to the stated blood group. For use the plasma is thawed by immersion in a water bath at a temperature not exceeding $37°$; thawing takes about 45 min.

Uses. In fresh frozen plasma labile clotting factors are preserved. It is used, in particular, as a source of Factor VIII for treating minor haemorrhage in mildly affected haemophiliacs.

DRIED HUMAN SERUM, BP

Blood collected without the addition of an anti-coagulant from donors who meet the requirements specified for Whole Human Blood is allowed to clot, and the separated fluid pooled, bottled and freeze-dried. The ratio of blood groups in the pool, and the pool size, are as for Dried Human Plasma, and all other requirements are identical with those for this product, with the exceptions that the protein content must not be less than 65 g/l, and that the test for coagulation with calcium chloride does not apply. Its uses are similar to those of dried plasma, except that it cannot be used as a source of fibrinogen.

THE FRACTIONATION OF PLASMA

By precipitation, individual protein components of human plasma can be separated from each other and prepared in concentrated form for use in the prophylaxis or treatment of certain conditions. The principal preparations of this type are concentrates of blood coagulation factors, concentrates of the plasma antibodies or immunoglobulins, and albumin preparations.

The fractionation procedures used make use of the following facts: (i) proteins are selectively precipitated from solutions without denaturation by the addition of organic solvents such as diethyl ether or ethanol, provided there is efficient mixing and the temperature is maintained at or below $0°$; (ii) the different proteins are minimally soluble at different pH values; and (iii) solubility in presence of organic solvents is differentially affected by variations in the salt concentration. In a series of precipitation steps in which these factors are carefully controlled, various components are separated from a single pool of plasma. At each stage the precipitate is separated by centrifugation. If reproducible separations are to be obtained, precise control must be maintained throughout over temperatures of solutions, protein concentrations, rates of addition of reagents, stirring speeds, equilibration times, and centrifugation speeds and temperatures.

The final sedimented paste of proteins containing the desired component in concentrated form is dissolved in a suitable solvent, the composition of which is carefully controlled with respect to pH and salt content. The solutions obtained are usually at this stage sterilized by filtration and freeze-dried. Freeze-drying removes residual organic solvent, and gives a stable product, suitable for storage and transport. Immunoglobulin and albumin are however sufficiently stable to be dispensed in solution, which is prepared by redissolving the freeze-dried material, adjusting the protein concentration to the desired value, filtering and bottling.

For the preparation of the more labile coagulation factors it is necessary to start with fresh plasma, separated from blood within a few hours of collection, and to complete the fractionation without delay.

At all stages precautions must be taken to prevent bacterial contamination, the introduction of pyrogens, and denaturation of protein. In the case of some fractions large volumes may be administered intravenously, and it is essential that the solutions are free from pyrogens, toxic substances, particulate matter and biological material from non-human sources.

In addition to routine tests for sterility, pyrogenicity, identity, solubility, protein and moisture contents, the quality of the plasma protein fractions is controlled by: (i) electrophoretic, immunoelectrophoretic, ultracentrifugal and chromatographic analysis; (ii) assay of specific activities, such as coagulation factor or antibody activity; and (iii) tests of heat stability.

The scheme for the fractionation of plasma by ethanol was originally developed in the United

States by Cohn and his co-workers (Cohn et al. 1946; Oncley et al. 1949) and that by ether by Kekwick and Mackay (1954) in the U.K. The ethanol fractions obtained are sometimes called Cohn fractions, e.g. Cohn Fraction I. In many laboratories a simpler modification of the original procedure, first described by Deutsch et al. (1946), and later applied on a large scale by Kistler and Nitschmann (1962), is now used. The properties of human plasma proteins, and methods for their fractionation have been reviewed by Schultze and Heremans (1966).

COAGULATION FACTORS

Shed blood clots because of the polymerization of fibrinogen, a soluble plasma protein with a molecular weight of 340 000. The fibrinogen molecules are elongated, and when clotting occurs they interact irreversibly to form a three-dimensional network of a semi-solid polymer, called fibrin. The polymerization of fibrinogen is brought about by the action of an enzyme, thrombin, which in turn results from the activation of prothrombin, another high molecular weight substance present in human plasma.

Substances liberated from damaged tissues, or exposure of blood to 'foreign' surfaces initiate a complex series of reactions which leads ultimately to the activation of prothrombin to thrombin. These reactions require the presence of platelets, calcium, and a number of plasma factors, which are proteins. They are designated Factors V, VII, VIII, IX, X, XI and XII. In a number of hereditary, congenital or acquired conditions, a deficiency of one of these factors may occur, resulting in impaired clotting function and a tendency to bleeding. Concentrates of some of these factors can now be prepared, and are used to arrest haemorrhage or to prevent it when surgery is necessary in patients with such deficiencies. The products available are fibrinogen and Factor VIII concentrates; concentrates of Factors II (prothrombin), VII, IX and X are at present under development. Preparations of thrombin and fibrinogen derivatives are made for use as local haemostatic agents (see Biggs & Macfarlane 1966; Biggs 1972).

DRIED HUMAN FIBRINOGEN, BP

Fibrinogen is one of the least soluble of the plasma proteins and is precipitated when ethanol is added to plasma at 0° and neutral pH to give a final concentration of 8 per cent v/v. After further purification, the fraction, obtained in the form of a centrifuged deposit, is dissolved in a citrate-saline solution. The citrate binds calcium ions and prevents spontaneous clotting of the product. The solution is freeze-dried, yielding a white powder or friable solid.

To reconstitute for use, the stated volume of Water for Injection at not less than 15° is added to the container and the contents mixed gently so as to avoid frothing. Solution is slow. The cloudy solution obtained after 15 to 30 min contains between 10 and 15 g/l of fibrinogen, and the fibrinogen comprises at least 70 per cent of the total protein present. The fibrinogen content is determined by adding thrombin to a known volume of solution and measuring the protein content of the separated and washed clot. The electrophoretic mobility of the main component in aqueous phosphate buffer at pH 8.0 lies between that of human β- and γ-globulin.

Storage. Under dry conditions; protected from light; below 25°.

Labelling. Additional to general requirements: (i) the amounts of fibrinogen clottable by thrombin, of sodium chloride and of sodium citrate contained in it; (ii) the quantity of Water for Injection required for reconstitution; (iii) that it be used immediately after reconstitution; and (iv) that it be administered through a recipient set fitted with a filter.

Uses. For the treatment of fibrinogen deficiency, particularly that associated with pregnancy. In conjunction with thrombin it may be used to repair severed nerves and to aid the adhesion of grafts.

Fibrinogen may transmit hepatitis B.

RADIO-IODINATED HUMAN FIBRINOGEN

Human fibrinogen which meets the BP requirements for clinical use, and also certain other requirements relating to stability, is labelled with the radioactive isotope ^{125}I or ^{131}I. It is an aid to the diagnosis of deep-vein thrombosis by external monitoring. Such fibrinogen is prepared from the blood of donors specially selected and tested to reduce the risk of transmitting hepatitis B.

CONCENTRATES OF HUMAN COAGULATION FACTOR VIII (ANTIHAEMOPHILIC FACTOR)

Clotting Factor VIII is absent or deficient in the blood of persons suffering from haemophilia A, i.e. haemophiliacs or 'bleeders'. Concentrates of the missing protein are prepared from pooled normal plasma: Kekwick and Wolf (1957) have described an ether-fractionated, and Blombäck et al. (1958) and Jorpes et al. (1962) an ethanol-fractionated material. A glycine precipitated fraction is also made (Webster et al. 1965).

The product is a freeze-dried protein, white in colour. On reconstitution its activity is at least three times that of fresh liquid plasma. Its protein composition is similar to that of human fibrinogen, fibrinogen being the principal constituent, and Factor VIII a trace component. Quality is controlled by assay of Factor VIII, and of total and clottable protein. Temperature requirements for storage have not yet been fully established. For prolonged storage of the dried product a temperature below $-20°$ is desirable. However for some weeks a temperature of $4°$ to $6°$ is safe, and the product can be transported unrefrigerated. Reconstitution is in Water for Injections at $20°$ to $30°$ and may be slow. The solution should be transfused without delay as activity may be lost on standing. The product is normally available only for specialized teams which have facilities for assaying Factor VIII in the patient's blood and in the products transfused.

Factor VIII concentrates may transmit hepatitis B.

Recent papers have described large scale procedures and the preparation of concentrates which can be given in small volumes by syringe (Brinkhous et al. 1968; Newman et al. 1971; Wickerhauser 1971).

HUMAN PLASMA CRYOPRECIPITATE

A protein fraction containing Factor VIII is obtained by freezing fresh plasma and then thawing it under controlled conditions (Pool & Shannon 1965). Plasma proteins which are sparingly soluble in the cold separate during thawing; these contain much of the Factor VIII. Products prepared in this way are now widely used. Because of the simplicity of preparation the cryoprecipitate can be made in transfusion centres and blood banks without highly specialized facilities. After separation from the supernatant plasma, the cryoprecipitate, suspended in a small amount of plasma, is frozen and stored at $-30°$. It is possible to recover red cell concentrates at the same time and the residual plasma can be used for the preparation of other therapeutic protein fractions.

FACTOR VIII CONCENTRATE DERIVED FROM ANIMAL PLASMA

Concentrates of Factor VIII made from bovine or porcine plasma are commercially available. They are prepared by methods similar to those used for the human fractions and are distributed freeze-dried in ampoules (Bidwell 1955). Because of the high content of Factor VIII in bovine and porcine plasma, concentrates with a very high specific activity can be prepared but they have the serious disadvantage that, after a limited period of treatment, the recipient becomes sensitized to the foreign protein and cannot thereafter be given the preparation concerned. The use of these animal products is thus confined to circumstances in which they are deemed to be life-saving. Like the human fractions, they are labile and expensive, and their use should be controlled by assays carried out on the patient's blood during treatment.

CONCENTRATES OF HUMAN COAGULATION FACTORS II, VII, IX AND X*

Concentrates containing these factors are prepared (Bidwell et al. 1967; Dike et al. 1972) and are generally available for patients with congenital absence of Factor IX (Christmas disease). Soulier et al. (1964) in France have made a similar product, as have Wickerhauser and Sgouris (1972) in the USA.

It should be noted that patients with a deficiency of Factor IX cannot be treated successfully with concentrates of human or animal Factor VIII. Specific concentrates should not therefore be used in patients with a bleeding tendency until the diagnosis has been confirmed by laboratory investigation.

DRIED HUMAN THROMBIN, BP

The active enzyme thrombin is prepared from a prothrombin-containing protein fraction precipitated from fresh plasma by organic solvents. The prothrombin is then activated by human tissue thromboplastin in the presence of calcium ions. The solution is clarified, sterilized by filtration and dried from the frozen state. The potency of the fraction is defined in terms of 'clotting doses', or 'units', one unit being the quantity of thrombin required to produce a visible clot in 1 ml of 1.0 g/l saline solution of fibrinogen at pH 7.2 in 15 s at $37°$.

Storage. Under dry conditions; protected from light; below $20°$.

Labelling. Besides general requirements; the number of clotting doses present.

---

* Synonyms: II = prothrombin; VII = stable factor; IX = Christmas factor or antihaemophilic factor B; X = Stuart-Prower factor.

Use. Thrombin has a limited use as a local haemostatic agent, usually applied by impregnating fibrin or other foam that is absorbed by the tissues, with the solution obtained by reconstituting the dried product.

Thrombin must not be injected intravenously; the label normally bears the words Do Not Inject in bold type. The product must be carefully distinguished from prothrombin-containing preparations intended for intravenous use. Thrombin may transmit hepatitis B.

HUMAN FIBRIN FOAM

To prepare this material thrombin is added to a solution of fibrinogen and the mixture immediately and rapidly made to foam. The semi-solid foam of fibrin is then freeze-dried; and the freeze-dried material fixed and sterilized by dry heat at 130°. It is issued in suitably sized and shaped pieces in sealed sterile containers and should be stored below 20° protected from light. For use as an absorbable surgical haemostatic agent it is usually impregnated with human thrombin and applied locally. It is however not widely used, alternative materials such as oxidized cellulose or gelatin sponges now being preferred.

HUMAN IMMUNOGLOBULIN

The antibodies formed in man may be composed of any or all of the three classes of serum proteins designated as IgG, IgM and IgA immunoglobulins respectively. The antibodies associated with two other, more recently described, classes, IgD and IgE, are under investigation.

Human immunoglobulin is the name given to that fraction, separated from human plasma, which consists almost entirely of IgG immunoglobulin i.e. the slowest moving group of proteins in plasma analysed by moving boundary electrophoresis. This fraction was previously known as γ-globulin or immune serum globulin. When the fraction is prepared from random pools of human plasma it is named *human normal immunoglobulin*. Preparations containing specified amounts of particular antibodies are called 'human immunoglobulin anti-' followed by the name of the appropriate antigen (x). More often the name used is 'human anti-(x) immunoglobulin'. This name replaces the terms 'hyperimmune γ-globulin' or 'convalescent γ-globulin'. The human specific immunoglobulins are prepared from plasma obtained at the optimum time from convalescent patients or immunized donors or from donations found to be rich in the required antibody. (For a discussion of nomenclature of human immunoglobulin see *WHO Bulletin* 1964 **30**, 447.)

The antibodies in the IgG immunoglobulin are almost exclusively those against viruses and bacterial toxins. Thus human normal immunoglobulin usually contains significant amounts of antibodies against the viruses causing measles, rubella, hepatitis and poliomyelitis. According to the circumstances of the population from which the starting plasma was obtained it may also contain useful amounts of tetanus and diphtheria antitoxin, and antibody against α-staphylolysin, streptolysin and mumps. Since human normal immunoglobulin contains little or no IgM, it does not contain antibodies against Gram-negative bacteria and is therefore valueless against infection due, for example, to *Pseudomonas aeruginosa* or *Escherichia coli*. The prophylactic uses of the various preparations of immunoglobulin are described below; it is true to say that, in general, immunoglobulin has been shown to be of little value in treatment.

The different antibodies in human plasma have closely similar solubilities and it is not yet feasible to separate antibodies of different specificities during fractionation.

For reviews on the clinical use of immunoglobulins see Janeway et al. (1967), Pollock (1969) and WHO Technical Report (1966).

HUMAN NORMAL IMMUNOGLOBULIN INJECTION, BP

This preparation is a solution of IgG immunoglobulin separated from random pools of plasma. Each pool is derived from not less than 1500 individual donations of blood. To obtain the immunoglobulin in its final form, the paste obtained by solvent precipitation is freeze-dried and then dissolved to give a solution which is adjusted to the required pH, salt concentration, and protein concentration, usually 15 per cent w/v for the standard product. Other concentrations may be used in order to give the required dose of a particular antibody in suitable volume. The solutions contain 0.9 per cent w/v sodium chloride, 0.01 per cent w/v of Thiomersal, or other bactericide in suitable concentration, and are adjusted to pH 6.8 ± 0.4. In some countries they may contain 2.25 per cent w/v glycine, which is thought to improve stability on storage. The Therapeutic Substances Regulations include specifications relating to analysis in the ultracentrifuge, both on the original solution and after incubation at 37° for 1 month. The quality is also controlled by electrophoresis, at least 90 per cent of the protein being required to have the mobility of γ-globulin. Antibody assays with respect to certain antibodies are carried out. The solution should contain not less than 4 to 8 i.u. measles antibody per ml. It is clear and pale yellow or light brown in colour. A trace of flocculent protein may precipitate during storage.

It has been shown empirically that human immunoglobulin prepared by the cold ethanol or ether technique or by cold ammonium sulphate precipitation does not transmit hepatitis. It cannot be assumed that material prepared by other fractionation methods will be safe. Thus immunoglobulin prepared by procedures such as ion exchange chromatography or preparative-scale electrophoresis should not be used until shown to be free of hepatitis virus.

Labelling. Additional to general requirements: (i) the amount of immunoglobulin as total protein; (ii) the nature and amount of preservative; and (iii) 'not for intravenous injection'.

Uses

Measles. To prevent or attenuate the disease. When the subject is in good health, the dose is selected to bring about attenuation only so that active immunity will ensue. In debilitated infants and others in whom an attack of measles would be dangerous, the dose used is one which will prevent the disease. If it is desired to prevent infection immunoglobulin should be given within 4 days of exposure to infection.

To prevent complications of vaccination against measles in infants and children suffering from certain pulmonary and cardiac conditions a dose of 4 to 8 I.U. is given at the same time as the vaccine.

Rubella. To prevent the disease. When a woman contracts rubella in the first 4 months of pregnancy, her child may be born with certain abnormalities. For many years in the U.K. women in the first 4 months of pregnancy, exposed to rubella, were given 750 mg normal immunoglobulin since this preparation contains considerable amounts of rubella antibody. Evidence suggests however, that this dose is ineffective (Public Health Laboratory Service Report 1968a). Whether a larger dose would be effective is not yet known. When immunoglobulin is given, it should be given as soon as possible after exposure.

Infectious hepatitis. Normal immunoglobulin is effective in preventing clinical disease and is particularly useful in nurseries, mental institutions and other situations where the risk of spread is great. In day schools only classmates are usually protected. A single dose will protect for 6 months. Travellers who intend to visit countries where the incidence of hepatitis is greater than in Western Europe or the United States should be given immunoglobulin (Public Health Laboratory Service Report 1968b; WHO Technical Report 1964).

Hepatitis B. The value of normal immunoglobulin in preventing the disease is not yet defined.

Chickenpox. Normal immunoglobulin will modify the disease but not protect against it. Its use is confined to prophylaxis or treatment in subjects at special risk, e.g. premature and newborn infant contacts.

Hypogammaglobulinaemia (M.R.C. Report 1969). Patients with this condition are particularly susceptible to bacterial infections, particularly with Gram-positive bacteria. The regular administration of normal immunoglobulin lessens the incidence of infection but does not necessarily protect against chronic infection of the respiratory or gastrointestinal tracts.

HUMAN ANTI-VACCINIA IMMUNOGLOBULIN

This specific immunoglobulin is prepared from the blood of donors revaccinated against smallpox during the previous three months. The method of preparation is the same as for human normal immunoglobulin. It should contain not less than 500 I.U. per ml.

It is used (i) to prevent complications of vaccination in children with eczema or in eczematous children accidentally exposed to vaccinia, and (ii) to provide immediate passive protection in previously unvaccinated smallpox contacts who have just been vaccinated to produce active immunity. It is also used to treat eczema vaccinatum, generalized vaccinia and progressive vaccinia. It is of no value for treating post-vaccinial encephalitis.

HUMAN ANTI-TETANUS IMMUNOGLOBULIN

Prepared from the blood of donors who have been immunized against tetanus. The method of preparation is the same as for human normal immunoglobulin. The preparation is of special value for protecting persons known to be sensitive to animal tetanus antitoxin. An injection of 250 I.U. will give a serum level of 0.01 to 0.05 I.U. per ml which is usually regarded as protective.

HUMAN ANTI-D IMMUNOGLOBULIN

Anti-D immunoglobulin is used to suppress sensitization of Rh-negative mothers to the Rh(D) antigen. This may occur when an unsensitized Rh-negative mother gives birth to an Rh-positive infant. Rh(D) positive foetal cells may escape across the placenta into her circulation during labour. If this occurs the mother becomes permanently sensitized, so that any further Rh-positive infant will suffer from haemolytic disease of the newborn.

If anti-D immunoglobulin is given to the mother within 60 h of delivery, it interacts with the foetal Rh(D) positive cells, causes them to disappear from her circulation and prevents them from stimulating her antibody-forming tissues to produce anti-D immunoglobulin (Clarke 1968).

The specific immunoglobulin is prepared from plasma obtained from Rh-negative persons whose blood contains incomplete antibody to the Rh(D) antigen. At present the most numerous donors of such plasma are Rh-negative mothers who have been sensitized to the Rh(D) antigen derived from an Rh positive pregnancy. Suitable plasma is also obtained from Rh-negative volunteers who have been deliberately sensitized to this Rh(D) antigen. The method of preparation is the same as for human normal immunoglobulin (WHO Technical Report 1971; Woodrow 1970).

ANTI-HB$_s$ IMMUNOGLOBULIN

A preparation of immunoglobulin containing antibody to hepatitis B surface antigen is under investigation. This antigen has been found to be associated with the carrier-state in hepatitis B, and the specific immunoglobulin, prepared from selected donors who have been found by testing to have the antibody, may be of value in preventing or modifying serum hepatitis—for example, in laboratory or hospital staff accidentally exposed to infection with the virus, or possibly in patients inadvertently transfused with hepatitis B surface antigen-positive blood.

ALBUMIN PREPARATIONS

An important function of the plasma protein is to contribute to the maintenance of blood volume. The protein which is present in plasma in greatest amount is albumin and in purified form it can be used as an alternative to whole plasma as a volume expander.

The albumin preparations for clinical use have been heated in solution for 10 h at 60°, which inactivates the virus of hepatitis B. They thus have an important advantage over whole plasma, but the disadvantage that their preparation is complex and the yield poor. A less pure albumin fraction, made by a simplified fractionation procedure, has been developed which gives a better yield at lower cost (Hink et al. 1957; Mealey et al. 1962; Kistler & Nitschmann 1962). It contains up to 10 per cent of proteins other than albumin but these are sufficiently stable to withstand heating for 10 h at 60°, without serious denaturation.

HUMAN ALBUMIN FRACTION (SALINE), BP (PLASMA PROTEIN FRACTION, BP)

This product is dispensed in liquid form. The total protein concentration is about 45 g/l, and it exerts an osmotic pressure equivalent to that of ACD plasma recovered from whole human blood. Albumin, as determined electrophoretically, forms at least 90 per cent of the protein present. The pH is 7.0 ± 0.3 and sufficient sodium chloride is added to make the solution isotonic. It contains in addition a stabilizing agent, such as 0.004 M sodium caprylate, which improves the heat stability of the albumin and other proteins present.

Storage.   Protected from light; 2° to 25°.

Labelling.   Additional to general requirements: (i) the total amount of protein; (ii) the concentrations of sodium, potassium and citrate ions; (iii) the nature and concentration of any protein stabilizer or other substance added; and (iv) that the contents should not be used if the solution is turbid or contains a deposit.

Human Albumin Fraction (Saline) may also be distributed in freeze-dried form.

Uses.   Similar to those of dried plasma except that it cannot be used as a source of fibrinogen.

HUMAN ALBUMIN (PURIFIED)

Purified albumin contains less than 5 per cent globulins as determined by moving boundary electrophoresis. It is prepared in the U.K. as a salt-poor freeze-dried product, usually in 25 g quantities. The fraction obtained by solvent precipitation techniques is made up without the addition of sodium chloride. The sodium content of the product must not exceed 12 mg sodium per g protein. For clinical use the freeze-dried powder is reconstituted with Water for Injection, or, at protein concentrations below 15 per cent Dextrose Injection, 5 per cent, giving a clear solution in less than 10 min. In many countries purified albumin is distributed as a salt-poor solution containing 20 or 25 per cent protein.

Storage and labelling requirements are similar to those for Human Albumin Fraction (Saline), BP.

The label must include particulars of the total sodium content.

Uses. (i) As for Human Albumin Fraction (Saline) and (ii) plasma volume or protein replacement in any patients in whom sodium intake is being restricted, for example in renal failure not responding to diuretic therapy.

IODINATED (^{125}I) HUMAN ALBUMIN INJECTION BP

IODINATED (^{131}I) HUMAN ALBUMIN INJECTION BP

Human albumin labelled with a radioactive iodine isotope is used for the determination of blood volume and for localizing tumours and the placenta. The albumin used for radio-iodination must meet the requirements for Human Albumin BP and must in particular have been treated for 10 h at 60° to inactivate the virus of serum hepatitis. The *British Pharmacopoeia* monograph for the product specifies a maximum concentration of free radioactive iodide, and that the label must state total radioactivity in microcuries or millicuries, with the date of determination.

PLASMA SUBSTITUTES

Certain obvious limiting factors and disadvantages are inseparable from the use of human blood and plasma and their derivatives. As a result many attempts have been made to find substances, mostly not of human origin, which could be used to restore a depleted blood volume. Such a substance would among other things, have to be non-antigenic, non-toxic, completely excreted or metabolized and possess the property of exerting a colloid osmotic pressure. Many substances have been investigated, including gum acacia, modified globin (derived from human haemoglobin), synthetic polymers such as polyvinyl pyrrolidone, hydroxyethyl starch, modified gelatin and dextran. Dextran and, to a lesser extent, gelatin have been more widely used than any of the others.

Fluids in use or proposed as blood volume expanders, including plasma and albumin preparations in addition to the substitutes listed above, have been reviewed by Gruber (1969).

Since Grönwall and Ingelman (1944) suggested that certain· polysaccharides of bacterial origin, known as dextrans, might be used as volume expanders, these substances have been extensively examined (see Squire et al. 1955; Grönwall 1957; Segal 1964). The dextrans are long chain polymers of dextrose (D-glucose) in which the sub-units are joined mainly through α 1:6 glucosidic linkages. Dextran for clinical use is produced commercially (Foster 1968) by large-scale fermentation, using a strain of the bacteria *Leuconostoc mesenteroides* (National Collection of Industrial Bacteria No. 8710) specified in the *British Pharmacopoeia*. Dextran, precipitated from the fermentation medium, and purified to remove pyrogenic and antigenic substances, provides a clinically useful volume expander similar to plasma in its colloid properties.

DEXTRAN 110 INJECTION, BP

For therapeutic use it is desirable to have a dextran with a relatively homogeneous molecular size and an average molecular weight of 110 000. In the fermentation process a polymer with a higher molecular weight is produced, which is subjected to controlled hydrolysis, followed by fractionation with ethanol or acetone. The final product should not contain much material with a molecular weight above 240 000 as this tends to aggregate and 'sludge' the erythrocytes in the patient's veins. On the other hand, dextran with too low a molecular weight, below the renal threshold, will be excreted rapidly. The distribution of molecular weight in Dextran 110 Injection is controlled by the following *British Pharmacopoeia* tests:

(1) Determination of the intrinsic viscosity of the material precipitated by the addition of 4 volumes of 95 per cent ethanol (intrinsic viscosity values are related to mean molecular weight). A value within the range 0.27 to 0.32 is required.

(2) Determination of the intrinsic viscosity of the 'top 10 per cent', i.e. of the material in the first 10 per cent of the total dextran present to be precipitated when the ethanol concentration is progressively increased. The intrinsic viscosity for this fraction or 'cut' should not exceed 0.40.

(3) A urinary excretion test in the rabbit. A high excretion rate indicates an excessive content of material of too small a molecular size.

Dextran 110 Injection is a solution of the polymer in Dextrose Injection 5 g/l, or in Sodium Chloride Injection, which has been sterilized either by autoclaving or filtration. It is an almost colourless, slightly viscous solution, which should not be used if it is cloudy, or if a deposit is present. Further tests listed in the *British Pharmacopoeia* specify (i) the permitted pH range, (ii) maximum permitted contents for heavy metals, acetone, ethanol, nitrogen and reducing sugars, and (iii) maximum sulphated ash. Tests for foreign protein and pyrogens are also required.

Storage. Dextran 110 Injection in 5 g/l dextrose stored below 25° will retain its properties for at least 5 years. In Sodium Chloride Injection, Dextran 110 stored at temperatures up to 40° will retain its properties for at least 5 years.

Labelling. Additional to general requirements: (i) concentration of dextran; (ii) the name of the solvent; and (iii) the strain of *Leuconostoc mesenteroides.*

Use. Emergency restoration of blood volume.

Large infusions of dextran have been reported to interfere with blood coagulation; caution should therefore be exercised if Dextran 110 is given to patients with a bleeding tendency.

Rouleaux formation may occur after large infusions of dextran and complicate blood group and compatibility tests. There are various ways of overcoming these difficulties (Ricketts 1966).

DEXTRAN 40 INJECTION, BP

This preparation has an average molecular weight of 40 000. Small molecular weight dextran of this size has a specific action in diminishing red cell aggregation (Gelin & Thorsen 1961). Because of its small molecular size it exerts a considerable osmotic pressure but the consequent expansion of blood volume is brief, 75 per cent of the dextran being excreted in 24 h. Small molecular weight dextran is used to promote blood flow in circumstances where this is endangered, as in thromboembolic conditions.

The method of preparation, the appearance of the product and the required control tests are similar to those described for Dextran 110. Dextran 40 Injection should be stored at a temperature not exceeding 25°; temperature fluctuations should be avoided. Under these conditions it may be expected to retain its properties for at least 5 years.

A dextran solution with an average molecular weight of 70 000 is also used in the U.K. and in certain other countries. Its properties in general are similar to those of Dextran 110.

GELATIN

Gelatin from bone or hides is subjected to controlled hydrolysis to produce a material with a suitable molecular weight. Gelatin solutions have been used on a limited scale as volume expanders in the U.S.A. and have also been introduced in some European countries.

REFERENCES

BERG, R., BJÖRLING, H., BERNTSEN, K. & ESPMARK, Å. (1972) *Vox Sang.* **22**, 1.

BIDWELL, E. (1955) *Brit. J. Haemat.* **1**, 35, 386.

BIDWELL, E., BOOTH, J. M., DIKE, G. W. R. & DENSON, K. W. E. (1967) *Brit. J. Haemat.* **13**, 568.

BIGGS, R. (ed.) (1975) *Human Blood Coagulation, Haemostasis and Thrombosis.* 2nd Edn. Oxford: Blackwell Scientific Publications.

BIGGS, R. & MACFARLANE, R. G, (eds.) (1966) *Treatment of Haemophilia and other Coagulation Disorders,* Oxford: Blackwell Scientific Publications.

BLOMBÄCK, M. (1958) *Ark. Kemi* **12**, 387.

BLUMBERG, B. S., SUTNICK, A. I. & LONDON, W. T. (1969) *J. Am. med. Ass.* **207**, 1895.

BOWLEY, C. C. & DUNSFORD, I. (1967) *Techniques in Blood Grouping.* 2nd Edn, Edinburgh: Oliver & Boyd.

BRINKHOUS, K. M., SHANBROM, E., ROBERTS, H. R., WEBSTER, W. P., FEKETE, L. & WAGNER, R. H. (1968) *J. Am. med. Ass.* **205**, 613.

CAYSER, I., DANE, D. S., CAMERON, C. H. & DENNING, J. V. (1974) *Lancet* **i**, 947.

CLARKE, C. A. (1968) *Lancet* **ii**, 1.

COHN, E. J., STRONG, L. E., HUGHES, W. L., Jr., MULFORD, D. J., ASHWORTH, J. N., MELIN, M. & TAYLOR, H. L. (1946) *J. Am. chem. Soc.* **68**, 459.

DEUTSCH, H. F., GOSTLING, L. J., ALBERTY, R. A. & WILLIAMS, J. W. (1946) *J. biol. Chem.* **164**, 109.

DIKE, G. W. R., BIDWELL, E. & RIZZA, C. R. (1972) *Brit. J. Haemat.* **22**, 469.

FOSTER, F. H. (1968) *Process Biochem.* **3**, 15, 55.

GELIN, L. E. & THORSEN, A. K. A. (1961) *Acta chir. scand.* **122**, 303.

GREAVES, R. I. N. (1946) *Medical Research Council Special Report Series No. 258.* London: HMSO.

GRÖNWALL, A. (1957) *Dextran and Its Use in Colloidal Infusion Solutions.* Stockholm: Almquist & Wiksell, Oxford: Blackwell Scientific Publications.

GRÖNWALL, A. & INGELMAN, B. (1944) *Acta physiol. scand.* **7**, 97.

GRUBER, U. F. (1969) *Blood Replacement,* translated by Oxtoby, L. & Armstrong, R. F. Berlin: Springer-Verlag.

HINK, J. H., Jr., HIDALGO, J., SEEBERG, V. P. & JOHNSON, F. F. (1957) *Vox Sang.* **2**, 174.

JANEWAY, C. A., ROSEN, F. S., MERLER, E. & ALPER, C. A. (1967) *The Gamma Globulins.* London: Churchill.

JORPES, J. E., BLOMBÄCK, B., BLOMBÄCK, M. & MAGNUSSON, S. (1962) *Acta med. scand.* **171**, Suppl. 379, 7.

KEKWICK, R. A. & MACKAY, M. E. (1954) *Medical Research Council Special Report Series No. 286.* London: HMSO.

KEKWICK, R. A. & WOLF, P. (1957) *Lancet* **i**, 647.

KISTLER, P. & NITSCHMANN, H. (1962) *Vox Sang.* **7**, 414.

LING, C. M. & OVERBURY, L. R. (1972) *J. Immunol.* **109**, 834.

MEALEY, E. H., LARSEN, L. H., DWYER, R. C. & MULFORD, D. J. (1962) *Vox Sang.* **7**, 406.

MEDICAL RESEARCH COUNCIL REPORT (1969) *Lancet* **i**, 163.

MOLLISON, P. L. (1972) *Blood Transfusion in Clinical Medicine,* 5th Edn. Oxford: Blackwell Scientific Publications.

NEWMAN, J., JOHNSON, A. J., KARPATKIN, M. H. & PUSZKIN, S. (1971) *Brit. J. Haemat.* **21**, 1, 21.

ONCLEY, J. L., MELIN, M., RICHERT, D. A., CAMERON, J. W. & GROSS, P. M., Jr. (1949) *J. Am. chem. Soc.* **71**, 541.

POLLOCK, T. M. (1969) Human Immunoglobulin in Prophylaxis, *Brit. med. Bull.* **25**, 202.

POOL, J. G. & SHANNON, A. E. (1965) *New Engl. J. Med.* **273**, 1443.

PRINCE, A. M. (1968) *Proc. natl. Acad. Sci., Wash.* **60**, 814.

PUBLIC HEALTH LABORATORY SERVICE REPORT (1968a) *Brit. med. J.* **3**, 203.

PUBLIC HEALTH LABORATORY SERVICE REPORT (1968b) *Brit. med. J.* **3**, 451.

REESINK, H. W., DUIMEL, W. J. & BRUMMELHUÏS, H. G. J. (1973) *Lancet* **ii**, 1351.

RICKETTS, C. R. (1966) *Brit. med. J.* **2**, 1423.

SCHULTZE, H. E. & HEREMANS, J. F. (1966) *Molecular Biology of Human Proteins,* Vol. 1. Amsterdam: Elsevier.

SEGAL, A. (1964) *The Clinical Use of Dextran Solutions.* New York and London: Grune & Stratton.

SIMSON, L. R., LIEN, D. M., WARNER, C. L. & OBERMAN, H. A. (1966) *Am. J. clin. Path.* **45**, 367.

SOULIER, J. P., BLATRIX, Ch. & STEINBUCH, M. (1964) *Presse med.* **72**, 1223.

SQUIRE, J. R., BULL, J. P., MAYCOCK, W. d'A. & RICKETTS, C. R. (1955) *Dextran. Its Properties and Use in Medicine.* Oxford: Blackwell Scientific Publications.

WEBSTER, W. P., ROBERTS, H. R., THELIN, G. M., WAGNER, R. H. & BRINKHOUS, K. M. (1965) *Am. J. med. Sci.* **250**, 643.

W.H.O. (1964) *Expert Committee on Hepatitis.* Second Report, Technical Report Series No. 285.

W.H.O. (1971) *Prevention of Rh Sensitization,* Technical Report Series No. 468.

W.H.O. (1966) *The Use of Immunoglobulin,* Technical Report Series No. 327.

WICKERHAUSER, M. (1971) *Thromb. Diath. haemorrh., suppl.* **43**, 165.

WICKERHAUSER, M. & SGOURIS, J. T. (1972) *Vox Sang.* **22**, 137.

WOODROW, J. C. (1970) *Series Haematologica* **3**, No. 3.

36

Sutures and Ligatures

The use of strings made by twisting vegetable and animal materials is described in the most ancient of surviving records of the history of mankind. Animal skins, intestines and sinews were used for musical instruments, bows and many other items. Vegetable fibres, spun and woven, date back to pre-historic times. Linen as spun strand was well known by 5000 B.C. and probably was first prepared long prior to this date.

In surgery Susruta (1500 B.C.) records the use of ligatures for tying umbilical cord and Celsus in the first century A.D. described the ligature as of ancient origin. In the highly developed civilization of ancient Egypt surgeons closed wounds with sutures. Galen (c. A.D. 200) used silk and hemp cords as ligatures and also recommended the use of animal gut. The term 'catgut' is said to be derived from the gut used to string a musical instrument known as a kit, an Arabic word for a dancing master's fiddle, hence 'kitgut'. The Arabian surgeon Rhazes (c. A.D. 900) used harp strings made from sheep intestine to repair abdominal wounds, but the use in surgery of twisted animal intestines was not generally practised as the patients nearly always became infected.

Ambroise Paré (1517–90) appears to have revived the use of ligatures and there are numerous references in his works to their use, particularly in amputations where he preferred them to the cautery. His valuable work, however, appears not to have been generally recognized and surgeons continued with the old methods of the hot knife and searing iron.

The credit for the reintroduction of catgut is given to P. S. Physick (1816) house surgeon to J. Hunter, and later Professor of Surgery in Philadelphia, but his observations, and publications of other workers of the same period, did not persuade surgeons to adopt the material.

It was not until 1869 that Joseph Lister, as a result of his *Observations on the Ligature of Arteries on the Antiseptic System* opened the way to the modern surgical suture techniques. The first step had been to show that sepsis was due to the growth of microorganisms from the site of infection. From that time onwards the search to find means of preventing infection has not ceased. The history of this work applied to surgical sutures and ligatures during the past seventy years is too large a subject for this chapter but the investigations by a host of dedicated workers into hundreds of different procedures has led to the highly efficient methods being employed today.

For further details on the historical aspect, see Fandre (1944).

Although the terms 'ligature' and 'suture' are often used in the same sense, and they are of the same material, there is nevertheless a technical difference. A ligature is a thread used to constrict and seal off a blood vessel, vein or artery—hence to ligate. The thread is a suture when it is used to stitch together the edges of various tissues, e.g. skin, fascia, muscle, tendon, peritoneum, etc. Hence a needle is always used for a suture (sewing) but not for a ligature.

Sutures and ligatures are classified as absorbable, or non-absorbable, depending on the materials from which they are made.

ABSORBABLE

Absorbable sutures and ligatures are absorbed by the tissues in which they are implanted and the time taken for complete disappearance is dependent on a number of factors which will be treated more fully later in this chapter. Absorbable materials are catgut (non-boilable and boilable), reconstituted collagen, synthetic absorbable polymers, kangaroo tendon, ribbon gut and fascia lata.

NON-ABSORBABLE

Non absorbable sutures and ligatures are not absorbed by tissue and, unless they are on the surface, remain in the body after the wound has healed. Some, notably silk, fragment after a long period of time; others are encapsulated by fibrous tissue, while others remain as inert implants. The most commonly used are silk, linen, nylon (polyamides), polyester, polyolefines and stainless steel wire, and to a very small extent: cotton, horsehair, human hair, silkworm gut and wires of other metals, e.g. tantalum, silver, phosphor bronze, etc.

The polymeric materials are also used in the form of woven meshes particularly for hernia repair and silk and nylon in floss form have specialist uses also.

Mention should also be made of the use of clips (Michel, Kifa, etc.) for surface application and the past few years have seen a good deal of development, particularly in Russia and the USA, in the use of small wire staples (usually stainless steel) which are implanted by means of stapling guns.

STANDARDS AND LEGAL REQUIREMENTS FOR SUTURES AND LIGATURES

Although the National Pharmacopoeias of most countries publish monographs on surgical sutures, the standards nowadays for EEC countries, Denmark, Sweden, and Switzerland, i.e. the signatories to the Convention, are established by the European Pharmacopoeia. Volume II of the first edition published in 1971 contained monographs for Sterile Catgut, Sterile Reconstituted Collagen Strings and Sterile Non-absorbable strands including Braided Silk, Braided Polyester, Braided Polyamides 6 and 6/6, Monofilament Polyamides 6 and 6/6 and Linen Thread. Some amendments were introduced in Volume III published in 1975 to approximate to the USP XIX (1975).

Both these compendia have adopted a metric numbering system whereby the gauge number applied to the suture represents the actual diameter in tenths of a millimetre. Previously a so-called conventional system was used and, although in the case of the UK and the USA the sizes represented were comparable, the values for diameter differed between absorbable and non-absorbable materials. The conventional systems employed by other countries themselves differed and there was a lack of flexibility as finer sutures were developed for modern surgical techniques. (See table.)

Metric Number	Former Conventional Size	
	Catgut/Collagen	Non-absorbables Synthetic Absorbables
0.1	–	–
0.2	–	10/0
0.3	9/0	9/0
0.4	–	8/0
0.5	8/0	7/0
0.7	7/0	6/0
1	6/0	5/0
1.5	5/0	4/0
2	4/0	3/0
3	3/0	2/0
3.5	2/0	0
4	0	1
5	1	2
6	2	3 & 4
7	3	5
8	4	6

Sutures have always been the odd man out as far as legislation is concerned and have been classed sometimes as 'drugs' and sometimes as 'devices'. In the UK the manufacture and sterilization of catgut and other products of animal origin became subject to control by licensing under the Therapeutic Substances Act in 1929 largely as a result of the reports of T. J. Mackie and of Bulloch, Lampitt and Bushill. This control now extends to various 'Surgical Materials' of animal origin and to synthetic materials capable of being absorbed.

The Medicines Act is in process of taking over from the Therapeutic Substances Act. Anomalies still remain however that in the meantime non-absorbable materials of vegetable or synthetic origin are not subject to such control.

ABSORBABLE MATERIALS

SURGICAL CATGUT

Sterilized surgical catgut consists of a strand prepared from collagen derived from healthy mammals purified and sterilized. The most widely used

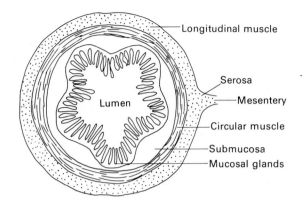

FIG. 36.1. Diagrammatic section of intestine.

source is the submucosa of the small intestine from sheep or lambs and to a lesser extent, the serosa from beef cattle. The length of ovine intestine is about 20 m and it is desirable in the preparation of surgical catgut that the diameter of the intestine should not be more than 18 mm. A number of factors are important in the selection of suitable intestinal material. Obviously intestines will vary considerably depending on the age of the animal, the pasture, climate, etc., and it is not uncommon to find that intestines from some animals have been affected by scar tissue and are not suitable for preparing surgical catgut. Generally speaking the younger the animal the smaller its intestine, and less likely to be affected by feed.

A number of manufacturers of catgut use only the first 8 m of intestine measured from the duodenum. In the meat trade such intestines are described as ligature casings or runners.

In the slaughterhouse the gut is removed from the animal by the gut pullers and is first of all cleaned to remove faecal matter after which it is inspected, measured and then preserved either in a frozen state or salted. The largest supplies of intestines come from Australia and New Zealand and the slaughterhouses in these countries are well equipped to deal with the vast number of animals involved. The intestine of any cadaver is the most vulnerable to bacterial attack and decomposition of this part of the body always begins earlier than any other. It is, therefore, vitally important that the slaughterhouse technique involves rapid cleaning and freezing or preservation by other methods in order to keep the bacterial growth as low as possible.

The ovine intestine consists of four layers (Fig. 36.1). The outermost is known as tunica serosa or serous layer, much of which is torn off in removal from the animal; next the tunica musculosa made up of two layers, one longitudinal and the other circular; the third layer is the tunica submucosa from which catgut is prepared and the innermost layer is the tunica mucosa or mucous coat which is the wall to the lumen of the intestine. The intestine receives its blood supply from the mesenteric artery and being some twenty-eight times the length of the sheep itself is twisted into a mass of convolutions until near its end where it ascends to join the colon.

The Medical Research Council report on the preparation of catgut contains interesting microphotographs of the submucosal layer.

The manufacturer of surgical catgut receives intestines either intact or rough scraped at the abbatoir, made up as knots or bundles which may be frozen, salted or in brine, and the first step is to soak these in water to thaw out or to remove salt and prepare them for splitting. It may be noted in passing that the intestines destined for sausage skins are not split but are cleaned and scraped in the tubular form and known as sausage casings. This cleaning usually takes place in the abbatoir and the product is marketed in barrels or casts.

Splitting

The splitting or cutting operation is carried out by inserting the curved horn of a cutting tool into the end of the intestine and pulling the runner over cutting blades (Fig. 36.2). The number of ribbons produced can be varied but is usually two or three. The horn follows the curvature of the intestine and therefore can be said to locate down the track of the mesenteric vein, which is often called the rough side as distinct from the upper part known as the smooth side. The two parts of the intestine are kept separate throughout the process as they behave in different ways physically and chemically.

Cleaning of Submucosa

The next step is to remove the mucosa, muscle and any remaining serosa, or, if the material has been cleaned in the abbatoir, the remnants of these layers, and this is facilitated by treatment with alkaline solution. The general method of scraping is to fix the ribbons in a frame or on suitable flat surfaces so that the submucosa can be cleaned of unwanted material (Fig. 36.3). Often this is carried out by hand and is a very skilled operation. In other cases an apparatus known as a sliming machine is employed.

When the ribbons are judged satisfactorily cleaned they are cut to a predetermined length and assembled in multiples of ribbons of the same type and mounted on to string loops at either end. The number of ribbons will determine the ultimate size of the spun strand.

Spinning

The apparatus used by manufacturers for spinning ribbons of catgut is largely dependent on the manufacturer's choice. The number of hooks on the machine to which the string loops are attached varies from 2 to 20. In some cases spinning takes place from both ends of the strand and may take place immersed in water or alkaline solution. The spinning of catgut destined for surgical use is a highly skilled operation. Multiples of ribbons which are overspun will tend to lack elasticity and will curl when dry. On the other hand, if they are

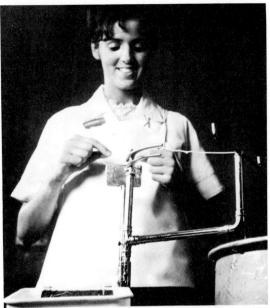

FIG. 36.2. Splitting of intestine (Ethicon Ltd, Edinburgh).

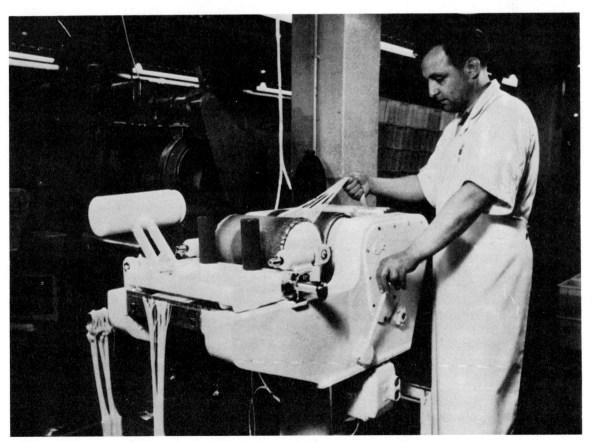

FIG. 36.3. Slimming machine for removal of mucosal and muscular coats from the submucosa of intestinal ribbon (Ethicon Ltd, Edinburgh).

underspun the elasticity will be too great and the tensile strength reduced. The angle of ply to the horizontal is to some extent a guide as to whether a string has been properly prepared, but many other factors can affect the ultimate quality of the catgut. Because catgut is a biological material it must of necessity vary considerably and no one animal intestine is exactly the same as another. The spinning of catgut is, therefore, still largely on art rather than a mechanical operation. After spinning, the catgut is mounted on drying frames, the conditions of drying time and humidity being carefully controlled. The resulting strand of dried catgut is known at this stage as raw catgut and is usually between 3 and 5 m long.

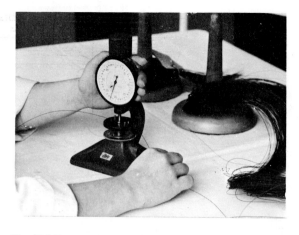

FIG. 36.4. Baty gauge (London Hospital Ligature Laboratories).

Polishing

Strands of catgut can be prepared with such care and attention to manufacturing detail that they will vary only slightly in diameter and need only a light manual polishing, but more usually the manufacturer employs a technique which produces an approximate size and then polishes or grinds the string to a predetermined diameter. This process is achieved by means of machines, either by rotating the strings while a carriage bearing an abrasive paper moves to and fro along their length, or by using a pair of grinding wheels similar to those employed by engineers and setting the wheels the required distance apart. Both methods have to be very carefully controlled to avoid damage to the plies of the strand with consequent loss in tensile strength. The finish, moreover, must be such that the gut is neither 'whiskery' nor so smooth that the surgeon's knots will slip and cause the wound to re-open.

Gauging

The methods of gauging carried out by various manufacturers vary with their own particular preferences, but the final control instrument for checking diameter is a gauge of the dial reading type, in which the details of pressor foot and weight loading are specified (Fig. 36.4). As the diameter of catgut will vary with the relative humidity of the atmosphere, the control test as laid down is the diameter in a relative humidity between 60 and 80 per cent and at a temperature between 16° and 21°.

The normal gauges used in British surgery vary from the finest size 1 in ophthalmic work to the

thickest, size 7, which is occasionally used for specialist surgery.

Standards

Length. This is determined immediately after removal of the strand from its container and is measured without stretching. The length must be not less than 90 per cent of the length stated on the label.

Tensile strength. The test is carried out on a machine of the deadweight type, having a movable jaw with a constant rate of traverse of 30 cm/min, and a capacity so that when the strand breaks, the angle which the pendulum arm makes with the vertical is not less than 9° and not more than 45°. The clamp heads are specially designed and any strands breaking within 12.5 mm of the clamps are disregarded. The strands are tested within 15 min of removal from their container and in a temperature between 16° and 21° and in an atmosphere in which the relative humidity is between 60° and 80°. As catgut is inevitably knotted in the patient, the test is always carried out on strands in which a surgeon's knot (Fig. 36.5) has been

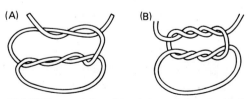

FIG. 36.5. (A) Surgeon's knot (simple knot tied on double knot); (B) nylon knot.

formed at a point midway between the two clamps. The knot strength is approximately half of the figure which would be obtained on an unknotted sample.

Labelling. The label on or in the container must state by indelible marking or perforation the length of the strand, the gauge number, whether the strand is plain, hardened or chromicized, and that the container should not be subjected to heat treatment. The label on the box must state the name and percentage of any bactericide in the fluid in which the sutures are immersed.

Storage. Sterilized surgical catgut should be protected from light and stored in a cool place.

Packaging. The *British Pharmacopoeia* states that sterilized surgical catgut is packed either in glass tubes sealed by fusion of the glass, or in other suitable containers which once opened cannot be resealed. Although glass tubes are probably the ideal method of packaging surgical sutures in that they are transparent, inert and impermeable, they are nevertheless regarded as a nuisance in the operating theatre because they have to be broken, and a large variety of flexible packages based on aluminium foil or plastic films which can be torn open, have in the past few years tended to replace glass. The bottle packs, which are still used to some extent in continental Europe, in which a continuous length in the form of a cocoon of catgut is packed in ingenious dispensing devices, is considered to introduce an element of risk of contamination, and this form of packing is no longer used in Great Britain.

Sterility testing. The Therapeutic Substances Act in Great Britain lays down the fundamental required for bacteriological testing of surgical catgut. Definitions are given of the term batch, the percentage of samples from each batch which are to be tested and broad definitions of the media and incubation times to be employed. The technique to be adopted where any bactericides present are liable to inhibit growth in the medium is specified. The medium is so designed that it will detect the presence both of aerobes and anaerobes. If after an incubation period of 14 days no growth or microorganism is found in any tube, the sample may be regarded as having passed the test. If growth of microorganisms is found in any tube a further sample may be taken from the batch and the test repeated. If no growth occurs the sample

shall be regarded as having passed the test, but if any microorganism is found the batch is treated as not sterile.

STERILIZATION OF CATGUT

Lister's work on catgut in 1869 using aqueous phenol and later phenol and olive oil was the forerunner of antiseptic technique applied to sutures. His experiments and resulting papers stimulated work in which a very large number of chemical compounds were investigated with varying success to bring about a reduction in the number of microorganisms present in surgical catgut.

The variety of substances employed was very numerous and is surveyed in detail in the Medical Research Council Report on *The Preparation of Catgut for Surgical Use* (Bulloch et al. 1929). Bulloch checked the efficacy of a large number and found most to be of very doubtful value. As with most newly presented ideas each substance had its adherents and at a time when a large number of hospitals preferred to sterilize their own catgut sutures there were bound to be failures and many patients became infected as a result. The preparation of bulk sterile material by present day skilled technological methods was, before 1929, in its infancy and the problems of inactivating microorganisms in catgut were not then fully appreciated.

Mammalian intestine in the living animal is normally relatively free of microorganisms but immediately after death growth of microorganisms proceeds at a very rapid rate. Conditions in slaughterhouses, however clean, are, moreover, not conducive to aseptic techniques and the intestines inevitably carry a large bacterial population. The freezing or salting of the material inhibits further growth but does not kill these organisms. Staphylococci, streptococci, with a large proportion of *Str. faecalis*, and *Escherichia coli* are commonly found in intestinal material but although a number may be pathologically significant they are relatively susceptible to sterilizing techniques. Even if they survive the manufacturing process, many would be killed by the alcohol in the final container. Sporing aerobes mostly nonpathogenic, such as *Bacillus subtilis* and its phage type which used to be known as *B. mesentericus ruber*, or the catgut bacillus, are very numerous, but the potentially dangerous organisms are *Bacillus anthracis* and the anaerobic spore bearing types, among them *Clostridium sporogenes*, *Cl. tetani*, and *Cl. welchii*. The spores of both aerobes and abaerobes are not easily killed, the aerobic types being generally more resistant. The fact that they revert to the spore form if conditions for growth are unsatisfactory further complicates the situation. The difficulty is exacerbated by the structure of the catgut strand where ribbons twisted together will carry any contamination throughout their whole cross-section and at the centre of the string any organisms are well insulated. The successful means of attack on these microorganisms is by either chemicals (liquid or gaseous), heat, or radiation. The choice of method must, however, be related to other desiderata. It is useless, for instance, to use a method to sterilize the material which will ruin its physical characteristics such as tensile strength and absorbability. Ideally, the aim will be to interfere as little as possible with the inherent structural advantages of collagen as a strong, flexible and elastic fibre that will be absorbed by the body in a surgically acceptable manner.

Chemical

The three methods will now be discussed in further detail.

The chemical method must employ a material which is sporicidal as distinct from bactericidal. Most inorganic or organic compounds in common use as antiseptics, disinfectants or bactericides are active against microorganisms in the vegetative phase. Certain products such as the quaternary ammonium compounds are even more limited in that they are specific, i.e. they will kill Gram-positive organisms and leave Gram-negative types unaffected. Other preparations will be effective against most organisms but certain genera will not be killed and, most important of all, none of these compounds are sporicidal and are therefore useless in bringing about sterility in catgut.

The available sporicidal compounds are, in fact, relatively few. The main substances are formaldehyde, hydrogen peroxide, hypochlorite, glutaraldehyde, ethyl iodide, methyl bromide, iodine, ethylene oxide and β-propiolactone. Of these still fewer are suitable for commercial sterilization of catgut.

Histological techniques employing formalin introduced about 1893 led to its application to catgut sterilization by Cunningham (1895). Although a number of workers demonstrated that formaldehyde solutions of the order of 5 per cent for prolonged periods were necessary to destroy anthrax spores and that this treatment seriously affected catgut, the 'formalin period' lasted for about 15 years and there is little doubt that a great deal of unsterile material was used. The resulting catgut, moreover, was so hardened that its absorption in the body was considerably delayed and its tensile strength much reduced.

Hydrogen peroxide will effectively sterilize catgut but results in a material which is of poor quality. The compound has, however, sometimes been used to improve the colour of catgut by treating the collagen in the ribbon form, i.e. before spinning.

Solutions of sodium or potassium hypochlorites although sporicidal, particularly in acid solution, are not suitable for catgut as their penetrative power is very poor and the catgut is unduly swollen and of poor tensile strength.

Glutaraldehyde behaves very much in the same way and is only active in sodium bicarbonate buffered solutions. The solution only retains its sporicidal activity for about two weeks.

Iodine remained, as the only suitable chemical for large scale commercial sterilizing of catgut. Ethyl iodide and methyl bromide in alcohol and mixtures of iodine and iodine trichloride have also been used.

Basically the process consisted of immersion of standard lengths of catgut wound on frames or reels in a carefully standardized aqueous solution of iodine, potassium iodide and potassium iodate, the pH being rigidly controlled. The catgut must absorb about 12 per cent of its own weight of iodine and when this has taken place the catgut is transferred from the solution and excess iodine removed by sterile solvent often containing a bacteriostatic. The sterile strands are then transferred under aseptic conditions to their final container, sterile fluid is added (usually 95 per cent ethanol or 90 per cent isopropanol) and the container sealed. Processes involving ethyl iodide or iodine and iodine trichloride are carried out in alcoholic solution but in other respects the process is similar to the aqueous method.

Ethylene oxide may be employed as a sterilizing agent in the gaseous form or in solution. The important factors to be controlled are concentration, moisture time and temperature employed. It is an explosive gas and is usually supplied mixed with carbon dioxide or freon. The process is usually monitored with spore strips of B. subtilis var. niger (B. globigii). Care must be taken to limit the residual ethylene oxide in the suture material. It is usually necessary to carry out an aseptic procedure for filling and sealing the final container.

Heat Sterilization

Raw catgut contains 12 per cent to 25 per cent by weight of combined moisture, depending on storage conditions. Heating above 80° will result in hydrolysis of the collagen and the resulting gelatine or glue would render it useless for surgical purposes. All heat sterilizing processes, therefore, are based on the fundamental necessity of removing this combined moisture before the strings can be raised to sterilizing temperature of 150° to 165°. The process varies with different manufacturers, but basically consists in inserting gauged standard lengths of coiled catgut into glass tubes which are then plugged, placed in ovens and the strings dehydrated by gradually raising the temperature. Baskets of tubes are then placed in a sterilizing chamber and the catgut covered with an organic fluid of high boiling point and the temperature raised to about 160°.

Alternatively, the tubes are subjected to the vapour of the organic fluid usually toluene or xylol under pressure, the temperature again being held at about 160° for a suitable time. Any condensed fluid is removed by a further heating period. Most variations in the methods have been aimed at reducing the fire and explosion hazards and at the same time producing a more acceptable catgut.

After sterilizing the tubes are allowed to cool and are then drained if necessary. The catgut is at this stage very brittle and could not be used in surgery. Under full aseptic conditions a suitably hydrated sterile alcoholic fluid is added in order to put back the necessary moisture and the tubes are sealed. This is the origin of the term tubing fluid, which is still used by many manufacturers even though the tube has been replaced with other forms of pack. After a few days the catgut is sufficiently rehydrated to be usable.

Boilable catgut. Although catgut in Great Britain is now all of the non-boilable type, up to a few years ago a boilable variety was prepared by some manufacturers. The term was used to indicate to operating theatre staff that the external surface of the tubes could be sterilized by boiling in water.

Boilable catgut was prepared by the heat sterilizing method outlined above but instead of adding a hydrated tubing fluid the strands were immersed in a non-aqueous compound such as toluene. The catgut, when removed from the tube, was hydrated by the operating theatre staff by soaking it in sterile saline or water some time before it was required for use.

Radiation Sterilization
Currently by far the most commonly employed method of sterilization for sutures is that of irradiation by electron particles or by gamma rays. More than 50 per cent of the suture companies in Europe use this process. Whilst the original commercial method in 1957 made use of electron machines, since 1961 most suture manufacturers now employ gamma radiation usually from cabalt 60 sources. The recognized sterilizing dose for sutures is 2.5 megarad. The method has the advantage that sterilization is effected in the final sealed container, indeed some manufacturers apply it to the complete sales package.

RECONSTITUTED COLLAGEN

The limitations on length imposed by the length of intestinal material combined with the natural biological variations in thickness and character have led manufacturers to search for many years for a means of overcoming these disadvantages. Collagen is available from a large number of sources. It is the major constituent of skin, tendon, ligament, etc. As a protein built up of some 11 amino acids, it is partially soluble in acids. The basic process has been to obtain an acidic solution of collagen prepared from hides or tendons which can be extruded into a coagulating solution and the resulting fibres oriented by stretching. The filaments can then either be spun or rolled to make up the necessary sizes of strand required. Reconstituted collagen is produced mainly in the finer sizes 0.5, 1 and 2 for ophthalmic and cuticular surgery.

SYNTHETIC ABSORBABLE MATERIAL

The search for evenness and continuous length has also been pursued among synthetic organic compounds. A number of patents have been obtained for filaments produced from the polymerization of certain lactides, hydroxy acids, etc., and two such products are gaining acceptance in surgery. The USP XIX describes Absorbable Surgical Suture as 'a sterile strand prepared from collagen derived from healthy mammals or from a synthetic polymer'.

KANGAROO TENDON

This absorbable material consists of the tail tendons of the wallaby. The tendons, which were usually preserved with naphthalene, were prepared and graded into various sizes, e.g. fine, medium, and stout. Lengths were 30–40 cm. They were sterilized as for catgut and their main use was for hernia repair and bone surgery. This material is virtually unobtainable today.

RIBBON GUT

Ribbon gut as its name suggests is in the form of ribbon approximately 12 mm wide and usually about 45 cm long. Its use is limited but is preferred by some surgeons for the repair of large ventral herniae and in the closure of the kidney after nephrotomy. The material is prepared from bovine oesophagus and is sterilized in the same way as catgut.

FASCIA LATA

This may be excised from the patient, or prepared from bovine thigh muscle, cleaned and sterilized. It is supplied in lengths of about 30 cm × 6 mm wide and is used surgically for hernia repair, urethral slings, etc.

ABSORPTION OF CATGUT IN THE BODY

Catgut is used in surgery because it is capable of being absorbed by animal and human tissues. This concept was propounded by Lister who recognized that the continued presence of a non-absorbable material presented a focus for infection. The term 'absorption' is often wrongly used to describe the loss of tensile strength of holding power of the suture in the wound and this is more rapid than the disappearance of the material itself. Formerly, terms such as '10 day', '20 day', '30 day', and even '40 day' were applied to catgut sutures. The basis for such claims was never stated and indeed in 1940 Holder showed that in the case of iodine sterilized catgut the terms were meaningless since the hardening effect of the iodine process was greater than that of any treatment applied to catgut. These dscriptions are now obsolete although they occasionally occur in surgical papers. When the term '20 day' is used it is taken to refer to the present day 'medium chromic material'. Medium chromic, now often abbreviated to 'chromic', or hardened material is catgut which has been subjected either in the ribbon form or as a string to a mild basic chrome tanning.

Lawrie (1955), working mainly with heat sterilized material implanted in the lumbar muscle of the rat, followed the rate of loss of tensile strength and evolved the concept of Half Strength Time (HST) which was the time required for the strength of the material to be reduced to 50 per cent of its original strength in vivo. Plain catgut was shown to possess a HST of 5–7 days and to reach zero strength in 3–4 weeks, while medium chromic catgut had a HST of 19 days and took about 5 weeks to reach zero strength.

The process which takes place in the body when catgut implants are made has been extensively studied by histological observation from the day after insertion of the material up to its complete disappearance in the tissue (Lawrie et al. 1959, 1960). It is undoubtedly the reaction of the tissues to the foreign body protein that brings about what is termed the absorption process. Although catgut prepared and sterilized by different methods tends to show different behaviour in the body, nevertheless the general histological picture is similar.

At first, around the site of the implant there is a fairly rapid gathering of polymorphonuclear leucocytes together with varying proportions of a fibrinous exudate. These cells are evident as early as one day after implantation of plain catgut which tends to excite a greater reaction in the tissue than chromicized material which does not begin to attract polymorph formations until up to 10 days after implantation. It should be understood that tissue reaction, i.e. inflammation, is the inevitable result of leucocytic concentrations (pus).

With plain catgut the polymorph phase begins to die down after about 5 days and there is an increasing accumulation of macrophages, by which time the catgut is considerably fragmented and any ultimate suture material is absorbed by phagocytosis.

With chromic catgut the mechanism is not necessarily exactly the same although with certain types of suture material very little difference can be observed. Where a difference is present the longer absorption usually involves fragmentation by phagocytes, histiocytes and foreign body giant cells. These observations do not, of course, explain why the catgut disappears and although a considerable amount of research has taken place the actual proteolytic enzymes responsible have not been isolated. At present the leucocytes or histiocytes themselves are believed to carry their own proteolytic enzyme system, and at one time this was thought to be very closely related to α-chymotrypsin. The cellular reaction varies somewhat in different animals but the process in the rat is very similar to that which occurs in human tissue although absorption periods are somewhat longer. Very many attempts have been made by manufacturers of surgical catgut to try to relate the in vivo absorption of catgut to a standardized in vitro control. These latter methods have generally been based on exposing catgut to standard solutions of proteolytic enzymes such as trypsin, pepsin, papain, etc., and although the results obtained are of some practical use, it has not been possible to incorporate them into a reliable system of evaluation.

NON-ABSORBABLE SUTURES

SILK

Silk consists of strands prepared from filaments of the cocoon spun by the silkworm of the Bombyx family before it enters the chrysalis stage. Three forms are used in surgery—twisted (sometimes known as Chinese twist), floss and plaited or braided silk. Silk in its natural state contains up to 25 per cent of natural gum and strands prepared from this are described as undischarged. Twisted silk suture material is prepared from unbleached, undischarged filaments spun in multiples to the *British Pharmaceutical Codex* range of diameters and may be dyed with non-toxic dyestuffs. The surgical use of twisted silk has very much declined in favour of the braided type.

Floss silk is prepared from the coarser filaments on the outer surface of the silkworm cocoon and is used in its spun glossy white form mainly in the repair of herniae. Its use is diminishing fast as the plastic polymer meshes gain in popularity.

Plaited or braided silk is the material in large scale use in modern surgery. It is prepared from discharged silk and the range of sizes is dependent on the number of strands braded together. As the gum has been removed it is not serum proof or non-capillary and for most surgical purposes it is therefore treated with proofing waxes or silicones.

Silk is identified chemically by warming with mercuric nitrate solution when a brick-red colour is produced and it is stained yellow by trinitrophenol solution. Silk, because of its strength, softness and general ease of handling is used in many sites of surgical operation, the fine strands being particularly suited to ophthalmic and neurosurgery. Silk sutures are classified as non-absorbable in the body and are normally encapsulated by fibrous tissue. However, many cases have been reported where after a considerable length of time the silk has fragmented or even migrated from the original site of implantation.

Silk is sterilized either by autoclaving, which causes a certain loss in its tensile strength, or by radiation or ethylene oxide sterilization.

It is normally supplied by suture manufacturers to comply with the monographs published in the *British Pharmaceutical Codex*.

LINEN

Linen sutures consist of selected fibres made into a twisted strand from flax (*Linum usitatissinum*).

The strand is normally prepared by spinning three cords together, the size of the cords being chosen to produce the ultimate desired gauge of thread. For surgical use it must be firmly and evenly spun and free from fuzziness. Identification is by microscopic examination.

Linen may be dyed with any non-toxic dyestuff but although a certain amount of black thread is used the majority of surgeons prefer off-white or ivory colour.

It is extensively used in many surgical techniques and frequently needs to be rendered non-capillary and serum proof by treatment with suitable proofing agents similarly to braided silk.

It can be sterilized by autoclaving or ethylene oxide. Radiation sterilization does however cause a considerable loss of strength.

It is the subject of a monograph in the *British Pharmaceutical Codex* to which all British manufacturers conform.

POLYAMIDES

In the U.K. these polymers are better known by the word Nylon but as this is a registered trademark in certain European countries, it is likely that the word polyamide will be used in the future. These compounds are formed from the polymerization of the reaction product of an acid and an amine. Hitherto, they have been known by suffixing the word Nylon with a number, e.g. Nylon 6, Nylon 66, Nylon, 10, 11, 12, etc. Polyamide 66 is formed by the combination of hexamethylenediamine and adipic acid. Polyamide 6 is formed by the polymerization of caprolactam.

All the polyamides and suture materials are produced by an extrusion process, the size of the orifice on the extruder head determining the size of the filament. The bulk of the material used in surgery is produced in the form of monofilament. Its main use is in skin suturing although it is sometimes used internally. Polyamide mesh finds a use in hernia repair.

Finer filaments of polyamide are braided together to form braided nylon on non-absorbable surgical sutures. Monofilament polyamide is normally coloured with distinctive non-toxic dye-stuffs or pigments in order to improve its visibility. It may be sterilized by autoclaving, by ethylene oxide or by radiation treatment, but is incompatible with phenol and its homologues and other phenolic substances. The knotting of polyamide requires a special knot (Fig. 36.5).

POLYESTER

This suture material is usually prepared in the plaited or braided form and consists of filaments prepared by polymerizing the ester formed by a combination of ethylene glycol and terephthalic acid. In its commercial form it is known under the trade marks Terylene (I.C.I.) and Dacron (Du Pont). The number of filaments in the braid determines the size of the completed strand.

The polymer has a softening temperature of not less than 255° and may be sterilized by autoclaving, ethylene oxide or radiation treatments. In order to improve its visibility in tissue it is often dyed or pigmented with non toxic materials.

STAINLESS STEEL WIRE

Stainless steel wire has largely replaced the various wires which have been used in surgery in past years, such as silver, tantalum, phosphor bronze, etc. It is supplied for surgical purposes in three forms, namely, monofilament, twisted and plaited or braided. The *British Pharmaceutical Codex* includes monographs on all three types and lays down standards for diameter and tensile strength.

In all three cases the wire is prepared from austenitic chromium–nickel stainless steel and is fully annealed. The austenitic steels are non-magnetic and only capable of being hardened by cold working. The wire is made to British Standards Specification 4106: 1967.

It may be sterilized by dry heat, autoclaving, ethylene oxide or radiation but it is important that the wire should be fully degreased when heat treatment is used.

Its main use is in orthopaedic work, but very fine wire is also used in plastic surgery and for repair of tendons.

SUTURE CLIPS

Michels and Kifa clips are used to some extent for long skin wound approximations and find a considerable use in research work on animals where they are less irritating in the skin surface than sutures.

WIRE STAPLES

A considerable amount of experimental and clinical work is now being carried out, particularly in the U.S.S.R. and the U.S.A., on the use of very small wire staples, usually of stainless steel. The field of investigation is very wide and papers have been published on their use in orthopaedic, cardiovascular and arterial work and in the U.S.S.R. the results of many thousands of cases of gastric resection have been reported.

SURGICAL NEEDLES

Whenever a suture is required to close a wound, needles to arm the suture material are necessary. The number of sizes and the variety of different shapes of needles run into many thousands. The range supplied by manufacturers is usually classified into types for specific surgery, as for example, arterial, general purpose, intestinal, obstetric, ophthalmic, plastic, retention. Shapes are designated as: straight, curved, $\frac{1}{2}$-circle, $\frac{5}{8}$-circle, etc. and the sections as round bodied, triangular cutting edge, triangular reverse cutting, cutting point, trocar point. In addition the length of the needle from point to hilt is specified in millimetres and the hilts are designed to take the various diameters of suture material employed. Needles are chosen by the surgeon to suit his operating technique and it is largely because of the surgeons interest in improving suture efficiency that the development of surgical needles has taken place. In very many cases the surgeon himself has caused needles to be made to his own design and a large number of commonly used needles are referred to by the name of the inventing surgeon.

Surgical needles are of two types; those which have an eye through which the suture is threaded, and eyeless needles where the suture is inserted into the hollow hilt and held in position by swaging the metal around it. The first patent on an eyeless needle was obtained by the late Sir Henry Souttar in 1921, but in the U.K. their use has only increased appreciably in the past few years. In the U.S.A. 70 per cent of the suture needles are of the eyeless type.

The needles themselves are made either of stainless steel or of carbon steel, the latter usually being plated to resist corrosion. At one time the carbon steel needle had a better resistance to bending than its counterpart in stainless steel, but recent technological advances have improved stainless steel needles and they now compete in strength with carbon steel and have the added advantage that they will not corrode and do not present the surgeon with the dreaded emergency of having to locate and extract the broken point of a needle embedded somewhere in the tissues of an unfortunate patient.

REFERENCES

BULLOCH, W., LAMPITT, L. H. & BUSHILL, J. H. (1929) *The Preparation of Catgut for Surgical Use*. Medical Research Council Special Report, No. 138.

CUNNINGHAM, R. H. (1895) *New York med. J.* **61**, 494.

DAWSON, J. O., ROYLANCE, T. W. & SMITH, T. (1964) *J. Pharm. Pharmacol.* **16** Suppl., 121T.

FANDRE, A. (1944) *Le Catgut*. Paris: Masson et Cie.

HOLDER, E. J. (1946) *Desirable Factors in Surgical Sutures*. Edinburgh: William Blackwood & Sons Ltd.

LAWRIE, P. (1955) *Studies in the Absorption of Surgical Catgut*. Edinburgh: William Blackwood & Sons Ltd.

LAWRIE, P., ANGUS, E. A. & REESE, A. J. M. (1959) *Br. J. Surg.* **46**, 638.

LAWRIE, P., ANGUS, E. A. & REESE, A. J. M. (1960) *Br. J. Surg.* **47**, 551.

LISTER, J. (1869) *Lancet* 1869, **i**, 451.

MACKIE, T. J. (1928) *An Inquiry into Post-operative Tetanus*—A Report to the Scottish Board of Health.

Part VI

FORMULATION AND PACKAGING

37

Formulation

It is only on relatively few occasions that a drug, as such, may be directly administered to a patient. Usually, the medicament must be mixed with adjuvants, stabilizers, preservatives, etc. and subjected to various processes to give a practical dose-form: in other words the medicament must be formulated. The practising pharmacist is ethically and legally required to supply medicines complying with accepted specifications and for this reason must be aware of the relevant formulation and storage requirements for those medicines. These requirements are likely to be particularly stringent for the complex, more recently developed, medicaments, but care is needed even with apparently simple products such as aspirin tablets if all the main aims of formulation are to be satisfied. These aims, not in order importance, are that the product shall be:

(a) economical for large scale manufacture,
(b) acceptable,
(c) chemically and physically stable,
(d) correctly packaged,
(e) preserved against microbial contamination,
(f) able to provide correct dose of drug, and
(g) therapeutically effective.

ECONOMIC LARGE-SCALE MANUFACTURE

Earlier formulation studies will have established the main product requirements and possible means by which these may be achieved. Difficulties may arise when bench or even pilot scale methods are translated to full commercial production; Oldshue (1961), for instance, has discussed scale-up problems for solid/liquid mixing processes. Particular attention must be given to those processes which are prolonged on the industrial scale. It may be necessary, for instance, to pass a stream of nitrogen or other inert gas through an industrial comminutor if the drug is heat or oxygen sensitive and its transit time in the equipment is long. Heat-up and cool-down times for a manufactured batch may be increased by a large factor compared with bench experiment, and a degradative reaction that may be ignored during initial studies may assume crucial importance on the large scale. Theoretical treatment of the problem leads to mathematical difficulties (see Eriksen et al. 1958) but even a small additional loss, regardless of cause, could be significant within the context of the overall degradation during the life of the product and it may be necessary, for instance, to install cooling coils within the processing vessel. Alternatively, new equipment might be purchased or a completely original production facility designed. These points require a good knowledge of pharmaceutical engineering and the resources available to the particular organization, as well as an awareness that equipment and manufacturing costs must bear a reasonable relation to the expected throughput and selling price of the product.

ACCEPTABILITY

A product must be acceptable to those who handle or use it. The doctor, for instance, will note those features of a product that facilitate its administration to the patient. An injection that is so viscous that it cannot readily be drawn into the syringe is unlikely to attract continued use if an alternative more readily administered product is available. Ultimately, it is the patient who uses a product. The success of a treatment often depends on strict adherence to a given dose regimen that may extend over a considerable period of time. The patient may well find, for example, a gritty ointment or an unpalatable mixture, completely unacceptable, and may abandon treatment or ask the physician for an alternative form of the drug.

Flavour and Perfumes

These are available to the formulator as concentrated extracts and alcoholic or aqueous solutions, or they may be adsorbed on powder carriers or micro-encapsulated. They are usually mixtures of natural and synthetic materials; concentrated fruit extracts or juices are used to prepare fruit syrups. Volatile oils still find use although their solubility tends to be limited by the terpene fractions. These may be removed and the deterpenated oil is more soluble in water and dilute alcohols, has a finer flavour lacking the terpene overtones, and is some 2 to 8 times stronger than the original oil. Short (1960) makes the point that removal of terpenes leads to a less readily oxidized oil. Some flavours, and most perfumes, tend to 'disappear' when first added to a product but develop their full effect later. When deciding the optimum level at which to use these materials, products having a range of concentrations should be prepared and assessed after a short period of storage.

Only the bitter, sweet, salt or acid elements of a flavour are perceived by the taste buds of the tongue, all other flavours and perfumes being recognized by smell. A heavy cold causes almost complete obliteration of taste and smell. As water-insoluble materials have little or no taste, unpleasant drugs may be rendered more acceptable by administration as a water-insoluble derivative—a classical example is chloramphenicol palmitate—although acceptability obtained in this way may cause problems of sedimentation, bio-availability, etc. If an insoluble derivative cannot be used, a strong perfume or flavour may be required to mask an unpleasant drug but there is the high probability that a strong identifiable perfume or flavour, initially acceptable, may eventually be actively disliked if the treatment is prolonged. It must be remembered that the preferences of the sick adult or child do not necessarily coincide with, and are likely to be more capricious than those of the healthy subject. Where possible it is probably better to use a neutral but nevertheless pleasant and effective flavour or perfume that is not recognized

by the patient. The problems of flavouring are most acute for paediatric preparations where a very strong flavour may itself cause nausea and vomiting. Few situations are more difficult than the firmly shut mouth of a child refusing to take a medicine.

There are associations between colours and flavours e.g. yellow with lemon, red with cherry, etc. and between flavours e.g. acids with citrus flavours. It is generally true that lime flavour, for instance, is more appropriate to a pale green, faintly acid product than to one which is neutral and coloured red. With the wide range of flavours available to the formulator it is not surprising that there has been a tendency for the traditional materials to be ignored but there is still a case for the judicious use of pharmaceutical substances such as oils of dill and caraway, and oleoresins of capsicum and ginger, particularly in those situations where their carminative action may be useful in allaying any gastric upset caused by the drug. A persistent flavour of the chocolate type, or the local anaesthetic action of menthol, pure or in peppermint oil, is particularly effective in covering bitter unpleasant tastes—a combination of both may be tried if the taste of ferrous salts must be masked. Charnicki and Kober (1957), in describing all stages of the flavouring trials for an aqueous oral penicillin/sulphonamide product, noted that a flavouring agent may also adversely affect product stability. Vanillin accelerated decomposition, whereas clove and aniseed were without effect. As will be seen, sulphur dioxide used to preserve fruit juices and syrups against microbial spoilage has been implicated in the fading of colouring substances.

Apart from flavouring it may be necessary to cover a bitter taste by means of a sweet vehicle. While sucrose is likely to remain the most widely employed sweetening agent, glycerin and chloroform may be of value and have preservative action in sufficient concentration. Alternatively, given suitable preparations, honey, liquorice and treacle have useful sweetening action. Soluble saccharin (the sodium salt) is said to have a less obtrusive bitter after-taste than saccharin itself and, depending on concentration, is about 200 to 700 times sweeter than sugar; it is best used in conjunction with sugar at trial concentrations of 0.02–0.05 per cent. The cyclamates are 20 to 30 times sweeter than sugar but until their freedom from toxicity has been completely established it would be wise to avoid their use in formulation. Sorbitol is recommended as a replacement for sugar in diabetic preparations but has only half the sweetening power, is more expensive and is said to have some laxative action. It is converted to fructose in the liver and is contra-indicated where there is intolerance to that sugar. It may be noted also that lactose used in tablets may give trouble with galactosaemic patients. These problems are most acute for children where the dose of carbohydrate related to body weight is higher than for adults. A useful review is given by Leach (1970).

Colours
These may be derived from natural sources (Cochineal) or made synthetically (Tartrazine). They may be soluble in water (Amaranth), in oil (Scarlet Red) or insoluble in both solvents. In the latter group those of pharmaceutical interest include a few pigments (Bole) and the lakes which are insoluble calcium or aluminium complexes of water-soluble dyes. Carmine is the aluminium lake of the colouring matter from cochineal. Lakes are included in tablets and tablet coating because of their greater light stability compared with the corresponding water-soluble dye. Opacification of the shell of capsules of Chlordiazepoxide and some other drugs by lakes etc., is carried out where it is necessary to exclude light and avoid photodecomposition.

The majority of dyes used in formulation are synthetically produced and are usually salts. The coloured ion may react with substances of opposite polarity; thus both Tartrazine and Amaranth give insoluble salts with solutions containing nicotine. Dyes vary in their stability to pH, light and reducing agents as discussed by Swartz and Cooper (1962). Non-ionic surfactants may promote accelerated fading due possibly to interaction between the ethylene oxide moiety of the surfactant and the chromophoric group of the dye (Scott et al. 1962). The effect of such variables should be checked in the formulated product for the proposed range of dyes.

Dyes are used to standardize or improve an existing colour, to mask an innocuous colour change, to complement a flavour or odour or for identification purposes. Unfortunately there is evidence that some dyes may act as carcinogens or are otherwise undesirable and for this reason are not permitted in foodstuffs or, by implication, in drugs or cosmetics. Dyes must be selected with care as there is no internationally recognized list of permitted colours; a colour which is allowed in one country may be totally banned in another. A useful summary of the situation is given in the Extra Pharmacopoiea (Martindale) (1972). In Great Britain the colouring agents which may be used are given in the Colouring Matter in Foods Regulations, 1966 (S.I. 1966: No. 1203) and for Scotland in S.I. 1966: No. 1384. If it is imperative to include a dye in the formulation, the lowest concentration should be used, especially for paediatric products, since children are likely to vomit with consequent staining of clothes.

STABILITY

The main causes of physical and chemical instability have been discussed elsewhere in this volume. Here only a number of details in the use of anhydrous vehicles and in the formulation of suspensions will be discussed.

Anhydrous Vehicles
If these are needed for the formulation of water sensitive drugs in oral products, either a water miscible or an oily vehicle may be considered. The former could comprise various mixtures of ethyl or isopropyl alcohols, glycerol, propylene glycol or the low molecular weight polyoxyethylene glycols. Ethylene glycol must *not* be used as it is metabolized to oxalic acid which is toxic. Generally, vehicles based on alcohols and glycols have an unpleasant burning taste but are much more acceptable if diluted with water immediately prior to administration. If the stability of the medicament is such that it will have a reasonable shelf-life in the presence of a limited amount of water, a combination of the alcohols with a suitable syrup produces an acceptable vehicle of the type used for the official elixirs.

As well as olive and arachis oils, a number of other oils are suitable for the formulation of oily vehicles. Cottonseed, soyabean and corn oils are all used for culinary purposes and are sufficiently bland for consideration as oily vehicles for oral preparations. Fractionated coconut oil is virtually colourless, odourless and tasteless; it is used as a diluent for Phenoxymethylpenicillin Mixture BPC. Such vehicles are rather difficult to flavour except with vanillin, volatile oils or other oil-soluble flavours. Sweetness may be improved by the addition of saccharin.

Anhydrous vehicles are also much used for the formulation of ointments, suppositories and parenteral solutions. In the first two types of product a suitable consistency is obtained by the inclusion or exclusive use of fats and waxes. Absorption from topical preparations and the pharmacological basis of topical therapy are discussed by Wagner (1961) and D'Arcy (1965) respectively. Systemic medication per rectum is convenient where oral administration may induce nausea or vomiting, onset of action is usually faster than by the oral route and (in common with buccal absorption) enterohepatic recycling is avoided. The lower efficiency of rectal absorption may dictate a dose larger than that given by mouth. The formulation of suppositories and related matters are discussed by Senior (1969a & b) and Wagner (1971). Anhydrous injection vehicles have been reviewed by Speigel and Noseworthy (1963), who note that care is needed in selecting the vehicle if unwanted modification of drug activity is to be avoided. Polyoxyethylene glycol vehicles markedly increase the toxicity of nitrofurantoin and are incompatible with many phenolic substances. If the drug is only partially soluble in the vehicle, temperature fluctuation may cause a coarsening of the particle size of the undissolved portion. For completely soluble drugs it is necessary to check that this condition also obtains at a suitably low temperature, say $-5°$, as material deposited at a lower than normal temperature may not readily redissolve when the temperature rises again.

Suspensions
The stability of these depends both on the properties of the dispersed solid and on those of the vehicle. Apart from gravitational sedimentation which is a function of particle size, the behaviour of the solid may be determined by the zeta potential. If this is small, say in the range $+25$ to -25 mV, nett attractive forces cause particles to aggregate and settle rapidly to form a high volume loosely packed sediment which is readily redispersed on shaking. At larger zeta potentials repulsive forces predominate and particles sediment individually and slowly to form a densely packed, clay-like, dilatant sediment which is not easily redispersed by shaking. From the point of view of product formulation neither system is satisfactory but, as discussed by Haines and Martin (1961), it may be possible to adjust the zeta potential of the suspended particles by addition of electrolytes to give the optimum compromise between the slow sedimentation of the deflocculated state and the ready redispersion of sediment that is characteristic of the flocculated system. For this purpose, polyvalent ions are usually most efficient; for example, sodium citrate controls the degree of flocculation of the bentonite in Calamine Lotion, and hence its consistency; it will also deflocculate a 100 per cent w/w barium sulphate paste to give

a thin pourable suspension. Matthews and Rhodes (1968a & b) reported that satisfactory griseofulvin suspensions may be prepared by zeta potential control with Al^{3+} ions.

Even with correct control of the zeta potential, the size or density of the particles may be such that they still settle too rapidly for the proper quantity of medicament to be poured out, drawn into a syringe or topically applied. For *dilute* suspensions the rate v at which a particle of density D and radius r settles in a liquid of viscosity η and density d is given by Stokes' equation in the form:

$$v = \frac{2r^2(D-d)g}{9\eta} \qquad (37.1)$$

In general, for more concentrated dispersions crowding and other effects will reduce the rate of settling. The densities of the particles and vehicle are fixed by product requirements while processing methods, therapeutic requirements, etc. may determine the optimum particle size in which case it is only by increasing the viscosity of the vehicle that the sedimentation rate may be decreased. For this purpose, as well as traditional suspending agents such as tragacanth and acacia, the alginates and cellulose derivatives should also be considered. As noted elsewhere in this volume, modification of the naturally occurring cellulose chain produced the first commercial plastics; it is also a fruitful starting material for a large number of hydrophilic colloids. Cellulose is an extended open chain some 1000 to 3000 anhydro-β-glucose units long (Fig. 37.1). Steric hindrance near the -O-linkages limits rotation of the glucose units relative to one another. This, together with the rigidity of the glucose units restricts the flexibility of the chain. Interchain attraction is very high due to hydrogen bonding between neighbouring -OH groups and as a result cellulose is not thermoplastic, cannot be plasticized and is insoluble in all but very acid or alkaline aqueous media. If the -OH is modified by the formation, of an ester, e.g. cellulose acetate, or ether, e.g. methyl cellulose, hydrogen bonding is much reduced and the properties of the resultant product

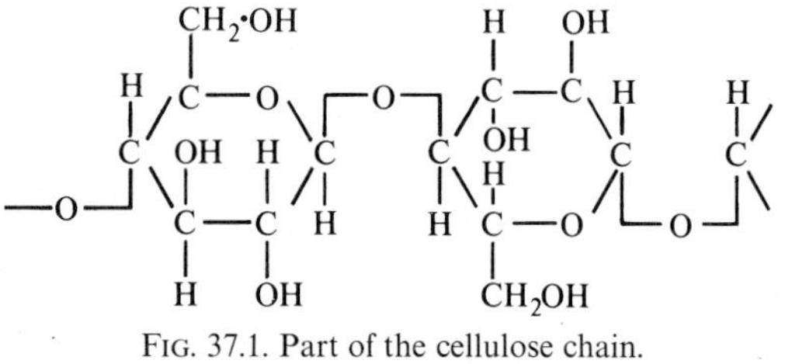

FIG. 37.1. Part of the cellulose chain.

will depend on the degree of substitution, the average chain length and the distribution of chain lengths. In general the degree of substitution controls the solubility (Table 37.1) while the chain

TABLE 37.1

THE EFFECT OF SUBSTITUION ON THE SOLUBILITY OF
CELLULOSE ESTERS

Derivative	Alkoxyl groups/glucose unit		Soluble in
Methyl–	1.6–1.8	$-OCH_3$	Water
Ethyl–	0.5	$-OC_2H_5$	10 per cent NaOH solution
	0.8–1.3		Water
	1.4–2.5		Alcohol
	2.5–2.8		Non-polar solvents
Sodium carboxy-methyl–	0.7–0.8	$-OCH_2COONa$	Water
Hydroxy-propyl-methyl–	1.6–1.8 0.1–0.2	$-OCH_3$ $-OC_3H_7OH$	Water—low to medium viscosity
	1.1–1.4 0.1–0.3	$-OCH_3$ $-OC_3H_7OH$	Water—medium to high viscosity

length and distribution determines the viscosity grade. The propoxyl group is sufficiently hydrophobic for propyl cellulose to be insoluble in water at all levels of substitution. The viscosity grade is indicated by a number after the name, i.e. Hypromellose 20 BPC would be that grade of hydroxypropylmethylcellulose which, at a concentration of 2 per cent in water gives a solution with a viscosity of 20 centistokes. A 2 per cent solution is also used for standardizing methylcellulose but the concentration is 1 per cent for sodium alginate and sodium carboxymethylcellulose. Sodium alginate is a purified substance extracted from *Laminaria* type seaweeds. Alginic acid is a D-mannuronic acid polymer; solutions of the sodium salt at a given concentration become more viscous as the degree of polymerization of the acid is increased. A wide variety of viscosity grades is available but only one (30–60) is official. Carboxypolymethylene is a totally synthetic vinyl polymer with a high degree of carboxyl substitution. The acid powder is dispersed in water and then neutralized with a base to give a viscous solution that is most stable between pH 6 and pH 11. Unless protected by an antioxidant the solutions lose viscosity on exposure to sunlight.

Substances that desolvate the polymer chain of suspending agents reduce the viscosity of their solutions and may, eventually, precipitate the polymer. Typical of such substances are inorganic salts and high concentrations of such hydrophilic materials as alcohol, glycerol and sucrose. Heating solutions of the polymers changes their viscosity reversibly thus solutions of methylcellulose or hydroxypropylmethylcellulose gel at a certain temperature, the so-called gel-point, which is lower for methyl- than for hydroxypropylmethyl cellulose. Above the gel-point the polymer is precipitated. Prolonged heating, however, of most natural and synthetic suspending agents leads to depolymerization and permanent loss of viscosity. This loss of viscosity may amount to some 25 per cent when, for instance, sodium carboxymethylcellulose solutions are sterilized by autoclaving.

Sodium alginate, –carboxymethylcellulose and –carboxypolymethylene give insoluble salts with a number of multivalent metal ions and the acids are precipitated at a sufficiently low pH. Hypromellose is the preferred polymer for thickening ophthalmic solutions as these are clearer and have fewer undispersed fibres. The official preparation is used for the replacement of lachrymal secretion where this is deficient.

The availability of a wide range of viscosity grades permits the selection of the grade and type of polymer best suited to the needs of the product. Assume, for instance that it is required to suspend a powder of 50 μm maximum diameter and density 1.5 g/cm³. If the mixture is to be taken every four hours an arbitrary decision might be taken that the largest particles must not sediment more than 1 cm in that time. The density of the vehicle may be taken as 1.0 g/cm³. Substituting in equation (37.1):

$$\frac{1}{4 \times 60 \times 60} = \frac{2 \times (25 \times 10^{-4})^2 \times (1.5 - 1.0) \times 981}{9\eta}$$

(37.2)

whence $\eta \approx 10$ poise

From Fig. 37.2 it would appear that the most economical materials for providing a vehicle of this viscosity would be Tragacanth or Sodium carboxymethylcellulose 3500 at a concentration of about 0.7 per cent. Smoother pouring characteristics might result from using a lower viscosity grade suspending agent at a higher concentration. Additionally, less suspending agent than is implied by the above calculation would probably achieve the desired performance as the majority of particles would have a diameter less than 50 μm. In any case their concentration is likely to be greater than

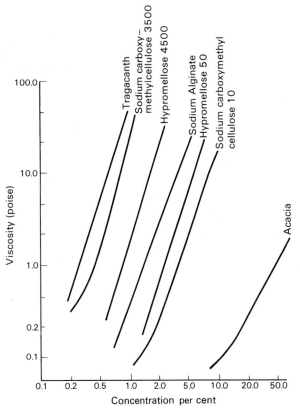

FIG. 37.2. Viscosity of some solutions of hydrocolloids as a function of concentration. These curves should be used as a guide only as the viscosity is very dependent on the method of measurement and the technique used to prepare the solutions.

that for which Stokes' equation is strictly applicable and sedimentation would be hindered by crowding and other effects. Clearly, the foregoing effects would need to be investigated by direct experiment.

For lotions and related products it may be possible to thicken the product with bentonite or related materials that form structured gels with water. The intention is that vigorous shaking would break the structure to give a thin pourable product but on standing the structure would reform and so prevent sedimentation of dispersed solids.

(*Packaging* is considered in Chapter 39.)

PRESERVATION AGAINST MICROBIAL SPOILAGE

In the strictest sense microbial spoilage is another form of product instability but is conveniently discussed here as a separate issue. There is an obvious connection with the addition of bacteriostatics to multidose quantities of injections to prevent the development of microorganisms accidentally introduced during use; indeed, this is a specific instance of the general problem of preventing microbial spoilage where failure may have particularly serious consequences. The addition of antimicrobial substances to non-sterile preparations is intended to stop the multiplication of microorganisms present when the product was manufactured as well as those subsequently introduced. It is important that preservative measures should have a broad spectrum of activity because of the wide range of the likely contaminants both bacterial and fungal, the impossibility of predicting the kind of contamination that may occur during the life of the product, and the nutrient properties of many pharmaceutical products.

Physical Methods of Protection

These include sterilization and pasteurization, low moisture content, unfavourable pH, low temperature, minimum nutrient content and high osmotic pressure. It may be noted that a number of *Aspergillus* and *Penicillium* spp will grow at a pH as low as 2.0 while osmophilic yeasts are found in honey. However, the major disadvantage with physical methods of protection is that they become inoperative as soon as the particular constraint is removed, for example, the product is stored in a warm rather than cool place or the closure is taken out of a vial of sterile product. It is generally preferable to use a method that is largely independent of the environmental conditions namely the addition of a chemical substance that will kill contaminating organisms or at least prevent their multiplication in the product during storage and use.

Chemical Methods of Preservation

In addition to the specific requirement that an antimicrobial substance shall have a wide range of activity against contaminating organisms it must also comply with the more general requirements for all pharmaceutical adjuvants. It should be:
(a) effective in low concentration,
(b) non-toxic, non-irritant and non-sensitizing,
(c) odourless, tasteless, colourless and soluble in the proposed vehicle,
(d) stable and effective, unaffected by pH,
(e) inert, non-volatile, readily prepared in a pure state, easily standardized, and
(f) compatible with all other product constituents.
A list of commonly used preservatives is given in Table 37.2.

TABLE 37.2
SUBSTANCES USED AS ANTIMICROBIAL PRESERVATIVES

Substance	Usual concentration per cent w/v	Remarks
For oral use:		
Ethyl alcohol	At least 10	These hydroxylic materials probably act by increased osmotic
Isoprpyl alcohol	At least 10	pressure. Ethylene glycol is toxic and must *not* be used (see text)
Glycerol	At least 25	
Propylene glycol	At least 25	
Sugar	At least 65	
Sulphur dioxide and sulphites	400 ppm.	Used in foodstuffs
e.g. sodium metabisulphite	0.1	Oxidizes and loses efficiency; may reduce dyes
Benzoic acid	0.1	Rapid loss of effectiveness above pH 5.0. Soluble about 0.3 per cent in water at room temperature
Dehydroacetic acid	0.1	More effective in acid products
Sorbic acid	0.1	More effective in acid products. Soluble about 0.15 per cent in water at room temperature
Methyl *p*-hydroxybenzoate	0.2	Less effective above pH 8.0. Soluble about 0.3 per cent in water at room temperature
Propyl *p*-hydroxybenzoate	0.02	Less effective above pH 8.0. Soluble about 0.03 per cent in water at room temperature Mixtures of these esters have a wider range of action. May be used as carbon source by one species of *Ps.aeruginosa* (Hugo & Foster 1964) Solutions of the sodium salts are strongly alkaline
Chloroform	0.25 0.5	Chloroform water Double strength chloroform water Has warm sweet taste. Is very volatile and is easily lost from the product
For other uses:		
Alcohols and glycols Benzoic, dehydroacetic and sorbic acid *p*-hydroxybenzoic acid esters		See above. Sorbic acid may cause skin irritation.
Formaldehyde		Very effective and highly reactive—may cause skin irritation. Rarely used in pharmaceutical products but 0.05 per cent may be used in shampoos
Benzyl alcohol	1.0	Has weak local anaesthetic action
Phenylethyl alcohol	0.5	Has been used in ophthalmic preparations
β-Phenoxyethyl alcohol	1.0	Very little action against Gram-positive organisms
Chlorbutol	0.8	Soluble about 0.8 per cent—action is erratic due to losses by volatilisation and hydrolysis—HCl is produced and may acidify the product
Phenol	0.5	
Cresol	0.3	
Chlorocresol	0.1	
Thiomersal	0.01	Unstable at pH lower than 7
Phenylmercuric salts	0.001	Maximum solubility about 0.1 per cent depending on salt used. The highly insoluble chloride may be precipitated if product contains chloride ions.
Chorhexidine salts	0.01	Has been used for ophthalmic preparations. Salts of low solubility formed with many anions particularly of the anionic surfactants
Quaternary ammonium salts e.g. Benzalkonium chloride	0.01	Incompatible with anionic surfactants, alkali hydroxides and carbonates. Benzalkonium chloride has been used in ophthalmic preparations

Selection of Anti-Microbial Preservatives

In addition to the simple sub-division into oral and other use (Table 37.2) there may be other restrictions that narrow the range of choice when selecting a preservative. Apart from gross incompatibilities there are a number of situations in which activity may be impaired. Either the proportion of the the active form of the preservative may be reduced (as with the effect of unfavourable pH) or (as occurs with hydrocolloids, surfactants and oil phases) the active form may be bound and not available for action.

Adjustment of the pH of a solution may affect both the chemical stability and the activity of the preservative. The former effect is, however, usually slight. If it is accepted that most pharmaceutical products will have a pH in the range 3–8, the only commonly used preservative for which serious chemical instability problems are likely to arise is thiomersal which degrades in acid media. Within the assumed pH range there will, however, be a marked variation in the activity of the ionized preservatives. In general, it is the *unionized* form of these that has antimicrobial activity and the proportion of that form at any pH may be calculated by means of the Henderson-Hasselbalch equation arranged as follows:

Proportion of unionized preservative

$$= \frac{1}{1 + \text{antilog}(\text{pH} - \text{pK}_a)} \quad (37.3)$$

Bandelin (1958) examined the effect of pH on the activity of a number of ionizable preservatives against *Chaetomium globosum*, *Alternaria solani*, *Penicillium citrinum* and *Aspergillus niger*. The substances chosen for the study were benzoic, sorbic and dehydroacetic acids and the esters of *p*-hydroxybenzoic acid. As expected, he found that the activity decreased as the pH increased. In general, *A.niger* was the organism most resistant to the antifungal action of the preservatives. His data for that organism is summarized in Fig. 37.3. Winsley and Walters (1965) also grew *A.niger* in media of differing pH in the presence of benzoic acid and determined the concentration of this that just stopped growth—see also Fig. 37.3. By multiplying the minimum inhibitory concentration by the proportion of unionized molecules at the particular pH they were able to calculate the minimum inhibitory concentration for the completely unionized acid. The constancy of this value (0.0169–0.0185) argues strongly in favour of the view that it is the unionized form of the benzoic acid which

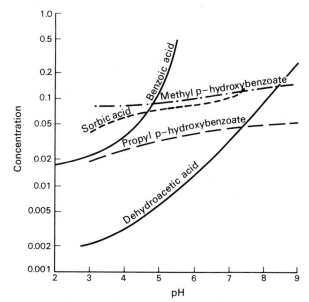

FIG. 37.3. Effect of pH on the minimum inhibitory concentration of some acid preservatives against *Aspergillus niger*. (Winsley & Walters, 1965, Bandelin 1958).

is responsible for antifungal action. With a knowledge of the pKa and the minimum inhibitory concentration for the unionized form it is possible to calculate the minimum inhibitory concentration at any pH. Suppose it is required to preserve a product of pH 4.7 with benzoic acid and that *A.niger* is a likely challenge organism. The pKa of benzoic acid is 4.2 and substituting in equation (37.3):

Proportion of unionized benzoic acid at pH 4.7

$$= \frac{1}{1 + \text{antilog}[4.7 - 4.2]}$$

$$= \frac{1}{1 + 3.16} = 0.24$$

Preservative concentration of acid at pH 4.7

$$= \frac{0.0185}{0.24} \text{ per cent} = 0.07 \text{ per cent}$$

It would be good practice to allow a safety margin and use, say, 0.1–0.15 per cent of the preservative in the product.

The activity of preservatives is reduced if these are bound by another substance. Hydrophilic colloids of the type used for suspending insoluble solids are particularly liable to cause trouble. The hydroxybenzoate esters, for instance, are indifferent to the presence of tragacanth and sodium carboxy-methylcellulose but show loss activity in the presence of methylcellulose, polyvinylpyrrolidone and gelatin (Miyawaki et al. 1959). On the other hand, methylcellulose diminishes the activity of cetylpyridinium chloride (Delucca & Kostenbauder 1960). As there is no simple rule by which interaction may be predicted it is advisable directly to check antimicrobial activity where hydrocolloids are employed in a formulation.

In their active form many preservatives are predominantly lipophilic and tend to partition between the hydrophilic and lipophilic phases of a two-phase system. The absorption of preservatives by rubber and plastics is discussed elsewhere but it must be remembered that absorption may also occur with any other lipophilic solid. A solution of water-soluble surfactant may be regarded as another type of two-phase system with an aqueous and a lipophilic micellar pseudophase between which the preservative may partition; the effect is well known in the field of phenolic disinfectants. In the presence of polyoxyethylene sorbitan oleate loss of activity has been shown to occur with sorbic acid (Blaug & Ahsan 1961a), cetylpyridinium chloride (Delucca & Kostenbauder 1960) and the p-hydroxy-benzoic acid esters (Pisano & Kostenbauder 1959). The foregoing surfactants at a 5 per cent concentration, caused a four-fold increase in the amount of methyl p-hydroxybenzoate required for effective preservative action (Blaug & Ahsan 1961b). It is possible to determine the amount of preservative in the aqueous phase of a surfactant solution; this allows comparison of the activity of solutions with and without surfactant, but having the same concentration of preservative in the aqueous phase. Humphreys et al. (1968) found a higher than predicted activity for benzoic acid/non-ionic surfactant systems which they ascribed to micelles acting as reservoirs for preservative and to other effects.

Emulsions are more obvious examples of two-phase systems. In the simplest model, a mechanical dispersion of oil in water, lipophilic antimicrobial substances will partition between the oil and water until:

$$\frac{\text{Concentration of preservative in oil}}{\text{Concentration in water}}$$

$$= \frac{C_o}{C_w} = \text{the partition coefficient } (K)$$

The weight of preservative in the system is

$C(V_o + V_w) = C_w V_w + V_o C_o$ where C is the concentration of preservative in the whole system and V_w and V_o are the volumes of water and oil respectively. If $V_o/V_w = \phi$

$$C(\phi V_w + V_w) = C_w V_w + \phi V_w K C_w$$

and $$C_w = \frac{C(\phi + 1)}{\phi K + 1} \qquad (37.4)$$

The effect of partitioning in a simple oil–water system is described in a paper by Bean & Heman-Ackah (1964). For a liquid paraffin–water system at 15° the partition coefficient of phenol is 0.062. If ϕ is 1.0—i.e. a 50 per cent v/v dispersion and the overall concentration (C) of phenol in the preparation is 0.5 per cent, the concentration of that substance in the aqueous phase is:

$$C_w = \frac{0.5(1.0 + 1.0)}{0.062 \times 1.0 + 1.0} = 0.94 \text{ per cent.}$$

This is due to the fact that the partition coefficient as defined above is less than 1.0. The efficiency (E) of an antimicrobial substance is given by:

$$E = pC_w^m \qquad (37.5)$$

where p is a constant and n is the concentration exponent; for phenol and chlorocresol n may be put equal to 6. If, arbitrarily, the efficiency of a 0.5 per cent phenol solution is set at 1.0 the relative activity of a 0.94 per cent solution is:

$$\frac{E}{1.0} = \frac{p(0.94)^6}{p(0.5)^6} = (1.88)^6 = 44.2$$

The foregoing enhanced activity may be compared with the decrease that occurs when chlorocresol is employed under similar circumstances. The partition coefficient is 1.34 at 15° and a suitable value for C is 0.1 per cent. The concentration of preservative in the aqueous phase of a 50 per cent v/v dispersion may be calculated as 0.086 per cent and the efficiency is reduced to 0.41, that is, less than half the value for the corresponding simple aqueous solution having the same overall concentration of chlorocresol.

Bean and Heman-Ackah point out that the partition coefficient usually changes in favour of the oil as the temperature is raised and this may explain the failure of products in a warm climate that have proved satisfactory in a more temperate environment. Thus, if the temperature of the above dispersion were raised to 35° (when the partition coefficient for chlorocresol at 35° is 1.78) the concentration of preservative in the aqueous phase is only 0.072 per cent and a relative efficiency 0:14 as compared with 0.41.

A real emulsion might include an emulgent which could provide a micellar pseudophase into which the antimicrobial substance would partition. The behaviour of a preservative in a real emulsion is therefore more complex than in the two-phase system described above and a full theoretical treatment would reflect this. By finding experimentally the ratio (R) of the total preservative in the aqueous phase to the free preservative in that phase Bean et al. (1969) were able to simplify the theoretical treatment and derived the expression:

$$C_w = \frac{C(\phi + 1)}{K\phi + R} \qquad (37.6)$$

where the symbols have the previously defined meanings. Extending the previous example with chlorocresol as the preservative ($\phi = 1.0$, $K = 1.34$ and $C = 0.1$ per cent) with $R = 3$ that is, three quarters of the total amount of preservative in the aqueous phase is locked in micelles:

$$C_w = \frac{0.1(1.0 + 1.0)}{1.34 \times 1.0 + 3.0} = \frac{0.2}{4.34} = 0.046 \text{ per cent.}$$

and

$$\frac{E}{1.0} = \frac{p(0.046)^6}{p(0.1)^6} = (0.046)^6 = 0.01$$

It will be clear from the above calculation why it is so difficult to preserve emulsions against microbial contamination. In general, the oil and emulgent concentration should be kept to as low a value as possible, the selected antimicrobial substance should have a low concentration exponent and all components should be chosen to minimize the value of K and R. The amount of preservative in the aqueous phase will, of course, be raised by substances that increase its solubility in that phase. Hibbott and Monks (1961), for example, reported that the partition coefficient of methyl hydroxybenzoate is changed in favour of the aqueous phase if this contains glycerol or propylene glycol. These and many other factors that affect the preservation of emulsified preparations are discussed in considerable detail by Wedderburn (1964). It should be noted that many countries now require creams to be supplied in a sterile condition, or at least with a very low level of contamination; this is the main purpose of official instructions for the preparation and packaging of creams. For complete assurance of sterility it may be necessary to heat the cream in which case there will be problems of physical stability superimposed upon those associated with preservative activity.

Assessment procedures usually reveal the minimum concentration needed to protect the product against specific organisms. A safety margin must, however, be provided to take account of manufacturing tolerances. By way of illustration assume that 0.3 per cent phenol is found to be the best preservative for a given lotion. It may be considered that 90 to 110 per cent of the nominal amount of preservative is a reasonable manufacturing tolerance. By substitution in equation 37.5, however, it can be shown that reduction of the concentration of phenol to 90 per cent of the nominal value will have a very marked effect on the bactericidal efficiency of the preparation. Thus for phenol $n = 6$ and:

$$\frac{E}{1.0} = \frac{p(90)^6}{p(100)^6} = 0.53$$

A reduction of the phenol concentration of 10 per cent has therefore reduced the bactericidal efficiency to 53 per cent of its original value. Clearly, to provide for the worst conditions of manufacture, the amount of phenol must be increased to:

$$\frac{0.3 \times 100}{90} = 0.33 \text{ per cent}$$

In practice an even higher concentration, perhaps 0.5 per cent, would be used to ensure efficient protection during the whole life of the product.

Testing preservative efficiency. There is no standard method for testing the activity of a preservative in a product. Although details vary there is general agreement that performance should be compared in normal and sterilized products when challenged by a variety of bacteria and fungi. These should also include a mixed culture obtained at the manufacturing unit, organisms isolated from failed samples and any special organisms relevant to the end use of the product, e.g., it is advisable to challenge eye-drops with several pseudomonad species and in particular with *Pseudomonas aeruginosa*. This organism is exceptionally resistant to the action of most preservatives which are acceptable for use in ophthalmic preparations (Brown & Norton 1965).

Inoculated samples should be incubated for at least 10 weeks at a variety of temperatures between 20° and 40°. Samples must be examined at intervals appropriate to the product, e.g. an hour or less for ophthalmic preparations as a rapid kill is required, whereas less frequent sampling would be more appropriate to mixtures. If possible the test should be carried out in such a way that quantitative results may be obtained.

Correct Dose

Although every care may be taken in the manufacture of a drug preparation the patient will not receive the correct dose if the product has deteriorated in storage. Chemical degradation leads to a reduction in the amount of the active constituent and low dose follows directly from this. If the product is physically unstable then the correct total amount of drug may be present but this may be unevenly distributed throughout the product. In this way the patient may receive a variable dose of drug. This situation is potentially dangerous in those cases where the drug forms a dilatant sediment which is not easily dispersed by shaking the full container. Early doses might contain less than the correct amount of drug. Later, because shaking may be more efficient with a partially emptied container, the sediment may become dispersed and the patient could be exposed to an overdose.

Uneven distribution may also arise from unsuspected faults in the manufacturing process, particularly if this involves the dispersion of one solid phase with another. The difficulties in obtaining even distribution of a small amount of drug in a much larger quantity have been discussed in the sections concerned with mixing, and with tablets and capsules, in Chapters 17 and 19 respectively. It should be noted that, even if the correct manufacturing procedures have been employed, bulk powders may demix during storage and transport and every care should be taken at the formulation stage to foresee and eliminate this possibility.

Finally, the correct amount of drug in a product, as determined by analysis, does not guarantee that the desired clinical response will be elicited in the patient. This matter is considered in the next section.

THERAPEUTIC EFFECTIVENESS

With very few exceptions a drug must be in aqueous solution to exert its therapeutic action.

Often the site of action is remote from the site of administration and therefore a transport system is required; this is provided by the circulation of blood (Fig. 37.4). When administered by buccal, rectal, intramuscular, or subcutaneous routes, the drug directly diffuses into the blood from the absorbing tissue. Onset of action from this route will, therefore, be somewhat slower than by intravenous administration where the drug is directly injected into the blood. Onset of action is even longer by the oral route. This is partly due to the transit time of the drug to that part of the gastro-intestinal tract from which it is best absorbed, to the nature of the absorbing tissue, hepato-enteric recycling and to the nature of the oral product. Simple solutions tend to act faster than suspensions as time will be required for the suspended solid to dissolve so that it can exert its effect. Similarly, suspensions (fine particles) will act faster than powders (coarse particles) which in turn act faster than capsules and tablets. As far as the body is concerned all drugs are foreign substances and mechanisms are available for their elimination. The drug may be excreted in the faeces, urine or saliva, etc. either unaltered or as metabolites. The therapeutic response is often related to the amount of drug in the blood which in turn is determined by the nett effect of the absorption, transport and elimination processes. Products may therefore be ranked in order of promptness of response and duration of action as in Table 37.3. Each type of product will have a characteristic response, thus without considering the relevant theory at this stage, the graph for the time course of action for an oral product may be sketched as in Fig. 37.5. If the characteristic response of any product is to be modified for whatever purpose, there are three main ways in which this may be done:

Biological—a classic example is the co-administration of adrenalin with local anaesthetics to cause local vasoconstriction which minimizes leakage of anaesthetic from the injection site and therefore prolongs its action.

Chemical—the compound diethylaminoacetanilide (I) is clearly related to lignocaine (diethylaminoacet-2,6-xylidide) (II), and yet has only transient local anaesthetic action. This is due to the absence

I

II

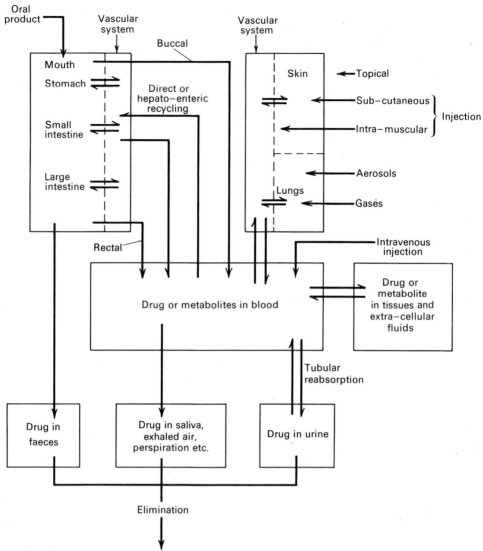

FIG. 37.4. Distribution of drugs in the body.

of methyl groups in the 2,6 positions that allows hydrolytic enzymes to gain access to the –NH.CO– group which is rapidly hydrolysed and the activity of the drug destroyed.

Pharmaceutical—by embedding a drug in wax, the rate of release of the drug may be slowed down and the activity prolonged in suitable cases.

Most frequently the formulator will use the third method to modify drug action but there are occasions where the second method may be more applicable. Two examples will be quoted here. Above a certain dose level, the duration of action of

oestradiol by deep intramuscular injection is independent of the dose. The diproprionate ester is the preferred form of the medicament for depot injections as, in vivo, hydrolysis of the ester controls the release of the hormone and the duration of the action is dose dependent. Basic drugs form insoluble tannates from which the base is released in the body at a controlled rate by hydrolysis. The tannates of pheniramine, mepyramine and phenylephrine have been combined in both tablet and suspension formulations to provide a sustained action product. Regardless of the method chosen, the formulator may be concerned either with

TABLE 36.3

THERAPEUTIC EFFECTIVENESS OF PHARMACEUTICAL PRODUCTS

Type	Product	Onset	Duration
Conventional	i/v injection	Immediate—seconds	Normal for drug by that route—usually some four to six hours
	i/m injection. Subcutaneous injection. Buccal tablet. Suppository. Aerosol. Gases	Rapid—up to a few minutes	Normal for drug by that route
	Oral preparations Solution. Suspension. Powder. Capsule. Tablet	Prompt to slow—a few minutes to more than an hour	Normal for drug by that route
	Topical products	Varies	Varies
Modified	Prolonged action tablets, capsules and short term depot injections	Prompt to slow—a few minutes to over an hour	Longer than normal for drug by that route—up to twelve hours
	Enteric coated preparations	Delayed up to a few hours	Normal for drug after onset of action
	Long term depot injections	Up to a few days	Several weeks
	Solid implants	Up to a few days	Several months

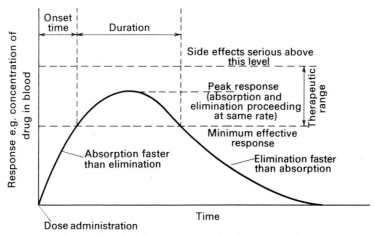

FIG. 37.5. Typical time course of action for a dose of drug.

correcting unintentional deficiencies in an existing product of conventional type or with the design of a modified dose-form with defined performance. In general these objectives may be attained by attention to the biological availability of the drug. Often, this is defined with reference to a 'standard' preparation but in quantifying this parameter it is also necessary to take account both of the total amount and rate of release of drug, particularly in relation to the nature of the required therapeutic action. The definition is best illustrated by reference to Fig. 37.6. For product A the onset is rapid and the response is maintained above the minimum effective level for a suitable period of time, i.e., the biological availability is high. Although the same amount of drug is released by product B, at no

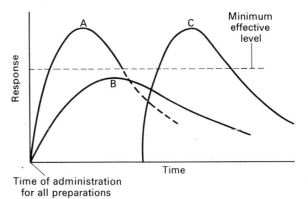

FIG. 37.6. Time course of action characteristics for conventional and modified products. A, effective conventional product; B, non-effective conventional product; C, modified product.

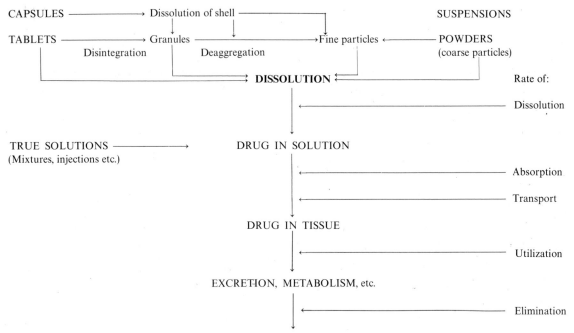

FIG. 37.7. Course of drug utilization for conventional products.

time is the minimum effective level attained and therefore the biological availability is low. On occasion it may be desirable to delay the release of drug because, for instance, it is inactivated by acid gastric secretions. The curve for product C best expresses the type of response that is required for high biological availability under these circumstances.

Biological Availability of Drugs from Conventional Preparations

It is axiomatic that a drug preparation shall be therapeutically effective yet only in the past decade or so has it been realized how wide may be the margin between potential activity as inferred from the known drug content and the actual activity observed in clinical use. For example, Anderson (1966) related the low therapeutic activity of a chloramphenicol palmitate preparation to the use of the wrong polymorph (q.v.). As noted earlier, the formulator's efforts are best directed at securing the correct rate of release of drug from the product. Although solutions usually give the highest rate of release, care should be taken to ensure that precipitation of active substance does not occur due to dilution of the vehicle or pH changes. When sodium phenylbutazone solution is injected intramuscularly the drug is precipitated at the injection site due to pH changes and the rate of release is limited by the dissolution rate of the solid material.

Apart from such examples, biological availability problems are most likely to occur if the product is a solid or a dispersion of a solid in a liquid. In these circumstances there is a high probability that the dissolution rate is the key factor (Fig. 37.7).

In the Noyes and Witney (1897) model of dissolution, diffusion of solute from the interface to the bulk solution across the stationary film at the surface of the solid was the rate determining step. Alternative models assume that the dissolution process is rate determining or that macroscopic packets of solvent transport solute to the bulk solvent. Each model requires a different mathematical treatment (see Higuchi 1967), but in all cases the rate of dissolution may be related to the difference between the concentration (C_s) of the solute in solution adjacent to the interface—often assumed to be saturated—and that in the bulk solvent (C), the surface area (S) exposed to attack and other factors (K) such as the viscosity and the degree of agitation of the solvent. The generalized equation may be written:

$$\text{Dissolution rate} = (C_s - C) \cdot F(S) \cdot f(K) \quad (37.7)$$

If C is small and is only a small fraction of C_s then $(C_s - C) \approx C_s$ and the dissolution is then said to be proceeding under sink conditions and:

$$\text{Solubility dissolution rate} = C_s \cdot F(S) \cdot f(K)$$

The parameter C_s is temperature dependent and is

affected by those factors that determine the intrinsic solubility of a solid such as its chemical and physical state. Generally, the salts of weak acids or bases are more soluble and better absorbed than the parent weak acids or bases; phenoxymethylpenicillin, for instance, gives lower blood levels than the corresponding potassium salt. It is not always the most soluble form of drug that is preferred. The soluble sodium salt of tolbutamide has a rapid onset and an intense but short action that may put the patient into a transient state of hypoglycaemia. As the diabetic patient will be on a permanent dose regimen, rapid onset is of secondary importance and the less soluble tolbutamide is the drug of choice.

The physical form of a drug also affects its solubility. In the amorphous condition the atoms or molecules lack the regular arrangement of a lattice that is characteristic of a crystal; some drugs, e.g., penicillin, insulin, novobiocin can exist in both amorphous and crystalline states. For many crystalline drugs there is also the possibility of different lattice arrangements and these amorphous and different crystalline forms are known as polymorphs. Only one polymorph is stable under given physical conditions and all other forms tend to revert more or less rapidly to that stable form. The life-time of some polymorphic forms may be so long that the polymorphs appear to have a separate existence and are said to exist in a metastable state. From the formulator's point of view it is an unfortunate fact that the most stable form is also the least soluble and thereby is potentially the least active. In the case of novobiocin, the amorphous form of the acid is an effective antibiotic whereas the less soluble crystalline variety is inactive at the same dose level (Mullins & Macek 1960). The crystalline sodium salt is converted to the amorphous state under the acid conditions of the stomach and the calcium salt is amorphous; both forms are active in-vivo. Chloramphenicol palmitate exists in an amorphous and three crystalline forms. Aguiar et al. (1967) showed that administration of 1.5 g of the most stable form of the ester to adults produced a mean peak blood level of about 2.5 μg/ml whereas the most soluble variety of the drug gave a peak concentration nearly ten times higher.

Polymorphic forms of drugs occur more frequently than is generally realized and lack of awareness of their existence can lead to unwelcome therapeutic effects even though chemical analysis would reveal nothing amiss. The low potency of some chloramphenicol palmitate preparations which have been marketed was due to the selection of the most stable but least active polymorph (Anderson 1966). Equally dangerous is the higher activity and incidence of side effects that might occur if a product formulated on the basis of clinical trials with the stable variety was inadvertantly manufactured with the metastable polymorph. The problem is further complicated by the possibility that the metastable variety may revert to the stable state during the lifetime of the product. Such changes may often be prevented by added substances, such as hydrocolloids and surface active agents, that poison the crystal lattice. Mullins and Macek found that benzalkonium chloride increased the rate of crystallization of solutions of amorphous novobiocin. Methylcellulose, on the other hand, had the reverse effect and increased the time for crystals to appear in the solution from 22 days at 37° to more than 365 days at the same temperature. Calcium novobiocin, although amorphous, did not revert to the crystalline form at 37° even after storage for two years.

Surface area. Particle size reduction is a familiar pharmaceutical operation employed to secure better dispersion of a drug in its vehicle. The process also increases the surface area per given weight of material (the specific surface area) and can therefore affect the biological availability. As originally submitted to clinical trial, griseofulvin had a specific surface area of 0.4 m²/g, a particle diameter of about 10 μm and a recommended dose of 250 mg. Subsequently the manufacturing procedure was changed and yielded a powder with a specific surface area of 1.5 m²/g and a particle diameter of 2.7 μm. The more rapid dissolution rate of the finer powder allows the dose to be halved. The official description 'a white to pale cream powder the particles of which are generally up to 5 micrometres in maximum dimension' is framed to give a powder with an average particle size smaller than this to ensure the correct biological availability for the antibiotic. Modern insulin preparations provide a further example of the importance of particle size and polymorphic form as factors controlling the biological availability of a drug. An insulin–zinc complex can be precipitated either as 10–40 μm crystals or as amorphous particles up to 2 μm in size. If a mixture of both types is injected the amorphous particles dissolve rapidly for prompt response which is maintained by the slower dissolution of the crystals. The proportions of each type of particle determine the release profile of the preparation and may be varied to suit the individual needs of the patient.

As was the case with tolbutamide it is not always the most rapidly absorbed form of the drug that is most satisfactory for clinical use. A similar situation has arisen with nitrofurantoin where the 10 μm powder, in suitable dose forms, gives a satisfactory concentration in the urine at an oral dose level of 50–100 mg but nausea and vomiting is a problem for a significant number of patients. It has been shown (Paul et al. 1967) that although side effects rarely occur if the coarser 100–150 μm powder is used, neither the urinary concentration nor the amount of drug absorbed are markedly changed. It may also be necessary to avoid a small particle size powder if local action in the distal parts of the gastrointestinal tract is required and the drug has appreciable water solubility. Premature dissolution and absorption of the drug in, say, the stomach might give rise to toxic effects and would certainly reduce the amount available for the required local action.

The Variable (K)

For the three types of dissolution mechanism that have been proposed K will include a factor for viscosity and degree of agitation as well as for specific effects peculiar to the particular type of preparation. The viscosity is important in that it determines the speed with which the molecules move away from the interface to the bulk dissolution medium. Hydrocolloids are often included in the formulae of pharmaceutical products to suspend solids, to prevent polymorphic changes or to act as binders during the moist granulation of powders for tableting. At best the hydrocolloid may mix with the dissolution medium, increase viscosity and slow down diffusion of the dissolving molecules: at worst it may adsorb onto the solid surface to form a thin layer having an extremely high viscosity which will considerably delay diffusion. If adsorption occurs, the effect is out of all proportion to the actual concentration of hydrocolloid in the product. Instead of being adsorbed, these materials may be precipitated on to the particle surface by interaction with the contents of the gastrointestinal contents. Whatever the cause the effect is well illustrated by the following data from Davidson et al. (1961).

The degree of agitation is important both from the point of view of drug dissolution in vivo and also for possible tests for dissolution rate in vitro. In any static dissolution system there is a

Dose: 0.72 millimoles of 'salicylate' per kg administered orally to rats

Preparation	Peak level after 30 minutes in:	
	plasma (μg/ml)	brain (μg/g)
Aspirin suspended in 2 per cent methylcellulose solution	132	11.6
Sodium acetylsalicylate solution	201	19.6
Sodium salicylate	208	21.1
Sodium salicylate in 2 per cent methylcellulose solution	162	13.3

tendency for a stagnant pool of solution to form in the vicinity of the dissolving solid. As a consequence, the concentration gradient is reduced and further dissolution of the solid is inhibited. Such evidence as is available (Levy 1963) suggests that the degree of agitation in the gastrointestinal tract is only moderate. It will be recalled that large doses of rapidly soluble materials such as the alkali metal halides must be dissolved in water before administration to avoid the nausea and vomiting that would arise from high local concentrations of solute in the stomach. Furthermore, if the density of the product is unusually high it may become lodged in lower parts of the stomach and in the case of iron preparations this has led to gastric erosion. In normal situations however the degree of agitation in the stomach is probably sufficient to ensure that the rate of dissolution is not limited by poor mixing.

Apart from viscosity and agitation effects it is convenient to include in the variable K a number of factors peculiar to certain types of dose form. Suspensions should be free from effects other than those that may be attributed to factors already discussed above. Nevertheless, as an instance of the way quite minor changes may influence the time course of action of griseofulvin it was noted by Duncan et al. (1962), that a suspension prepared by dispersing the antibiotic directly in a solution of wetting agent gave a lower peak blood level than a product containing the same concentration of adjuvant added as a solid to the drug prior to dispersion with water.

The simplest model of a hard capsule comprises a powder mass enveloped in a water-soluble shell. It might be thought that such a system would be free from dissolution problems. The work of Aguiar and co-workers (1968) suggests that this is far from the truth; their examination of four nominally identical brands of chloramphenicol capsules showed peak plasma levels in adults varying from 2.2–9.5 μg/ml. The observed differences were related to the rate of deaggregation of the drug during dissolution. In the wider range of chloramphenicol capsules examined by Withey and Mainville (1969) the time for dissolution of 50 per cent of the dose of drug (t_{50}) varied from 2.4 to 20 minutes and with one brand, a soft capsule, only a quarter of the drug had dissolved in 30 minutes as compared with 60 to 90 per cent for the hard capsule preparations. Several experimental capsules were also studied and confirmed earlier reports that the capsule shell interferes with the initial stages of dissolution. Many hard capsule formulations contain lactose in addition to the drug and in high concentrations this may also depress the dissolution rate. For drug mixtures containing 43 per cent of the sugar t_{50} was about 4 minutes but was increased to about 13 minutes with 80 per cent of the adjuvant in the mixture. On the other hand, when lactose was substituted for calcium sulphate in manufactured batches of phenytoin capsules, enhanced activity and a much higher incidence of side effects were noted. Tyrer et al. (1970) have reported blood serum concentrations (20 to 25 μg/ml) for the formulation with lactose and only about a third of this value for the product with calcium sulphate.

There are so many variables in the production of tablets that it is difficult to disentangle the many possible interactions that may have a bearing on biological availability. One such attempt has been described by Ganderton et al. 1967. In studies with phenylindione tablets they reported a maximum dissolution rate at compaction pressures in the range 400 to 800 kg/cm^2 within which range it is known from other studies that there is also a maximum in the internal surface area of the tablets. At less than about 800 kg/cm^2 compaction pressure the dissolution rate is increased by small granule size, surfactant to promote wetting by the dissolution medium, and starch to aid disintegration. Conversely, the hydrophobic nature of magnesium stearate used as the lubricant has the effect of decreasing dissolution rate. It is shown elsewhere that this effect can be put to good use in the formulation of sustained action tablets.

Dissolution Rate Tests

When designing test apparatus means must be provided for agitating the dissolution medium, supporting the sample without impeding the flow of liquid and estimating the quantity of drug that has dissolved. Closed circuit systems have been devised,

by e.g., Marshall and Brook (1969), to take advantage of the methods that now exist for continuously monitoring the concentrations of solutes in liquids. Provision may also be made for replacing part of the dissolution medium from time to time or for changing its nature; both modifications are intended to give a closer simulation of actual conditions within the gastrointestinal tract. A more intractable problem is that of ensuring the right degree of agitation and it would appear that this is probably less than is commonly assumed by designers of test apparatus. Often the dissolution rate becomes sensibly constant above a certain (high) level of agitation—see, for instance, Flanagan et al. (1969). If a high level of agitation is accepted for the sake of experimental reproducibility, it must be recognized that the dissolution may be proceeding under conditions quite different from those which are thought to obtain in vivo. Some workers, for example, have used the official tablet disintegration test apparatus with a finer mesh to retain all particles in the oscillating tube. According to Levy (1963) these conditions are too severe, as this method did not distinguish between tablets shown to be different by other methods and by trial in vivo.

That no universally acceptable apparatus has so far been designed is evidenced by the large number of devices that have been described in the literature; Hersey (1969) has provided a useful review. With proper attention to operating conditions dissolution tests provide valuable in vitro data for the development of pharmaceutical products, an indication of relative potential in vivo performance and means for quality control. Certainly, there is now considerable evidence to show that in a given series of products, the one with the highest dissolution rate will probably produce the most rapid and intense response in vivo. It is not even necessary for the products to be all of the same type: Bates et al. (1969), for example, compared suspension and tablet formulations of salicylamide and demonstrated that their in vivo behaviour ran parallel to their in vitro dissolution rates. It is now also clear that the tablet disintegration time is, in most cases, a poor guide to the biological availability of the drug. In the series of aspirin tablets examined by Levy (1961), the one with the longest disintegration time gave the highest rate of excretion. There was however an obvious correlation between the amount (E) of drug excreted in the first hour after the administration of 600 mg of aspirin to adults and the dissolution rate (D) expressed as the weight of drug dissolved from the tablets in 10 minutes under stated conditions. In two series of experiments (A & B) the data were described by the equations:

$$E = 0.074D + 6.2 \qquad (A)$$

and

$$E = 0.084D + 1.0 \qquad (B)$$

The nearly identical slopes indicated that the mechanisms of absorption and excretion were identical in both series but the author attributed the different values of the constant (6.2 and 1.0) to the fact that in the series A experiments, a glass of water was taken half an hour before the administration of the tablets and 200 ml with the dose, whereas in series B a glass of water was taken one hour before and only 100 ml when the tablets were taken. The higher liquid intake for the first series of experiments probably caused more rapid gastric emptying and absorption of the aspirin.

Modification of the Onset, Intensity and Duration of Therapeutic Action

It was noted earlier that the time course of action curve for a drug is a composite of the absorption transport and elimination processes. Frequently, it is found that once the peak response is past, a plot of the logarithm of response e.g., concentration in the blood, is, for all practical purposes, a linear function of time (Fig. 37.8). By analogy with chemical kinetics theory this is a first order process that is, the rate of elimination is effectively proportional to the concentration of drug in the blood,

thus:

$$\frac{dC_B}{dt} = kC_B \qquad (37.8)$$

which when integrated gives

$$C_B = C_{B_o} e^{-kt} \qquad (37.9)$$

C_B is the response at time t, C_{B_o} is the response that would be required to produce the observed data in the absence of other processes and k is the elimination constant, which has the dimensions of time^{-1}. The elimination rate is more easily visualized however, in terms of the time taken to eliminate half the drug originally present in the blood. This is called the biological half-life ($t_{1/2}$) and is related to the elimination constant as follows:

$$C_B = C_{B_o} e^{-kt} \qquad (37.9)$$

$$\therefore \qquad \log e \frac{C_{B_o}}{C_B} = \log e2 = 0.693 = kt_{1/2}$$

or

$$t_{1/2} = \frac{0.693}{k} \qquad (37.10)$$

The biological half-life may be short (benzylpenicillin, 30 minutes), a few hours (theophylline, 3 hours) or even longer (tetracycline, 8 hours). It is important to ensure, where data are used for calculation of the required dose or for other purposes, that the measured parameter e.g. blood concentration, from which the biological half-life is calculated is positively related to the therapeutic effect. Reserpine activity, for instance, persists for about two days even though the apparent biological half-life (calculated from blood level data) is less than half an hour. This is because reserpine probably acts by interfering with the amine binding mechanisms associated with the biogenic amines and these take a day or so to return to normal after a single dose of the drug.

In most cases, treatment with drugs involves administration of doses at fixed intervals of time. The activity will, therefore alternately rise and decline as reported, for example, by Drain et al. (1959) for doses of *p*-aminosalicylic acid and its esters. To ensure continuous therapeutic effect each dose must be given at a time when there is still an effective response from the previous administration. Each peak will be higher than its predecessor but will ultimately attain an equilibrium value as the rate of decline of response is proportional to, and therefore increases with, the peak value of the response. If the correct dose and timing is chosen,

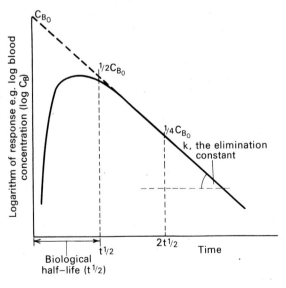

FIG. 37.8. Biological half-life of a drug.

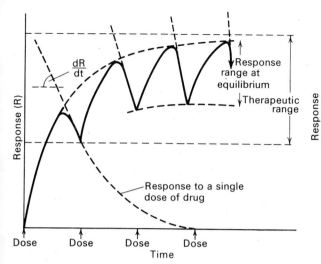

FIG. 37.9. Time course of action for several doses of drug.

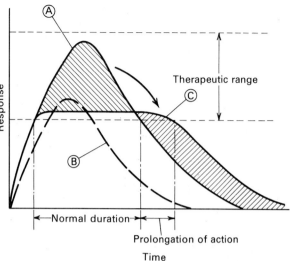

FIG. 37.10. Prolongation of drug action.

the peaks and troughs of response will fall within the upper and lower limits for effective therapy (Fig. 37.9). When doses are too widely spaced, the troughs will fall below the level required for proper treatment but, on the other hand, if they are administered too frequently the peaks may exceed the level for acceptable incidence of side effects.

When thinking of preparations with modified time course of action it is easy to forget that there are situations in which shortened, rather than prolonged, drug action is required. Numerous medium to long-acting general anaesthetics are known and yet it is only recently that safe short-acting general anaesthetics for use in dentistry and minor surgery have become available. It is worth recalling also that it is not always easy or convenient to administer medicaments by the intravenous route in very young or very old patients. If large volumes of liquid must be given parenterally in these circumstances, it is possible to inject subcutaneously at up to about 10 ml/minute provided hyaluronidase is used to increase tissue permeability (Wilson 1959). There are also occasions (the treatment of diabetes by insulin is an obvious example), where a reduction in the frequency of dose administration would be a great convenience to the patient; but for dose-forms other than injections the argument for reducing the frequency of dose administration is more tenuous. Nevertheless, in suitable cases, there are other good reasons for increasing the duration of action of individual dose units.

For reasonable duration with a normal dose, the response to the drug is likely to be in excess of that necessary for effective therapeutic action (Fig. 37.10, curve A); if the dose is reduced to avoid

this situation, the period of effective action is reduced (curve B). The amount of drug in excess of that strictly necessary for effective therapy would be more usefully employed in stretching the period of activity as shown in the shaded portions of curves A and C. The benefits are obvious; curative action has been extended without increasing the total amount of drug while the reduced peak response will probably lower the incidence of side effects. It is unlikely, however, that these factors would extend the useful period of activity by more than about a third; thus, assuming the normal effective period of action to be some four hours, it would be extended to just over five hours.

For a worthwhile prolongation of drug action it is necessary to combine a prompt dose for rapid onset with a maintenance dose or doses to obtain therapeutic action for about twelve hours (Fig. 37.11), but the total amount of drug in the dose unit will be several times the normal dose. In addition to the advantages noted above, such a system would eliminate deficiencies in treatment due to incorrect timing of individual doses.

Prolonged action preparations are not without disadvantages. No matter how well formulated and manufactured, there is always the chance, however small, that the unit will fail to release the drug in the correct manner. It is shown later that a prolonged action preparation may contain 2 to 5 times the normal dose of drug, so that in the event of failure the patient is either deprived of drug or exposed to a serious overdose for a long period. This problem is particularly serious with very potent short half-life medicaments which are

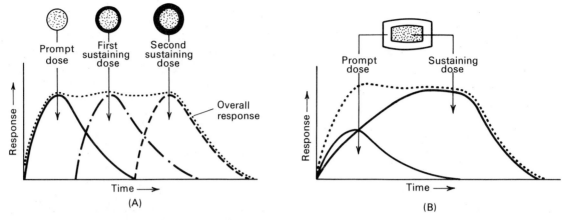

FIG. 37.11. Types of prolonged action oral dose forms. A, repeat action preparation; B, sustained action preparation.

probably unsuitable for formulation as sustained action preparations. If the half-life is very long there is very little point in attempting to extend the duration of action, at least for oral products.

The maximum practical size for a solid dose unit is 1 to $1\frac{1}{2}$ g depending on the density of the product. This value could easily be exceeded with

a prolonged action preparation if the normal dose is large, perhaps 0.5 g, and the biological half-life is short. Finally, although products have been specifically designed to release drugs under specific physiological states or at specific sites in the body, this is not a universally applicable product design philosophy as it is well known that there is always

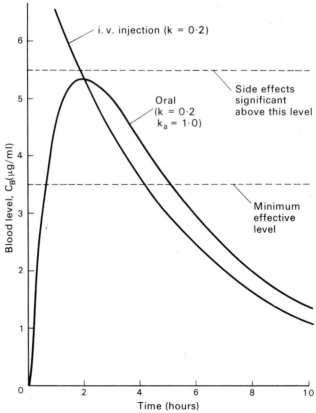

FIG. 37.12. Time course of action curves for intravenous and oral administration of 80 mg of drug having biological half-life of 3.46 hours.

considerable inter-patient variation in the response to medication and also variation from day to day for a particular patient.

Formulation of Prolonged Action Preparations

Oral sustained action products are of two kinds depending on the way in which the maintaining dose is released (Fig. 37.11). For the so-called repeat action and timed release products the maintaining doses become available at discrete time intervals. If the maintaining drug is continuously released, the product is of the prolonged action or sustained release type. Although other names are used for branded products there is no widespread agreement on nomenclature; the terms used in the text should be self-explanatory. In spite of the diversity of names the formulator may use coatings, erosion, diffusion or a limited combination of these to control drug release from oral products. Additionally there is a group of miscellaneous products where biological availability is controlled by the dissolution rate, partitioning, chemical reaction within the body and by other means.

Coatings. Enteric and barrier coatings are used. *Enteric* coatings are intended to resist the acid gastric secretions but dissolve in the intestinal fluids. Cellulose acetate phthalate and some other polymeric films avoid most of the problems associated with earlier materials and provide reliable enteric action. Their use in the formulation of sustained action products is less clearly defined. Once the coating has dissolved, the release of drugs is identical with that of the uncoated dose-form but is displaced by a period equivalent to the transit time from the mouth to the stomach or intestine and by the time taken for the coating to dissolve. The latter is a primary function of coating thickness, as above pH 6.0 the dissolution rate of the coating is not markedly affected by the reaction of the solvent.

It is not possible to control the transit time, however, as this is dependent on the stomach emptying rate. An average value for the stomach emptying time is 4 hours but is longer if the stomach is empty and less if the drug is taken with plenty of fluid. The emptying rate is also affected by the posture of the patient; it is less if the patient lies on the left side as this requires the gastric contents to follow the natural uphill curve of the stomach towards the duodenum.

In general, the foregoing problems do not arise with permeable barrier coatings; for these the only requirement is that water shall be available for diffusion through the barrier to provide solvent for the drug so that it may diffuse outwards through the barrier, to the gastrointestinal tract. Ethylcellulose, nylon and acrylic plastics modified by hydrophilic groups are polymeric materials that have been used to give permeable films that are applied in much the same way as cellulose acetate phthalate. These coatings may be applied to whole tablets or to pellets formed by coating preformed sucrose seeds with drug dissolved or suspended in an adhesive solution. Alternatively, drug crystals may be coated by mechanical micro-encapsulation (Nack 1970) or coacervation (Nixon et al. 1968). Sustained action tablets prepared by compressing polymer film coated crystals have been evaluated (Bell et al. 1966).

As an alternative to polymers, lipophilic coatings comprising paraffin waxes, fatty alcohols and acids, glyceryl monostearate and distearate may also be used to form permeable barriers. For a given coating composition the release rate is decreased if the thickness is increased or, for a given coating thickness, the more polar materials allow water to penetrate more rapidly and this results in a faster release of drug (Jack 1961). Release is delayed by the time taken for water to penetrate to the solid and for this to diffuse outwards. In one product using this method of controlling release, the drug is formed into small pellets as described above and these are treated with a wax composition dissolved in a suitable solvent. Normal pan coating is used. The batch of pellets will have a mean value for the delay and release rate. Due to the nature of the pan coating process the values of these parameters will vary by a greater or lesser extent about the mean values for the batch. A typical sustained action preparation consists of a capsule containing untreated drug pellets together with pellets that have been given different thicknesses or compositions of wax coatings. On ingestion the capsule shell dissolves and the uncoated drug pellets provide a prompt dose which is maintained by release from the different coated pellets at timed intervals. The release profile is shown in Fig. 37.11. The statistical release of drug from each batch of pellets smoothes out the peaks and troughs in the response. A dextamphetamine product of this type behaves in the expected manner (Beckett & Tucker 1966).

It is worth noting that if product performance is to be assessed by urinary excretion data, it is necessary in the case of ionized drugs to control the pH of the urine so that tubular reabsorption is avoided.

Erosion control. The finely powdered medicament is embedded in a wax formed from one or more of the following—stearic acid, hydroxystearic acid, hardened castor oil and fatty alcohols. If necessary, water penetration may be controlled by the inclusion of a hard polyethylene glycol in the wax. The drug is dispersed in molten wax, rapidly solidified on a cold drum or in trays and the flakes passed through a swing-hammer granulator. The granules are compressed in the normal manner to give a sustained action core onto which is compressed a dose of the same drug formulated for prompt release. When administered, the coating disintegrates to provide the prompt dose which is maintained by gradual erosion of the core that constantly exposes fresh surface from which drug may be dissolved. Wax embedment has been used to produce sustained action liquid oral products containing sulphaethidole. The molten mixture is either spray congealed (Raghunathan & Becker 1968) or dispersed in dilute surfactant solution to form a mechanical emulsion and chilled (Robinson & Becker 1968). The wax spheres containing drug formed by these processes are very small and it is likely that a diffusion, rather than erosion, mechanism is responsible for the sustained action properties.

Diffusion control. This may be exerted by a gelled layer of hydrophilic colloid, a plastic matrix or by ion exchange resins. In the first of these methods the drug is mixed with inert filler, hydrophilic colloid and lubricant and compressed in the normal way at high compaction pressure. Tragacanth, hydroxypropylmethyl cellulose and a number of other gums have been used as the gelling agent. The lubricant is usually employed in a higher than normal concentration to raise the contact angle of the pores and thereby control penetration of liquid into the tablet. The initial release of drug is rapid as it is dissolved from the surface but the rate subsequently slows down as the colloid hydrates to form the gelled layer through which drug must diffuse to provide the maintenance dose. It is possible that in vivo there may be some erosion of the gelled layer.

Diffusion governed drug release from an insoluble plastic matrix is also used to provide sustained action products. Polythene, polyvinyl acetate or chloride, ethylcellulose and other plastics have been used. Tablets are prepared by mixing the drug with powdered plastic and compressing in the normal way or, alternatively, the mixed powders may be moist granulated with a solution of the plastic in a suitable organic solvent.

Higuchi (1963) derived equations for the release of drug from matrices and showed that for a range of conditions the amount of drug (Q) released should vary as the square root of time, that is:

$$Q = m.t^{1/2} \qquad (37.11)$$

where m is a constant relating to the matrix and elution conditions. In vitro tests have shown that equation 37.11 applies to a wax matrix under non-eroding conditions (Schwartz et al. 1968) and to plastic matrices (Desai et al. 1966 a & b) provided the dissolution fluid contains a surfactant to promote pore wetting and air is removed by vacuum treatment. The plastic matrix does not disintegrate but is excreted unchanged.

Ion-exchange resins provide a means for binding ionized drugs inside a diffusion controlling insoluble matrix. The maximum size of the molecule that may be accommodated within the molecular mesh of the resin is determined by the degree of cross-linking. This factor and the size of the resin beads determines the rate of release, which is slower for partially saturated resins (Chaudry & Saunders 1956). Drug is released regardless of the nature of the gastrointestinal fluids; taking the case of a cationic drug bound to an anionic sulphonic acid resin the appropriate reactions in the stomach and intestine are:

Stomach:
$$R\text{–}SO_3'X^+ + H^+Cl' \rightarrow R\text{–}SO_3'H^+ + X^+Cl'$$

Intestine:
$$R\text{–}SO_3'X^+ + Na^+Cl' \rightarrow R\text{–}SO_3'Na^+ + X^+Cl'$$

The utility of ion-exchange resins for the formulation of sustained action products is limited in that only ionic drugs are suitable and the capacity of the resin for the drug is small. There is also the possibility that the body electrolyte balance may be disturbed by absorption of ions by the resin. An example of this type of medication is afforded by an anti-tussive mixture, formulated by suspending the ion-exchange resin complexes of pholcodine and phenyltoloxamine in a syrupy vehicle.

Other Long-acting Preparations
It is often possible to extend the duration of activity by forming a derivative of the drug that has low solubility. The utility of this approach in the case of insulin preparations has been described already. Deep injection into muscle and the use of an oily vehicle may also help to prolong action provided the latter is viscous enough to form a localized depot rather than spread along the muscle fascia.

Early penicillin injections used oil thickened with beeswax but were difficult to use unless thinned by gentle warming prior to administration. According to Buckwalter and Dickison (1958) oily depot injections of procaine penicillin gelled with aluminium stearate give higher and more prolonged blood levels than corresponding products with beeswax or plain oil. Ober et al. (1958) investigated aqueous depot injections of the same antibiotic derivative. Using a high (40 to 70 per cent w/v) concentration of the drug together with sodium citrate as deflocculating agent they produced a series of injections having as a characteristic rheological property a spur in the shear stress/shear rate curve. Suitable products were obtained when the spur had a value which, on their rotational viscometer, was equivalent to a torque in the range 10^5 to 10^6 dyne cm. The shear stress in the needle exceeds the upper value and the product can be withdrawn from the vial and injected into the patient. In muscle, where the shear stress is less than the lower value, structure build-up takes place and the injected material sets to form a depot.

A broad range of particle size is desirable to provide immediate response by the dissolution of fine particles and a sustained effect lasting several days by the less rapid dissolution of the coarser particles.

It is also possible to control the release of drug by adsorption onto insoluble carriers such as zinc or aluminium hydroxides or phosphates. Corticotrophin depot injections are produced in this way: zinc phosphate carriers tend to crystallize on storage and must be produced by precipitation of the carrier in the container just prior to injection. This procedure is not necessary with the zinc hydroxide carrier as the latter does not crystallize when stored.

With suitable drugs it is possible to produce depot injections with an effective duration of several weeks while even longer periods are possible with implants. Preparations of these types are only feasible with drugs that are effective in very low dosage and which are also very insoluble in water. This combination of therapeutic and physico-chemical requirements limits the range of medicaments that are worthwhile formulating as ultra long-acting drugs to the steroid hormones and a few other substances. They also form esters that hydrolyse in vivo at rates convenient for formulation purposes, as discussed earlier. Depots of drug are formed by deep intramuscular injection of aqueous suspensions of the drug or oily solutions of these. Oestradiol, testosterone, methylpredni-

solone and fluphenazine are examples of drugs available as depot injections.

If a longer period of therapy is required the drug may be fused or compressed into a pellet (implant) and inserted into the muscle by a minor surgical operation. The use of additives for the production of implants is prohibited. Obviously, the surface area of the implant will decrease as the drug dissolves. Nevertheless, for the purpose of dose calculation, Edkins (1959) has shown that the average daily dose over a given period may be related to the initial surface area of the implant. Thus, for deoxycortone acetate implants:

Weight (mg)	Surface area (mm^2)	Average daily dose (mg)	Duration (days)
25	49	0.3	83
300	222	1.3	230

If an average daily dose of 1.2 mg for 83 days is required then 4×25 mg would be implanted in the muscle. Generally, as in the case of testosterone, the release is sufficiently limited by the dissolution rate that there is no need to employ the ester. It will be appreciated that the complete prohibition of additives and the need for rigorous aseptic precautions during manufacture pose formidable technical problems.

Calculation of doses for sustained action products. The total dose of drug, D_t, in a prolonged action preparation comprises the normal (prompt) dose, D_n, and the sustaining dose D_s i.e.,

$$D_t = D_n + D_s \qquad (37.12)$$

If the first order elimination rate constant is k, the rate at which drug is eliminated when a normal dose is given is $D_n k$ which is the rate at which drug must be replaced if the peak blood level is to be maintained. Given a maintenance period t the maintenance dose (D_s) is $D_n kt$. The total dose is therefore:

$$D_t = D_n + D_s$$
$$= D_n + D_n kt$$
$$= D_n(1 + kt)$$
$$= D_n(1 + 0.693 \, t/t_{1/2}) \qquad (37.13)$$

Suppose the biological half-life is 1.73 hours, D_n is 80 mg and t is 10 hours, substituting in equation 13:

$$D_t = 80\left(1 + \frac{0.693 \times 10}{1.73}\right) = 80 + 320 = 400 \text{ mg}$$

For a $t_{1/2}$ of 3.46 hours

$$D_t = 80 + 160 = 240 \text{ mg}$$

The use of the normal dose does not take into account the fact that to obtain a reasonable duration of action it may be necessary to accept a peak response near that at which side effects become noticeable. Nelson (1957) suggested that a factor (f) should be used in calculation to adjust the amount of drug such that lower but still therapeutically effective blood levels are attained. Fig. 37.12 shows the calculated response curve for an 80 mg oral dose of drug having a biological half-life of 3.46 hours and it is assumed that the upper and lower limits of blood concentration for effective therapy are 3.5–5.5 μg/ml respectively. The peak blood level is 5.35 μg/ml, the onset about 35 minutes and the duration about $4\frac{1}{2}$ hours. If a reasonable blood level is 4.0 μg/ml the value of D_n for equation 37.13 must be reduced by the factor (f) equal to 4.0/5.35 = 0.75. The total dose may be recalculated as follows:

$$D_t = 0.75 \times 80\left(1 + \frac{0.693 \times 10}{3.46}\right)$$

$$= 60 + 120 = 180 \text{ mg}$$

Even with these reduced amounts of drug the concentration in the blood may be higher than intended due to the simultaneous release from both the prompt and maintenance forms. There is also the possibility (Rowland & Beckett 1964) that there may be an initial peaking of the blood level, particularly for drugs with short biological half-lives. It must be stressed that some products, for example those of the repeat action type, are not subject to this particular problem. Similarly, the problem may be avoided if the release of drug from the maintenance form is deliberately delayed by, say, the use of film coating.

Further sophistication of the calculations for the amounts of the prompt and sustaining doses requires more elaborate theoretical treatment than has been used so far. A fundamental theory of the time course of action of drugs relies on a knowledge of the effective concentration of drug at the ultimate site of action but this is not accessible. One approach, widely used, is that of compartmental analysis due to Teorell (1937). A compartment may be regarded as a transferable reservoir of drug the amount of which changes with time. Strictly, a compartment is a convenient mathematical device for simplifying calculations and need not be identified with a particular part of the body but it is often

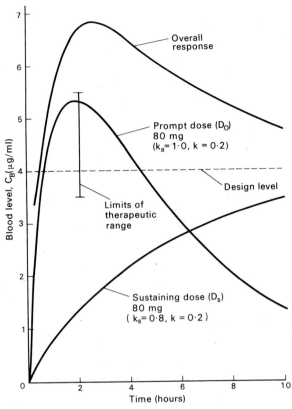

FIG. 37.13. Combined effect of 80 mg of prompt and sustaining doses of drug having a biological half-life of 3.46 hours.

convenient to do so. The method may be illustrated by a model that comprises a single compartment (equivalent to the blood, tissues and extravascular fluids) into which the drug is rapidly introduced and from which it is eliminated by first order processes. The model mimics rapid intravenous injection in those cases where it can be assumed that equilibrium between the blood and tissues is so rapid relative to other processes that it has negligible effect on the time course of action.

Dose D_O by rapid intravenous injection at time $t = 0$

Compartment equivalent to blood, tissues and extravascular fluids

$$D_B = V_D C_B \xrightarrow{\ \ k\ \ } \text{Elimination}$$

$$\frac{dD_B}{dt} = -kD_B$$

By integration, $\qquad D_B = D_O e^{-kt} \qquad (37.14)$

where D_O is the total dose given by rapid intravenous injection, D_B is the amount of drug present in the body at time t and k is the rate constant for elimination. D_B cannot be determined directly— only the body fluids are accessible and these will have a concentration C_B of drug. The term V_D is the apparent volume of distribution such that $D_B = V_D \cdot C_B$ it too is a mathematical device used to account for the mass of drug in each part of the model and should not be identified with the total body fluids. The value of V_D is calculated from the data obtained in each particular study of drug action but an acceptable value for the purposes of these calculations is 10 litres (10 000 ml). Substitution gives:

$$C_B = \frac{D_0}{V_D} = e^{-kt} \qquad (37.15)$$

Clearly, equations (37.14) and (37.15) are alternative forms of equation (37.9). Assume the dose of 80 mg (80 000 micrograms) used in the previous calculations and a biological half-life of 3.46 hours, that is $k = 0.2$ hours^{-1}. The blood level after 1 hour is:

$$C_B = \frac{80\,000}{10\,000} e^{-0.2 \times 1.0} = 8 \times 0.8187 = 6.55 \ \mu g/ml.$$

and for other times is shown in Fig. 37.12.

It must be emphasized that compartmental analysis is applied to the results of in vivo investigations to obtain the mathematical model that best fits the experimental data. Apart from providing information about the mechanisms of absorption metabolism and excretion the model allows the effects of dose size, rate of release, dose frequency and other factors to be calculated. Subsequent in vivo experiments to determine the optimum values for those parameters are thereby reduced and this is of the greatest importance if tests are to be conducted with human volunteers.

Applying the method to the formulation of a sustained action tablet, assume that a single compartment model is known to provide a good fit to the available in vivo data. The model is:

Prompt dose (D_0) $\xrightarrow{k_a}$

$D_B = V_D C_B$ $\xrightarrow{k}$ elimination

Sustaining dose D_s $\xrightarrow{k_s}$

Zero order release from the sustaining dose ensures a constant level of drug in the blood; the rate constant is k_s. If, as before, $k = 0.2$ hr^{-1} the design value of C_B is 4 μg per ml and the drug is completely absorbed, i.e. $F = 1$

$$k_s = FkC_B = 1 \times 0.2 \times 4.0 = 0.8 \ \mu g \text{ per hour.}$$

If $V_D = 10$ litres and the sustaining time (T) is 10 hours the sustaining dose D_s is

$$k_s V_D t = 0.8 \times 10\,000 \times 10 = 80 \text{ mg}$$

For the zero-order sustaining process

$$\frac{dC_B}{dt} = k_s - kC_B \qquad (37.16)$$

Which on integration gives:

$$C_B = \frac{k_s}{k}(1 - e^{-kt}) \qquad (37.17)$$

The release and absorption of drug from the prompt dose is first order overall and rate constant is k_a. The appropriate rate equation is:

$$\frac{dD_B}{dt} = Fk_a D_o - kD_B \qquad (37.18)$$

Which, on integration, gives:

$$C_B = \frac{Fk_a D_o}{(k_a - k) V_D} (e^{-kt} - e^{-k_a t}) \qquad (37.19)$$

For $F = 1$, $k_a = 1.0$ hr^{-1}, $D_o = 80$ mg, $k = 0.2$ hr^{-1} and $V_D = 10$ litres the blood concentration at, say, 2 hours is:

$$\frac{1.0 \times 1.0 \times 80\,000}{(1.0 - 0.2) \times 10\,000} (e^{-0.2 \times 2} - e^{-1 \times 1})$$

$$= 5.35 \ \mu g \text{ per ml.}$$

The complete curve is given in Fig. 37.12.

Clearly, when the additional drug released from the maintenance dose is also taken into account, at, say, 2 hours after administration of the sustained action tablet, the blood level would be very much in excess of the design level. Calculation shows that a peak level of the order of 6.8 μg per ml would be produced thus the level beyond which side effects become serious would also be exceeded as shown in Fig. 37.13. By reducing the amount of prompt dose these problems may be avoided and it has been suggested that a suitable value would be:

$$D_o = \frac{D_s}{Tk} \qquad (37.20)$$

which for the preparation considered here is:

$$\frac{80}{10 \times 0.2} = 40 \text{ mg}$$

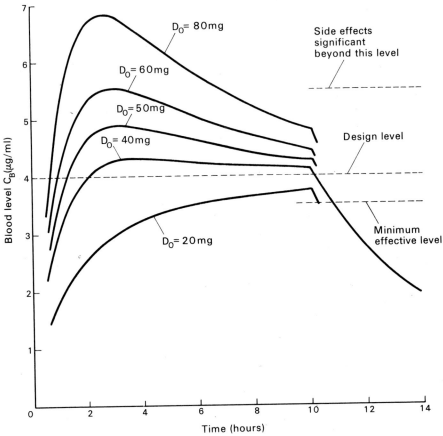

FIG. 37.14. Calculated effect of size of prompt dose (D_o) on blood levels attained by a sustained action preparation for which $D_s = 80$ mg, $k = 0.2$ hr^{-1}, $k_a = 1.0$ hr^{-1}, $k_s = 0.8$ mg hr^{-1}.

Equations 37.17 for the sustaining dose and 37.19 for the prompt dose may be combined to give equation 37.21.

$$C_B = \frac{Fk_aD_o}{(k_a-k)V_D}(e^{-kt} - e^{-k_at}) + \frac{k_s}{k}(1-e^{-kt})$$

(37.21)

This may be solved for different values of prompt dose (D_o) until the desired release profile is obtained as shown in Fig. 37.14.

At the end of the sustaining period the normal exponential decline in the value of C_B occurs. If the concentration of drug in the blood at the end of the sustaining period is C_T, for this part of the time course of action curve:

$$C_B = C_T e^{-k(t-T)}$$

(37.22)

From these calculations it would appear that a tablet comprising a prompt dose of 40 mg and a sustaining dose of 80 mg should meet the design specification. In practice several trial formulations would be made and then tested in vivo.

REFERENCES

AGUIAR, A. J., KRC, J. Jr., KINKEL, A. W. & SAMYN, J. C. (1967) *J. pharm. Sci.* **56**, 847.

AGUIAR, A. J., WHEELER, L. M., FUSARI, S. & ZELMER, J. E. (1968) *J. pharm. Sci.* **57**, 1844.

ANDERSON, C. M. (1966) *Austr. J. Pharm.* **47**, 544–546.

BANDELIN, F. J. (1958) *J. Am. pharm. Ass. (Sci. Edn)* **47**, 691.

BATES, T. R., LAMBERT, D. A. & JOHNS, W. H. (1969) *J. pharm. Sci.* **58**, 1468.

BEAN, H. S. & HEMAN-ACKAH, S. M. (1964) *J. Pharm. Pharmacol.* **16**, 58T.

BEAN, H. S., KONNING, G. H. & MALCOLM, S. A. (1969) *J. Pharm. Pharmacol.* **21**, 173S.

BECKETT, A. H. & TUCKER, G. T. (1966) *J. Pharm. Pharmacol.* **18**, 72S.

Bell, S. A., Murray, B. & Holliday, W. M. (1966) *J. new Drugs* **6**, 284.

Blaug, S. M. & Ahsan, S. S. (1961a) *J. pharm. Sci.* **50**, 138; (1961b) *J. pharm. Sci.* **50**, 441.

Brown, M. R. W. & Norton, D. A. (1965) *J. Soc. cosmet. Chem.* **16**, 369.

Buckwalter, F. H. & Dickison, H. L. (1958) *J. Am. pharm. Ass. (Sci. Edn)* **47**, 661.

Charnicki, W. F. & Kober, M. L. (1957) *J. Am. pharm. Ass. (Sci. Edn)* **46**, 481.

Chaudry, N. C. & Saunders, L. (1956) *J. Pharm. Pharmacol.* **8**, 975.

Davison, C., Guy, J. L., Levitt, M. & Smith, P. K. (1961) *J. Pharmacol. exp. Ther.* **134**, 430.

D'Arcy, P. F. (1965) *Pharm. J.* **194**, 637–643.

Delucca, P. P. & Kostenbander, H. B. (1960) *J. Am. pharm. Ass. (Sci. Edn)* **49**, 430.

Desai, S. J., Singh, H., Sunonelli, A. P. & Higuchi, W. I. (1966a) *J. pharm. Sci.* **55**, 1230; (1966b) *J. pharm. Sci* **55**, 1235.

Drain, D. J., Lazare, R., Poulter, G. A., Tattersal, K. & Urbanska, A. (1959) *J. Pharm. Pharmacol.* **11**, 139T.

Duncan, W. A. M., Macdonald, G. & Thornton, M. J. (1962) *J. Pharm. Pharmacol.* **14**, 217.

Edkins, R. P. (1959) *J. Pharm. Pharmacol.* **11**, 54T.

Eriksen, S. P., Paul, J. F. & Swintosky, J. V. (1958) *J. Am. pharm. Ass. (Sci. Edn)* **47**, 697.

Flanagan, T. H., Broad, R. D., Rubinstein, M. H. & Longworth, A. R. (1969) *J. Pharm. Pharmacol.* **21**, 129S.

Ganderton, D., Hadgraft, J. W., Rispin, W. T. & Thompson, A. G. (1967) *Pharm. Acta Helv.* **42**, 152.

Haines, B. A. & Martin, A. N. (1961) *J. pharm. Sci.* **50**, 753.

Hersey, J. A. (1969) *Mfg. Chem. & Aerosol News* **40**, 32.

Hibbott, H. W. & Monks, J. M. (1961) *J. Soc. Cosmet. Chem.* **12**, 2.

Higuchi, T. (1963) *J. pharm. Sci.* **52**, 1145.

Higuchi, W. I. (1967) *J. pharm. Sci.* **56**, 315.

Hugo, W. B. & Foster, J. W. S. (1964) *J. Pharm. Pharmacol.* **16**, 209.

Humphries, K. J., Richardson, G. & Rhodes, C. T. (1968) *J. Pharm. Pharmacol.* **20**, 4S.

Jack, D. (1961) *J. mond. Pharm.* **4**, 10.

Leach, R. H. (1970) *Pharmaceut. J.* **205**, 227.

Levy, G. (1961) *J. pharm. Sci.* **50**, 388.

Levy, G. (1963) *J. pharm. Sci.* **52**, 1039.

Marshall, K. & Brook, D. B. (1969) *J. Pharm. Pharmacol.* **21**, 790.

Martindale (1972) *The Extra Pharmacopoeia.* London: Pharmaceutical Press.

Matthews, B. A. & Rhodes, C. T. (1968a) *J. Pharm. Pharmacol.* **20**, 204S; (1968b) *J. pharm. Sci.* **57**, 569.

Miyawacki, G. M., Patel, N. K. & Kostenbauder, H. B. (1959) *J. pharm. Sci.* **48**, 315.

Mullins, J. D. & Macek, T. J. (1960) *J. Am. pharm. Ass. (Sci. Edn)* **49**, 245.

Nack, W. (1970) *J. Soc. Cosmet. Chem.* **21**, 85.

Nelson, E. (1957) *J. Am. pharm. Ass. (Sci. Edn)* **46**, 572.

Nixon, J. R., Khalil, S. A. H. & Carless, J. E. (1968) *J. Pharm. Pharmacol.* **20**, 528.

Noyes, A. A. & Witney, W. R. (1897) *J. Amer. chem. Soc.* **19**, 930.

Oker, S. S., Vincent, H. C., Simon, D. E. & Frederick, K. J. (1958) *J. Am. pharm. Ass. (Sci. Edn)* **47**, 667.

Oldshue, J. J. (1961) *J. pharm. Sci.* **50**, 523.

Paul, H. E., Hayes, K. J., Paul, M. F. & Borgman, A. R. (1967) *J. pharm. Sci.* **56**, 882.

Pisano, F. D. & Kostenbauder, H. B. (1959) *J. Am. pharm. Ass. (Sci. Edn)* **48**, 310.

Raghunathan, Y. & Becker, C. H. (1968) *J. pharm. Sci.* **57**, 1748.

Robinson, I. C. & Becker, C. H. (1968) *J. pharm. Sci.* **57**, 49.

Rowland, M. & Beckett, A. H. (1964) *J. Pharm. Pharmacol.* **16**, 156T.

Schwarz, J. R., Sunonelli, A. P. & Higuchi, W. I. (1968) *J. pharm. Sci.* **57**, 274.

Scott, M. W., Goudie, A. J. & Huetteman, A. J. (1960) *J. Am. pharm. Ass. (Sci. Edn)* **49**, 467.

Senior, N. (1969a) *Pharm. J.* **203**, 703; (1969b) *Pharm. J.* **203**, 732.

Short, G. R. A. (1960) *Pharm. J.* **185**, 565.

Speigel, A. J. & Noseworthy, H. M. (1963) *J. pharm. Sci.* **52**, 917.

Swartz, C. J. & Cooper, J. (1962) *J. pharm. Sci.* **51**, 89.

TEORELL, T. (1937) *Arch intern. Pharmacodyn.* **57**, 205.

TYRER, J. H., EADIE, M. J., SUTHERLAND, J. M. & HOOPER, W. D. (1970) *Br. med. J.* **4**, 271.

WAGNER, J. C. (1961) *J. pharm. Sci.* **50**, 359.

WAGNER, J. C. (1971) Biopharmaceutics and relevant Pharmacokinetics, Drug Intelligence Publications Hamilton, Illinois, U.S.A.

WEDDERBURN, D. L. (1964) *Advances in Pharmaceutical Sciences* (I), Ed. Bean, H. S., Beckett, A. H. & Carless, J. E. London: Academic Press.

WILSON, A. (1959) *J. Pharm. Pharmacol.* **11**, 44T.

WITHEY, R. J. & MAINVILLE, C. A. (1969) *J. pharm. Sci.* **58**, 1120.

38

Pharmaceutical Aerosols

Aerosols or pressurized packs have been in use since the 1940s by which time they had been developed for the dissemination of insecticides. The term aerosol has a specific meaning denoting a fine dispersion of liquid or solid particles in a gas where the particle size is less than 50 μm in diameter, as for example, a mist or smoke. In the packaging sense however, aerosol is generally understood to refer to a self-contained sprayable product operating under the pressure of a liquefied or compressed gas known as the propellant. The range of such products has developed rapidly, particularly in the household field where convenience of use has offset the increased cost of this form of packaging.

In the pharmaceutical field the advance has not been so rapid. To some extent this may be due to a shortage of personnel in the pharmaceutical industry suitably trained in pressurized packaging and to the time required to assimilate the ideas and possibilities of such a comparatively new technology. Also the capital cost of setting up aerosol development laboratories and filling equipment has in many cases resulted in manufacturers using contract specialists to produce their products.

The administration of medicines by aerosols probably poses greater problems in stability, toxicity and particularly formulation, than the more traditional methods of presentation and certainly medicinal aerosols require more stringent attention · and perhaps a more conservative approach than other forms of aerosol. Even so, an impressive number of pharmaceutical and veterinary preparations are at present available. These fall into a number of categories according to their use.

CATEGORIES

Topical preparations. These are intended for application to the external surfaces of the body.

Local analgesics. The refrigerant effect of the evaporating propellant is used to produce surface analgesia. Ethyl chloride spray is an early example. The ethyl chloride acts both as propellant and analgesic agent.

Local anaesthetics. These usually contain benzocaine or xylocaine.

Antiseptic and skin sterilizers. Chlorhexidine, benzalkonium chloride, surgical spirit, etc., may be used for pre-operative skin sterilization and in the treatment of burns where swabbing with antiseptic is minimized or obviated. This results in less discomfort to the patient and prevents the transfer of microorganisms to other areas. Care is required here since, in contradistinction to local anaesthetics, the refrigerant effect of the evaporating propellant may cause trauma when applied to the damaged skin. Surgical spirit is easily formulated into an aerosol for the prevention of bed sores. In at least one hospital this has resulted in a saving of spirit over the usual swabbing technique on cotton wool, which more than covered the increased cost of aerosol presentation with less discomfort to the patient.

Skin dressings. Based on polymers (e.g. acrylic resins), these may be sprayed on to serve as surgical dressings. They provide a flexible water resistant and microorganism-proof barrier applied with less discomfort, more easily and quickly than traditional dressings.

Fungicidal agents. Undecylenic acid derivatives and 3-*p*-chlorophenoxypropane 1:2 diol are used for the treatment of such conditions as atheletes' foot.

Antiparasitic agents. These are used in the treatment of scabies.

Antibiotics. Neomycin, polymyxin, tyrothricin and gramicidin are used as powder aerosols. They give good coverage in micronized suspension and some have been used as spray-on ointments in oleaginous bases.

Anti-inflammatory agents, e.g. hydrocortisone and its derivatives.

Anti-pruritics, e.g. fluocinolone acetonide.

Preparations for administration to body cavities.
   Ear. The treatment of *otitis media* by the local application of an aerosol is said to be more successful than older methods.
   Nose. Nasal decongestants such as quinine, camphor, menthol, chlorbutol, thymol, oil of eucalyptus, methyl salicylate and ephedrine hydrochloride are used, either singly or combined, for the treatment of nasal congestion. The inclusion of various germicides is said to give cold relief.
   Throat. Similar preparations traditionally given by atomizer give relief in sore throats. A benzocaine preparation is available for use in preparing the patient for laryngoscopy.
   Oral. Antiseptic and odoriferous agents are used for mouth hygiene and halitosis. Amethocaine hydrochloride and benzocaine are included in an aerosol for use in dentistry.
   Oral inhalation. A number of preparations are available for oral inhalation which are intended to produce either a local or a systemic effect. The problems associated with these and their formulation are discussed later.
   Local action in the lungs. Isoprenaline, noradrenaline, adrenaline and atropine salts are used for the treatment and relief of bronchospasm in asthma, chronic bronchitis and emphysema. Accurate dosage is applied through a metered valve and suitable oral inhalation adaptor. The greater convenience and facility in use of the aerosol method

of presentation over traditional inhaler methods has led to some fatalities due to too frequent usage. Lobeline hydrochloride is used as an anti-smoking inhalant. Radiological diagnostic agents such as propyliodone have also been formulated as aerosols for X-ray examination of the respiratory tract.
   Systemic action via the lungs. Many drugs are readily absorbed systematically through the tracheo-bronchial tree. Systematic rather than local effects may be achieved by suitable formulation.

Veterinary products. The vast majority of these are for topical application and consist of antiparasitics (pyrethrum, pybuthrin, lindane), shampoos, preparations to protect bitches in season, poultry pecking preventatives, ear tick treatments, cat and dog repellants, sheep foot-rot treatments, lamb fosterage aids, ringworm treatments (dichlorophen, undecylenic acid), post-surgical antiinfectives, spray bandages.

THE ADVANTAGES AND DISADVANTAGES OF AEROSOLS

The number and variety of aerosol packs clearly indicates that they possess some advantages over the more traditional methods of presentation. The advantages are many and the disadvantages few, though not negligible.

Advantages
1. Convenience, speed and ease of application.
2. Efficient dispersion.
3. Avoidance of manual contact with the medicament.
4. Immediate local application.
5. High concentration of the medicament over a limited area.
6. Application without manual contact with the patient thus producing minimum irritation of painful areas.
7. Rapid response to the medicament.
8. Controlled and uniform dosage produced by metered valves.
9. By changing the pressure in the pack or using special valves the spray characteristics may be varied from a coarse wet spray to a fine dry mist.
10. A fine mist is easily formed for inhalation purposes.
11. Insufflation of pressurized powders is available.
12. If the drug is soluble in the propellant few formulation difficulties are encountered.
13. No contamination of the product from the environment since the system is pressurized.
14. The sterility of sterile products is maintained since no organisms can enter the pack when the valve is opened.

15. The exclusion of light by all but clear glass containers protects photolabile constituents.

16. Absence of air in the container prevents oxidation of susceptible drugs.

17. Hydrolysis of ingredients can be prevented since propellants contain no water.

18. Drugs given by oral inhalation are less liable to decomposition since they do not pass through the gastrointestinal tract.

Disadvantages

1. Cost. The container, valves, propellants and filling methods are more expensive than traditional packs.

2. Disposal may be difficult. Residual amounts of propellants in exhausted packs continue to exert a pressure and may constitute a hazard in disposal through the usual methods. The number of aerosol packs however is small compared with the total amount of domestic refuse disposed of and local authorities seem not to have experienced any special difficulties.

3. Aerosol packs must not be subjected to heat since high pressures can develop. Most pharmaceuticals should not be exposed to heat in any case.

4. Where the drug is not soluble in the propellant, co-solvent, emulsion, or suspension systems must be used. This may result in formulation difficulties greater than those met in conventional packs.

5. The toxicity of propellants, though very small, may cause problems where inhalation therapy takes place over a considerable period of time. There is some present disquiet that heart patients may be at risk if propellants are inhaled.

6. The refrigerant effect of highly volatile propellants may cause discomfort on injured skin.

7. Catalytic oxidation of drugs such as ascorbic acid and epinephrine has been caused by traces of metal from valve parts or container.

8. It is necessary to test the formulation against *all* parts of the container and valve, including gaskets, for stability.

BASIC AEROSOL TECHNOLOGY

AEROSOL SYSTEMS

All aerosols or pressurized packs consist of a container and valve together with a propellant or mixture of propellants and the active ingredient. The propellants supply the pressure required to eject the product from the pack when the valve is opened and may also form the solvent for the active ingredient. Fig. 38.1 shows the simplest form,

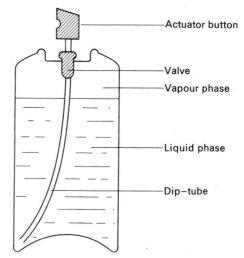

FIG. 38.1. Diagram of a simple form of aerosol package.

namely, a *two-phase system*. The liquid phase consists of the propellant or propellant mixture with the active principle in solution. The vapour phase consists of the vapour of the propellant(s). Since the vapour pressure of the propellant(s) is high, the contents exert a pressure against the walls of the container. When the valve is opened by pressing the actuator button this internal pressure forces the liquid contents up the dip-tube or stand pipe through a valve orifice, valve stem and actuator button orifice into the atmosphere where the propellant instantly vapourizes leaving a fine dispersion of the active principle. Where the active principle is not soluble in the propellant, modifications are necessary. Co-solvents may be used to achieve solution but these will affect the vapour pressure of the system. Solution of the active principle in a suitable solvent which is immiscible with the propellant gives rise to *three phase systems* consisting of the propellant liquid phase, the solution liquid phase and the vapour phase. If the propellant is lighter than the solution, the dip-tube must reach to the bottom of the container as in Fig. 38.2A. If it is heavier the dip-tube must be shortened as in Fig. 38.2B so as to avoid spraying propellant and not product. The two liquid phases may also be emulsified to produce an *emulsion system* which may be oil–in–water or water–in–oil, the propellant representing the oil phase. The characteristics of these two forms of emulsion are quite different. The oil–in–water system produces a foam whilst the water–in–oil system generally produces a coarse wet spray or stream. Suspended powder aerosols are examples of three-phase systems. They consist of a solid phase (the powder)

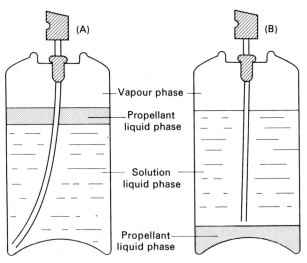

FIG. 38.2. Aerosol three-phase systems A and B.

suspended in a liquid phase (the propellant), the vapour phase consisting of propellant vapour. The inclusion of lubricants and close control of particle size of the powder are usually necessary. Aerosols consistings of the powder as the ingredient, and a compressed gas as the propellant, are examples of *solid-gas two phase systems*.

PROPELLANTS

The propellants used in aerosol systems may be classified into liquified gases; (a) fluorinated hydrocarbons, and (b) hydrocarbons, and compressed gases; (a) insoluble in water, i.e. nitrogen, argon, and (b) soluble in water, i.e. carbon dioxide, nitrous oxide.

Liquefied Gases
Fluorinated hydrocarbons. A large number of fluoromethanes and fluoroethanes are available under the trade names of *Arctons*, *Algofrenes*, *Freons*, *Genetrons*, *Isceons*, *Isotrons* and *Ucons*. The most commonly used in practice by far are trichlorofluoromethane, dichlorodifluoromethane and dichlorotetrafluoroethane. A numbering system used by the refrigeration industry has been generally adopted to designate these propellants. Reading the number from *right to left* the first digit is the number of fluorine atoms in the compound, the second digit is the number of hydrogen atoms plus one and the third digit is the number of carbon atoms minus one. If the latter digit is zero, it is omitted. The number of chlorine atoms is determined by subtracting the sum of hydrogen and fluorine atoms from the total number of atoms

which can be attached to the carbon atoms. When one carbon atom is present this sum is four, when six carbon atoms are present it is six. Where isomers occur the same number is given to all but the letters a, b, c, etc., are appended to indicate increasing asymmetry (see Table 38.1).

TABLE 38.1

FLUORINATED HYDROCARBONS

Name	Formula	Designation
		Propellant
Trichlorofluoromethane	$C.Cl_3F$	11
Dichlorodifluoromethane	$C.Cl_2F_2$	12
Dichlorotetrafluoroethane symmetrical	$C.ClF_2C.ClF_2$	114
Dichlorotetrafluoroethane asymmetrical	$C.Cl_2FCF_3$	114a

Each propellant exerts its own absolute vapour pressure. The gauge pressure which is found by substracting one atmosphere is that pressure exerted by the propellant alone when enclosed in the container. It can be measured by suitably applying a pressure gauge to the pack. The gauge pressures exerted by the commonly used propellants at 21.1° are as follows.

Propellant 11   2.64 inches of mercury vacuum.
Propellant 12   70.2 pounds per square inch (psig)
Propellant 114   12.9 psig

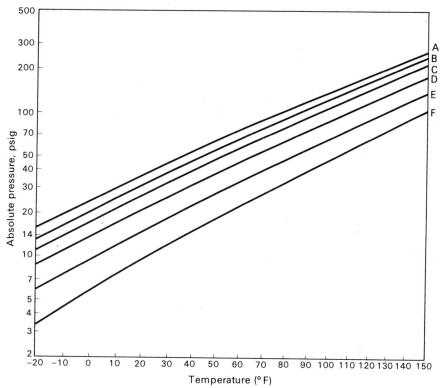

FIG. 38.3. The effect of temperature on the absolute pressure (in psig for kg/cm² conversion factors is 0.070308) of mixtures of propellants 12 and 114. A, 100 per cent propellant 12; B, 20 per cent propellant 12; C, 60 per cent propellant 12; D, 40 per cent propellant 12, E, 20 per cent propellant 12, F, 100 per cent propellant 114 (for gauge pressure subtract 14.7).

Comparative figures and conversion factors are—

One atmosphere = 14.696 psig

= 1.0333 kg/cm²

One lb per square in = 0.070308 kg/cm²

Since these propellants are miscible it is clear that suitable mixtures will provide an infinite variety of pressures up to about 70 psig (4.92 kg/cm²). The use of chlorodifluoromethane can extend this range to 122.5 psig (8.613 kg/cm²). This is a very useful facility, since pressure plays a large part in determining the spray characteristics of the finished product. Most aerosol formulation and testing is done at 21.1°, hence most data are provided for that temperature. Fig. 38.3 shows the pressures of mixtures of propellants 12 and 114 and also the effect of temperature on these. Fluctuations in temperature of more than a few degrees may affect the satisfactory operation of the aerosol pack.

Calculation of vapour pressure of a mixture of liquefied gases.

If the solution is ideal the resultant vapour pressure of a mixture of two liquefied gases may be calculated according to Raoult's Law by multiplying the sum of the mole fraction of each component present by its vapour pressure, for example—

From the following data calculate the gauge pressure of a mixture of 30 ml propellant 114 and 70 ml propellant 12, assuming atmospheric pressure to be 1.033 kg/cm².

	Propellant 114	Propellant 12
Molecular weight	170.9	120.9
Vapour pressure at 21.1°	1.9 kg/cm²	6.0 kg/cm²
Density of liquid at 21.1°	1.468 g/ml	1.325 g/ml
Convert to weight		
30 ml propellant 114 =	30 × 1.468	= 44.04 g
70 ml propellant 12 =	70 × 1.325	= 92.75 g

Percentage of 114 = $\dfrac{44.04}{92.5+44.04} \times 100$ = 32.2

Percentage of 12 = $\dfrac{92.5}{92.5+44.04} \times 100$ = 67.8

Moles of 114 in liquid = $\dfrac{32.2}{170.9}$ = 0.188

Moles of 12 in liquid =	$\dfrac{67.8}{120.9}$	= 0.561
Total moles =	0.188 + 0.561	= 0.749
Mole fraction of 114 =	$\dfrac{0.188}{0.749}$	= 0.251
Mole fraction of 12 =	$\dfrac{0.561}{0.749}$	= 0.749
Partial pressure of 114 =	0.251 × 1.9	= 0.477 kg/cm^2
Partial pressure of 12 =	0.749 × 6.0	= 4.494 kg/cm^2
Total pressure of mixture =	0.477 + 4.494	= 4.971 kg/cm^2 absolute
Gauge pressure of mixture =	4.971 − 1.033	= 3.938 kg/cm^2 gauge

Since the solution of the two liquefied gases is not usually ideal, the calculated pressure usually falls below the measured pressure by up to about 10 per cent. Aerosol propellant manufacturers can usually supply nomograms from which the resultant pressure of mixtures of propellants can easily be read for different temperatures.

Hydrocarbons. Fluorinated hydrocarbon propellants are themselves non-flammable. Paraffin hydrocarbons such as propane, butane, pentane and hexane however, which may have found greater use in some countries because of their comparative cheapness, have been limited to some extent by their flammability. They are largely used to replace part of the fluorinated hydrocarbons in order to lower the price of the pack. They may also be used in three-phase systems where the propellant and product are immiscible. The low density hydrocarbons form the upper layer and are not sprayed until the whole of the product has been dispersed. Fig. 38.4 shows the vapour pressure-temperature relations of the hydrocarbon propellants. Mixtures may be used.

Since the pressure in an aerosol pack is determined mainly by the vapour pressure of the liquefied propellant or propellant mixture and not by the amount present, it follows that this pressure will be sensibly maintained so long as a drop of propellant remains. This is a great advantage over the use of compressed gases where the pressure falls as the product is used.

Excess pressure—the presence of air in an aerosol pack gives rise to a pressure in excess of that calculated for the propellant-product system. This can be quite appreciable as indicated in Fig. 38.5. For this reason, air must be removed either by the

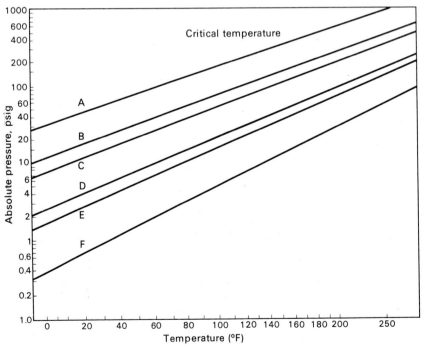

FIG. 38.4. A, hexane; B, pentane; C, isopentane; D, butane; E, isobutane; F, propane. The vapour pressure-temperature relationships of hydrocarbon propellants (adapted from Pressurized Packaging (Aerosols), Herzka and Pickthall, Butterworths Scientific Publications).

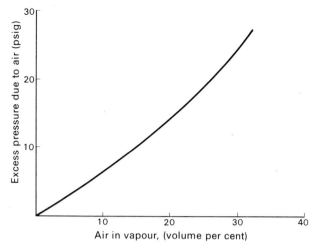

FIG. 38.5. Excess pressure due to presence of air. Propellants 11 and 12 equal parts in mixture.

application of a vacuum which is broken by the propellant fill, or by purging with a small amount of propellant.

Toxicity—The classification of toxicity groups of common refrigerants (some propellants are used as refrigerant gases), Table 38.2, has been used to

TABLE 38.2
TOXICITY CLASSIFICATION

| Group | Lethal effects or serious injury at | |
	Concentration in air volume per cent	Exposure time
1	0.5–1.0	5 min
2	0.5–1.0	30 min
3	2.0–2.5	1 hour
4	2.0–2.5	2 hours
5	Considerably less toxic than group 4, more toxic than group 6	
6	20.0	No harmful effects after exposure for 2 hours

From Nuckolls, A. H., *The Comparative Life, Fire and Explosion Hazards of Common Refrigerants.* M.H. 2375, 1933, 106. Underwriters Laboratories, Chicago.

assess the life hazard of propellants when present in air in the absence of flame or hot surfaces. Thus inhalation toxicity classification places propellants 12 and 114 in Group 6 and propellant 11 in Group 5. However, decomposition of fluorohydrocarbons at high temperatures in the presence of moisture, which may occur if they are sprayed into a flame or on a red-hot surface, results in the formation of hydrogen chloride, hydrogen fluoride and some

phosgene. Care should therefore be taken that flame extension tests for flammability are carried out in a suitably ventilated environment. There is some indication that persons suffering from heart conditions may have a sudden collapse as a result of inhaling propellants.

Compressed Gases
Insoluble gases. Nitrogen and argon being substantially insoluble in the product, pose problems when used as propellants. As the product is used the gas expands with the increasing headspace and the pressure falls. This can result in changing spray characteristics and even failure to deliver the whole contents of the pack. Higher initial pressures are necessary and suitable one-or-two-piece containers required to withstand the pressures involved. Assume that 30 psig (2.11 kg/cm^2) pressure is required to produce a satisfactory spray from a product filled two-thirds full with one-third headspace when the last of the product is being dispersed. At this point the gas will have expanded to three times its volume, hence an initial pressure of 90 psig (6.33 kg/cm^2) would be necessary. For liquid preparations the output is usually in the form of a wet-stream rather than a spray and special break-up spray actuators are necessary.

Soluble gases. Nitrous oxide and carbon dioxide are soluble in aqueous products. The gas in solution is in equilibrium with the gas in the head space and dependent upon the pressure of the gas in the container. As the head space increases this equilibrium is re-established by gas coming out of solution. There is a fall in pressure but it is less pronounced than that observed with insoluble gases. With suitably formulated products and using a foam actuator, foams may be produced as the gas in solution expands on leaving the nozzle.

CONTAINERS

Aerosol containers may be composed of tin plate, aluminium, glass, plastic-coated glass, plastics or stainless steel.

Tin plate containers are three-piece being composed of a cylindrical body and a top and bottom. The body consists of a rectangular sheet of tin plate formed into a cylinder by means of, usually, a soldered joint or seam. The tin plate is composed of a rolled sheet of mild steel plate or black plate which has been coated with tin usually by an electrolytic process, more exceptionally by a process of hot-dipping, where the steel plate is plunged into a bath of molten tin. The former process produces a more even coat more cheaply. Tin plate thus produced has a complete tin coating over both surfaces and also over the edges. When such a large sheet is cut into suitably sized rectangular areas from which to form a cylinder, the cut edges will be raw, not plated. The exposed raw edges present a source of corrosion especially as they are lapped and soldered to form the walls of the container. Such joints consisting of tin, mild steel plate and solder can form the electrodes of electrolytic cells. Corrosion can be minimized by coating both surfaces of the finished container with a suitable lacquer. The outer surface usually consists of the decoration of the container. The inner surface is especially at risk when propellant 11 is used, resulting in acid products or where the product includes alcohol, resulting in the production of alcoholates. From an economic point of view the coating should be as thin as possible. Pinholes in the lacquer may occur resulting in concentrated points of attack which may even puncture the container. The top and bottom of the containers are jointed with a suitable elastomeric material between them to form a seal. Because of these top, bottom and side seams such containers are usually limited in practice to pressures of about 45 to 50 psig (3.16–3.52 kg/cm^2), these pressures being suitable for products contained therein.

Aluminium containers may be two-piece or mono-bloc. Two-piece containers have the sides of the cylinder and the top formed in one piece from a plug of aluminium suitably extruded and formed with, usually, a tin-plate base attached. Since there is only one joint at the base these will withstand higher pressures. The base is usually dome-shaped inwards the better to withstand the pressure. Mono-bloc containers are formed in one piece by extrusion from a plug of aluminium, the top being subsequently formed to accept the one-inch cup valve. Such containers will withstand even higher pressures and are often used when the propellant consists of insoluble or soluble gases.

Glass containers are moulded so as to accept 13, 15, 18 or 20 mm bottle valves. Since the strength of the walls depends upon the condition of the glass surfaces, low pressures of some 15 psig (1.06 kg/cm^2) are maximal.

Plastic-coated glass containers are glass containers as above, dipped in molten plastic so as to form a coat. The plastic coating is complete up to the neck so that when the valve is crimped on, the joint encloses the plastic. A single large or a number of smaller holes in the plastic coating on the base allows the more gentle escape of the contents in the event of the fracture of the glass, the glass fragments being contained by the plastic coat. (Fracture of an uncoated glass container will result in an explosion scattering gragments of glass). Such plastic-coated containers can be filled to pressures of some 25 psig (1.76 kg/cm^2).

Plastic containers are now formed with thick walls of acetal resins or polypropylene and will withstand somewhat higher pressures. Possible loss of contents to the plastics container and leaching of contents from the compounded plastics to the product must be considered in formulation.

Stainless steel containers are also available in small sizes, suitable for use with bottle valves. They are strong and also reduce corrosion problems.

VALVES

These consist basically of two types. One inch cup valves where the valve cup has a diameter of one inch and is swaged into the container via a gasket of elastomeric material and 13, 15, 18 or 20 mm bottle valves where the valve is crimped over the neck of the usually glass, plastic coated, glass, plastics or stainless steel container. The former are usually in more common use in the wide field of aerosols, whereas the latter are usually used on smaller containers. The parts of a simple one-inch cup valve are shown in Fig. 38.6. An actuator

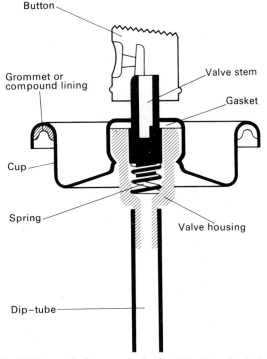

FIG. 38.6. A one-inch cup aerosol valve (Metal Box Co. Ltd.).

button is fitted to the top of such a valve. When this is depressed against the valve spring the contents enter the dip-tube and valve and are extruded from the container via the actuator button. The explosive effect of the propellant produces a spray. Within the confines of these two valves a vast number of variations are available. Variations in the dimensions of the valve parts can affect spray pattern and delivery rates. Similarly variations in design of the actuator button can affect these parameters and mechanical break-up buttons with baffles, and foam heads are used with suitable formulations.

Metered valves are usually fitted to pharmaceutical preparations when a definite volume of the product is released in one operation of the valve button. Such valves contain a reservoir of defined volume. These are of two types. Depression of the valve button may release the contents of the reservoir which refills on release of the button, or depression of the valve button may fill the reservoir the contents of which are ejected on release of the button. Other variations are available.

BASIC AEROSOL FORMULATION

The basic principles of aerosol formulation depend upon the solubility of the active principle in the propellant or propellant mixture. This determines the form in which the constituent is presented.

1. *The active principle is soluble in the propellants.* In this case the active principle is dissolved directly in the propellant or propellant mixture. Usually a mixture of propellants is used, their relative proportions being adjusted to produce the desired pressure (see Fig. 38.3).

2. *The active principle is not soluble in the propellants but is soluble in a co-solvent.* Assuming for example, that the active principle is not soluble in propellants 11 or 12 but is soluble in ethanol, the ternary diagram ethanol/propellant 11/propellant 12 is used in selecting the proportions of these three liquids (Fig. 38.7). This diagram has been prepared by measuring the pressures exerted by various mixtures and plotting the different isobars. Spray characteristics have also been examined and areas of satisfactory spray pattern shaded on the diagram. Points may be selected on the diagram so as to formulate for suitable pressures and spray patterns. Each point represents a different proportion of the three liquids by weight. The nearer to propellant 12 on the diagram, the greater the proportion of

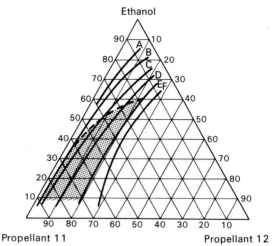

FIG. 38.7. Ternary system, propellants 11, 12 and ethanol.

Vapour pressure contour	psig	kg/cm²
A	5	1.38
B	10	1.74
C	15	2.09
D	20	2.44
E	25	2.79
F	30	3.14

the high pressure propellant 12, and the higher the pressure and the finer the spray. The nearer to propellant 11, the greater the proportion of the low pressure propellant 11, and the lower the pressure and the coarser the spray. The nearer to alcohol on the diagram on any isobar, the wetter the spray. Within these confines a number of test preparations may be made and the most satisfactory selected. One difficulty experienced in formulation is that when the filled test preparations are produced, since most containers are opaque, the contents cannot be seen and the presence of two liquid phases instead of one not easily determined. This may be obviated in either of two ways. Naarden compatibility testers consist of thick resistance glass containers to which valves can be fitted. These can be filled by any of the normal methods and the contents inspected. Alternatively, and more cheaply, small glass bottles such as are used for pressurized drinks may be cold filled and crown caps fixed on. These are usually placed for safety in boxes with transparent plastic fronts through which they may be examined for phase relationships and deposits after raising to 21.1°. They are subsequently emptied by cooling to −30° and removing the cap.

3. *The active principle is not soluble in the propellant nor in a co-solvent, but is soluble in water.* Since water and propellants are immiscible two possibilities exist.

(a) The container is filled with an aqueous solution of the active principle and the propellant introduced. Two liquid and one vapour phase are produced. If the propellant phase is lighter than water (e.g. hydrocarbons, propane, butane, hexane, etc.) the propellant phase will float on the aqueous phase (Fig. 38.2A). The dip-tube should therefore reach the bottom of the container. If the propellant phase is heavier than the aqueous phase (e.g. fluorohydrocarbons) it will sink to the bottom and the dip-tube must be cut short or propellant phase only will be ejected (Fig. 38.2B). With such systems even higher pressures will still result in unsatisfactory spray patterns since the propellant is not ejected and its explosive effect at the outlet is non-existent. Mechanical break-up actuators fitted with baffles are required to produce a finer spray.

(b) An emulsion is formed, the propellant being the oily phase and the solution of the active principles in water being the aqueous phase. Using appropriate emulgents and phase-volume relationships such an emulsion may be water–in–oil or oil–in–water. Since the propellant in oil–in–water emulsions is the internal phase its expansion on release from the valve tends to produce a foam and a foam actuator should be fitted. Water–in–oil emulsion however can be sprayed, since the propellant here is the external phase. Generally speaking, larger quantities of propellant are required for emulsion systems and they should be vigorously shaken before use.

4. *The active principle is an insoluble solid.* Here the active principle in a suitable form of subdivision is presented as a suspension in the propellant mixture. In contradistinction to all previous methods the particle size of the active principle depends upon its size reduction before adding to the formulation. Too large particles may clog the valve. The smallest valve orifices are of the order of 400 μm diameter. Agglomeration of particles however, occurs and much smaller particles may cause clogging. Particles passing a 325 mesh sieve possess a maximum diameter of 43 μm. Such particles can be sprayed in suitable formulations up to 5 per cent, exceptionally 10 per cent, by weight. Recommended sizes are 5 to 10 μm, none greater than 50 μm. Formulation should be directed towards preventing agglomeration. Particles should be thoroughly wetted by the liquid phase and a dispersing agent may be required. Impaction of the solid phase on standing may require mechanical aids such as ceramic balls to disperse it. The inclusion of a fraction per cent of a mineral oil ensures maximum powder impaction on the target area.

Factors Affecting Spray Characteristics
A number of factors affect the spray characteristics of the finished product and these must be considered during the development of the formulation.

Viscosity. As the viscosity of the formulation increases, so does the particle size of the spray which therefore becomes coarser. Further increase in viscosity may produce a stream instead of a spray.

Vapour pressure of the propellants. The higher the vapour pressure of the propellant or propellant mixture the smaller the particle size produced and the finer the spray. This is due to the increase in the disruptive forces of the propellants as the pressure increases.

Propellant product ratio. The greater the proportion of propellant in the formulation the finer and drier the spray. Adjustment of this ratio of propellant to product and adjustment of the relative proportions of the two propellants are the two factors having greatest immediate effect on spray characteristics. A given product may therefore be presented in all variations between a coarse wet spray and a fine dry one. A single propellant of an intermediate pressure gives a finer spray than a mixture of two propellants having the same vapour pressure.

Presence of solvents. The solvents or co-solvents frequently used in aerosol formulations may affect the pressure. Such effects may be determined from the appropriate ternary diagrams. The vapour pressure of the solvent may also affect the lifetime of the particles in the spray. Low pressure solvents evaporate more slowly and produce particles with longer lifetimes than high pressure ones.

Temperature. Figs 38.3 and 38.4 indicate the rapid change in vapour pressure of propellants with temperature. Formulation should take into account the temperature at which the aerosol product is likely to be used since the spray characteristics change with the resulting change in vapour pressure. Most formulation and testing is done at 21.1° and this is usually satisfactory for temperate climes although changes of more than a few degrees either way may alter the spray pattern between coarse and fine. The expected ambient temperature must therefore be considered in the formulation of products for overseas markets.

AEROSOL FILLING

The machinery used for aerosol filling ranges from simple laboratory apparatus through semi-automatic to automatic equipment. There are two basic filling methods, *pressure filling* and *cold filling*.

Pressure Filling with Hydrocarbon and Fluorohydrocarbon Propellants

The procedure is as follows, using the laboratory burette filler (Fig. 38.8). The same principles apply on larger machines.

1. The product is filled into the container.
2. A short burst of low pressure propellant is introduced into the container to purge the air.
3. The valve and cup are immediately swaged on with a swaging machine. This exerts a downward pressure on the valve cup gasket forming an effective seal and at the same time expands the vertical sides of the valve cup under the can opening to

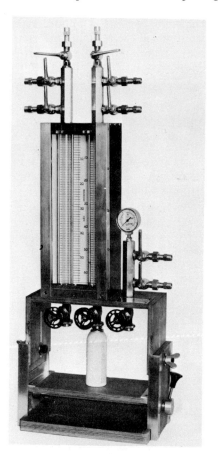

Fig. 38.8. Laboratory burette filler (by courtesy of Aerofill Ltd.).

form a secure closure. Some commercial machines use a vacuum to purge the air at this stage.

4. The valve orifice is offered up to the filling head of the machine and the valve opened by gentle pressure. The needle valve of the filling machine is opened and the appropriate volume of low pressure propellant run in. Due to the low pressure such filling is often slow. It may be speeded up by previously immersing the container in ice, warming the cylinder of propellant slightly or applying pressure to the liquid from a cylinder of inert gas. This is usually necessary because as soon as one drop of the propellant enters the container the vapour pressure exerted is the same as that in the propellant cylinder. Commercial machines push the propellant into the container via a piston operated by compressed air.

5. The container is then removed and offered up to the filling head of the high pressure propellant which is similarly filled. Due to its higher pressure no difficulty is usually experienced.

6. The container is removed and shaken to homogenize the contents.

Using such a method and employing a laboratory burette filler, varying amounts of two propellants may be filled into each successive container. This is necessary during formulation experiments. Commercial apparatus is adjusted to fill definite volumes of the propellants or of a propellant mixture and will produce a repetitive series of containers filled to the same condition. *Transfer filling* is a useful method for use during formulation experiments and is also adaptable to small scale filling in a hospital dispensary. It is a form of pressure filling. A series of large aerosol containers is charged with different propellants or propellant mixtures. Such containers may be purchased ready filled from the propellant manufacturers or filled from the appropriate machines. The product is filled, the air purged and the valve swaged on to the container as before. The propellant container without a dip-tube is inverted over the product container and the contents expelled to weight through a transfer button which connects the two valves together. Slight pressure is required to open both valves.

Cold Filling with Hydrocarbon and Fluorohydrocarbon Propellants

In this method the propellants are refrigerated to a temperature at least 5° below their boiling points when they emerge from the plant as liquids. Propellant 12 has a boiling point of about −30° hence refrigeration should be to −35°. The cold filling plant consists of a tank filled with spirit which is cooled by the addition of solid carbon-dioxide to the required temperature. Electrical methods of refrigeration may also be used. The propellants are fed via cooling coils in the tank to taps from which the filling is done. Asbestos gloves should be worn and care taken not to let any of the refrigerated propellants touch the skin as serious cold burns can ensue. The procedure is as follows:

1. The (often pre-cooled) product is placed in the container.
2. The appropriate amount of low pressure propellant is run in to weight.
3. The appropriate amount of high pressure propellant is run in to weight. During this process air is purged by the natural evaporation of the propellants.
4. The valve and cup are quickly swaged on and the container shaken to homogenize the contents.

Cold filling is unsuitable for products whose active principle is destroyed by low temperatures.

Soluble and insoluble compressed gases are filled by pressure filling until the correct pressure has been reached as indicated on the gauge. The rate of solution of soluble gases is increased by using shaker-gassing equipment where the containers are shaken as the gas is applied.

THE TESTING OF AEROSOLS

A number of testing procedures has been evolved to ensure the safe and satisfactory operation of the finished product. Most testing is carried out after the containers have been equilibrated to 21.1°.

Leakage. Each individual container is passed completely immersed through a bath of hot water so that the contents reach a temperature of 54.4°, and examined for leakage. The bath is often illuminated for easier inspection and covered by a grill for safety. The points examined are the valve itself, the valve cup and the top, bottom and side seams. Leakage at the valve cup gasket indicates unsatisfactory swaging and the collets of the swaging machine may require adjustment. Some pharmaceuticals aerosols may be exempted from this test if the contents are thermolabile.

Internal pressure. This is measured with a pressure gauge having a suitable adaptor to fit the valve orifice. The actuator button is removed from the valve stem, the container shaken vigorously and the adaptor offered up to the valve orifice. On depression of the valve with the gauge the pressure is recorded by inverting the container, clearing the dip-tube by depressing the valve, and

applying the gauge in the inverted position. For more accurate pressure determinations three readings are taken with two minutes re-equilibration to 21.1° between each. These usually show a slightly diminishing series which can be plotted and extrapolated to give the true pressure. Barometric corrections should be applied.

Spray pattern. Spray pattern is largely determined by the internal pressure, the product–propellant ratio and the viscosity of the product. The spray may be examined visually on depression of the valve actuator but a closer and more permanent record can be made by determining the spray pattern. One technique (Root 1956) is to mix a water or oil soluble dye appropriate to the solvent in the pack with talc and brush it on to vellum paper. The product is then sprayed on to the paper from a fixed distance for a fraction of a second in a closed box and the patterns thus produced are photographed. Some difficulty may be experienced in accurately timing the length of time of the burst. Dixon's (1959) method has proved more satisfactory. The target consists of a photographic quarter plate from which the backing and emulsion have been washed and a coating applied from burning magnesium ribbon. This is placed behind a shutter

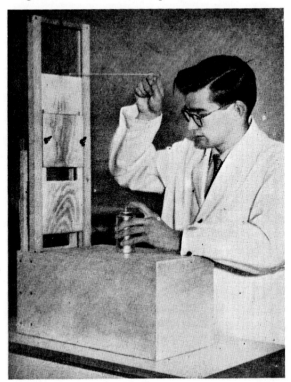

Fig. 38.9. Apparatus for the determination of spray pattern (from Dixon, 1959).

with an adjustable slot. The container is placed at a fixed distance from the shutter. As the actuator button is depressed the shutter is also released thus slicing through the spray and allowing a representative sample of spray to impinge on the target *via* the slot (Fig. 38.9). A permanent record, is obtained by placing the target, coated side downwards, on to photographic paper and printing.

Discharge rates. The determination of discharge rates gives an indication of the number of operations required to empty the container and hence the most suitably sized container for the particular product. It is also useful in the determination of doses delivered by medicinal aerosols. The container is immersed in a water bath at 21.1° for half an hour (or such time as is required for the contents to reach that temperature), removed from the bath, discharged for approximately five seconds to remove water and non-homogeneous mixtures from the valve and dip-tube, wiped dry and weighed. The valve is held open for $10 \pm 1/5$ seconds and the container reweighed. The difference in weight, or discharge rate, is expressed in gm per second. Three such determinations are made unless the results differ by more than 0.1 gm/second when a fourth and fifth determination is made. The average discharge rate is calculated for each container and the arithmetic mean, standard deviation and standard error of the mean of these averages calculated.

Flammability. Although fluorohydrocarbon propellants are not inflammable the inclusion of co-solvents such as ethanol may result in a flammable product. In the *flame extension test* the valve is operated for about 15 to 20 seconds 18 cm from the flame of a standard candle. The length of any flame produced is measured with the standard candle as zero. Flame extensions of over 20 cm indicate that the product is combustible and over 45 cm, flammable. Any containers which flash back to the valve are classed as flammable.

The *modified Tagliabue open cup test* gives an indication of the flammability of the product alone if there has been a leak resulting in loss of propellant and where the residual contents are heated to cause excessive evaporation or boiling. The top of the dispenser is punctured with a fine hole so as to allow the propellant to escape. The hole is enlarged, the contents warmed to 15.56° and transferred to the Tagliabue open cup in the apparatus up to the test line. The contents are now heated at the rate of 1.11° a minute and the gas flame testing burner applied until the contents flash completely across the top of the cup or the

volume falls 6 mm from the original level. In the latter case if there is no flash the contents are recorded as having no flash under the conditions of the test. Products which flash below 37.78° are considered flammable and those which flash between 37.78° and 148.9° combustible.

The *drum test* gives an indication of the hazards which may result if excessive quantities are sprayed into a confined space where a flame is present. The equipment consists of a 55-gallon drum placed on its side, one end consisting of a top hinged cover which will open at 5 psig (0.35 kg/cm²) pressure. The closed end has three 2.5 cm diameter shuttered openings each 5 cm from the circumference, one at the top, one at the bottom and one mid-way between. In the centre is a 15 cm square opening of safety glass for visual inspection of the container. A plumber's candle is placed on the bottom midway between the two ends. In the *open* drum test the drum is placed outside at a temperature of 15.56° to 26.67°. The dispenser is discharged for approximately one minute into the upper half of the drum with the hinged cover held in the open position. Any propagation of flame away from the source of ignition is regarded as positive, while unsustained burning in the vicinity of that source is negative. In the *closed* drum test the hinged cover is allowed to rest freely against the end of the drum. Each of the three shutters is opened in turn and a burst of about 1 minute duration directed into the drum. Any explosion or raising of the hinged cover is regarded as a positive result and the product is considered flammable.

Particle size analysis. Particle size is of major importance for inhaled medical aerosols to ensure that the particles reach deep down into the respiratory tract and are not exhaled. With insecticidal space sprays too large particles may fall out of the atmosphere too quickly, whereas too small particles may slipstream around the insect without impact upon it. Most of the usual methods of particle size analysis may be used but the cascade impactor is less laborious than many. This consists of a series of tubes of diminishing diameters arranged at right angles to each other with a glass slide across each corner and a standard rate of air flow through the apparatus. Because of this standard rate of air flow, the diminishing diameters of the successive tubes causes increasing velocities therein. This results in the inertial deposition of successively smaller particle sizes on each slide as the discharged aerosol spray passes through the apparatus. The slides are coated with a suitable medium to collect the particles which are then sized with a microscope. Light scattering methods have also been used.

Moisture determination. The presence of moisture in pressurized packs can give rise to corrosion problems especially when propellant 11 is used. Where the pack can be sacrified, it is punctured to allow the low boiling point propellants to evaporate. Moisture is determined in the residue by the standard Karl Fischer method. Where the pack is to be retained a sample may be introduced into the moisture determination apparatus by inserting a sawn-off hypodermic needle into the actuator orifice. If a dip-tube is fitted the dispenser is held in the normal vertical position. The vapour phase or head-space is introduced by first inverting the dispenser and clearing the dip-tube and valve.

Analysis of propellant mixtures. This is carried out by gas-liquid chromatography using kieselguhr packed columns impregnated with dionylphthalate the apparatus being maintained at 100°. The sample is introduced into a nitrogen stream.

AEROSOLS FOR ORAL INHALATION

The administration of drugs by oral inhalation is a method which has long been used in the treatment of certain diseases and conditions. For example, asthma has been alleviated by the inhalation of smoke from burning stramonium and lobelia herb. Preparations of compound tincture of benzoin added to hot water and the vapours inhaled have been useful in the symptomatic relief of bronchitis and hay fever and menthol and eucalyptus oil suitably formulated have been used in nebulizers as sprays for similar conditions. Accurate dosage is difficult to obtain with these methods. With the aerosol metered valve, however, the correct dose of medicament can be given accurately and with greater facility. Small containers of the more active substances can be carried on the person for use when required. The ease of such administration has resulted in a number of fatalities due to over-use. The propellants themselves are inhaled directly into the lungs and this has recently raised the problem of cardiotoxic responses in those suffering from cardiac conditions. Nevertheless, such preparations have been used with great effect. The fact that a suitable aerosol is readily available has relieved stress in asthmatic patients and possibly resulted in the reduced onset of attacks. Although most preparations are formulated for local action in the respiratory tract, this route offers the possibility of general systemic absorption of potent drugs, and could, in certain circumstances, replace injection

TABLE 38.3

PERCENTAGE RETENTION OF INHALED AEROSOL PARTICLES IN VARIOUS REGIONS OF THE RESPIRATORY TRACT

	Percentage retention									
	Tidal air 450 cm³					Tidal Air 1500 cm³				
Particle size, μm	20	6	2	0.6	0.2	20	6	2	0.6	0.2
Region										
Mouth	15					18	1			
Pharynx	8					10	1			
Trachea	10	1				19	3			
Pulmonary bronchi	12	2				20	5	1		
Secondary bronchi	19	4	1			21	12	2		
Tertiary bronchi	17	9	2	1	1	9	20	5		
Quaternary bronchi	6	7	2	1	1	1	10	3	1	1
Terminal bronchioles	1	19	6	4	6	1	9	3	2	4
Respiratory bronchioles	0	11	5	3	4	0	3	2	2	4
Alveolar ducts	0	25	25	8	11	0	13	26	10	13
Alveolar sacs	0	5	0	0	0	0	18	17	6	7
Totals	93	83	41	16	22	99	95	59	21	29

From Goldstein et al. (1968) *Principles of Drug Action*, Harper and Row, N.Y., p. 118.

resulting in greater comfort and convenience. Table 38.3 shows the retention of particles of different sizes in various regions of the respiratory tract and indicates that particle size is of prime importance in deciding the place of deposition. Certain conclusions can be drawn. Impaction and retention of the larger particles takes place in the upper regions of the respiratory tract. Smaller particles reach deeper into the lungs but may also be exhaled. Hence the total amount of drug retained is less than for larger particles. The total retention of very small particles increases again probably due to the effect of gravimetric sedimentation, diffusion and Brownian motion. Particles of all sizes are carried deeper into the lungs before impacting on deeper inspiration (increased tidal volume) even though the respiratory rate remains the same. There is probably an increase in total retention and in transpulmonary absorption on holding the breath after inspiration, since this increases the time in which the forces of deposition can act. Drug impaction in the respiratory tract depends upon inertial forces, gravitational forces and Brownian motion.

Inertial forces. When an air current changes direction, the particle tends to continue along its original path. Deposition therefore increases with particle size and is of more significance in the upper regions of the respiratory tract. *Gravitational forces* cause the sedimentation of particles and this effect is more noticeable in the deeper regions of the lungs where the air is more still. *Brownian motion* causes sub-micronic particles to deposit in the alveoli. Retention in the respiratory tract is approximately proportional to the particle diameter. Where hygroscopic substances are present in the formulation the particles increase in size as they pick up moisture and rate of impaction increases. For this reason particle size measurements made in comparatively dry air may be inadmissible.

In general, the *formulation* and *testing* of aerosols for oral inhalation follow the precepts previously mentioned under these headings, but additional problems arise.

Where *local pulmonary action* is required the drug is used in dilute solutions. Careful control of the particle size distribution can result in the introduction of a minute quantity of a potent substance sufficient to produce a local effect but not large enough to produce a systemic effect by trans-pulmonary absorption.

It has been calculated that one litre of air emanating from a particle generator producing particles of 0.3 μm in diameter contained 15 billion such particles. Assuming that the human lung contains 700 million alveoli, one breath would introduce more than 150 particles into every alveolus for a few microgrammes of drug. The inclusion in the formulation of pneumodilators and vasoconstrictors enhances this local activity. Some single drugs such as phenylephrine and cyclopentamine act in both capacities. The *general systemic actions* of most drugs can be produced by providing a suitable dose of larger particle size since most drugs are readily absorbed from all regions of the respiratory tract. The inclusion of vasodilators increases this effect and the amount of drug found in the blood depends upon the amount deposited in the tract.

Once the formulation has been produced consideration must be given to stability and packaging. Loss of active principle due to leaching of reactive materials from the whole container or its absorption by the container, especially where plastics are concerned, could give rise to serious results. Such problems may be considered under the following headings.

The stability of the formulation with respect to the components of the aerosol package. Each in-

gredient in the formulation may come into contact with plastics (valve components, gaskets, containers), glass (container), or metals (container, valve components). Loss or change in any of these ingredients may cause breakdown of the formulation and/or failure of the pack to operate correctly. It is preferable to test each individual ingredient against all components of the package as well as the completed formulation, under different temperature conditions. Such tests should include an assay for the final activity of the active principle chemically, physically or biologically, as appropriate. Leaching of alkali from a glass container may cause an undesirable change in pH. The active principle or any other component of the formulation may be absorbed by plastics resulting in breakdown or loss of activity.

Additives in the plastics composition may result in inactivation of the active principle. The nature of the elastomeric material may change, causing leaks at gaskets. Metal ions may catalyse a degradative reaction in the formulation or the metal valve parts may rust and malfunction.

Since air or oxygen is not present in the pack, oxidation is not usually a problem. The propellants themselves do not support microbial growth and may even be self-sterilizing. Microbial decomposition is not usual although it should be considered. Exposure to light only occurs in glass containers.

The *compatibility* of the active principle and ingredients in the formulation with the propellant system should be examined, including the solubility of the active principle in such propellants. This is usually limited and in the majority of systems a co-solvent is used. This will usually depress the vapour pressure of the formulation and result in increased particle size and coarser sprays. The co-solvent is also inhaled and may give rise to taste problems.

A *suspension* of the drug in the propellants is often desirable to obviate these effects. Attention must be given to the initial particle size reduction of the drug to obtain the desired effect. Particle growth may take place on storage, hence, particle size distribution should be examined over a period of time under different temperature conditions. Subsequent valve clogging may occur. Sedimentation and impaction of solid particles may be apparent and attention to the difference in densities between the drug particles and the supporting medium can reduce these effects. The closer the densities of the two phases the less the problem.

The *metered valve* must reproduce accurate doses

throughout the life of the package regardless of the amount of product left in the container. This is not usually a problem where hydrocarbons or fluorohydrocarbons are used, since the pressure remains sensibly the same. The time and type of shaking required to produce a homogeneous dispersion must be examined. On storage, sedimentation of the larger particles takes place, the finer ones being deposited last. Inadequate shaking may give rise to a dispersion of finer particles from the upper layers in the first instance, and subsequently of the coarser particles. Variation in the dose of active principle in the same delivered volume could thus occur.

Uniformity of dosage through the adaptor. The mouthpiece used for inhalation may itself impact particles of the drug resulting in reduced dosage. Studies should be made of the actual dose delivered by the mouthpiece.

Uniformity of valve delivery. This can be tested by discharging the metered dose into a quantity of reagent and assaying for the active principle.

REFERENCES

ROOT, M. J. (1956) *J. Soc. cosmet. Chem.* **7**, 153.

DIXON, K. (1959) *J. Soc. cosmet. Chem.* **10**, 220.

GENERAL READING

Pressurised Packaging (Aerosols), Herska, A. & Pickthall, J. London: Butterworth and Co.

Aerosols: Science and Technology. Ed. Shepherd, H. R. New York: Interscience.

39

Packaging

A product is not correctly formulated unless it is properly packaged, and in some cases the major part of the formulation process may be concerned with selecting the right package for the product. The stability of a pharmaceutical may be totally dependent on proper functioning of the package, for example there must be rigorous exclusion of light and oxygen from oily vitamin preparations if loss of potency due to oxidation is to be avoided.

A package consists of:

the *container* in which the product is placed,

the *closure* which seals the container to exclude oxygen, carbon dioxide, moisture, bacteria, etc., and equally important, prevents the loss of water and other volatile substances from the product,

the *carton or outer*, constructed from a variety of materials such as carboard, moulded wood pulp or expanded polystyrene, which gives secondary protection against mechanical and other environmental hazards, and also serves for the display of written information,

the *box* in which multiples of the product are packed. The box provides primary defence against external hazards and usually incorporates suitable shock absorbing features.

Cartons and boxes will not be dealt with here; the reader is referred to Paine (1962) for an introductory text.

The suitability of the container and closure for their particular purpose depends on:

(a) their ability to contain the product without loss by spillage or permeation,

(b) the protection they afford against environmental hazards,

(c) whether they are suited to the function of the product both in form and size, for example a volume of injection intended to provide several doses for use on different occasions should not be packed in an ampoule,

(d) freedom from interaction between product and container,

(e) reasonable cost in relation to the cost of the product and that of alternative packages which may offer some marginal advantages.

This technically formidable specification is derived, in large measure, from the concept of an ideal package. To match this as closely as possible is a function of the materials from which the package is formed and these must first be discussed.

PACKAGING MATERIALS

With very few exceptions containers and closures are fabricated from metals, rubber, plastic, glass or a combination of these. These materials may be divided into two groups. On the one hand the metals are polycrystalline, that is, composed of a large number of small, randomly orientated, crystalline structural units (grains) separated by a grain boundary, about two or three atomic distances wide, in which the atoms do not belong precisely to either of the adjacent lattices (Fig. 39.1). On the other hand plastics, rubber and glass, are all polymers formed by the bonding together of a large number of molecular units. The basic structural elements in polymers are therefore long chains of repeating molecular units which intertwine to form a three dimensional network.

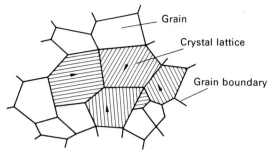

FIG. 39.1. Polycrystalline structure of metals.

METALS

There are over seventy metals in the periodic table but of these only tin, lead, aluminium and iron are of significance in pharmaceutical packaging. In use, small stresses sufficient to cause only elastic deformation are accommodated by changes in the distances between the atoms in the crystal lattices of the grains. Larger stresses bring about relative slippage of the crystal planes (dislocation) and the deformation is permanent.

Tin

This metal is very resistant to chemical attack and readily coats a number of other metals. Tin-coated lead tubes combine the softness of lead with the inertness of tin and for this reason were formerly used for packaging fluoride toothpaste. The high cost of lead has resulted in the use of the much less expensive lacquered aluminium tubes for this purpose. Currently, some eye ointments are still packaged in pure tin ointment tubes.

Iron

Although iron as such is not used for pharmaceutical packaging, large quantities of tin-coated steel are employed for the fabrication of drums, screw-caps and aerosol cans. Tin-coated steel, popularly called 'tin', combines the strength of steel with the corrosion resistance of tin. The performance of tin-coated steel is dependant on the uniformity of the coating. If an aqueous liquid can penetrate a pinhole or other fault in the layer of tin, what is virtually a short-circuited galvanic cell is set up and the intense chemical action which results brings about rapid failure of the underlying steel. As a further protection measure tinned steel packaging components may be given a thin coating of lacquer.

Aluminium

This metal has a very low atomic weight implying that it should be very reactive. The surface, however, reacts with atmospheric oxygen to form a thin, tough, coherent, transparent coating of the oxide, of atomic thickness, which protects the metal from further oxidation. Any substance which reacts with the oxide coating can cause corrosion, e.g., products of high or low pH, those which complex aluminium, mercurials, etc. As a result of the corrosion process hydrogen may be evolved. Aluminium ointment tubes (Pharmaceutical Journal 1957), containers for tablets and other unit-dose products (Glowacki 1966) and screw-caps, are widely used in pharmaceutical packaging. Some official creams such as those containing Cetrimide, Neomycin or Hydrocortisone may be packed in aluminium tubes provided a phosphate buffer is included in the formulation to inhibit corrosion and evolution of hydrogen. Alternatively an internally lacquered tube may be suitable but care must be taken to ensure that the coating is of sufficient thickness and satisfactory composition, and is free from pinholes and other faults.

POLYMERS

The polymer chains may be free to glide independently over one another or may be partially constrained in relation to neighbours by chemical cross-links as is shown for silicone rubber in Fig. 39.2. The cross-link is formed, in the example given, from methyl groups attached to silicon atoms in adjacent chains.

The similar form of the molecular structures of plastics, rubber and glass, leads to similarities in their physical behaviour. All three materials have a glass transition temperature (T_g) below which they become hard, rigid, brittle solids and are said to be in the glassy state. In this condition they are not crystalline but are supercooled liquids of high viscosity as explained in the section on glass. If rubber is cooled in liquid air below its glass transition temperature it becomes brittle and shatters like glass if subjected to mechanical shock. Above T_g there is a progressive loss of rigidity. The familiar properties of polymers depend therefore on whether T_g is greater (glass: about $1000°$; polymethylmethacrylate: $110°$) or less (polypropylene: $-27°$; rubber: about $-60°$) than the normal ambient temperature. *Thermoplastics*, such as polyethylene, soften and melt if heated to a high enough temperature. Other plastics are very highly cross-linked and for these *thermosetting* plastics T_g is so high that decomposition takes place before the material can soften and melt; urea-formaldehyde plastics are of this type. Below T_g the

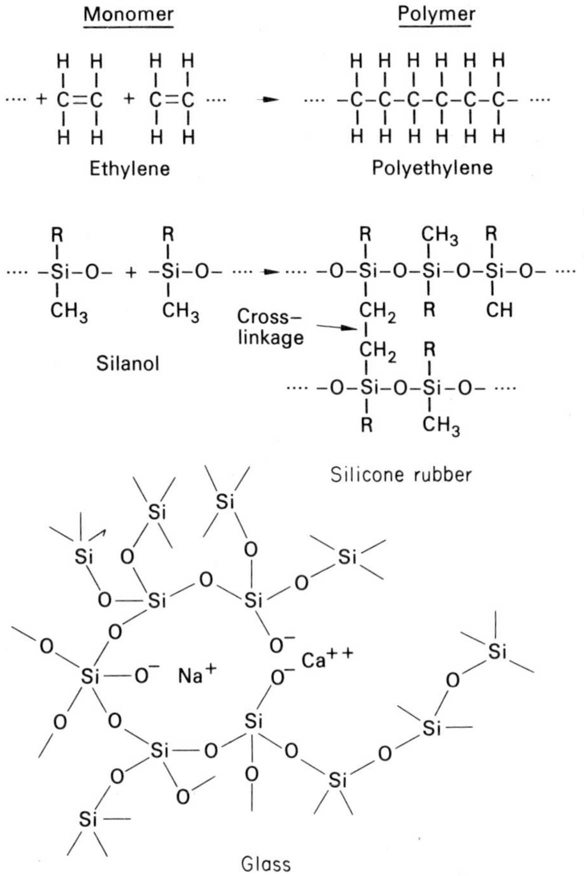

Monomer

$$\cdots + \underset{\underset{H}{|}}{\overset{\overset{H}{|}}{C}} = \underset{\underset{H}{|}}{\overset{\overset{H}{|}}{C}} + \underset{\underset{H}{|}}{\overset{\overset{H}{|}}{C}} = \underset{\underset{H}{|}}{\overset{\overset{H}{|}}{C}} \cdots$$

Ethylene

Polymer

$$\cdots -\underset{\underset{H}{|}}{\overset{\overset{H}{|}}{C}}-\underset{\underset{H}{|}}{\overset{\overset{H}{|}}{C}}-\underset{\underset{H}{|}}{\overset{\overset{H}{|}}{C}}-\underset{\underset{H}{|}}{\overset{\overset{H}{|}}{C}}-\underset{\underset{H}{|}}{\overset{\overset{H}{|}}{C}}-\underset{\underset{H}{|}}{\overset{\overset{H}{|}}{C}}- \cdots$$

Polyethylene

$$\cdots -\underset{\underset{CH_3}{|}}{\overset{\overset{R}{|}}{Si}}-O- + -\underset{\underset{CH_3}{|}}{\overset{\overset{R}{|}}{Si}}-O- \cdots \quad \rightarrow$$

Silanol

Cross-linkage →

$$\cdots -O-\underset{\underset{CH_2}{|}}{\overset{\overset{R}{|}}{Si}}-O-\underset{\underset{R}{|}}{\overset{\overset{CH_3}{|}}{Si}}-O-\underset{\underset{CH}{|}}{\overset{\overset{R}{|}}{Si}}-O- \cdots$$
$$\underset{CH_2}{|}\qquad\underset{R}{|}$$
$$\cdots -O-\underset{\underset{R}{|}}{\overset{\overset{CH_2}{|}}{Si}}-O-\underset{\underset{CH_3}{|}}{\overset{\overset{R}{|}}{Si}}-O- \cdots$$

Silicone rubber

Glass

FIG. 39.2. Polymer structure.

rotational freedom of the bonds and relative movement of the molecular chains of thermoplastics are severely restricted. Near the glass transition temperature there are, in addition to greater freedom of movement for the chains, changes in density, refractive index and other physical parameters. Above T_g the molecular chains are able continuously to move about, change their shape and intertwine with neighbours. Nevertheless, there is evidence from X-ray diffraction studies that disorder is not complete and that zones exist wherein the chains are more regularly aligned than elsewhere (Fig. 39.3). Such zones are said to be 'crystalline' but it must be clearly understood that the term in this context refers to the regular arrangement of molecular chains, not of atoms. Some polymers, polypropylene for example, can be prepared in a highly crystalline form, and the crystalline polymer has a higher density than the truly amorphous variety because of closer packing of the chains. Other polymers, such as rubber, attain a higher state of order when placed in

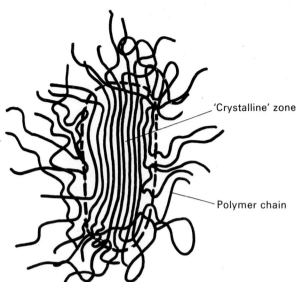

FIG. 39.3. Crystalline zone in a polymer.

tension, as this causes the molecular chains to align themselves in the direction of the applied force. With thermoplastics the stretching force may overcome the relatively weak bonds holding the chains together and permanent deformation follows. There is sufficient cross-linking with rubbers to prevent interchain slip, elastic deformation occurring up to very high stress levels.

Fig. 39.4 shows diagrammatically the effect of temperature on the modulus of elasticity for amorphous, lightly cross-linked, and partially crystalline varieties of a thermoplastic such as polystyrene. Above the glass transition temperature the cross-linked variety exhibits a rubbery behaviour which is barely discernible with the amorphous form of the plastic. The partially crystalline

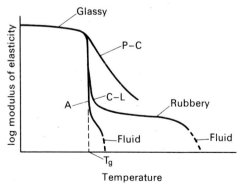

FIG. 39.4. Effect of temperature on elasticity of a polymer. A, Amorphous; C–L, lightly cross-linked; P–C, partially crystalline.

form has a glass transition temperature but this is obscured by the modifying influence of the crystalline regions.

PLASTICS

Plastics are high molecular weight polymers, usually based on a carbon 'backbone': they are good thermal and electrical insulators and their density falls in the range 0.9 to 1.5. The polymerization process may generate non-functional side-chains that hinder close packing of the polymer molecules. High pressure polymerization of ethylene gives a polyethylene of lower density (0.92 to 0.94) than that made by the low pressure process (density about 0.96). These varieties are known as low and high density polyethylene respectively. Depending on type, plastics may be useable at temperatures as low as $-100°$ or as high as $350°$ but individual materials have a more restricted useable temperature range. Although less rigid,

they are as strong as metals on a weight to weight basis. Generally, they show a high degree of resistance to attack by inorganic reagents but are usually softened or dissolved by organic solvents (Childs 1955).

The first plastic, celluloid, was obtained by nitrating cellulose. Many different cellulose polymers have been made since and are still important today. If dissolved and reprecipitated, the chain length is shortened and this modified cellulose is suitable for the production of textile products such as rayon dressings—see the BPC 1973. Nitration yields an explosive (gun cotton), a plastic (celluloid) or a lacquer (the official Collodions), depending on the reaction conditions. Other pharmaceutically important polymers derived from cellulose are the water soluble suspending agents such as methyl cellulose (see Chapter 37) and film forming agents like Cellulose Acetate Phthalate (see Chapter 19) which is employed for enteric coating.

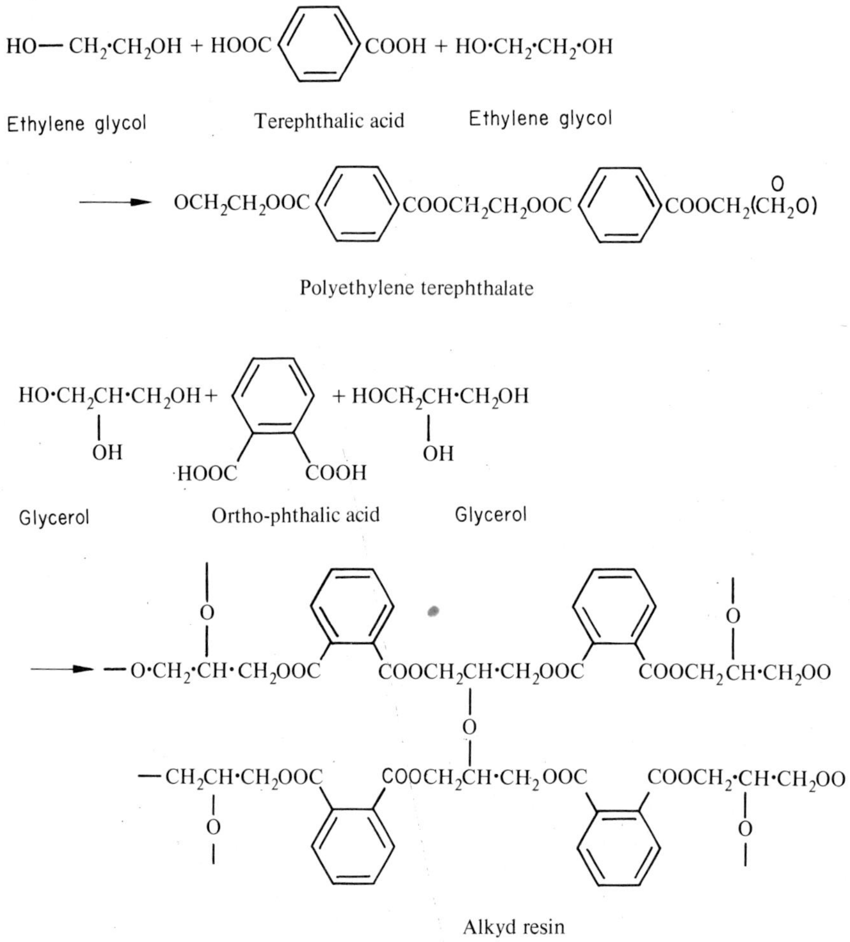

FIG. 39.5. Effect of functionality on polymer type.

For large scale direct synthesis of plastic a catalyst is added to the monomer to initiate the growth of chains. Polymerization may take place in the gas phase (polyethylene), in bulk (polystyrene), as a mechanical dispersion in water (polyvinyl chloride, PVC) or as an emulsion (polyvinyl acetate). Thermoplastics are formed from monomers with only two functional groups which, in theory, can only form long linear chains. Reaction of ethylene glycol with terephthalic acid (Fig. 39.5) gives polyethylene terephthalate, variously known as Terylene or Dacron and used as a suture material. Tri-functional glycerol has a 'spare' –OH group for cross-linking and with orthophthalic acid gives an alkyd resin of the type used in lacquer and paint manufacture. The chemical structures of some plastics are given in Fig. 39.6.

Compounding Plastics
Although some plastics may be used directly to form the finished article, it is usual to add other substances for improved stability, processing behaviour, or in-use performance. Stabilizers are often necessary because side reactions during polymerization produce a proportion of unsaturated, potentially unstable compounds while high processing temperatures may degrade the polymer molecule. Under certain conditions polyvinyl chloride loses a molecule of hydrogen chloride with the formation of a double bond; considerable darkening of the plastic occurs at the same time. Many PVC stabilizers are, therefore, basic substances capable of removing HCl although one of the most efficient stabilizers, octyl tin, seems not to act in this way. Plastics are also vulnerable to oxidation. The antioxidants added to provide protection combine with free radicles much in the manner of their counterparts used to prevent rancidity in oils. The most efficient antioxidants for plastics (and rubber) are sterically hindered phenols and secondary amines e.g. NN'-di-β-naphthyl-p-phenylenediamine:

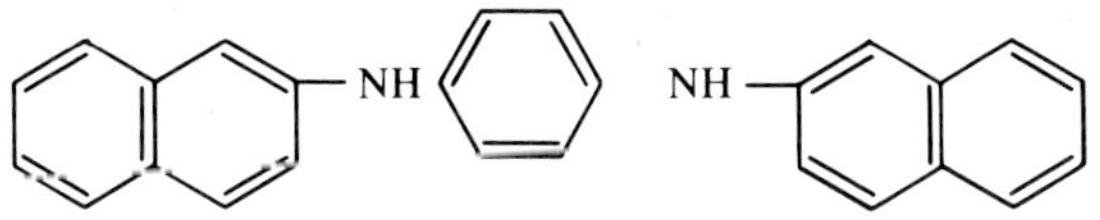

Pigments are sometimes included: apart from their decorative use they may absorb in the u.v. region and thereby reduce photodegradation. For clear plastics organic absorbers such as 4-biphenylsalicylate are used. Fillers are often employed to cheapen the product but in some cases may be essential for correct product performance. Bakelite,

a phenol-formaldehyde resin, is a brown brittle material quite unsuited for the manufacture of screw-caps unless mixed with a filler such as wood flour. Among other fillers are whiting, asbestos and mica. Plasticizers are added to lower the glass transition temperature by directly reducing the attractive physical forces between polymer chains, and by increasing the interchain distance. As a result the plastic is softened, it can be processed at a lower temperature and the final product has greater flexibility. Camphor is used as a plasticizer for celluloid, and castor oil for collodion. More generally, high boiling esters are employed as these have low volatility and do not evaporate from the product. Dibutyl sebacate, tritolyl phosphate and dioctyl phthalate are among the many esters employed for this purpose. Cellulose acetate phthalate, used as a film forming agent for enteric coating, may be plasticized with substances such as castor oil or butyl stearate. Thermosetting plastics are compounded by mixing a suitable precursor with a cross-linking agent. For Bakelite the precursor is a phenol-rich partially cross-linked condensate with formaldehyde which when mixed with filler and hexamine (a source of further formaldehyde) may be placed in a suitable mould and heated to complete the cross-linking reaction. One of the curing agents for the epoxy resins is triethylamine tetramine. Activators and accelerators may be added to lower the temperature at which the 'cure' takes place and to reduce the time for its completion. In this way degradation and darkening due to overheating may be avoided. The similarities with the compounding of rubber will be noted.

The substances required for the rough mix of thermoplastics are passed through two or three heated rollers to complete the dispersion process. The resultant crude sheet is chopped up into small cubes or flakes ready for the forming process. Rods, tubes or films are made by heating the compounded plastic to a temperature at which it has the consistency of dough, when it may be extruded under pressure through a suitable nozzle, rather like squeezing ointment out of a tube. If individual articles are required the dough may be squeezed into a closed mould (injection moulding) or extruded tubing may serve as the feedstock for blow moulding whereby a portion of tube is trapped in a hot mould and blown to shape. Extruded sheet may be heated and forced to take the shape of a suitable jig (thermoforming); for thermosetting plastics the compounded material is fed into a mould, compressed and heated to complete the cross-linking

Thermoplastics

$-CH_2-CH_2-CH_2-CH_2$ Polyethylene ($-120°C$)

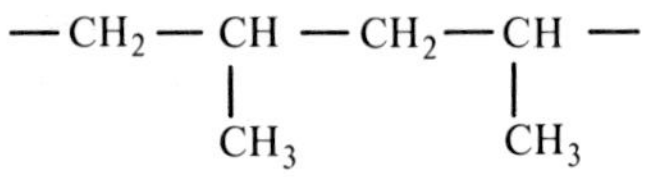

$-CH_2-CH-CH_2-CH-$ with CH_3 substituents Polypropylene ($-27°C$)

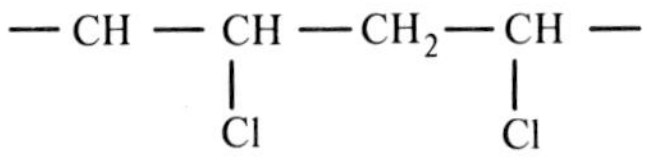

$-CH-CH-CH_2-CH-$ with Cl substituents Polyvinylchloride (PVC) ($80°C$)

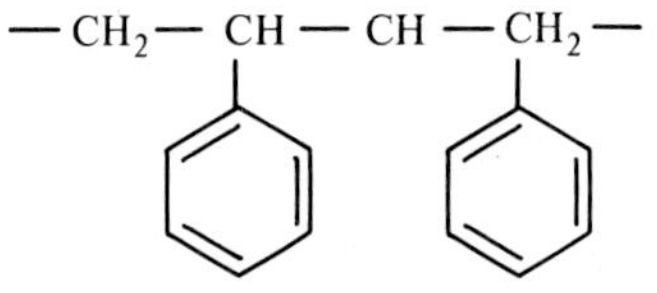

$-CH_2-CH-CH-CH_2-$ with phenyl substituents Polystyrene ($100°C$)

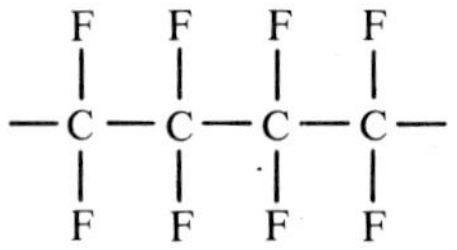

$-C-C-C-C-$ with F substituents Polyfluortetraethylene (PTFE)($126°C$)

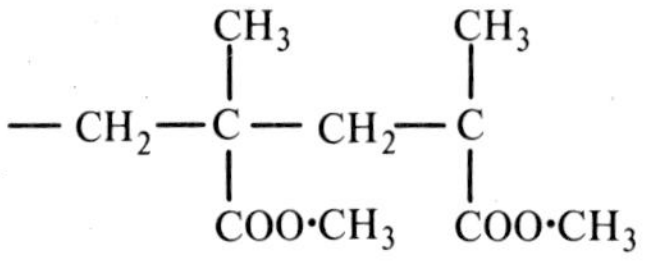

$-CH_2-C-CH_2-C$ with CH_3 and $COO·CH_3$ substituents Polymethylmethacrylate ($110°C$)

Thermosetting plastics

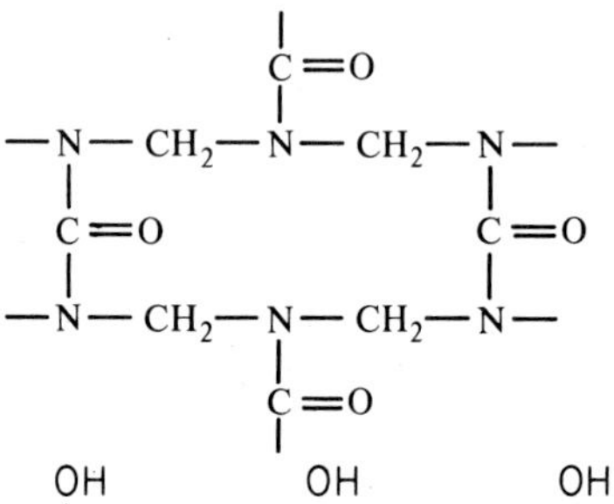

$-N-CH_2-N-CH_2-N-$ network with $C=O$ groups Urea-formaldehyde

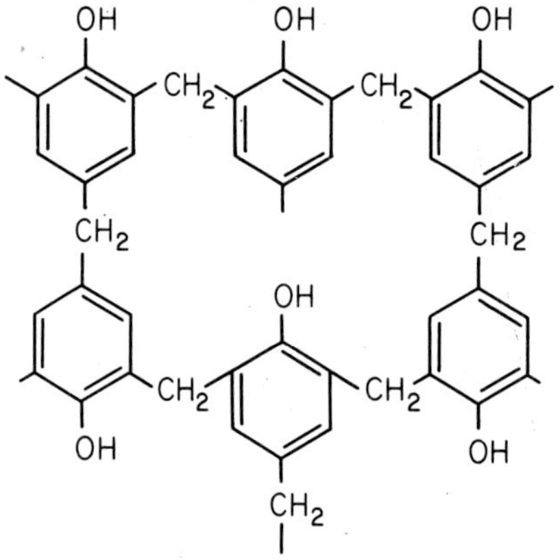

Phenol formaldehyde network with OH and CH_2 groups

Fig. 39.6. Some common plastics (glass transition temperature in brackets).

(compression moulding). (See Paine 1967 for an introductory text.)

Moulds must be made to very rigid tolerances if given dimensions are to be maintained throughout a batch. A faulty cavity in a multiple mould would produce a small proportion of faulty articles which might not be detected if the quality control sample was too small, an identical problen is encountered in tabletting. Long (1961) has reported the sporadic failure of polyethylene plug closures due to a fault of this type.

Toxicity

Plastics are probably inert physiologically—it is the additives which give rise to toxicity problems. As noted earlier, octyl tin is an excellent stabilizer for PVC but is known to be toxic (Cooper 1966). Biological tests on extractives prepared with different solvents, and implantation of pieces of plastic in animals are among the control procedures proposed. Simpson (1969) has commented that the solvents and the amounts injected into the animal may themselves give rise to biological effects. He suggested that an aqueous extract of the plastic should be examined for pyrogenicity as some of the chemicals used for compounding purposes are known to be pyrogenic. The British Pharmacopoeia 1973 requires that the additives to plastics for pharmaceutical packaging shall be non-toxic and prescribes a test with which containers must comply to ensure freedom from toxic extractives in use, particularly if a sterilization procedure is involved. In particular, autoclaving accelerates the leaching process and represents the most rigorous in-use condition to which the plastic container is ever likely to be exposed.

Permeability

When using plastics for packaging it is necessary to consider not only the permeability to oxygen, water vapour and carbon dioxide but also the permeation or absorption of product constituents. For a flexible pack of dusting powder containing camphor it is the loss of this latter to the environment that is important. On the other hand, if the product is an oxygen sensitive steroid, it is the permeation of oxygen from the environment into the product via the container wall that must be considered.

Assuming there are no cracks or other defects, and that the plastic is not heavily 'filled', the passage of gases and vapours occurs by diffusion. Above the transition temperature the polymer chains are in continuous thermal motion and the

spaces between them constantly form and disappear. If a high concentration is established at one surface of the plastic, diffusing molecules will move from space to space to the low concentration side. Applying Fick's Law:

$$Q = -\frac{ADt}{l} \cdot \frac{dc}{dx} \qquad (39.1)$$

Q is the quantity of gas diffusing in time t under the influence of a linear concentration gradient dc/dx. The plastic has a thickness l, area A and diffusion constant D. According to Henry's Law, $c = pS$ where p is the partial pressure of the diffusing species and S its solubility coefficient for the plastic. Integrating (39.1), making the appropriate substitutions and rearranging:

$$P = DS = \frac{lQ}{At(p_1 - p_2)} \qquad (39.2)$$

where p_1 and p_2 are the partial pressures at the surfaces of the plastic and P is the permeability constant. If, as was assumed in deriving (39.2), the diffusing gas obeys the gas laws reasonably well, the effect of temperature is given by an Arrhenius type equation:

$$P = P_o e^{-E/RT} = D_o S_o e^{-E/RT}$$

D_o may be regarded as a measure of the number of interchain 'spaces' in the plastic at a given moment in time. Fewer spaces will be available for diffusion in the crystalline or cross-linked plastic than in the corresponding amorphous form. This is in line with Flück's (1966) observations that amorphous forms of a particular plastic are usually more permeable than the crystalline or cross-linked varieties. Plasticizing also increases permeability— it is well known, for instance, that moist gases permeate nylon films more rapidly than dry gases, as water is adsorbed and acts as plasticizer. The factor S_o is a function of the relationship of the affinity of the diffusing molecules for plastic molecules to their affinity for each other In general, low molecular weight, highly polar molecules permeate less rapidly than lipophilic molecules having structural similarities to those of the polymer.

It will be appreciated, therefore, that the physical properties of a given plastic will vary markedly according to the nature of the additives and the treatment it has undergone in manufacture—see, for instance Busse and Hughes (1969). The data in Table 39.1 must be regarded as approximate, but

TABLE 39.1

PERMEABILITY CONSTANT (P) OF PLASTICS TO OXYGEN AND
WATER VAPOUR POLYETHYLENE
(P in units of $cm^3/cm^2/mm/sec/cm\ Hg \times 10^{10}$)

	Low density	High density	Poly-propylene	Poly-styrene	Rigid PVC
Water vapour	400	130	250	12 000	1600
Oxygen	50	11	23	30	4

Note that water vapour best permeates the more polar plastics whereas the reverse is true for oxygen. The more open molecular structure of low density polythene as compared with the high density variety is reflected in the lower value of P for the latter with both gases.

will serve as a comparative guide to the permeability of a number of plastics to oxygen and water vapour.

Plastics in the Packaging of Pharmaceutical Products

Compared with glass, plastics offer the obvious advantages of lightness, resistance to mechanical hazards and low cost. There is also the possibility that a particular property of a plastic, flexibility say, may be exploited to obtain greater package functionality. Against these advantages must be set the problems of permeability and toxicity, neither of which arise with glass, and of disposal. In selecting plastic containers it is necessary to check that:

(a) toxic substances are not leached from the plastic into the product,

(b) product constituents are not lost by absorption or permeation,

(c) loss or gain of moisture or permeation by oxygen takes place at an acceptable rate,

(d) no other interactions can occur between product and container.

Large numbers of plastic containers are now employed for dispensing mixtures, tablets, capsules, ointments, etc. Although polyethylene and polypropylene were used for some of the containers examined by Jolly et al. (1970) the majority were fabricated from high impact polystyrene. This is a polystyrene/styrene–butadiene rubber formulation which is as rigid but less brittle than polystyrene. Perfusion fluids and retention enemas are now packaged in plasticized PVC 'sachet' packs. These have the merit of collapsing as fluid is withdrawn and with perfusion fluids this obviates the use of an air bleed which was necessary on the older type of giving set with glass transfusion bottle. Water loss by permeation from sachet type containers can

be as much as 10 per cent per annum but may be reduced to a quarter of this value by a polythene wrapper. Single applications of some eye drops are now packed in low density polythene sachets, container and contents being sterilized by γ-radiation. A further advantage of the sachet type packages for applications such as these is the reduced amount of particulate matter shed from the container surface, which is a particular problem with the corresponding glass containers. Metal particles are sometimes found in ointments packed in metal tubes in spite of careful cleansing of the tube prior to filling—a difficulty which does not arise with plastic ointment tubes. Because its walls remain in opposition as the contents are removed, it has been said that a metal ointment tube is the only container that is completely full until it is completely empty. The same comment could not be made of the early plastic ointment tubes, which regained their original shape—sucked back—after each removal of contents, leading possibly to oxidation and microbial contamination problems. Suck-back is less of a problem with the modern plasticized PVC tubes. Considerable economies are now possible in the manufacture of suppositories since the introduction of a machine that uses a preformed plastic package which also serves as the mould. Suitable grades of polypropylene (and some other plastics) may be autoclaved. This is possible because the viscosity of the plastic at the autoclaving temperature, which is about 150° above T_g, is still high enough for the article to resist the deforming effect of its own weight. As described in the section on glass, this viscosity is of the order of 10^{13} poises or more.

Finally, two other methods of packaging which do not rely on a primary container and closure should be noted. In strip packaging, the tablet is sandwiched between two layers of foil or paper coated with a thermoplastic material such as polyethylene. This is fused together around the periphery of each tablet. Each strip is usually two tablets wide and several tablets long depending on requirements. Water vapour resistance normal to the surface is excellent but is lower round the edges. Where tablets are to be taken in a given sequence, they are deposited into a pocket thermoformed in a sheet of PVC and sealed in position with a foil laminate. The tablet is released by pushing it through the foil.

RUBBER

Rubber is an elastic polymer (elastomer), and may be obtained from natural sources or by synthetic methods. It has a glass transition temperature well below the normal ambient temperature; for natural rubber T_g is about $-60°$.

Natural Rubber

The basic material is a colloidal dispersion (latex) obtained from the rubber tree *Hevea braziliensis*, containing about 30 to 35 per cent rubber hydrocarbons and up to 5 per cent overall of resins, proteins, sugars and salts, the rest being water. The solids may be precipitated by the addition of acid and the coagulum dried in the smoke of a wood fire when it acquires a dark brown colour and

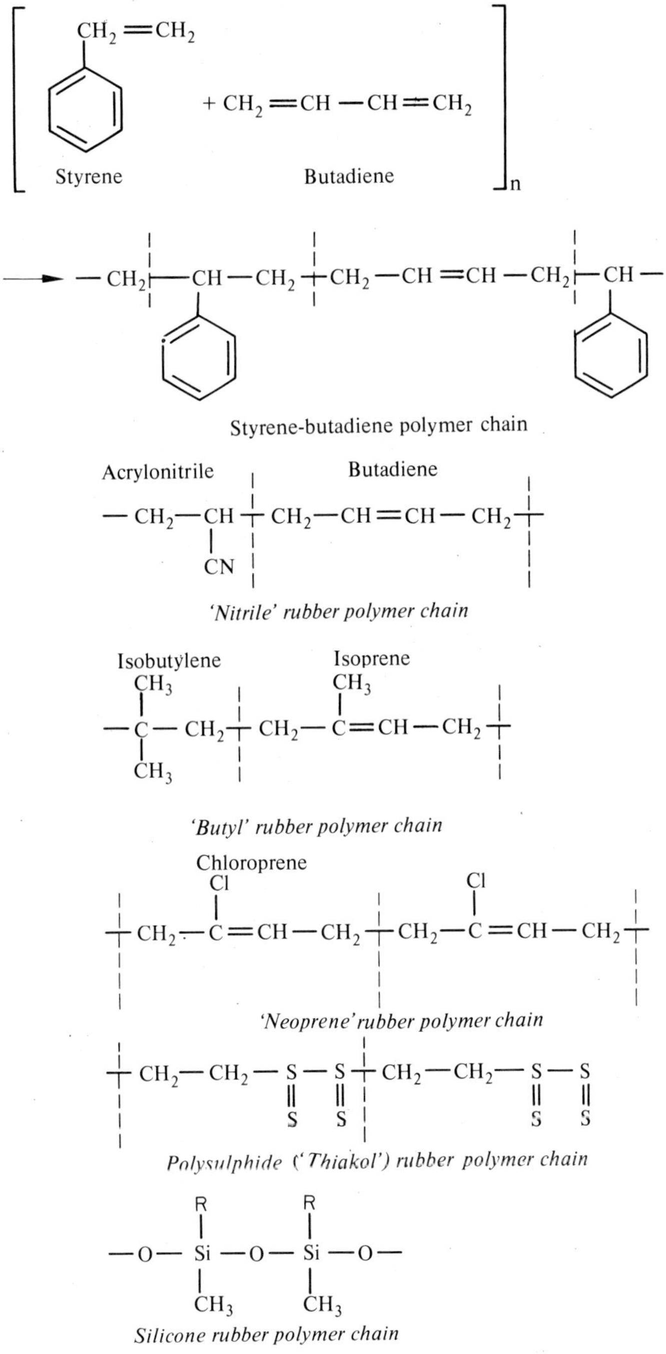
Styrene
Butadiene
Styrene-butadiene polymer chain
Acrylonitrile
Butadiene
'Nitrile' rubber polymer chain
Isobutylene
Isoprene
'Butyl' rubber polymer chain
Chloroprene
'Neoprene' rubber polymer chain
Polysulphide ('Thiakol') rubber polymer chain
Silicone rubber polymer chain

FIG. 39.7. Synthetic rubbers.

absorbs sufficient phenolic substances to prevent microbial spoilage during shipment. If pale crepe rubber is required, bisulphite is added prior to precipitation and the coagulum is dried at air temperature. The bisulphite stops oxidative discoloration and inhibits mould growth. For a number of purposes it is convenient to maintain the rubber in a 'liquid' state. To avoid the expense of shipping water the crude latex is either creamed by the addition of common salt or concentrated by evaporation or centrifugation. Preservative is added to inhibit subsequent microbial spoilage.

Synthetic Elastomers
These are manufactured by polymerization of the reactants while emulsified in a soap solution. For styrene–butadiene rubber (SBR) the reactants are styrene and butadiene (Fig. 39.7). The dispersed polymer (latex) is either concentrated by the addition of salt which causes creaming, or solid obtained by addition of acid. The compositions of a number of other synthetic rubber polymer chains are also given in Fig. 39.7.

Further Processing
The polymer chains of natural rubber consist of some 1000–40 000 isoprene units (Fig. 39.8A). In common with synthetic rubber polymer chains they possess double bonds that readily oxidize on exposure to air and light. Furthermore, although the coiled and intertwined molecules unravel when the polymer is placed in tension there is slip between

the chains and therefore a considerable deformation, which remains when the tension is released. The familiar elastic properties of rubber are obtained by providing sufficient cross-links per chain such that the product is not rigid but the chains may still uncoil although constrained in their movement relative to one another when the rubber is stretched. The cross-links ensure that the rubber returns, more or less, to its original shape when the stretching force is released.

The cross-links between silicone rubber chains are formed from the methyl groups attached to the silicon atoms, whereas natural and synthetic rubbers are cross-linked by heating with sulphur. Polysulphide rubber has 'built in' sulphur which can be caused to cross-link by heating with zinc oxide. The cross-linking, curing or vulcanization process (Fig. 39.8) when applied to natural rubber gives a tough material with reduced sensitivity to oxidation, which is swelled but not dissolved by organic solvents and which has a high degree of elasticity. As originally developed some 8 to 30 per cent of sulphur was needed for the vulcanization process and the high temperatures used brought about inevitable degradation of the rubber. Nowadays accelerators (Fig. 39.9) are added to speed up the cross-linking process, reduce the amount of sulphur required (0.5 to 3.0 per cent is now typical) and lower the temperature at which vulcanization is carried out. Activators raise the efficiency of the accelerators—zinc oxide, stearic acid or zinc stearate are commonly employed. The vulcanized

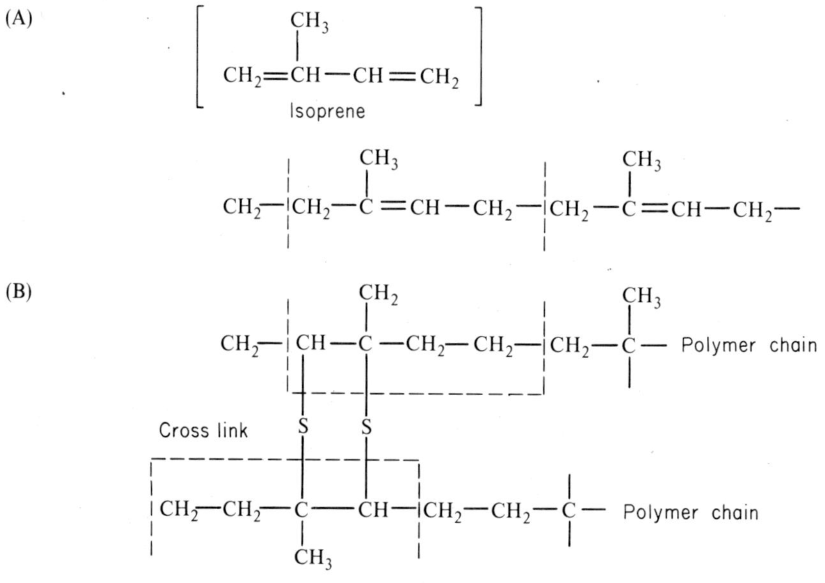

FIG. 39.8. Natural rubber: A, polymer chain from latex; B, cross-linked polymer chain after vulcanization.

Accelerators

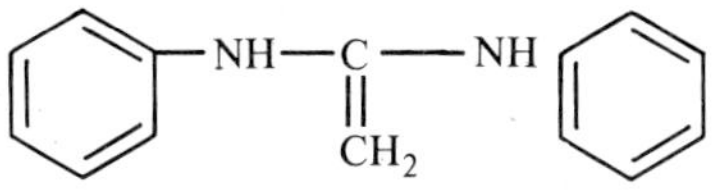

Diphenyl guanidine

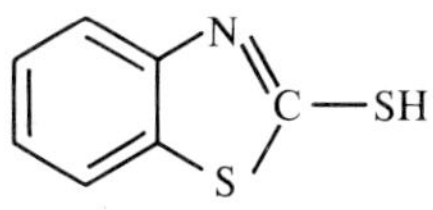

2-mercaptobenothiazole

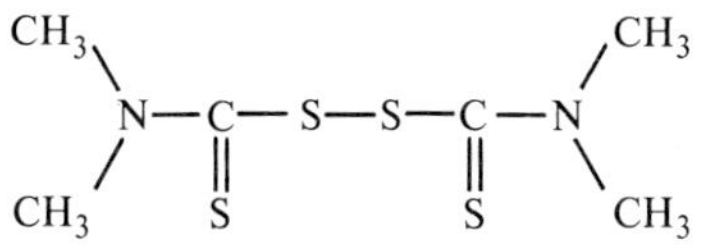

tetramethylthiuram disulphide

Antioxidant

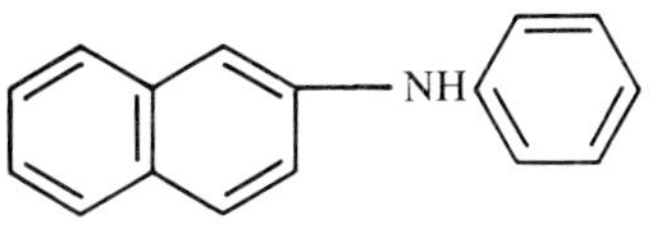

phenyl-β-naphthylamine

Sequestering agent and antioxidant

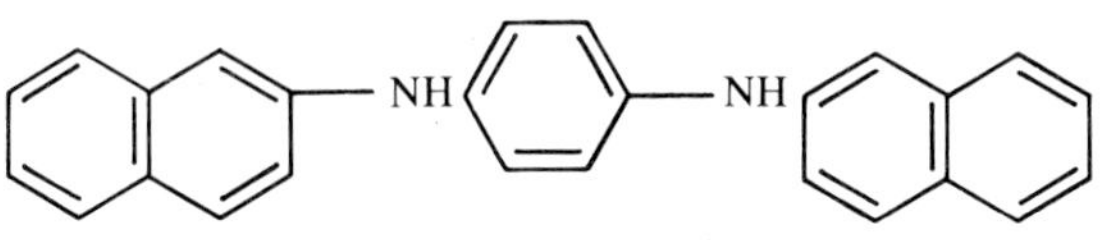

NN′-di-β-naphthyl-*p*-phenylene diamine

FIG. 39.9. Some rubber additives.

rubber still possesses unsaturated bonds therefore antioxidants, which persist in the final product, are added to minimize oxidation both during and subsequent to vulcanization. Traces of manganese or copper are known to catalyse the oxidation of rubber, and a sequestering agent, which may also act as an antioxidant, may be added to the compounded rubber mix prior to vulcanization. The cost of a rubber article may be reduced by using a proportion of reclaimed rubber or an extending filler such as whiting or talc. To modify the hardness or other mechanical properties, reinforcing fillers such as clays, magnesium carbonate or further quantities of zinc oxide are added as necessary to the rubber mix. These fillers are believed to combine in some way with the polymer chains (Haworth 1953; Reznek 1953b). Pigments may be added both for decorative purposes and to absorb ultraviolet radiation which promotes oxidation.

If the article is to be made by moulding, rubber solids are finely minced in a masticator and the other compounding ingredients added. The rollers of the masticator are heated to soften the rubber but it may also be necessary to add a softener such as pine oil or tar, petroleum or coal tar fractions to obtain even dispersion. For some synthetic rubbers a plasticizer may be required. The mix has the characteristics of a dough. For dipping compounds the concentrated latex (about 60 per cent solids) is mixed with accelerators and a stabilizer to control the viscosity of the liquid so as to give the required film thickness. Foam rubber is produced by the addition to the mix of a blowing agent which decomposes during vulcanization to evolve gas (usually nitrogen). Wood and other resins may be added to provide surface stickiness or 'tack'. Small amounts of waxes that migrate to the rubber surface during vulcanization can be added to improve resistance both to water absorption and to oxidation.

To produce moulded articles a mould of the required shape and size is filled with the rubber dough which is then vulcanized by heating. It is usual to dust the surface of the dough with a mould release agent such as talc or zinc stearate so that the rubber is easily removed from the mould after vulcanization. Dipping is used where the thickness of rubber is small e.g. surgeons gloves, rubber teats. A glass or porcelain former is dipped into the compounded latex and the film coagulated in an acid bath. The process is repeated until the required thickness of rubber is built up and this is then vulcanized by heating in hot air. The composition of the moulding and dipping compounds given in Table 39.2 are illustrative of those used for the manufacture of vaccine bottle caps and rubber teats respectively. The rubber mix for closures to be used in less demanding situations would contain less rubber and a much higher proportion of filler.

TABLE 39.2

RUBBER MOULDING AND DIPPING FORMULATIONS

Function	Material	Per cent dry weight for stated use:	
		moulding	dipping
Rubber	Pale crepe rubber	88.4	—
	Latex (60 per cent solids)	—	97.6
Vulcanizer	Sulphur	1.0	1.0
Accelerator	2-mercaptobenzothiazole diphenylguanidine mixture	0.3	—
	Zinc diethyldithiocarbamate	—	1.0
Activator	Zinc oxide	1.5	0.2
	Stearic acid	0.4	—
Antioxidant	Phenyl-β-naphthylamine	0.4	—
Filler	Zinc oxide	7.0	—
Special ingredient	Paraffin wax	1.0	—
	Film thickness stabilizer	—	0.2

For the majority of purposes natural rubber, or natural rubber with a proportion of styrene–butadiene gives the best all round performance. Synthetic rubbers are used in high proportion where special properties are at a premium. Nitrile rubber, for instance is not as resilient as natural rubber but has a very high solvent resistance that is only surpassed by the polysulphide rubbers. Butyl rubber exhibits high resistance to attack by oxygen, ozone and chemical reagents as well as very low permeability to oxygen and water vapour. Trials with butyl rubber wads (Bloom & Drennan 1957) were disappointing due to the low resilience of the rubber which led to permanent deformation and poor reseal performance. Neoprene combines good general rubber qualities with a high order of resistance to solvent and chemical attack; it is also flame resistant due to the chlorine atoms in the polymer chain. Silicone rubbers are completely saturated, inert and may be autoclaved many times, an in-use condition that would result in the rapid failure of normal rubber. They retain their resilience over a very wide range of temperature.

Rubber in the Packaging of Pharmaceuticals

Rubber is used exclusively as a closure and wad material. The specification of the B.P. 1973 is based on British Standard 3263: 1960 with certain ammendments. The specification excludes reclaimed rubber which is known to yield inferior closures and sets standards for dimensional tolerances. The force required to penetrate the closure with a hypodermic needle must not be excessive and a value for this parameter is specified. A further test limits the number of fragments of rubber detached during penetration by the hypodermic needle. Finally, if the contents of a multidose container are to remain free from microbial contamination the rubber must have good reseal properties and a test is described to assess this characteristic.

Like plastics, rubber may be regarded as a solid organic solvent and it is necessary in evaluating a particular closure to determine the oxygen and water vapour permeability, the leaching of substances from the rubber and the absorption of constituents from the product. An average value for the permeability constant P, as previously defined, is 230 for oxygen and 25 000 for moisture vapour, the units being $cm^3/cm^2/mm/sec/cm \, Hg \times 10^{10}$. Since the performance of a closure probably depends more on its fit in the container (hence the standard for dimensional tolerances) than on its permeability, the British Standard describes a practical test of performance. In this test, the gain in weight of a desiccant sealed in a container by the test closure is compared with the gain in weight where the closure is one which has previously been found to be acceptable.

The process of compounding rubber suggests that two types of material which persist after the vulcanization process may be extracted, namely zinc and organic substances. Reznek (1953 a & b) studied the extraction of zinc from rubber used as the plunger in dental anaesthetic cartridges. Generally, the amount extracted from the plunger increased with the acidity of the solution, storage time and temperature and content of zinc in the rubber. With 16.1 cm^2 of rubber surface exposed to 50 ml of 0.1 N HCl for 56 days at 50° the final concentration of zinc in the solution varied from 14 to 78 ppm as the zinc oxide content of the rubber was increased from 0.41 to 1.01 per cent by weight. Direct experiment will show that zinc is readily extracted from closure rubber by solutions of both high and low pH and also at more neutral pH values if the leaching solution contains a substance such as citrate which is capable of complexing the zinc. Some of the organic compounds used for compounding rubber are virtually insoluble in water, while many accelerators are destroyed during the vulcanization process. Nevertheless, leaching of thiuram disulphide and other organic substances was noted by Lachman et al. (1963b) during studies of preservative uptake by rubber closures. The toxicological significance of zinc and organic substances extracted from rubber is not clear. The British Standard limits the amount of water soluble extractive and also describes a test for the compatibility of product and closure. Natural rubber contains a proportion of protein and this has caused allergic reactions in sensitive individuals. Non-allergenic rubber is now available.

Absorption of substances from the product is, of course, very important. It may be expected that lipophilic substances are more likely to be taken up than those more polar in nature. Unfortunately, the former group includes a high proportion of the antimicrobial preservatives which depend on lipophilic properties to pass the microbial cell wall. If these are absorbed by the closure, the product is left without protection against microbial contamination. Wing (1955 & 1956) examined some thirty rubber formulations for preservative uptake and found that the initial rapid absorption slowed down with time and eventually reached an equilibrium situation. The rate of uptake increased with temperature but often the partition coefficient was less favourable to the rubber at the higher temperatures. Wing noted extremes of partition coefficient, for instance from 0.3 to 1.7 for phenol and 7 to 47 for chlorocresol depending on the rubber composition. Silica fillers and some softeners increased the partition coefficient in favour of the rubber, the former presumably by physical adsorption and the latter by providing a more favourable solvent for the preservative (Royce & Sykes 1957). Sykes (1958) and Lachman et al. (1962, 1963 a & b) have reported studies which are in general agreement if the inevitable variations in the compositions of the rubbers used by these workers are taken into account. Contact of rubber with phenol, cresol or methyl p hydroxybenzoate solutions results in the uptake of about a third of the preservative. Under similar conditions up to 90 per cent of chlorocresol, chlorbutol, cetrimide and phenylmercuric nitrate would be lost from solution. As the cetrimide would be completely ionized, adsorption rather than absorption is the most likely mechanism whereby that substance is removed from solution. The phenylmercuric nitrate is probably inactivated by

–SH groups in the rubber. For the same reason specially formulated rubber caps are used for penicillin preparations. If the preservative is volatile—for example cresol—it may evaporate from the rubber surface into the atmosphere, a process that would continue until almost all the preservative has been removed from solution. Rubber also interacts with sodium metabisulphite.

Attempts to mitigate the undesirable effects that attend the use of rubber closures have involved the application of a wax or lacquer coating. Although these give short term protection they eventually flake off, or perhaps worse, may block the hypodermic needle. The most successful approach is to presaturate the rubber with those absorbable substances with which it is to come into contact. This is the official method and the reader is referred to the official monographs for details. It is sufficient here to note that the closures must be carefully washed to remove mould lubricant and dust, and that both the quantity and concentration of solution to be used for soaking is specified to ensure correct saturation of the closures.

GLASS

Structure and Composition

Even the weak bonds between the molecules of a liquid will effectively permit a random disordered structure; the viscosity of a liquid is a measure of the amount of energy which must be available for disrupting the inter-molecular bonds during flow. If the viscosity exceeds some 10^{13} poises the liquid deforms so slowly under the influence of its own weight that for all practical purposes it behaves like a solid. For a liquid to crystallize, energy must also be available to break the intermolecular bonds so that these can subsequently reform to give the ordered lattice configuration of the crystal. In the case of very viscous liquids the energy required may be so large that the initial bond cleaving step is unlikely to occur and the liquid may remain more or less permanently in the supercooled state at or below the normal crystallization temperature. Technically, 'glasses' may be defined as liquids which may be supercooled to temperatures at which the viscosity exceeds 10^{13} poises, in which condition they exhibit the properties of a solid while retaining the disordered internal structure of a liquid. A large number of substances can be obtained as glasses, e.g., sulphur, many plastics, arsenic trisulphide, and these all have in common a well developed molecular network. In everyday usage, however, the term glass is applied to the hard, brittle, transparent material, based on a network of silicon and oxygen atoms, that is widely used for making products as diverse as electric light bulbs, windows and bottles.

Silica melts at about 1700°C and on cooling yields a glass commonly known as fused silica. This material is very resistant to the attack of all chemicals except strong alkalis, hydrofluoric acid and related substances and, since the coefficient of linear expansion is low (0.5×10^{-6}), silica ware can be subjected to sudden large temperature changes (thermal shock) without breaking. Fused silica lacks the regular crystal lattice of quartz but possesses instead an open random three- dimensional network in which each silicon atom is surrounded by four oxygen atoms, each of the latter being shared by two silicon atoms (Fig. 39.10). The

(A)

(B)

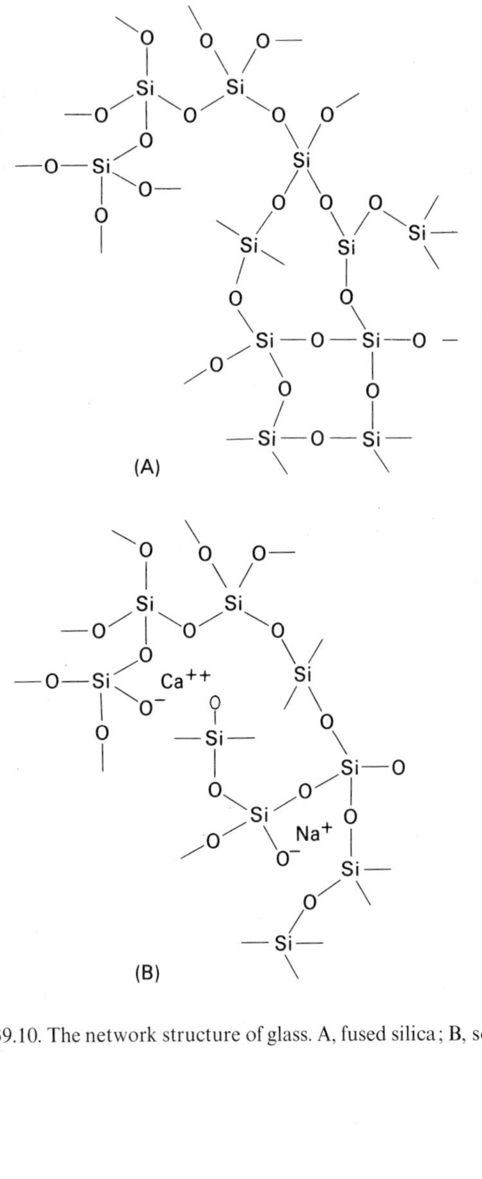

FIG. 39.10. The network structure of glass. A, fused silica; B, soft glass.

high melting temperature of silica derives from the strong covalent Si–O bonds which may be pictured as radiating from the central silicon atom and directed towards the four corners of a tetrahedron so that the bond angle is fixed at about 108° (cf. carbon). The angle between the two bonds associated with each oxygen atom is not so rigidly fixed and this provides the flexibility necessary for the formation of the network. Both the extreme viscosity of molten silica and the high temperature at which it must be worked preclude the widespread use of fused silica. More useful glasses result from the addition of modifiers to the silica, which have the effect of lowering the working temperature and viscosity, though not without some loss of mechanical strength, resistance to thermal shock and chemical durability. Monovalent metals, e.g. Na^+ and K^+, disrupt the silica network and have the most marked effect on the working properties, but the glass has too low a resistance to chemical attack to be of any practical value. Calcium, magnesium, barium and other divalent metals can take part in the network by sharing two oxygen atoms. The structural distortion and replacement of a strong covalent bond by two weaker electrovalent bonds results in a useful reduction of working temperature without sacrificing too much chemical durability. Suitable combinations of both mono- and divalent metals yield glasses which are readily worked and yet possess adequate strength and chemical durability for use in non-critical situations (Fig. 39.10). 'Soft' or lime-soda glass is of this type and is employed in the production of many of the containers used in pharmacy. The performance of such containers falls short of the ideal when exposed to the more severe conditions encountered in, for instance, sterilization by autoclaving. In these circumstances it may be necessary to use a 'harder' glass, in which the content of mono- and divalent metals has been reduced and replaced by multivalent elements such as aluminium and boron. These elements are called network formers because they can take part in the network by covalent bonding in much the same way as silicon itself. The chemical durability, resistance to thermal shock and mechanical strength are thereby much improved but the glass is more expensive.

Four main types of glass are in common use for the production of the containers used in pharmacy. Table 39.3 gives an approximate composition, in terms of the appropriate oxide, that is representative of each type. The low values of some elements is due to their presence as contaminants in the raw materials, e.g., magnesium in limestone. It is necessary to use a high grade sand as the source of silica, as ordinary grades contain large amounts of iron, which produces a green tinge in the glass and decolorizers, usually selenium compounds, are ineffective if the ferric iron content is greater than about 0.1 per cent. Certain elements may be deliberately added to produce a coloured glass, the following being of pharmaceutical interest:

amber: carbon and sulphur or iron and manganese
green: chromium with some iron and manganese
blue: cobalt with, occasionally, some copper.

The light absorption curves for these glasses are given on page 148. At one time arsenic was used as a decolorizer. Alkaline preparations were known to dissolve glass and, to avoid contamination, arsenic free glass containers, distinguishable by their blue colour, were used to package such preparations. In this way a blue glass container has become associated with Mixture of Magnesium Hydroxide, and is still used, even though the glass employed for the fabrication of pharmaceutical containers is now arsenic (and lead) free.

TABLE 39.3

APPROXIMATE COMPOSITIONS OF SOME GLASSES USED FOR THE PRODUCTION OF CONTAINERS USED IN PHARMACY

	Soft (lime-soda)	Neutral (for containers)	Neutral (for ampoules)	Hard (boro-silicate)
SiO_2	73	73	67	80
Na_2O	13	7	8.5	4
K_2O	0.5	1.5	4	—
CaO	10	—	4	0.2
MgO	0.3	—	0.3	—
BaO	—	3	—	—
Al_2O_3	0.5	5	8.5	2.5
B_2O_3	—	8.5	7.5	13

Container Production

Furnaces for large scale glass production are typically rectangular in shape, about a metre deep and 100 m^2 in area. For the production of soft glass, high grade sand, soda, limestone and alumina together with waste glass of the same kind are continuously fed into the furnace and heated to about 1400°. The bubbles of carbon dioxide and other gases formed during the reaction rise to the surface as the glass approaches the furnace outlet where the temperature is higher and the viscosity of the melt much reduced. A 'bridge' across the outlet skims off impurities as the melt flows into a fore-hearth at which point the temperature is about 1000° and the viscosity is suitable for the start of container manufacture. Full details of the methods used are given by Moody (1963), but in each case a preformed blank or 'parison' is blown into the final form inside a mould. A small gap between the halves of the mould allows air to escape as the container is blown to shape—its position is revealed by a fine ridge seam on the outer surface of the finished container. Careful design of the mould is necessary to ensure that the quantity of glass in the blank mould gives container walls of the correct thickness at the blowing stage.

By the time the container has been formed its external surface has cooled to approximately 300° and is rigid enough to maintain the final shape. The inside, however, is still hot and the stresses set up by uneven cooling would lead to early failure of the container in service. To overcome this problem the temperature is raised to about 550° in an annealing kiln or *lehr* so that stress dissipation by internal flow can take place. Subsequently, further stress formation is avoided by allowing the container to cool slowly and uniformly as it travels towards the exit of the kiln. Prior to entering the lehr it is usual for the moulding ridges on the rim of the neck to be removed by local heating (fire polishing).

Mechanical Strength

As the covalent Si–O bond is very strong, this should be reflected in the mechanical strength of glass. Freshly drawn fibres can support loads of the order of 1500 MNm^{-2} (15 000 kg cm^{-2}) but the tensile strength of bulk glass varies from about 200 MNm^{-2} when new, to about a fifth of this value after being used for some time. The variable low value for the strength of bulk glass as compared with freshly drawn fibres is attributed to the presence of sub-microscopic cracks on the surface of bulk specimens and these will tend to be more numerous on the surface of used specimens, due to damage in service. These cracks open up under tension and, since the glass is a liquid, there are no internal boundaries to inhibit their propagation. The cracks do not open up when compressive loads are applied and glass is found to be some ten times stronger in compression than in tension.

Glass containers are subject to a number of mechanical hazards both on the filling line and in service. If they rub together abrasion scars are formed that seriously weaken the glass as described above. They are prone to fracture on impact, particularly if full of liquid and for this reason must be packed for transport and handling in cartons with shock absorbent partitions around each container. The filling and capping head may impose a vertical load on the container and this condition also obtains when the cartons of filled containers are stacked for storage or transport. The vertical load which a bottle will support without fracture is roughly proportional to the radius of curvature of the neck.

As glass is weaker in tension than in compression, the aim of modern design is to ensure that the shoulder and sides are evenly compressed by vertical loading, and tensile stresses reduced as much as possible by using the largest radius of curvature for the shoulder that is appropriate to the particular size and function of the container. In this way it has been possible to increase the vertical load resistance from some 200 kg for the older, square shouldered 'winchester' to ten times this value for its modern more rounded counterpart (Fig. 39.11). Similar changes may be seen in the shape of most modern glass containers used for packaging pharmaceutical products. The modern shape also facilitates mould design to secure uniform thickness of glass at the shoulder. Finally, the shape must be considered in terms of the internal pressure that the bottle must withstand in use. The cooling of a full transfusion bottle, for instance, usually lags behind that of the autoclave. As a consequence the bottle may still be under pressure when the chamber of the autoclave has reached atmospheric pressure.

Where mechanical strength is of paramount importance it may be necessary to employ a hard glass container, but the mechanical strength of soft glass containers may be improved by a process known as titanizing. After the container has been reheated at the start of the annealing process, the outer surface is sprayed with a tin or titanium compound. This decomposes to leave an oxide film which dissolves in the glass to give a thin surface layer that significantly reduces glass–to–glass friction and the tendency to form sub-microscopic cracks. The process allows wall thickness to be reduced and yet, with suitable designs, the resistance to breakage from impact, abrasion scars and vertical loading can be better than that of similar untreated containers.

Resistant to Thermal Shock

The outside of a hot glass container cools and contracts if exposed to a cold environment, that is, to downwards thermal shock. The thicker the container wall the lower the rate of heat transfer from the warm interior and in any case this rate is low, due to the poor thermal conductivity of glass. Thus the transient temperature difference which is rapidly established between the inner and outer surfaces of the glass is greater for thick than for thin walled containers. The outer wall cannot contract to the full extent implied by the decrease in temperature and the coefficient of linear expansion, because it is constrained by the warmer glass to which it is attached. Thus, the outer surface is placed in tension while the inner surface is placed in compression but, since glass is much stronger in compression than in tension, it is the cooled surface that determines the subsequent behaviour of the container. If the tensile stress in that surface is greater than the tensile strength of the glass, the container will shatter.

A number of factors determine the resistence of a particular container to thermal shock, for example, tensile strength and coefficient of linear expansion of the glass, wall thickness and variations of wall thickness. Shape is also very important, particularly where the base joins the side-walls and the small radius of curvature at that point imposes severe bending stresses on the glass under conditions of thermal shock. Where possible these stresses are minimized by a gentle insweep of the container wall that increases the effective radius of curvature near the base. It will be clear that the calculation of the resistance to thermal shock of a given container is a matter of some complexity but an approximate value for the maximum temperature jump (T_{max} in degrees C) that may be safely imposed on a soft glass cylindrical container by chilling the

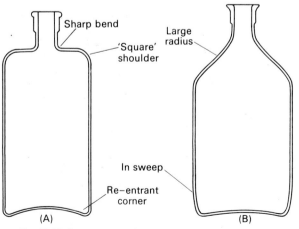

FIG. 39.11. Improvements in container design: A, old; B, new.

outer surface is given by

$$T_{\max} = 32d^{-1/2}$$

where d is the wall thickness in centimetres. The wall thickness of a container is inevitably a compromise between the opposing requirements of strength (thick wall) and resistance to thermal shock (thin wall). In some cases it may be necessary to use the mechanically stronger neutral or borosilicate glasses; the latter has the particular advantage that its coefficient of linear expansion is only a third of that of soft or neutral glass. In practice, 'winchesters' (2 litre) will survive a temperature drop of at least 30°, large (half-litre) containers about 50° and small thin-wall containers about 70°; these values may be doubled for thermal shock provided by rising temperature increments of the same order. These factors emphasize the great care that should be taken when handling hot glassware. The most serious condition arises when products which have been sterilized are prematurely removed from the autoclave. The resultant thermal shock when the container is exposed to the much colder environment outside the autoclave often leads to explosive shattering of the glass, as the container and contents will still be under pressure.

Chemical Durability

Ideally, product and package should not interact and material derived from the package that finds its way into the product must be regarded as a contaminant. Nevertheless, even the silicate glasses which are probably the most inert materials likely to be used for the fabrication of containers are attacked at all pH levels by aqueous liquids and it is necessary to apply realistic tests to ensure that the amount of contamination is within acceptable limits. Attack by alkaline solutions leads to the steady dissolution of glass, often without apparent change in appearance (Dimbleby 1953). The only visual evidence of such attack may be the formation of insoluble silicates in the product. Hydrofluoric acid and a few related fluorine containing substances also dissolve glass, but for all other acidic or neutral aqueous solutions the attack proceeds by an ion exchange process in which monovalent and, later, divalent cations in the surface are replaced by hydroxonium ions. The layer of hydrated silica formed by this process affords some protection for the glass if the attacking liquid is acidic and neutralizes the cations as they diffuse from the surface. Under conditions of severe attack by water the extracted alkali may cause dissolution of the hydrated silica layer thus exposing the glass beneath to attack. The deterioration of a glass surface under adverse storage conditions involves both kinds of action. If the humidity is high, moisture condenses on the surface and extracts cations. Subsequently the film may dry to leave behind a white deposit which contains a high proportion of sodium carbonate. When moisture again condenses on the surface the deposit dissolves and the concentrated alkaline solution attacks the silica network. The resultant loss of surface brilliance is known as weathering. In severe cases the surface acquires a white etched appearance that cannot be improved by normal washing procedures; a similar effect may be noted with soft glass containers that have been autoclaved many times.

The rate at which a glass surface is attacked depends on the type of glass and any surface treatment to which it may have been subjected, the wetted area, the type and temperature of the attacking solution and the time it has been in contact with the surface. For alkaline solutions the rate of attack falls off with time due to the accumulation of silica and other components of glass in the attacking solution. If M is the amount of material dissolved in time t from unit surface area and the amount of silica etc. accumulating in the attacking solution is proportional to M then:

$$dM/dt = K/(r+kM)$$

where K, k, and r are constants. Under neutral conditions the attack is diffusion controlled by a hydrated silica layer of thickness d proportional to the amount of cations M leached from the surface that is:

$$d = k'M$$

and

$$dM/dt = P/d = P/k'M$$

where P and k' are constants. Actually, the process involves outward diffusion of Na^+ ions and inward diffusion of H_3O^+ ions but if, as seems likely, only one of these processes is the rate controlling step, the foregoing treatment is valid. As with attack by alkaline solutions the rate decreases with time, in this case because of the increasing thickness of the hydrated silica layer. Both fundamental rate equations lead to a parabolic time law ($M^2 \propto t$) of attack. Furthermore, as both chemical reaction leading to dissolution of the glass and loss of surface alkali by diffusion are activated processes, the Arrhenius relation may be applied, that is:

$$\log \frac{M}{\sqrt{t}} = -\frac{E}{RT} + C$$

where E is the activation energy, R the gas constant and C a constant. Hubbard and Hamilton (1941) and Douglas and Isard (1949) have confirmed that this relationship applies to the attack on a number of glasses by alkalis and by water respectively.

Surface treatment of soft glass offers a possible means for reducing the interaction with aqueous fluids. Silicones appeared to be suitable agents as they are chemically related to glass and produce water repellant films. With these substances protection was good initially, but the film tended to detach on storage or autoclaving. A more satisfactory treatment is based on the early observation that the outer surfaces of glass containers that had been annealed in a coal or gas fired lehr were more resistant to attack by water than the inner surfaces. Sulphur dioxide and other acidic components of the furnace gases had reacted with the Na^+ ions in the surface to form salts which were removed on washing the containers. The annealing process ensured that the silica rich layer which was left behind was compacted and firmly bonded to the underlying glass. Unfortunately, furnace gases do not readily penetrate the interior of a container, hence its lower resistance to attack by aqueous liquids, and in any case some lehrs are now heated electrically. To overcome these problems an acidic atmosphere is artificially formed by placing an ammonium sulphate pellet in the container prior to annealing. The process is known as *sulphating*.

Flake and Spicule Formation

The chemical durability of glass is assessed by exposing it to attack by appropriate chemical reagents and measuring the effect on that reagent or on the glass itself. The BP 1973 has adopted the tests of the European Pharmacopoeia (Vol. II) 1971. The hydrolytic resistance test sets a limit on the amount of alkali that may be extracted from the containers used to package injectable products. The containers are filled with the nominal volume of freshly distilled water and autoclaved. The alkali leached by the water from the glass and is then titrated with $N/100$ HCl. According to the provisions of the test for 1 ml ampoules, the extracted alkali must not exceed that equivalent to 0.02 ml of $N/100$ HCl. As about 5 cm^2 of internal surface is wetted by the nominal contents of 1 ml ampoules in current use the foregoing corresponds to an extraction rate of;

$$\frac{0.02}{5} \times \frac{23}{100} \times \frac{106}{1000} = 0.92 \; \mu g \; cm^{-2} \; Na^+$$

Similar calculations for 10 ml (28 cm^2 wetted surface) and 50 ml (78 cm^2 wetted surface) give extraction rates of 0.82 and 0.88 $\mu g \; cm^{-2}$ respectively. Thus, the hydrolytic resistance test relates the amount of extracted alkali to the internal surface area of the container. In this way it differs from the test for alkalinity of glass in the BP 1968 which limited the concentration of extracted alkali in the container contents irrespective of the size.

A further set of tests, not previously described in a British Pharmacopoeia, but having affinities with tests in the United States is intended to distinguish between neutral, surface treated and soft glass. A crushed glass test is used to determine whether the container has been fabricated from neutral or soft glass. A further test in which the internal surface is exposed to the action of hydrofluoric acid to remove for example, the silica rich layer of a sulphated container, allows the latter to be differentiated from similar components made from neutral glass.

There is one further effect due to the reaction between the glass surface and acidic or neutral solutions. When the cations are replaced by hydroxonium ions, additional water molecules are also carried into the surface. To accommodate the hydroxonium ions and water molecules, the surface layer swells and in some cases may rupture the bonds at the interface with the unattacked glass below, so that silica rich laminae (flakes) or needle-like fragments (spicules) detach from the surface. If the attack takes place at room temperature a considerable period may elapse before flake or spicule formation becomes visible. If the temperature of the container and its contents is raised, additional stresses due to differential expansion of the glass and the hydrated silica layer causes more prompt rupture of interfacial bonds and the detachment of flakes or spicules. It is known that nearly neutral solutions containing citrates, phosphates, tartrates and bicarbonates are most prone to trouble from flake and spicule formation. Presumably, this is due to some attack of the silica network itself, in addition to the swelling and thermal effects noted above. Such products may often be packed and sterilized in new sulphated lime-soda bottles, but have a tendency to flake and spicule contamination if the bottle has been in use for some time. Although Groves and Major (1964) have confirmed the previously held view that the rubber closure, rather than the glass container, was the major source of contamination in commercially available transfusion fluids, the presence of particles of any kind should be suspect as even particles smaller than 1 μm in diameter have given rise to adverse physiological effects (Stehbens & Florey 1960). Sterile pharmaceutical solutions completely free of particles could probably not be manufactured on a commercial scale.

Groves (1966) proposed a limit of not more than 50 particles greater than 5 μm in size per ml of product (see also Cooper & Barrett 1970). The BP 1973 requires that all injections must be free from particulate matter that can be observed by visual inspection. Additionally, specified products must conform to a limit for 2 to 5 μm particles and for particles larger than 5 μm. Such products include large volume perfusion fluids containing, for example, sodium chloride and sodium lactate.

The European Pharmacopoeia distinguishes between three types of glass: type I has high hydrolytic resistance due to its composition and includes the neutral glasses; type II derives its hydrolitic resistance from surface treatment e.g. sulphating; type III includes soft glass and has only moderate hydrolytic resistance. Type III glass may be used to package a wide variety of products such as ointments, lotions, mixtures, powders for the preparation of injections and non-aqueous injections. All other parenteral products must be packaged in type I or II glass containers. Sufficient alkali could be extracted from soft glass to cause the precipitation of basic substances. Thus, strychnine has a pK_b of 6.0 and a solubility (S_o) in water of only 1 in 7000 (0.0143 per cent) at room temperature. For an aqueous injection containing, say 1 mg per ml (S = 0.1 per cent) of the alkaloid as a salt the pH at which that alkaloid will just precipitate (pH′) is given by:

$$pH' = pK_w - pK_b + \log\left[\frac{S_o}{S-S_o}\right]$$
$$= 14 - 6 + \log\left[\frac{0.0143}{0.1-0.0143}\right]$$
$$= 7.22$$

Direct experiment shows that occasionally enough alkali may be leached from the inner surface of a soft glass ampoule to raise the pH of the contents to or above this level. Formerly, the liberation of narcotine from its salts was used in Germany as a performance test for glass containers. Many bases are sufficiently soluble in water at high pH that precipitation is unlikely to occur. Thus, with atropine, adrenaline and procaine accelerated decomposition in alkaline conditions rather precipitation is the problem. Some medicaments such as Adrenaline Acid Tartrate have inherent buffering capacity in the pH range which is optimum for stability. For Chloramphenicol Eye Drops the balance between solubility and stability is maintained by a pH 7.0 borate/boric acid buffer (Heward et al. 1970).

Another example where the extraction of alkali must be limited by the use of hard glass containers is in the packaging of Insulin Injection. The isoelectric point of this polypeptide is 5.5 to 5.6 and, although the injection is adjusted to pH 3.0 to 3.5, sufficient alkali could be extracted from unsatisfactory containers to bring the pH to the isoelectric point thus causing precipitation of insulin. The major danger with this medicament is, however, the very much accelerated degradation of the polypeptide that occurs if the pH exceeds 7.5. Borosilicate glass is too expensive for widespread use as a container material. The cheaper neutral glasses provide an acceptable alternative and are available in two grades (Table 39.1), one of which is formulated for a low fusion temperature to facilitate the sealing of ampoules (B.S. 795: 1961). Although the coefficient of linear expansion is similar to that of soft glass, thermal shock is rarely a problem as the ampoule walls are thin. The container grade of neutral glass is employed for the production of multidose injection containers antibiotic vials, etc. Transfusion bottles (B.S. 2463: 1962) can be made of neutral glass but sulphated lime-soda glass provides a cheaper alternative which is now much used for eye drop bottles (B.S. 1679: 1965). To avoid the danger of flaking with repeated use, surface treated eye drop bottles are employed once only and are therefore known as 'one-trip' eye drop bottles. Some injections such as those containing apomorphine, ascorbic acid or papaveretum are light sensitive, and amber coloured ampoules have been much used for packaging them. However visual evidence of deterioration, e.g. flaking, colour changes, etc., should be readily discernible and it is now more usual to pack the product in colourless containers and exclude light by means of the ampoule box. Another reason for using colourless containers is that the product might be contaminated by the elements used to colour the glass, and Girard and Kemy (1950) have reported that iron extracted from amber glass may interfere with the stability of adrenaline solutions. For non-parenteral products the packaging requirements are less stringent and as amber containers are no more expensive than the colourless variety, the majority of chemicals, galenicals, etc. are now routinely packed in amber glass bottles regardless of the light sensitivity of the packaged material.

CLOSURES

An ideal closure will seal the container to prevent loss of product and ingress of gases or other substances. Where necessary the closure should withstand sterilizing conditions and prevent subsequent contamination by microorganisms. The closure and product must not react together. Finally, if only part of the contents of the container is to be used at a time, it should be easy to remove and replace the closure, and the reseal properties must be adequate for this purpose.

Except for this last requirement, a glass fusion seal is as perfect a seal as it is possible to make; all other seals are less satisfactory. If the product absorbs water vapour, the partial pressure for that substance inside the container will be lower than that in the enviroment. This provides a concentration gradient across any imperfection in the closure and leads to continuous diffusion into the container and hence into the product. Additionally, any change in ambient temperature or pressure will result in a flow of air into or out of the container via the imperfections in the closure—the container is said to 'breathe'. Over a period of storage the combined effects of breathing and diffusion may lead to the transfer of considerable quantities of water to the product and may result in instability.

The basic types of closure are folded, push-on, bung, screw-cap and fusion.

Folded Seals

These will be familiar both as the seam down the side of tinned-steel containers and as the folded end of ointment tubes. If the product inside the tube is very viscous there will be a considerable back pressure as the product is forced out of the nozzle

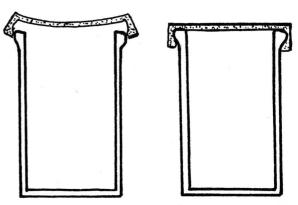

FIG. 39.13. Push-on closure.

and this will tend to unfold the seal. In commercial practice, when the folds have been formed they are crimped by corrugated jaws and this prevents unfolding of the seal (Fig. 39.12). Seepage via the folded seal may be prevented by the use of latex sealing compounds.

Push-on Seals

These are often used for tubes of lozenges and rely on the resilient distortion of the closure both for pushing the cap over the retaining ring at the rim of the tube and also for maintaining a tight seal between the neck and the rim (Fig. 39.13).

Bung Seals

These are among the oldest known closures. They are conical and can be inserted for about half their length into the neck of the container (Fig. 39.14A). Sideways pressure due to distortion of the bung on insertion provides a seal the perfection of which depends both on the bung material and finish of the neck. Cork usually gives a good seal for general purposes but eventually becomes permanently distorted with consequent loss of reseal properties. Rubber is an excellent material for bung closures but cannot be used for oils or solvents due to swelling, or for lubricant products as the bung tends to eject from the neck of the container. There are many varieties of this type of closure. With vaccine bottle caps, bung action is assisted by a 'skirt' that folds over the outside of the neck of the bottle. A wire loop round the skirt ensures that the bung is not ejected during heat sterilization. Another type of bung closure, now much used, is that used for vials of penicillin powder. The bung is held in place by a thin aluminium cap which is spun round a retaining ring on the neck of the vial (Fig. 39.14B).

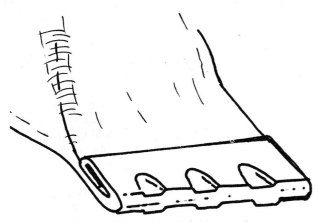

FIG. 39.12. Crimped end of ointment tube.

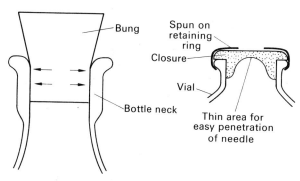

FIG. 39.14. Bung seals.

Screw-cap

The essential features (Fig. 39.15) are a cap with thread matching that of the container, and a tough liner behind which is placed a resilient wad. When the cap is screwed down the liner makes contact with the rim, distortion of the wad maintaining the liner in close contact with the rim. For efficient sealing, the thread on the cap must match that on the container; the rim of the container must be square and free from moulding imperfections. Although formerly a source of trouble, moulding imperfections have virtually been eliminated by the fire polishing process before entry of the glass container into the lehr as described in the section on glass. The performance of plastic containers in this respect has yet to be determined. The depth of the cap must be such that it does not foul the annulus on the neck of the bottle. Over-tightening must be avoided as this may crack or distort the cap. If a rubber wad is used (a liner is not required) elastic recovery from over-tightening may lead effectively to loosening of the closure. Finally, the screw-cap must be dimensionally stable. Should an aluminium cap be over-tightened the free edge may stretch and will not properly fit the screw thread on the container. Phenol-formaldehyde

bottle caps are often filled with wood-flour. If the cap is basically of poor quality the wood-flour swells in contact with moisture from alkaline products with an effect similar to that described for over-tightened aluminium caps. Aluminium hydroxide gel and magnesium hydroxide mixture have both been implicated in cap distortion of this type. At one time, tinned-steel screw-caps were much used but tended to rust where friction with the thread damaged the tin coating. Both thermoplastics and thermosetting plastics are now much used for screw-cap production.

Liners for screw-caps must be tough. Ceresine impregnated paper, aluminium foil and plastics such as polythene are much used. Rubber is a good wad material provided it is not over-tightened; it is inert to most materials, except as described elsewhere, and does not support mould growth. Plastics share most of the properties of rubber but lack its resilience. For cheaper closures, wood pulp and felt board wads are employed but resilience is low and the reseal properties poor. Glue or resin bonded cork chips are also used but the former disintegrate in contact with aqueous liquids and support mould growth. The resin bonded variety is much better in these respects but distorts readily. Labour costs can be reduced if the wad and liner are bonded together to give for instance, a polythene-faced resin-bonded cork wad. For some modern dispensing bottles the wad and the liner are replaced by a lip moulded into the screw-cap (Fig. 39.16). Rolled-on screw-caps avoid the problem of matching cap and container thread by using a straight-sided blank cap which is held firmly against the rim of the neck while a rotating head forms the thread on the cap against that on the neck. A particular advantage of the rolled on type of seal is that provision can be made for an extended perforated skirt to fit over the annulus. The

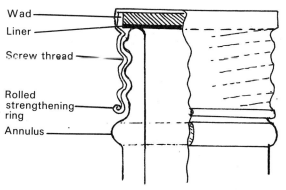

FIG. 39.15. Conventional screw-cap closure.

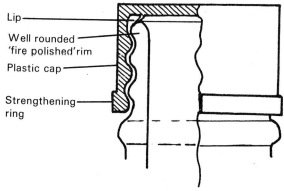

FIG. 39.16. Modern screw-cap closure.

perforations must be broken before the cap may be removed. This particular system provides a pilfer-proof closure.

Fusion Seals
This type of seal is used for ampoules and when properly made is hermetic. Products of the sachet type use a plastic fusion seal.

PACKAGE TESTING

Each product has its own particular packaging problems, and some typical examples are discussed by Stephenson (1953). In general, it is necessary to establish:
(i) the amount, kind and toxicity of any materials that may be extracted from the package by the product and how this may be avoided,
(ii) whether any of the product constituents are being absorbed and how this may be prevented or minimized,
(iii) the amount, size and kind of any particulate matter that may appear in the product and the steps necessary to prevent this,
(iv) the light transmission characteristic if the product is photosensitive,
(v) closure efficiency: this is best achieved by placing the product in the proposed package and noting, say, weight changes over a period. An unfilled control will establish weight changes due to the package alone.
(vi) any specific interactions, how these arise and how they may be minimized, and,
(vii) whether the package satisfies legal require-ments both in the country of origin and in those to which the product may be exported.

FILLING

Packaging does not finish with the selection of a suitable container for the product; the latter must be filled into the container. This involves further processing and handling procedures which themselves may have an effect on the long-term stability of the product. If the batch is small, hand filling may be appropriate but on an industrial scale a batch may consist of thousands of product units, requiring for economic filling semi-automatic or automatic equipment. Such equipment would assemble the containers and closures, dispense the medicament into the container, apply the closure and label and carry out such other operations as may be necessary such as placing the product into a carton. As filling operations are common to many industries, a wide variety of equipment is available to the pharmaceutical manufacturer. Different organizations therefore are unlikely to adopt the same system for a given operation. Nevertheless, there are problems basic to the filling of liquids, semi-solids, powders and unit-dose products, regardless of the production method, and these are briefly discussed here.

Liquids
There are obvious problems in filling suspensions, particularly official preparations of kaolin, magnesium trisilicate, etc., which do not contain a suspending agent. If a product of the correct

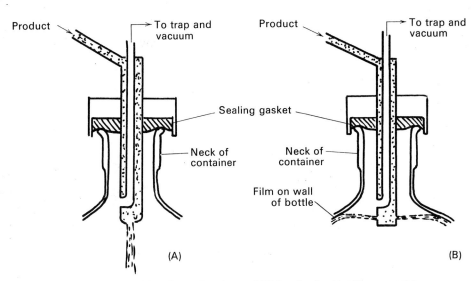

FIG. 39.17. Filling head for (A) non-foaming, and (B) foaming liquids (diagrammatic).

composition is to be packaged, the bulk must be continuously and thoroughly stirred throughout the entire filling operation with particular attention to the corners of the main container where stirring is relatively ineffective and where solid may accumulate. Furthermore, the transit time of the product from the bulk to the final container must be short to minimize sedimentation in the filling head. Apart from inaccuracies in the composition of the filled product, accumulating solid may jam the head mechanism. Even solutions present filling problems if the surface tension is low and the foam stability high. The liquid from the filling head (Fig. 39.17A) jetting into the product already in the bottle causes considerable agitation and build-up of a persistent froth. It is necessary for the vacuum line to suck off to the trap a large volume of froth before the bottle is properly filled with liquid product. A variant of the standard head, that is normally successful in avoiding this problem, is shown in Fig. 39.17B. The liquid jets onto the wall of the container and gently flows as a thin film without frothing. As these types of head fill to a given distance below the rim of the neck, volumetric accuracy of filling is entirely dependent on the observance of rigid tolerances during manufacture of the container. Furthermore, it is, not easy significantly to vary the filling volume from the nominal value for the container. Machine driven automatic syringes are employed if greater versatility is required, a method which finds considerable use in large scale ampoule filling. The syringe size and plunger stroke determine the volume transferred to the container.

Semi-solids

The filling of extracts, pastes, ointments, creams and other semi-solids is sometimes facilitated by warming the product to reduce viscosity. The technique must be applied with care as it may accelerate a degradative chemical reaction or have an effect on physical characteristics or stability. Sedimentation of suspended solids may occur if the viscosity of the vehicle is excessively reduced by heating, while permanent changes in consistency resulting from the breakdown of gel structure when creams are stirred or heated must be allowed for at the formulation stage. Viscous products, particularly those containing surfactants, are prone to aeration. Apart from the fact that aeration may accelerate oxidation, the entrained air bubbles are highly compressible and interfere with pumping when the product is homogenized or filled. Finally, it may

not be possible to get the required amount of aerated product into the selected container.

Powders

It is often possible to resolve a powder filling problem into a powder flow problem—the subject is discussed in Chapter 17. It is worth bearing in mind, however, that the filling machine may demix the powder by stirring, may cause some particle size reduction by attrition in the feed-screw and may expose the powder to atmospheric oxygen or water vapour. If the product is particularly water sensitive, for example ampicillin, it may be necessary to provide low humidity filling conditions; it is generally accepted that, for stability, 1 per cent represents the maximum water content that may be permitted for penicillin formulations in powder form. There is often a dust hazard associated with the filling of powders and this must be carefully controlled to avoid toxic effects on the operatives and contamination of other products.

Unit-dose Products

These are usually packed in sub-multiples or multiples of a hundred. The tablets or capsules are placed in the filling machine and each unit separately interrupts a light beam or other mechanism that actuates a counting device whereby the product feed is shut off as soon as the correct number of units have been placed in the container. The filling process subjects the product to tumbling action and for this reason tablets should be formulated for high resistance to abrasion, particularly at the edges. To minimize abrasion when the tablet is in the container, the head-space is filled with 'necking' material. Formerly, cotton wool was much used but unless thoroughly dried its normal moisture content is sufficient to promote the degradation of sensitive products. Preformed polyurethane foam is now used for necking; it is easier to insert and has a very low moisture content.

REPACKAGING

After manufacture a product may undergo one further packaging process if prescription requirements do not match available pack sizes. The repackaging process often affects stability and poses other problems as well as those specifically associated with the correct choice of dispensing container. It might seem that these difficulties would be mitigated by the shorter period of further storage typical of dispensed items, but the prescribed quantity of drug may be intended to last the patient several months e.g. Tolbutamide or Primidone, and this factor must be assessed and taken into account. For most official preparations the packaging and storage requirements are stated in the relevant monographs. It should be noted that there are now precise meanings attached to such familiar phrases as light-resistance, freshly prepared etc.

Official directions for the preparation of creams are intended to minimize microbial contamination of the product, and this must not be increased during the repackaging operation. Additional problems are the possible interaction between the new container and the product and the selection of the correct diluent (if required) for the avoidance of incompatibilities and significant change in rheological behaviour. The latter is also a factor to be considered in the provision of dispensing containers for mixtures and lotions. Although the original pack may serve as a guide, it is worth remembering that, even when thinned by shaking, thixotropic products such as Aluminium Hydroxide Gel and Mixture of Magnesium Hydroxide are more readily poured from a container with a wide neck. As discussed earlier, some wood-flour filled phenol-formaldehyde screw caps may swell or distort in contact with products of this type. Very thorough shaking of suspensions before dispensing is essential if the original composition is to be maintained in both the dispensed and remaining material. If the product is to be supplied in a diluted form, care must be taken that specific stabilizers and preservatives are present in sufficient quantity for efficient protective action. The oxygen permeability of a plastic container may be crucial to the stability of the product if absorption or dilution of the antioxidant has taken place.

Tablets are often repacked from bulk supplies, and the danger exists that progressive abrasion will occur as the tablets are tumbled when taken from the bulk container. The latter is frequently an aluminium or tinned-steel container or an amber glass bottle, all of which provide protection against light. The container selected for repackaging must also possess this property if the product is photo-sensitive. A high proportion of the moisture sensitive drugs exhibit adequate stability if stored and dispensed in a well sealed container. More sensitive preparations—Effervescent Potassium Tablets, for example—require a much higher level of moisture exclusion. In commercial packs the tablets are sealed in a polythene bag with a desiccant sachet, enveloped in a further polythene bag and then issued in a sealed aluminium screw-capped container. Unless this order of moisture protection can be maintained in repackaging, it is probably best to obtain the prescribers agreement for the supply of the nearest size commercial pack.

It cannot be too strongly stated that thoughtful repackaging may be ruined if appropriate directions for storage and use are not given and explained to the patient.

REFERENCES ·

BLOOM, C. & DRENNAN, M. (1957) *Pharmaceut. J.* **178**, 416.

BRITISH STANDARD 3263: 1960, Rubber Closures for Injectable Products. British Standards Institution, London.

BRITISH STANDARD 795: 1961, Ampoules. British Standard Institution, London.

BRITISH STANDARD 2463: 1962, Transfusion equipment for medical use. British Standards Institution, London.

BRITISH STANDARD 1679: 1965, Eye dropper bottles. British Standards Institution, London.

BUSSE, M. J. & HUGHES, D. A. (1969) *Pharmaceut. J.* **203**, 338.

CHILD, C. L. (1955) *J. Pharm. Pharmacol.* **7**, 793.

COOPER, D. & BARRETT, C. W. (1970) *Pharmaceut. J.* **205**, 186.

COOPER, J. (1966) *Pharmaceut. J.* **197**, 391.

DEMBLEBY, V. (1953) *J. Pharm. Pharmacol.* **12**, 969.

DOUGLAS, R. W. & ISARD, J. O. (1949) *J. Soc. Glass Technol.* **33**, 289.

FLÜCK, H. (1966) *Pharmaceut. J.* **197**, 393.

GIRARD, P. & KEMY, G. (1950) *Ann. Pharm. Franc.* **8**, 462.

GLOWACKI, E. Z. (1966) *Pharmaceut. J.* **197**, 428.

GROVES, M. J. (1966) *J. Pharm. Pharmacol.* **18**, 161.

GROVES, M. J. & MAJOR, J. F. G. (1964) *Pharmaceut. J.* **193**, 227.

HAWORTH, J. (1953) *J. Pharm. Pharmacol.* **12**, 990.

HEWARD, M., NORTON, D. A. & RIVERS, S. M. (1970) *Pharmaceut. J.* **204**, 386.

HUBBARD, D. & HAMILTON, E. H. (1941) *J. Res. Nat. Bur. Stand.* **27**, 143.

JOLLY, S. C., LUND, W. & JOHN, E. G. (1970) *Pharmaceut. J.* **204**, 291.

LACHMAN, L., WEINSTEIN, S., HOPKINS, G., SLACK, S., EISMAN, P. & COOPER, J. (1962) *J. pharm. Sci.* **51**, 224.

LACHMAN, L., WEINSTEIN, S., URBANYI, T., EBERSOLD, E. & COOPER, J. (1963a) *J. pharm. Sci.* **52**, 241.

LACHMAN, L., URBANYI, T. & WEINSTEIN, S. (1963b) *J. pharm. Sci.* **52**, 244.

LONG, W. R. (1961) *Pharmaceut. J.* **187**, 165.

MOODY, B. E. (1963) *Packaging in Glass.* London: Hutchinson.

PAINE, F. A. (1962) *Fundamentals of Packaging.* London: Blackie.

PAINE, F. A. (1967) *Packaging Materials and Containers.* London: Blackie.

PHARMACEUTICAL JOURNAL (1957) **178**, 424.

REZNEK, S. (1953a) *J. Am. pharm. Ass. (Sci. Edn)* **42**, 288.

REZNEK, S. (1953b) *J. Am. pharm. Ass. (Sci. Edn)* **42**, 291.

ROYCE, A. & SYKES, G. (1957) *J. Pharm. Pharmacol.* **9**, 814.

SIMPSON, B. J. (1969) *Pharmaceut. J.* **203**, 335.

STEHBENS, W. E. & FLOREY, H. W. (1960) *Q. J. exp. Physiol.* **45**, 252.

STEPHENSON, D. (1953) *J. Pharm. Pharmacol.* **12**, 999.

SYKES, G. (1958) *J. Pharm. Pharmacol.* **10**, 40.

WING, W. T. (1955) *J. Pharm. Pharmacol.* **7**, 648.

WING, W. T. (1956a) *J. Pharm. Pharmacol.* **8**, 734.

WING, W. T. (1956b) *J. Pharm. Pharmacol.* **8**, 738.

Index